Retina-
Vitreous-
Macula

Retina-
Vitreous-
Macula

DAVID R. GUYER, M.D.

Director, Residency Training
Manhattan Eye, Ear & Throat Hospital
Clinical Associate Professor of Ophthalmology
Cornell University Medical Center
New York, New York

LAWRENCE A. YANNUZZI, M.D.

Vice-Chairman and Director of Retinal Services
Manhattan Eye, Ear & Throat Hospital
Professor of Clinical Ophthalmology
Columbia University College of Physicians and Surgeons
New York, New York

STANLEY CHANG, M.D.

Edward S. Harkness Professor
Chairman, Department of Ophthalmology
Columbia University College of Physicians and Surgeons
New York, New York

JERRY A. SHIELDS, M.D.

Director of Oncology Service
Wills Eye Hospital
Professor of Ophthalmology
Thomas Jefferson University
Philadelphia, Pennsylvania

W. RICHARD GREEN, M.D.

International Order of Odd Fellows Professor of Ophthalmology
Professor of Pathology
The Johns Hopkins University School of Medicine
Baltimore, Maryland

1999

W.B. SAUNDERS COMPANY
A Division of Harcourt Brace & Company
Philadelphia ■ London ■ Toronto ■ Montreal ■ Sydney ■ Tokyo

W. B. SAUNDERS COMPANY
A Division of Harcourt Brace & Company

The Curtis Center
Independence Square West
Philadelphia, Pennsylvania 19106

Library of Congress Cataloging-in-Publication Data

Retina, vitreous, macula / [edited by] David R. Guyer — [et al.]. —
1st ed.
    p.   cm.
   ISBN 0–7216–6756–2
   1. Posterior segment (Eye)–Diseases. I. Guyer, David R.
  [DNLM: 1. Retinal Diseases. 2. Vitreous Body. 3. Macula Lutea.
4. Choroid Diseases. WW 270 R43806 1999]
RE475.R48 1999
617.7′3—dc21
DNLM/DLC   97-16250

RETINA-VITREOUS-MACULA

Volume 1 0–7216–7607–3
Volume 2 0–7216–7608–1
Set ISBN 0–7216–6756–2

Printed in the United States of America.

Last digit is the print number: 9   8   7   6   5   4   3   2   1

To my mother and father for all their great support and encouragement.
David R. Guyer

*To all of my teachers, my partners, my students, my friends, my family.
My eternal gratitude for your encouragement and support.*
Lawrence A. Yannuzzi

To Jean, Jonathan and Gregory

Stanley Chang

*To my loving wife Carol and our six wonderful children—Jerry, Patrick,
Billy Bob, Maggie Mae, Dinger, and Charlotte Nellie.*
Jerry A. Shields

To Janet, Parke and Gordon

W. Richard Green

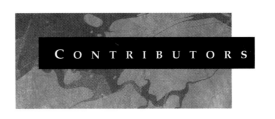
THOMAS M. AABERG, SR., M.D., F.A.C.S.
Chair, Department of Ophthalmology, Emory School of Medicine; F. Phinizy Calhoun Senior Professor, Emory University; Chief, Section of Ophthalmology, Emory Clinic, Atlanta, Georgia
Intermediate Uveitis (Pars Planitis); Surgical Management of Proliferative Vitreoretinopathy

ALBERT L. AANDEKERK, F.O.P.S.
Institute of Ophthalmology, University of Nijmegen, Nijmegen, The Netherlands
Benign Concentric Maculopathy

GARY W. ABRAMS, M.D.
Professor and Chairman, Department of Ophthalmology, Kresge Eye Institute, Wayne State University, Detroit, Michigan
Vitrectomy

DAVID H. ABRAMSON, M.D., F.A.C.S.
Clinical Professor of Ophthalmology, Cornell Medical Center; Director, Ophthalmic Oncology, The Robert M. Ellsworth Ophthalmic Oncology Center at New York Hospital, New York, New York
Age-Related Macular Degeneration: Radiation Therapy for Choroidal Neovascularization

ANTHONY P. ADAMIS, M.D.
Associate Professor of Ophthalmology, Harvard Medical School; Research Associate, Surgical Research Laboratory, Children's Hospital; Associate Surgeon, Massachusetts Eye and Ear Infirmary, Boston, Massachusetts
Antiangiogenic Therapy

LLOYD M. AIELLO, M.D.
Associate Professor of Ophthalmology, Harvard Medical School; Director, Beetham Eye Institute, Joslin Diabetes Center, Boston, Massachusetts
Diabetic Retinopathy

LLOYD P. AIELLO, M.D., PH.D.
Assistant Professor of Ophthalmology, Harvard Medical School; Investigator, Joslin Diabetes Center, Boston, Massachusetts
Diabetic Retinopathy

NANCY C. ARBOUR, PH.D.
Post Doctoral Research Associate, University of Iowa, Iowa City, Iowa
Best's Disease: Molecular and Clinical Findings

GAETANO R. BARILE, M.D.
Assistant Professor of Clinical Ophthalmology, Columbia University College of Physicians and Surgeons; Assistant Attending Ophthalmologist, Edward S. Harkness Eye Institute; St. Luke's-Roosevelt Hospital Center, New York, New York
Parafoveal Telangiectasis; Disseminated Intravascular Coagulopathy

ROBERT G. BARONE, M.D.
Clinical Assistant Professor of Ophthalmology, Cornell University Medical College, New York, New York
Surgical Management of Retinal Detachments Due to AIDS

CAROLINE R. BAUMAL, M.D., F.R.C.S.C.
Assistant Professor, Tufts University School of Medicine; Attending Physician, Department of Vitreoretinal Surgery, New England Eye Center, Boston, Massachusetts
New Diagnostic and Therapeutic Approaches to Retinal Disease

MYLES M. BEHRENS, M.D., D.M.SC
Professor of Clinical Ophthalmology, Columbia University College of Physicians and Surgeons; Attending Ophthalmologist, Presbyterian Hospital, New York, New York
Optic Disc Drusen

GEORGE W. BLANKENSHIP, M.D.
Professor and Chairman of Ophthalmology, Penn State University College of Medicine; Penn State Geisinger Health System, The Milton S. Hershey Medical Center, Hershey, Pennsylvania
Proliferative Diabetic Retinopathy

MARK S. BLUMENKRANZ, M.D.
Professor of Ophthalmology, Chairman, Department of Ophthalmology, Stanford University, Stanford, California
Acute Retinal Necrosis; Fungal Diseases

ROSARIO BRANCATO, M.D.

Chairman and Professor, Department of Ophthalmology, University of Milan; Department of Ophthalmology and Visual Sciences, San Raffaele Hospital, Milan, Italy

The Rheumatic Retinal Diseases

NEIL M. BRESSLER, M.D.

Professor of Ophthalmology, The Johns Hopkins University School of Medicine; Retinal Vascular Center, Wilmer Ophthalmological Institute, The Johns Hopkins Hospital, Baltimore, Maryland

Neovascular (Exudative) Age-Related Macular Degeneration

SUSAN B. BRESSLER, M.D.

Associate Professor of Ophthalmology, Johns Hopkins University School of Medicine; Wilmer Eye Institute, The Johns Hopkins Hospital, Baltimore, Maryland

Nonneovascular (Nonexudative) Age-Related Macular Degeneration

W.Z. BRIDGES, JR., M.D.

Southern Vitreoretinal Associates, Tallahassee, Florida

Viral Syndromes

ROY D. BROD, M.D.

Clinical Associate Professor of Ophthalmology, Penn State University College of Medicine, Hershey Medical Center; Active Staff, Lancaster General Hospital, Lancaster, Pennsylvania

Endophthalmitis Management

NEIL D. BROURMAN, M.D.

Instructor in Ophthalmology, UCLA; Attending Physician, Cedars-Sinai Hospital, Los Angeles, California

Fungal Diseases

DAVID M. BROWN, M.D.

Clinical Instructor, Baylor College of Medicine, Houston, Texas

Best's Disease: Molecular and Clinical Findings

GARY C. BROWN, M.D.

Professor of Ophthalmology, Thomas Jefferson School of Medicine; Director, Retina Vascular Unit, Wills Eye Hospital, Philadelphia, Pennsylvania

Retinal Arterial Occlusive Diseases; Ocular Ischemic Syndrome; Congenital Pits of the Optic Nerve Head; Congenital Retinal Arteriovenous Communications (Racemose Hemangiomas)

JEREMIAH BROWN, JR., M.D.

Vitreoretinal Fellow, Department of Ophthalmology, University of Iowa Hospital, Iowa City, Iowa

Multifocal Choroiditis, Punctate Inner Choroidopathy, and Other Related Conditions

ALEXANDER J. BRUCKER, M.D.

Professor of Ophthalmology, University of Pennsylvania School of Medicine; Attending Ophthalmologist, Scheie Eye Institute and Hospital of the University of Pennsylvania, Philadelphia, Pennsylvania

Chorioretinal and Retinal Folds

SVEN-ERIK BURSELL, PH.D.

Assistant Professor, Department of Ophthalmology, Harvard Medical School; Investigator, Joslin Diabetes Center, Boston, Massachusetts

Diabetic Retinopathy

NORMAN E. BYER, M.D.

Clinical Professor of Ophthalmology, University of California, Los Angeles School of Medicine, Los Angeles, California

Peripheral Retinal Lesions Related to Rhegmatogenous Retinal Detachment

ANTONIO CAPONE, JR., M.D.

Associate Professor, Emory University, Atlanta, Georgia

Intermediate Uveitis (Pars Planitis); Surgical Management of Proliferative Vitreoretinopathy

RONALD E. CARR, M.D., M.SCI. (OPHTHAL)

Professor of Ophthalmology, New York University Medical Center, New York, New York

Retinitis Pigmentosa and Allied Diseases; Cone Dystrophies

JERRY D. CAVALLERANO, O.D., PH.D.

Associate Professor, New England College of Optometry; Staff Optometrist, Beetham Eye Institute, Joslin Diabetes Center, Boston, Massachusetts

Diabetic Retinopathy

ANDREW A. CHANG, M.B.B.S., F.R.A.C.O., F.R.A.C.S.

Consultant Retinal Surgeon, Sydney Eye Hospital, Sydney, Australia

Ophthalmic Contact B-Scan Ultrasonography; Three-Dimensional Ophthalmic Ultrasonography of the Posterior Segment; Postsurgical Cystoid Macular Edema

BENJAMIN CHANG, M.D.

Attending Surgeon, Manhattan Eye, Ear & Throat Hospital, New York, New York

Acute Retinal Pigment Epitheliitis

STANLEY CHANG, M.D.

Edward S. Harkness Professor, Chairman, Department of Ophthalmology, Columbia University College of Physicians and Surgeons, New York, New York

Vitreous Substitutes; Surgical Management of Giant Retinal Tears

DEVRON H. CHAR, M.D.
Professor of Ophthalmology, Radiation Oncology, and Francis I. Proctor Foundation, University of California Medical Center, San Francisco, California
Intraocular Lymphoid Tumors

STEVE CHARLES, M.D.
Clinical Professor of Ophthalmology, University of Tennessee, College of Medicine, Memphis, Tennessee
Epimacular Membranes

ANTONIO P. CIARDELLA, M.D.
Retina Fellow, Manhattan Eye, Ear & Throat Hospital, New York, New York
Ophthalmic Contact B-Scan Ultrasonography; Three-Dimensional Ophthalmic Ultrasonography of the Posterior Segment; Central Retinal Vein Occlusion: A Primer and Review; Plasma Protein Risk Factors for Retinal Vascular Occlusive Disease; The Rheumatic Retinal Diseases; Multiple Evanescent White Dot Syndrome (MEWDS); Ocular Sarcoidosis; Diffuse Unilateral Subacute Neuroretinitis; Myiasis

JOHN G. CLARKSON, M.D.
Dean, University of Miami School of Medicine; Professor of Ophthalmology, University of Miami School of Medicine; Anne Bates Leach Eye Hospital, Miami, Florida
Central Retinal Vein Occlusion: A Primer and Review

MICHAEL J. COONEY, M.D.
Senior Ophthalmology Resident, The Wilmer Eye Institute, The Johns Hopkins Hospital, Baltimore, Maryland
Combined Hamartoma of the Retina and Retinal Pigment Epithelium

GABRIEL COSCAS, M.D.
Professor of Clinical Ophthalmology, Eye University Clinic or Créteil, University of Paris-XII; Hôpital de Créteil, Créteil, France
Angioid Streaks; Myopia

PATRICK DE POTTER, M.D.
Professor of Ophthalmology, School of Medicine, University Catholic of Louvain; Chairman of the Ophthalmology Department, Cliniques Universitaires St-Luc, Brussels, Belgium
Choroidal Hemangioma

AUGUST F. DEUTMAN, M.D., E.B.O.D.
Chairman, Institute of Ophthalmology, University of Nijmegen, Nijmegen, The Netherlands
Benign Concentric Maculopathy

SANDER DUBOVY, M.D.
Resident, Department of Pathology, College of Physicians and Surgeons, Columbia University, New York, New York
Tuberculosis

JAY S. DUKER, M.D.
Associate Professor of Ophthalmology, Tufts University School of Medicine; Director, Vitreoretinal Surgery, New England Eye Center, New England Medical Center, Boston, Massachusetts.
Birdshot Retinochoroidopathy

DEAN ELIOTT, M.D.
Assistant Professor, Department of Ophthalmology, Kresge Eye Institute, Wayne State University, Detroit, Michigan
Bietti's Crystalline Dystrophy

SHARON FEKRAT, M.D.
Assistant Chief of Service, Director, Ocular Trauma; Instructor, Wilmer Ophthalmological Institute, Johns Hopkins Medical Institutions, Baltimore, Maryland
Hemoglobinopathies

AARON FENSTER, PH.D., F.C.C.P.M.
Professor, University of Western Ontario; Director, Robarts Research Institute, London, Ontario, Canada
Three-Dimensional Ophthalmic Ultrasonography of the Posterior Segment

PHILIP J. FERRONE, M.D.
Assistant Clinical Professor of Biomedical Sciences, Eye Research Institute, Rochester, Michigan; Medical Staff Physician, William Beaumont Hospital, Royal Oak, Michigan
Retinopathy of Prematurity: Stages 1 Through 3; Retinopathy of Prematurity: Stages 4 and 5

STUART L. FINE, M.D.
Professor and Chairman, Department of Ophthalmology, University of Pennsylvania School of Medicine; Director, Scheie Eye Institute, University of Pennsylvania, Philadelphia, Pennsylvania
Clinical Examination of the Posterior Segment of the Eye

DANIEL FINKELSTEIN, M.D.
Professor of Ophthalmology, The Wilmer Institute, The Johns Hopkins University School of Medicine, Baltimore, Maryland
Branch Retinal Vein Occlusion

YALE L. FISHER, M.D.
Clinical Professor of Ophthalmology, Cornell Medical Center-New York Hospital; Surgeon Director, Manhattan Eye, Ear & Throat Hospital, New York, New York
Ophthalmic Contact B-Scan Ultrasonography; Three-Dimensional Ophthalmic Ultrasonography of the Posterior Segment

HARRY W. FLYNN, JR., M.D.
Professor of Ophthalmology, Bascom Palmer Eye Institute, University of Miami School of Medicine, Miami, Florida
Endophthalmitis Management

JAMES C. FOLK, M.D.
Professor, Department of Ophthalmology, College of Medicine, The University of Iowa, Iowa City, Iowa
Multifocal Choroiditis, Punctate Inner Choroidopathy, and Other Related Conditions

BRADLEY S. FOSTER, M.D.
Clinical Fellow in Ophthalmology, Harvard Medical School; Vitreoretinal Fellow, Massachusetts Eye and Ear Infirmary, Boston, Massachusetts
Choroidal Metastasis

GREGORY FOX, M.D.
Allegheny University Hospital, MCP Clinical Instructor, Philadelphia, Pennsylvania
Acute Retinal Necrosis

K. BAILEY FREUND, M.D.
Instructor in Clinical Ophthalmology, College of Physicians and Surgeons of Columbia University; Assistant Attending Surgeon, Manhattan Eye, Ear & Throat Hospital; Assistant Ophthalmologist, Edward S. Harkness Eye Institute, New York, New York
Principles of Indocyanine-Green Angiography; Leber's Idiopathic Stellate Neuroretinitis

DOROTHY NAHM FRIEDBERG, M.D., PH.D.
Clinical Associate Professor of Ophthalmology, New York University School of Medicine; Attending Physician; New York Eye & Ear Infirmary, New York, New York
The Retina and Choroid in HIV Infection

ALAN H. FRIEDMAN, M.D.
Clinical Professor of Ophthalmology and Pathology, Mount Sinai School of Medicine; Attending Ophthalmologist Pathologist, Mount Sinai Hospital, New York, New York
Sympathetic Ophthalmia; Ocular Cysticercosis

THOMAS W. GARDNER, M.D.
Associate Professor of Ophthalmology and Cellular Physiology, Penn State University College of Medicine; Penn State Geisinger Health System, The Milton S. Hershey Medical Center, Hershey, Pennsylvania
Proliferative Diabetic Retinopathy

J. DONALD M. GASS, M.D.
Professor of Ophthalmology, Vanderbilt Medical School, Nashville, Tennessee
Vogt-Koyanagi-Harada Syndrome

RONALD C. GENTILE, M.D.
Fellow, Vitreoretinal Diseases and Surgery, Kresge Eye Institute, Wayne State University, Detroit, Michigan
Vitrectomy

MORTON F. GOLDBERG, M.D.
William Holland Wilmer Professor of Ophthalmology, The Johns Hopkins University School of Medicine; Director, The Wilmer Eye Institute, The Johns Hopkins Hospital, Baltimore, Maryland
Hemoglobinopathies

EVANGELOS S. GRAGOUDAS, M.D.
Professor of Ophthalmology, Harvard Medical School; Director of the Retina Service, Massachusetts Eye and Ear Infirmary, Boston, Massachusetts
Radiation Retinopathy; Bone Marrow Transplant Retinopathy; Choroidal Metastasis

W. RICHARD GREEN, M.D.
International Order of Odd Fellows Professor of Ophthalmology, Professor of Pathology, The Johns Hopkins University School of Medicine, Baltimore, Maryland
Retinal Histology

DAVID R. GUYER, M.D.
Director, Residency Training, Manhattan Eye, Ear & Throat Hospital; Clinical Associate Professor of Ophthalmology, Cornell University Medical Center, New York, New York
Clinical Examination of the Posterior Segment of the Eye; Principles of Fluorescein Angiography; Principles of Indocyanine-Green Angiography; Central Serous Chorioretinopathy; Central Retinal Vein Occlusion: A Primer and Review; Plasma Protein Risk Factors for Retinal Vascular Occlusive Disease; Disseminated Intravascular Coagulopathy; Myiasis

LISABETH S. HALL, M.D.
Assistant Professor of Ophthalmology, New York Medical College; Assistant Director, Pediatric Ophthalmology and Strabismus, New York Eye and Ear Infirmary, New York, New York
Central Serous Chorioretinopathy

PRUT HANUTSAHA, M.D.
Assistant Professor, Department of Ophthalmology, Ramathibodi Hospital, Mahidol University, Bangkok, Thailand
Three-Dimensional Ophthalmic Ultrasonography of the Posterior Segment

J. WILLIAM HARBOUR, M.D.
Assistant Professor of Ophthalmology and Director, Center for Ocular Oncology, Washington University School of Medicine, St. Louis, Missouri
Intraocular Lymphoid Tumors

SOHAN SINGH HAYREH, M.D., PH.D., D.SC., F.R.C.S., F.R.C.OPHTH.
Professor of Ophthalmology, Director, Ocular Vascular Division, College of Medicine, University of Iowa, Iowa City, Iowa
Hypertensive Fundus Changes

JOHN R. HECKENLIVELY, M.D.
Professor of Ophthalmology, Jules Stein Eye Institute, UCLA Medical Center, Los Angeles, California
Stargardt's Disease and Fundus Flavimaculatus

MURK-HEIN HEINEMANN, M.D.
Assistant Professor of Ophthalmology, Cornell University Medical College; Chief, Ophthalmology Service, Memorial Sloan Kettering Cancer Center, New York, New York
Surgical Management of Retinal Detachments Due to AIDS

ALLEN C. HO, M.D.
Assistant Professor of Ophthalmology, University of Pennsylvania School of Medicine; Scheie Eye Institute Retina Service, Philadelphia, Pennsylvania
Clinical Examination of the Posterior Segment of the Eye; Macular Hole; Ocular Syphilis

NANCY M. HOLEKAMP, M.D.
Instructor, Department of Ophthalmology and Visual Sciences, Washington University School of Medicine; Barnes Retina Institute, St. Louis, Missouri
Subretinal Surgery; Surgical Managment of CNV

MICHAEL HUMAYUN, M.D.
Surgeon, Vitreoretinal Staff, Washington Hospital Center, Washington, D.C.
Congenital Hypertrophy of the Retinal Pigment Epithelium

GLENN J. JAFFE, M.D.
Associate Professor of Ophthalmology, Duke University Medical Center, Durham, North Carolina
Diagnostic Vitrectomy

LEE M. JAMPOL, M.D.
Louis Feinberg Professor and Chairman, Department of Ophthalmology, Northwestern University; Chief of Ophthalmology, Northwestern Memorial Hospital, Chicago, Illinois
Posterior Scleritis

MARK W. JOHNSON, M.D.
Associate Professor of Ophthalmology, W.K. Kellogg Eye Center, University of Michigan School of Medicine, Ann Arbor, Michigan
Uveal Effusion

ROBERT N. JOHNSON, M.D.
Assistant Clinical Professor of Ophthalmology, University of California, San Francisco, San Francisco, California
Acute Multifocal Posterior Placoid Pigment Epitheliopathy (AMPPPE)

PETER K. KAISER, M.D.
Associate Staff, Division of Ophthalmology, The Cleveland Clinic Foundation Eye Institute, Cleveland, Ohio
Radiation Retinopathy; Bone Marrow Transplant Retinopathy

ROBERT E. KALINA, M.D.
Professor of Ophthalmology, University of Washington, Seattle, Washington
Acute Macular Neuroretinopathy

NEIL E. KELLY, M.D.
Retina Consultants, Sacramento, California
Macular Hole Surgery

JUDY E. KIM, M.D.
Clinical Instructor, Medical College of Wisconsin, Milwaukee, Wisconsin; Staff, Eye Surgeons Assocations, PC, Davenport, Iowa
Drug-Induced Toxic Retinopathies

INGRID KREISSIG, M.D.
Professor and Chairman of Ophthalmology, University of Tuebingen, Tuebingen, Germany; Adjunct Professor of Clinical Ophthalmology, New York Hospital-Cornell Medical center, New York, New York
Balloon Buckles for Repair of Retinal Detachment

DAGMAR KUHN, M.D.
Teaching Fellow, University of Paris-XII; Fellow, University Eye Clinic of Créteil, Créteil, France
Myopia

BRIAN L. LEE, M.D.
Jules Stein Eye Institute, University of California, Los Angeles, Los Angeles, California; Presently Fellow, Department of Ophthalmology, University of California, San Diego, San Diego, California
Systemic Genetic Disorders Associated with Retinal Dystrophies; Stargardt's Disease and Fundus Flavimaculatus

HILEL LEWIS, M.D.
Professor and Chairman, Division of Ophthalmology; Director, Cleveland Clinic Eye Institute, The Cleveland Clinic Foundation, Cleveland, Ohio; Professor of Ophthalmology, Ohio State University School of Medicinek, Columbus, Ohio
Vitreoretinal Surgery for Ocular Trauma

HARVEY LINCOFF, M.D.
Professor of Ophthalmology, Cornell University Medical School; Attending Surgeon, The New York Hospital, New York, New York
Balloon Buckles for Repair of Retinal Detachment

ANAT LOEWENSTEIN, M.D.
Assistant Professor, Tel Aviv University; Head of Retina Unit, Ichilov Hospital, Tel Aviv, Israel
Retinal Histology; Neovascular (Exudative) Age-Related Macular Degeneration

MONICA LORENZO-LATKANY, M.D.
Clinical Instructor in Ophthalmology, New York University School of Medicine; Attending Physician, New York Eye and Ear Infirmary, New York, New York
The Retina and Choroid in HIV Infection

GERARD LUTTY, PH.D.
Associate Professor, The Johns Hopkins Hospital, Baltimore, Maryland
Hemoglobinopathies

ALICE T. LYON, M.D.
Instructor in Ophthalmology, Northwestern University Medical School; Northwestern Memorial Hospital, Chicago, Illinois
Posterior Scleritis

ALBERT M. MAGUIRE, M.D.
Assistant Professor of Ophthalmology, University of Pennsylvania, Scheie Eye Institute, Philadelphia, Pennsylvania
Ocular Toxocariasis

MARTIN A. MAINSTER, M.D., PH.D.
Professor and Vice Chairperson, Department of Ophthalmology, University of Kansas Medical Center, Kansas City, Kansas
Laser Photocoagulation

NARESH MANDAVA, M.D.
Assistant Professor of Ophthalmology, University of Colorado Health Sciences Center, Denver, Colorado
Principles of Fluorescein Angiography; Coats' Disease

ERIC S. MANN, M.D., PH.D.
Assistant Professor of Ophthalmology, St. Louis University of Medicine, St. Louis, Missouri
Ocular Histoplasmosis

FILIPPO MARANO, M.D.
Staff member, University of Catania, Sicily, Italy
Benign Concentric Maculopathy

H. RICHARD MCDONALD, M.D.
Associate Clinical Professor of Ophthalmology, University of San Francisco, San Francisco, California
Acute Multifocal Posterior Placoid Pigment Epitheliopathy (AMPPPE)

MARY E. MENDELSOHN, M.D.
Attending Ophthalmologist, Pascock Valley Hospital, Westwood, New Jersey
Age-Related Macular Degeneration: Radiation Therapy for Choroidal Neovascularization

TRAVIS A. MEREDITH, M.D.
Clinical Professor of Ophthalmology, Barnes Retina Institute, Washington University School of Medicine, St. Louis, Missouri
Ocular Histoplasmosis

WILLIAM F. MIELER, M.D.
Professor of Ophthalmology and Chief of the Vitreoretinal Service, Eye Institute, Medical College of Wisconsin, Milwaukee, Wisconsin
Posterior Segment Manifestations of Blunt Trauma; Drug-Induced Toxic Retinopathies; Management of Posterior Segment Intraocular Foreign Bodies

ELENA MIER-TROTTER, M.D.
Senior Fellow in Uveitis, National Eye Institute, National Institutes of Health, Bethesda, Maryland
Subretinal Fibrosis and Uveitis Syndrome

GOLNAZ MOAZAMI, M.D.
Instructor in Clinical Ophthalmology, Attending Ophthalmologist, Columbia University College of Physicians and Surgeons; Lenox Hill Hospital, New York, New York
Optic Disc Drusen

SUMIT K. NANDA, M.D.
Clinical Assistant Professor, Vitreoretinal Service, Dean A. McGee Eye Institute; Department of Ophthalmology, University of Oklahoma, Oklahoma City, Oklahoma
Photic Retinopathy

JAMI NICHOL, BFA
Research Photographer, Wills Eye Hospital, Philadelphia, Pennsylvania
Principles of Fluorescein Angiography

JOHN H. NIFFENEGGER, M.D.
Instructor, University Hospitals, Cleveland, Ohio
Other Causes of Choroidal Neovascular Membranes

KENNETH G. NOBLE, M.D.
Associate Professor of Clinical Ophthalmology, New York University Medical Center, New York, New York
Retinitis Pigmentosa and Allied Diseases; Congenital Stationary Night Blindness; Choroidal Dystrophies; Pattern Dystrophy of the Retinal Pigment Epithelium; Sorsby's Fundus Dystrophy

ROBERT B. NUSSENBLATT, M.D.
Scientific Director, National Eye Institute, National Institutes of Health, Bethesda, Maryland
Subretinal Fibrosis and Uveitis Syndrome; Toxoplasmosis

JEFFREY G. ODEL, M.D.
Associate Clinical Professor of Ophthalmology, Columbia University, Edward S. Harkness Eye Institute, New York, New York
Optic Disc Drusen

DENNIS ORLOCK, CRA
Retinal Research, Lu Esther T. Mertz Retinal Research Unit, Manhattan Eye, Ear & Throat Hospital, New York, New York
Principles of Fluroescein Angiography; Principles of Indocyanine-Green Angiography

DONALD W. PARK, M.D.
Retinal Consultants of Arizona, Phoenix, Arizona
Acute Multifocal Posterior Placoid Pigment Epitheliopathy (AMPPPE); Best's Disease: Molecular and Clinical Findings

ARUN C. PATEL, M.D.
Retina Consultants, Sacramento, California
Macular Hole Surgery

SAMIR C. PATEL, M.D.
Assistant Professor, University of Chicago; Director of Vitreoretinal Service, Chicago, Illinois
Tuberculosis

DANTE J. PIERAMICI, M.D.
Assistant Professor of Ophthalmology, Vitreoretinal Section, Department of Ophthalmology and Visual Science, Yale University School of Medicine, New Haven, Connecticut
Surgical Management of Proliferative Vitreoretinopathy

ALFRED J.L.G. PINCKERS, M.D.
Lecturer in Ophthalmology, University of Nijmegen, Nijmegen, The Netherlands
Benign Concentric Maculopathy

ERIC A. POSTEL, M.D.
Assistant Professor of Ophthalmology, Vitreoretinal Service Duke Eye Center, Durham, North Carolina
Posterior Segment Manifestations of Blunt Trauma; Management of Posterior Segment Intraocular Foreign Bodies

CARMEN A. PULIAFITO, M.D.
Professor of Ophthalmology and Health Management, Tufts University School of Medicine; Chair, Department of Ophthalmology, New England Eye Center, Boston, Massachusetts
New Diagnostic and Therapeutic Approaches to Retinal Disease

MADDALENA QUARANTA, M.D.
Fellow, University Eye Clinic of Créteil, Créteil, France
Angioid Streaks

DAVID A. QUILLEN, M.D.
Assistant Professor of Ophthalmology, Penn State University College of Medicine; Penn State Geisinger Health System, The Milton S. Hershey Medical Center, Hershey, Pennsylvania
Proliferative Diabetic Retinopathy

ALI M. RAMADAN, M.D.
Visiting Associate, National Eye Institute, Lab of Immunology, National Institutes of Health, Bethesda, Maryland
Toxoplasmosis

CARL D. REGILLO, M.D.
Associate Professor of Ophthalmology, Thomas Jefferson University Hospital; Associate Surgeon, Wills Hospital, Philadelphia, Pennsylvania
Familial Exudative Vitreoretinopathy

REEM Z. RENNO, M.D.
Resident, Manhattan Eye, Ear & Throat Hospital, New York, New York
Central Retinal Vein Occlusion: A Primer and Review

VINCENT REPPUCCI, M.D.
Assistant Professor of Clinical Ophthalmology, Columbia University College of Physicians and Surgeons; Adjunct Assistant Professor of Ophthalmology, Cornell University Medical College, New York, New York
Surgical Management of Giant Retinal Tears

DANIEL F. ROSBERGER, M.D., PH.D.
Assistant Professor of Ophthalmology, Cornell University Medical College; Assistant Professor of Ophthalmology, The New York Hospital-Cornell Medical Center, New York, New York
Nonneovascular (Nonexudative) Age-Related Macular Degeneration

PATRICK E. RUBSAMEN, M.D.
Associate Professor, Bascom Palmer Eye Institute, University of Miami School of Medicine, Miami, Florida
Vogt-Koyanagi-Harada Syndrome

CHANDER N. SAMY, M.D.
Harvard Medical School, Massachusetts Eye and Ear Infirmary, Boston, Massachusetts
Choroidal Metastasis

ARTURO SANTOS, M.D.
Professor of Ophthalmology, Centro Universitario de Ciencias de la Salud, Universidad de Guadalajara; Active Medical Staff, Servico de Oftalmologia, Hospital Civil de Guadalajara, Guadalajara, Jalisco, Mexico
Retinal Diseases in Pregnancy

DAVID A. SAPERSTEIN, M.D.
Assistant Professor, Emory University, Atlanta, Georgia
Intermediate Uveitis (Pars Planitis)

ANDREW P. SCHACHAT, M.D.
Professor of Ophthalmology, Johns Hopkins University; Director, Ocular Oncology Service, The Johns Hopkins Hospital, Baltimore, Maryland
Combined Hamartoma of the Retina and Retinal Pigment Epithelium; The Ophthalmic Manifestations of Leukemia

HOWARD SCHATZ, M.D.
Clinical Professor of Ophthalmology, University of California, San Francisco; Director, Retina Research Fund of St. Mary's Medical Center, San Francisco, California
Acute Multifocal Posterior Placoid Pigment Epitheliopathy (AMPPPE)

WILLIAM SCHIFF, M.D.
Instructor of Clinical Ophthalmology, Columbia University College of Physicians and Surgeons; Assistant Attending in Ophthalmology, Roosevelt/St. Luke's Hospital Center; Assistant Ophthalmologist, Harkness Eye Institute, The Presbyterian Hospital; Associate Adjunct, Department of Ophthalmology, The New York Eye and Ear Infirmary, New York, New York
Surgical Management of Giant Retinal Tears

HERMANN D. SCHUBERT, M.D.
Professor of Clinical Ophthalmology and Pathology, Columbia University College of Physicians and Surgeons; Attending Surgeon, Director of Retina Clinic, Edward S. Harkness Eye Institute, Columbia Presbyterian Hospital, New York, New York
Eales' Disease

ROBERT SELKIN, M.D.
Resident, Lenox Hill Hospital, New York, New York
Sympathetic Ophthalmia

CAROL L. SHIELDS, M.D.
Assistant Professor, Department of Ophthalmology, Thomas Jefferson University; Surgeon, Oncology Service, Wills Eye Hospital, Philadelphia, Pennsylvania
Choroidal Osteoma; Retinal Capillary Hemangioma; Vasoproliferative Tumors of the Ocular Fundus

JERRY A. SHIELDS, M.D.
Director of Oncology Service, Wills Eye Hospital; Professor of Ophthalmology, Thomas Jefferson University, Philadelphia, Pennsylvania
Choroidal Nevus; Posterior Uveal Melanoma; Differential Diagnosis of Posterior Uveal Melanoma; Myogenic and Neurogenic Tumors of the Posterior Uvea; Tumors and Related Lesions of the Retinal Pigment Epithelium; Acquired Neoplasms of the Nonpigmented Ciliary Epithelium; Intraocular Medulloepithelioma; Retinoblastoma; Differential Diagnosis of Retinoblastoma; Retinal Cavernous Hemangioma; Retinal Astrocytoma; Melanocytoma of the Optic Nerve

LAWRENCE J. SINGERMAN, M.D.
Clinical Professor of Ophthalmology, Case Western Reserve University; Director, Retinal Institute, Mt. Sinai Medical Center, Cleveland, Ohio
Other Causes of Choroidal Neovascular Membranes

JASON S. SLAKTER, M.D.
Assistant Clinical Professor of Ophthalmology, College of Physicians and Surgeons of Columbia University; Attending Surgeon, Vitreoretinal Service, Manhattan Eye, Ear & Throat Hospital, New York, New York
Principles of Indocyanine-Green Angiography; Three-Dimensional Ophthalmic Ultrasonography of the Posterior Segment; Ocular Sarcoidosis; Diffuse Unilateral Subacute Neuroretinitis

M. MADISON SLUSHER, M.D.
Professor and Chairman, Bowman Gray School of Medicine, Wake Forest University; Director, Wake Forest University Eye Center, Wake Forest University, Winston-Salem, North Carolina
Retinal Arterial Macroaneurysms

KENT W. SMALL, M.D.
Associate Professor, Jules Stein Eye Institute, University of California, Los Angeles, Los Angeles, California
Systemic Genetic Disorders Associated with Retinal Dystrophies

JOHN A. SORENSON, M.D.
Assistant Clinical Professor of Ophthalmology, College of Physicians and Surgeons of Columbia University; Attending Surgeon, Vitreoretinal Service, Manhattan Eye, Ear & Throat Hospital, New York, New York
Principles of Indocyanine-Green Angiography; Multiple Evanescent White Dot Syndrome (MEWDS)

GISÈLE SOUBRANE, M.D., PH.D.
Professor of Clinical Ophthalmology, Eye University Clinic of Créteil, University of Paris-XII; Ophthalmologiste des Hopitaux de Paris, Directeur de Recherche, U INSERM, Cretéil, France
Angioid Streaks; Myopia

RICHARD F. SPAIDE, M.D., F.A.C.S.
Assistant Clinical Professor in Ophthalmology, New York Medical College, Valhalla, New York
Principles of Indocyanine-Green Angiography; Postsurgical Cystoid Macular Edema; Frosted Branch Angiitis

JANET R. SPARROW, PH.D.
Associate Professor of Ophthalmic Science, Department of Ophthalmology, Columbia University College of Physicians and Surgeons, New York, New York
Vitreous Substitutes

PAUL STERNBERG, JR., M.D.
Thomas M. Aaberg Professor of Ophthalmology, Emory University School of Medicine: Director, Vitreoretinal Service, Emory Eye Center, Atlanta, Georgia
Viral Syndromes

GLENN L. STOLLER, M.D.
Clinical Assistant Professor, Cornell University Medical College; Assistant Attending, The New York Hospital, New York, New York
Balloon Buckles for Repair of Retinal Detachment

EDWIN M. STONE, M.D., PH.D.
Professor, Department of Ophthalmology, University of Iowa College of Medicine, Iowa City, Iowa
Best's Disease: Molecular and Clinical Findings

JANET S. SUNNESS, M.D.
Associate Professor of Ophthalmology, The Wilmer Ophthalmological Institute, The Johns Hopkins University School of Medicine, Baltimore, Maryland
Retinal Diseases in Pregnancy

ANGELO P. TANNA, M.D.
Resident in Ophthalmology, The Wilmer Ophthalmological Institute, The Johns Hopkins Hospital, Baltimore, Maryland
The Ophthalmic Manifestations of Leukemia

WILLIAM TASMAN, M.D.
Professor and Chairman, Department of Ophthalmology, Thomas Jefferson Medical College; Ophthalmologist-in-Chief, Wills Eye Hospital, Philadelphia, Pennsylvania
X-Linked Retinoschisis

MATTHEW A. THOMAS, M.D.
Assistant Professor, Department of Ophthalmology and Visual Sciences, Washington University School of Medicine; Barnes Retina Institute, St. Louis, Missouri
Subretinal Surgery

DAVID TOM, M.D.
Assistant Attending Surgeon, Vitreoretinal Service, Manhattan Eye, Ear & Throat Hospital, New York, New York
Serpiginous Choroiditis

PAUL E. TORNAMBE, M.D., F.A.C.S.
Scripps Hospital System, Mericose Eye Institute, La Jolla, California
Pneumatic Retinopexy

WILLIAM A. TOWNSEND-PICO, M.D.
Clinical Faculty, Vitreoretinal Surgery, Veterans Administration Hospital, San Juan, Puerto Rico
Vitreoretinal Surgery for Ocular Trauma

ELIAS I. TRABOULSI, M.D.
Head, Department of Pediatric Ophthalmology, Director, The Center for Genetic Eye Disease, The Cleveland Clinic Foundation, Cleveland, Ohio
Congenital Hypertrophy of the Retinal Pigment Epithelium

MICHAEL T. TRESE, M.D.
Clinical Associate Professor, Kresge Eye Institute, Wayne State University, Detroit, Michigan; Clinical Associate Professor of Biomedical Sciences, Eye Research Institute, Oakland University, Rochester, Michigan
Retinopathy of Prematurity: Stages 1 Through 3; Retinopathy of Prematurity: Stages 4 and 5

SANDRO VERGANI, M.D.
Clinical Researcher, Department of Ophthalmology and Visual Sciences, University of Milan, S. Raffaele Hospital, Milan, Italy
The Rheumatic Retinal Diseases

KEITH A. WARREN, M.D.
Assistant Professor, Department of Ophthalmology, University of Kansas Medical Center, Kansas City, Kansas
Laser Photocoagulation

DAVID V. WEINBERG, M.D.
Assistant Professor of Ophthalmology, Director of the Vitreoretinal Service, Northwestern University Medical School, Chicago, Illinois
Progressive Outer Retinal Necrosis

DAVID J. WEISSGOLD, M.D.
Assistant Professor, University of Vermont College of Medicine; Attending Ophthalmologist, Fletcher Allen Health Care, Burlington, Vermont
Chorioretinal and Retinal Folds

ROBERT T. WENDEL, M.D.

Clinical Faculty, University of California, Davis, Davis, California

Macular Hole Surgery

C.P. WILKINSON, M.D.

Professor of Ophthalmology, Johns Hopkins University; Chairman, Department of Ophthalmology, Greater Baltimore Medical Center, Baltimore, Maryland

Scleral Buckling Techniques: A Simplified Approach

DAVID T. WONG, M.D.

Lecturer, University of Toronto; Attending Staff, St. Michaels Hospital, Toronto, Ontario, Canada; Courtesy Staff, Mississauga Hospital, Mississagua, Canada

Surgical Management of Giant Retinal Tears

LAWRENCE A. YANNUZZI, M.D.

Vice-Chairman and Director of Retinal Services, Manhattan Eye, Ear & Throat Hospital; Professor of Clinical Ophthalmology, Columbia University College of Physicians and Surgeons, New York, New York

Principles of Fluorescein Angiography; Principles of Indocyanine-Green Angiography; Central Serous Chorioretinopathy; Postsurgical Cystoid Macular Edema; Central Retinal Vein Occlusion: A Primer and Review; Coats' Disease; Parafoveal Telangiectasis; Plasma Protein Risk Factors for Retinal Vascular Occlusive Disease; Serpiginous Choroiditis; Multiple Evanescent White Dot Syndrome (MEWDS); Myiasis

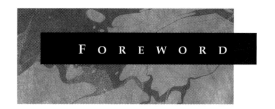

The importance of the retina is highlighted by current epidemiologic evidence showing that the two most prevalent blinding diseases in the United States involve this tissue; namely, age-related macular degeneration (AMD) and diabetic retinopathy. Regrettably, age-related macular degeneration is rapidly assuming epidemic proportions in the senior citizen population of North America. In one representative community of the United States, Beaver Dam, Wisconsin, for example, the prevalence of AMD in all persons 43 to 86 years of age was a remarkably high 17%, and epidemiologic studies have shown that it may be even higher in another representative community, Salisbury, Maryland. The prevalence figures for diabetic retinopathy in Beaver Dam were as high as 71% in type 1 diabetics and 39% in type 2 diabetics. Blindness from diabetes costs the United States approximately $500 million per year in lost income and expenses associated with public welfare. Despite major technical advances in both diagnosis and therapy, exemplified by fluorescein angiography, laser photocoagulation, and vitreoretinal surgery, both AMD and diabetic retinopathy remain major sources of visual disability in most developed countries.

It is fascinating to realize that a tissue as small as the retina (only about 260 sq mm) and as tiny as the macula (only about 2 millimeters in diameter) generates so much disease, intellectual curiosity, and clinical effort. With the burgeoning knowledge offered by the fields of molecular genetics (for AMD, for example), and growth factor physiology (for diabetic retinopathy, for example, and other diseases characterized by leaky blood vessels and neovascularization), it is apparent that attempts at understanding and treating these two major diseases will intensify substantially beyond the impressive activities that have already occurred.

The transparent media of the eye allow unparalleled opportunities to visualize a multitude of other blinding disorders of the retina, macula, and vitreous, in addition to those caused by diabetes and AMD. Many of these diseases are well-defined clinically, but several others represent "new" and/or poorly understood entities. There remain, therefore, numerous opportunities for more precise diagnostic techniques and more specific therapeutic interventions. Many of these procedures are yet to be invented, but, as has been true in the past, the creative minds of vitreoretinal specialists will, no doubt, rise to the occasion.

This comprehensive text, edited and written by expert diagnosticians and surgeons, is a timely, useful, and logical sequel to the valuable atlas of fundus disease compiled recently by several of the same specialists.[1] In addition to outstandingly educational illustrations in the initial atlas and in this text, the current pair of volumes also provide informative textual and clinicopathologic materials.

The beautifully hand-illustrated and clinically influential Wilmer atlas of the fundus was published in 1934,[2] setting the stage for heightened interest in retinal diseases in this country. Thereafter, the exponential rate of accretion of new knowledge regarding the retina, macula, and vitreous has been impressive. At increasingly short durations and in increasingly large volumes, key articles, texts, and atlases have appeared; for example, the refinements of scleral buckling by Schepens and many others, beginning in 1957,[3] the development of photocoagulation, first by Meyer-Schwickerath with the xenon arc in 1960[4]; the introduction of fluorescein angiography by A.E. Maumenee in 1960[5]; the fluorescein angiography atlas by Shikano and Shimizu in 1968[6]; the experience of L'Esperance, Zweng, Patz, and others[7–9] with the argon laser and slit lamp delivery system in 1968 and thereafter; the first edition of the Gass atlas of macular diseases in 1970[10]; and the advent of motorized vitrectomy surgery by Machemer and Peyman in 1971.[11,12] Most importantly, validation of several therapeutic interventions has occurred for photocoagulation and vitreoretinal surgery through numerous well-performed clinical trials from 1976[13] to the present, for such diseases as diabetic retinopathy, age-related macular degeneration, retinal vein occlusion, sickle cell retinopathy, retinopathy of prematurity, proliferative vitreo-retinopathy, endophthalmitis, and others.

No doubt the last half century has been characterized by an explosive efflorescence of new vitreoretinal knowledge, allowing a book of this size simultaneously to be both feasible and necessary. It would be understandable for an observer to view the developments of the last part of the twentieth century as a golden era in the understanding and treatment of retinal, macular and vitreous diseases. In truth, the next several years promise to be even more exciting and gratifying.

MORTON F. GOLDBERG, M.D.
Director and William Holland Wilmer Professor
  of Ophthalmology
The Wilmer Ophthalmological Institute
The Johns Hopkins University School of Medicine
Baltimore, Maryland

REFERENCES

1. Yannuzzi LA, Guyer DR, Green DR: The Retina Atlas. St. Louis. Mosby, 1995.
2. Wilmer WH: Atlas Fundus Oculi. New York. The MacMillan Company, 1934.
3. Schepens CL, Okamura ID, Brockhurst RJ: The scleral buckling procedures. I. Surgical techniques and management. Arch Ophthalmol 58:797–811, 1957.
4. Meyer-Schwickerath G. Light Coagulation. Trans. by SM Drance. St. Louis. Mosby, 1960.
5. Maclean AL, Maumenee AE: Hemangioma of the choroid. Am J Ophthalmol 50:3–11, 1960.
6. Shikano S, Shimizu K: Atlas of Fluorescence Fundus Angiography. Tokyo, Iguku Shoin Ltd., 1968.
7. L'Esperance FA Jr: An ophthalmic argon laser photocoagulation system: design, construction, and laboratory investigations. Trans Am Ophthalmol Soc 66:827–904, 1968.
8. Zweng HC, Little HL, Peabody RR: Laser photocoagulation of macular lesions. Trans Am Acad Ophthalmol Otolaryngol 72:377–388, 1968.
9. Patz A, Maumenee AE, Ryan SJ: Argon laser photocoagulation. Trans Am Ophthalmol Otolaryngol 75:569–579, 1971.
10. Gass JDM: Stereoscopic Atlas of Macular Diseases, 4 ed. St. Louis, Mosby, 1997.
11. Machemer R, Buetner H, Norton EWD, Parel J-M: Vitrectomy: a pars plana approach. Trans Am Acad Ophthalmol Otolaryngol 75:813–820, 1971.
12. Peyman GA, Dodich NA: Experimental vitrectomy: instrumentation and surgical technique. Arch Ophthalmol 86:548–551, 1971.
13. The Diabetic Retinopathy Study Research Group. Preliminary report on effects of photocoagulation therapy. Ophthalmology 81:383–396, 1976.

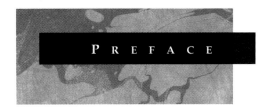

When it comes to the accessibility of an internal tissue . . . from the vitreoretinal interface through the retinal circulation and pigment epithelium to the uveal scleral junction . . . for critical and dynamic clinical study, the fundus has no equal. Armed with an array of special examining instruments such as the direct and indirect ophthalmoscope, and the slit lamp biomicroscope with a contact lens, the ophthalmologist can view the retina and adjacent structures with unparalleled clarity and accuracy to correlate clinical manifestations to known histopathological changes. Given that no other organ can be examined in such a fashion, it is understandable that many ophthalmologists have a fascination . . . a passion . . . for viewing and studying the retina.

Furthermore, relatively simple observations of the fundus can now be enhanced for even more meaningful clinical information through the use of sophisticated diagnostic adjuncts, including ultrasonography, fluorescein and indocyanine-green angiography, digital imaging, ocular coherent tomography, scanning laser ophthalmoscopy and even endoscopy.

These unique images have sustained a high level of interest on the part of retinal specialists over the years to record and to publish their findings in a series of important textbooks. Many of these educational editions have been very successful with widespread, if not universal, acceptance. So, why another text? In this text we hope to combine high quality color photography and histopathological correlations within a comprehensive textbook. In addition, in recent years there has also been a steady stream of biophysiological advances from ophthalmologists as well as allied specialists, particularly molecular biologists, immunologists, and geneticists. Their discoveries have led to a better understanding of the pathogenesis of many chorioretinal diseases and, in some instances, their treatment. In tandem with these developments, there has also been the introduction of new therapeutic instrumentation beginning more than 35 years ago with the Zeiss xenon photocoagulator, the forerunner of ophthalmic lasers. Cryosurgery, an array of creative vitreoretinal surgical devices aided by innovative microsurgical instruments and supplemental adjuncts such as gas, silicon and superb, well-illuminated binocular viewing systems followed with sometimes daring and phenomenal applications. These changes have set the occasion for radical new approaches to the diagnostic and treatment of retinal disease. Coinciding with these advances has been clinical research which has elevated patient assessment and care from anecdotal-based impressions to acceptable scientific dogma due to prospective clinical trials, most notably the legendary series of national collaborative clinical trials funded by the National Institutes of Health (NIH) for the treatment of medical and surgical diseases of the retina. Based on initial impressions by experienced retinal specialists, these NIH trials were exquisitely designed, and their results were stringently evaluated within very strict and disciplined scientific environments. Recommendations for treatment of common disorders associated with severe vision loss –such as diabetic retinopathy, age-related macular degeneration, and retinal branch vein occlusion– were among the first to be disseminated to the ophthalmic public for patient management. The ethical ophthalmic literature is now enframed with these guidelines which have established new standards in patient care for the ensuing 21st Century.

One of these recent trials with multiple arms is devoted to the management of ocular melanoma. The retinal specialist of the present is not just a vitreoretinal surgeon, he or she also devotes time to ocular oncology in addition to traditional subjects such as hereditary disorders, immunologically based inflammatory diseases, infections, retinal vascular disease and degenerative conditions of the retinal and choroidal circulations. Finally, to best serve their patients, the retinal specialist of today must not only be able to recognize the clinical manifestations of each of these entities, he or she must also be well versed in the associated histopathology and mechanisms of diseases of the ocular fundus. It is the intent of this text to incorporate these important new changes and discoveries in the clinical evolution of the retinal specialist.

Given this multidisciplinary spectrum of today's retinal specialist (medical retina, vitreoretinal surgery, oncology, and pathology) one of us (DG) serving as coordinator, catalyst and conceptualizer of the text, assembled four of the leading experts in these subspecialties (LY, SC, JS, and WRG, respectively) to edit and embellish, where possible, the material in hope of producing a single work dedicated to the retina in a relatively comprehensive and authoritative fashion. Numerous contributions were also recruited from an elite corps of other international specialists in visual science, medical retina, oncology, and vitreoretinal surgery. Given these multiple authors, there is an expected variation in literary style. The editors have accordingly sought, where possible, to provide a level of organizational conformity without compromising the originality and style of the individual contributor. In most instances, chorioretinal disorders are reviewed with reference to their clinical findings, natural course, histopathological features where known, and the accepted forms of treatment. The final product is intended primarily for residents and retinal fellows in ophthalmology, for ophthalmologists who have had little formal training in retinal disease, and also for some retinal specialists who have had little opportunity to examine the less commonly encountered disorders.

On a personal level, the five authors have enjoyed a close friendship, in some instances for nearly 30 years, originating from a common interest in diseases of the retina. Over the years we have enjoyed working with and learning from each other, and it has indeed been a pleasure for us to collaborate on this volume. The contributing authors are not merely retinal experts but also good friends. We owe a great deal to them and to many others, including the physicians who referred patients to us, for management and our residents and fellows who have been a constant source of inspiration through their inquisitive and provocative thoughts. We owe special thanks to William Comstock who worked faithfully and diligently for many hours editing the text, verifying and standardizing the bibliography, and coordinating the materials submitted by the contributors.

DAVID R. GUYER, M.D.
LAWRENCE A. YANNUZZI, M.D.
STANLEY CHANG, M.D.
JERRY A. SHIELDS, M.D.
W. RICHARD GREEN, M.D.

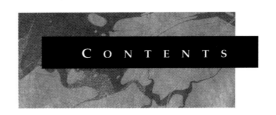

CONTENTS

VOLUME I

Section I
Anatomy, Clinical Examination,
Diagnostic Techniques, and
Laser Therapy 1

Chapter 1
Retinal Histology.. 3
    Anat Loewenstein, W. Richard Green

Chapter 2
Clinical Examination of the Posterior Segment
of the Eye 21
    Allen C. Ho, David R. Guyer, Stuart L. Fine

Chapter 3
Principles of Fluorescein Angiography 29
    Naresh Mandava, David R. Guyer,
    Lawrence A. Yannuzzi, Jami Nichol,
    Dennis Orlock

Chapter 4
Principles of Indocyanine-Green Angiography 39
    David R. Guyer, Lawrence A. Yannuzzi,
    Jason S. Slakter, John A. Sorenson,
    Richard F. Spaide, K. Bailey Freund,
    Dennis Orlock

Chapter 5
Ophthalmic Contact B-Scan Ultrasonography 47
    Andrew A. Chang, Antonio P. Ciardella,
    Yale L. Fisher

Chapter 6
Three-Dimensional Ophthalmic Ultrasonography
of the Posterior Segment.................................... 55
    Yale L. Fisher, Antonio P. Ciardella,
    Jason S. Slakter, Andrew A. Chang, Prut Hanutsaha,
    Aaron Fenster

Chapter 7
Laser Photocoagulation.. 61
    Martin A. Mainster, Keith A. Warren

Chapter 8
New Diagnostic and Therapeutic Approaches to
Retinal Disease... 69
    Caroline R. Baumal, Carmen A. Puliafito

Section II
Macular Disorders 77

Chapter 9
Nonneovascular (Nonexudative) Age-Related
Macular Degeneration 79
    Susan B. Bressler, Daniel F. Rosberger

Chapter 10
Neovascular (Exudative) Age-Related Macular
Degeneration... 94
    Anat Loewenstein, Neil M. Bressler

Chapter 11
Antiangiogenic Therapy 122
    Anthony P. Adamis

Chapter 12
Age-Related Macular Degeneration: Radiation
Therapy for Choroidal Neovascularization 126
    Mary E. Mendelsohn, David H. Abramson

Chapter 13
Subretinal Surgery... 131
    Nancy M. Holekamp, Matthew A. Thomas

Chapter 14
Other Causes of Choroidal Neovascular
Membranes 137
    John H. Niffenegger, Lawrence J. Singerman

Chapter 15
Angioid Streaks.................................163
    Gabriel Coscas, Gisèle Soubrane,
    Maddalena Quaranta

Chapter 16
Ocular Histoplasmosis.......................178
    Eric S. Mann, Travis A. Meredith

Chapter 17
Myopia 189
    Gisèle Soubrane, Gabriel Coscas,
    Dagmar Kuhn

Chapter 18
Central Serous Chorioretinopathy 206
    Lisabeth S. Hall, David R. Guyer,
    Lawrence A. Yannuzzi

Chapter 19
Macular Hole 217
    Allen C. Ho

Chapter 20
Epimacular Membranes 230
    Steve Charles

Chapter 21
Postsurgical Cystoid Macular Edema ...238
    Andrew A. Chang, Richard F. Spaide,
    Lawrence A. Yannuzzi

Chapter 22
Chorioretinal and Retinal Folds 256
    David J. Weissgold, Alexander J. Brucker

Section III
Retinal Vascular Diseases 269

Chapter 23
Retinal Arterial Occlusive Diseases 271
    Gary C. Brown

Chapter 24
Central Retinal Vein Occlusion: A Primer
and Review......................................286
    Antonio P. Ciardella, John G. Clarkson,
    David R. Guyer, Reem Z. Renno,
    Lawrence A. Yannuzzi

Chapter 25
Branch Retinal Vein Occlusion 308
    Daniel Finkelstein

Chapter 26
Diabetic Retinopathy 316
    Lloyd M. Aiello, Jerry D. Cavallerano,
    Lloyd P. Aiello, Sven-Erik Bursell

Chapter 27
Hypertensive Fundus Changes 345
    Sohan Singh Hayreh

Chapter 28
Ocular Ischemic Syndrome 372
    Gary C. Brown

Chapter 29
Retinal Arterial Macroaneurysms 383
    M. Madison Slusher

Chapter 30
Coats' Disease 390
    Naresh Mandava, Lawrence A. Yannuzzi

Chapter 31
Parafoveal Telangiectasis..................398
    Gaetano R. Barile, Lawrence A. Yannuzzi

Chapter 32
Retinopathy of Prematurity: Stages 1
Through 3..407
    Philip J. Ferrone, Michael T. Trese

Chapter 33
Eales' Disease.................................415
    Hermann D. Schubert

Chapter 34
Familial Exudative Vitreoretinopathy ...421
    Carl D. Regillo

Chapter 35
Frosted Branch Angiitis 431
    Richard F. Spaide

Chapter 36
Hemoglobinopathies.........................438
    Sharon Fekrat, Gerard Lutty,
    Morton F. Goldberg

Contents

Chapter 37
Plasma Protein Risk Factors for Retinal Vascular
Occlusive Disease...459
    Antonio P. Ciardella, David R. Guyer,
    Lawrence A. Yannuzzi

Chapter 38
Disseminated Intravascular Coagulopathy...........473
    Gaetano R. Barile, David R. Guyer

Chapter 39
Radiation Retinopathy..477
    Peter K. Kaiser, Evangelos S. Gragoudas

Chapter 40
Bone Marrow Transplant Retinopathy.................488
    Peter K. Kaiser, Evangelos S. Gragoudas

Chapter 41
Retinal Diseases in Pregnancy............................498
    Janet S. Sunness, Arturo Santos

Chapter 42
The Rheumatic Retinal Diseases.........................514
    Rosario Brancato, Sandro Vergani,
    Antonio P. Ciardella

Section IV
Inflammatory Disorders.................................535

Chapter 43
Acute Multifocal Posterior Placoid Pigment
Epitheliopathy (AMPPPE)..................................537
    Donald W. Park, Howard Schatz,
    H. Richard McDonald, Robert N. Johnson

Chapter 44
Serpiginous Choroiditis.....................................553
    David Tom, Lawrence A. Yannuzzi

Chapter 45
Birdshot Retinochoroidopathy...........................565
    Jay S. Duker

Chapter 46
Sympathetic Ophthalmia...................................569
    Alan H. Friedman, Robert Selkin

Chapter 47
Vogt-Koyanagi-Harada Syndrome......................573
    Patrick E. Rubsamen, J. Donald M. Gass

Chapter 48
Multiple Evanescent White Dot Syndrome
(MEWDS)...584
    Antonio P. Ciardella, John A. Sorenson,
    Lawrence A. Yannuzzi

Chapter 49
Acute Macular Neuroretinopathy.......................593
    Robert E. Kalina

Chapter 50
Acute Retinal Pigment Epitheliitis.....................597
    Benjamin Chang

Chapter 51
Intermediate Uveitis (Pars Planitis)...................599
    David A. Saperstein, Antonio Capone, Jr.,
    Thomas M. Aaberg, Sr.

Chapter 52
Multifocal Choroiditis, Punctate Inner
Choroidopathy, and Other
Related Conditions..614
    Jeremiah Brown, Jr., James C. Folk

Chapter 53
Subretinal Fibrosis and Uveitis Syndrome...........631
    Elena Mier-Trotter, Robert B. Nussenblatt

Chapter 54
Posterior Scleritis...635
    Alice T. Lyon, Lee M. Jampol

Chapter 55
Ocular Sarcoidosis...643
    Antonio P. Ciardella, Jason S. Slakter

Chapter 56
Uveal Effusion..658
    Mark W. Johnson

Section V
Infectious Disorders......................................669

Chapter 57
Toxoplasmosis...671
    Ali M. Ramadan, Robert B. Nussenblatt

Chapter 58
Ocular Toxocariasis...697
    Albert M. Maguire

Chapter 59
Ocular Cysticercosis 709
　Alan H. Friedman

Chapter 60
The Retina and Choroid in HIV Infection.............714
　Dorothy Nahm Friedberg,
　Monica Lorenzo-Latkany

Chapter 61
Viral Syndromes...............................749
　W.Z. Bridges, Jr., Paul Sternberg, Jr.

Chapter 62
Acute Retinal Necrosis.......................760
　Mark S. Blumenkranz, Gregory Fox

Chapter 63
Progressive Outer Retinal Necrosis 766
　David V. Weinberg

Chapter 64
Fungal Diseases...............................772
　Neil D. Brourman, Mark S. Blumenkranz

Chapter 65
Ocular Syphilis.................................793
　Allen C. Ho

Chapter 66
Tuberculosis 801
　Samir C. Patel, Sander Dubovy

Chapter 67
Diffuse Unilateral Subacute Neuroretinitis............806
　Jason S. Slakter, Antonio P. Ciardella

Chapter 68
Myiasis 813
　Antonio P. Ciardella, David R. Guyer,
　Lawrence A. Yannuzzi

Section VI
Traumatic Disorders 829

Chapter 69
Posterior Segment Manifestations of
Blunt Trauma 831
　Eric A. Postel, William F. Mieler

VOLUME II

Chapter 70
Photic Reinopathy 844
　Sumit K. Nanda

Section VII
Drug Toxicities.................................853

Chapter 71
Drug-Induced Toxic Retinopathies 855
　Judy E. Kim, William F. Mieler

Section VIII
Optic Nerve Diseases.......................873

Chapter 72
Congenital Pits of the Optic Nerve Head 875
　Gary C. Brown

Chapter 73
Optic Disc Drusen 880
　Golnaz Moazami, Jeffrey G. Odel,
　Myles M. Behrens

Chapter 74
Leber's Idiopathic Stellate Neuroretinitis..............885
　K. Bailey Freund

Section IX
Hereditary Chorioretinal Disorders:
Generalized and Localized 889

Chapter 75
Retinitis Pigmentosa and Allied Diseases 891
　Ronald E. Carr, Kenneth G. Noble

Chapter 76
Systemic Genetic Disorders Associated with
Retinal Dystrophies 924
　Brian L. Lee, Kent W. Small

Chapter 77
Congenital Stationary Night Blindness.................934
　Kenneth G. Noble

Chapter 78
Cone Dystrophies...............................942
　Ronald E. Carr

Contents

Chapter 79
Choroidal Dystrophies.....................................949
   Kenneth G. Noble

Chapter 80
Stargardt's Disease and Fundus
Flavimaculatus...978
   Brian L. Lee, John R. Heckenlively

Chapter 81
Best's Disease: Molecular and
Clinical Findings..989
   Donald W. Park, Nancy C. Arbour,
   David M. Brown, Edwin M. Stone

Chapter 82
Pattern Dystrophy of the Retinal Pigment
Epithelium..1006
   Kenneth G. Noble

Chapter 83
X-Linked Retinoschisis...................................1013
   William Tasman

Chapter 84
Sorsby's Fundus Dystrophy..............................1018
   Kenneth G. Noble

Chapter 85
Benign Concentric Maculopathy........................1025
   Filippo Marano, August F. Deutman,
   Alfred J.L.G. Pinckers, Albert L. Aandekerk

Chapter 86
Bietti's Crystalline Dystrophy..........................1037
   Dean Eliott

Section X
Tumors..1051

Chapter 87
Choroidal Nevus...1053
   Jerry A. Shields

Chapter 88
Congenital Hypertrophy of the Retinal
Pigment Epithelium......................................1058
   Michael Humayun, Elias I. Traboulsi

Chapter 89
Posterior Uveal Melanoma...............................1067
   Jerry A. Shields

Chapter 90
Differential Diagnosis of Posterior Uveal
Melanoma...1074
   Jerry A. Shields

Chapter 91
Choroidal Hemangioma..................................1083
   Patrick De Potter

Chapter 92
Choroidal Osteoma.......................................1092
   Carol L. Shields

Chapter 93
Choroidal Metastasis.....................................1103
   Bradley S. Foster, Chander N. Samy,
   Evangelos S. Gragoudas

Chapter 94
Myogenic and Neurogenic Tumors of the
Posterior Uvea...1110
   Jerry A. Shields

Chapter 95
Tumors and Related Lesions of the Retinal
Pigment Epithelium......................................1116
   Jerry A. Shields

Chapter 96
Combined Hamartoma of the Retina and
Retinal Pigment Epithelium.............................1123
   Michael J. Cooney, Andrew P. Schachat

Chapter 97
Acquired Neoplasms of the Nonpigmented
Ciliary Epithelium.......................................1130
   Jerry A. Shields

Chapter 98
Intraocular Medulloepithelioma.........................1134
   Jerry A. Shields

Chapter 99
Retinoblastoma...1139
   Jerry A. Shields

Chapter 100
Differential Diagnosis of Retinoblastoma...............1151
   Jerry A. Shields

Chapter 101
Retinal Capillary Hemangioma..........................1159
   Carol L. Shields

Chapter 102
Retinal Cavernous Hemangioma........................1168
   Jerry A. Shields

Chapter 103
Congenital Retinal Arteriovenous
Communications (Racemose
Hemangiomas)...1172
    Gary C. Brown

Chapter 104
Vasoproliferative Tumors of the Ocular
Fundus 1175
    Carol L. Shields

Chapter 105
Retinal Astrocytoma 1182
    Jerry A. Shields

Chapter 106
Melanocytoma of the Optic Nerve 1188
    Jerry A. Shields

Chapter 107
The Ophthalmic Manifestations of Leukemia......1194
    Angelo P. Tanna, Andrew P. Schachat

Chapter 108
Intraocular Lymphoid Tumors 1204
    J. William Harbour, Devron H. Char

Section XI
Surgical Retina...1217

Chapter 109
Peripheral Retinal Lesions Related to
Rhegmatogenous Retinal Detachment 1219
    Norman E. Byer

Chapter 110
Scleral Buckling Techniques: A Simplified
Approach..1248
    C.P. Wilkinson

Chapter 111
Pneumatic Retinopexy 1272
    Paul E. Tornambe

Chapter 112
Balloon Buckles for Repair of Retinal
Detachment..1288
    Harvey Lincoff, Ingrid Kreissig,
    Glenn L. Stoller

Chapter 113
Vitrectomy 1298
    Gary W. Abrams, Ronald C. Gentile

Chapter 114
Vitreous Substitutes..1320
    Stanley Chang, Janet R. Sparrow

Chapter 115
Surgical Management of Giant Retinal Tears 1338
    William Schiff, Stanley Chang,
    Vincent Reppucci, David T. Wong

Chapter 116
Surgical Management of Proliferative
Vitreoretinopathy..1350
    Dante J. Pieramici, Antonio Capone, Jr.,
    Thomas M. Aaberg, Sr.

Chapter 117
Vitreoretinal Surgery for Ocular Trauma 1370
    William A. Townsend-Pico, Hilel Lewis

Chapter 118
Management of Posterior Segment
Intraocular Foreign Bodies................................1395
    Eric A. Postel, William F. Mieler

Chapter 119
Proliferative Diabetic Retinopathy......................1407
    David A. Quillen, Thomas W. Gardner,
    George W. Blankenship

Chapter 120
Macular Hole Surgery 1432
    Robert T. Wendel, Arun C. Patel,
    Neil E. Kelly

Chapter 121
Surgical Management of CNV 1449
    Nancy M. Holekamp, Matthew A. Thomas

Chapter 122
Retinopathy of Prematurity: Stages 4 and 5........1459
    Michael T. Trese, Philip J. Ferrone

Chapter 123
Endophthalmitis Management 1466
    Roy D. Brod, Harry W. Flynn, Jr.

Chapter 124
Surgical Management of Retinal Detachments
Due to AIDS 1478
    Robert G. Barone, Murk-Hein Heinemann

Chapter 125
Diagnostic Vitrectomy.......................................1487
    Glenn J. Jaffe

Index i

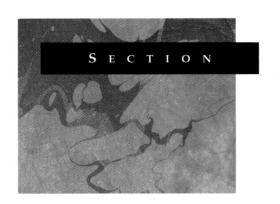

*Anatomy,
Clinical
Examination,
Diagnostic
Techniques,
and Laser
Therapy*

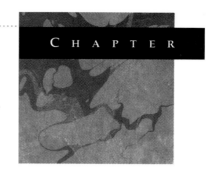

CHAPTER 1

Retinal Histology

Anat Loewenstein, M.D.
W. Richard Green, M.D.

The retina is composed of the tissues arising from the optic vesicle and consists of a pigment epithelial layer, derived from the outer layer of the optic cup, and a complex sensory layer, derived from the inner layer of the optic cup.

The sensory retina extends to the ora serrata, where it is continuous with the nonpigmented ciliary epithelium of the pars plana. The ora serrata is 2.1 mm wide temporally and 0.7 to 0.8 mm wide nasally. It is located more anteriorly on the nasal than on the temporal side; the nasal ora is about 6 mm posterior to the limbus, and the temporal ora is about 7 mm posterior to the limbus. The equator is located 6 to 8 mm posterior to the ora serrata and the macula is located 18 to 20 mm posterior to the equator. The average distance from the ora serrata to the optic nerve head is 32.5 mm temporally, 27 mm nasally, and 31 mm superiorly and inferiorly.

The term "macula" (macula lutea) refers to the deposition of a pigment, carotenoid, in a horizontal oval pattern (2.00 × 0.88 mm) in the posterior pole of the retina. The nature of this pigment, the "macular yellow," as well as the theories on its origin were summarized by Nussbaum et al.[1] The posterior pole of the retina is the *area centralis* and has four components based on histologic features (Fig. 1–1). In referring to the macula, most ophthalmologists consider the area inclusive of the parafoveal area (about 2.85 mm in diameter). Some, however, equate the macula to the foveal area (about 1.8 mm in diameter).[2] The fovea is a 1.5-mm depression in the center of the macula. The center of the fovea is located about 4 mm temporal and 0.8 mm inferior to the center of the horizontal plane of the optic disc. The inner retinal surface of the fovea is concave due to the more peripheral location of the inner retinal layers. The average thickness of the fovea is about 0.25 mm, roughly half that of the adjacent parafoveal area. The central 0.35 mm of the fovea is the foveola and is located within the capillary-free zone, which measures about 0.5 mm in diameter. A small protuberance in the center of the foveola is called the umbo, where there is a great concentration of cell bodies of elongated cones. A 0.5-mm-wide ring zone surrounding the fovea, where the ganglion cell, intranuclear layer, and the outer plexiform layer of Henle are the thickest, is called the parafoveal area. This is surrounded by a 1.5-mm ring zone called the perifoveal area where the ganglion cell layer is reduced from five to seven layers to a single layer of nuclei as seen elsewhere in the peripheral retina. Clinically, the anatomic subdivisions of the macula are ill defined. The foveal light reflex is due to reflection of light from the slanted margins (clivus) of the fovea. The capillary-free zone normally measures about 500 μm in diameter and is an important landmark to consider in laser photocoagulation.

HISTOLOGY

Retinal Pigment Epithelium

The retinal pigment epithelium (RPE) is a monolayer of cuboidal shaped cells (Fig. 1–2).[3–5] The estimated number of pigment epithelial cells is 4.2 to 6.1 million per eye. It extends from the margin of the optic disc to the ora serrata, where it continues as the pigmented ciliary epithelium and finally as the anterior layer of iris epithelium. At the margin of the disc, the pigment epithelial layer gradually becomes thinner, ending slightly before the termination of Bruch's membrane. In the posterior part of the eye, the RPE cells are narrow, tall, highly uniform in size and shape, and measure about 16 μm in diameter. In the midperiphery and equato-

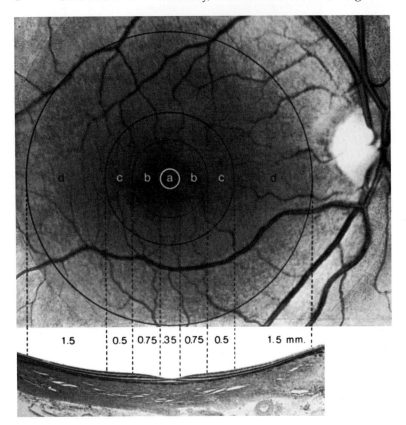

1.5 | 0.5 | 0.75 | .35 | 0.75 | 0.5 | 1.5 mm.

FIGURE 1-1 A fundus photograph matched with a horizontal section of the macular area delineates the (a) foveola, (b) fovea, (c) parafovea and (d) perifovea. (From Hogan MJ, Alvarado JE, Weddell JE: Histology of the Human Eye. Philadelphia, WB Saunders, 1971, p 491, with permission.)

rial areas, the cells are thinner. In the far periphery, the cells are wider (up to 60 μm in diameter), low, irregular, and variable in size, a variability that increases with age.[6,7] Robb[8] observed that the RPE cell density gradually increased in the macular area until 6 months of age and dropped in all other areas during the first 2 postnatal years. Like all epithelial cells, the pigment epithelial cells have apexes and bases. The basal surface has a convoluted cell membrane with infoldings of 1 μm or more. Adjacent to this convoluted cell membrane is a basal lamina (basement membrane), which is separated from the convoluted infoldings by a narrow space. This

basement membrane is the inner layer of Bruch's membrane. The apical surface of each cell possesses villous processes that extend internally and surround the external portion of the outer segments of the photoreceptors (Fig. 1-3). The outer segments of the rods extend to the surface of the cell, where they are surrounded by the retinal pigment epithelium villi. This is in contrast to the cones, which terminate at a greater distance from the cell surface so that the villi that extend internally to surround

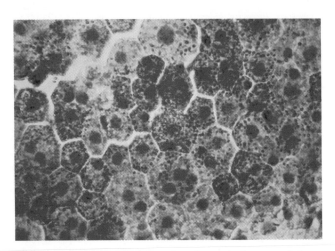

FIGURE 1-2 Tangential section shows the hexagonal shape of the RPE cells.

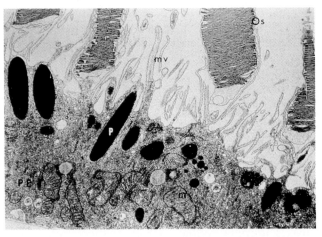

FIGURE 1-3 Ultrastructural appearance of RPE with apical villous processes (mv) that envelopes the photoreceptor outer segments (OS), melanin pigment granules (P), junctional complexes near apex, mitochondria (m), and lipofuscin granules. (Courtesy of Dr. T. Kuwabara.)

their outer segments are much longer and more complex that those of the rods.[9] Near the apexes, pigment epithelial cells are attached to one another by tight junctions. These consist of both zonula occludens and zonula adherens and comprise the outer blood-ocular barrier. At the optic nerve head the external limiting membrane of the retina becomes continuous with a zone of RPE junctional complexes (Verhoeff's membrane).[10]

The RPE cells have a round nucleus that is situated close to the base in the cell; in the peripheral area, some cells may contain two or more nuclei. Mitoses have not been observed in the RPE cells and it is believed that upon cell death or removal adjacent cells slide laterally to fill the space created.[11-13] The cytoplasm in the outer part of the RPE cells contains mainly mitochondria and the prominent infoldings of the plasma membrane. The cytoplasm in the inner part of the cell contains most of the melanin granules, which often extend into the apical villi around the outer segments of the photoreceptor. In the periphery there is a high concentration of melanin granules that gradually increases with age.[14,15] The inner part of the pigment epithelial cell also contains a few ribosomes lying freely in small clusters or attached to short segments of rough endoplasmic reticulum. With increasing age, other pigment granules, composed of lipofuscin, are found in the cytoplasm.[16] The increase in lipofuscin is most marked in the first and second decades but continues to increase with advancing age,[17,18] particularly in the macular area. Increase in the number of lipofuscin granules can occur also from mild acute or chronic insult caused by choroidal or RPE disease. When lipofuscin granules are present, they occupy most of the center part of the cell, which is otherwise relatively free of cell organelles. The existence of lipofuscin within the pigment epithelial cells of the macular region as contrasted with their relative sparseness in peripheral RPE cells suggests an anatomic basis for the macular area being darker during fluorescein angiography. Namely, the yellow-orange lipofuscin effectively acts as a filter in the macular area and screens out the underlying normal choroidal fluorescence.[19] Also present in the cytoplasm of the RPE cells are structures known as phagosomes, which are produced by the apical villi by phagocytosis of groups of discs from the outer segments of the rods and cones by the apical villi. Feeney observed that the melanin often becomes incorporated into the lysosomal system, where it is modified or degradated.[20] These phagosomes are gradually digested by enzymes that are derived from organelles in the cytoplasm of the RPE cells, and their products are often cast off into Bruch's membrane or are retained in the cytoplasm to become lipofuscin granules.

The RPE has numerous functions: storage of vitamin A and its conversion to a form that can be utilized by the photoreceptors for synthesis of rhodopsin; production of glycosaminoglycans that envelope the photoreceptors; phagocytosis and degradation of shed lamellar discs of the photoreceptors; promotion of retinal adhesion; and absorption scattered light.[16,21-24]

Sensory Retina

The sensory retina is a thin, transparent tissue. It is thickest near the optic disc, where it measures 0.56 mm. It thins to 0.18 mm at the equator and to 0.1 mm at the ora serrata. At the foveal area it is thinned to about 0.2 mm. Anatomically, the retina gradually terminates at the optic disc by reduction of the Müller cells and the nuclear and synaptic layers and by disappearance of the photoreceptors. The nerve fiber layer, however, increases in thickness at the edge of the disc and is the only retinal structure that continues into the disc and becomes the optic nerve. The internal aspect of the retina is in contact with the vitreous body and its external aspect is adjacent to the RPE between which is a potential space (the subretinal space). It is firmly attached to the RPE only at two points: posteriorly, at the optic disc, and anteriorly, at the ora serrata. Elsewhere, the attachment to the underlying RPE is weak and is maintained by the intraocular pressure, contact between the photoreceptor outer segments and the RPE villi, the mucopolysaccharide-cementing substance surrounding the photoreceptors, and active transport from internal to external. The internal surface of the retina is adjacent to the vitreous at the internal limiting lamina (internal limiting membrane [ILM]) of the retina.

The Nine Layers of the Sensory Retina

The sensory retina is composed of nine layers (Fig. 1–4). The retinal layers are connected to each other by synaptic connections between axons and den-

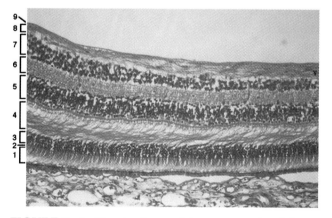

FIGURE 1–4   The nine layers of the sensory retina. *1,* Layer of the outer and inner segments of the photoreceptors of the rods and cones. *2,* The external limiting membrane. *3,* Outer nuclear layer. *4,* Outer plexiform layer. *5,* Inner nuclear layer. *6,* Inner plexiform layer. *7,* Ganglion cell layer. *8,* Nerve fiber layer. *9,* Internal limiting membrane (hematoxylin and eosin, × 100).

drites in the inner and outer plexiform layers and to the ganglion cells.[25,26] The neuronal cells are supported by fibers of Müller cells and the astrocytes in the inner portion of the retina.

From outside inward:

1. The photoreceptor layer is comprised of the outer and inner segments of the photoreceptors (Fig. 1–5). These, as well as the villi of the RPE, are surrounded by an extracellular substance composed of mucoprotein substance.

2. The external limiting membrane is not a true membrane but is formed by junctional complexes that unite the Müller cells with the photoreceptor cell inner segments. Occasionally, the connections are between Müller cells themselves or between neurons. The Müller cells extend fine fibrils externally between the inner segments of the rod and cone photoreceptors for a short distance. These fibrils are believed to play a part in the formation of the complex mucopolysaccharides that lie in this region.

3. The outer nuclear layer is composed of eight or nine layers of the cell bodies of the photoreceptor cells. Smaller, more densely staining nuclei belong to the rods and larger, more weakly stained, belong to the cones. Occasionally, cone nuclei are found to be displaced into the inner photoreceptor layer as a normal variation.[27] Others have considered this cone nuclei displacement to be an aging change.[28] Axons extend from both types of outer nuclear cells into the outer plexiform layer where they synapse with the rod and cone bipolar cells and also with horizontal cells and with adjacent bipolar cells. The rod axons terminate in a somewhat teardrop-shaped expansion termed spherule, and the cone axons terminate in a pedicle or foot with small branches called a peduncle. These expansions are filled with many small vesicles called synaptic vesicles, believed to contain acetylcholine, which is released at the cell surface upon appropriate stimulation. The Müller cells fill out all the space between the processes of the rods and cones and also between the bipolar and horizontal cells.

4. The outer plexiform layer consists of axons from the rod and cone cells that form synaptic junctions with dendrites from the bipolar cells and horizontal cells. The fibers in this layer are loosely arranged and form a delicate network. In the macular region, the axons and dendrites of the outer plexiform layer are greatly elongated and radiate outward from the foveal region, to form the fiber layer of Henle (Fig. 1–6).

5. The inner nuclear layer, which contains nuclei of bipolar cells, horizontal cells, amacrine cells, and Müller cells, is generally thinner than the outer nuclear layer. The bipolar cells have dendrites that are in contact with the axons of the rod and cone cells in the outer plexiform layer. Their axons extend into the inner plexiform layer, forming synapses with the dendrites of the ganglion cells and with the amacrine cells. The horizontal cells lie at the external aspect of this layer and have long and complex arborizing processes in the outer plexiform layer that synapse with the spherules and peduncles of the rod and cone axons and also with adjacent bipolar cells. Occasional processes extend from the horizontal cells into the inner plexiform layer. The amacrine cells are pear shaped and lie at the inner aspect of the inner nuclear layer. They have processes that extend into the internal plexiform layer, where they synapse widely with the dendrites of the ganglion cells and with the bipolar axons. The Müller cells send fibers

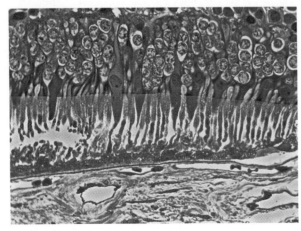

FIGURE 1–5 Area illustrates thin outer segments and the thicker and more darkly staining cone inner segments of the photoreceptors (paraphylenediamine, phase contrast, × 160).

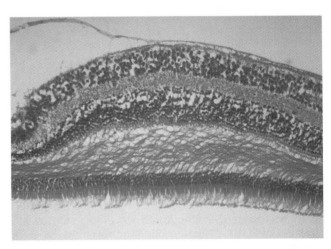

FIGURE 1–6 Parafoveal area with tangential orientation of the fibers in the outer plexiform layer and the thick ganglion cell and inner and outer nuclear layers (hematoxylin and eosin, × 100).

externally to form the zonulae adherens that compose the external limiting membrane.

6. The inner plexiform layer consists of the axons of the bipolar and amacrine cells and their synapses, and the dendrites of the ganglion cells.

7. The ganglion cell layer consists of the cell bodies of ganglion cells separated from each other by the processes of Müller cells and neuroglia. The ganglion cell layer forms a single layer throughout most of the retina. In the macular region of the retina, the ganglion cells are much more numerous, forming a layer two to eight cells deep.

8. The nerve fiber layer is composed almost entirely of the axons of the ganglion cells. These axons are aggregated into nerve fiber bundles that pass through the arcades formed by the columns and footplates of Müller cells. This layer is thickest near the disc because of the accumulation of the fibers from the retina as they converge on the disc. In the human retina the axons are unmyelinated because during embryonic development myelination ceases abruptly when it reaches the lamina cribrosa of the optic nerve head after proceeding from the chiasm down to the optic nerve head. Myelination may rarely extend into the retina.

9. The ILM consists mostly of basal lamina of the Müller cells. Its inner (vitreal) surface is smooth, whereas its outer surface follows closely the uneven surface of the Müller cell basal plasma membranes with a variable thickness topographically. Foos[29] found the internal limiting membrane to be thin at the vitreous base (51 nm), and to progressively thicken posteriorly to measure 306 nm at the equator and 1887 nm posteriorly. The internal limiting membrane becomes attenuated or is absent in the foveola, over major retinal vessels, and at the optic nerve head. It is attached to and blends with the cortical vitreous.

At the ora serrata the nine layers of the sensory retina resolve themselves into a single layer of cells that continues into the ciliary body as the nonpigmented epithelium. The external segments of the rods and cones disappear, and the inner segments persist as deformed and swollen structures. The nuclear layers blend into one, and the ganglion cells and fiber layer end, whereas the neuroglia and Müller cells increase.

The Macular Region

The structure of the macular region affords maximal visual acuity, and thus several modifications in retina architecture have been made. No retinal vessels exist in the fovea to hinder photic reception or to cast shadows. No rods exist in the foveola, but the cones have become so modified that they re-

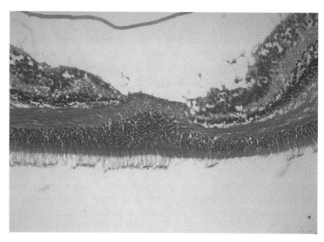

FIGURE 1–7 The accumulation of elongated cone cells in the foveola causes a slight bowing internally—the *umbo* (hematoxylin and eosin, × 100).

semble rods in form. The external segments of the cones are long and approach the apical side of the RPE cells. The accumulation of a large number of these specialized cones in the foveola causes a forward, bow-shaped configuration—the umbo (Fig. 1–7). At the edge of the fovea and extending away from it, the ganglion cell layer and the inner nuclear layer thicken, but both layers disappear within the fovea. In the foveola area, only photoreceptor cells and Müller cell processes are present. Each cell is united with a single bipolar cell and possibly with a single ganglion cell, thus yielding maximal transmission of the stimulus.

Individual Cells

Neuronal Cells

The *photoreceptor cells* are highly specialized neuroepithelial cells. The cone cell body is much larger that of the rod. Each rod and cone is composed of an outer and inner segment. The difference in size is also carried over into the rod and cone inner segments and axons. The outer segments contain the discs, and the inner segments contain the mitochondria and other enzyme-producing organelles. The inner segments of the cones are large and are filled with mitochondria, whereas the rods are longer, more cylindric, and contain fewer mitochondria. The outer segment of the rod is long and extends to the apical side of the RPE, whereas that of the cone is shorter and terminates earlier. Projecting from the apex of the inner segment is a highly modified cilium, with nine filaments forming a ring, but lacking the usual centrally located filament.

Bipolar cells possess typical dendrites that make up most of the truly plexiform portion of the outer plexiform layer. These dendrites are filled with a considerable number of mitochondria, smooth endoplasmic reticulum, and neurotubule-like structures or microtubules. The cell body is scanty and the axonal extensions have an axial arrangement of its cytoplasmic components.

The *horizontal cells* have a peculiar body in their cytoplasm, composed of special tubules and ribonucleoprotein.

Amacrine cells lack such a special structure and are identified by a lobulated nucleus.

The *ganglion cells* are multipolar, with large nuclei and prominent aggregates of rough endoplasmic reticulum (Nissl's granules). Their numerous dendrites end in the inner plexiform layer, and their long axons extend along the nerve fiber layer of the retina to the optic nerve and lateral geniculate body.

Glial Cells

Müller fibers form a framework throughout the thickness of the retina to support and surround the nerve cells and their axons and dendrites (Fig. 1–8); these fibers also contribute to the internal and external limiting membranes.

There is a large number of *astrocyte-like cells* that have processes in the nerve fiber, ganglion cell, and inner plexiform layers. The branching processes of these cells run in a plane at right angles to Müller fibers and have no close connection with them.

Occasionally, *astrocytes* are present in the ganglion cell and inner plexiform layers. They are star shaped, with round nuclei and numerous slender processes. They also are arranged horizontally and surround the vessels with a dense network of fibers. They form an arch-like, honeycomb structure that surrounds and supports the nerve axons derived from the ganglion cells. They frequently have strong attachment to the surfaces of the blood vessels.

Retinal Blood Vessels

The human retina is vascularized in its inner layers outward to the inner third of the inner nuclear layer. The choriocapillaris layer is responsible for nourishing the outer part of the retina. The retinal blood vessels are derived from the central retinal artery. As it enters the retina, the central retinal artery divides into four main branches: the upper and lower nasal and the upper and lower temporal. These arterioles divide into smaller arterioles and the circulation further includes precapillary arterioles, capillaries, postcapillary venules, and veins. There is a capillary-free zone in the peripheral 1 mm near the ora serrata and around the arterioles. The capillaries drain into venules that form a pattern similar to the arteries, joining larger venules distributed parallel to the main arteriolar branches and finally the central retinal vein at the optic disc. The major vessels lie near the internal limiting membrane or not far beneath it. Where the vessels

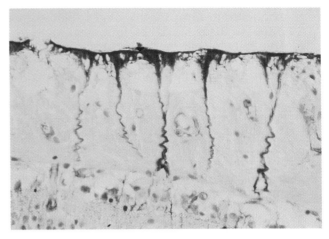

FIGURE 1–8 Müller cells broaden, forming footplates that are continuous with the internal limiting membrane (periodic acid–Schiff, × 400).

approach the surface, the internal limiting membrane may be extremely attenuated or absent. In the parafoveal area there are up to four strata of capillaries. A radially oriented layer of capillaries is present in the nerve fiber layer around much of the optic disc. Elsewhere in the retina, the capillaries are diffusely distributed and do not seem to form definite strata.

The retinal blood vessels are lined by an endothelium with tight cellular junctions—the site of the blood-ocular barrier of the inner circulation. In the normal eye, the capillaries have a 1:1 ratio of pericytes and endothelial cells. The retinal circulation extends into the retina as far as the inner portion of the inner nuclear layer. Consequently, the inner portion of the retina derives its nutrition from the retinal arterial system, and the outer layers, including the outer portion of the inner nuclear layer, derive their nutrition from the choriocapillaris of the choroid.

DEVELOPMENTAL VARIATIONS

Peripherally, the sensory retina extends to the ora serrata, where it is continuous with the nonpigmented ciliary epithelium of the pars plana. Early in embryologic development, the retina is contiguous with the pars plicata. As the eye enlarges and further develops the retina recedes posteriorly to the ora serrata. This process does not occur equally and leads to serrations, dentate processes, meridional folds, meridional complexes, ora bays, enclosed ora bays, and peripheral retinal tufts.

The term "ora serrata" refers to the serrated appearance of this zone. The retinal termination is serrated, forming *dentate processes*, or teeth, that persist on the pars plana, and intervening bays of the pars plana, that lie between the teeth and have their convexities posteriorly. The *dentate processes* are more prominent and more numerous on the nasal side of the eye.

An *enclosed ora bay* is defined as a posterior indentation in the retina that is separated from the pars plana by retinal tissue (Fig. 1–9). A *partially enclosed ora bay* is a posterior indentation in the retina that extends more than 0.5 mm posterior to the adjacent retina on both sides and has a width anteriorly that is less than half its maximum width posteriorly. Enclosed ora bays have been observed in 4% of autopsy eyes, and partially enclosed in 0.6%.[30] These lesions have been associated with meridionally aligned retinal tears at the posterior border of the vitreous base in 16.7%. All such tears occurred at the posterior border of the vitreous base and were a consequence of posterior vitreous detachment (PVD).

Meridional folds are radially oriented linear elevations of the peripheral retina aligned with a dentate process, an ora bay, or a meridional complex.[31,32] It is caused by excess of retinal tissue in relation to the other tissue coats of the eye and includes thickened retina with variable cystic degeneration and occasional hyperplasia of the RPE and glial cells (Fig. 1–10). These lesions have been observed in 26% of autopsy eyes, in 55% are bilateral, and are mainly located in the superonasal quadrant. The incidence in all age groups is similar.

A *meridional complex* is defined by the alignment of an elongated dentate process with a ciliary process in the same meridian (Figs. 1–9 and 1–10). These lesions have been observed in 16% of autopsy cases, in 58% are bilateral, and are mainly located in the nasal periphery. These lesions are not associated with retinal tears.

An *ora pearl* is a lesion that is a darkly pigmented or glistening small white nodule within a retinal dentate process extending over the pars plana (Fig. 1–11). Pearls have been observed in 20% of patients.[33,34]

Retinal tufts occur in the vitreous base, have sev-

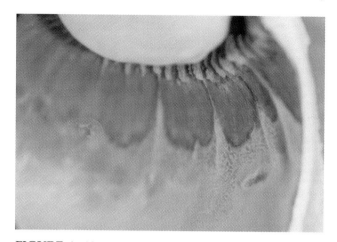

FIGURE 1–10   Area with four meridional folds—the two in the middle are aligned with dentate processes and the outer two are aligned with meridional complexes.

eral anatomic variations, and are important because of the tendency for associated holes and tears.[35–40]

A *retinal tuft (tag)* is an internal projection of peripheral retinal tissue located within the area of the vitreous base. Foos and Allen[35] have classified tufts into noncystic, cystic, and zonular traction types. A *noncystic retinal tuft* is a short, thin strand of retina and glial tissue that extends into the vitreous base (Figs. 1–12 and 1–13). Noncystic tufts were found in 72% of adult autopsy cases, were bilateral in 50% of cases, and were most commonly located in the inferonasal quadrant. These lesions are not associated with retinal tears or detachment. A *cystic retinal tuft* consists of an area of retinal thickening caused by cystic changes and glial cell proliferation. Cystic retinal tufts are located at the posterior portion of the vitreous base or just posterior to it (Figs. 1–14 and 1–15). Retinal tears may occur at sites of cystic retinal tufts (Fig. 1–16) and have been associated with retinal detachment, with the risk calculated by Byer to be less than 1%.[40]

A *zonular traction retinal tuft* consists of a thin strand of fibroglial tissue or embryonal epithelium

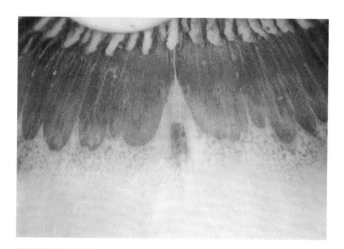

FIGURE 1–9   Area shows serrations, small dentate processes, and enclosed ora bay in line with a meridional complex.

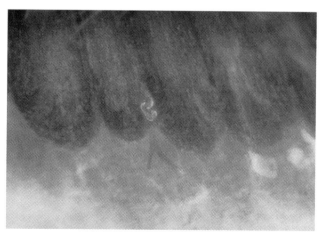

FIGURE 1–11   Irregular ora pearl in a short dentate process.

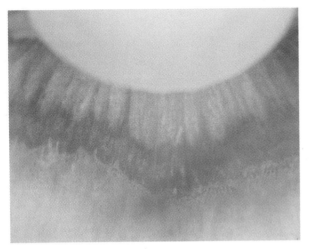

FIGURE 1-12 Gross appearance of noncystic peripheral retinal tufts.

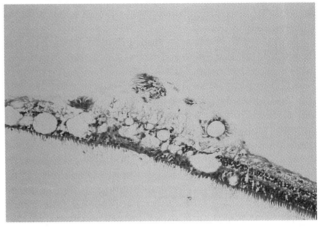

FIGURE 1-15 Cystic retinal tuft is composed of glial cells that extend internal to the retina that has cystic degeneration. Vitreous is adherent to the tuft (periodic acid–Schiff, × 100).

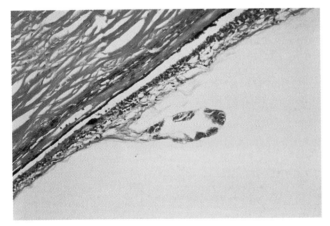

FIGURE 1-13 Noncystic retinal tuft is composed of glial cells (periodic acid–Schiff, × 100).

that extends anteriorly to be continuous with a thickened zonule at the apex (Figs. 1–17 and 1–18). These lesions were seen in 15% of autopsy eyes and in 15% were bilateral.[41] The most common location is nasal. With manipulation of the lens, zonular traction retina tufts may lead to direct traction and production of small holes at the vitreous base. This may lead to a characteristic type of aphakic detachment.

AGING CHANGES

Macular Thinning

Histologic changes in the macula consisting of thinning of the outer nuclear layer fragmentation of the external limiting membrane, atrophy of photoreceptors, and cystic degeneration of Henle's layer were observed in a third of eyes of patients older than 65 years examined postmortem by Kornzweig.[42] Clinically, the macula appears to be

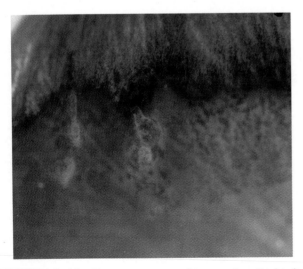

FIGURE 1-14 Gross appearance of two cystic retinal tufts.

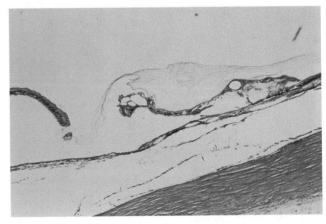

FIGURE 1-16 Posterior vitreous detachment with a retinal tear at a cystic retinal tuft (periodic acid–Schiff, × 40).

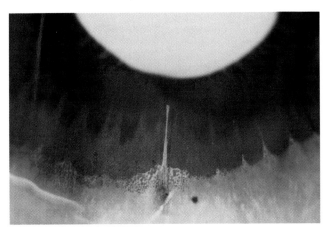

FIGURE 1–17 Gross appearance of zonular traction tuft.

thinned and mildly atrophic. These changes may predispose to idiopathic macular hole formation.[43,44]

Attrition of Ganglion Cells, Photoreceptor Cells, and Retinal Pigment Epithelium

Retinal Pigment Epithelium

Commencing at the age of 20 years, the RPE cells show changes that result from its constant activity over the years. This aging is manifested by depigmentation with migration of pigment granules into the basal portion of the cell. In addition, there is an increase in lipofuscin granules and in granules containing both melanin and lipofuscin, which are partly the result of phagocytosis of the rod and cone outer segments and their enclosure in phagosomes. Within the phagosomes, gradual digestion of the discs of the outer segments occurs, eventually producing residual bodies. Many incompletely digested discs and phagosomes are extruded into Bruch's membrane and between the basal cell membrane of the RPE cell and its basement membrane. Large amounts of residual bodies can be seen in most eyes at about the age of 40 to 60 years, increasing significantly by the age of 80. These changes are more extensive in the macula than in the equatorial and peripheral areas,[45] and are presumed to have a detrimental effect on the RPE cell by making it more vulnerable to light and free radical damage.[46] It has also been demonstrated that foveal RPE cells are significantly more dense and more hexagonal in eyes from younger persons. With increasing age, loss of hexagonality was observed in the fovea. The foveal RPE cells lose their unique morphologic characteristics and resemble nonfoveal cells.[47] In addition, a physiologic age decline in the number of RPE cells was found in many studies in the past.[45,48,49] An average annual loss of about 17 RPE cells per square millimeter of retina per year or 0.3% of an original RPE cell population of 5232 cells/mm² of retina per year was found by Panda-Jonas et al.[50] They calculated that about 30% of all RPE cells are lost over a lifespan of 100 years. This is associated with an age-related loss of about 3000 to 5000 optic nerve fibers, or about 0.3% per year of 1.4 million fibers at birth[51,52] and a decrease in the rod and cone densities of 0.3 to 0.5% per year related to the photoreceptor density of the newborn.[48] These observations indicate a reduced anatomic reserve capacity in older patients compared with younger individuals. It can be the reason for declining visual functions even when there is no active disease process.

Ganglion Cells

The optic nerve fiber count decreases with age, indicating an age-related physiologic optic nerve atrophy.[51–57] This suggests a predominant loss of small optic nerve fibers. This fact can be important in patients with Alzheimer's disease and glaucoma in whom the large axons have been shown to be lost preferentially.[53,58–62] All these changes suggest that a continuing loss of visual function need not be necessarily a result of progression of the disease but may be caused only by the natural ongoing age-related changes.

Sub-RPE Deposits

Diffuse thickening of the inner aspect of Bruch's membrane is a commonly observed aging change that is considered to be a form of drusen associated with vision loss in age-related macular degeneration. Two types of deposits are recognized: basal laminar deposit and basal linear deposit. *Basal laminar deposit* is composed mostly of wide-spaced collagen and some granular material located between the plasma membrane and basement membranes of the RPE cells (Fig. 1–19). It has been shown to also contain laminin, vesiculoid elements, membrane-bound structures, and fibronectin.[63,64]

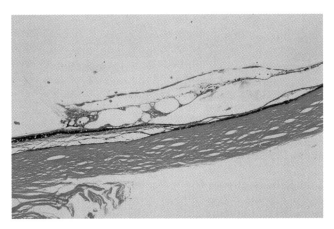

FIGURE 1–18 Zonular traction tuft consists of a strand of glial cells that extends over the pars plana from the peripheral retina (periodic acid–Schiff, × 40).

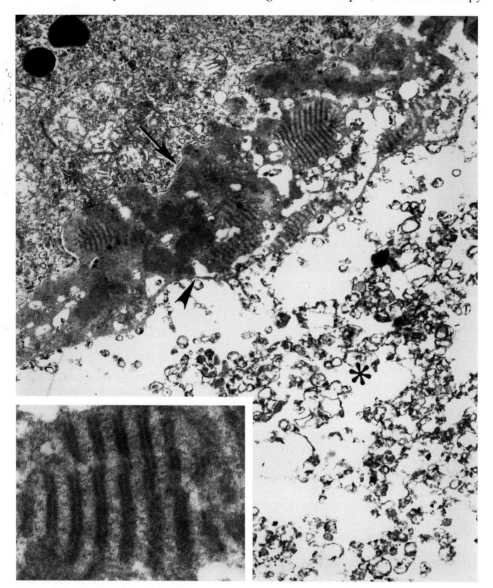

FIGURE 1–19   Macular area of an 84-year-old woman with basal laminar deposit mostly composed of wide-spaced collagen located between the plasma membrane (*arrow*) and basement membrane (*arrowhead*) of the retinal pigment epithelium (main figure and *inset*). A thick layer of vesicles and amorphous material (basal linear deposit) (*asterisk*) is located external to the retinal pigment epithelial basement membrane in the inner aspect of Bruch's membrane ($\times$ 11,000; inset, $\times$ 58,000). (From Bressler NM, Silva JC, Bressler SB, et al: Clinicopathologic correlation of drusen and retinal pigment epithelial abnormalities in age-related macular degeneration. Retina 14:130–142, 1994, with permission.)

Basal linear deposit (diffuse drusen, diffuse thickening of the inner aspect of Bruch's membrane) is the material that is located external to the basement membrane of the RPE—that is, in the inner collagenous layer of Bruch's membrane (Fig. 1–20). This deposit is rich in phospholipids and consists of granular and vesicular material with some widespaced collagen and linear profiles. This material is suspected to be released from the RPE through its basement membrane.[65]

Both deposits are clinically detected only by associated secondary changes: RPE hypopigmentation and pigment clumps, RPE atrophy, soft (large) drusen, serous detachments of the RPE, choroidal neovascularization, and disciform scarring.

RPE Hypertrophy and Hyperplasia

The RPE is one of the most reactive tissues in the eye. It reacts by undergoing atrophy, hypertrophy, hyperplasia and migration.

RPE hypertrophy is an aging and degenerative change that commonly occurs in the periphery and in association with numerous disease states. The

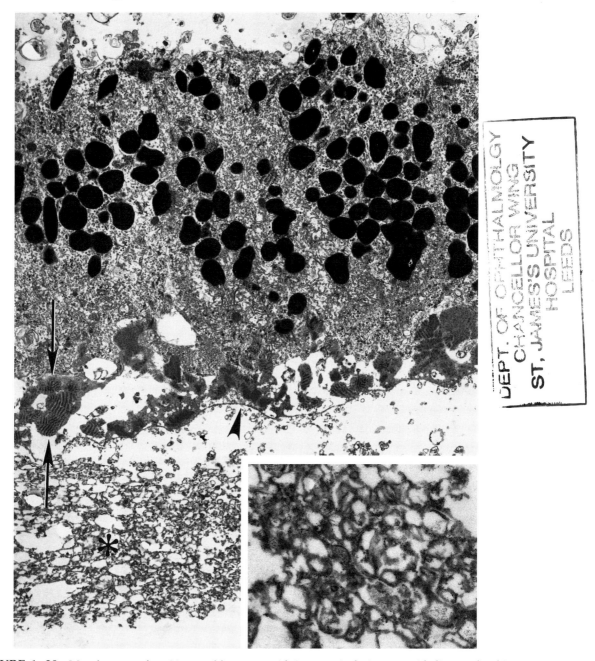

FIGURE 1–20   Macular area of an 84-year-old woman with intact retinal pigment epithelium and a thin layer of basal laminar deposit composed mostly of wide-spaced collagen (between *arrows*) located between the plasma membrane and the basement membrane (*arrowhead*) of the retinal pigment epithelium. The thick layer of electron-dense vesicular and membranous material (basal linear deposit) (*asterisk* and *inset*) is located external to the RPE basement membrane in the inner aspect of Bruch's membrane ($\times$ 5700; *inset*, $\times$ 58,000). (From Bressler NM, Silva JC, Bressler SB, et al: Clinicopathologic correlation of drusen and retinal pigment epithelial abnormalities in age-related macular degeneration. Retina 14:130–142, 1994, with permission.)

RPE cells become somewhat thicker than normal. In addition, the usual small and oval-shaped melanin granules become large and spheric. This gives the RPE cell a much darker brown or black appearance. Such hypertrophy can be localized (Figs. 1–21 and 1–22) or multifocal. It is often located just posterior to the ora serrata (Fig. 1–23) and around the optic disc.

RPE hyperplasia is a relatively common change observed in older persons. The spiculate appear-ance of pigment at the ora serrata may be caused by chronic vitreous base traction. Nodules of proliferated pigmented epithelium in the posterior aspect of the pars plana may be also associated with chronic vitreous base traction. *Localized hyperplasia* of the RPE is usually nonspecific (Figs. 1–24 and 1–25). It has a dark appearance and is associated with retinal vessels. In some instances the hyperplastic RPE remains under the retina, where it has a laminated appearance, with alternate layers of

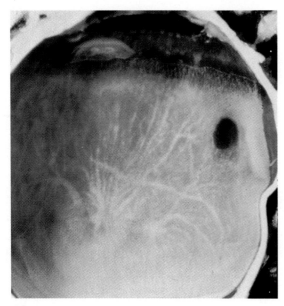

FIGURE 1–21   Gross appearance of a 3-mm solitary area of RPE hypertrophy.

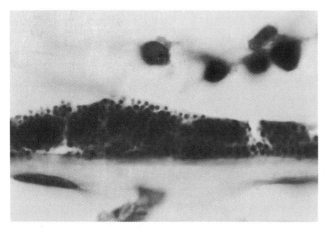

FIGURE 1–22   The hypertrophic RPE cells are distended by large, spherical melanin pigment granules (partial bleach, periodic acid–Schiff, × 400).

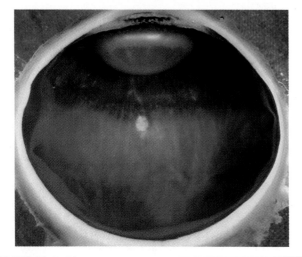

FIGURE 1–23   A 4-mm band of RPE hypertrophy located posterior to the ora serrata.

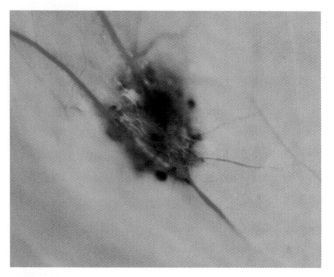

FIGURE 1–24   Gross appearance of localized area of RPE hyperplasia.

RPE, basement membrane, and collagen production. *Diffuse hyperplasia* of the RPE occurs throughout the retina in perivascular locations in traumatic retinopathy and retinitis pigmentosa.

Peripheral reticular pigmentary degeneration is a change due to aging characterized by a reticulated pattern of increased pigmentation in the periphery of the fundus.[32,41,66-69] It includes various combinations of atrophy, hypertrophy, and hyperplasia of the RPE in various intensities and patterns. It is frequently associated with nodular drusen. This pigmentary degeneration may have an association with age-related macular degeneration.[70,71]

Cystic Degenerations of the Retina

With increasing age the normal architecture of the retina is altered at the ora serrata and posteriorly for a variable distance. The ILM increases in thick-

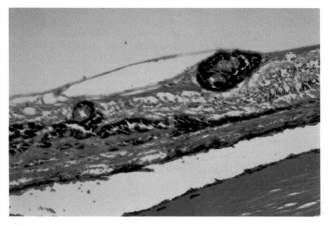

FIGURE 1–25   Lesion in Figure 1–24 consists of hyperplastic RPE under and within retina in a perivascular location (periodic acid–Schiff, × 100).

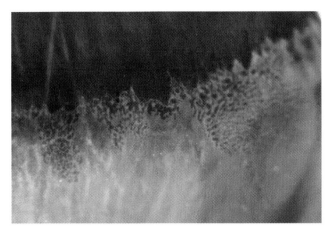

FIGURE 1–26 Gross appearance of typical peripheral cystoid degeneration of the retina.

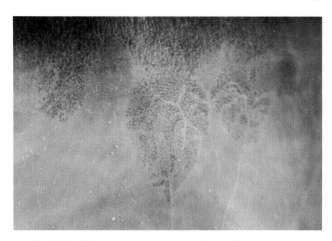

FIGURE 1–28 Gross appearance of reticular peripheral cystoid degeneration.

ness. The retina exhibits two types of cystoid spaces, typical and reticular, the former arising in the outer plexiform layer and the latter in the nerve fiber layer. These changes are seen in virtually all adults and were found in 86.8% of autopsy cases of all age groups, increasing in severity until the seventh decade.[72] The first type, *typical peripheral cystoid degeneration (TPCD) (Blessig-Iwanoff cysts)*, is characterized by cysts in the outer plexiform layer that contain hyaluronic acid, that also may coalesce, giving the appearance of lobulated, irregularly branching tortuous channels (Figs. 1–26 and 1–27). Complications resulting from TPCD are rare. Retinal holes do not result in retinal detachment, since the vitreous is usually intact over the lesion. Extension posteriorly to the equator is rare. It can lead to typical degenerative retinoschisis. The second type, *reticular peripheral cystoid degeneration*, is almost always continuous with and posterior to areas of typical and reticular peripheral cystoid degeneration and is usually in the inferior temporal quadrant. It has a reticular pattern corresponding to retinal vessels in the inner layers. A finely stippled internal surface corresponds to points of attachment of pillars of tissue to the inner layer. The cystic spaces are located in the nerve fiber layer. This process is present in 18% of adults, bilateral in 41%. It might develop into reticular degenerative retinoschisis[73,74] (Figs. 1–28 and 1–29).

Retinoschisis

Two degenerative forms of retinoschisis are recognized; both most commonly occur in the inferotemporal quadrant and both develop from pre-existing peripheral cystoid degeneration. Typical peripheral cystoid degeneration may lead to typical degenerative retinoschisis and both typical and reticular peripheral cystoid degeneration may lead to reticular degenerative retinoschisis.[73] *Typical degenerative retinoschisis* produces a smooth elevation in 1% of adults, bilateral in 33%. Typical peripheral cystoid degeneration typically surrounds the lesion (Figs. 1–30 and 1–31). The retinal splitting occurs at the

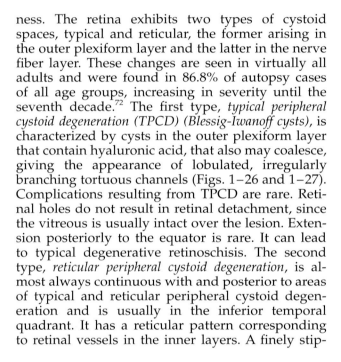

FIGURE 1–27 Typical peripheral cystoid degeneration with cystic spaces in the outer plexiform layer (hematoxylin and eosin, × 40).

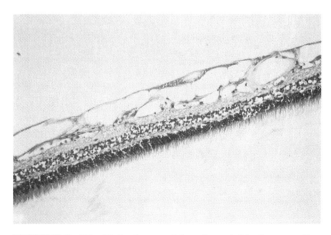

FIGURE 1–29 Reticular peripheral cystoid degeneration with cystic spaces in the nerve fiber layer (hematoxylin and eosin, × 100).

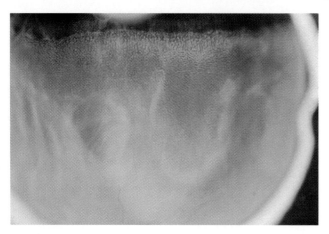

FIGURE 1–30 Gross appearance of two areas of typical degenerative retinoschisis just posterior to typical peripheral cystoid degeneration.

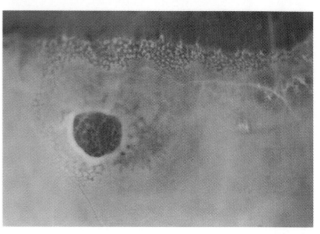

FIGURE 1–32 Gross appearance of reticular degenerative retinoschisis with a hole with rounded margins in the outer layer.

outer plexiform layer. Thus, the inner layer can contain the ILM, the nerve fiber layer, the retinal vessels, the ganglion cells, and the inner plexiform and inner nuclear layers. However, usually only the ILM, the nerve fiber layer, and portions of the inner nuclear layer are evident. The outer layer is thicker, scalloped, and consists of the outer nuclear and the photoreceptor layers. *Reticular degenerative retinoschisis* develops from the concurrent presence of typical and reticular peripheral cystoid degeneration of the retina.[73,75] It is characterized by round or oval areas of retinal splitting in which a bullous elevation of an extremely thin inner layer was found in 1.6% of adults, bilateral in 15% (Figs. 1–32 and 1–33). Typical peripheral cystoid degeneration is usually present anterior to this lesion, and reticular cystoid degeneration is usually evident adjacent to it. The splitting occurs in the nerve fiber layer, with the thin inner layer containing only the ILM, some retinal vessels and variable portions of the nerve fiber layer. The outer layer contains the relatively intact remaining retinal layers. Occasion-

ally, typical and reticular retinoschisis occur together. Byer noted that the differentiation between typical and reticular degenerative retinoschisis cannot always be made clinically, unless there is a bullous appearance, presence of outer layer holes, or posterior extension, features that are more common in the reticular than in the typical type.[76] Treatment of degenerative retinoschisis may be indicated if posterior extension threatens the macular area, if there is an associated nonrhegmatogenous retinal detachment, and if breaks exist in both layers.[41] According to Byer, treatment is indicated only when there is symptomatic progressive retinal detachment.[76]

Lattice Degeneration (A Vitreoretinal Degenerative Process)

The prevalence of lattice degeneration was reported to be 8% in a large clinical series[77] and 10.7% in

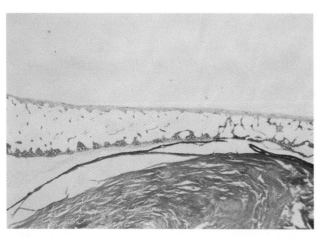

FIGURE 1–31 Typical degenerative retinoschisis with splitting of the retina at the outer plexiform layer (hematoxylin and eosin, × 10).

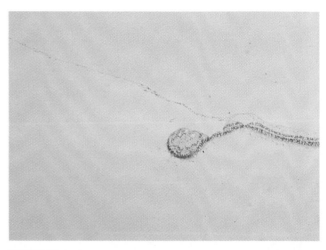

FIGURE 1–33 Section of reticular degenerative retinoschisis depicted in Figure 1–32 shows the thin inner layer and hole with typical rolled margin in the outer layer (hematoxylin and eosin, × 10).

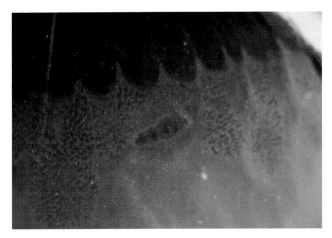

FIGURE 1–34 Gross appearance of retinal thinning in an area of lattice degeneration.

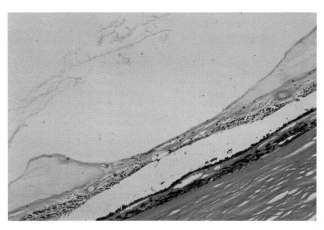

FIGURE 1–36 Lattice degeneration with a pocket of fluid vitreous, condensed vitreous adherent at the margin, and retinal thinning (hematoxylin and eosin, × 10).

autopsies.[78] The lesions were found to be bilateral and highly symmetric in 48.1%. It was found the lattice degeneration increases in frequency after the second decade. It is not clear whether lattice degeneration is more common in myopic eyes. Most lesions are situated in the pre-equatorial region, are circumferential in orientation, and are more common in the vertical meridians. Lattice lesions have the appearance of retinal thinning (Fig. 1–34), may have a wicker appearance from sclerotic vessels (Fig. 1–35), and may have variable pigmentation from hypertrophy and hyperplasia of the RPE. Histologic features include a pocket of overlying fluid vitreous; absence of the ILM, condensation of vitreous at the margin (Fig. 1–36); glial and RPE hyperplasia at the margin in some, retinal thinning and hole formation in center of lesion, sclerosis of larger vessels, sclerosis and acellularity of the capillaries, and RPE hypertrophy and hyperplasia. With development of posterior vitreous detachment, a tear may occur at the point of lattice because of more firm vitreoretinal adherence. The pig-

mentary changes are often the feature that ophthalmoscopically brings the lesion to one's attention. The lattice "wicker" is due to the sclerosis of the larger vessels and is present in about 11% of lesions. It has been suggested that retinal circulatory disturbances are the primary cause of lattice degeneration.[78] However, the pattern of overlapping lesions is inconsistent with ischemia. Rather, the process may be related to a defect in Müller cells.

Cobblestone Degeneration

This common chorioretinal degenerative process is present in up to 27% of persons over the age of 20 years.[72] It is located between the ora serrata and the posterior aspect of the equator, which is the watershed area between the posterior choroidal and the anterior ciliary circulation. Ophthalmoscopically, it appears as a small, discrete, yellowish white area with prominently visible choroidal vessels, sometimes with dark, hypertrophic RPE at the margin.

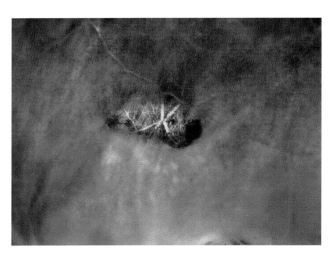

FIGURE 1–35 Gross appearance of lattice degeneration with associated RPE hypertrophy and a wicker pattern of sclerotic blood vessels.

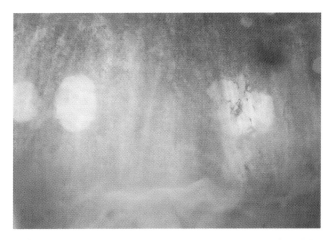

FIGURE 1–37 Gross appearance of three areas of cobblestone degeneration.

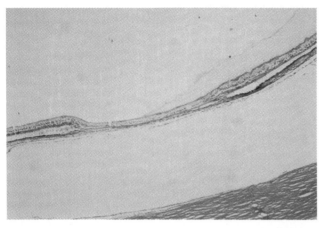

FIGURE 1–38   View of one of the lesions in Figure 1–38 shows loss of the RPE and outer retinal layers (periodic acid–Schiff, × 10).

These lesions may occur singularly or in groups (Fig. 1–37) and may become confluent, producing a band of depigmentation just posterior to the ora serrata. Histopathologic studies show signs of outer retinal ischemic atrophy including an attenuation or absence of choriocapillaris, and loss of RPE and outer retinal layers up to and including the outer portion of the inner nuclear layer (Figs. 1–38 and 1–39). The changes are limited to the portion of the retina that is supplied by the choriocapillaris and can be produced in rabbits by ligation of choroidal blood supply.[79] Cobblestone degeneration is a feature pointing to peripheral vascular disease and can be extensive in carotid occlusive disease.[80]

COMMENT ON RETINAL PHYSIOLOGY

During recent years there has been a great increase in knowledge concerning the functional pathways underlying processing of the visual image in the retina. In summary, vision begins in the rod and cone receptors of the retina. The surface membrane of the outer segment of these cells has ion channels that are open in darkness and are permeable to Na^+, which steadily enters the outer segment in darkness, constituting a "dark current." This current causes depolarization of the cell, thus maintaining a high steady release of neurotransmitter from the synaptic terminal.[81] This neurotransmitter is thought to be glutamate.[82] The Na^+ channels are light sensitive and close upon absorption of photons by the visual pigment in the outer segment.[83] This in turn stops the dark current and results in a slow, sustained hyperpolarization response. In the rods, the visual pigment is situated in discs within the outer segment and a cytoplasmic messenger probably mediates between the light absorption and the closure of the cation channels. In the cones, the disc membranes are continuous with surface membranes, and a second messenger is not necessary but probably exists.[84] It has been hypothesized that this second messenger is either Ca^{2+}, which directly blocks the cation channels[85] or a decrease in cGMP.[86] The light-induced hyperpolarization of the cell membrane influences second-order visual neurons (the bipolar cells) by modulating the rate of neurotransmitter release from the synaptic terminal of the photoreceptor.[87,88] The response of the bipolar cells to light can be either slow, sustained hyperpolarization or slow, sustained depolarization. Horizontal cells respond, too, with slow, sustained hyperpolarization as well as by lateral inhibitory feedback to the photoreceptor cell.[26] This feedback signal consists of summed information from a network of horizontal cells connected over a wide area of the outer plexiform layer. Another local circuit occurs in the inner plexiform layer at the bipolar to amacrine or ganglion cell synapse.[26] Using intracellular recording from horseradish peroxidase–stained neurons as well as complex tracing of serial electron micrographs, such circuits have identified mediating contrast, red and green color pathways, and pathways underlying night vision as summarized by Kolb in her Proctor lecture.[26]

Acknowledgments: This work was supported in part by The International Order of Odd Fellows, Winston-Salem, NC, and Core Grant EYO 1765-21 from the National Eye Institute, Bethesda, MD.

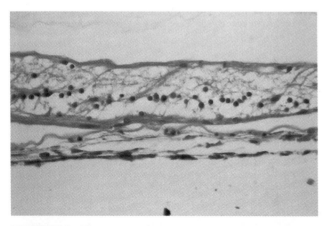

FIGURE 1–39   Central area of cobblestone lesion with loss of RPE and outer retinal layers. The remaining inner portion of inner nuclear layer rests against Bruch's membrane (periodic acid–Schiff, × 100).

REFERENCES

1. Nussbaum JJ, Pruett RC, Delori FC: Historic perspectives. Macular yellow pigment. The first 200 years. Retina 1:296–310, 1981.
2. Orth DH, Fine BS, Fagman W, Quirk TC: Clarification of foveomacular nomenclature and grid for quantitation of macular disorders. Trans Am Acad Ophthalmol Otolaryngol 83:OP506–514, 1977.
3. Spitznas M, Hogan MJ: Outer segments of photoreceptors

and the retinal pigment epithelium. Interrelationship in the human eye. Arch Ophthalmol 84:810–819, 1970.

4. Spitznas M: The fine structure of the chorioretinal border tissues of the adult human eye. Adv Ophthalmol 28:78–174, 1974.

5. Zinn KM, Benjamin-Henkind JV: Anatomy of the human retinal pigment epithelium. In Zinn KM, Marmor MF (eds): The Retinal Pigment Epithelium. Cambridge, Harvard University Press, 1979 pp 3–31.

6. Friedman E, Tso MO: The retinal pigment epithelium. II. Histologic changes associated with age. Arch Ophthalmol 79:315–320, 1968.

7. Hogan MJ, Alvarado JA, Weddell JE: Histology of the Human Eye: An Atlas and Textbook. Philadelphia, WB Saunders Co, 1971, pp 393–606.

8. Robb RM: Regional changes in retinal pigment epithelial cell density during ocular development. Invest Ophthalmol Vis Sci 26:614–620, 1985.

9. Fine BS, Yanoff M: Ocular Histology. A Text and Atlas. New York, Harper & Row, 1972, p 61.

10. Verhoeff FH: A hitherto undescribed membrane of the eye and its significance. Boston Med Surg J 149:456–458, 1903.

11. Heriot WJ, Machemer R: Pigment epithelial repair. Graefes Arch Clin Exp Ophthalmol 230:91–100, 1992.

12. Valentino TL, Kaplan HJ, Del Priore LV, et al: Retinal pigment epithelial repopulation in monkeys after submacular surgery. Arch Ophthalmol 113:932–938, 1995.

13. Hsu JK, Thomas MA, Ibanez H, Green WR: Clinicopathologic studies of an eye after submacular membranectomy for choroidal neovascularization. Retina 15:43–52, 1995.

14. Schmidt SY, Peisch RD: Melanin concentration in normal human retinal pigment epithelium. Regional variation and age-related reduction. Invest Ophthalmol Vis Sci 27:1063–1067, 1986.

15. Weiter JJ, Delori FC, Wing GL, Fitch KA: Retinal pigment epithelial lipofuscin and melanin and choroidal melanin in human eyes. Invest Ophthalmol Vis Sci 27:145–152, 1986.

16. Feeney-Burns L, Berman ER, Rothman H: Lipofuscin of human retinal pigment epithelium. In Davson H (ed): Current Topics in Eye Research. New York, Academic Press, 1980, pp 119–178.

17. Feeney-Burns L, Hilderbrand ES, Eldridge S: Aging human RPE: morphometric analysis of macular, equatorial, and peripheral cells. Invest Ophthalmol Vis Sci 25:195–200, 1984.

18. Wing GL, Blanchard GC, Weiter JJ: The topography and age relationship of lipofuscin concentration in the retinal pigment epithelium. Invest Ophthalmol Vis Sci 17:601–607, 1978

19. Fine BS, Yanoff M: The retina. In Fine BS, Yanoff M (eds): Ocular histology. A Text and Atlas. New York, Harper & Row, 1972, pp 47–107.

20. Feeney L: Lipofuscin and melanin of human retinal pigment epithelium. Fluorescence, enzyme cytochemical, and ultrastructural studies. Invest Ophthalmol Vis Sci 17:583–600, 1978.

21. Stramm LE: Synthesis and secretion of glycosaminoglycans in cultured retinal pigment epithelium. Invest Ophthalmol Vis Sci 28:618–627, 1987.

22. Bok D: Processing and transport of retinoids by the retinal pigment epithelium. Eye 4:326–332, 1990.

23. Clark VM: The cell body of the retinal pigment epithelium. In Adler R, Farber D (eds): The Retina. A Model for Cell Biology Studies: Part II. Orlando, FL, Academic Press, 1986, pp 129–168.

24. Young RW, Bok D: Participation of the retinal pigment epithelium in the rod outer segment renewal process. J Cell Biol 42:392–403, 1969.

25. Werblin F: Synaptic connections, receptive fields, and patterns of activity in the tiger salamander retina. A simulation of patterns of activity formed at each cellular level from photoreceptors to ganglion cells (the Friedenwald lecture). Invest Ophthalmol Vis Sci 32:459–483, 1991.

26. Kolb H: The architecture of functional neural circuits in the vertebrate retina. The Proctor Lecture 35:2385–2404, 1994.

27. Green WR: Retina. In Spencer WH (ed): Ophthalmic Pathology. An Atlas and Textbook, Vol 2. Philadelphia, WB Saunders Co, 1996, pp 667–1376.

28. Gartner S, Henkind P: Aging and degeneration of the human macula. Outer nuclear layer and photoreceptors. Br J Ophthalmol 65:23–28, 1981.

29. Foos RY: Vitreoretinal juncture; topographical variations. Invest Ophthalmol 11:801–808, 1972.

30. Spencer LM, Foos RY, Straatsma BR: Enclosed bays of the ora serrata: relationship to retinal tears. Arch Ophthalmol 83:421–425, 1970.

31. Spencer LM, Foos RY, Straatsma BR: Meridional folds, meridional complexes, and associated abnormalities of the peripheral retina. Am J Ophthalmol 70:679–714, 1970.

32. Rutnin U, Schepens CS: Fundus appearance in normal eyes. Peripheral degenerations. Am J Ophthalmol 64:1040–1062, 1967.

33. Lonn LI, Smith TR: Ora serrata pearls. Clinical and histological correlation. Arch Ophthalmol 77:809–813, 1967.

34. Daicker B, Eisner G: The drusen of the ora serrata; their clinical and pathological anatomy [Die Drusen der Ora serrata, ihre Klinik und pathologische Anatomie]. Graefes Arch Clin Exp Ophthalmol 174:336–343, 1968.

35. Foos RY, Allen RA: Retinal tears and lesser lesions of the peripheral retina in autopsy eyes. Am J Ophthalmol 64:643–655, 1967.

36. Foos RY: Zonular traction tufts of the peripheral retina in cadaver eyes. Arch Ophthalmol 82:620–632, 1969.

37. Foos RY, Simons KB: Vitreous in lattice degeneration of retina. Ophthalmology 91:452–457, 1984.

38. Foos RY, Spencer LM, Straatsma BR: Trophic degenerations of the peripheral retina. In Symposium on Retina and Retinal Surgery, Trans New Orleans Acad Ophthalmol. St Louis, CV Mosby Co, 1969, pp 90–102.

39. Spencer LM, Straatsma BR, Foos RY: Tractional degenerations of the peripheral retina. In Symposium on retina and retinal surgery, Trans New Orleans Acad Ophthalmol. St Louis, CV Mosby Co, 1969, pp 103–127.

40. Byer NE: Cystic retinal tufts and their relationship to retinal detachment. Arch Ophthalmol 99:1788–1790, 1981.

41. Straatsma BR, Foos RY, Feman SS: Degenerative diseases of the peripheral retina. In Duane TD (ed): Clinical Ophthalmology, Vol 3. Philadelphia, Harper & Row, 1980, pp 1–27.

42. Kornzweig AL: The eye in old age. V. Diseases of the macula: a clinicopathologic study. Am J Ophthalmol 60:835–843, 1965.

43. Guyer DR, Green WR: Idiopathic macular holes and precursor lesions. In Franklin RM (ed): Proceedings of the Symposium on Retina and Vitreous. New Orleans, Amsterdam, Kugler Publications, 1993, pp 135–162.

44. Morgan CM, Schatz H: Involutional macular thinning. A premacular hole condition. Ophthalmology 93:153–161, 1986.

45. Feeney-Burns L, Burns RP, Gao CL: Age-related macular changes in humans over 90 years old. Am J Ophthalmol 109:265–278, 1990.

46. Dontsov AE, Sakina NL, Ostrovski MA: Comparative study of lipid peroxidation in the eye of pigment epithelium of pigmented and albino animals. Biokhimiia 45:923–928, 1980.

47. Watzke RC, Soldevilla JD, Trune DR: Morphometric analysis of human retinal pigment epithelium: correlation with age and location. Curr Eye Res 12:133–142, 1993.

48. Dorey CK, Wu G, Ebenstein D, et al: Cell loss in the aging retina. Relationship to lipofuscin accumulation. Invest Ophthalmol Vis Sci 30:1691–1699, 1989.

49. Gao H, Hollyfield JG: Aging of the human retina. Differential loss of neurons and retinal pigment epithelial cells. Invest Ophthalmol Vis Sci 33:1–17, 1992.

50. Panda-Jonas S, Jonas JB, Jakobczyk-Zmija M: Retinal pigment epithelial cell count, distribution, and correlations in normal human eyes. Am J Ophthalmol 121:181–189, 1996.

51. Mikelberg FS, Drance SM, Schulzer M, et al: The normal human optic nerve. Axon count and axon diameter distribution. Ophthalmology 96:1325–1328, 1989.

52. Jonas JB, Muller-Bergh JA, Scholtzer-Schrehardt UM, Naumann GO: Histomorphometry of the human optic nerve. Invest Ophthalmol Vis Sci 31:736–744, 1990.

53. Jonas JB, Schmidt AM, Muller-Bergh A, et al: Human optic nerve fiber count and optic disc size. Invest Ophthalmol Vis Sci 33:2012–2018, 1992.

54. Balazsi AG, Rootman J, Drance SM, et al: The effect of age on the nerve fiber population of the human optic nerve. Am J Ophthalmol 97:760–766, 1984.

55. Sanchez RM, Dunkelberger GR, Quigley HA: The number and diameter distribution of axons in the monkey optic nerve. Invest Ophthalmol Vis Sci 27:1342–1350,1986.

56. Dolman CL, McCormick AQ, Drance SM: Aging of the optic nerve. Arch Ophthalmol 98:2053–2058, 1980.

57. Johnson BM, Miao M, Sadun AA: Age-related decline of human optic nerve axon populations. Age 10:5–9, 1987.

58. Mikelberg FS, Yidegilgne HM, White VA, Schulzer M: Relation between optic nerve axon number and axon diameter to scleral canal area. Ophthalmology 98:60–63, 1991.

59. Repka MX, Quigley HA: The effect of age on normal human optic nerve fiber number and diameter. Ophthalmology 96:26–32, 1989.

60. Quigley HA, Sanchez RM, Dunkelberger GR, et al: Chronic glaucoma selectively damages large optic nerve fibers. Invest Ophthalmol Vis Sci 28:913–920, 1987.

61. Quigley HA, Dunkelberger GR, Green WR: Chronic human glaucoma causing selectively greater loss of large optic nerve fibers. Ophthalmology 95:357–363, 1988.

62. Sadun AA, Bassi CJ: Optic nerve damage in Alzheimer's disease. Ophthalmology 97:7–8.63, 1990.

63. Loeffler KU, Lee WR: Is basal laminar deposit unique for age-related macular degeneration (Letter). Arch Ophthalmol 110:15–16, 1992.

64. Loeffler KU, Lee WR: Basal linear deposit in the human macula. Graefes Arch Clin Exp Ophthalmol 224:493–501, 1986.

65. Killingsworth MC: Age-related components of Bruch's membrane in the human eye. Graefes Arch Clin Exp Ophthalmol 225:406–412, 1987.

66. Daicker B: Lineare degenerationen des peripheren retinalen pigmentepithels; Eine patholgisch-anatomische Studie. Graefes Arch Clin Exp Ophthalmol 186:1–12, 1973.

67. Lewis H, Straatsma BR, Foos RY, Lightfoot DO: Reticular degeneration of the pigment epithelium. Ophthalmology 92:1485–1495, 1985.

68. Kanski JJ: Peripheral retinal degenerations. Trans Ophthalmol Soc UK 95:173–179, 1975.

69. Bastek JV, Siegel EB, Straatsma BR, Foos RY: Chorioretinal juncture. Pigmentary patterns of the peripheral fundus. Ophthalmology 89:1455–1463, 1982.

70. Lewis H, Straatsma BR, Foos RY: Chorioretinal juncture. Multiple extramacular drusen. Ophthalmology 93:1098–1112, 1986.

71. Humphrey WT, Carlson RE, Valone JA Jr: Senile reticular pigmentary degeneration. Am J Ophthalmol 98:717–722, 1984.

72. O'Malley PF, Allen RA: Peripheral cystoid degeneration of the retina. Incidence and distribution in 1,000 autopsy eyes. Arch Ophthalmol 77:769–776, 1967.

73. Foos RY: Senile retinoschisis: Relationship to cystoid degeneration. Trans Am Acad Ophthalmol Otolaryngol 74:33–51, 1970.

74. Foos RY, Feman SS: Reticular cystoid degeneration of the peripheral retina. Am J Ophthalmol 69:392–403, 1970.

75. Straatsma BR, Foos RY: Typical and reticular degenerative retinoschisis. XXVI Francis I Proctor Memorial Lecture. Am J Ophthalmol 75:551–575, 1973.

76. Byer NE: Long-term natural history of senile retinoschisis with implications for management. Ophthalmology 93:1127–1137, 1986.

77. Byer NE: Long-term natural history of lattice degeneration of the retina. Ophthalmology 96:1396–1402, 1989.

78. Straatsma BR, Zeegan PD, Foos RY, et al:Lattice degeneration of the retina (XXX Edward Jackson Memorial Lecture). Am J Ophthalmol 77:619–649, 1974.

79. Nicholls JVV: The effect of section of the posterior ciliary arteries in the rabbit. Br J Ophthalmol 22:672–687, 1938.

80. Michelson PE, Knox DL, Green WR: Ischemic ocular inflammation. A clinicopathologic case report. Arch Ophthalmol 86:274–280, 1971.

81. Hagins WA, Penn RD, Yoshikami S: Dark current and photocurrent in retinal rods. Biophys J 10:380–412, 1970.

82. Massey SC: Cell types using glutamate as a neurotransmitter in the vertebrate retina. Prog Ret Res 9:399–425, 1990.

83. Tomita T: Electrophysiological study of the mechanism subserving color coding the fish retina. Cold Spring Harb Symp Quant Biol 30:559–566, 1965.

84. Baylor DA, Fuortes MG: Electrical responses of single cones in the retina of the turtle. J Physiol (Lond) 207:77–92, 1970.

85. Hagins WA: The visual process: excitatory mechanisms in the primary receptor cells (Review). Ann Rev Biophys Bioeng 1:31–158, 1972.

86. Hubbell WL, Bownds MD: Visual transduction in vertebrate photoreceptors (Review). Ann Rev Neurosci 2:17–34, 1979.

87. Baylor DA, Fettiplace R: Transmission from photoreceptors to ganglion cells in turtle retina. J Physiol (Lond) 271:391–424, 1977.

88. Yau KW: Phototransduction mechanism in retinal rods and cones. The Friedenwald lecture. Invest Ophthalmol Vis Sci 35:9–32, 1994.

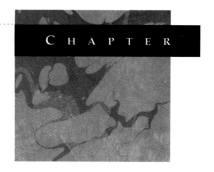

CHAPTER 2

Clinical Examination of the Posterior Segment of the Eye

Allen C. Ho, M.D.

David R. Guyer, M.D.

Stuart L. Fine, M.D.

Examination of the posterior segment of the eye is a technically demanding and challenging task. To examine these structures—vitreous, retina, subretinal layers, pars plana, and optic nerve—one must combine excellent observational skills, clinical experience, as well as a facility with the instruments and lenses used to illuminate and magnify the posterior structures of the eye. The basic principle of ophthalmoscopy is the focusing of light rays from the patient's fundus onto the examiner's fundus (Fig. 2–1). In this chapter we will discuss the various methods of ophthalmoscopy as well as the many types of tools that are used to examine the posterior ocular structures.

Examination of the entire posterior segment requires pupillary dilation. Dilation of the pupil permits adequate illumination of the vitreous and retina and allows one to examine peripheral retina. Our standard dilating drops are 1% tropicamide (Mydriacyl) and 2.5% neosynephrine (Mydrifin) drops, which are instilled into an eye anesthetized with topical proparacaine hydrochloride 0.5% (Ophthetic) (Fig. 2–2). Dilation is generally achieved within 20 or 30 minutes and is often more rapid in eyes with light-colored irides. Darker irides may require a second set of dilating drops.

METHODS OF OPHTHALMOSCOPY

There are three main methods of ophthalmoscopy: direct ophthalmoscopy, indirect ophthalmoscopy, and slit lamp contact or non–contact lens biomicroscopic ophthalmoscopy.

Direct Ophthalmoscopy

Historically, direct ophthalmoscopy was performed using candlelight. The examiner viewed the fundus monocularly through a small peephole. Purkinje first described the technique of ophthalmoscopy in 1823 and subsequently Von Helmholtz first introduced the direct ophthalmoscope in 1850. Since that time, illuminating sources for direct ophthalmoscopy have evolved from candlelight to gaslight to external and built-in electric light.

Direct ophthalmoscopy is the simplest way to examine the fundus and is the method most commonly used by medical students and nonophthalmologists. It is the least technically demanding form of ophthalmoscopy, although it does require practice. Modern direct ophthalmoscopes are often portable and afford various levels of illumination along with green, red, blue, or other filters (Fig. 2–3). The light source illuminates the patient's fundus through the pupillary axis and an upright and virtual image of the retina is produced with approximately 15 × magnification for the emmetropic eye. If a patient is myopic, then the eye has effective plus power and the ophthalmoscope requires a minus neutralizing lens. This resultant lens system is a Galilean telescope, which thus increases the magnification of fundus details. The opposite is true for hyperopic eyes whereby the image of fundus structures may be reduced in size. The observer creates

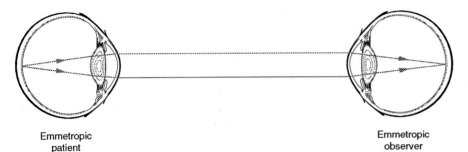

Emmetropic
patient

Emmetropic
observer

FIGURE 2–1 Conjugate retinal points are shown with an emmetropic observer and emmetropic patient, but inadequate illumination precludes visualization of posterior segment detail.

a crisp image by using neutralizing lenses that are present on the headpiece of the instrument.

One major limitation of direct ophthalmoscopy is that only a small field of view is produced. One can only visualize approximately 8 to 10 degrees of the fundus. It is important to position the direct ophthalmoscope very close to the patient's eye in order to maximize the limited field of view (Figs. 2–4 and 2–5). It is analogous to peering into a room through a keyhole: the closer one gets to the aperture or keyhole, the wider the field of view. As in most forms of ophthalmoscopy, it is helpful to have the patient use his opposite eye to fixate on an object to reduce wandering eye motion. The peripheral retina is not well visualized because of the restricted field of view. Another limitation of direct ophthalmoscopy is that only a monocular image is produced. In contrast, indirect ophthalmoscopy and slit lamp ophthalmoscopy permit stereoscopic viewing of the retina, which is very important in the examination of the retina and subretinal layers. finally, significant media opacities such as cataract will greater limit the resolution of the image with this instrument.

Although the direct ophthalmoscope is relatively inexpensive and portable and can be used without

pupillary dilation, indirect and slit lamp biomicroscopic ophthalmoscopy are generally favored by ophthalmologists because they offer a wider field of view and superior resolution of posterior segment details.

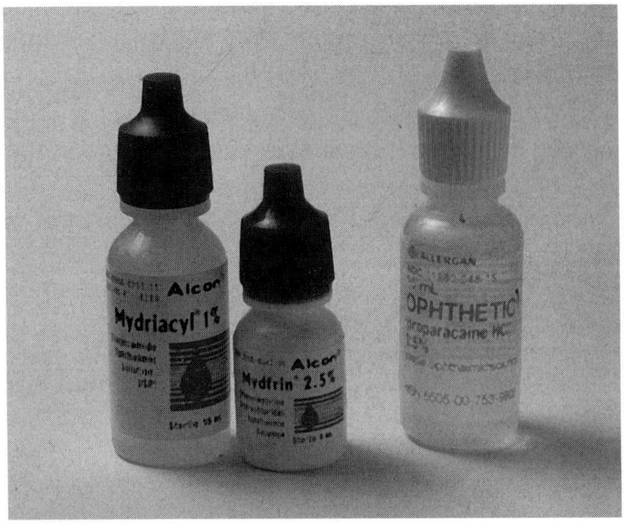

INDIRECT OPHTHALMOSCOPY

Schepens first introduced his binocular indirect ophthalmoscope in 1947, and since then the binocular indirect ophthalmoscope has become a standard ophthalmic instrument to examine the posterior structures of the eye.

The binocular indirect ophthalmoscope is portable, particularly with a mobile energy source, although it is not as small as the direct ophthalmoscope (Fig. 2–6). It traditionally has been comprised of an illuminating headpiece and modified oculars, although recently more portable eyeglass-style indirect ophthalmoscopes have become available. Examination of posterior segment structures requires a handheld condensing lens, most commonly 20 diopters in power, which is placed in front of the dilated eye (Fig. 2–7). The traditional headpiece incorporates an illuminating light source as well as condensing optics that effectively narrow the interpupillary distance, thereby affording binocular images of the posterior segment (Fig. 2–8). This also permits stereoscopic viewing of the fundus through a dilated pupil with a typical field of view of 30

FIGURE 2–2 Standard dilating drops are tropicamide 1% (Mydriacyl) and phenylephrine hydrochloride 2.5% (Mydfrin). These are instilled after topical anesthesia is achieved with proparacaine hydrochloride 0.5% (Ophthetic).

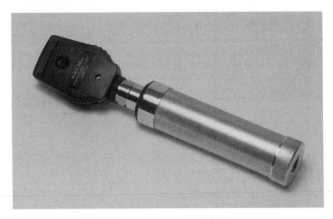

FIGURE 2–3 Direct ophthalmoscope.

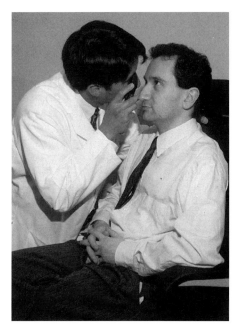

FIGURE 2–4   Direct ophthalmoscopy is best achieved by allowing the patient to fixate on a distant object and by bringing the ophthalmoscope close to the observed eye.

degrees or more, depending on the type of condensing lens placed in front of the eye.

The indirect ophthalmoscope adheres to Gullstrand's principle, whereby illuminating and viewing beams must be totally separated through the cornea, pupillary aperture, and lens (to avoid reflections), but must coincide on the retina to permit viewing. The viewing oculars of an indirect ophthalmoscope reduce the effective interpupillary distance, thereby permitting illuminating light and binocular stereoscopic views through a dilated pupil. An indirect ophthalmoscope permits adjustments in the position of the illuminating light beam as well as the effective interpupillary distance.

Further narrowing of the effective interpupillary distance on the headpiece of an indirect ophthalmoscope allows the examiner to perform funduscopy through a smaller pupil; however, the proximity of the illuminating and viewing beams increases distracting reflections. Increasing the effective interpupillary distance improves stereopsis, while decreasing this distance has the opposite ef-

fect. A pinhole light diaphragm can produce a narrower beam of light, which can reduce reflections.

Neutralization of a patient's refractive error is achieved by moving the condensing lens toward or away from the examined eye and/or accommodation by the examiner's eyes. The indirect ophthalmoscope produces a real inverted image for the observer that can be disorienting for the novice, since the field of view is upside down and backwards. To use this instrument properly requires considerable practice and experience. Simulated model eyes are available to practice the examining adjustments required to use properly the indirect ophthalmoscope.

In order to use the indirect ophthalmoscope properly, the headpiece and eyepieces must first be adjusted. The knob that adjusts the location of the illumination should be set such that the light fills the superior part of the field of view. The examiner checks the alignment of each ocular by closing one eye at a time. The condensing lens should be held 2 to 3 inches from the patient's eye with its most convex side facing the examiner (white line on the lens towards the patient) between the thumb and the first finger. The examiner's other hand may be used to hold open the patient's eyelids, since the intense illuminating light elicits a natural response to close the eyelids.

The observer then systematically examines the retinal periphery and finally the posterior pole. The examiner orients his eyes with the condensing lens and the patient's retina in each field of gaze such that an imaginary straight line could be placed between the point midway between the eye pieces, center of the condensing lens, center of the pupil, and the area of the retina to be examined (Fig. 2–9). This alignment then allows one to view the retinal area of interest. For example, to examine the superior nasal quadrant of the right eye, the physician should first tell the patient to look up and to the left. The observer should then orient his eyes with the lens and the patient's retina in order to obtain a clear image of this region by moving the condensing lens slowly toward or away from the patient's eye in order to allow the entire retinal image to fill the lens. The examiner may also change the distance between the headpiece and the condensing lens to achieve the same effect. Because the

FIGURE 2–5   Direct ophthalmoscopy performed by an illuminating hand-held light source and the focusing lenses of the direct ophthalmoscope.

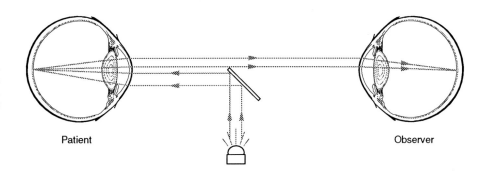

Patient   Observer

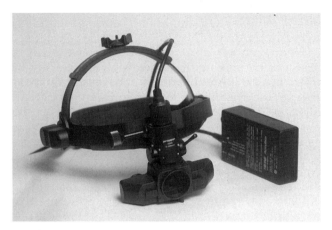

FIGURE 2–6 An indirect ophthalmoscope and portable energy pack.

bright illuminating light is disorienting, it may be helpful to give the patient an object of regard to look at with the nonexamined eye, even the patient's own outstretched hand, in order to help the patient maintain the direction of gaze.

A major advantage of the binocular indirect ophthalmoscope is that it allows one to view the peripheral retina. To increase the field of view of the peripheral retina, it is often helpful to slightly pivot the base of the condensing lens in the direction of the patient's gaze as well as to turn one's head so that the axis between the examiner's eyes is aligned with the patient's direction of gaze (Fig. 2–10 and 2–11). By turning one's head, the image is monocular and not stereoscopic but permits illumination and viewing of peripheral structures (Fig. 2–12). In this fashion, one can often observe the ora serrata without any further manipulation of the well-dilated eye. If the peripheral retina is not visualized using this lens and head-tilt technique, one can perform scleral depression to completely evaluate the peripheral retina.

Scleral depression is traditionally performed with a handheld metal instrument with a dilated end (Fig. 2–13). The scleral depressor indents the eye to bring the peripheral retina into view while performing indirect ophthalmoscopy. Other objects such as cotton-tip applicators are also often used as scleral depressors. It is helpful to apply topical anesthesia, although this is not essential. A depressor

may be placed on the eyelid in order to indent the globe or may be used directly on the surface of the globe when topical anesthesia is performed. The external aspect of the globe corresponding to the peripheral retinal area of interest is gently depressed inward using the scleral depressor. Excessive pressure is not necessary and should be avoided in order to avoid patient discomfort. The examiner should move the depressor around the eye for 360 degrees and observe each area using indirect ophthalmoscopy. This is done with the patient in the supine position, and the examiner often moves around the patient in order to perform ophthalmoscopy with scleral depression. Scleral depression requires considerable skill and practice.

Scleral depression is a dynamic process and movement of the scleral depressor underneath a lesion of interest can often be helpful in determining, for example, whether a retinal lesion is truly a retinal hole or not. Dynamic scleral depression beneath a true retinal tear or hole will elevate edges of the retinal defect. Dynamic scleral depression also allows the process to be more efficient, since sweeps of peripheral retina with the scleral depressor allow one to cover areas more efficiently than individual placement and adjustment of the scleral depressor tip.

There are different condensing lenses that can be used with the indirect ophthalmoscope. Although the 20-diopter condensing lens is the most common, other lenses may be used to broaden the field of view, to examine through a small pupil, or to examine the posterior segment when there is intraocular gas. For difficult views, (e.g., due to a small pupil or intraocular gas), a 28- or 30-diopter lens can be used, but the compromise will be a loss of magnification; 28- or 30-diopter lenses also increase the field of view. Examination of the posterior segment in the presence of intraocular gas is difficult because of increased reflections at different interfaces of fluid, gas, and tissue—28- or 30-diopter lenses can be helpful in this situation. It is also helpful to increase the distance between the patient's eye and the condensing lens as well as between the condensing lens and the examiner's eyes when examining an eye containing intraocular gas.

Finally, some ophthalmoscopes as well as slit lamps have colored filters that can be useful in cer-

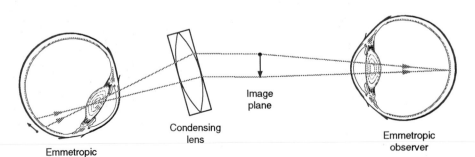

FIGURE 2–7 Indirect ophthalmoscopy is performed with a handheld condensing lens that produces a real and inverted 30-degree image on the observer's side of the condensing lens.

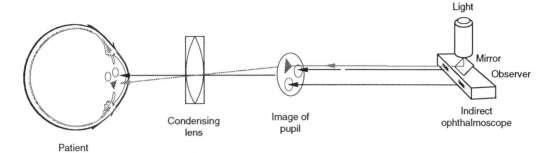

FIGURE 2–8   A binocular indirect ophthalmoscope effectively narrows the observer's interpupillary distance, thus permitting placement of the illuminating and viewing beams within the patient's pupillary aperture.

tain circumstances. A red filter absorbs red light and therefore red objects appear black. This can be helpful when examining retinal vascular abnormalities and retinal hemorrhages. Nerve fiber layer loss and retinal thickening are also highlighted by red-free light because a greater proportion of shorter visible wavelengths are scattered by superficial retinal layers. Blue filters highlight fluorescein during fluorescein angiography and can enhance autofluorescence of optic nerve had drusen.

The Retinal Drawing

Most retinal surgeons have been trained to create formal retinal drawings of the fundus. Retinal drawings are useful to document pathology, although many now prefer to document pathology with fundus photographs. The process of a retinal drawing can be a powerful way to improve observational skills of retinal lesions. Standard retinal drawing paper is used and various lesions are drawn with colored pencils in relation to the optic nerve, retinal vessels, and the three-dimensional boundaries of the fundus depicted on the retinal drawing paper. Some observers place the retinal drawing paper upside down (12 o'clock position towards the feed) on the supine patient's chest so that the drawing can represent what is visualized in the condensing lens and can be sketched during the examination process. Standard left and right retinal drawings are marked by meridional clock hours and concentric circles. The inner circle marks the equator of the globe and the two outermost circles delimit the pars plana. The middle circle thus represents the ora serrata. Retinal drawings on two-dimensional paper are hampered by problems similar to those that cartographers encounter; lesions in the retinal periphery are larger in size due to peripheral Cartesian distortion.

Colors on a conventional retinal drawing are standardized, with red representing attached retina or retinal hemorrhages, blue representing detached retina or subretinal fluid, green representing vitreous opacities, brown representing pigmented lesions or choroidal elevations, and yellow representing lipid exudation or fibrovascular scars.

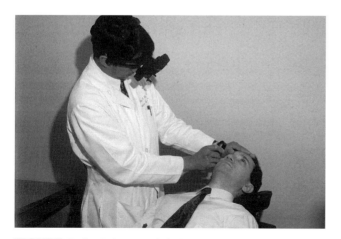

FIGURE 2–9   Indirect ophthalmoscopy performed on supine patient. To view the superonasal peripheral retina of the right eye, the patient fixates back and to the left with the examiner positioned opposite the direction of gaze.

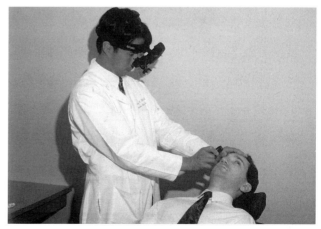

FIGURE 2–10   The peripheral retina is not well visualized because the examiner has not adopted a head tilt to view the nasal peripheral retina of the right eye.

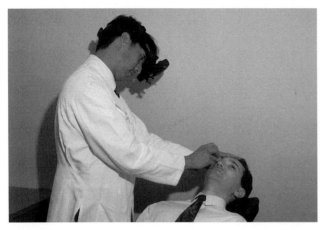

FIGURE 2–11 The peripheral retina is better visualized when the examiner tilts his head and rotates the base of the condensing lens in the direction of gaze.

Retinal Slit Lamp Biomicroscopic Ophthalmoscopy

Retinal slit lamp biomicroscopic ophthalmoscopy affords the high magnification and illumination necessary to evaluate in detail the vitreous, optic nerve, and macula as well as small peripheral retinal lesions such as retinal tears. The slit lamp is used with either a noncontact or a contact examining lens in this technique. The image is highly magnified and stereoscopic. The biomicroscopic capabilities of the slit lamp can be applied to examination of preretinal, intraretinal, and subretinal lesions. Furthermore, a detailed examination of the vitreous can be performed looking for features such as pigmented cells or inflammatory cells in the anterior or posterior vitreous. Status of the posterior vitreous attachment can also be assessed, although various cleavage planes within the vitreous body itself can mimic a true posterior vitreous detachment.

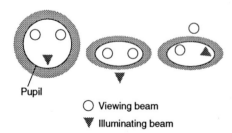

Pupil

○ Viewing beam
▼ Illuminating beam

FIGURE 2–12 The principle of head tilt to examine the fundus through an elliptical pupil. An effectively elliptical pupil is created when the patient fixates in extreme gaze to permit visualization of peripheral retina. In situation *A*, both viewing beams and illuminating beam are well accommodated to provide a view of the posterior fundus with the patient looking directly at the observer. In situation *B*, the examiner has not adopted a head tilt to accommodate the elliptical pupil and thus there is no view because the illuminating beam is blocked by the iris. In situation *C*, the examiner has tilted his head, which permits entry of the illuminating beam and only one viewing beam (nonstereoscopic image).

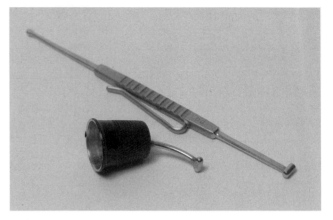

FIGURE 2–13 A thimble and a handheld scleral depressor.

Non–Contact Lens Slit Lamp Biomicroscopy

A non–contact lens biomicroscopic evaluation of the retina can be performed with a Hruby lens, which is present on many slit lamp ophthalmoscopes. This lens is a plano concave lens of high negative power that produces an upright, vertical image. The lens is swung into place on the slit lamp stage and a magnified image of vitreous, retina, or optic nerve can be obtained. A focused image is achieved by manipulating a lever attached to the lens that moves the lens toward or away from the patient's eye. This lens is useful for studying the optic never in detail and also for examining the posterior vitreous for inflammatory cells. To observe the posterior vitreous it is helpful to narrow the slit lamp light beam as well as to turn the incident light slightly off axis to retroilluminate the posterior vitreous cells, which will then appear black against the illuminated fundus background.

Non–contact lens biomicroscopic evaluation is more commonly performed with aspherical 60-diopter, 78-diopter, and 90-diopter lenses (Fig. 2–14). These non–contact lenses produce a real, inverted, high-quality image for the examiner. The ophthal-

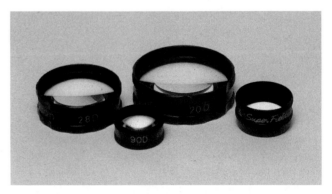

FIGURE 2–14 Twenty-eight– and 20-diopter condensing lenses for indirect ophthalmoscopy. A 90-diopter and wide-field macular lens for non–contact lens biomicroscopy.

mologist holds the lens in one hand and places it a few centimeters in front of the patient's eye. The physician may also hold open the patient's eyelids with the same hand. The slit lamp is then used to create a vertical beam to illuminate and examine the retina. A 90-diopter lens produces the widest field of view at the expense of magnification. A 78-diopter lens affords a nice compromise between field of view and magnification. The 60-diopter lens provides the greatest magnification. These lenses are often used to examine the optic nerve and posterior pole. The non–contact lens technique is especially useful prior to angiography, as the lenses do not disturb the cornea. When using handheld lenses in conjunction with the slit lamp, the examiner will often encounter distracting light reflections. It is useful to angle the incident light of the slit lamp slightly off center through the vertical axis or the horizontal axis of the slit lamp apparatus so that reflected light passes obliquely rather than directly back to the examiner.

Contact Lens Slit Lamp Biomicroscopy

The "gold standard" for examining the posterior or peripheral retina is contact lens slit lamp biomicroscopic ophthalmoscopy. Because a contact lens is used, topical anesthesia and a contact lens coupling gel are required. The coupling gel is typically a clear viscous liquid such as methylcellulose (Goniosol) or less viscous solutions such as Celluvisc. Saline may be used and is advisable if high-quality fundus photography or angiography is subsequently planned. The lenses are applied to an anesthetized eye by having the patient first look up with placement of the contact lens and coupling agent on the surface of the eye centered on the inferior limbus. The patient then directs his gaze towards the examiner to center the lens on the cornea thus providing a view of the posterior structures of the eye centered on the posterior pole.

There are several different types of contact lenses suitable for viewing the retina. The Goldmann three-mirror lens is comprised of a central viewing area for the posterior retina surrounded by three

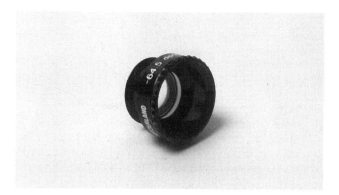

FIGURE 2–16   A contact macular lens.

mirrors of different size and angle orientation to view specific parts of the eye (Fig. 2–15). The smallest thumbnail-shaped mirror allows visualization of the anterior chamber structures as well as the far retinal periphery. Because this is a mirror, the location of the area that is examined is 180 degrees opposite from the position of the mirror. The middle sized mirror has a different angle of orientation and allows visualization of the retina anterior to the equator. The larger mirror is used to study the retina between the equator and the macula. A Goldmann lens can be rotated 360 degrees so that all areas of the retina and the anterior chamber can be observed. It is helpful to understand that if the patient looks toward a mirror, then a more posterior region of the retina will be seen by the observer. A high-quality, magnified view of the peripheral retina can be obtained using the Goldmann three-mirror lens combined with scleral depression. The technique is challenging and many retina specialists prefer depression of peripheral lesions with indirect ophthalmoscopy.

Specific macular lenses have also been designed that feature flanges on the ocular contact surface that are compressed against the globe by the patient's eyelids (Fig. 2–16). This type of design makes it harder for the patient to dislodge a contact lens. These specialized macular lenses are placed on the eye in a similar fashion to the Goldmann

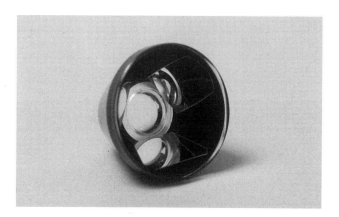

FIGURE 2–15   A Goldmann three-mirror contact lens.

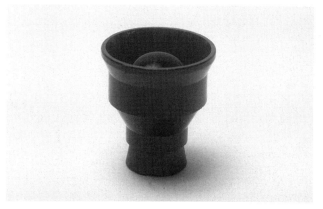

FIGURE 2–17   A Rodenstock panfunduscopic contact lens.

lens and also provide a high-quality, magnified stereoscopic macular view but do not allow the clinician to observe peripheral retina.

Another very useful contact lens for fundus biomicroscopy is the panfunduscopic or Rodenstock lens (Fig. 2–17). This lens is comprised of a meniscus lens and a spherical lens. The image produced is real, inverted, and minified. This lens is especially useful to obtain a wide-angle view of the retina, particularly in eyes with poor pupillary dilation. The disadvantage of this lens is the small image size and lower resolution views of the retinal periphery. It is, however, very useful for peripheral or panretinal laser photocoagulation. There are other panfunduscopic lenses available such as the Mainster lens, which produces less magnification than the panfunduscopic lens with only a slightly reduced field of view. More peripheral areas of the retina can be viewed with the panfunduscopic lens

by tilting the lens slightly and having the patient direct his gaze slightly away from the area of interest.

SUMMARY

Clinical examination of the posterior structures of the eye requires specialized equipment, a facility with this equipment, and active observational processes. Direct ophthalmoscopy permits a limited field of view but is generally the most easily mastered method of examination. In direct ophthalmoscopy is more challenging but affords the most efficient views of the peripheral retina. Slit lamp contact or non–contact lens ophthalmoscopy provides the highest resolution of the posterior structures of the eye.

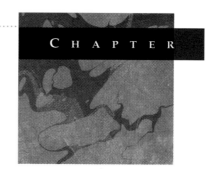

CHAPTER 3

Principles of Fluorescein Angiography

Naresh Mandava, M.D.

David R. Guyer, M.D.

Lawrence A. Yannuzzi, M.D.

Jami Nichol

Dennis Orlock

Over 100 years ago, fundus photography of rabbits was first attempted by Henry Noyes with limited results. It was not until 1926 when Nordensen and Carl Zeiss produced the first reliable commercial fundus camera that clinical photographs of the human ocular fundus were possible. It was in 1955 when Zeiss introduced the electronic flash that the modern fundus camera was born.

Sodium fluorescein was first synthesized in 1871 by Von Baeyer and one of its early uses was to study the water flow of the Danube River. MacLean and Maumenee performed angioscopy in humans with a slit lamp and cobalt blue filter in 1960.[1] They were able to use this technique for diagnostics but were unable to document and/or study the fluorescein angioscopy. Flocks attempted angiography with motion picture film with limited success.[2] It was not until the advent of the electronic flash that Novotny and Alvis were able to perform the first successful fluorescein angiogram on a human.[3] Using the combination of matched filters, Zeiss optics and high-speed high-resolution film, careful study of the retinal circulation was possible. In the past three decades of clinical use, this procedure has greatly expanded our knowledge and treatment of chorioretinal diseases. Today, with digital imaging and computer analysis, the technique and our understanding of fluorescein angiography are still expanding.

PROPERTIES OF SODIUM FLUORESCEIN DYE

Sodium fluorescein is yellow-red in color with a molecular weight of 376.67, a spectrum of absorption at 465 to 490 nm (blue), and excitation at 520 to 530 nm (yellow-green wavelength). Sodium fluorescein dye is usually available as 2 to 3 ml of 25% concentration or 5 ml of 10% sodium fluorescein. Many institutions prefer injecting the smaller volume of the 25% solution. There has been no evidence of increased side effects with the higher concentration of solution.[4,5] The dye is usually injected as a bullous into the antecubital vein to maximize the contrast of the early filling phase of the angiogram. Care should be taken not to extravasate the dye, since infiltration is painful.

Once injected, 80% of the dye binds with plasma proteins, particularly to albumin. It is metabolized by the liver and kidney and within 24 to 36 hours is eliminated in the urine, which is discolored a bright orange hue. The skin may also turn a slight yellow hue, especially in lightly pigmented individuals, for a few hours. Patients have increased photosensitivity when the skin is yellow and must be cautioned regarding skin protection from ultraviolet light. Although there has been no reported adverse reaction or apparent risk to the pregnant

TABLE 3–1 Frequency of Adverse Reactions*

Mild	
87% of respondents estimated a 0–5% incidence	
Nausea	
Vomiting	
Pruritus	
Moderate	
Urticaria	1:82
Syncope	1:337
Other	1:769
Overall	1:63
Severe	
Respiratory	1:3800
Cardiac	1:5300
Seizures	1:13,900
Death	1:221,781
Overall	1:1900

* From Yannuzzi LA, Rohrer MA, Tindel LJ, et al: Fluorescein angiography complication survey. Ophthalmology 93:611–617, 1986, with permission.

woman or the fetus, we do not use fluorescein angiography during pregnancy unless it is absolutely crucial to the management of the patient.[6,7]

Adverse reactions to intravenous fluorescein angiography have ranged from mild to severe.[5,8–12] Mild reactions are classified as those with a transient effect that resolves completely not requiring treatment. They most commonly include nausea (3 to 15%), vomiting (0 to 7%), and pruritus. Moderate adverse reactions resolve with medical intervention. They include urticaria, syncope, thrombophlebitis, pyrexia, local tissue necrosis, and nerve palsy. Severe reactions are those requiring intensive intervention with variable recovery. Severe reactions include laryngeal edema, bronchospasm, anaphylaxis, shock, myocardial infarction, cardiac arrest, tonic-clonic seizures, and death.[5] The incidence of adverse reactions have been reported in a multicenter collaborative study (Table 3–1).

TECHNIQUE OF FUNDUS PHOTOGRAPHY AND FLUORESCEIN ANGIOGRAPHY

Spare parts for your fundus camera cannot be obtained from your local photo supply store. It is necessary to keep certain supplies and replacement parts on hand at all times. These include illumination bulbs, a spare flash tube, and an extra camera body. Routine maintenance should be performed yearly, and at that time, the fluorescein filters should be inspected and replaced if necessary. The objective lens should be cleaned periodi-

cally by an experienced technician, but it is good preventive maintenance and common sense to keep the lens covered with the lens cap between photography sessions.

Modern fundus cameras are reliable and relatively easy to operate, but the photographer must be knowledgeable of the various camera controls to obtain high-quality photographs. The most common cause of poorly focused fundus photographs is operator error. The fundus camera produces an aerial image, which exists at infinity. There are cross hairs in the eyepiece reticle that allow the photographer to correct for their spherical refractive error. To produce a well-focused fundus photograph, the photographer must see both the cross hairs and the fundus in good focus at the same time. The focusing wheel is then used for fine focus of the retinal pathology.

Unlike the slit lamp, the joy stick of the fundus camera is used to critically align the camera to the patient's eye only. The photographer will look for even illumination of the image to determine proper alignment of the camera. Misalignment causes peripheral or central artifacts in the images. Small, careful lateral movements with the joystick should be used to eliminate these before the photographs are taken. Many cameras provide variable magnification of 20, 30, and 50 degrees. It is important to select a magnification that is appropriate to the pathology being photographed.

Maximal dilation is critical for optimal images. A pupil of at least 4 to 5 mm is necessary for fundus photography or fluorescein angiography. Pupil size can influence exposure and it may be necessary to increase the flash setting with a very small pupil. When in doubt, "bracket" exposures. It may also be necessary to increase the exposure for a "dark" fundus or highly pigmented pathology.

The patient must also be prepared for the procedure to improve cooperation during the angiogram. The photographer should try to help the patient through a photographic procedure with a minimum of anxiety and discomfort. This requires communication, patience, and good photographic technique. Ninety per cent of successful ophthalmic photography is patient management.

The best way to avoid the common errors or pitfalls of fundus photography is to develop and follow a standard photographic protocol. Following a protocol will help the photographer to avoid making mistakes in a busy clinical setting. A sample "photographic procedure" follows:

1. Proper camera back and film—color (fundus photography), black and white (fluorescein angiography).
2. Proper flash setting for film used.
3. Viewing intensity (as low as possible for patient comfort but adequate to focus).
4. Focus cross hairs.
5. Photograph patient identification label.
6. Position patient at camera (adjust camera height and chin rest).

7. Adjust camera in relation to patient's eye.
8. Fixate eye using a fixation target.
9. Choose correct field size based upon pathology to be evaluated.
9. Focus on retina (remember to visualize cross hairs).

Normal Fluorescein Angiogram

After rapid injection into the antecubital vein, fluorescein dye enters the short posterior ciliary arteries and is visualized in the choroid and optic nerve head in 10 to 15 seconds. The speed of injection, age, and the cardiovascular condition of the patient will influence the rapidity of fluorescence. The *choroidal flush* is the hallmark of choroidal filling. The mottled fluorescence of the choriocapillaris is attributed to variable blockage by the retinal pigment epithelium. *Patchy filling* of the choroid anatomically represents perfusion of choriocapillaris lobules sequentially, rather than simultaneously. In the early angiogram, leakage of dye from the choriocapillaris and staining of Bruch's membrane eclipse choroidal vessel detail. In 10 to 15% of patients, a cilioretinal artery (choroidal circulation) is present and will fluoresce simultaneously with the choroid.

Retinal circulation filling begins at 10 to 15 seconds, approximately 1 to 3 seconds after the onset of *choroidal filling*. After the dye is seen in the central retinal arteries, the fluorescein travels into the precapillary arterioles, the capillaries, the postcapillary venules, and then exits the eye through the veins in a laminar pattern. The *early arteriovenous phase* is followed by the *late arteriovenous phase*, which is characterized by the maximal fluorescence of the arteries and the capillary bed, with early laminar filling of the veins. Laminar filling of veins is caused by the preferential concentration of unbound fluorescein along the vessel walls. This has been attributed to the faster flow of blood as well as the higher concentration of erythrocytes in the central vascular lumen.

The juxtafoveal capillary network achieves maximal fluorescence at 20 to 25 seconds. A dark background in the macula, created by blockage of choroidal fluorescence by xanthophyll pigment and a high density of retinal pigment epithelial cells, enhances capillary detail. The normal capillary free zone or foveal avascular zone (FAZ) is 300 to 500 μm.

At 30 seconds, the first pass of fluorescein through the retinal and choroidal vasculature is complete. This is followed by *recirculation phases* in which there is intermittent mild fluorescence. At 10 minutes, both circulations are generally devoid of fluorescein. The late angiogram is characterized by staining of Bruch's membrane, the choroid, and sclera, which is more visible in patients with light retinal pigment epithelium. Staining of the disc margin and the optic nerve head is independent of the degree of retinal pigment epithelium (RPE) pigmentation.

INTERPRETATION OF ABNORMAL FLUORESCEIN ANGIOGRAPHY

The localization of abnormal areas of fluorescence and the identification of *hypofluorescence* and *hyperfluorescence* is crucial in the interpretation of fluorescein angiograms.[13–19] Fluorescein angiograms are dynamic, so the characteristics of specific anatomic areas can change over the course of the angiogram. Hypofluorescence is a reduction or absence of normal fluorescence, while hyperfluorescence is increased or abnormal fluorescence (Tables 3–2 and 3–3).

TABLE 3–2 Hypofluorescence

Blocked retinal fluorescence
  Media opacity
  Vitreous opacification (hemorrhage, asteroid hyalosis, vitritis)
  Subhyaloid hemorrhage
  Intraretinal pathology (hemorrhage [vein occlusion], edema)
Blocked choroidal fluorescence
  All entities causing blocked retinal fluorescence
  Outer retinal pathology (lipid, hemorrhage, xanthophyll [normal pigment])
  Subretinal pathology (hemorrhage, lipid, melanin, lipofuscin, fibrin, inflammatory material)
  Sub-RPE pathology (hemorrhage)
  Choroidal pathology (nevus, melanoma)
Vascular filling defects
  Retinal
    Occlusion or delayed perfusion
      Central or branch artery occlusions
      Capillary nonperfusion secondary to diabetes, vein occlusion, radiation, etc.
    Atrophy or absence of vessels or retina
  Choroidal
    Occlusion of large choroidal vessels or choriocapillaris (sectoral infarct [wedge-shaped], malignant hypertension, toxemia, lupus choroidopathy, renal disease)
    Atrophy or absence of choroidal vessels or choriocapillaris (choroideremia, AMPPPE)
  Optic disc
    Occlusion (ischemic optic neuropathy)
    Atrophy or absence of tissue (coloboma, optic nerve pit, optic nerve hypoplasia or optic atrophy)

RPE, retinal pigment epithelium; AMPPPE, acute multifocal posterior placoid pigment epitheliopathy.

TABLE 3–3 Hyperfluorescence

Pseudofluorescence
Autofluorescence
Transmitted fluorescence
  Geographic atrophy
  Bull's eye maculopathy
  Macular Hole
  Atrophic chorioretinal scar
Abnormal vessels
  Retina
    Angioma/Wyburn-Mason
    Cavernous hemangioma
    Vascular tumor
    Retinoblastoma
  Choroid
    Melanoma
    Plaque/CNV
    Choroidal hemangioma
  Optic nerve
    Peripapillary vascular loops
Leakage
  Retinal vessels—venous occlusive disease,
    frosted angiitis, phlebitis
  Neovascularization
Pooling
  Neurosensory detachment—CSC, optic nerve pit
    (slow filling), Best's disease
  Subretinal neovascularization
  RPE detachment (serous, fibrovascular)
Staining
  Staphyloma, disc, sclera, chorioretinal scar

CNV, choroidal neovascularization; CSC, central serous
choroidopathy; RPE, retinal pigment epithelium.

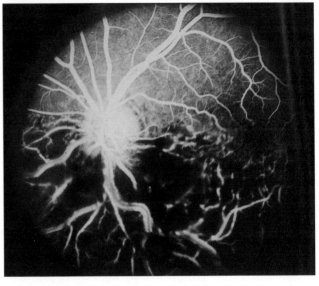

FIGURE 3–1 Blocked fluorescence localizes the level of the blocking material. An acute hemiretinal vein occlusion with hemorrhages within the inner retina blocking retinal vascular detail. Note that superficial larger retinal vessels fluoresce where hemorrhages are slightly deeper within the retina.

Hypofluorescence

Hypofluorescence can be categorized into blockage (masking of fluorescence) or vascular filling defects. *Blocked fluorescence* can give us clues to the level of the blocking material (i.e., vitreous, retinal, or subretinal). Blocked retinal fluorescence can be caused by any element that diminishes the visualization of the retina and its circulation. Media opacity secondary to corneal pathology or cataract can block or reduce retinal fluorescence. In addition, hemorrhage on the surface of the retina (preretinal) or debris in the vitreous cavity (inflammatory cells, hemorrhage) can mask fluorescence.

Blockage of retinal fluorescence may localize the pathology to the inner retina. It is crucial to understand that large retinal vessels and precapillary (first-order) arterioles lie in the nerve fiber layer while capillaries and postcapillary venules are located in the inner nuclear layer. As such, a flame-shaped hemorrhage (nerve fiber layer) will block all

retinal vascular fluorescence, while a deeper dot or blot hemorrhage or intraretinal lipid will block capillary fluorescence but will not block larger vessels (Fig. 3–1). Inner retinal edema caused by central retinal artery occlusions will block retinal fluorescence; however, the vascular filling defects in this entity will also contribute to the hypofluorescence.

Blockage of choroidal fluorescence can occur with any of the previously described pathologic entities located anterior to the choroid. In addition, subretinal material in pathologic states such as lipid, fibrin, inflammatory material, hemorrhage, lipofuscin, and melanin can block choroidal fluorescence (Fig. 3–2). It is also important that the normal

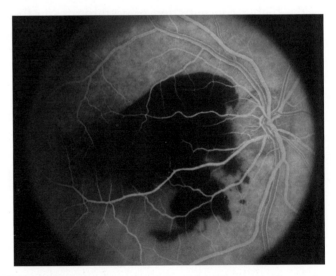

FIGURE 3–2 Blockage of choroidal fluorescence by a subretinal hemorrhage secondary to neovascularization in a patient with age-related macular degeneration.

fluorescein angiogram displays blockage of choroidal fluorescence as evidenced early by patchy
choroidal filling and throughout the angiogram by
a dark macular region. Xanthophyll and a high
density of RPE (melanin) are responsible for this
blockage of fluorescence in the posterior pole. Also,
material within and beneath the RPE may block
choroidal fluorescence. Melanin can accumulate in
retinal pigment epithelial cells in many disease processes from the common retinal pigment epithelial
hypertrophy surrounding a scar to the less common
congenital hypertrophy of the retinal pigment epi-

thelium (CHRPE). Fundus flavimaculatus and
Best's disease have lipofuscin deposits that block
choroidal fluorescence. Subpigment epithelial hemorrhage is also a common source of masked fluorescence. Finally, blocking material can be located
within the choroid itself such as in a choroidal nevus (melanin).

Vascular filling defects cause hypofluorescence
because of decreased or absent perfusion of tissues.
Retinal vascular filling defects producing hypofluorescence can involve large-, medium- or small-
caliber vessels. Central or branch artery occlusions

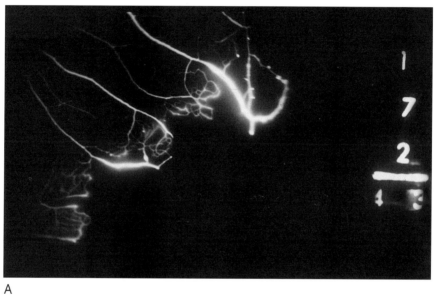

A

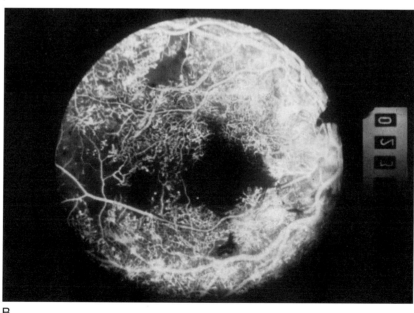

B

FIGURE 3–3   Vascular filling defects demonstrate hypofluorescence. *A*, Peripheral capillary nonperfusion
in a patient with sickle cell retinopathy. *B*, Capillary nonperfusion (ischemia) in the posterior pole of a severe
diabetic. The "peak phase" of the fluorescein angiogram demonstrates the peak of fluorescence in the arteriovenous phase. Parafoveal capillary detail is best seen in this frame of the angiogram. *Illustration continued
on following page*

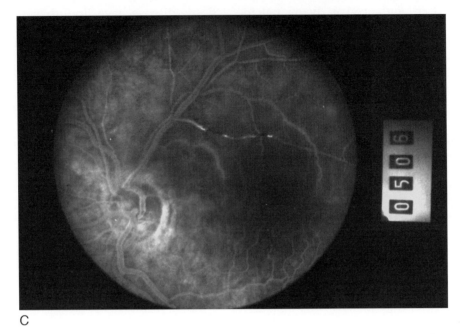

C

FIGURE 3–3   *Continued   C,* Relative hypofluorescence of the retinal vasculature in a central retinal artery occlusion. Over 50 seconds into the angiogram, there is only scattered, segmental filling of the arteries with fluorescein dye.

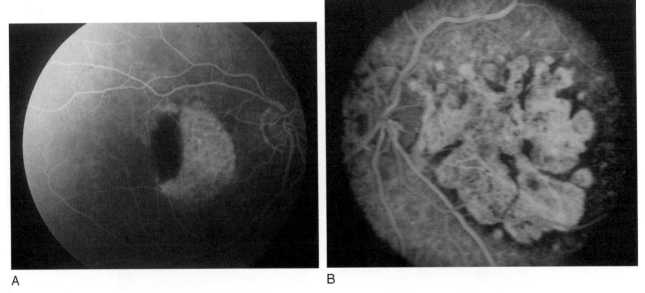

A   B

FIGURE 3–4   Transmitted fluorescence. *A,* Retinal pigment epithelial rip. The well-demarcated area of choroidal fluorescence represents a window defect created by the "scrolling" of retinal pigment epithelium temporally. The area of hypofluorescence in the temporal aspect of the lesion is secondary to blockage by redundant retinal pigment epithelium. *B,* Geographic atrophy in age-related macular degeneration. The serpiginoid pattern of choroidal fluorescence is an uncommon presentation of this common disease. The geographic area of transmission hyperfluorescence is created by retinal pigment epithelial atrophy. The boundary of the lesion is hypofluorescent secondary to a rim of retinal pigment epithelial hyperplasia.

will show hypofluorescence of the entire involved arterial tree, while zones of capillary nonperfusion or ischemia will demonstrate hypofluorescence in the distribution of the involved capillaries (Fig. 3–3). "Pruning" of vessels is seen in zones of capillary nonperfusion.

Choroidal vascular filling defects are more difficult to visualize, as the native RPE produces variable blockage of fluorescence depending upon its degree of pigmentation. The anatomy of the choroidal circulation is less well understood than that of the retinal vasculature. In general, occlusive disease involving isolated larger vessels will manifest as sectoral, wedge-shaped areas of hypofluorescence. More commonly choroidal hypoperfusion will exhibit diffuse involvement of the choriocapillaris. Systemic diseases including malignant hypertension, toxemia of pregnancy, and lupus choroidopathy will produce zones of hypofluorescence. Neighboring perfused choriocapillaris may leak into the areas of hypofluorescence in the late angiogram. Atrophy or degeneration of the chorio-

capillaris is the pathogenesis of choroideremia and has been purported to contribute to the angiographic findings in acute mutifocal posterior placoid pigment epitheliopathy (AMPPPE), although this is an area of controversy. Interestingly, vascular filling defects of the optic nerve head (disc) are visualized by fluorescein angiography. Sectoral or complete disc hypofluorescence is seen with ischemic optic neuropathy. In addition, many atrophic or hereditary anomalies of the optic nerve head can manifest with hypofluorescence. Congenital anomalies presenting with hypofluorescence include optic nerve colobomas, optic nerve hypoplasia, and optic pits. Atrophy of the optic nerve head secondary to optic atrophy or end-stage glaucomatous cupping may also display hypofluorescence.

Hyperfluorescence

Hyperfluorescence is caused by an increase in normal fluorescence or an abnormal presence of fluores-

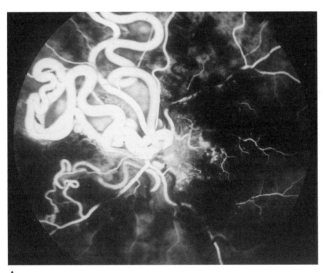

A

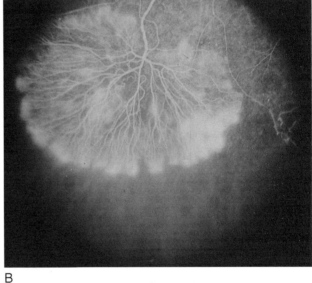

B

FIGURE 3–5 Hyperfluorescence secondary to abnormal blood vessels. *A*, These large-caliber dilated vessels represent a congenital retinal arteriovenous malformation (AVM) called the Wyburn-Mason anomaly. Interestingly, this large AVM has caused a secondary retinal vein occlusion as evidenced by intraretinal hemorrhages that block fluorescence. *B*, "Sea fan" in sickle cell retinopathy. Retinal neovascularization can be demonstrated sometimes even in the early angiogram by hyperfluorescence of pathologic new blood vessels as seen in this patient with proliferative sickle cell disease. Characteristically, the large sea fan is at the edge of a large zone of capillary nonperfusion. *C*, Choroidal hemangioma. This highly vascular choroidal lesion fluoresces in the early angiogram. This frame illustrates the very early laminar filling phase of the fluorescein angiogram. Note the lesion extends under the fovea.

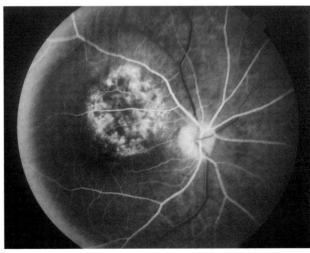

C

cence. Normally, a blue exciter filter allows the passage of blue wavelength light into the eye, while the green barrier filter allows fluoresced yellow-green light to return to the fluorescein camera. When there is overlap of the wavelength of light allowed to pass (filter mismatch), white and brighter structures in the fundus will reflect and cause "false" fluorescence or *pseudofluorescence*. Barrier filters and excitation filters must periodically be evaluated and changed if mismatch exists. *Autofluorescence* is a natural phenomenon caused by very few pathologic entities, including optic nerve head calcified drusen, astrocytic hamartomas, and large deposits of lipofuscin. These lesions act physiologically like fluorescein dye in that when blue light reflects from their surface, yellow-green light is emitted.

In routine fluorescein angiography, hyperfluorescence is frequently seen with *transmission win-dow defects* and the presence of *abnormal blood vessels*. A *window defect* refers to choroidal fluorescence produced by a relative decrease or absence of pigment in the RPE or an absence of RPE. *Transmitted fluorescence* is seen with common pathologic processes such as the geographic atrophic form of macular degeneration, drusen, chorioretinal atrophic scars, and full-thickness macular holes (Fig. 3–4). Hyperfluorescence attributed to the presence of *abnormal blood vessels* is seen in the retina, choroid, and optic disc. Retinal congenital and acquired vascular malformations include capillary angiomas, arteriovenous malformations, and Coats' disease (Fig. 3–5A). Common abnormalities of native blood vessels in pathologic states include telangiectasias, aneurysms, anastomoses, dilation, and tortuosity. A myriad of diseases in medical retina produce these vascular findings, including venous obstructive disease and diabetes. Neovascularization within the

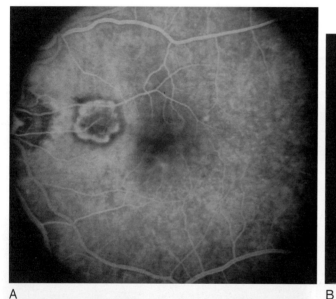

A

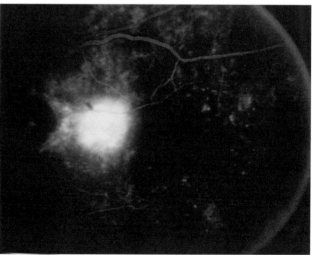

B

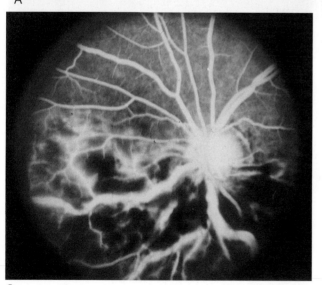

C

FIGURE 3–6 Hyperfluorescence secondary to leakage of fluorescein dye. *A*, Classic choroidal neovascularization in age-related macular degeneration. The arteriovenous phase of the angiogram demonstrates a well-demarcated zone of choroidal hyperfluorescence in the papillomacular bundle. *B*, Over 4 minutes into the fluorescein angiogram, the abnormal neovascular lesion demonstrates late leakage with blurring of its margins. *C*, Hemiretinal vein occlusion. Late leakage of the dilated venous system in this patient with acute vein occlusion. Blockage of venous outflow has caused incompetence of vessel walls as illustrated by perivascular leakage of fluorescein dye. Note there is also hyperfluorescence of the vessel walls themselves. This is termed "staining" as there is deposition of fluorescein dye into the tissues of the vessel walls. The fluorescein picture is similar to that seen in retinal vasculitis or frosted-branch angiitis.

retina and choroid is a common end point to many retinal diseases including diabetic retinopathy and age-related macular degeneration. Hyperfluorescence of these new pathologic blood vessels is often seen on fluorescein angiography, although late leakage of fluorescein dye is a more common presentation of hyperfluorescence in neovascularization (Fig. 3–5B). Finally, vascularized tumors of the choroid such as melanoma or choroidal hemangioma and of the retina such as retinoblastoma can hyperfluoresce on fluorescein angiography (Fig. 3–5C).

Leakage of fluorescein dye into the extravascular space leads to hyperfluorescence. Late leakage into the vitreous cavity is a hallmark of retinal neovascularization and is often located adjacent to an area of capillary nonperfusion. In addition, subretinal neovascularization secondary to age-related macular degeneration may well demonstrate a well-defined area of leakage (classic choroidal neovascularization) (Fig. 3–6A, B). By fluorescein angiogram, subclinical neovascularization (not identified by ophthalmoscopy) may sometimes be identified on the optic disk or elsewhere. Vasculitis or inflammatory lesions can leak fluorescein into the retina or vitreous because of the increased permeability of vessel walls (Fig. 3–6C). Intraretinal leakage is most commonly seen with macular edema. Angiographically, diabetic macular edema presents with leaking focal parafoveal microaneurysms, while cystoid macular edema as seen after cataract surgery (Irvine-Gass) or in the uveitic patient demonstrates leakage into the cystoid spaces

of the outer plexiform layer often in a petalloid pattern. The normal optic disc has minimal leakage along its margins secondary to leakage from adjacent choroidal capillaries. Papilledema and ischemic optic neuropathy will produce more profound disc leakage late in the angiogram as a result of capillary leakage on the disc surface. The early angiogram may display only capillary dilation and vessel tortuosity.

Hyperfluorescence secondary to subretinal and choroidal pathology has been more difficult to correlate histopathologically. However, the timing, pattern, and location of hyperfluorescence are reproducible in many diseases. *Pooling* refers to dye accumulation into an anatomic space, while *staining* is the deposition of fluorescein into involved tissues. Pooling is seen in both neurosensory and pigment epithelial detachments (Fig. 3–7A). The rapidity and pattern of pooling in these entities is important in their differentiation. For example, neurosensory detachments in central serous chorioretinopathy fluoresce slowly if at all because fluorescein must pass through small leaks in the RPE. By contrast, retinal pigment epithelial detachments in macular degeneration are characterized by rapid pooling of fluorescein under the dome of the detachment, as their is no barrier to choriocapillaris permeability. Some use the term "pooling" when referring to the accumulation of dye in the outer plexiform layer in cystoid macular edema, as this is also an accumulation of dye into an anatomic space (Fig. 3–7B). Staining of ocular tissues by fluorescein occurs in normal and pathologic states.

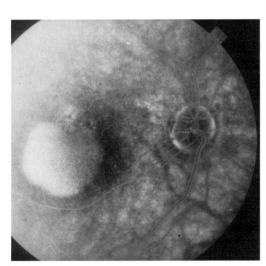

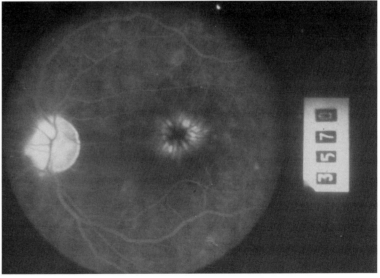

A   B

FIGURE 3–7   Pooling of fluorescein dye. *A,* Late fluorescein angiogram of a serous pigment epithelial detachment (PED) in age-related macular degeneration. The retinal vasculature is devoid of fluorescein dye. There is some hyperfluorescence of the choriocapillaris with hypofluorescence of larger choroidal vessels. Most importantly, fluorescein dye has pooled in the sub-RPE space. A notch in the PED at the superior margin of the lesion represents choroidal neovascularization, which is a probable cause of the present pathology. *B,* Late angiogram demonstrating a petalloid pattern of pooling of fluorescein dye intraretinally. Histopathologically, pooling occurs in the potential spaces of the outer plexiform layer.

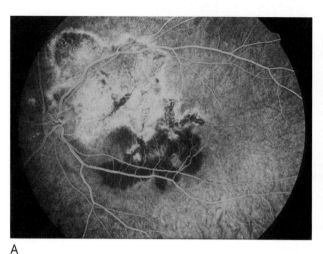

A

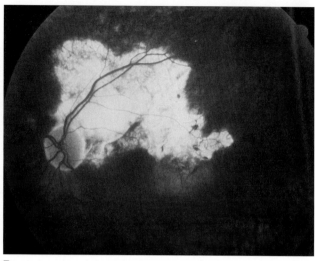

B

FIGURE 3-8   Staining of ocular tissues by fluorescein dye. *A,* This is an arteriovenous phase fluorescein angiogram of a patient with serpiginous choroidopathy. The hyperfluorescent zone in the superior aspect of the lesion is secondary to severe atrophy of the retinal pigment epithelium with a concomitant partially intact choriocapillaris. *B,* The late angiogram illustrates scleral staining in the same distribution as the zone of early hyperfluorescence.

Damaged Bruch's membrane or RPE, and disciform scars may stain late in the angiogram. Normal structures such as the optic disc and sclera may also stain. Scleral staining is more easily seen in high myopes (especially with staphylomas) and patients with lightly pigmented fundi because of enhanced transmission through the RPE. Patients with severe atrophic diseases involving wipeout of the RPE such as gyrate atrophy, serpiginous choroidopathy, and severe chorioretinal atrophy secondary to posterior uveitis will demonstrate significant scleral staining (Fig 3–8). Atrophy or loss of choriocapillaris may diminish the degree of staining.

Fluorescein angiography has remained a constant, priceless tool for the retinal specialist. Not only has it aided us in the identification of the pathophysiology and diagnosis of disease, but it also has enhanced our treatment and management of patients. More descriptive explanations of fluorescein angiography for specific retinal diseases are discussed in the appropriate chapters.

REFERENCES

1. MacLean AL, Maumenee, AE: Hemangioma of the choroid. Am J Ophthalmol 50:3–11, 1960.
2. Flocks M, Miller J, Chao P: Retinal circulation time with the aid of fundus cinematography. Am J Ophthalmol 48:3 –6, 1959.
3. Novotny HR, Alvis DL: A method of photographing fluorescence in circulating blood in the human retina. Circulation 24:82–86, 1961.
4. Justice J Jr, Paton D, Beyrer CR, Seddon GG: Clinical comparison of 10% and 25% intravenous sodium fluorescein solutions. Arch Ophthalmol 95:2015–2016, 1977.
5. Yannuzzi LA, Rohrer MA, Tindel LJ, et al: Fluorescein angiography complication survey. Ophthalmology 93:611–617, 1986.
6. Halperin LS, Olk J, Soubrane G, Coscas G: Safety of fluorescein angiography during pregnancy. Am J Ophthalmol 109:563–566, 1990.
7. Greenberg F, Lewis RA: Safety of fluorescein angiography during pregnancy (Letter to the editor). Am J Ophthalmol 110:323–325, 1990.
8. Amalric P, Biau C, Fenies MT: Incidents et accidents au cours de l'angiographie fluoresceinique. Bull Soc Ophtalmol Fr 68:968–972, 1968.
9. Stein MR, Parker CW: Reactions following intravenous fluorescein. Am J Ophthalmol 72:861–868, 1971.
10. Levacy R, Justice J Jr: Adverse reactions to intravenous fluorescein. Int Ophthalmol Clin 16(2):53–61, 1976.
11. Butner RW, McPherson AR: Adverse reactions in intravenous fluorescein angiography. Ann Ophthalmol 15:1084–1086, 1983.
12. Marcus DF, Bovino JA, Williams D: Adverse reactions during intravenous fluorescein angiography. Arch Ophthalmol 102:825, 1984.
13. Delori F, Ben-Sira I, Trempe C: Fluorescein angiography with an optimized filter combination. Am J Ophthalmol 82:559–566, 1976.
14. Gass JDM: Stereoscopic Atlas of Macular Diseases: Diagnosis and Treatment, 4th edition. St Louis, Mosby-Year Book, Inc, 1997.
15. Gitter KA, Schatz H, Yannuzzi LA, McDonald HR (eds): Laser Photocoagulation of Retinal Disease. San Francisco, Pacific Medical Press, 1988.
16. Justice J Jr (ed): Ophthalmic Photography. Boston, Little, Brown & Co, 1982.
17. Rabb MF, Burton TC, Schatz H, Yannuzzi LA: Fluorescein angiography of the fundus: a schematic approach to interpretation. Surv Ophthalmol 22:387–403, 1978.
18. Schatz, H: Flow sheet for the interpretation of the fluorescein angiograms. Arch Ophthalmol 94:687, 1976.
19. Schatz H, Burton TC, Yannuzzi LA, Rabb MF: Interpretation of fundus fluorescein angiography. St Louis, Mosby-Year Book, Inc. 1978.

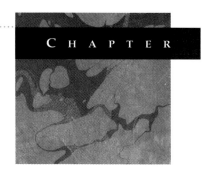

Principles of Indocyanine-Green Angiography

David R. Guyer, M.D.

Lawrence A. Yannuzzi, M.D.

Jason S. Slakter, M.D.

John A. Sorenson, M.D.

Richard F. Spaide, M.D.

K. Bailey Freund, M.D.

Dennis Orlock

Digital indocyanine-green videoangiography (ICG-V) is a new diagnostic technique to image the choroid and its associated pathology. This procedure is useful in the clinical management of occult or poorly defined choroidal neovascularization secondary to age-related macular degeneration (AMD).[1,2] It is also a useful technique to learn more about the pathogenesis of other chorioretinal disorders. In this chapter we will review the properties of the dye, as well as the use of this technique in the diagnosis and study of various disorders. Although ICG angiography has been available since the 1970s[3-7] it has not been until the technological advance of combining digital imaging systems or scanning laser ophthalmoscopes to ICG cameras that this technique has achieved high enough resolution such that the technique is now of clinical relevance.[2,8]

SPECIAL PROPERTIES OF ICG

ICG is a tricarbocyanine dye that has several special properties that give it certain advantages over sodium fluorescein as a dye for ophthalmic imaging. The dye is highly protein bound and is active

in the infrared range. These properties make ICG useful in imaging occult or poorly defined choroidal neovascularization secondary to AMD in which the neovascular complex is not well defined due to blockage by overlying blood and/or serosanguineous fluid during fluorescein angiography. The dye also allows enhanced visualization of the choroid and its associated pathology in other conditions such as choroiditis, tumors, and central serous chorioretinopathy.

HISTORY OF ICG ANGIOGRAPHY

In 1970 Kogure and associates[9] performed choroidal absorption angiography using intra-arterial injection in monkeys. David[10] and Flower[4-7] were early pioneers in performing the first ICG angiograms in humans. Choroidal absorption angiography was performed in cats using intravenous injection in 1971 by Hochheimer.[11] Flower and Hochheimer performed intravenous absorption ICG angiography in a human 1 year later.[4] This same group then described ICG fluorescence angiography, which was a major breakthrough.[6,7] Flower and co-workers were responsible for several other improvements and studies throughout the 1970s.[3-6] The major problem, however, was that infrared film did not have the necessary sensitivity to capture the low-intensity ICG fluorescence.

In the 1980s Hayashi's group,[12-14] as well as Puliafito and co-workers[8] described ICG-V, which improved the resolution to some degree. In 1989 Scheider and Schroedel reported on high-resolution ICG-V using a scanning laser ophthalmoscope.[15] Digital high-resolution ICG-V was introduced in 1992 by Guyer et al[8] and Yannuzzi and co-workers.[2] These researchers combined 1024-line digital imaging systems to ICG cameras and noted very-high-resolution ICG angiograms.

PHARMACOLOGY[16-19]

ICG is a water soluble tricarbocyanine dye with an empiric formula of $C_{43}H_{47}N_2NaO_6S_2$. The dye is an anhydro-3,3,3,3,-tetramethyl-1,1-di(4-sulfobutyl)-4, 5,4,5-dibenzoindotricarbocyanine hydroxide sodium salt. It has a molecular weight of 775 daltons. The dye has been thought to bind predominately to albumen in the serum, but 80% of ICG in the blood is actually bound to globulins such as lipoproteins. ICG is active between 790 and 805 nm. It is excreted via bile by the liver.

TOXICITY

The dye is relatively safe and appears to be safer than sodium fluorescein. Nausea and vomiting are extremely uncommon, unlike with fluorescein angiography.[20]

The dye should not be used in patients with shellfish allergies, since it contains iodine. In addition, it should not be used in uremic patients or in those with liver disease. Emergency equipment should be readily available.

TECHNIQUE[2]

The fundus camera systems that are used today for ICG-V are essentially original retinal fundus cameras that have been modified to allow the maximum infrared wavelength transmissions. Compared to other types of fundus imaging, maximum pupillary dilatation is as important or even more critical when doing ICG angiography. This requirement is most critical in the early and late stages of the study when the available dye in the fundus is at a minimum.

It is generally accepted that approximately 25 to 50 mg dissolved in 1 to 2 ml of distilled water, or an average of 40 mg is adequate. We have found with the ICG-V systems available today that for the average patient, 25 mg of ICG dissolved in 2 ml of aqueous solvent provides high contrast images. For patients who are poorly dilated or with a darkly pigmented fundus, a higher concentration of 50 mg of ICG dissolved in 3 ml of aqueous solvent is used.

ICG angiography is a dynamic study of which all phases are used for diagnosis. Images are usually taken during the filling phase and at 3, 5, 10, and 30 minutes. Valuable information is obtained from all of these phases.

CLINICAL APPLICATIONS

Age-Related Macular Degeneration

The most useful clinical application for digital ICG-V is with occult or poorly defined choroidal neovascularization secondary to AMD (Fig. 4–1). Under fluorescein guidance, only approximately 13% of patients with exudative maculopathy are found to have a well-defined or classic neovascular membrane that is amenable to laser treatment.[21] Indocyanine green angiography increases the resolution of the neovascular complex and thus allows us to potentially treat more patients with laser photocoagulation.

We recently studied 1000 consecutive eyes with occult neovascularization secondary to AMD using ICG-V.[22] Three morphologic types of choroidal neovascularization may be seen with ICG angiography. These lesions include focal spots, plaques, and combination lesions (in which both focal spots and plaques are noted). There are three subtypes of combination lesions: marginal spots (focal spots at the edge of plaques of neovascularization); overlying spots (hot spots overlying plaques of neovascularization); or remote spots (a focal spot remote from a plaque of neovascularization).

In studying these 1000 consecutive eyes, we determined the relative frequency of these various lesions to be as follows:

Focal spots	283 cases/29%
Plaques	597 cases/61%
Combination lesions	84 cases/8%
Marginal spots	35 cases/3%
Overlying spots	37 cases/4%
Remote spots	12 cases/1%

In seven additional cases (1%) a mixture of these lesions was noted. In an additional 13 eyes (1%), no hyperfluorescence was noted on the ICG angiogram. Sixteen eyes had unreadable or unobtainable ICG angiograms.

Focal Spots

Focal spots (hot spots) (Figs. 4–2, 4–3, and 4–4) are areas of clinical subretinal exudation that appear as

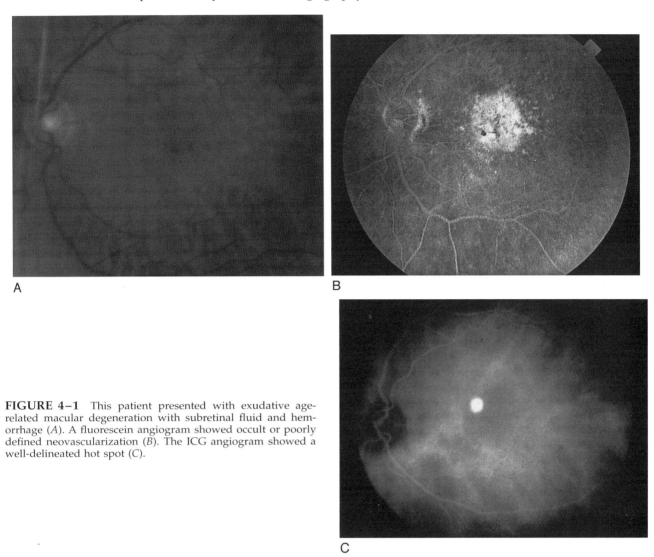

FIGURE 4–1 This patient presented with exudative age-related macular degeneration with subretinal fluid and hemorrhage (A). A fluorescein angiogram showed occult or poorly defined neovascularization (B). The ICG angiogram showed a well-delineated hot spot (C).

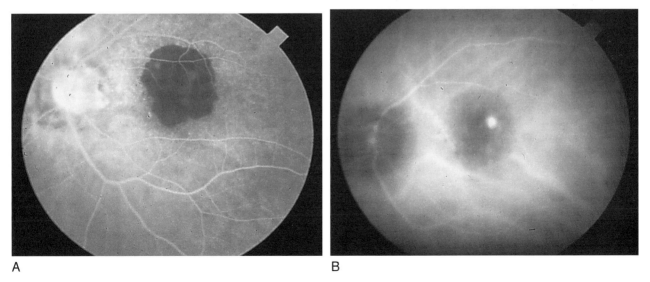

FIGURE 4–2 This patient presented with subretinal hemorrhage secondary to age-related macular degeneration (A). The ICG was able to penetrate through the blood and revealed a hot spot (B).

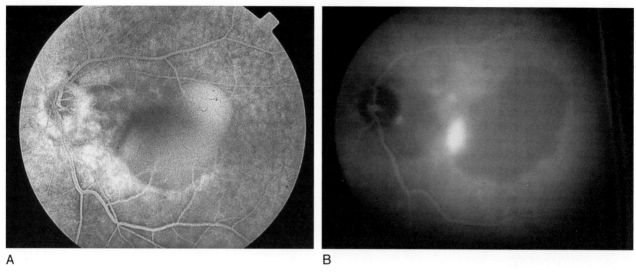

A   B

FIGURE 4–3   This patient presented with the characteristic fluorescein angiographic findings of a pigment epithelial detachment secondary to age-related macular degeneration. No definitive neovascularization was noted (*A*). The ICG angiogram, however, separated the hyperfluorescent neovascularized component of the pigment epithelial detachment from the hypofluorescent serous portion of the detachment (*B*).

occult choroidal neovascularization by fluorescein angiography. During ICG-V, a hyperfluorescent lesion less than 1 disc area in size is noted. In our study of 1000 consecutive eyes, we found focal spots in 283 (29%) of our cases. The lesion is usually noted to be outside the foveal avascular zone, and is thus potentially treatable by ICG-guided laser photocoagulation.

We have had very encouraging preliminary results in uncontrolled studies of ICG-guided laser photocoagulation of these focal spots. In one study of 79 eyes, 44 (56%) showed obliteration of the neovascularization.[23] This study had a median follow-up of 23 weeks. More recently we have looked at our 1-year data of ICG-guided laser photocoagulation. We found that 48% of eyes with occult choroidal neovascularization without a pigment epithelial detachment (PED) and 23% of eyes with occult choroidal neovascularization with a PED were successfully treated at 1-year follow-up (in preparation for publication).

Thus, although these preliminary studies are uncontrolled, our preliminary experience with ICG-guided laser photocoagulation of focal spots suggests that this modality may be a useful way to treat these patients. Further natural history as well as controlled clinical trials of ICG-guided laser photocoagulation of focal spots or hot spots are necessary to confirm these exciting preliminary studies.

Plaques

The most common pattern of neovascularization on the ICG angiogram is a plaque (Fig. 4–5). A plaque is a hyperfluorescent area greater than 1 disc area in size on the ICG angiogram. These lesions are

usually subfoveal. In our study of 1000 consecutive eyes, plaques were noted in 597 (61%) of the eyes. Plaques may be well defined or poorly defined. ICG-guided laser photocoagulation is probably not advisable for these plaques due to their size and subfoveal location. However, we do not have sufficient clinical experience yet to definitively know whether any of these lesions may benefit from laser photocoagulation.

A preliminary study of the natural history of these plaques of choroidal neovascularization suggests that there is progressive growth of these lesions at 1 year associated with decreased visual acuity and a deteriorating clinical picture. Of six eyes studied at 1 year, the plaques in all increased in size. The median initial size of the plaque was 7.1 mm^2 and the median final size of the plaque at 1 year was 15.3 mm^2. Of these six eyes, four (67%) lost 2 to 3 more lines of vision at 1 year, and the degree of exudation was noted clinically to have increased during this time as well.

We have one histopathologic correlation of a plaque of choroidal neovascularization.[24] Serial sections were obtained through the plaque, and histopathologic examination demonstrated choroidal neovascularization. This study demonstrates, at least in this case, that a plaque on the ICG angiogram appears to represent choroidal neovascularization on histopathologic examination.

Combination Lesions

The third and least common type of neovascularization on the ICG angiogram is a combination lesion (Fig. 4–6). In these cases, both a focal spot and plaque are noted. Three such subtypes exist depending upon the relationship between the focal

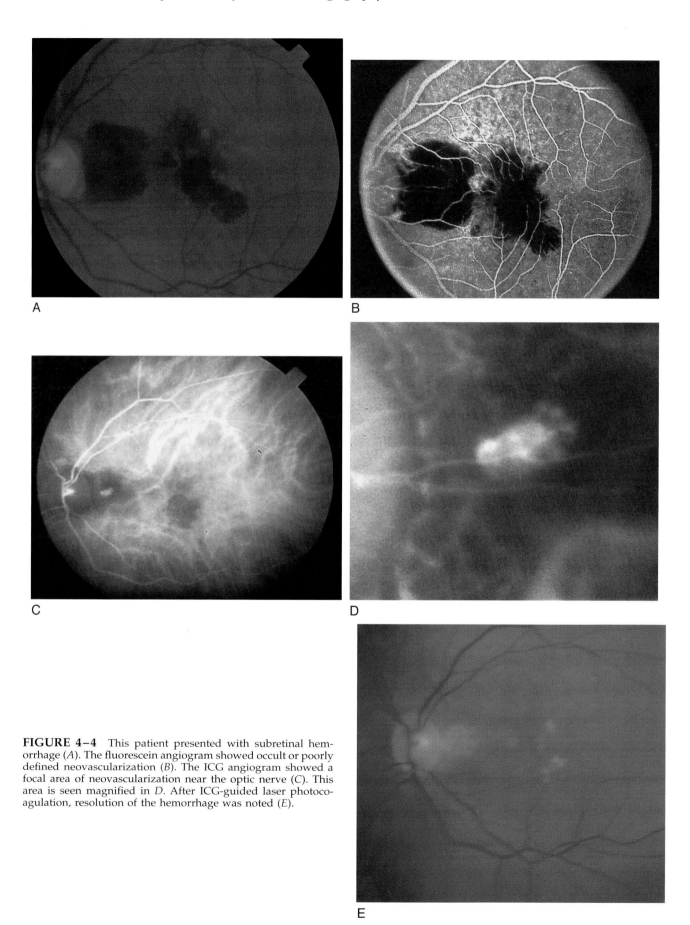

FIGURE 4-4 This patient presented with subretinal hemorrhage (*A*). The fluorescein angiogram showed occult or poorly defined neovascularization (*B*). The ICG angiogram showed a focal area of neovascularization near the optic nerve (*C*). This area is seen magnified in *D*. After ICG-guided laser photocoagulation, resolution of the hemorrhage was noted (*E*).

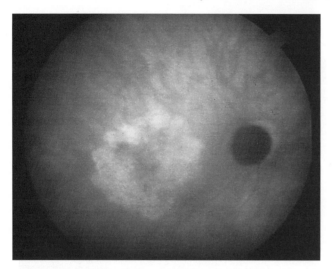

FIGURE 4–5 The most common type of choroidal neovascularization seen by ICG angiography is a plaque.

spot and plaque. A marginal spot is a focal spot at the edge or margin of a plaque of neovascularization. Such spots were noted in 35, or approximately 3%, of the eyes in our study. We have recently published a pilot study on ICG-guided laser photocoagulation to the focal spot of this marginal lesion.[25] In this technique we do not treat the plaque but only the focal spot. In our preliminary uncontrolled study of 19 eyes at 1 year, we were able to successfully obliterate 13 (68%). In 9 (69%) of 13 successfully treated eyes at 1 year, the visual acuity was stabilized or improved. A prospective randomized controlled clinical trial is warranted for this group of patients as is further study of the natural history of this lesion.

The second type of combination spot is the overlying spot in which the focal spot is on top or over-lies the plaque of neovascularization. The overlying spot always is on top of the plaque, and never is on one of its edges. Such a lesion was noted in 37, or approximately 4%, of the eyes in our study. Limited natural history information as well as treatment data exist for this group of eyes.

Finally, 12 eyes (1%) had remote spots on the ICG angiogram in which the focal spot and plaque were not contiguous with each other. Minimal information is presently known concerning this rare lesion.

In summary, digital ICG-V is an important adjunctive technique for imaging occult choroidal neovascularization secondary to exudative AMD. Fluorescein angiography is always performed first and is superior for imaging classic or well-defined choroidal neovascularization. However, in the approximately 87% of cases in which fluorescein imaging does not yield a treatable lesion, ICG angiography is helpful in better delineating the occult or poorly defined neovascularization in many cases.

From earlier studies we know that approximately 87% of patients have occult choroidal neovascularization.[21] In a more recent study, we have learned that 29% of eyes have potentially treatable focal spots or hot spots by the ICG angiogram.[22] Therefore, 87% × 29% or 25% of eyes with exudative maculopathy may potentially be treatable by ICG-guided laser treatment. We have shown an overall success rate of ICG-guided laser treatment (combining PED and non-PED cases) of approximately 36% at 1 year. These findings suggest that we can potentially successfully treat an additional 9% of patients with ICG-guided laser photocoagulation. Fluorescein imaging has a success rate of only 6.5% (13% eligible lesions divided by a recurrence rate of 50%). Therefore, it appears that ICG

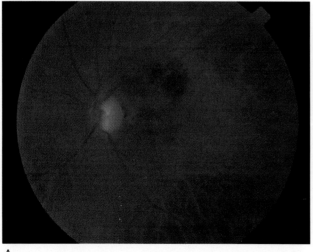

A

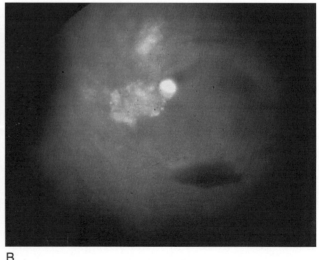

B

FIGURE 4–6 This patient presented with subretinal hemorrhage secondary to age-related macular degeneration (*A*). The ICG angiogram showed a marginal lesion, which is a type of combination lesion, where both a focal spot and plaque are present (*B*).

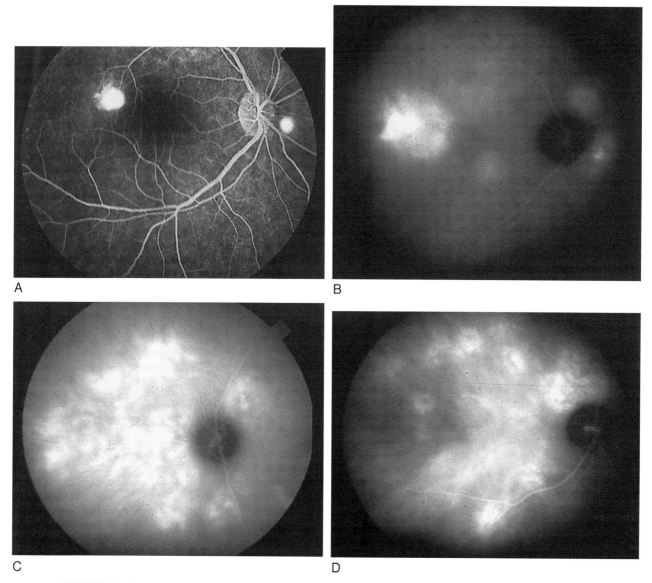

FIGURE 4–7 This patient shows the characteristic fluorescein angiographic findings of central serous chorioretinopathy (*A*). The ICG angiogram of the same patient, however, also showed two hyperfluorescent areas superior to the nerve and inferior to the optic nerve that were not seen on the corresponding fluorescein angiogram (*B*). Other patients with central serous chorioretinopathy demonstrate the characteristic multiple areas of hyperfluorescence seen in this disease (*C* and *D*).

angiography may allow us to potentially double the number of patients that we can treat with laser photocoagulation. It should be emphasized that controlled clinical trials are necessary to confirm our encouraging preliminary studies.

Other Disorders

Indocyanine-green angiography may be of important clinical use by improving imaging of occult choroidal neovascularization secondary to AMD. It has also become an important research tool in understanding the pathogenesis of other conditions such as central serous chorioretinopathy, various

chorioretinal inflammatory disorders (Fig. 4–7), and polypoidal vasculopathy. Some of these areas will be discussed in sections on ICG angiography under these individual conditions.

REFERENCES

1. Guyer DR, Yannuzzi LA, Slakter JS, et al: Digital indocyanine green videoangiography of occult choroidal neovascularization. Ophthalmology 101:1727–1737, 1994.
2. Yannuzzi LA, Slakter JS, Sorenson JA, et al: Digital indocyanine green videoangiography and choroidal neovascularization. Retina 12:191–223, 1992.
3. Flower RW: Infrared absorption angiography of the choroid and some observations on the effects of high intraocular pressures. Am J Ophthalmol 74:600–614, 1972.

4. Flower RW, Hochheimer BF: Clinical infrared absorption angiography of the choroid (Letter). Am J Ophthalmol 73: 458–459, 1972.
5. Flower RW, Hochheimer BF: A clinical technique and apparatus for simultaneous angiography of the separate retinal and choroidal circulations. Invest Ophthalmol 12: 248–261, 1973.
6. Flower RW, Hochheimer BF: Indocyanine green dye fluorescence and infrared absorption choroidal angiography performed simultaneously with fluorescein angiography. Johns Hopkins Med J 138:3–42, 1976.
7. Hyvärinen L, Flower RW: Indocyanine green fluorescent angiography. Arch Ophthalmol 58:528–538, 1980.
8. Guyer DR, Puliafito CP, Monés JM, et al: Digital indocyanine green angiography in chorioretinal disorders. Ophthalmology 99:287–290, 1992.
9. Kogure K, David NJ, Yamanouchi U, Choromokos E: Infrared absorption angiography of the fundus circulation. Arch Ophthalmol 83:209–214, 1970.
10. David NJ: Infrared absorption fundus angiography. In Proceedings of International Symposium on Fluorescein Angiography, Albi, France, 1969. Basel, Karger, 1971, pp. 189–192.
11. Hochheimer BF: Angiography of the retina with indocyanine green. Arch Ophthalmol 86:564–565, 1971.
12. Hayashi K, DeLaey JJ: Indocyanine green angiography of neovascular membranes. Ophthalmologica 190:30–39, 1985.
13. Hayashi K, Hasegawa Y, Tazawa Y, Delaey JJ: Clinical application of indocyanine angiography to choroidal neovascularization. Jpn J Clin Ophthalmol 33:57–68, 1989.
14. Hayashi K, Hasegawa Y, Tokoro T, Delaey JJ: Value of indocyanine green angiography in the diagnosis of occult choroidal neovascular membrane. Jpn J Clin Ophthalmol 42:827–829, 1988.
15. Scheider A, Schroedel C: High resolution indocyanine green angiography with scanning laser ophthalmoscope. Am J Ophthalmol 108:458–459, 1989.
16. Cherrick GR, Stein SW, Leevy CM, et al: Indocyanine green: observation on its physicial properties, plasma decay, and hepatic extraction. J Clin Invest 39:592, 1960.
17. Fox IJ, Wood EH: Applications of dilution curves recorded from the right side of the heart or venous circulation with the aid of a new indicator dye. Proc Mayo Clin 32:541, 1957.
18. Fox IJ, Wood EH: Indocyanine green: physical and physiological properties. Mayo Clin Proc 35:732, 1960.
19. Baker KJ: Binding of sulfobromophthalein (BSP) sodium and indocyanine green (ICG) by plasma α_1-lipoproteins. Proc Soc Exp Biol Med 122:957, 1966.
20. Hope-Ross M, Yannuzzi LA, Gragoudas ES, et al: Adverse reactions due to indocyanine green. Ophthalmology 101: 529, 1994.
21. Freund KB, Yannuzzi LA, Sorenson JA: Age-related macular degeneration and choroidal neovascularization. Am J Ophthalmol 115:786–791, 1993.
22. Guyer DR, Yannuzzi LA, Slakter JS, et al: Classification of occult choroidal neovascularization by ICG angiography. Ophthalmology (in press) 1996.
23. Slakter JS, Yannuzzi LA, Sorenson JA, et al: A pilot study of indocyanine green videoangiography-guided laser treatment of occult-choroidal neovascularization in age-related macular degeneration. Arch Ophthalmol 112:465–472, 1994.
24. Chang TS, Freund KB, Delacruz Z, et al: Clinico-pathological correlation of choroidal neovascularization demonstrated by indocyanine green angiography in a patient with retention of good vision for almost four years. Retina 14:114–124, 1994.
25. Guyer DR, Yannuzzi LA, Ladas I, et al: Indocyanine green-guided laser photocoagulation of focal spots at the edge of plaques of choroidal neovascularization. Arch Ophthalmol 114:693–697, 1996.

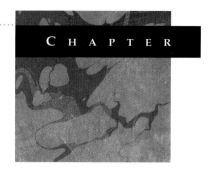

Ophthalmic Contact B-Scan Ultrasonography

Andrew A. Chang, M.B.B.S.

Antonio P. Ciardella, M.D.

Yale L. Fisher, M.D.

Contact B-scan ultrasound offers the clinician a safe, noninvasive, dynamic tool with instant feedback for the evaluation of vitreoretinal disorders. Ultrasound examination is indicated when opacification of the ocular media precludes adequate clinical examination of the posterior segment. This may be due to corneal opacification, anterior chamber hyphema or hypopyon, small pupil, cataract, vitreous hemorrhage, or inflammation. In the presence of clear media, it is useful for evaluation of the state and position of the vitreous.

Ultrasound provides the clinician with a readily accessible means for diagnosing tumors, retinal detachments, hemorrhage, and intraocular foreign bodies. This chapter will cover the background of B-scan ultrasound, the basic physics of ultrasound, techniques of contact B-scan ultrasound, and clinical situations encountered in performing ultrasonography.

HISTORY OF ULTRASOUND

Historically, ultrasound began with the discovery of piezoelectricity in the 1880s. Quartz crystals were noted to emit electrical potentials when mechanically stimulated and conversely vibrate when exposed to electricity. During World War II, pulse echo-ultrasound principles were utilized in sonar detection devices.

Application of ultrasound for ocular diagnosis first occurred in 1956, when Mundt and Hughes reported using A-scan ultrasound technique to detect intraocular tumors.[1] During the 1950s, Oksala[2-4]

applied A-scan ultrasound to detect tumors, retinal detachments, vitreous hemorrhages, and intraocular foreign bodies.

Baum and Greenwood[5] were the first to introduce B-scan ultrasound to ophthalmology. A water bath was used as a coupling device between the ultrasound transducer and the globe. Immersion techniques were subsequently developed by Purnell,[6] Ossoinig,[7] and Coleman et al.[8-10]

In 1972, Bronson introduced the first handheld unit, which was applied directly to the closed eyelid without a water bath.[11] Following this, B-scan ultrasonography became more appealing and practical, allowing the widespread clinical use of ultrasound.

Clinical applications for ultrasound have developed in many ophthalmic subspecialties including vitreoretinal, cataract, and orbital surgery.

PRINCIPLES AND TECHNICAL ASPECTS OF ULTRASOUND

Ultrasound is sound of high frequency, beyond that of human audition. In ophthalmology the frequencies used range from 7.5 to 15 MHz for most posterior globe and orbit evaluations. Recent developments with higher frequencies in the 40- to 60-MHz range have permitted high-resolution anterior segment examination.

Ultrasound is generated and returning echoes are detected by a single ultrasound transducer unit. The active element in the transducer is a piezoelectric material that emits a certain sound frequency when stimulated by an alternating electrical potential. The crystal is also capable of receiving echoes and converting them to electrical potentials that are processed for display on a oscilloscope screen. Electronic switching changes the transducer mode from "transmit" to "receive" in microseconds.

In clinical practice, high-frequency sound waves are projected into soft tissues by contact of the ultrasonic transducer to the skin of the lids or directly on the globe. Echoes occur at tissue interfaces with different acoustic interfaces with differences in acoustic impedances. The larger the difference, the stronger the echo. As the ultrasound waves advance they are attenuated by the distance from the probe head, differential absorption by different tissues within the eye, producing acoustic interfaces which reflect, refract, or scatter sound waves. The reflected waves are returned to the probe as echoes.

Once detected, the echoes are sent to a processor to be modified and amplified for display and interpretation.

The two most useful display modes are:

1. **A-scan** (time-amplitude). In this mode the echoes appear as amplitude spikes on a horizontal time axis. Common uses for this mode include tissue interpretation and intraocular lens calculation.
2. **B-scan** (intensity modulated). In this mode, a cross-section display is created from a family of A-scan to produce spots of light on the display screen. The brightness of the spots is a function of this echo amplitude.

Recording of the Information

There are a variety of means of recording the generated image. Videotape recording represents the superior method because ultrasound is a dynamic study. However, this is limited by expense and convenience. Polaroid photographs taken by a camera mounted to the unit with a hinged mechanism represents the most common method. Other methods of recording the image are 35-mm photographs or thermal prints.

A-SCAN ULTRASOUND

The A-scan mode is ideal for tissue interpretation. Some instruments that utilize A-scan are quantified in that comparisons are made between heights (amplitudes) of echoes to known normal structures such as sclera, retina, and orbital fat. Strong reflections from retina and sclera demonstrate high echo amplitudes (the vertical deflection from the horizontal baseline is high), whereas weaker reflectors from vitreous hemorrhage demonstrate lower vertical deflections. In most current instruments, A-scan imagery is displayed at the bottom of the ul-

trasound screen with a simultaneous B-scan image. A moveable tracer line (vector) on the B-scan image helps orient the examiner to the exact place in the B-scan image that is being depicted in the A-scan below.

Narrow beam A-scan measurements provide the most accurate means of measuring tissue thickness (biometry). The accuracy of resolution increases with the frequency used, but penetration decreases, limiting the range of useful frequencies. The most common transducer used is 10 MHz with resolution of about 0.1 mm. Precise alignment is required for accurate biometry.

CONTACT B-SCAN ULTRASOUND

In B-scan ultrasound, a rapidly moving ultrasonic transducer within a sealed water-filled case is held gently against the closed eyelids of a patient. An array of individual sound waves is sent into the eye as the transducer rocks back and forth through approximately 40 degrees of arc. A 10-MHz ultrasonic signal (10 million cycles/sec) is directed into the globe. Methylcellulose is used as a sound-coupling agent between the transducer head and the patient's skin. As sound passes through the tissues, echoes from the sweeping beam of sound occurs at each tissue interface with a different acoustic impedance. The echoes return and are detected by the probe transducer, changed into electric signals, amplified, and visualized as small dots on the display screen. Time is displayed along the horizontal axis of the display with the separate echo dots spreading out in a linear fashion depending on the time of detection. Echoes from the nearest reflections are seen to the left of the display, while those to the right are the farthest reflections. The display is also correlated to the transducer probe casing. A manufacturer's mark (usually a dot or line) corresponds to the top of the display screen; that is, the beginning of the B-scan cross-sectional image.

There are several concepts that are essential to the understanding of contact B-scan ultrasonography.[12,13] These concepts are real time, gray scale, and three-dimensional thinking.

Real Time

This refers to the quality of motion seen during B-scan imaging. Primary and secondary aftermovements of vitreous and retinal detachments are detectable. The quality of movement of intraocular tissues can be used to help differentiate one structure from another. For example, the rapid movements of vitreous hemorrhage differ greatly from the usual slower and undulating motion of a rhegmatogenous retinal detachment.

Gray Scale

The term "gray scale" refers to interpretation of echo amplitudes. In B-scan ultrasound, the brightness of the echo is represented in gray scale. Echoes with a higher amplitude (strong reflectors) appear as whiter images and those with lower amplitude (weaker reflectors) appear less bright. The gain setting (sensitivity), measured in decibels (dB), is constantly altered to allow interpretation of the echo strength. The object studied must be perpendicular to the examining beam so that the strongest possible echoes will be recovered by the B-scan transducer.

Building a Three-Dimensional Picture

Interpretation of the B-scan involves creating a composite image of the globe from two-dimensional B-scan cross sections. During the ultrasound examination, the transducer probe is constantly moved by the examiner, permitting multiple two-dimensional cross sections to be mentally reconstructed into a three-dimensional image.

The horizontal dimension on the screen is related to time and therefore distance. The echoes on the left-hand side of the screen are closest to the probe head. The echoes farthest from the probe appear towards the right side. The marker on the probe tip corresponds to the superior portion of the screen. Therefore, when the orientation of the probe is held vertically, the top of the screen represents the superior portion of the globe. When the probe is held horizontally with the marker towards the nose (by convention), the top of the screen represents the nasal part of the globe. The temporal part of the globe is seen along the bottom of the screen. Recognition

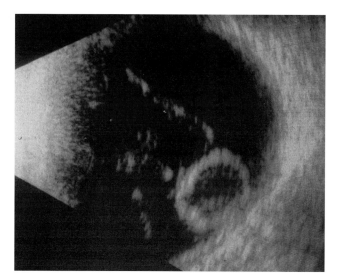

FIGURE 5–1 Crystalline lens posteriorly dislocated into the vitreous in a patient with Marfan's syndrome. The lens appears as a circular lesion in the inferior vitreous cavity.

of these spatial arrangements is critical to interpretation of abnormal intraocular structures.

In practice, the A- and B-scan modes are complementary, with the B-scan providing topographic information and the A-scan providing tissue interpretation. The B-scan image of the internal structure of intraocular tumors is cross-correlated with A-scan amplitudes. A combination of both topographic and tissue interpretation information is used to make ultrasound diagnoses.

Both A- and B-scan can be performed using a water immersion bath or more commonly a contact method. Immersion techniques are useful in scanning the anterior segment of the globe.

CLINICAL OCULAR CONTACT B-SCAN ULTRASONOGRAPHY

Lens

Ultrasound may be helpful in situations where anterior chamber media is opaque or semiopaque. With contact techniques, only the posterior lens capsule is usually visible. However, as the lens becomes cataractous more of it becomes visible and multiple intralenticular echoes can be seen. When completely liquified, the lens appears ultrasonographically homogenous and essentially echo-free, similiar to a water-filled cystic structure.

When the lens becomes dislocated into the vitreous, the lens may be detected by its biconvex shape and echogenicity. Figure 5–1 shows a posteriorly dislocated lens in a patient with ectopia lentis and Marfan's syndrome.

Vitreous Opacities

Vitreous opacification represents one of the most common indications for performing ultrasound. Vitreous hemorrhage and inflammatory debris are indistinguishable on ultrasound. Normal vitreous is almost ultrasonongraphically clear. Unclotted vitreous hemorrhage with no cellular clumps may not be ultrasonically visible. However, once cellular aggregates occur, ultrasound echoes are visible. With gray scale, the strongest reflectors are from the sonically densest opacities, which appear white, while the weaker echoes are of varying shades of gray. This allows some evaluation of the severity of the vitreous opacification.

Posterior vitreous hemorrhage may accumulate on the posterior surface of a separated posterior vitreous face and produces a sheet-like echo that may simulate a retinal detachment. Differentiation of these two conditions is possible on the basis of sonic reflectivity and architecture. The posterior vitreous hyaloid has a relatively weak reflection when compared to that of retina, usually disappearing when the sensitivity of the ultrasound gain is reduced below 70 dB. Clumped blood cells adherent to the hyaloid will increase echo strength but often not significantly. Attachment of a sheet-like interface to the optic nerve head suggests a retinal detachment rather the posterior vitreous hyaloid. However, when the posterior vitreous hyaloid is incompletely detached, further confusion with a retinal detachment may occur. "Kinetic scanning" in these situations with real time evaluation of movement is extremely helpful. The patient is asked to voluntarily move the eyes while the ultrasound scan is observed. Vitreous hyaloid usually demonstrates a jerking stacatic movement, while retinal tissue moves more smoothly, with an undulating pattern. Aftermovements are also helpful in assessing vitreoretinal ultrasonic abnormalities.

Ultrasound aids in estimating the prognosis. For example, the degree of intravitreal hemorrhage can often be correlated to the time required for spontaneous resolution. Repeat ultrasound examination can be used to trace absorption or new hemorrhage. Severe hemorrhage involving formed vitreous often means that the time required for spontaneous clearing will be longer.

Asteroid hyalosis may be confused with vitreous hemorrhage on ultrasound. Vitreous hemorrhage will disappear as the gain is reduced while reflectivity from the intravitreal calcium salt deposits do not. The reflective particles can be visualized as bright stars hanging in the vitreous (Fig. 5–2). Using real time evaluation, the particles move in a flowing motion with after motion.

Posterior Vitreoretinal Interface

Ultrasound allows the reliable evaluation of the posterior vitreoretinal interface that is important in the natural history and preoperative evaluation of a number of disorders.[14] In vitreomacular traction

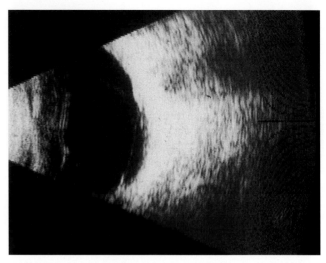

FIGURE 5–3 Vitreomacular traction syndrome. There is persisting vitreous attachment to the macula.

syndrome, the incomplete vitreous detachment with persisting attachment to the macula may be visualized (Fig. 5–3).

In the evaluation of macular holes, ultrasound allows determination that the fellow eye with separation of the posterior hyaloid membrane in the foveal region is usually protected from further macular hole development.[15] Figure 5–4 shows the small elevation of the retina at the site of an impending macular hole.

Retinal Tears

With careful ultrasound examination, even small retinal tears can be detected using ultrasound. The attached vitreous can be seen to insert onto the flap of a horseshoe tear (Fig. 5–5). Dynamic vitreoretinal interface examination is possible using scleral depression at the time of ultrasonic evaluation.

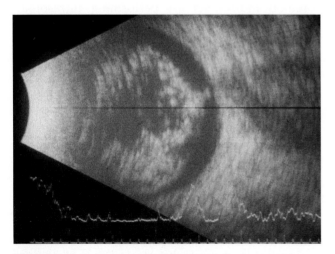

FIGURE 5–2 Asteroid hyalosis. The reflective particles are clearly visible. The clear vitreous gel between the retina and the asteroid opacities may simulate a detachment of the posterior hyaloid of the vitreous.

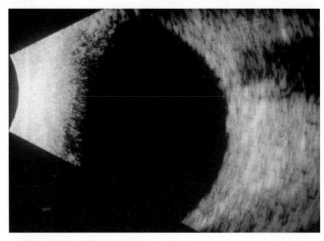

FIGURE 5–4 Impending macula hole. Note the small "nub" that represents the site of vitreoretinal traction to the macula.

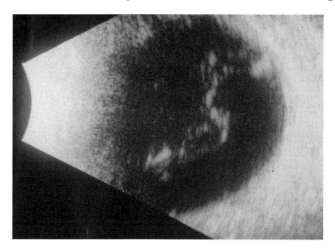

FIGURE 5–5   Retinal horseshoe tear. Note the strand of vitreous attached to the apex of the flap of a retinal horseshoe tear.

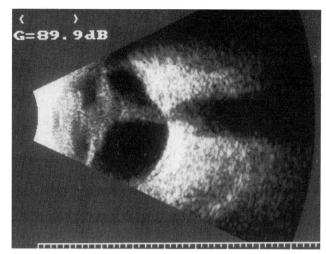

FIGURE 5–7   Funnel retinal detachment on axial scanning. Note the detachment extending to the optic nerve head.

Retinal Detachment

Detached retina appears as a highly reflective membrane within the vitreous cavity (Fig. 5–6). In retina detachment the echo persists as the sensitivity is reduced below 70 dB. To maximize the strength of the signal, the probe must be held perpendicular to the detached retinal tissue.

Attachment to the optic nerve suggests retinal detachment. Real time evaluation of retinal detachment has less aftermovement when compared with posterior vitreous detachment. The appearance varies with the duration of the detachment. Fresh bullous detachments may be highly mobile. Long-standing detachments may become stiff with development of proliferative vitreoretinopathy. Ultrasound allows the configuration of the detachment to be determined. It may be shallow or bullous. The funnel of the retinal separation may be open or closed.

Ultrasound examination of a funnel retinal de-

tachment may have dramatically different appearance depending on the direction of ultrasound scanning. Figure 5–7 demonstrates a funnel retinal detachment on axial scanning. The same eye on scanning transversely (Fig. 5–8) reveals a circular lesion in the vitreous corresponding to the stalk of the funnel detachment.

Retinoschisis can be mistaken for partial retinal detachments, which are indistinguishable on the basis of echo strength. They appear as smooth and dome-shaped and do not insert onto the disc. Retinoschisis is often bilateral and more commonly located inferotemporally. In addition, retinoschisis does not usually move during real time testing.

Traction Retinal Detachment

Assessment of diabetic fibroproliferative disease is one of the most challenging aspects of clinical ul-

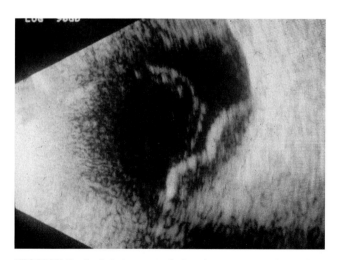

FIGURE 5–6   Inferior retinal detachment. Note the higher sound signal of the retinal detachment when compared to the posterior vitreous face.

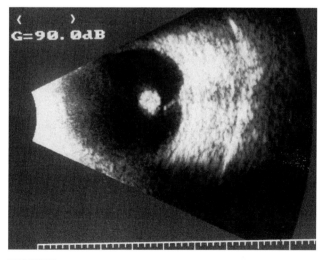

FIGURE 5–8   Funnel retinal detachment on transverse scanning. The stalk of the detachment appears as a circular echodense lesion within the vitreous cavity.

trasonography. Often a combination of tractional and/or rhegmatogenous retinal detachment exists along with hemorrhage and fibrovascular bands, making interpretation difficult (Fig. 5–9). With experience, however, accurate ultrasound-derived drawings of the diabetic globe are possible. To gain experience, ultrasonic examination of patients with clear media is suggested, permitting correlation of the ultrasound drawing with the ophthalmoscopic appearance.

Choroidal detachments may be a result of hemorrhage or effusion. On B-scan, these present as smooth convex elevations. Figure 5–10 shows the ultrasound of a patient with large, almost touching choroidal hemorrhage. The choroidal detachment is thicker than retina and inserts anteriorly near the lens and posteriorly near the equator of the globe. In choroidal hemorrhage, ultrasound is often effective in determining liquefaction of blood clot, aiding surgical timing decisions for drainage.

Tumors

The ultrasound evaluation of intraocular tumors involves topographic localization of solid-mass echoes and interpretation of internal acoustic gray scale characteristics.

While ultrasound is able to detect tumors as small as 0.4 mm in height, only those larger than 1.5 mm can be evaluated for ultrasonic tissue characteristics. Songraphy is particularly useful when there is no view of the fundus due to to media opacities such as lens changes or vitreous hemorrhage. Ultrasound is also able to define neoplasms under a serous retinal detachment. With experience, topographic and height measurements are reproducible and accurate.[16]

In practice, however, it is often difficult to make

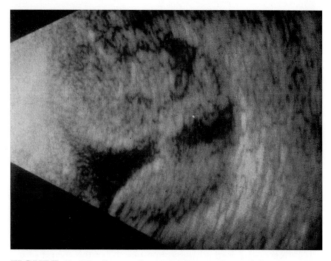

FIGURE 5–10   Large choroidal hemorrhage following cataract extraction. The choroidal elevations are almost touching each other.

tissue diagnosis based on the ultrasound characteristics alone. Tissue characteristics are more difficult to interpret, as they are based upon interpretation of accoustic impedence mismatch of cellular elements that can differ from lesion to lesion and even within the same tumor mass. General characteristics are discernible.

Choroidal malignant melanoma has a fairly reproducible pattern (Fig. 5–11). The high initial spike of the A-scan is due to the vitreoretinal interface from retinal tissue over the tumor. The surface has a smooth convex anterior surface. A collar stud appearance may result from tumor rupture through Bruch's membrane (Fig. 5–12). Other acoustic characteristics include the low internal acoustic reflectivity, which correlates with the cellular tumor pattern of small, tightly packed homogenous cells. However, small lesions (<1.5 mm) may appear highly reflective. Tumor-infiltrated choroid pro-

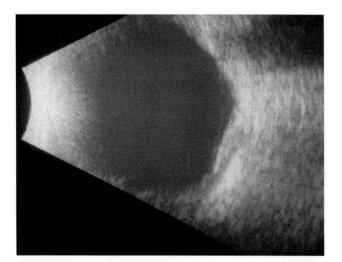

FIGURE 5–9   Diabetic tractional detachment and fibrovascular membrane.

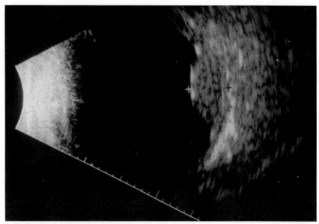

FIGURE 5–11   Choroidal melanoma. Note the high ultrasound signal at the surface of the lesion and the low internal acoustic reflectivity within the tumor.

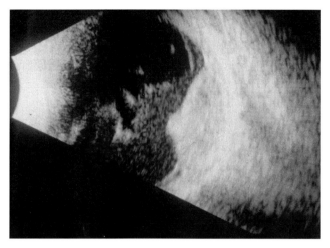

FIGURE 5–12 Rupture of choroidal melanoma through Bruch's membrane. Note the collar-stud appearance.

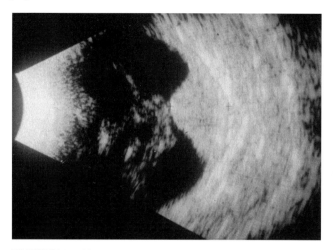

FIGURE 5–13 Metastatic carcinoid tumor with overlying vitreous hemorrhage. The small elevation on the surface of the lesion represents a transvitreal biopsy site.

duces an apparent disappearance of the normal choroidal pattern. This "missing" choroid has been called "choroidal excavation," which is a misnomer, as the choroid is infiltrated not excavated. Orbital shadowing refers to loss in intensity of the orbital fat pattern secondary to signal attenuation within the tumor. Other ocular findings seen may include vitreous hemorrhage and serous retinal detachment.

Metastatic tumors involve the choroid in the posterior pole and may be bilateral and multiple. They characteristically are broad-based and solid with internal echoes that are moderate in intensity. Figure 5–13 shows an example of metastatic carcinoid tumor. Metastatic tumors may have an associated serous retinal detachment.

Choroidal hemangiomas have significant acoustic heterogeneity due to the vascular channels and vessels within these masses. They have a broader base and shallow elevation. Internal echoes are strong and the tumors appear solid ultrasonically.

Ocular calcification produces high-amplitude A-scan patterns and intense B-scan images. Shadowing of the sclera and orbital fat occurs behind areas of calcification. Calcification may be due to dystrophic deposition as well as tumors such as choroidal osteoma and retinoblastoma.

Trauma

Ultrasound provides an accurate means of assessing eyes after penetrating eye trauma, provided great care is used to prevent globe compression or contamination. Ultrasound can be used to detect intraocular foreign bodies and is most useful to detect secondary damage such as retinal detachment, vitreous and choroidal hemorrhage, and posterior scleral wounds in the presence of media opacity.[17,18]

Intraocular Foreign Body

Ultrasound is helpful in the management of intraocular foreign bodies. The presence of hemorrhage, cataract, or inflammation may obscure visualization of the foreign body. A high index of suspicion is required and often the history may be misleading. Ultrasound is complementary to other investigations such as x-ray and computed tomography (CT) scanning. Associated ocular injuries such as retinal detachment can be determined. The location of the foreign body and its relation to the wall of the eye using ultrasound is of great value in planning the surgical approach.

Intraocular foreign bodies are readily seen when they are lying free in the vitreous. Because of their different acoustic properties they are strong reflectors of sound and often give trailing shadows. The location of an intraocular foreign body is only relative to ocular structures. Precise assessment of size is not possible, although some estimation of the size can be made. When the intraocular foreign body is situated close to the wall of the eye, it is much more difficult to locate. If the intraocular foreign body is small and linear, then it may be missed if the beam is not directed perpendicular to it. Therefore, examination of the intraocular foreign body should take place from different angles and with alteration of the sensitivity of the scan. Figure 5–14 shows an intraocular foreign body located anteriorly on the pars plana region.

Metallic, glass, stone, and plastic intraocular foreign bodies may all be visible on ultrasound. Metallic foreign bodies demonstrate the phenomenon of "ringing" due to reverberation of sound. This is an artifact caused by multiple reflections of sound. Shadowing is usually seen behind the intraocular foreign body.

A number of structures in the eye may mimic an intraocular foreign body. Optic nerve head drusen and choroidal calcification may produce strong ech-

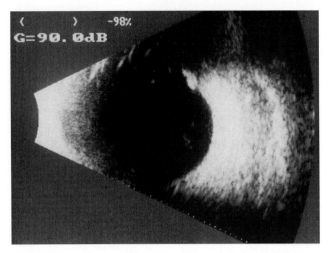

FIGURE 5–14 Intraocular foreign body. The metallic foreign body is seen to be located anteriorly in the pars plana region.

ogenic signals, suggesting an intraocular foreign body. Small bubbles of air that entered the globe at the time of the injury may simulate a foreign body.

Globe Shape

Ultrasound is particularly useful in evaluating the shape of the globe. Staphylomas in myopes are clearly visible as in Figure 5–15. Knowledge of the size and shape of the globe is important in avoiding complications of globe perforation by needles when administering parabulbar injections.

In phthisis bulbi, the hypotonous globe is smaller and has a squarer appearance due to distortion of the soft globe exerted by the extraocular muscles.

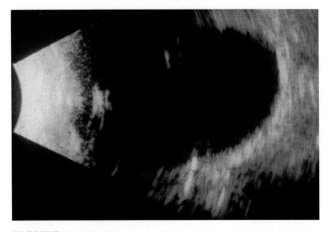

FIGURE 5–15 Myopic staphyloma. Note the posterior bowing of the globe wall corresponding to the staphyloma.

SUMMARY

Contact B-scan ultrasound provides the clinician with a convenient noninvasive means of evaluating intraocular structures in situations where clinical examination is not possible due to opaque ocular media. The vitreoretinal relationships can be evaluated using dynamic examination. Ultrasound examination should be used in conjunction with detailed clinical examination and other investigational modalities such as x-ray and CT scanning in the diagnosis of intraocular mass lesions and intraocular foreign bodies.

REFERENCES

1. Mundt GH, Hughes WF: Ultrasonics in ocular diagnosis. Am J Ophthalmol 41:488–498, 1956.
2. Oksala A, Lehtinen A: Diagnostic value of ultrasonics in ophthalmology. Ophthalmologica 134:387–395, 1957.
3. Oksala A: The clinical value of time-amplitude ultrasonography. Am J Ophthalmol 57:453–460, 1964.
4. Oksala A, Lehtinen A: Diagnostics of detachment of the retina by means of ultrasound. Acta Ophthalmol 35:461–467, 1957.
5. Baum G, Greenwood I: The application of ultrasonic locating techniques to ophthalmology. Part 2. Ultrasonic visualization of soft tissues. Arch Ophthalmol 60:263–279, 1958.
6. Purnell EW: Intensity modulated (B scan) ultrasonography. In Goldberg RE, Sarin LK (eds): Ultrasonics in Ophthalmology: Diagnostic and Therapeutic Applications, Philadelphia, WB Saunders Co, 1967.
7. Ossoinig KC: Clinical echo-ophthalmology. In Blodi FC (ed): Current Concepts in Ophthalmology, Vol 3. St Louis, CV Mosby, 1972, pp 101–130.
8. Coleman DJ: Reliability of ocular and orbital diagnosis with B scan ultrasound. 1. Ocular diagnosis. Am J Ophthalmol 73:501–516, 1972.
9. Coleman DJ, Koenig WF, Katz L: A hand-operated ultrasound scan system for ophthalmic evaluation. Am J Ophthalmol 68:256–263, 1969.
10. Coleman DJ, Lizzi FL, Jack RL: Ultrasonography of the Eye and Orbit. Philadelphia, Lea & Febiger, 1977.
11. Bronson NR: Quantitative ultrasonography. Arch Ophthalmol 81:400–472, 1969.
12. Bronson NR, Fisher YL, Pickering NC, Traynor EH: Ophthalmic Contact B-scan Ultrasonography for the Clinician. Baltimore, Williams & Wilkins, 1980.
13. Fisher YL: Contact B scan ultrasonography: a practical approach. Int Ophthalmol Clin 19:103–125, 1979.
14. Fisher YL, Slakter JS, Friedman RA, Yannuzzi LA: Kinetic ultrasound evaluation of the posterior vitreoretinal interface. Ophthalmology 98:1135–1138, 1991.
15. Fisher YL, Slakter JS, Yannuzzi LA, Guyer DR: A prospective natural history study and kinetic ultrasound evaluation of idiopathic macular holes. Ophthalmology 101:5–11, 1994.
16. Char DH, Stone RD, Irvine AR, et al: Diagnostic modalities in choroidal melanoma. Am J Ophthalmol 89:223–230, 1980.
17. Rubsamen PE, Cousins SW, Winward KE, Byrne SF: Diagnostic ultrasound and pars plana vitrectomy in penetrating eye trauma. Ophthalmology 101:809–814, 1994.
18. Restori M, McLeod D: Ultrasonic examination of the traumatized eye. Trans Ophthalmol Soc UK 98:38–42, 1978.

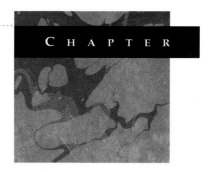

CHAPTER

6

Three-Dimensional Ophthalmic Ultrasonography of the Posterior Segment

Yale L. Fisher, M.D.

Antonio P. Ciardella, M.D.

Jason S. Slakter, M.D.

Andrew A. Chang, M.B.B.S.

Prut Hanutsaha, M.D.

Aaron Fenster, Ph.D.

Interest in three-dimensional ultrasound (3D US) imaging has increased since the development of modern computers.[1-6]

Any ophthalmologist knows the importance and the difficulty in ophthalmic ultrasonography of mentally reconstructing bidimensional B-scan images of the eye in a three-dimensional model. Although the ability and expertise of the examiner are usually sufficient to obtain correct image interpretation, accurate volume measurement of intraocular structures is not easily calculated, particularly important when overall volume is desired for such pathologic entities as intraocular tumors or myopic staphylomas. For this reason we have recently introduced a new three-dimensional contact B-scan ultrasound system for clinical practice that is capable of evaluation and volume measurement.

Our system consists of a conventional B-mode ultrasound system (i-Scan, Ophthalmic Technologies Inc., Downsview, Canada) adapted and coupled to a microcomputer (MAC 7500/100, Apple Computer, Cupertino, CA) (Fig. 6–1). A motorized, handheld transducer rotation assembly completes the hardware package (Fig. 6–2). A software package permits three-dimensional acquisition and display (3D i-Scan, Ophthalmic Technologies Inc., Downsview, London, Ontario, Canada).[7,8]

To obtain the sharp-bordered images necessary for reproducible measurements, ultrasound gain is adjusted to 70 decibels (dB). The contact ophthalmic ultrasound transducer is inserted into the motorized rotation assembly and held gently against the patient's lid in a standard ultrasound examination fashion. Methylcellulose solution (1%) is used as a sound coupling agent on the transducer tip. Once the area of interest is displayed centrally on the ultrasound screen, the examiner activates the computer acquisition mode, causing the ultrasound transducer to rotate axially through 200 degrees in 8 seconds. During acquisition, 200 conventional B-mode two-dimensional images are collected and stored by the microcomputer using a video-based digitizer. For best acquisition results, the transducer/handheld assembly must be held motionless by the examiner, and the patient's globe must not move. A fixation light may be used to help the patient to maintain a steady fixation. The area of the globe and/or orbit displayed depends upon the operator's choice of ultrasound probe position as well as the mechanical sector scan of the ultrasound device. The i-Scan transducer scanning angle is 50 degrees. At 25 mm from the transducer, the area scanned during ultrasound probe axial rotation is 3.75 cm^2.

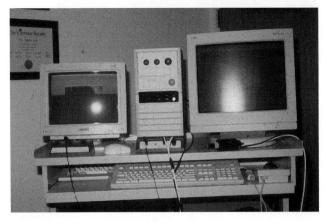

FIGURE 6–1 Three-dimensional contact B-scan ultrasound system. A conventional B-mode device is coupled to a microcomputer.

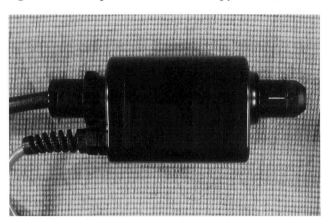

FIGURE 6–2 Conventional B-scan ultrasound probe is inserted into a motorized, handheld transducer rotation assembly.

The sequence of 200 stored images is reconstructed into a single three-dimensional image using an algorithm that generates the correct Cartesian geometry by placing each acquired image into its proper location in three dimensions. The reconstruction process requires 120 seconds.

One reconstructed, the 3D image can be viewed and manipulated interactively using a "multislicing texture mapping" technique that displays the three-dimensional image as a multisided object (cube) (Fig. 6–3), with the appropriate anatomy "painted" on each side. The display program allows viewing of the 3D image in coronal, horizontal, sagittal, and oblique planes. Any of the planes can be activated and moved by manipulating a computer mouse (Fig. 6–4).

The operating program of the computer requires 2.5 megabytes (MB). Acquired data can be stored prior to (17.2 MB required) or following three-dimensional reconstruction (23.1 MB required). Hard and optical disc data storage are possible.

MEASUREMENT TECHNIQUES

Linear Measurement Technique

Linear measurements of reconstructed images are made with a special software display entitled "image brightness profile." Utilizing the computer mouse, the examiner places two mobile icon markers on any "cut" face of the three-dimensional image. The computer draws a line between these markers and plots the image brightness as a function of distance, which is displayed as a line graph beneath the three-dimensional image (Fig. 6–5). By

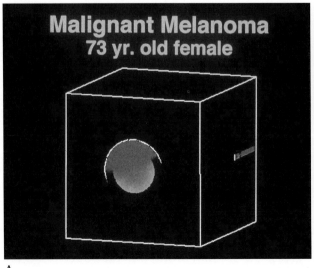

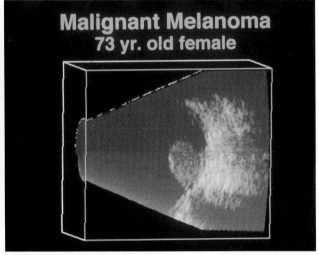

A

B

FIGURE 6–3 The 3D display presented as a cube (*A*). 3D images "painted" on the sides of the cube (*B*).

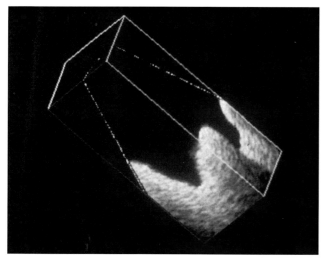

FIGURE 6–4   Rotation of the 3D image permits us to study the intraocular tumor with a completely new perspective.

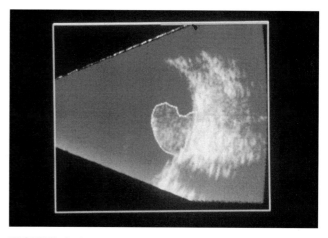

FIGURE 6–6   The operator moves a cursor to outline the border of a lesion. Area measurement is calculated by the computer. Total volume of the lesion is estimated by measurements of sequential parallel 0.5-mm slices.

moving calibrating bar markers on this linear brightness graph, the examiner measures the distance between these markers. Although the linear graph is reminiscent of A-scan, there is no cross correlation.

Area Measurement Technique

Area calculations are performed using the trace/area calculation software. The borders of the markers are outlined on the display screen. The computer automatically determines the traced area for each marker (Fig. 6–6).

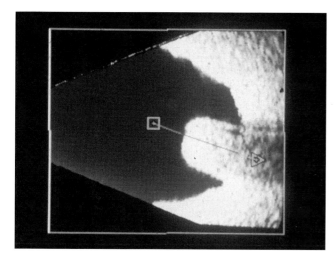

FIGURE 6–5   Rectangular and triangular icons are positioned for linear measurement. An image brightness profile graph connects the icons. Fine linear measurement is performed by moving the vertical bars on the line graph to superimpose the lesion borders (phantom eye).

Volume Measurement Technique

Volumetric measurements are performed utilizing the tracing/area calculation software. The examiner outlines the tumor in sequential parallel planes at predefined distances (0.5 mm in this case). Volume measurements are obtained by automatic computer summation of these outlines.

IN VITRO TESTING

We have performed linear, area, and volume measurements using phantom devices to test the accuracy and reproducibility of the ultrasound system.

Volume measurements of intraocular tumors were performed with a specially designed, solid, ocular-shaped phantom (Imaging Research Laboratories, Ontario). The model consisted of a five-sided plexiglass cube filled with solid agar material shaped to simulate the posterior portion of the globe. A "tumor" constructed of the same solid agar was simulated at the center of the posterior pole of the model. The phantom was filled with water and covered anteriorly by a thin membrane. Actual volume of the "tumor" by water-displaced technique was 270 mm^3. A similarly constructed phantom eye, but with a posterior staphyloma, was also used. Two examiners performed ten scans of each phantom, and linear, area, and volume measurements were calculated for each scan. Then, a single scan was measured ten times by the two examiners. A high degree of accuracy and reproducibility was found.

CLINICAL EXPERIENCE

Ten patients with choroidal melanomas and ten pathologic myopic eyes have been examined with

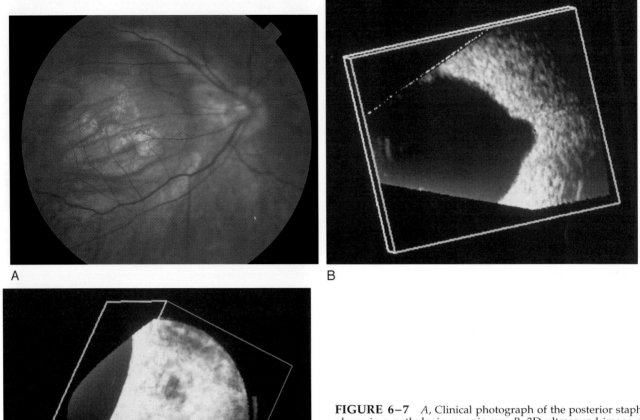

A

B

C

FIGURE 6–7   *A*, Clinical photograph of the posterior staphyloma in a pathologic myopic eye. *B*, 3D ultrasound image of a sagittal view of the posterior staphyloma. *C*, Further rotation of the image permits examination of the globe from a posterior approach. With this view we can determine the relationship of the staphyloma (inferior) to the optic nerve (superior).

3D US. Linear, area, and volume measurements have proven to be both accurate and reproducible.

Tumor volume is one of the most important considerations for clinical prognosis and treatment.[9–11] Direct volume measurements derived from 3D US, rather than conventional volume estimations, may prove useful in all clinical management phases of tumor patients. Pathologic myopia remains one of the leading causes of blindness worldwide. In spite of the fact that over 2% of the population in the Western world are estimated to suffer from this condition, little is known about its pathogenesis and virtually nothing is known about its treatment. The exact role that the posterior staphyloma itself plays has not yet been explored. It is our hypothesis that the nature of the posterior staphyloma (i.e., its location, size, morphology, and volume) may be implicated in the overall visual prognosis. These

structural features of the staphyloma can be best studied utilizing this three-dimensional ultrasound system (Figs. 6–7 and 6–8).

LIMITATIONS AND ARTIFACTS

Since this 3D system is based upon contact two-dimensional B-scan images, limitations and artifacts are in part similar to conventional contact B-scan ultrasonography. In addition, maintaining perpendicularity to the area of interest is slightly more difficult, especially for more anterior examinations, due to the increased size of the handheld rotation assembly. Image movement artifacts (Fig. 6–9) induced by the examiner or patient during the acquisition mode (8 seconds) create initial difficul-

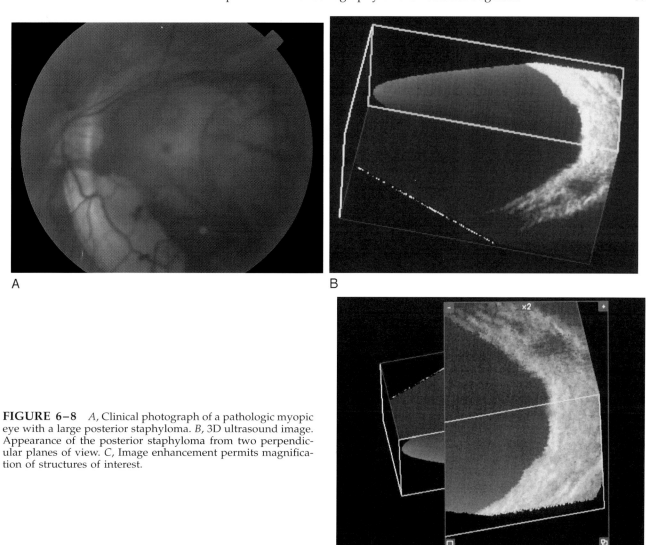

FIGURE 6–8   *A*, Clinical photograph of a pathologic myopic eye with a large posterior staphyloma. *B*, 3D ultrasound image. Appearance of the posterior staphyloma from two perpendicular planes of view. *C*, Image enhancement permits magnification of structures of interest.

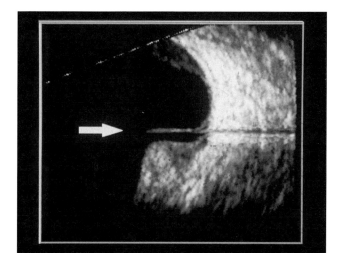

FIGURE 6–9   An example of image movement artifact (*arrow*).

ties for 3D reconstruction and measurement, since these motions affect spatial relationships. With examiner experience, patient education, and cooperation, these artifacts can be quickly reduced, permitting excellent image reconstruction. While the software learning curve is short, most examiners require volume tracing experience to produce consistent and reproducible results.

REFERENCES

1. Gosbell AD, Barry WR, Favilla I: Computer-aided volume measurement of choroidal melanomas. Aust N Z J Ophthalmol 15:349–357, 1987.
2. Basset O, Gimenez G, Mestas JL, et al: Volume measurement by ultrasonic transverse or sagittal cross-sectional scanning. Ultrasound Med Biol 17:291–296, 1991.
3. Silverman RH, Coleman DJ, Lizzi FL, Rondeau MJ: In vivo volume determination by ultrasound (Abstract). Invest Ophthalmol Vis Sci 32(Suppl):1194, 1991.

4. Hansen MK, Jensen PK: Ultrasonographic, three-dimensional scanning for determination of intraocular tumor volume. Acta Ophthalmol 69:178–186, 1991.

5. Silverman RH, Coleman DJ, Rondeau MJ, et al: Measurement of ocular tumor volumes from serial cross-sectional ultrasound scans. Retina 13:69–74, 1993.

6. Rankin RN, Fenster A, Downey DB, et al: Three-dimensional sonographic reconstruction: techniques and diagnostic application. Am J Roentgenol 161:695–702, 1993.

7. Fenster A, Miller JM, Tong S: Three Dimensional Ultrasound Imaging. U.S. Patent Application. No. 08/158, 267, 1993.

8. Fenster A, Dunne S, Chan T: Method and System for Constructing and Displaying Three-dimensional Ultrasound Images. U.S. Patent Application. No. 08/264, 800, 1994.

9. McLean MIW, Foster WD, Zimmerman LE: Prognostic factors in small malignant melanomas of choroid and ciliary body. Arch Ophthalmol 95:48–54, 1977.

10. Thomas JF, Green WR, Maumenee AE: Small choroidal melanomas, a long-term follow-up study. Arch Ophthalmol 97:861–864, 1979.

11. Shields JA, Shields CL, Donoso LA: Management of posterior uveal melanoma. Surv Ophthalmol 36:161–195, 1991.

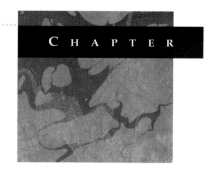

CHAPTER 7

Laser Photocoagulation

Martin A. Mainster, M.D., Ph.D.
Keith A. Warren, M.D.

Retinal photocoagulation is widely used in ophthalmic practice. Laser light absorption produces a brief localized increase in chorioretinal temperature that causes immediate inflammation and delayed therapeutic scarring. Effective photocoagulation requires a basic understanding of certain optical and thermodynamic principles. This chapter presents a practical analysis of laser light, tissue optics, and clinical photocoagulation.

LASER EFFECTS

Laser Light

The electromagnetic spectrum includes ultraviolet, visible, and infrared radiation. Radiation interacts with biologic materials in different ways depending on its wavelength and the optical properties of individual tissues. For example, the cornea transmits radiation between 300 and 1300 nm, but is opaque to ultraviolet radiation below 300 nm.[1] Potentially phototoxic near-ultraviolet radiation that penetrates the cornea between 300 and 400 nm is blocked by the crystalline lens but transmitted by intraocular lenses that don't have ultraviolet-absorbing chromophores.[2-3]

Electromagnetic radiation has wave- and particle-like properties. Its wave-like properties account for large-scale phenomena such as refraction and interference. Its particle-like properties account for atomic-level phenomena such as light absorption and emission by atoms or molecules. Particles of light are termed photons. A laser's resonant cavity amplifies only photons traveling along its axis, so a laser beam is directional and has less divergence than light from an incandescent source.[4,5]

Laser light is composed of one or several individual wavelengths. This monochromaticity occurs because there are only a limited number of efficient electronic transitions between excited electron energy levels in an atom or molecule and lower-lying electron energy levels. Irradiance at a particular wavelength from a laser is millions of times greater than that from an incandescent or arc lamp. Monochromaticity permits wavelength selection for specific applications or tissue targets.

Laser light has spatial and temporal coherence.[4,5] Coherence means that there is a predictable correlation between the amplitude and phase of different points of a light wave. Spatial (or transverse) coherence characterizes the quality of this correlation perpendicular to the laser beam's direction of travel. Temporal (or longitudinal) coherence describes the quality of this correlation at different times at a particular location in space. Coherence of laser light is responsible for interference patterns that cause speckle when a laser beam illuminates a rough surface. Spatial and temporal coherence are important considerations in diagnostic laser techniques such as interferometric visual acuity testing and optical coherence tomography, but coherence is not needed for contemporary clinical laser photocoagulation.

Laser light can be focused into a small spot size, producing a high level of power per unit area (power/area), termed irradiance. Retinal temperature rise from a laser beam is proportional to irradiance for a particular spot size and exposure duration.[6-9] Since retinal irradiance is equal to laser power delivered to the retina divided by the area of the laser beam on the retina, a 50-μm retinal spot produces four times more retinal irradiance than a 100-μm spot for a particular laser power setting (the 50-μm spot has an area that is four times smaller than the 100-μm spot).

The smallest spot size into which a laser beam can be focused is proportional to its wavelength and the focal length of the focusing lens. Argon laser 514-nm green light can be focused into a smaller spot than neodymium:yttrium-aluminum-garnet (Nd:YAG) laser 1064-nm infrared radiation. It can also be focused into a smaller spot size with a short- rather than with a long-focal-length lens. Light scattering by ocular media or chorioretinal tissues also increases spot size.

Tissue Optics

A light beam striking the surface of a biologic tissue is either reflected or refracted. Refracted light passing through the tissue may be scattered or absorbed. Scattering and absorption affect photon distribution in tissue targets ("tissue optics"), but absorption is required for the tissue heating responsible for photocoagulation.

Light Scattering

Light scattering is the process by which some of the photons in a beam of light are redirected without an appreciable change in their wavelength. Light scattering depends on the size of the particles that cause it.

Light scattering by particles less than one tenth the wavelength of light is known as Rayleigh scattering.[10-12] In Rayleigh scattering, light is scattered equally well in all directions, but blue light is scattered more readily than longer wavelengths. Rayleigh scattering is responsible for the sky's blue color. Since blue light is scattered preferentially, light reaching an observer from any point in the sky other than the sun's disc itself is mostly blue light scattered in atmospheric transit (the sky would appear black without atmospheric scattering). Rayleigh scattering is also responsible for the blue color of lightly pigmented irides. Since short-wavelength light is scattered more than longer wavelengths in intraocular transit, yellow or red light has an advantage over blue-green or green laser light for clinical photocoagulation in eyes with hazy media.[7,8]

Light scattering by particles larger than one tenth the wavelength of light is known as Mie scattering.[10-12] In Mie scattering, light is preferentially scattered forward in its direction of propagation, but the scattering is independent of wavelength. Mie scattering from large water droplets is responsible for white clouds (no wavelength dependence) and deep shadows around lights on foggy nights (forward scattering). Mie scattering by melanin granules in the retinal pigment epithelium (RPE) and choroid probably increases retinal image contrast by decreasing side-scattered light. Light scattering in retinal photocoagulation is a poorly understood process that involves scattering by multiple foci of many sizes.

Light Absorption

Photon absorption increases the energy of electrons in biologic molecules. Excited molecules can convert this excess electronic energy into an increase in average vibrational motion, producing heat and a temperature increase. Thus light absorption converts photon energy into heat. Vibrating molecules transfer this thermal energy to neighboring molecules, diffusing the heat outside the irradiated area in a process known as heat conduction.

Light absorption depends on the wavelength of incident laser photons and the type of light-absorbing molecules in a tissue target.[8,13-16] If a tissue were perfectly transparent, no photon energy would be deposited in it, and laser irradiation would not increase its temperature (enormous laser irradiances can transfer energy even to transparent media by nonlinear effects such as photodisruption).[7,9] The excellent absorption of visible light by melanin in the trabecular meshwork and RPE makes these tissues excellent targets for laser photocoagulation. The poor absorption of visible light by the cornea helps make it an effective window for vision and for retinal photocoagulation. Melanin, hemoglobin, and macular xanthophyll are the three most significant chorioretinal light absorbers.[8]

Melanin is the best chorioretinal light absorber. Its light absorption gradually decreases with increasing wavelength, one of the main reasons that longer laser wavelengths such as krypton red and diode infrared produce deeper chorioretinal lesions than argon green laser light.[8,15-18]

Hemoglobin is the next most effective light absorber. Hemoglobin absorption also decreases with increasing wavelength except for two peaks in the absorption spectrum of oxyhemoglobin (542 nm, green; 577 nm, yellow) and one absorption peak for reduced hemoglobin (555 nm, yellow).[8,14] Hemoglobin absorbs blue, green, and yellow light well but has poor red light absorption. Reduced hemoglobin has better red light absorption than oxyhemoglobin, the reason that retinal veins are more prominent than arteries in monochromatic red ophthalmoscopy.

Xanthophyll in the inner and outer plexiform layers of the macula is the least effective light absorber. Macular xanthophyll absorbs blue light well, green light minimally, and yellow and red light negligibly. If argon blue laser light were used for macular photocoagulation, inner retinal light absorption could cause undesirable neurosensory retinal damage in addition to a therapeutic RPE-choroidal lesion.[19] On the other hand, contemporary protocols for treating macular choroidal neovascularization produce such intense chorioretinal lesions that inner retinal damage occurs even with longer wavelength photocoagulation.[8]

Thermal Effects

Mathematical models of chorioretinal heat conduction provide valuable clinical insights, showing that threshold retinal photocoagulation is associated with an RPE temperature rise of 10° to 20°C[6,20,21] and that solar maculopathy is due to phototoxicity rather than photocoagulation because solar observation causes less that a 4°C elevation.[22] Retinal temperature increases are computed from the heat conduction equation after initially determining chorioretinal thermal source strength. Heat conduction depends on chorioretinal density, thermal conductivity, and specific heat, which are similar to the properties of water.

Chorioretinal thermal source strength characterizes the amount and distribution of thermal energy deposited in the retina and choroid by the absorption of laser light. Source strength is highest at the inner edge of the RPE (at the photoreceptor-RPE border), decreasing exponentially into the RPE and choroid according to the Beer-Lambert law.[6,15] Source strength is highest and decreases slowest for large absorption coefficients, the reason that short-wavelength lasers produce higher temperatures at the photoreceptor-RPE junction than long-wavelength lasers for a particular retinal irradiance.[8,15–18] Absorption coefficients characterize the amount of light of a particular wavelength that is absorbed per centimeter as the light penetrates a particular tissue.

Retinal photocoagulation occurs when laser light absorption produces a transient 10° to 20°C temperature increase in the RPE.[6,20,21] The overlying neurosensory retina is initially opacified, diffusely scattering ophthalmoscopic white light back at the observer, and producing a whitish lesion known as a "retinal burn." The overlying retina regains its transparency postoperatively. The thermally damaged area undergoes postoperative inflammation and subsequent scarring. Burns are less distinct in areas of diabetic retinal edema because the difference between light scattering by the burn and by surrounding unexposed tissues is less prominent than in normal retina. Thus, caution must be exercised to avoid excessive treatment of edematous areas of the central retina, which could cause unnecessary postoperative chorioretinal scarring.

The extent of a thermal injury to tissue depends on the magnitude and duration of the temperature increase to which the tissue is exposed (Arrhenius integral).[7,23] Some reciprocity exists between temperature rise and exposure time so that a longer exposure to a lower temperature may produce a lesion similar to that from a shorter exposure to a higher temperature.

Typical clinical photocoagulation causes retinal temperature rises far in excess of 20°C in order to produce retinal lesions that are visible immediately. Subthreshold burns can occur with much lower temperature elevations, however, and these lesions may not be apparent for several hours after treatment. Excessive irradiances can produce mechanical or explosive effects (thermoacoustic damage) due to rapid tissue expansion or water vaporization. Thermoacoustic damage can occur even at clinical irradiances in areas of dense pigmentation, however, so caution must be exercised in such areas to reduce the risk of a retinal hemorrhage or hole.

For brief laser exposures less than 1 msec in duration, lateral temperature profiles (across the retina) are the same as retinal irradiance profiles.[6] That is, if a photocoagulator produces a uniform laser beam with the same power at its center as its edge, there will be a uniform retinal temperature profile within the irradiated area, and a negligible temperature rise outside the irradiated area (in the absence of significant light scattering). For exposures longer than 1 msec, however, heat conduction spreads energy outside the irradiated area.[6]

Heat conduction becomes significant for exposures of 0.1 second or longer. For example, if the RPE temperature rise is 50°C in the center of a uniform, 200-μm, 0.1-second retinal lesion, it will be 10°C in the RPE 50 μm from the edge of the lesion, 5°C in the RPE 100 μm from the edge of the lesion, and 25°C in the neurosensory retina 50 μm anterior to the center of the lesion.[6] Heat conduction and laser light scattering in intraocular and intraretinal transit account in part for postoperative retinal burn "spreading."[8] Spreading also results from postoperative inflammation and scarring adjacent to the primary thermal lesion.[8]

Retinal temperature patterns depend on heat conduction and intraocular light scattering. Lateral retinal temperature profiles depend on the profile of the laser beam, while axial temperature profiles depend on the laser wavelength because light absorption depends on tissue absorption coefficients.[6,15] Since melanin in the RPE in the most effective light absorber, temperature rise initially is highest at the photoreceptor-RPE junction, where thermal source strength is highest. After 1 msec of exposure, temperature profiles flatten out laterally and axially due to heat conduction. As noted above, melanin absorption decreases with increasing wavelength, so RPE temperature rise for a particular retinal irradiance is higher for shorter laser wavelengths such as argon green than longer ones such as diode infrared.[15,16]

CLINICAL PHOTOCOAGULATION

Clinical laser photocoagulators consist of a laser source and a delivery system that couples the laser source to an ophthalmoscope or treatment probe. The laser source provides one or more treatment wavelengths, and has controls for selecting power and exposure duration. The delivery system has a telescopic lens system for selecting laser spot size and safety filters to protect the operator against laser flashback.

Laser Sources

The ophthalmoscopic appearance and intensity of a burn depend on laser power, spot size, exposure duration, and laser wavelength. As noted above, light absorption by melanin decreases with increasing wavelength. Thus, more radiation is transmitted through the RPE into the choroid with longer wavelengths such as krypton red or diode infrared than with shorter wavelengths such as argon green.[15-18] Longer laser wavelengths tend to produce deeper chorioretinal lesions that are less prominent ophthalmoscopically and more painful. If burns of similar ophthalmoscopic appearance are produced with an argon and a diode laser, choroidal damage will be more extensive with the diode than the argon laser.

Modern ophthalmic laser photocoagulators use argon, krypton, dye, diode, or frequency-doubled Nd:YAG laser sources. The theoretical advantages and disadvantages of different laser wavelengths for macular photocoagulation have been presented previously,[8] but no controlled trial has convincingly demonstrated a significant therapeutic advantage of one laser wavelength over another for the high irradiance treatment protocols used in contemporary retinal photocoagulation.

Argon photocoagulators use an argon-ion plasma tube to produce blue (488.0 nm) plus green (514.5 nm) or green-only (514.5 nm) laser light. Argon lasers have been used in most of the large clinical trials that demonstrated the efficacy of retinal photocoagulation. They continue to be the most widely used ophthalmic photocoagulators.

The original argon laser photocoagulators used a blue-green laser source, but a green-only option was added in the early 1980s when disadvantages of argon blue light were widely recognized. The primary disadvantages of argon blue light are that it is scattered more than longer wavelengths in intraocular and intraretinal transit, it has higher potential retinal phototoxicity than longer laser wavelengths, and it is a poor choice for macular photocoagulation because of its absorption by inner retinal xanthophyll.[8]

Argon-krypton photocoagulators use separate argon-ion and krypton-ion plasma tubes. Krypton tubes typically produce red laser light of 647 nm (some 676-nm red light may also be produced). Krypton red photocoagulation was introduced because of the disadvantages of argon blue laser light discussed above. The main difference between argon green and krypton red photocoagulation is that green light is well absorbed by hemoglobin but red light is relatively poorly absorbed by it.[8] Argon green and krypton red both produce the desired RPE-choriocapillaris lesion, but krypton red lesions

are somewhat deeper because of the lower melanin absorption of red light. Neither laser has enough light absorption in retinal capillaries to damage them directly.

Krypton red light is scattered less in intraocular transit than shorter wavelengths, so it is potentially useful for treating patients with hazy ocular media. On the other hand, the retina is viewed in white light from a slit lamp or indirect ophthalmoscope, and treatment in hazy media is usually limited by poor ophthalmoscopic visualization of the retina rather than by the inability to deliver a laser beam to a visible treatment site. Multiwavelength krypton photocoagulators can produce 531-nm (green), 568-nm (yellow), or 647-nm (red) laser light.

Commercial dye laser photocoagulators use an argon laser to excite an organic dye, usually rhodamine-6G. Users can choose between argon blue-green, argon green, or dye laser output. Dye laser output is tuned by a birefringent filter that permits laser light selection at 1-nm increments between 575- (yellow) and 630-nm (red) photocoagulation wavelengths.

Dye laser yellow light at 577 nm is a useful laser wavelength for general retinal applications because 577 nm is a peak in the oxyhemoglobin absorption spectrum. The theoretical advantages of 577-nm yellow laser light include negligible absorption in macular xanthophyll, low light scattering in intraocular and intraretinal transit, negligible retinal phototoxicity, good lesion visibility, limited patient pain, the highest ratio of oxyhemoglobin to melanin absorption for treatment of vascular structures with a minimum of damage to adjacent pigmented tissues, and a high ratio of oxyhemoglobin to reduced hemoglobin absorption for treating depigmented fibrovascular tissue through thin subretinal hemorrhage.[8]

Semiconductor diode (GaAlAs) laser photocoagulators produce infrared radiation at 810 nm. Their compact size and portability are useful in the operating room and neonatal intensive care unit, and they are widely used for treating retinopathy of prematurity.[24-27] The primary difference between diode infrared and visible light photocoagulation is that chorioretinal melanin has lower infrared radiation absorption. Thus, diode laser lesions require more power and tend to be deeper, less prominent, and more painful than argon green or dye yellow laser lesions. Since 810-nm light is invisible, however, patients do not notice the distracting flashes of light that occur during visible laser light photocoagulation.

Frequency-doubled, Nd:YAG crystal lasers (FD-YAG) have been introduced as an alternative to visible light argon or dye lasers. Frequency doubling uses a nonlinear crystal to halve the wavelength of 1064-nm Nd:YAG infrared laser radiation to 532-nm green light. FD-YAG 532-nm green light is close to the 542-nm peak of the oxyhemoglobin absorption spectrum, so continuous-wave 532-nm green light has theoretical advantages similar to 577-nm dye laser yellow photocoagulation. High power is needed for efficient frequency doubling, however, so pulsed, high-repetition-rate Q-switched Nd:YAG lasers may be used in FD-YAG systems.[4,5] Pulsed FD-YAG photocoagulators may have marked differences between their peak and average laser power so they may differ in clinical performance from ordinary continuous-wave argon, krypton, dye, or diode photocoagulators.

Delivery Systems

Laser delivery systems can be divided into fiberoptic probe or ophthalmoscopic systems. In a fiberoptic probe system, the tip of the fiberoptic cable is placed adjacent to or in contact with target tissues. Intraocular fiberoptic delivery systems are convenient for applications such an diabetic vitrectomy, but they are absolutely necessary when media around a target are opaque to laser radiation. For example, vitreous is opaque to erbium 2.9-μm infrared radiation, and a flexible, fiberoptic cable is needed for intraocular erbium vitreous surgery.

An ophthalmoscopic delivery system consists of a fiberoptic cable, telescope, and micromanipulator. The telescope is used to change laser spot size. It is mounted on a slit lamp or the headband of an indirect ophthalmoscope. In a slit lamp system, a micromanipulator is used to position the laser's aiming beam on the retina. Its control lever is usually located on the slit lamp's joystick or just below its oculars. The telescopic spot size changer and slit lamp are separate optical devices. Thus, changing slit lamp magnification alters the appearance of the aiming beam but does not change the retinal size of the aiming or treatment beam.

Slit lamp telescopic spot size selectors can be divided into defocus or parfocal devices.[7,9,28] In a defocus system, the focal point of the laser beam is located posterior (toward the patient) to the "working distance" of the slit lamp. Slit lamp working distance is determined by using the slit lamp alignment bar as discussed below. Laser spot size is increased by moving the laser beam's focal point *toward* the patient, increasing the area that the laser beam intercepts at the slit lamp's working distance and at patient's cornea, crystalline lens, and retina. The advantage of a defocus laser delivery system is that an experienced user can quickly change spot size by moving the slit lamp joystick forward or backward. Defocus systems provide the lowest possible crystalline lens irradiances during retinal photocoagulation with an indirect ophthalmoscopy contact lens and a large spot size.

In a parfocal laser delivery system, the laser beam is focused at the slit lamp's working distance. Spot size is increased by reducing the laser beam's convergence, without changing the location of its focal point. The system is called parfocal because the axial location of the beam's focal point doesn't change with changes in laser spot size. The advantage of a parfocal delivery system is that the spot size that has been selected is the smallest retinal spot size that can be obtained. Moving the slit lamp joystick forward and backward can't produce a spot size smaller than one that's selected, it can only make a larger spot size with lower target tissue irradiance. Thus, parfocal systems offer security against spot sizes smaller or irradiances higher than the one that has been selected. Parfocal laser delivery systems also provide aiming spots with sharper borders than defocus systems, an advantage in visualizing the aiming beam in hazy ocular media.

Regardless of the type of telescopic spot size selector on a slit lamp photocoagulator, spot size settings are valid only when the ophthalmoscopic image is located at the working distance of the slit lamp. Since physicians can accommodate and the slit lamp itself has a considerable depth of field, it is important that individuals use their proper ocular settings and that each photocoagulator be aligned properly.[7,9]

Proper ocular settings may be determined by placing the slit lamp alignment bar in its holder, fogging each eye separately by adding excess plus power to the ocular, and decreasing excess plus power until the surface of the alignment bar initially comes into focus. With proper ocular settings for each eye, the physician's unaccommodated retina is conjugate with the working distance of the slit lamp. With the slit lamp alignment bar removed and the slit lamp moved forward until the retina initially comes into focus, the retina will be at the slit lamp's working distance, and spot size settings will be valid.[7,9]

If improper ocular settings are used, difficulties could arise when slit lamp movement inadvertently reduces spot size and increases focal irradiance. Proper photocoagulator calibration may be checked by using the correct ocular settings and placing a piece of cardboard at the working distance of the slit lamp. With the aiming beam on its smallest setting, usually 50 μm, forward or backward joystick movement should only increase spot size if the photocoagulator is properly aligned. Burn paper may also be used to check proper photocoagulator alignment.

Treatment Parameters

Photocoagulators have controls for selecting exposure duration, laser power, and spot size. These settings can be varied to change the intensity of a retinal burn or the severity of a patient's pain. As noted earlier, thermal injury depends on the magnitude and duration of retinal temperature rise. Retinal temperature rise itself depends on retinal irradiance (which is laser power at the retina divided by retinal spot size of the laser beam) and the efficiency of converting laser energy into heat energy at the target site (which depends upon light absorption coefficients and thus laser wavelength).[6,9,15] Dye, multiwavelength krypton, and argon-krypton lasers also have controls for wavelength selection as is discussed under laser sources above.

Burn intensity can be reduced by decreasing exposure duration and power or by increasing spot size. A patient's pain can be reduced by decreasing power, spot size, exposure duration or burn repetition rate, or by using a shorter wavelength. Decreasing exposure duration and spot size are common ways to localize laser effects in a variety of procedures. If both parameters are decreased, so much laser energy can be delivered in such a short period of time to such a small tissue volume that target tissues can be ablated, perforating or reshaping them.[29] Ablation is used in erbium laser vitreous surgery as well as excimer laser photorefractive keratectomy and Nd:YAG laser photodisruption, but thermomechanical effects are undesirable complications in conventional retinal photocoagulation.

Decreasing exposure duration can minimize the role of heat conduction in clinical photocoagulation, localizing thermal effects in the retina both laterally and axially.[6,8,9,30] Contemporary treatment protocols require retinal lesions that are immediately apparent, however, so very high power settings would be needed if very short exposures were used. Other ophthalmoscopic or angiographic markers could be developed for lower power laser photocoagulation not requiring an immediately visible retinal lesion. High power settings with brief exposures (0.01 to 0.05 second) are useful for reducing pain in panretinal photocoagulation. Smaller diameter retinal lesions are needed for treating macular problems, however, and if an area of increased subretinal pigmentation were unexpectedly treated with a very high power setting, thermomechanical damage and hemorrhage could occur.[8,31,32] In general, for argon laser photocoagulation, the safety margin between retinal burn and retinal hemorrhage becomes narrower as pulse duration is decreased, particularly for small-diameter lesions and exposure durations less than 0.05 second.[32]

Ophthalmoscopy

Photocoagulator spot size settings are affected by ophthalmoscopic lens selection. Ophthalmoscopic lenses may be divided into direct and indirect lenses.[33] In direct ophthalmoscopy, a slit lamp is used to view an erect, virtual image of a patient's retina located just posterior to the patient's crystalline lens. In indirect ophthalmoscopy, a slit lamp or head-mounted ophthalmoscope is used to view a real, inverted image of the patient's retina produced by a contact or noncontact ophthalmoscopic lens. The ophthalmoscopic image is located within the indirect ophthalmoscopy lens or between it and the observer.

The Goldmann flat-surfaced contact lens is the most widely used direct ophthalmoscopy lens for slit lamp photocoagulation. It provides excellent magnification for viewing the posterior pole, and its internal reflecting surfaces permit detailed examination of the peripheral retina. It also provides very low crystalline lens irradiance during retinal photocoagulation. The chief disadvantage of Goldmann-type lenses is their limited field of view. Numerous lens manipulations are needed for panretinal photocoagulation, and less experienced users may become disoriented when using peripheral mirrors and inadvertently encounter the macula. Indirect ophthalmoscopy contact lenses were introduced to provide a broader field of view to facilitate clinical photocoagulation.

Indirect ophthalmoscopy lens performance is a balance between magnification and field of view.[33] Lenses designed for focal laser treatment have magnification comparable to or greater than the Goldmann lens but a field of view that is three times larger. Lenses designed for midperipheral scatter photocoagulation have lower magnification than a Goldmann lens but a six to nine times greater field of view. Ametropia has little effect on direct ophthalmoscopy magnification, but the magnification of indirect ophthalmoscopy lenses slightly decreases in myopia and increases in hyperopia.[33] The field of view of indirect ophthalmoscopy lenses increases in myopia and decreases in hyperopia.[33]

Reflections from indirect ophthalmoscopy lenses are a difficult problem. Since illumination can't be separated from observation in the patient's pupil with conventional slit lamp photocoagulators, ophthalmoscopic lens surfaces have optical coatings to reduce light reflections. The coatings are used to improve observation, not because they're needed for photocoagulation. Typical lenses have a broad-spectrum antireflection coating that reduces light reflection in the visible spectrum from roughly 4% to less than 1% for normal incidence.

Lens manufacturers should be consulted on how their indirect ophthalmoscopy lenses alter photocoagulator spot size.[28,33] Higher magnification lenses for focal laser treatment produce a retinal spot size close to photocoagulator spot size settings (e.g., Ocular Instruments Standard and Volk Area Centralis lenses). Retinal spot size for panretinal photocoagulation lenses can be estimated by multiplying the photocoagulator spot size setting by 1.5 for wide-field lenses (e.g., Ocular Instruments Wide Field and Rodenstock Panfundoscope) or by 2 for very-wide-field lenses (e.g., Ocular Instruments UltraField PRP and Volk QuadraAspheric).

Anterior segment irradiance may exceed retinal irradiance for large photocoagulator spot size settings when using wide- or very-wide-field indirect ophthalmoscopy lens, particularly for photocoagulators equipped with a parfocal telescopic spot size selector.[33] Anterior segment irradiance typically increases as the field of view of an indirect ophthalmoscopy lens increases. For example, for a 500-μm parfocal spot size setting, crystalline lens irradiance is five times higher than retinal irradiance for a Rodenstock Panfundoscope lens and 11 times higher for a Volk QuadraAspheric lens.[28] If media opacities are present, high pupillary irradiance can cause local light absorption and damage. Cornea and crystalline lens damage were first reported after Panfundoscope photocoagulation in 1983,[34,35] but all wide-field indirect ophthalmoscopy contact lenses share this potential problem. In general, photocoagulator spot size settings should be kept below 500 μm to reduce the risk of ocular media damage.

Ocular media opacities can scatter light, diminishing the contrast of ophthalmoscopic images. In hazy media, the clarity of retinal images is improved most effectively by changing the orientation or reducing the height and width of the slit lamp beam, not by increasing slit lamp brightness. Increasing slit lamp brightness increases veiling backscattered light, decreasing ophthalmoscopic image contrast. Media scattering can also increase retinal spot size, a problem that can be countered by decreasing photocoagulator spot size. It is important to recognize that spot size can decrease and retinal irradiance can markedly increase when areas of clearer media are encountered. Photocoagulation with an indirect ophthalmoscope or with a slit lamp using a noncontact ophthalmoscopic lens is useful in patients with intraocular gas after vitreous surgery, but reflections from intraocular gas can cause lesions remote from the intended treatment site.[36]

Safety

Photocoagulation produces brilliant light reflections from ophthalmoscopic lenses. The operator's eyes are protected against potential light injury by safety filters that must be in place in the viewing system before photocoagulating power levels can be delivered to the patient's eye. Safety filters are fixed or switched into place.

With a fixed safety filter, aiming and treatment laser beams are produced by separate lasers with different wavelengths.[37] The aiming beam is usually a red helium-neon or diode laser. A filter is fixed in place to block treatment beam reflections but to transmit the rest of the visible spectrum for ophthalmoscopy and aiming beam localization. Some ophthalmoscopic detail is lost when protection is needed for a treatment beam in the visible portion of the spectrum, but fixed filters are silent and secure.

Switched operator safety filters are required when the same laser source is used for aiming and treatment beams. When the photocoagulator's foot switch is depressed, switched protective filters swing into place before laser power is increased

from aiming to treatment levels. Ophthalmoscopy is unimpaired prior to treatment and the operator is completely protected from treatment beam flashback,[38] but filter operation may be noisy and distracting with older photocoagulators.

Safety filters fully protect photocoagulator operators, but adjacent personnel are potentially vulnerable to reflections from ophthalmoscopic lenses, even with antireflection coatings. For example, during argon laser photocoagulation with a Goldmann-type lens, specular reflections from the flat surface of the lens can exceed maximum permissible levels for an individual standing behind the operator, within 1.6 m of the lens.[39] Personnel should avoid the conical reflection zone behind the lens and operator, or wear safety goggles appropriate for the treatment wavelength. No injury of this type has ever been reported.

Safety filters protect clinicians against treatment beam flashback, but aiming beams are usually viewed without protection. Aiming beam reflexes can be dazzling and annoying, but they are well below maximal permissible exposure levels for brief exposures.[38] Very subtle defects in blue color contrast sensitivity have been demonstrated in long-term users of argon blue-green laser photocoagulators, however, presumably due to the blue component of the argon blue-green aiming beam which has a greater potential retinal phototoxicity than longer wavelengths.[40,41] No retinal abnormalities were documented in those studies and their clinical significance remains uncertain. Nonetheless, it makes good sense to use the lowest effective aiming beam intensities for both clinician and patient safety. Many modern photocoagulators are equipped with green-only or red aiming beams to minimize the risk of phototoxicity during blue-green photocoagulation.[37]

REFERENCES

1. Boettner EA, Wolter JR: Transmission of the ocular media. Invest Ophthalmol 1:776–783, 1962.
2. Mainster MA: Spectral transmittance of intraocular lenses and retinal damage from intense light sources. Am J Ophthalmol 85:167–170, 1978.
3. Mainster MA: The spectra, classification, and rationale of ultraviolet-protective intraocular lenses. Am J Ophthalmol 102:727–731, 1986.
4. O'Shea DC, Callen WR, Rhodes WT: Introduction to Lasers and Their Applications. Reading, MA, Addison-Wesley, 1978.
5. Hecht J: The Laser Guidebook, 2nd edition. Blue Ridge Summit, PA, Tab, 1992.
6. Mainster MA, White TJ, Tips JH, Wilson PW: Retinal temperature increases produced by intense light sources. J Opt Soc Am 60:264–270, 1970.
7. Mainster MA: Ophthalmic laser surgery: principles, technology and technique. In Klein EA (ed): Symposium on the Laser in Ophthalmology and Glaucoma Update, New Orleans Academy of Ophthalmology. St Louis, CV Mosby Co, 1985, pp 81–101.
8. Mainster MA: Wavelength selection in macular photocoagulation: tissue optics, thermal effects and laser systems. Ophthalmology 93:952–958, 1986.

9. Mainster MA: Laser light, interactions, and clinical systems. In L'Esperance FA Jr (ed): Ophthalmic Lasers: Photocoagulation and Surgery, 3rd edition. St Louis, CV Mosby Co, 1989, pp 61–77.
10. Overheim RD, Wagner DL: Light and Color. New York, Wiley, 1982.
11. Minnaert M: Light and Color in the Outdoors. New York, Springer-Verlag, 1993.
12. Meyer-Arendt JR: Introduction to Classical and Modern Optics, 2nd edition. Englewood Cliffs, NJ, Prentice-Hall, 1984.
13. Mainster MA: Ophthalmic applications of infrared lasers—thermal considerations. Invest Ophthalmol Vis Sci 18:414–420, 1979.
14. Bursell SE, Mainster MA, Sliney DH: Spectral properties of ocular pigments. Unpublished data.
15. Mainster MA, White TJ, Allen RG: Spectral dependence of retinal damage produced by intense light sources. J Opt Soc Am 60:848–855, 1970.
16. Vogel A, Birngruber R: Temperature profiles in human retina and choroid during laser coagulation with different wavelengths ranging from 524 to 810 nm. Lasers Light Ophthalmol 5:9–16, 1992.
17. Schmidt-Erfurth U, Vogel A, Birngruber R: The influence of wavelength on the laser power required for retinal photocoagulation in cataractous human eyes. Lasers Light Ophthalmol 5:69–78, 1992.
18. Benner JD, Huang M, Morse LS, et al: Comparison of photocoagulation with the argon, krypton and diode laser indirect ophthalmoscopes in rabbit eyes. Ophthalmology 99:1554–1563, 1992.
19. Marshall J, Hamilton AM, Bird AC: Intra-retinal absorption of argon laser irradiation in human and monkey retinae. Experientia 30:1355–1357, 1974.
20. Mainster MA, White TJ, Tips JH, Wilson PW: Transient thermal behavior in biological systems. Bull Math Biophys 32:303–314, 1970.
21. Priebe LA, Cain CP, Welch AJ: Temperature rise required for the production of minimal lesions in the Macaca mulatta retina. Am J Ophthalmol 79:405–413, 1975.
22. White TJ, Mainster MA, Wilson PW, Tips JH: Chorioretinal temperature increases from solar observation. Bull Math Biophys 33:1–17, 1971.
23. Birngruber R: Thermal modeling in biological tissues. In Hillenkamp F, Pratesi R, Sacchi CA (eds): Lasers in Biology and Medicine. New York, Plenum, 1980, pp 77–97.
24. McNamara JA, Tasman W, Vander JF, Brown GC: Diode laser photocoagulation for retinopathy of prematurity. Arch Ophthalmol 110:1714–1716, 1992.
25. Hunter DG, Repka MX: Diode laser photocoagulation for threshold retinopathy of prematurity. Ophthalmology 100:238–244, 1993.
26. Bandello F, Brancato R, Trabucchi G, et al: Diode versus argon-green laser panretinal photocoagulation in proliferative diabetic retinopathy—a randomized study in 44 eyes with a long follow-up time. Graefes Arch Clin Exp Ophthalmol 231:491–494, 1993.
27. McHugh D, England C, van der Zypen E, et al: Irradiation of rabbit retina with diode and Nd:YAG lasers. Br J Ophthalmol 79:672–677, 1995.
28. Dewey D: Corneal and retinal energy density with various laser beam delivery systems and contact lenses. SPIE Proc 1423:105–116, 1991.
29. Mainster MA: Classification of ophthalmic photosurgery. Lasers Light Ophthalmol 6:65–67, 1994.
30. Roider J, Michaud NA, Flotte TJ, Birngruber R: Response of the retinal pigment epithelium to selective photocoagulation. Arch Ophthalmol 110:1786–1792, 1992.
31. Mainster MA, Sliney DH, Belcher CD III, Buzney SM: Laser photodisruptors—damage mechanisms, instrument design and safety. Ophthalmology 90:973–991, 1983.
32. Obana A, Lorenz B, Gassler A, Birngruber R: The therapeutic range of chorioretinal photocoagulation with diode and argon lasers—an experimental comparison. Lasers Light Ophthalmol 4:147–156, 1992.
33. Mainster MA, Crossman JL, Erickson PJ, Heacock GL: Retinal laser lenses: magnification, spot size and field of view. Br J Ophthalmol 74:177–179, 1990.
34. Birngruber R, Lorenz B, Weinberg W, et al: Komplikationen bei der laserkoagulation durch das panfunduskop. Fortschr Ophthalmol 79:434–437, 1983.
35. Gamel JW, Eiferman RA: Cataracts produced by argon laser photocoagulation. Arch Ophthalmol 101:665, 1983.
36. Whitacre MM, Mainster MA: Hazards of laser beam reflections in eyes containing gas. Am J Ophthalmol 110:33–38, 1990.
37. Whitacre MM, Manoukian N, Mainster MA: Argon indirect ophthalmoscope photocoagulation: reduced potential phototoxicity with a fixed safety filter. Br J Ophthalmol 74:233–234, 1990.
38. Sliney DH, Mainster MA: Potential laser hazards to the clinician during photocoagulation. Am J Ophthalmol 103:758–760, 1987.
39. Sliney DH: Biomedical laser safety. In Goldman L (ed): The Biomedical Laser. New York, Springer-Verlag, 1982, pp 11–24.
40. Gunduz K, Arden GB: Changes in colour contrast sensitivity associated with operating argon laser. Br J Ophthalmol 73:241–246, 1989.
41. Arden GB, Berninger T, Hogg, CR, Perry S: A survey of color-discrimination in German ophthalmologists—changes associated with the use of lasers and operating microscopes. Ophthalmology 98:567–575, 1991.

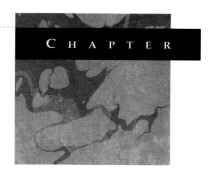

CHAPTER 8

New Diagnostic and Therapeutic Approaches to Retinal Disease

Caroline R. Baumal, M.D.
Carmen A. Puliafito, M.D.

NEW MODALITIES FOR DIAGNOSIS OF RETINAL DISEASE

Optical coherence tomography (OCT) is a new imaging modality that produces high-resolution, cross-sectional images of ocular structures in vitro and in vivo.[1] Developed by researchers from Tufts University and the Massachusetts Institute of Technology, OCT produces detailed two-dimensional images of the retina and measures retinal thickness with a longitudinal image resolution of approximately 10 μm. This resolution is superior to other imaging techniques such as B-scan ultrasound and the scanning laser ophthalmoscopy, which have image resolutions of 150 and 300 μm, respectively. Ultrasound biomicroscopy (UBM) is capable of image resolution up to 20 μm with a high-frequency 100-MHz transducer; however, the depth of penetration is limited to 4 mm, preventing posterior segment applications.[2,3]

The principles of OCT are similar to B-mode ultrasound; however, OCT utilizes the reflection of light waves from different structures in the eye rather than sound. When light is directed into the eye, it is reflected at the boundaries of tissues with different optical properties, as well as scattered and absorbed. Low-coherence interferometry is used to measure the time-of-flight delay of light reflected from structures within the retina. The low-coherence light is produced by a continuous-wave superluminescent diode source, which is coupled into a fiberoptic Michelson interferometer; 200 μW of 830 nm probe light is incident on the fundus, which is within the exposure limit for permanent intrabeam viewing recommended by the American National Standards Institute.[4] The interferometer splits the light source into a probe beam and a reference beam. The probe beam is directed into the eye and is reflected from retinal structures at different distances. The reflected probe beam is composed of multiple echoes that give information about the distance and thickness of the retinal structures. The reference beam is reflected from a reference mirror at a known variable position. The two beams recombine at a detector where an interference signal only occurs when the propagation distances of both the probe and reference beams match to within the source coherence length. The coherence length of the source light defines the longitudinal resolution of the OCT system. This was experimentally measured to be 14 μm in air and 10 μm in the retina after accounting for the difference in refractive index between air and tissue.[5] The transverse resolution is determined by multiple factors, including the probe beam diameter and the separation of individual A scans, and may be up to 13 μm.

Microstructural features of retinal tissue are determined by measuring the "echo" time it takes for the light to reflect from the different structures at varying longitudinal distances, analogous to ultrasound A-scan. Two-dimensional B-mode images are created by performing successive longitudinal scans in the transverse direction. Each tomogram is composed of a sequence of 100 A-scans, obtained in 2.5 seconds. The beam is focused onto the retina with a +78-diopter condensing lens. An infrared camera is used to view the fundus and probe beam location. Ocular fixation is achieved with either a computer-controlled light fixating the scanned eye or an externally mounted light on the slit lamp to fixate the fellow eye when the scanned eye has vision below 20/300. The position of a scan and the coordinates of the fixation light are automatically recorded by the computer to permit future OCT scanning at the same location. Computer algorithms adjust for the effect of longitudinal but not transverse eye movement. The resultant OCT image of optical reflectivity is displayed in false color. Dark colors such as blue and black represent regions of minimal relative optical reflectivity, while bright colors such as red and white represent regions of high optical reflectivity.

As OCT is an optical technique, it can be performed without physical contact with the eye and minimal patient discomfort. The use of short coherent light as opposed to sound waves allows higher spatial resolution than achieved with other imaging methods. OCT is limited by intraocular media opacities such as vitreous hemorrhage and corneal edema, which attenuate the incident and reflected light, although retinal imaging may be achieved through early cataracts.

Assessment of retinal architecture requires knowledge of the OCT features of a normal eye as illustrated in Figure 8–1. The cross-sectional anat-

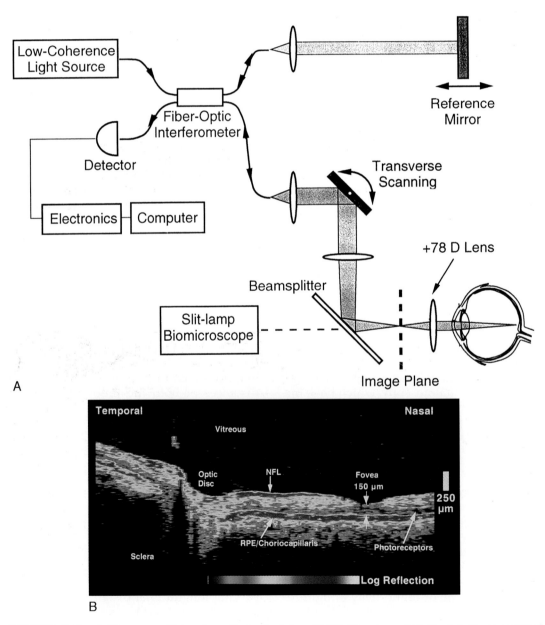

FIGURE 8–1   *A,* Diagram outlining the optical principles of OCT. (Courtesy of M. Hee.) *B,* Cross-sectional anatomy of the fovea and optic disc.

omy of the fovea and optic disc are evident as is the layered structure of the retina. A highly reflective red layer, measuring approximately 70 μm in thickness, corresponds to the retinal pigment epithelium (RPE) and choriocapillaris.[6] The contrast between this red layer and the neural retina creates a reproducible boundary for measurement of neurosensory retina thickness. The dark layer immediately anterior to the RPE/choriocapillaris likely represents the photoreceptor outer segments. The middle retinal layers exhibit moderate backscattering. Retinal blood vessels are noted by their shadowing of deeper retinal structures. The retinal nerve fiber layer corresponds to a bright red reflective layer at the inner retinal margin. The vitreoretinal interface is well defined due to the contrast between the nonreflective vitreous and the backscattering retina. Weak reflections appear from the deep choroid and sclera due to signal attenuation after passing through the retina. The fovea is recognized by its characteristic contour and the lateral displacement of the retina anterior to the photoreceptors and Henle's nerve fiber layer. In normal eyes, the mean ± standard deviation of central fovea thickness is 147 ± 17 μm.[7]

The optical properties of the eye and the accessibility of the retina make OCT particularly suitable for ophthalmologic use. As the technique of OCT imaging is performed in conjunction with slit lamp biomicroscopy, simultaneous viewing of the retina allows the OCT scan to be directed to the area of interest. OCT has proven useful in characterizing a wide variety of retinal pathology, including macular holes, epiretinal membranes, macular edema, central serous chorioretinopathy, and age-related macular degeneration (AMD).[8] High resolution imaging of anterior chamber structures and measurement of peripapillary nerve fiber layer thickness is also possible.[9-11] OCT may establish a diagnosis, monitor treatment efficacy, and evaluate the course of a disease.

Macular Holes

The cross-sectional image produced by OCT can distinguish true full thickness macular holes from partial thickness holes, macular pseudoholes, and cysts. OCT is able to stage idiopathic macular holes as classified by Gass, assess the vitreoretinal interface, measure hole diameter, and detect the presence and amount of surrounding intraretinal fluid.[5,12] A stage 1 macular hole demonstrates absence of the normal fovea depression. An area of decreased reflectivity is present beneath the fovea, consistent with a foveolar detachment. No breaks are seen in the inner foveal tissue. Vitreous traction may be noted in the foveal region. With OCT, a detached posterior vitreous is seen as a patchy, thin, reflective band anterior to the retina as seen in Fig. 8–2. A stage 2 hole reveals a break in retinal surface with a small, full-thickness loss of retinal tissue (Fig. 8–2). Stage 3 macular holes demonstrate a sharply defined, full-thickness loss of retinal tissue centrally. The margin of neurosensory retina is increased in thickness with decreased optical reflectivity, consistent with intraretinal edema. A prehole opacity may be visualized. Stage 4 reveals a full-thickness hole with complete separation of the posterior vitreous from the macula and optic disc. In contrast, lamellar holes exhibit a steepened foveal contour with an intact outer neurosensory retina. Macular cysts demonstrate localized intraretinal accumulation of optically clear fluid.

Up to 50% of stage 1 holes spontaneously abort

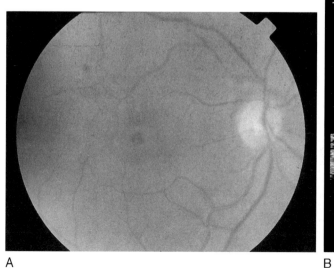

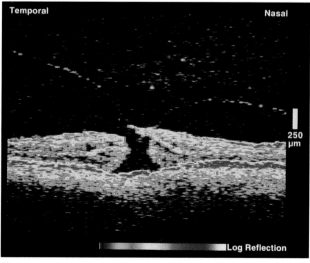

A   B

FIGURE 8–2   Stage 2 macular hole. *A*, Fundus photograph of a stage 2 macular hole. *B*, OCT demonstrates a full-thickness break in retinal tissue. The posterior hyaloid remains attached to the flap of dehisced retina. (Courtesy of Dr. E. Reichel.)

over time without substantial vision loss, while stage 2 holes almost always progress to stage 3 holes with additional loss of acuity.[13] As OCT can accurately stage macular holes, this modality may prove useful to identify potential surgical candidates. Vitreofoveal traction plays a role in the pathogenesis of macular holes.[14] OCT can reveal whether the vitreous is detached at the fovea; thus, it may identify eyes that are no longer at risk for future development of a macular hole. The size of the macular hole can be measured, which may prove to influence postsurgical visual outcome. In addition, hole resolution and macular thickness can be measured after surgery. OCT may be able to evaluate the risk of macular hole formation in the fellow eye of patients with a unilateral idiopathic macular hole. In one study, vitreofoveal abnormalities were observed in 21% of contralateral eyes.[15] Vitreous detachments as small as 150 μm can be detected by OCT.[8] The presence of vitreofoveal abnormalities may help predict the clinical course and select surgical candidates.

Epiretinal Membrane

Epiretinal membranes are visualized on OCT as a highly reflective tissue on the surface of the retina. Factors that may contribute to loss of vision such as neurosensory retinal disruption, macular edema, and membrane opacity may be identified on OCT. Retinal distortion is noted as irregularity in the cross-sectional retinal contour, while intraretinal areas of decreased reflectivity represent edema.[8] Membrane opacity is indicated by its thickness and increased reflectivity with OCT. As OCT may provide information regarding the thickness and adherence of preretinal fibrosis to the retina, this may have prognostic value for visual recovery after surgical removal.

Macular Edema

OCT is a highly sensitive tool for diagnosis and monitoring the course of macular edema. It has been used to assess patients with macular edema secondary to diabetes, retinal vein occlusion, uveitis, epiretinal membrane, and status following cataract extraction. It may also demonstrate resolution of edema after laser photocoagulation.[7] Macular edema is characterized on OCT as intraretinal areas of decreased reflectivity and retinal thickening. Round, optically clear regions within the neurosensory retina are noted in cystoid macular edema. Measurement of retinal thickness is easily performed between the two well-defined, highly reflective red layers of the nerve fiber layer and the RPE/choriocapillaris layer.

Advantages of OCT for assessment of macular edema include a high degree of accuracy and re-

producibility. Although slit lamp biomicroscopy can confirm the diagnosis of macular edema, OCT was shown to be more sensitive in detecting small changes in retinal thickness.[7] Fluorescein angiography may reveal vascular leakage, but does not provide quantitative information. It has been demonstrated that retinal thickness correlates better with visual acuity than the degree of fluorescein leakage in macular edema and increased retinal thickness.[16] In patients with diabetic retinopathy, measurement of central macular thickness by OCT correlated well with visual acuity.[7] OCT may eventually prove to be a sensitive test for early detection of macular thickening in diabetic patients.

Central Serous Chorioretinopathy

Central serous chorioretinopathy (CSR) is characterized by detachment of the neurosensory retina secondary to one or more areas of leakage at the level of the RPE. An associated RPE detachment may be present. Fluorescein angiography confirms the diagnosis by identifying leakage at the level of the RPE and excluding pathology such as choroidal neovascularization, which may present similarly. OCT can diagnose and objectively quantify the height of the neurosensory detachment. There is an area of decreased reflectivity between the neurosensory retina and the highly reflective RPE/choriocapillaris, corresponding to a neurosensory detachment. The height of this fluid-filled cavity measures 590 μm. A small detachment of the RPE is noted in the foveal center, corresponding to the hyperfluorescent leakage point on fluorescein angiogram. A small discontinuity in the RPE connects the RPE and neurosensory detachments.

OCT may be able to exclude choroidal neovascularization, which is noted as areas of disruption of the highly reflective band corresponding to the RPE and choriocapillaris. Hee and associates demonstrated that OCT may diagnose small neurosensory detachments that were clinically undetectable with slit lamp biomicroscopy.[17] Interval examinations are able to accurately detect changes in the height of the neurosensory detachment.

Age-Related Macular Degeneration

OCT has been used to evaluate choroidal neovascularization and other findings associated with AMD.[18] This may be useful when visualization of choroidal neovascularization is obscured on fluorescein angiography by a thin layer of fluid or hemorrhage. Typically, thickening or disruption of the RPE/choriocapillaris layer is observed. Choroidal neovascularization, which is well defined on fluorescein angiography, can be seen as a fusiform discrete area of increased reflectivity of the RPE/choriocapillaris layer, while occult neovascularization exhibits an irregular disrupted configuration. OCT may be able to define the boundary of choroidal neovascularization for laser photocoagulation and confirm complete closure after therapy. The dry scar after treatment is characterized by increased reflectivity deep to the choriocapillaris and a lack of intraretinal fluid.

OCT is presently the most sensitive tool to evaluate retinal architecture in vivo. In addition to a cross-sectional image, OCT provides a quantitative, objective measurement of retinal thickness with a longitudinal image resolution up to 10 μm. OCT images correspond with known histopathologic characteristics of retinal disorders. Present retinal applications include characterization of vitreomacular traction, macular holes, epiretinal membranes, and choroidal neovascularization. Other posterior segment disorders such as tumors, retinoschisis, cotton-wool spots, optic nerve pits, and retinal inflammatory disorders have a characteristic appearance. Accurate quantification of retinal thickness and measurement of neurosensory retinal and pigment epithelial detachments is possible. OCT is presently complementary to fundus photography and fluorescein angiography; however, in some cases, it may potentially replace these tests for diagnosis or monitoring retinal disorders.

NEW DEVELOPMENTS IN RETINAL LASER THERAPY

The effect of laser energy is dependent on the laser wavelength, and on the distribution of tissue chromophores and their absorption of laser energy. Laser photocoagulation has proven effective for treatment of retinal disorders such as choroidal neovascularization and proliferative diabetic retinopathy. During photocoagulation, laser energy is transformed into heat within the absorbing tissues and the thermal effects are temperature and time dependent. As the length of exposure increases, thermal effects are often not confined to the absorbing area and spread to surrounding tissues. At the exposure duration used for conventional retinal photocoagulation, the nonabsorbing neural retina may be thermally damaged due to its position adjacent to the RPE. However, selective damage to a specific retinal component may be desirable. For example, closure of choroidal neovascularization without damage to the neurosensory retina may lead to improved visual acuity.

Several methods have been investigated to increase the specificity and effectiveness of laser procedures. The rationale is to target specific retinal and/or choroidal structures with decreased energy requirements, thus minimizing damage to the adjacent neurosensory retina. Dye enhancement requires administration of an exogenous agent that concentrates in the target tissue. Localization of the laser effect is based on the similar wavelength of absorption for the exogenous agent and the emission from the laser. Photodynamic therapy depends on activation of an exogenous agent by low-intensity light to produce a photochemical reaction with subsequent tissue damage. Spatial confinement of thermal injury may be produced with repetitive exposure to short subthreshold laser pulses or by selective absorption of brief laser pulses by the target tissue.

Dye Enhancement

Exogenous dyes such as sodium fluorescein and indocyanine green (ICG) have been utilized to enhance retinal laser therapy. Fluorescein dye absorbs the blue wavelength emitted from the argon blue–green laser, decreasing the amount of laser energy required for closure of fluorescein-filled blood vessels. Fluorescein dye has been used to enhance argon laser therapy of retinal angiomas outside the macular region.[19] However, this technique is rarely used due to the potential ocular toxicity associated with blue laser wavelengths.

ICG is a water-soluble tricarbocyanine dye that is currently used for ophthalmic angiography. Due to its unique properties, ICG dye has proven superior to sodium fluorescein for visualization of the choroidal vasculature. ICG is approximately 98% bound and essentially a nondiffusible dye in the normal retinal circulation. ICG dye leaks less from the fenestrated choriocapillaris than fluorescein and has a predilection to concentrate in choroidal neovascular membranes.[20,21] The absorption (795 to 810 nm) and emission (835 to 850 nm) of ICG is in the near infrared range, while sodium fluorescein has peak absorption and emission (465 and 525 nm, respectively) in the visible spectrum. The infrared wavelength of ICG fluorescence allows improved delineation of the choroidal vasculature through overlying hemorrhage, fluid, or pigment. Clinically, ICG has been useful to characterize occult choroidal neovascularization and other choroidal disorders.[21–24] ICG videoangiography may convert occult choroidal neovascularization into well-defined, potentially treatable lesions in up to one third of patients with AMD.[23]

Selection of a laser whose wavelength matches the absorption characteristics of the target tissue should potentially maximize the laser effect. As the peak wavelength of ICG absorption (805 nm) is similar to that of diode laser emission (810 nm), ICG dye may act as a chromophore enhancing absorption of diode laser. The semiconductor diode laser emits at a longer wavelength than other conventional lasers used for photocoagulation. This infrared emission produces maximal damage to the outer retina and choroid with relative sparing of the inner retina and nerve fiber layer.[25–28] In addition, the diode laser has excellent penetration through serous fluid or retinal edema and minimal absorption by intraocular media opacities. ICG dye is selectively concentrated in choroidal neovascular membranes after being cleared from the adjacent choroidal vasculature.[21] Administration of ICG dye immediately prior to diode laser photocoagulation may permit selective ablation of ICG-filled choroidal neovascular membranes (CNVM) with lower energy requirements, thus limiting laser-induced damage to the adjacent normal retina.[23]

ICG dye-enhanced diode laser photocoagulation has been advocated for treatment of subfoveal occult choroidal neovascularization, which is deemed untreatable by the Macular Photocoagulation Study (MPS) group. The natural history of subfoveal choroidal neovascularization in AMD is poor without treatment.[29] Eyes treated with conventional subfoveal photocoagulation lose approximately three Snellen lines of vision immediately after treatment, most likely due to the thermal damage to the adjacent inner retina.[30] ICG-enhanced diode treatment may improve visual results by sparing the subfoveal neurosensory retina. In addition, this technique may be useful when ICG angiography shows superior demarcation of choroidal neovascularization when compared to fluorescein angiography. ICG-enhanced diode photocoagulation may enhance closure of choroidal neovascularization associated with an overlying serous pigment epithelial detachment or hemorrhage, due to the deeper penetration of the diode laser wavelength.

For this technique, preoperative fluorescein and ICG digital angiography are performed to diagnose and localize the area of choroidal neovascularization. ICG dye is contraindicated in patients with an allergy to iodine-based dye or liver insufficiency. Five milligrams per kilogram of weight of ICG dye is injected as a bolus into a peripheral arm vein, followed by a 10-ml flush of sterile normal saline. Diode laser photocoagulation is performed 1 to 5 minutes after ICG injection. Confluent burns are applied to the area of ICG hyperfluorescence until a deep, light gray burn is achieved. Some surgeons recommend treatment with a grid pattern to spare the center of the fovea when treating subfoveal choroidal neovascularization. The end point is a lighter color than the heavy white photocoagulative lesion achieved by the MPS, presumably representing minimal damage to the retinal pigment epithelium. Laser parameters are titrated to achieve the light gray end point. Typical diode laser settings range from a spot size of 200 to 500 μm, a duration of 0.2 to 0.5 seconds, and a power of 300 to 950 mW.[31] Fluorescein and ICG angiograms are repeated 2 to 3 weeks after treatment to assess for closure.

Preliminary results with this technique have been encouraging. In primates, ICG dye–enhanced diode therapy successfully closed choroidal neovascularization with lower energy requirements than for diode laser treatment alone.[32] Histopathologic studies in animals treated with ICG-enhanced diode photocoagulation revealed full-thickness choroidal damage with minimal neurosensory ret-

inal damage.[33] Reichel and associates used ICG dye–enhanced diode photocoagulation to treat ten eyes with poorly defined subfoveal CNVM secondary to AMD.[31] Stabilization of visual acuity within two lines of presenting vision was achieved in nine of ten patients with an average follow-up of 15 months. A variety of parameters, such as the timing of ICG administration with respect to laser therapy, the optimal laser parameters, and the effect of diode laser alone compared to diode laser with ICG enhancement, require further investigation. Evaluation of ICG dye–enhanced diode laser photocoagulation with prospective controlled clinical trials is necessary to assess its effect on the visual outcome and the natural history of choroidal neovascularization in AMD.

Photodynamic Therapy

Photodynamic therapy (PDT) requires administration of an exogenous photosensitizing agent that is activated upon absorption of low-intensity light of an appropriate wavelength. A photochemical interaction between the photosensitizer and light leads to in situ production of singlet oxygen and superoxide anions that interact with cellular components.[34] This results in cellular damage and vascular thrombosis and occlusion in the target tissue.[35] PDT produces selective tissue damage, as the photosensitizer preferentially concentrates and is retained longer in hyperproliferating and neoplastic tissues than in surrounding normal tissue.[36] Thermal damage to adjacent normal tissues is avoided by direct application of low-intensity light. The wavelength of light used depends on absorption spectrum of the photosensitizer.

PDT is currently being investigated to treat a variety of systemic and cutaneous malignancies. Most medical experience with PDT has been with the photosensitizer hematoporphyrin derivative (HPD) and its derivatives. HPD preferentially localizes in tumors and absorbs at 624 nm. New photosensitizers have been synthesized that are activated by longer wavelength light and potentially have more selective target tissue uptake with diminished cutaneous photosensitivity. The longer wavelength absorption may improve penetration through tissues, pigment, and blood and be activated by low-energy diode sources. These agents include chloroaluminum sulfonated phthalocyanine (CASPc), benzoporphyrin derivative monoacid (BPD-MA), and tin etiopurpurin (SnET2), which are activated by light of 675, 692, and 664 nm, respectively.[37]

PDT is well suited for ophthalmologic applications due to the optical properties of the eye and the accessibility of the eye to light irradiation by the transpupillary route. PDT has been used in humans to treat retinoblastoma and melanomas of the choroid, ciliary body, and iris. HPD has been utilized with variable success in small series of patients with choroidal, ciliary body, and iris melanomas. Clinical regression has been obtained in some patients with lightly pigmented small- and medium-sized melanomas.[38] Retinoblastomas without vitreous seeds initially responded to PDT; however, the therapeutic effect did not persist long term. Vitreous seeds of retinoblastoma did not respond to PDT, possibly due to lack of HPD concentration or insufficient oxygen availability.[39] CASPc and BPD-MA have successfully produced regression of experimental choroidal melanomas in rabbits.[40,41] It has been demonstrated that vascular injury plays a major role in tumor destruction following PDT, and endothelial cells are particularly sensitive to the effects of photosensitization.[37] This effect is potentially useful to permit selective treatment of ocular neovascularization. In animal models, PDT with SnET2, CASPc and BPD-MA has successfully produced closure of experimental choroidal neovascularization in primates.[42–44]

Short Pulse Lasers

Laser output may be delivered at a continuous power level, in a single pulse, or as a series of pulses. The pulse mode allows energy to be concentrated and delivered over a short time period, resulting in average and peak powers. The rate of energy delivery is equal to energy measured in joules divided by pulse duration in seconds. Short laser pulses can confine injury to absorbing structures at pulse energies below the threshold energy for single-pulse damage. To avoid the high peak temperature achieved by a single short pulse, multiple subthreshold pulses are applied to compensate for the lower pulse energy. Selective RPE damage was produced in rabbits using multiple subthreshold short laser exposures (514 nm, 5 μsec, 1 to 500 pulses at 500 Hz, 2 to 10 μJ pulse energy) with minimal effect on the adjacent neurosensory retina and choroid.[45] Lesions were often not visible clinically due to decreased damage to the adjacent neurosensory retina.[46] Ultrashort laser pulses in the femtosecond range (1 fsec = 10^{-15} second) produce extremely high peak laser intensity with minimal pulse energy. Retinal damage mechanisms and thresholds produced by a single 80-fsec laser pulse (625 nm) have been evaluated in rabbits.[47] The ultrashort pulse has lower energy and produced fewer nonspecific thermal effects due to nonlinear damage mechanisms.

Selective Photothermolysis

Selective photothermolysis describes a method where selective thermal injury is determined by the unique properties of the target tissue, rather than precise aiming of the laser beam.[48] After exposure to laser energy, the target tissue dissipates heat by conduction to surrounding tissues. Selective target heating may be achieved when the energy is deposited at a rate faster than the rate of cooling. In order to achieve this effect, the pulse duration must be equal to or less than the target's thermal relaxation time. The length of exposure is determined by the size of the target. A wavelength that reaches and is preferentially absorbed by the target structure and a fluence sufficient to cause thermal damage are also required. This method has produced selective damage to blood vessels (577 nm, 3.0 × 10^{-7} second) and melanocytes (351 nm, 2.0 × 10^{-8} second), and in principle, this technique may be applicable at the subcellular level.[49]

Further studies are required to evaluate the effect of different laser wavelengths for therapy of retinal diseases. New developments in laser technology may increase the specificity of tissue damage, possibly to the cellular or subcellular level. While the desired histopathologic result is selective destruction of retinal pathology without adjacent tissue damage, the significance with respect to visual acuity remains to be determined.

REFERENCES

1. Huang D, Swanson EA, Lin CP, et al: Optical coherence tomography. Science 254:1178–1181, 1991.
2. Pavlin CJ, Sherar MD, Foster FS: Subsurface ultrasound microscopic imaging of the intact eye. Ophthalmology 97: 244–250, 1990.
3. Pavlin CJ, Harasiewicz K, Sherar MD, Foster FS: Clinical use of ultrasound biomicroscopy. Ophthalmology 98:287–295, 1990.
4. The Laser Institute of America: American National Standard for the Safe Use of Lasers. Toledo, OH, The Institute. 186;34 (ANSI 136:1, 1986).
5. Hee MR, Puliafito CA, Wong C, et al: Optical coherence tomography of macular holes. Ophthalmology 102:748–756, 1995.
6. Hee MR, Izatt JA, Swanson EA, et al: Optical coherence tomography of the human retina. Arch Ophthalmol 113: 325–332, 1995.
7. Hee MR, Puliafito CA, Wong C, et al: Quantitative assessment of macular edema with optical coherence tomography. Arch Ophthalmol 113:1019–1029, 1995.
8. Puliafito CA, Hee MR, Schuman JS, Fujimoto JG: Macular diseases. In Optical Coherence Tomography of Ocular Diseases. New Jersey, SLACK Incorporated, 1996, pp 37–289.
9. Izatt JA, Hee MR, Swanson EA, et al: Micrometer-scale resolution imaging of the anterior eye in vivo with optical coherence tomography. Arch Ophthalmol 112:1584–1589, 1994.
10. Schuman JS, Pedut-Kloizman T, Hee MR, et al: Quantification of nerve fiber layer thickness in normal and glaucomatous eyes using optical coherence tomography. Arch Ophthalmol 113:586–596, 1995.
11. Schuman JS, Hee MR, Arya AV, et al: Optical coherence tomography. A new tool for glaucoma diagnosis. Curr Opin Ophthalmol 6:89–95, 1995.
12. Gass JDM: Reappraisal of biomicroscopic classification of stages of development of a macular hole. Am J Ophthalmol 119:752–759, 1995.
13. Gass JDM, Jooneph BC: Observations concerning patients with suspected impending macular holes. Am J Ophthalmol 109:638–646, 1990.
14. Gass JDM: Idiopathic senile macular hole: its early stages and pathogenesis. Arch Ophthalmol 106:629–639, 1988.

15. Duker JS, Puliafito CA, Wilkins JR, et al: Imaging fellow eyes in patients diagnosed with idiopathic macular holes using optical coherence tomography (OCT). American Academy of Ophthalmology Annual Meeting, Atlanta, GA, 1995, p 118.

16. Nussenblatt RB, Kaufman SC, Palestine AG, et al: Macular thickening and visual acuity. Ophthalmology 94:1134–1139, 1987.

17. Hee MR, Puliafito CA, Wong C, et al: Optical coherence tomography of central serous chorioretinopathy. Am J Ophthalmol 120:65–74, 1995.

18. Puliafito CA, Hee MR, Baumal CR, et al: Optical coherence tomography of age-related macular degeneration and choroidal neovasularization. Invest Ophthalmol Vis Sci 37 (Suppl):S956, 1996.

19. Gorin MB: Von Hippel-Lindau disease: clinical considerations and the use of fluorescein-potentiated argon laser therapy for treatment of retinal angiomas. Semin Ophthalmol 7:182–191, 1992.

20. Schneider A, Kaboth A, Neuhauser L: Detection of subretinal neovascular membranes with indocyanine green and an infrared scanning laser ophthalmoscope. Am J Ophthalmol 113:45–51, 1992.

21. Destro M, Puliafito CA: Indocyanine green videoangiography of choroidal neovascularization. Ophthalmology 96:846–853, 1989.

22. Guyer DR, Puliafito CA, Mones JM, et al: Digital indocyanine-green angiography in chorioretinal disorders. Ophthalmology 99:287–291, 1992.

23. Guyer DR, Yanuzzi LA, Slakter JS, et al: Digital indocyanine-green videoangiography of occult choroidal neovascularization. Ophthalmology 101:1727–1737, 1994.

24. Lim JI, Sternberg P Jr, Capone A Jr, et al: Selective use of indocyanine green angiography for occult choroidal neovascularization. Am J Ophthalmol 120:75–82, 1995.

25. Puliafito CA, Deutsch T, Boll J, To K: Semiconductor laser endophotocoagulation of the retina. Arch Ophthalmol 105:424–427, 1987.

26. McHugh JDA, Marshall J, Capon M, et al: Transpupillary retinal photocoagulation in the eyes of rabbit and humans using a diode laser. Lasers Light Ophthalmol 2:125–143, 1988.

27. Duker JS, Federman JL, Schubert H, Talbot C: Semiconductor diode laser endophotocoagulation. Ophthalmic Surg 20:717–719, 1989.

28. Balles MW, Puliafito CA, D'Amico DJ, et al: Semiconductor diode laser photocoagulation for retinal vascular disease. Ophthalmology 97:1553–1561, 1990.

29. Bressler SB, Bressler NM, Fine SL, et al: Natural course of choroidal neovascularization in the foveal avascular zone in senile macular degeneration. Am J Ophthamol 93:157–163, 1982.

30. Macular Photocoagulation Study Group: Laser photocoagulation of subfoveal neovascular lesions in age-related macular degeneration. Arch Ophthalmol 109:1220–1231, 1991.

31. Reichel E, Puliafito CA, Duker JS, Guyer DR: Indocyanine green dye-enhanced laser photocoagulation of poorly defined subfoveal choroidal neovascularization. Ophthalmic Surg 25:195–201, 1994.

32. Balles MW, Puliafito CA, Kliman GH, et al: Indocyanine green dye enhanced diode laser photocoagulation of subretinal neovascular membranes. Invest Ophthalmol Vis Sci 31(Suppl):282, 1990.

33. Matsumoto M, Miki T, Obana A, et al: Choroidal damage in dye-enhanced photocoagulation. Lasers Light Ophthalmol 5:157–165, 1993.

34. Weishaupt KR, Gomer CJ, Dougherty TJ: Identification of singlet oxygen as the cytotoxic agent in photo-inactivation of murine tumor. Cancer Res 36:2326–2329, 1976.

35. Nelson JS, Liaw LH, Orenstein A: Mechanism of tumor destruction following photodynamic therapy with hematoporphyrin derivative, chlorin and phthalocyanine. J Natl Cancer Inst 80:1599–1605, 1988.

36. Henderson BW, Dougherty TJ: How does photodynamic therapy work? Photochem Photobiol 55:145–157, 1992.

37. Fisher AMR, Murphree AL, Gomer CJ: Clinical and preclinical photodynamic therapy. Lasers Surg Med 17:2–31, 1995.

38. Favilla I, Barry WR, Gosbell A, et al: Phototherapy of posterior uveal melanomas. Br J Ophthalmol 75:718–721, 1992.

39. Murphee AL, Cote M, Gomer CP: The evolution of photodynamic therapy in the treatment of intraocular tumors. Photochem Photobiol 46:919–923, 1987.

40. Panagopoulos JA, Svitra PP, Puliafito CA, Gragoudas ES: Photodynamic therapy for experimental intraocular melanoma using chloroaluminum sulfonated phthalocyanine. Arch Ophthalmol 107:886–890, 1989.

41. Schmidt-Erfurth U, Bauman W, Gragoudas E, et al: Photodynamic therapy of experimental choroidal melanoma using lipoprotein-delivered benzoporphyrin. Ophthalmology 101:89–99, 1994.

42. Kliman GH, Puliafito CA, Stern D, et al: Phthalocyanine photodynamic therapy: new strategy for closure of choroidal neovascularization. Lasers Surg Med 15:2–10, 1994.

43. Miller JM, Walsh AW, Kramer M, et al: Photodynamic therapy of experimental choroidal neovascularization using lipoprotein-delivered benzoporphyrin. Arch Ophthalmol 113:810–818, 1995.

44. Baumal CR, Puliafito CA, Pieroth L, et al: Photodynamic therapy of experimental choroidal neovascularization with tin ethyl etiopurpurin. Invest Ophthalmol Vis Sci 37(Suppl):S122, 1996.

45. Roider J, Hillenkamp F, Flotte T, Birngruber R: Microphotocoagulation: selective effects of repetitive short laser pulses. Proc Natl Acad Sci USA 90:8643–8647, 1993.

46. Roider J, Michaud NA, Flotte TJ, Birngruber R: Response of the retinal pigment epithelium to selective photocoagulation. Arch Ophthalmol 110:1786–1792, 1993.

47. Birngruber R, Puliafito CA, Gawande A, et al: Femtosecond laser-tissue interactions: retinal injury studies. IEEE J Quantum Electronics QE-23:1836–1844, 1987.

48. Parrish JA, Deutsch TF: Laser photomedicine. IEEE J Quantum Electronics QE-20:1386–1396, 1984.

49. Anderson RR, Parrish JA: Selective photothermolysis: precise microsurgery by selective absorption of pulsed radiation. Science 220:524–527, 1983.

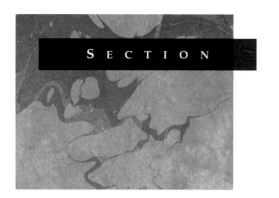

SECTION

II

*Macular
Disorders*

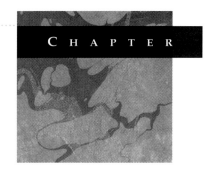

CHAPTER 9

Nonneovascular (Nonexudative) Age-Related Macular Degeneration

Susan B. Bressler, M.D.
Daniel F. Rosberger, M.D., Ph.D.

Age-related macular degeneration (AMD) is the most common cause of legal blindness in the United States among persons 60 years of age and older.[1] In the recently published Third National Health and Nutrition Examination Survey, the prevalence of any fundus manifestations associated with AMD among Americans 40 years of age and older was 9.2%. This suggests a minimum of 8.5 million Americans are presently affected with this disease. Some racial and ethnic differences were observed with prevalence rates of 9.3% among whites, 7.4% among blacks, and 7.1% among Mexican-Americans.[2]

AMD has been classified into nonneovascular (dry or atrophic) and neovascular (wet or exudative) forms of the disease. Nonneovascular AMD, the topic of this chapter, includes abnormalities at the level of the retinal pigment epithelium (RPE)–Bruch's membrane–choriocapillaris complex that lead to a variety of clinical appearances characterized by drusen and pigmentary abnormalities including focal hyperpigmentation, RPE degeneration, and geographic atrophy. When choroidal neovascularization (CNV) and/or disciform scarring accompanies these fundus abnormalities, neovascular AMD has developed. Neovascular AMD is far less common than nonneovascular AMD with prevalence rates of 1.2% for neovascular AMD and 15.6% for nonneovascular AMD among adults age 43 to 86 in Beaver Dam, Wisconsin.[3] It is estimated that the most severe manifestation of nonneovascular AMD, geographic atrophy, is present in 0.6% of adults[3] and is responsible for between 12 and 21% of the blindness caused by AMD,[4] whereas neovascular disease is responsible for the balance.[4–6] However, it is likely that the nonneovascular form of AMD accounts for a much greater percentage of the mild to moderate visual loss attributed to AMD.

Drusen, derived from the German word for nodules, were first described in 1855 by Donders.[7] Otto Haab is generally credited with first reporting the clinical appearance of atrophic pigmentary changes associated with central visual dysfunction in older patients.[8–10] In 1967, Gass proposed that drusen, atrophic macular degeneration, and disciform macular degeneration were a continuum of the same underlying disease.[11] Subsequent histopathologic studies have provided clinicopathologic confirmation of this concept. Unfortunately, a consensus definition and classification system of AMD has proved more elusive. Studies on AMD have lacked a uniform application of diagnostic criteria and nomenclature, and this has plagued the clinical, epidemiologic, and pathology literature. (Table 9–1). For example, the minimum age requirement for diagnosis has varied widely and different investigators have used a variety of diagnostic tools including visual acuity, perimetry, contrast sensitivity, scanning laser ophthalmoscopy, slit lamp biomicroscopy, black and white fundus photography, color fundus photography, and fluorescein and indocyanine-green (ICG) angiography to characterize the disease. This has led to significant variation between studies in the definitions and grading scales used for various stages in the disease process.[3,4,12–17]

Recently, an international classification and grading system for age-related maculopathy (ARM) and

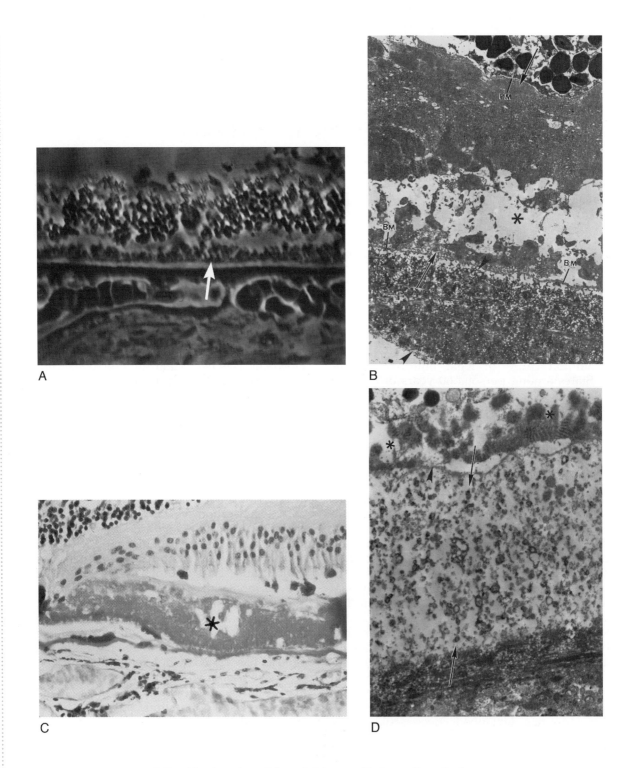

A

B

C

D

A, Basal laminar deposit (*arrow*), interposed between the retinal
pigment epithelium and Bruch's membrane, has an irregular
internal margin and is demonstrated here by phase contrast. *B*,
Ultrastructural appearance of a 9.6-μm-thick layer of basal laminar
deposit (*between arrows*) located between the plasma membrane
(PM) and basement membrane (BM) of the retinal pigment

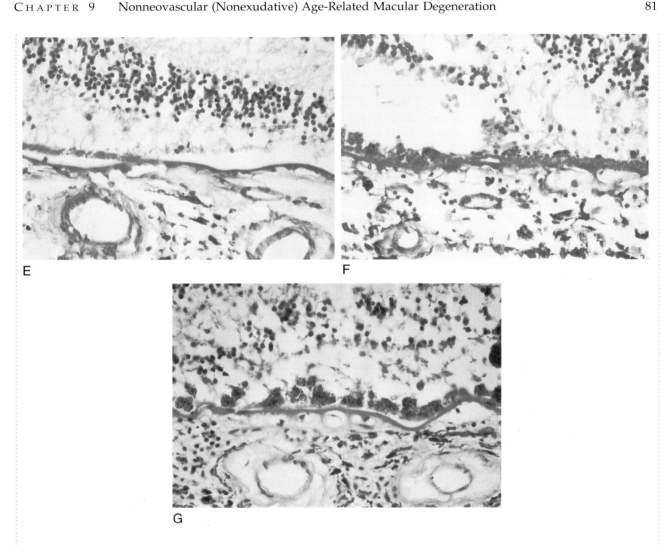

epithelium. A cleavage in this material (*asterisk*) has led to early detachment. Vesicular material (basal linear deposit) is present throughout Bruch's membrane (*between arrowheads*) (original magnification, × 9900). (From Green WR, Enger C: Age-related macular degeneration histopathologic studies. The 1993 Lorenz E. Zimmerman Lecture. Ophthalmology 100:1519–1535, 1993, with permission.) *C,* Basal linear deposit (diffuse drusen) (*asterisk*) is 25 µm thick and has associated atrophy of the retinal pigment epithelium and photoreceptor cell layer. *D,* Electron microscopic appearance of a 6.4-µm-thick basal linear deposit composed of vesicular material (*between arrows*) located between the retinal pigment epithelial basement (*arrowhead*) and the remainder of Bruch's membrane. A 2.2-µm-thick layer of wide-spaced collagen (basal laminar deposit) (*asterisks*) is present internal to the retinal pigment epithelial basement membrane (*arrowhead*) (original magnification, × 15,000). (From Green WR, Enger C: Age-related macular degeneration histopathologic studies. The 1993 Lorenz E. Zimmerman Lecture. Ophthalmology 100:1519–1535, 1993, with permission.) *E* through *G,* Age-related macular degeneration with areolar atrophy. Central area with loss of photoreceptor cell layer, retinal pigment epithelium, and basal laminar deposit (*E*). In the adjacent area there is loss of the photoreceptor cell layer and the retinal pigment epithelium but the basal laminar remains intact (*F*). All of the layers are intact peripheral to the above (*G*). (From Green WR, Enger C: Age-related macular degeneration histopathologic studies. The 1993 Lorenz E. Zimmerman Lecture. Ophthalmology 100:1519–1535, 1993, with permission.)

TABLE 9–1 Definitions of and Age Limits in ARM Used in Population-Based Studies*

1. *Framingham Eye Study*

An eye was diagnosed as having senile macular degeneration if its visual acruity was 20/30 or worse and the ophthalmologist designated the etiology of changes in the macula or posterior pole as senile.

Age limits: 52–85 years.

2. *National Health and Nutrition Eye Study*

Age-related macular degeneration: loss of macular reflex, pigment dispersion and clumping, and drusen associated with visual acuity of 20/25 or worse believed to be due to this disease.

Age-related disciform macular degeneration: choroidal hemorrhage and connective-tissue proliferation between retinal pigment epithelium and Bruch's membrane causing an elevation of the foveal retina (this condition should be differentiated from disciform degenerations of other causes, e.g., histoplasmosis, toxoplasmosis, angioid streaks, and high myopia).

Age-related circinate macular degeneration: perimacular accumulation of lipoid material within the retina.

Age limits: 1–74 years.

3. *Gisborne Study*

Senile macular degeneration: when the visual acuity in the affected eye was 6/9 (20/30) or worse and senile macular degeneration was identified as the probable cause of this visual loss.

Age: ≥65 years.

4. *Copenhagen Study*

Age-related macular degeneration (AMD): best corrected visual (Snellen) acuity (including pin hole improvement) of 6/9 or less, explained by age related morphologic changes of the macula.

Atrophic (dry) changes: disarrangement of the pigment epithelium (atrophy/clustering) and/or a small cluster of small drusen and/or medium drusen and/or large drusen and/or pronounced senile macular choroidal atrophy/sclerosis without general fundus involvement.

Exudative (wet) changes: elevation of the neurosensory retina and/or the pigment epithelium and/or hemorrhages, and/or hard exudates and/or fibrovascular tissue.

Age-related macular changes without visual impairment (AMCW) is defined as similar morphological lesions but without visual deterioration.

Age limits: 60–80 years.

5. *Chesapeake Bay Study*

No specific overall definition.

Geographic atrophy: an area of well-demarcated atrophy of the RPE in which the overlying retina appeared thin.

Chesapeake Bay Study, Continued

Exudative changes: choroidal neovascularization, detachments of the RPE, and disciform scarring.

Grading of AMD in 4 grades:

Grade 4: geographic atrophy of the RPE or exudative changes.

Grade 3: grade 4 or eyes with large or confluent drusen or eyes with focal hyperpigmentation of the RPE.

Grade 2: grade 4 or 3 or eyes with many small drusen (≥20) within 1500 μm of the foveal center.

Grade 1: Grade 4, 3, or 2 or eyes with at least five small drusen within 1500 μm of the foveal center or at least ten small drusen between 1500 and 3000 μm from the foveal center.

No visual acuity included.

Age limits: ≥30 years.

6. *Beaver Dam Eye Study*

Early age-related maculopathy was defined as the absence of signs of late age-related maculopathy as defined below and as the presence of soft indistinct or reticular drusen or by the presence of any drusen type except hard indistinct, with RPE degeneration or increased retinal pigment in the macular area. Late age-related maculopathy was defined as the presence of signs of exudative age-related macular degeneration or geographic atrophy.

The grade assigned for the participant was that of the more severely involved eye.

No visual acuity included.

Age limits: 43–86 years.

7. *Rotterdam Study*

All ARM changes had to be within a radius of 3000 μm of the foveola. No definition of early ARM, but separate prevalence figures for drusen and retinal pigment epithelial hyperpigmentations or hypopigmentations attributable to age-related causes.

Late ARM (is similar to AMD): the presence of atrophic AMD (well-demarcated area of RPE atrophy with visible choroidal vessels) and/or neovascular AMD (serous and/or hemorrhagic RPE detachment, and/or subretinal neovascular membrane and/or hemorrhage, and/or periretinal fibrous scar) attributable to age-related causes. In a participant the most severely involved eye was taken for the analysis.

No visual acuity included.

Age limits: ≥55 years.

* From Bird AC, Bressler NM, Bressler SB, et al: An international classification and grading system for age-related maculopathy and age-related macular degeneration. Surv Ophthalmol 39:367–374, 1995, with permission.

AMD has been proposed.[18] It defines ARM as a degenerative disorder of persons 50 years of age or older that is characterized by the following abnormalities in the macula: soft drusen 63 μm or larger, hyperpigmentation and/or hypopigmentation of the RPE, RPE and associated neurosensory detachment, (peri)retinal hemorrhages, geographic atrophy of the RPE, or (peri)retinal fibrous scarring in the absence of other retinal (vascular) disorders. Visual acuity is not a factor in the disease definition or classification scheme. Early ARM specifically applies to the presence of drusen and any of the aforementioned RPE abnormalities. The late stages of ARM, which include geographic atrophy, RPE detachment, choroidal neovascularization, and disciform scars, are also referred to as age-related macular degeneration (AMD). Extensive and specific standardization of grading methods and criteria were proposed to classify the condition when viewing stereoscopic color photographs of the macula (Table 9–2; Fig. 9–1). It is hoped that this internationally derived and accepted nosology will facilitate comparisons of future cross-sectional, longitudinal, and case-control epidemiologic studies in this field.

PATTERNS OF AGE-RELATED MACULOPATHY

A knowledge of the anatomic relationship of the choriocapillaris, Bruch's membrane, retinal pigment epithelium, and neurosensory retina is necessary to understand the clinical features and histopathology of macular degeneration. The neurosensory retina lies anterior to the RPE and is dependent upon it for nutrition, support, recycling, and disposal of waste products. Bruch's membrane is a five-layered structure interposed between the choroid and the RPE. The innermost layer is the basement membrane of the RPE and the outermost layer is the basement membrane of the choriocapillaris endothelium. The centermost layer consists of interrupted clumps of elastin that is sandwiched between two loose collagenous layers composed of typical fibrils in a random array. Posterior to Bruch's membrane is the choroid, with the choriocapillaris representing the innermost component of this vascular structure (see "Normal Anatomy" in Chapter 1).

Small, Hard Drusen

Small drusen have been alternatively defined as being less than 50 μm or less than 63 μm in diameter.[3,15,17,19] The latter definition has been adopted as the standard.[18] Typical small drusen appear as well-defined ("hard"), discrete, yellow-white deposits that are external to the RPE (Fig. 9–2). During fluorescein angiography, hard drusen behave as pin-point window defects. Histopathologic studies have demonstrated that small, hard drusen correspond to either single enlarged RPE cells with lipid accumulation[20] or represent focal deposits of periodic acid–Schiff (PAS)–positive hyaline material along the inner aspect of Bruch's membrane.[21] Ultrastructurally, they consist of aggregates of finely granular or amorphous material that contain tube-like structures, pale and bristle-coated vesicles, and sometimes abnormal collagen.[22] Given that these localized accumulations occur in the presence of otherwise histologically normal appearing Bruch's membrane argues that they are not a feature of a more generalized RPE–Bruch's membrane–choriocapillaris disease. The presence of small, hard drusen alone are not sufficient to diagnose early ARM or AMD because these deposits are ubiquitous. Small drusen are commonly present in adults of all ages by photographic identification,[3,15] they are noted in 87% of eyes examined postmortem in individuals older than 40 years of age,[23] and the new development of small drusen in an adult eye without prior evidence of hard drusen is not age dependent.[24] In contrast to large or soft drusen; small, hard drusen are not associated with an increased risk for the development of choroidal neovascularization[19] and they are not age related.[3,15]

Large, Soft Drusen

Large, soft drusen have been alternatively defined as greater than or equal to 50 μm or greater than or equal to 63 μm in diameter,[3,15,17,19] although the latter definition has been accepted as the standard.[18] Their borders are generally ill defined ("soft"), they vary in size and shape, and there may be decreasing density of the drusen noted from the center to the margin[15,18] (Fig. 9–3). Soft drusen have a tendency to cluster and merge with one another, demonstrating *confluence*. With fluorescein angiography, soft drusen hyperfluoresce early and either fade or stain in the late phase of the study. Persistent late staining, when it occurs, may correspond to pooling of dye within focal detachments of Bruch's membrane or staining of diffuse drusen material.

Three histopathologic types of soft drusen have been identified: (1) localized detachments of RPE and basal *linear* deposit (diffuse drusen) in eyes with diffuse basal *linear* deposit; (2) localized detachments of RPE and basal *laminar* deposit in eyes with diffuse basal *laminar* deposits; and (3) localized RPE detachment due to focal accumulation of basal *linear* deposit in eyes without diffuse basal *linear* deposit.[25,26] Basal *linear* deposits, also known as diffuse thickening of the inner aspect of Bruch's membrane, refers to material located external to the RPE basement membrane, lying within the inner collagenous zone of Bruch's membrane. Ultrastructurally, these deposits consist of granular and ve-

TABLE 9-2 Standardized Grading Criteria for AMD*

Grading of Drusen[†]

1.1 *Drusen morphology. Grade highest # present within outer circle.*
   0) absent
   1) questionable
   2) hard drusen (<C1, 125 μm)
   3) intermediate, soft drusen (>C0 ≤ C1; >63 μm ≤ 125 μm)
   4) large, soft distinct drusen (>C1, 125 μm)
   5) large, soft indistinctive drusen (>C1, 125 μm)
     5a) crystalline/calcified/glistening
     5b) semisolid
     5c) serogranular
   7) cannot grade, obscuring lesions
   8) cannot grade, photo quality

1.2 *Predominant drusen type within outer circle*
   0) absent
   1) questionable
   2) hard drusen (<C1, 125 μm)
   3) intermediate, soft drusen (>C0 ≤ C1; >63 μm ≤ 125 μm)
   4) large, soft distinct drusen (>C1, 125 μm)
   5) large, soft indistinct drusen (>C1, 125 μm)
     5a) crystalline/calcified/glistening
     5b) semisolid
     5c) serogranular
   7) cannot grade, obscuring lesions
   8) cannot grade, photo quality

1.3 *Number of drusen*
   0) absent
   1) questionable
   2) 1–9
   3) 10–19
   4) ≥20
   7) cannot grade, obscuring lesions
   8) cannot grade, photo quality

1.4 *Drusen size*
   1) <C_0 (<63 μm)
   2) ≥C_0 < C_1 (≥63 μm, <125 μm)
   3) ≥C_1 < C_2 (≥125 μm, <175 μm)
   4) ≥C_2 < C_3 (≥175 μm, <250 μm)
   5) ≥C_3 (≥250 μm)
   7) cannot grade, obscuring lesions
   8) cannot grade, photo quality

1.5 *Main location of drusen.* Drusen may not be central to indicated subfield, but may be more to periphery.
   1) outside outer circle (midperipheral subfield)
   2) in outer subfield
   3) in middle subfield
   4) in central subfield
     4a) outside fovea (center point)
     4b) in fovea
   7) cannot grade, obscuring lesions
   8) cannot grade, photo quality

1.6 *Area covered by drusen in subfield 1.5*
   1) <10%
   2) <25%
   3) <50%
   4) ≥50%

   7) cannot grade, obscuring lesions
   8) cannot grade, photo quality

Hyperpigmentation and Hypopigmentation of the Retina[†]

Hyperpigmentation
   0) absent
   1) questionable
   2) present <C_0 (<63 μm)
   3) present ≥C_0 (≥63 μm)
   7) cannot grade, obscuring lesions
   8) cannot grade, photo quality

Hypopigmentation
   0) absent
   1) questionable
   2) present <C_0 (<63 μm)
   3) present ≥C_0 (≥63 μm)
   7) cannot grade, obscuring lesions
   8) cannot grade, photo quality

Main location hyper/hypopigmentation. This may not be central to indicated subfield, but may be more to periphery. Choose most central location.
   1) outside outer circle (midperipheral subfield)
   2) in outer subfield
   3) in middle subfield
   4) in central subfield
     4a) outside fovea (center point)
     4b) in fovea
   7) cannot grade, obscuring lesions
   8) cannot grade, photo quality

Geographic Atrophy[†]

Presence
   0) absent
   1) questionable
   2) present: ≥C_2
   7) cannot grade, obscuring lesions
   8) cannot grade, photo quality

Location. Choose most central location.
   1) outside outer circle (midperipheral subfield)
   2) in outer subfield
   3) in middle subfield
   4) in central subfield
     4a) outside fovea (center point)
     4b) in fovea
   7) cannot grade, obscuring lesions
   8) cannot grade, photo quality

Area covered
   1) ≥C_2 < C_3 (≥175 μm < 250 μm)
   2) ≥C_3 < C_4 (≥250 μm < 500 μm)
   3) ≥C_4 and <1000 μm (~central circle of grid)
   4) ≥1000 μm and <3000 μm (~middle circle)
   5) ≥3000 μm and <6000 μm (~outer circle)
   6) >6000 μm
   7) cannot grade, obscuring lesions
   8) cannot grade, photo quality

Table continued on opposite page

TABLE 9–2 *Continued*

Neovascular AMD†

Presence
  0) absent
  1) questionable
  2) present
  7) cannot grade, obscuring lesions
  8) cannot grade, photo quality
Typifying features
  1) hard exudates
  2) serous neuroretinal detachment
  3) serous RPE detachment
  4) hemorrhagic RPE detachment
  5) retinal hemorrhage
    5a) subretinal
    5b) in plane of retina
    5c) subhyaloid
    5d) intravitreal
  6) scar/glial/fibrous tissue
    6a) subretinal
    6b) preretinal

  7) cannot grade, obscuring lesions
  8) cannot grade, photo quality
Location. Choose most central location.
  1) outside outer circle (midperipheral subfield)
  2) in outer subfield
  3) in middle subfield
  4) in central subfield
    4a) not underlying (in) fovea (center point)
    4b) underlying (in) fovea
  7) cannot grade, obscuring lesions
  8) cannot grade, photo quality
Area covered
  1) $\geq C_2 < C_3$ (≥ 175 µm < 250 µm)
  2) $\geq C_3 < C_4$ (≥ 250 µm < 500 µm)
  3) $\geq C_4$ and <1000 µm (~central circle of grid)
  4) ≥ 1000 µm and <3000 µm (~middle circle)
  5) ≥ 3000 µm and <6000 µm (~outer circle)
  6) >6000 µm
  7) cannot grade, obscuring lesions
  8) cannot grade, photo quality

* From Bird AC, Bressler NM, Bressler SB, et al: An international classification and grading system for age-related maculopathy and age-related macular degeneration. Surv Ophthalmol 39:367–374, 1995, with permission.
† In some categories, numbers are missing due to similar use of 7) and 8).

sicular lipid-rich material and may contain wide-spaced collagen. In contrast, basal *laminar* deposits are situated between the plasma membrane and the basement membrane of the RPE and mainly consist of wide-spaced collagen.[27] Differentiating basal *linear* and basal *laminar* deposit by light microscopy is difficult, although basal *laminar* deposit may be seen as a PAS-positive brush-like deposit along the inner aspect of the RPE basement membrane. These

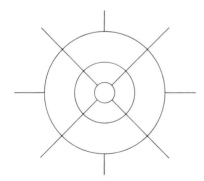

FIGURE 9–1 Standard grid for ARM/AMD classification. For a 30-degree fundus camera the diameter of the central, middle, and outer circle is 1000, 3000, and 6000 µm, respectively. These circles represent the central, middle, and outer subfields, respectively. The midperipheral subfield is outside the outer circle within field 2. The spokes may be of help in centering the grid on the macula and in estimating the length of a lesion. (From Klein R, Davis MD, Magli YL, et al: The Wisconsin age-related maculopathy grading system. Ophthalmology 98:1128–1134, 1991, with permission.)

diffuse histopathologic and associated electron microscopic abnormalities may not be visible clinically and can extend well beyond visible soft drusen. Clinically, soft drusen are identified whenever there is sufficient RPE hypopigmentation or atrophy overlying diffuse Bruch's membrane thickening, or, when there are focal detachments within this material. These findings suggest that the clinical identification of large or soft drusen identifies an eye with diffuse changes at the RPE–Bruch's membrane complex.

Soft drusen are present in 13 to 20% of American adults,[3,15] although the prevalence of soft drusen is significantly age related, with prevalence rates of 44% in individual age 75 and older as compared to 7% among those age 43 to 54.[3] Large drusen may also spontaneously regress or disappear over time.[24,28]

The presence of soft drusen alone is sufficient to make a diagnosis of AMD because both the incidence and prevalence of soft drusen are age related,[3,15,24,28] and the presence of soft drusen confers an increased risk for the subsequent development of RPE abnormalities,[24] geographic atrophy,[24] and CNV.[19,24,29] Similarly, elderly eyes with choroidal neovascularization or disciform scarring are often noted histopathologically to contain soft drusen with diffuse thickening of the inner portion of Bruch's membrane.[21,27,30,31]

The risk of severe vision loss in eyes with soft drusen is most closely related to the development

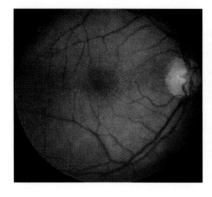 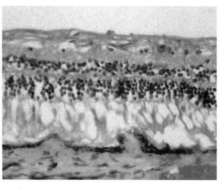

FIGURE 9-2   Hard drusen in this eye are characteristically small, well demarcated, and located primarily in the central macula. (From Bressler NM, Bressler SB, Fine SL: Age-related macular degeneration. Surv Ophthalmol 32:375–413, 1988, with permission.)

of choroidal neovascularization. Retrospective analyses of patients with bilateral drusen have suggested that eyes with large drusen are more apt to develop CNV as compared to eyes without large drusen. One prospective study of patients age 65 and older with bilateral drusen (nearly all of whom had large drusen) identified cumulative incidence rates of 6% at 1 year and 18% at 3 years for the development of neovascular AMD in at least one eye.[32] Geographic atrophy developed in 3% of these participants by 1 year and 8% by 3 years. However, the rate at which an eye with soft drusen progresses to CNV appears to be much faster if the contralateral eye of the patient manifests neovascular AMD. In a 5-year prospective study of fellow eyes of patients with unilateral neovascular AMD who participated in the extrafoveal AMD trial of the Macular Photocoagulation Study (MPS), eyes without large drusen or focal pigment had a 10% risk for the development of choroidal neovascularization, whereas eyes with large drusen had a 30% risk for developing CNV.[19] Subsequent analyses on a larger number of fellow eyes among the individuals participating in the juxtafoveal and subfoveal AMD trials of the MPS have confirmed the heightened risk associated with large drusen and permitted further quantification of that risk. In these later studies fellow eyes with large drusen had a 46% chance of developing CNV within 5 years.[29] Severe visual loss in fellow eyes with nonneovascular AMD at baseline occurred almost exclusively in those eyes that developed choroidal neovascularization during follow-up. Among the fellow eyes that did not develop choroidal neovascularization,

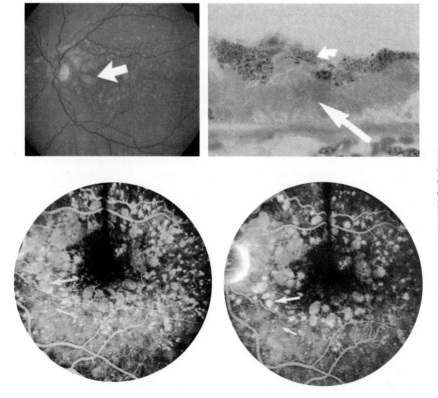

FIGURE 9-3   Soft drusen are larger; have amorphous, poorly demarcated borders that often merge into one another; and are occasionally accompanied by clumps of focal hyperpigmentation (arrow). (From Bressler NM, Bressler SB, Fine SL: Age-related macular degeneration. Surv Ophthalmol 32:375–413, 1988, with permission.)

the average visual acuity loss over the 5-year follow-up period was only 0.4 lines of vision.[33]

Nongeographic Atrophy of the RPE or RPE Degeneration

Nongeographic atrophy of the RPE or RPE degeneration is characterized by pigment mottling and stippled hypopigmentation with thinning of the overlying neurosensory retina (Fig. 9–4).[15] These abnormalities may precede geographic atrophy and have been referred to as "incipient atrophy."[10,34] Fluorescein angiography in areas of RPE degeneration reveals diffuse hyperfluorescence with a pattern of reticular or punctate blockage corresponding to the pigment clumping.[10] Histopathology demonstrates mottled areas of RPE hypopigmentation or atrophy overlying diffuse basal linear and basal laminar deposits.[26]

Nongeographic atrophy is reported to occur in 8 to 10% of adult Americans.[3,15] Incidence and prevalence rates of RPE depigmentation are age dependent,[3,24] and the likelihood of developing nongeographic atrophy is greater among eyes with large drusen.[24] Similarly, eyes that have nongeographic atrophy are more apt to develop other signs of AMD including soft drusen, geographic atrophy, and CNV.[24] Lastly, patients with unilateral neovascular maculopathy who undergo laser photocoagulation for CNV are more likely to manifest recurrent CNV following laser treatment if their fellow eye has nonneovascular AMD with areas of nongeographic atrophy.[35]

Focal Hyperpigmentation

Focal hyperpigmentation of the retinal pigment epithelium is defined as clinically evident pigment clumping at the level of the outer retina or subretinal space (Fig. 9–3). It may be punctate, linear, or reticular in shape and is present in 3 to 12% of adults.[3,15] During fluorescein angiography, these areas focally block background choroidal fluorescence. Although it has been suggested that focal hyperpigmentation identified on color fundus photographs may represent RPE disturbances overlying existing occult choroidal neovascularization,[36] clinicopathologic correlation has demonstrated intraretinal and subretinal pigment migration overlying diffuse thickening of the inner aspect of Bruch's membrane without evidence of choroidal neovascularization.[26]

Incidence and prevalence rates of focal hyperpigmentation increase with age,[3,24,28] and eyes with soft or large drusen are more likely to develop increased retinal pigment.[24] The presence of focal hyperpigmentation in an eye increases the probability that soft drusen or geographic atrophy will develop over time.[24] In addition, increased retinal pigment in an eye with nonneovascular AMD confers an increased risk for progression to the neovascular phase of the disease, particularly when present in conjunction with large drusen.[19,24,26,33,37] Fellow eyes of individuals with unilateral neovascular maculopathy have a 58 to 73% chance of developing CNV within 5 years if the macula has both large drusen and focal hyperpigment at presentation.[19,29]

Geographic Atrophy of the RPE

Geographic atrophy (GA) of the retinal pigment epithelium (also called areolar atrophy) represents an advanced form of nonneovascular AMD accounting for 12 to 21% of the cases of legal blindness attributed to AMD.[4–6] The term "geographic atrophy" was introduced by Gass and describes one or more discrete areas of absent or attenuated RPE forming an areolar pattern.[38] The neurosensory retina thins overlying areas of geographic atrophy, and there is atrophy of underlying choriocapillaris such that visualization of large-caliber choroidal vessels becomes prominent within these zones (Fig.

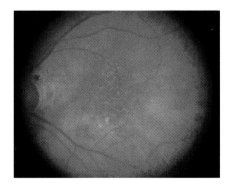

FIGURE 9–4   Nongeographic atrophy refers to a finding of tiny mottled areas of hypo- and hyperpigmentation that may show some thinning of the overlying sensory retina. (From Bressler SB, Bressler NM, Gragoudas ES: Age-related macular degeneration: drusen and geographic atrophy. In: Principles and Practice of Ophthalmology. Albert DM, Jakobiec FA [eds]: WB Saunders, Philadelphia, 1993, p 826–833, with permission.)

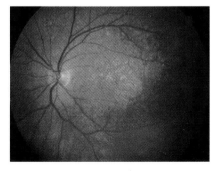

FIGURE 9–5   Fundus with geographic atrophy demonstrating well-demarcated areas of RPE atrophy through which the larger choroidal vessels may be seen. (From Bressler NM, Bressler SB, Fine SL: Age-related macular degeneration. Surv Ophthalmol 32:375–413, 1988, with permission.)

9–5).[30] A minimum area of involvement is recommended before classifying an area as geographic atrophy because lesions with a diameter of less than 175 μm are too small to confidently determine the loss of RPE and choriocapillaris.[18]

Fluorescein angiography reveals early bright and discrete hyperfluorescence within zones of geographic atrophy, as background choroidal fluorescence is easily transmitted through the absent or attenuated RPE. The choriocapillaris may fill slowly or be entirely absent within these zones and the size and shape of the area does not change during the study. In the late phase of the angiogram there is persistent hyperfluorescent staining within geographic atrophy because of increased visibility of choroidal and scleral tissue staining.

Clinically, geographic atrophy may arise from one of three fundus patterns of nonneovascular AMD.[34,39] Areas of confluent large, soft drusen may regress and leave behind irregularly shaped areas of geographic atrophy. These areas eventually enlarge and coalesce with other similarly derived areas and ring the fovea. Small foci of reticulated hypo- and hyperpigmented mottling of the RPE (nongeographic atrophy) within the macula may progress to a single area of geographic atrophy that then spreads contiguously in a horseshoe configuration, surrounding the fovea and later encompassing it. Lastly, spontaneous flattening of a pigment epithelial detachment can result in geographic atrophy.

Histopathologic examination of soft drusen has demonstrated replacement of drusen material by dystrophic calcification.[34] Dystrophic calcification has been identified clinically as bright, glistening yellow specks within drusen. Within these zones of dystrophic calcification the overlying RPE may progressively atrophy, the underlying choroidal vessels may become sclerotic with thickening of the intercapillary septae, and a zone of geographic atrophy may emerge.[21] Within areas of geographic atrophy there is also loss of the overlying photoreceptors, which accounts for the central visual field and acuity loss that occurs in these eyes.

Geographic atrophy is far less common than the other manifestations of nonneovascular AMD. In the Beaver Dam Eye Study, GA was identified in at least one eye of 0.6% of participants.[3] However, the prevalence of GA increases significantly with age, since 2 to 3% of participants age 75 and older had GA. The development of GA is also less common than the development of drusen and pigmentary abnormalities, with an incidence rate of 0.3% over a 5-year period.[24] Once again, these rates were significantly affected by age, as individuals 75 years of age or older were 17 times more likely to develop GA as compared to individuals who were younger.

Several authors have studied eyes with GA to learn more about the natural course of this manifestation of AMD and to quantify the rate of enlargement of the atrophic areas.[34,39,40] Schatz and McDonald studied 50 eyes with geographic atrophy among which 40% had multifocal areas of atrophy.[39] The average greatest horizontal linear dimension of the geographic atrophy was 509 μm at presentation, with a range of 200 to 5300 μm. The greatest horizontal linear dimension was shown to expand at an average rate of 139 μm/year (approximately 1/10 of a disc diameter). Atrophic areas in patients under age 75 tended to progress faster than those in patients aged 75 and over. However, great variability was demonstrated, making it impossible to predict the magnitude and direction of greatest progression in an individual case. Sarks et al reported on a series of 208 eyes with geographic atrophy.[34] In their series geographic atrophy tended to start in a parafoveal location with foveal sparing in the early stages of the disease. When the atrophy had progressed to within 750 μm of the foveal center, the total average area affected was approximately 1 disc area (DA). Total involvement of the fovea occurred only in the later stages, such that the average affected area in eyes with complete geographic atrophy of the fovea measured more than 7 DAs. Patients affected with geographic atrophy often have bilateral and symmetric disease, although there may be differences in onset and progression rates between the two eyes.[34,39,40] In a prospective natural history study of 74 patients with bilateral GA by Sunness and colleagues, the median total area of involvement was 4.4 DA at presentation (range, 0.1 to 27.7 DA). There was a strong correlation between the two eyes of a patient for the size of the atrophic area. The median rate of spread of GA was 0.73 DA per year taking into account changes in all dimensions of an atrophic area. The median absolute difference in rates of progression between eyes of a patient was 0.38 DA per year.

Visual acuity loss may be gradual and progressive in eyes with geographic atrophy, with the degree of visual acuity impairment directly related to foveal involvement.[41] Since GA involves the foveal center late in the course of the process, visual acuity is a poor guide of the extent of atrophy or visual impairment a patient may have. In a study on 83 patients with bilateral GA and median visual acuity of 20/54 in the better-seeing eye, the majority reported difficulty reading, a need to use low-vision devices, difficulty seeing in a dim environment, trouble recognizing faces, and an awareness of a blurry area.[42] These vision symptoms remained frequent even in a subgroup of 39 patients with visual acuity better than 20/50 (median, 20/35). All patients had dense scotomas by SLO testing; therefore, scotomas from GA, even those that do not involve the fovea, may have a significant impact on visual function.

The precise rate at which GA patients lose visual acuity has recently been investigated in a prospective study of 74 eyes with GA and good visual acuity (>20/50), at presentation. One half of the study group doubled their visual angle (a loss of ≥3 lines of acuity) and one quarter quadrupled their visual angle (a loss of ≥6 lines of acuity) by the 2-year follow-up examination.[43] Reading speed, which was compromised in most of these patients at baseline, deteriorated during this same time period. Therefore, all eyes with GA, even those with a parafoveal location, are at high risk of significant vision impairment within a few years of presentation.

Patients with GA report gradual progression of their vision loss, even when a more precipitous loss of visual acuity is documented between visits as an atrophic area enlarges and involves more of the foveal center. Generally, patients with GA will use central fixation if there is a small foveal region without atrophy and eccentric fixation when the fovea is totally involved; however, as the atrophy progressively encroaches on the foveal center, these patients may go through a transitional period in which they alternate between central and eccentric fixation, and this gradual transfer of the fixation focus may explain the lack of perception of a sudden alteration in acuity.[44] Alternatively, the explanation may lie within the nature of the residual central vision in eyes with preservation of small foveal islands. As the foveal island progressively decreases in size, the size of the central visual field gets progressively smaller such that fewer words or facets of the visual image fit into the functional region, even though relatively good acuity with letters may be preserved. At the point at which the patient transfers their fixation to an eccentric locus, the amount of useful functional central retina may not provide better vision than the eccentric region.

Geographic atrophy appears to act as a barrier for choroidal neovascularization, such that choroidal neovascularization does not begin within and rarely progresses through atrophic areas. However, CNV may occur contiguous to these regions and course along the external perimeter of the area. Since patients with progressive geographic atrophy rarely complain of abrupt changes in visual function, any such change should prompt an investigation for the development of choroidal neovascularization. Forty-five to 49% of the fellow eyes with nonneovascular maculopathy and zones of geographic atrophy at study entry into the MPS AMD trials of laser photocoagulation progressed to CNV within 5 years.[29,33] Among 45 patients with unilateral GA and a fellow eye with neovascular maculopathy followed prospectively for natural history of GA, 23% developed CNV at the edge of GA within 2 years, whereas CNV did not develop in any of 92 patients with bilateral GA during the same time interval, suggesting that patients with bilateral GA without evidence of CNV are at low risk for developing CNV.[45]

TREATMENT

Although nonneovascular AMD can cause progressive visual loss, the blinding consequences of AMD are primarily related to the development of neo-

vascular AMD. Fellow eyes of patients with unilateral neovascular maculopathy followed prospectively in the Macular Photocoagulation Study had an average decrease in vision of 0.4 lines of acuity over 5 years if CNV did not develop during that period.[33] On the other hand, an average loss of 8 lines of acuity occurred if an eye progressed to neovascular maculopathy. Although laser treatment has been demonstrated to be of benefit in comparison to observation in select cases of choroidal neovascularization, in most eyes it only limits or postpones severe vision loss. Since there is no current treatment that restores vision function within areas of geographic atrophy, disciform scarring, or photocoagulation, the major means of limiting vision loss from AMD lies in prevention of the development and/or progression of the earlier forms of nonneovascular AMD.

Light Exposure

There has been speculation that ultraviolet or visible light may lead to the generation of reactive oxygen species in the outer retina or choroid[46,47] which may, in turn, cause lipid peroxidation of photoreceptor outer segment membranes potentially contributing to the development of AMD. Clinical studies in humans, however, have failed to provide much support for the theory that cumulative sunlight exposure is associated with AMD. The Chesapeake Bay Waterman Study found no association between cumulative ultraviolet or visible light exposure and the presence of large drusen or retinal pigment epithelial abnormalities.[48] There was, though, a significantly higher exposure to blue light and all wavelengths in the visible spectrum within the 20-year period, immediately preceding study participation among the eight participants with advanced AMD in the cohort when compared to age-matched control subjects.[49] In the Eye Disease Case Control Study (EDCCS), no positive relationship could be demonstrated between lifetime sunlight exposure and the presence of neovascular AMD.[50] In the Beaver Dam Eye Study, there was a limited association between light and AMD with increased summertime outdoor exposure being associated with increased retinal pigment among male subjects and late ARM in male and female subjects.[51] The available data are inconsistent and inconclusive in regards to a relationship between light and AMD. Ultraviolet light has been shown to be associated with the development of lenticular opacities,[52] therefore, given that sunglasses are inexpensive and associated with few side effects, it seems reasonable not to discourage their use.

Antioxidants

Several observational epidemiologic studies have found an association between nonneovascular, neovascular, or both forms of age-related macular degeneration and cigarette smoking,[4,5,50,53-56] so possible prevention or amelioration of age-related macular degeneration would seem to be an additional reason to recommend that patients discontinue smoking. Similarly, although there are inconsistent data with regard to the association of age-related macular degeneration and hypertension, cardiovascular disease, and increased cholesterol and saturated fat intake,[5,12,50,53-55,57,58] it would seem reasonable to recommend that patients undergo routine regular medical examinations with a generalist physician to monitor blood pressure and cholesterol levels and screen for other treatable cardiovascular disease.

Cross-sectional and case-control epidemiologic investigations have explored the hypothesis that an enriched antioxidant status may be associated with a decreased risk of AMD. This hypothesis stems from the suggestion that AMD may be caused by cumulative oxidative insults. Data from the first National Health and Nutrition Examination Survey (NHANES I) found that individuals with diets rich in fruits and vegetables, particularly those substances containing vitamin A, were less apt to have AMD.[12] This study did not measure blood levels of carotenoids or other antioxidant micronutrients. Subsequent studies have determined serum or blood levels of antioxidant substances in age-matched individuals with and without AMD. The EDCCS compared 421 patients with neovascular AMD and 615 age-matched patients without evidence of AMD with respect to serum levels and dietary consumption histories of specific antioxidant micronutrients. No statistically significant association was found between serum levels of vitamin C, vitamin E, or selenium and AMD.[59] However, participants with medium and higher serum levels of carotenoids were less likely to have neovascular AMD as were individuals with a higher "antioxidant index" (a combination of measurements for carotenoids, vitamin C, vitamin E, and selenium). High dietary consumption of carotenoid food sources was also inversely associated with neovascular AMD in this study.[60] On the other hand, consumption of foods rich in vitamin E were not associated with any statistical risk reduction, whereas foods rich in vitamin C afforded a marginal risk reduction.

The Baltimore Longitudinal Study of Aging (BLSA) represents a cross-sectional evaluation of 976 participants enrolled in a study that investigates the normal or physiologic changes of aging. The relationship between fasting plasma levels of retinol, vitamin C, vitamin E, and betacarotene and AMD were explored in this cohort.[61] Individuals with higher levels of vitamin E were less likely to have any evidence of AMD. Additionally, an increased antioxidant index, composed of levels of vitamin C, vitamin E, and betacarotene, was also associated with a lower risk for AMD. No significant protective effect was seen for any of the micronutrients under investigation and advanced AMD (CNV and GA), although there were too few cases of severe AMD to address this question adequately. Participants with and without AMD were as likely to report use of dietary vitamin supplements.

In contrast to the findings of the EDCCS and the BLSA, a nested case-control study within the Beaver Dam population-based cohort found similar average carotenoid or vitamin E levels between participants with and without AMD. Only low levels of one serum carotenoid, lycopene, was related to an increased likelihood of AMD.[62]

In summary, the data from these various observational epidemiologic studies are compatible with a small to moderate protective role of micronutrient antioxidants on varying levels of AMD. However, the results for specific nutrients and specific AMD types have been inconsistent and, therefore, inconclusive. These studies also have several important limitations. Dietary consumption histories may be imprecise, blood levels may reflect recent behaviors rather than general stores, blood levels may not reflect tissue levels, and the likely effects of uncontrolled confounding. A cause-and-effect relationship cannot be concluded from these types of studies.

One small prospective study evaluated short-term oral zinc supplementation in patients with nonneovascular AMD as a means of decreasing vision loss. This study reported reductions in vision loss among treated patients when compared to an unusually high rate of vision loss among placebo-supplemented patients when followed for a period of up to 2 years.[63] Long-term results in a larger number of patients are needed to potentially confirm and extend these observations. Meanwhile, epidemiologic studies have been unable to demonstrate a relationship between serum zinc levels and signs of AMD.[50] Furthermore, a recently completed randomized prospective trial of oral zinc administration in patients with unilateral neovascular maculopathy failed to affect the natural course of the fellow eye with nonneovascular disease at study entry. Rates of CNV development, progression of drusen and RPE abnormalities, and change in visual acuity were similar in the zinc- and placebo-treated group during this 4-year study.[64]

Ultimately, the role of diet and nutritional supplementation in managing patients with nonneovascular AMD may be answered by the Age-Related Eye Disease Study (AREDS). AREDS is a multicenter, double-blind, placebo-controlled study supported by the National Institutes of Health (NIH) that is exploring rates of development and progression of AMD and age-related cataracts among Americans age 55 to 80. Combinations of antioxidant vitamins and minerals are being evaluated in this chemotherapeutic trial with careful monitoring of specific morphologic and vision end points, in addition to long-term morbidity and mortality data that may be associated with this in-

tervention. Two recently completed large randomized trials evaluating antioxidants as a means of
reducing lung cancer in patients at high risk found
that these agents, specifically betacarotene, were associated with a significantly greater risk of lung
cancer and mortality as compared to placebo.[65,66]
The widespread use of pharmacologic doses of antioxidants should be discouraged among AMD patients until their health claims have been substantiated and their long-term safety more firmly
established.

Photocoagulation

Another form of treatment presently under investigation in the management of eyes with nonneovascular AMD to potentially alter the course of the
disease is photocoagulation, either directly or adjacent to soft drusen. It had been observed that eyes
treated with laser photocoagulation for choroidal
neovascularization sometimes had drusen disappear in untreated macular areas.[67] In 1979, Cleasby
et al[68] described grid photocoagulation in the fellow
eyes of 29 patients with unilateral neovascular
maculopathy; 200 to 300 applications of 50 to 100
μm spots of argon laser were placed within a broad
ring around the fovea. During follow-up (average,
28.4 months), three patients developed CNV. The
same treatment technique was also applied in the
more advanced eye of 25 patients with bilateral
nonneovascular AMD. During follow-up (average,
27.3 months), no eye, treated or untreated, developed CNV and there was no difference in visual
acuity between treated and untreated eyes. All 25
treated eyes among the patients with bilateral nonneovascular AMD demonstrated a reduction in
drusen, whereas only five (25%) of the nontreated
fellow eyes of these patients demonstrated a similar
reduction.

In 1988, Wetzig presented a retrospective review
of 42 eyes of 27 patients in whom he had applied
laser treatment for extensive foveal soft drusen.[69]
Light scatter treatment of approximately 50 to 75
burns directly to drusen were applied with krypton, argon, or xenon laser. During an average
follow-up period of 3 years, 22 of 42 eyes (52%)
showed stabilization of vision and disappearance
of drusen. In 1994, Wetzig reported additional
follow-up on 39 of the original 42 eyes.[70] The mean
follow-up period for this subsequent report was 10
years. Snellen visual acuity remained within 1 line
of pretreatment vision in 13 eyes (33%), fell by 2 to
3 lines in 8 eyes (21%), and fell by 3 or more lines
in 18 eyes (46%). Progressive enlargement of the
laser scars and progressive retinal pigment epithelial atrophy in untreated areas was noted as a potential long-term negative consequence of treatment. In addition, at least four eyes developed
CNV over time.

Figueroa et al furthered investigations in this
area by applying argon green laser directly to soft
drusen located temporally within the macula of 20
patients.[71] These temporal drusen promptly disappeared in all patients. Untreated nasal drusen subsequently disappeared as well, on average 10
months after treatment. Drusen resorption extended from treated to untreated areas with treated
temporal drusen disappearing first, followed by
subfoveal drusen, and then nasal drusen. Visual
acuity improved by at least 1 line in 30% of patients, remained unchanged in 65%, and decreased
in 5%. Improvement in visual acuity coincided with
resorption of subfoveal drusen. During the 18
months of follow-up no treatment-related complications were noted and no eye developed CNV.
This prospective, uncontrolled study demonstrated
that light laser photocoagulation of nonfoveal drusen may safely promote resorption of macular drusen, but it did not resolve the question of whether
laser photocoagulation and disappearance of drusen alters the likelihood of development of choroidal neovascularization and severe visual loss.
Furthermore, as each of the above-reviewed case
studies omits control subjects, we are unable to determine if the drusen disappearance seen in these
treated eyes exceeds the natural rate of drusen
resorption.[24,28]

The mechanism by which laser treatment may
cause the disappearance of drusen is unclear. Studies of naturally occurring drusen in the eyes of rhesus monkeys, however, suggest that mild photocoagulation with argon green laser induces the
migration of phagocytic cells, perhaps derived from
choriocapillaris pericytes, which take up the drusen
material.[72]

Several clinical trials are presently underway in
which eyes with nonneovascular AMD are randomly being assigned to macular laser treatment or
observation.[73-76] A variety of treatment protocols
are being explored and short-term safety and efficacy data are being reviewed. One such study by
Bressler and colleagues demonstrated a significant
reduction in drusen number among treated eyes
when compared to control eyes, 6 months after randomization. No adverse vision outcomes were
identified but a few treated patients developed geographic atrophy at sites of laser application. No
patients in either group developed CNV by 6
months. Long-term data on morphologic features
and vision outcomes are needed in larger numbers
of patients to fully evaluate the potential merits,
limitations, and risks of this treatment.

Education

Presently, the most important aspect of patient
management remains education. Patients need to
be informed that macular degeneration does not in
the majority of cases cause legal blindness and that
even in the worst cases, peripheral vision is almost

always retained. Patients should be taught to monitor their central vision in a monocular fashion on a regular basis to detect symptoms that may herald the development of choroidal neovascularization. It must be emphasized that any changes should prompt an immediate visit to the ophthalmologist, since certain cases of neovascular AMD are presently managed with photocoagulation and other forms of therapy may be found beneficial for neovascular AMD in the years ahead. In addition, as some patients who progress to choroidal neovascularization may not appreciate any symptoms,[77] we also recommend surveillance examinations biannually to look for progression to neovascular AMD. Simultaneously, we search for atrophy-inducing vision loss, re-evaluate low vision needs, and re-educate the patient and family as to the natural course of the disease.

Consultation with low-vision specialists is of the utmost importance in maximizing a patient's ability to use the visual function that they currently retain and minimize the associated disability. We advise patients to maintain an ongoing dialogue with a low-vision specialist to discuss changes in their needs and new aids that may become available. Thoughtful counseling of elderly patients and their families as they confront the frightening loss of sight and its ramifications cannot be overemphasized.

REFERENCES

1. National Society to Prevent Blindness: Visual problems in the United States: Definitions, Data Sources, Detailed Data Tables, Analyses, Interpretation. New York, NY: National Society to Prevent Blindness, 1980, pp 1–46.
2. Klein R, Rowland ML, Harris MI: Racial/ethnic differences in age-related maculopathy. Third National Health and Nutrition Examination Survey. Ophthalmology 102:371–381, 1995.
3. Klein R, Klein BEK, Linton KLP: Prevalence of age-related maculopathy. The Beaver Dam Eye Study. Ophthalmology 99:933–943, 1992.
4. Leibowitz HM, Krueger DE, Maunder LR, et al: The Framingham Eye Study Monograph: VI. Macular degeneration. Surv Ophthalmol 24(Suppl):428–457, 1980.
5. Hyman LG, Lilienfeld AM, Ferris FL, Fine SL: Senile macular degeneration: a case control study. Am J Epidemiol 118:213–227, 1983.
6. Ferris FL, Fine SL, Hyman L: Age-related macular degeneration and blindness due to neovascular maculopathy. Arch Ophthalmol 102:1640–1642, 1984.
7. Donders FC: Beitrage zur pathologischen Anatomie des Auges. Arch Ophthalmol 1:106, 1855.
8. Haab O: Erkrankungen der Macula lutea. Centralblat Augenheilkd 9:384–391, 1885.
9. Duke-Elder S: Diseases of the uveal tract. In System of Ophthalmology, Vol 9. St. Louis, Mosby-Year Book, 1966, p 603.
10. Sarks SH, Sarks JP: Age-related macular degeneration: atrophic form. In Ryan SJ, Schachat AP, Murphy RB (eds): Retina, Vol 2. St Louis, Mosby-Year Book, 1994, pp 1071–1102.
11. Gass JDM: Pathogenesis of disciform detachment of the neuroepithelium. Am J Ophthalmol 63:573–711, 1967.
12. Goldberg J, Flowerdew G, Smith E, et al: Factors associated with AMD: analysis of the first NHANES. Am J Epidemiol 128:700–710, 1988.
13. Matinez GS, Campbell AJ, Reinken J, Allan BC: Prevalence of ocular disease in a population study of subjects 65 years old and older. Am J Ophthalmol 94:181–189, 1982.
14. Vinding T: Age-related macular degeneration. Macular changes, prevalence and sex ratio. Acta Ophthalmol 67:609–616, 1989.
15. Bressler NM, Bressler SB, West SK, et al: The grading and prevalence of macular degeneration in Chesapeake Bay watermen. Arch Ophthalmol 107:847–852, 1989.
16. Vingerling JR, Dielemans I, Hofman A, et al: The prevalence of age-related maculopathy in the Rotterdam Study. Ophthalmology 102:205–210, 1995.
17. Klein R, Davis MD, Magli YL, et al: The Wisconsin age-related maculopathy grading system. Ophthalmology 98:1128–1134, 1991.
18. Bird AC, Bressler NM, Bressler SB, et al: An international classification and grading system for age-related maculopathy and age-related macular degeneration. Surv Ophthalmol 39:367–374, 1995.
19. Bressler SB, Maguire MG, Bressler NM, Fine SL: The Macular Photocoagulation Study Group: relationship of drusen and abnormalities of the retinal pigment epithelium to the prognosis of neovascular macular degeneration. Arch Ophthalmol 108:1442–1447, 1990.
20. El Baba F, Green WR, Fleischmann J, et al: Clinicopathologic correlation of lipidization and detachment of the retinal pigment epithelium. Am J Ophthalmol 101:576–583, 1986.
21. Green WR, McDonnell PJ, Yeo JH.: Pathologic features of senile macular degeneration. Ophthalmology 92:615–627, 1985.
22. Hogan MJ: Role of the retinal pigment epithelium in macular disease. Trans Am Acad Ophthalmol Otolaryngol 76:64–80, 1972.
23. Coffey AJH, Brownstein S: The prevalence of macular drusen in postmortem eyes. Am J Ophthalmol 102:164–171, 1986.
24. Klein R, Klein BEK, Jensen SC, Meuer SM: The 5-year incidence and progression of age-related maculopathy: The Beaver Dam Eye Study. Ophthalmology 104:7–21, 1997.
25. Green WR, Enger C: Age-related macular degeneration histopathologic studies: the 1992 Lorenz E. Zimmerman Lecture. Ophthalmology 100:1519–1535, 1993.
26. Bressler NM, Silva JC, Bressler SB, et al: Clinicopathologic correlation of drusen and retinal pigment epithelial abnormalities in age-related macular degeneration. Retina 14:130–142, 1994.
27. Sarks SH: Aging and degeneration in the macular region: a clinicopathological study. Br J Ophthalmol 60:324–341, 1976.
28. Bressler NM, Munoz B, Maguire MG, et al: Five-year incidence and disappearance of drusen and retinal pigment epithelial abnormalities. Waterman study. Arch Ophthalmol 113:301–308, 1995.
29. Maguire MG, Bressler SB, Bressler NM, et al, for the Macular Photocoagulation Study Group: risk factors for choroidal neovascularization in the second eye of patients with juxtafoveal or subfoveal choroidal neovascularization secondary to age-related macular degeneration. Arch Ophthalmol 115:741–747, 1997.
30. Green WR, Key SN: Senile macular degeneration: a histopathologic study. Trans Am Ophthalmol Soc 75:180–254, 1977.
31. Sarks SH: Drusen and their relationship to senile macular degeneration. Aust J Ophthalmol 8:117–130, 1980.
32. Holz FG, Wolfensberger TJ, Piguet B, et al: Bilateral macular drusen in age-related macular degeneration. Ophthalmology 101:1522–1528, 1994.
33. Burgess DB, Hawkins BS, Jefferys J, et al: Macular Photocoagulation Study Group: five-year follow-up of fellow eyes of patients with age-related macular degeneration and unilateral extrafoveal choroidal neovascularization. Arch Ophthalmol 111:1189–1199, 1993.

34. Sarks JP, Sarks SH, Killingsworth MC: Evolution of geographic atrophy of the retinal pigment epithelium. Eye 2: 552–577, 1988.
35. Macular Photocoagulation Study Group: Persistent and recurrent neovascularization after krypton laser photocoagulation for neovascular lesions of age-related macular degeneration. Arch Ophthalmol 108:825–831, 1990.
36. Jampol LM: Discussion of prognosis of patients with bilateral macular drusen. Ophthalmology 91:276–277, 1984.
37. Smiddy WE, Fine SL: Prognosis of patients with bilateral macular drusen. Ophthalmology 91:271–277, 1984.
38. Gass JDM: Drusen and disciform macular detachment and degeneration. Arch Ophthalmol 90:206–217, 1973.
39. Schatz H, McDonald HR: Atrophic macular degeneration: rate of spread of geographic atrophy and visual loss. Ophthalmology 96:1541–1551, 1989.
40. Sunness JS, Bressler NB, Tian Y, et al: Invest Ophthalmol Vis Sci 37(3):S21, 1996.
41. Maguire P, Vine AK: Geographic atrophy of the retinal pigment epithelium. Am J Ophthalmol 102:621–625, 1986.
42. Applegate CA, Sunness JS, Haselwood DM: Visual symptoms associated with geographic atrophy from age-related macular degeneration. Invest Ophthalmol Vis Sci 37(3):S112, 1996.
43. Sunness J, Ruben G, Applegate C, et al.: Visual function abnormalities and prognosis in eyes with age-related geographic atrophy of the macula and good visual acuity. Ophthalmology 104:1677–1691, 1997.
44. Sunness JS, Bressler NM, Maguire MG: Scanning laser ophthalmoscopic analysis of the pattern of visual loss in age-related geographic atrophy of the macula. Am J Ophthalmol 119:143–151, 1995.
45. Sunness JS, Bressler NM, Marsh MJ, et al: The development of choroidal neovascularization in eyes with geographic atrophy from age-related macular degeneration. Invest Ophthalmol Vis Sci 38(4):S967, 1997.
46. Young RW: Solar radiation and age-related macular degeneration. Surv Ophthalmology 32:252–269, 1988.
47. Gottsch JD, Bynoe LA, Harlan JB: Light-induced deposits in Bruch's membrane of protoporphyric mice. Arch Ophthalmol 111:126–129, 1993.
48. West SK, Rosenthal FS, Bressler NM, et al: Exposure to sunlight and other risk factors for age-related macular degeneration. Arch Ophthalmol 107:875–879, 1989.
49. Taylor HR, West S, Munoz B, et al: The long-term effects of visible light on the eye. Arch Ophthalmol 110:99–104, 1992.
50. The Eye Disease Case Control Study Group: Risk factors for neovascular age-related macular degeneration. Arch Ophthalmol 110:1701–1708, 1992.
51. Cruickshanks KJ, Klein R, Klein BEK: Sunlight and age-related macular degeneration: the Beaver Dam Eye Study. Arch Ophthalmol 111:514–518, 1993.
52. Taylor HR, West SK, Rosenthal FS, et al: Effect of ultraviolet radiation on cataract formation. N Engl J Med 319:1429–1433, 1988.
53. Blumenkranz MS, Russell SR, Robey MG, et al: Risk factors in age-related maculopathy complicated by choroidal neovascularization. Ophthalmology 96:552–558, 1986.
54. Delaney WV, Oates RP: Senile macular degeneration: preliminary study. Ann Ophthalmol 14:21–24, 1982.
55. Maltzman BA, Mulvihill MN, Greenbaum A: Senile macular degeneration and risk factors: case-control study. Ann Ophthalmol 11:1197–1201, 1979.
56. Klein R, Klein BEK, Linton KLP, DeMets DL: The Beaver Dam Eye Study: the relationship of age-related maculopathy to smoking. Am J Epidemiol 137:190–200, 1993.
57. Klein R, Klein BEK, Franke T: The relationship of cardiovascular disease and its risk factors to age-related maculopathy. The Beaver Dam Eye Study. Ophthalmology 100:406–414, 1993.
58. Mares-Perlman JA, Brady WE, Klein R, et al: Dietary fat and age-related maculopathy. Arch Ophthalmol 113:743–748, 1995.
59. The Eye Disease Case-Control Study Group: Antioxidant status and neovascular age-related macular degeneration. Arch Ophthalmol 111:104–109, 1993.
60. Seddon JM, Ajani UA, Sperduto RD, et al: Dietary carotenoids, vitamins A, C, and E, and advanced age-related macular degeneration. JAMA 272:1413–1420, 1994.
61. West S, Vitale S, Hallfrisch J, et al: Are antioxidants or supplements protective for age-related macular degeneration? Arch Ophthalmol 112:222–227, 1994.
62. Mares Perlman JA, Brady WE, Klein R, et al: Serum antioxidants and age-related macular degeneration in a population-based case-control study. Arch Ophthalmol 113:1518–1523, 1995.
63. Newsome DA, Swartz M, Leone NC, et al: Oral zinc in macular degeneration. Arch Ophthalmol 106:192–198, 1988.
64. Stur M, Tittl M, Reitner A, Meisinger V: Oral zinc and the second eye in age-related macular degeneration. Invest Ophthalmol Vis Sci 37:1225–1235, 1996.
65. The Alpha-Tocopherol, Beta Carotene Cancer Prevention Study Group: The effect of vitamin E and beta carotene on the incidence of lung cancer and other changes in male smokers. N Engl J Med 330:1029–1035, 1994.
66. Omenn GS, Goodman GE, Thornquist MD, et al: Effects of a combination of beta carotene and vitamin A on lung cancer and cardiovascular disease. N Engl J Med 334:1150–1155, 1996.
67. Gass JMD: Drusen and disciform macular detachment and degeneration. Arch Ophthalmol 90:206–217, 1973.
68. Cleasby GW, Nakanishi AS, Norris JL: Prophylactic photocoagulation of the fellow eye in exudative senile maculopathy. Mod Probl Ophthalmol 20:141–147, 1979.
69. Wetzig PC: Treatment of drusen-related aging macular degeneration by photocoagulation. Trans Am Ophthalmol Soc 86:276–290, 1988.
70. Wetzig PC: Photocoagulation of drusen-related macular degeneration. A long-term outcome. Trans Am Ophthalmol Soc 92:299–306, 1994.
71. Figueroa MS, Regueras A, Bertrand J: Laser photocoagulation to treat macular soft drusen in age-related macular degeneration. Retina 14:391–396, 1994.
72. Duvall J, Tso MOM: Cellular mechanisms of resolution of drusen after laser photocoagulation. Arch Ophthalmol 103:694–703, 1985.
73. Frennesson IC, Nilsson SE: Effects of argon (green) laser treatment of soft drusen in early age-related maculopathy: a six month prospective study. Br J Ophthalmol 79:905–909, 1995.
74. Bressler SB, Vitale S, Hawkins BS, et al: Laser to Drusen Trial: an assessment of short term safety within a randomized prospective, controlled clinical trial. Invest Ophthalmol Vis Sci 36(4), S225, 1995.
75. Frennesson IC, Nilsson SEG: Significant decrease in exudative complications after prophylactic laser treatment of soft drusen maculopathy in a randomized study. Invest Ophthalmol Vis Sci (38)4, S18, 1997.
76. Ho AC, Javornik N, Maguire MG, and the CNVPT Study Group: The Choroidal Neovascularization Prevention Trial (CNVPT): assessment of macular risk factors for CNV through 1 year. Invest Ophthalmol Vis Sci (38)4, S17, 1997.
77. Moisseiev J, Bressler NM: Asymptomatic neovascular membranes in the second eye of patients with visual loss from age-related macular degeneration (AMD). Invest Ophthalmol Vis Sci 31:462, 1990.

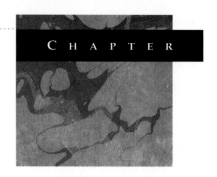

CHAPTER 10

Neovascular (Exudative) Age-Related Macular Degeneration

Anat Loewenstein, M.D.
Neil M. Bressler, M.D.

Although most patients with age-related macular degeneration (AMD) manifest only drusen or abnormalities of the retinal pigment epithelium (RPE) (nonneovascular AMD), the majority of patients who experience severe visual loss from AMD do so because of the development of neovascular AMD, namely choroidal neovascularization (CNV) and related manifestations such as subretinal hemorrhage, detachment of the RPE, and disciform scarring (fibroglial and fibrovascular tissue). This chapter will review the definitions, clinical and fluorescein angiographic manifestations, risk factors and natural history, as well as proven treatments of neovascular AMD.

PATHOGENESIS

Experimental and Clinicopathologic Studies

The pathogenesis of neovascular AMD is poorly understood. Diffuse thickening of the inner aspect of Bruch's membrane predisposes to the development of breaks in this tissue through which ingrowth of new vessels from the choriocapillaris may occur.[1-5] Other cellular processes may participate in the development of the CNV, since in some eyes with AMD, breaks in Bruch's membrane can be identified in areas in which no CNV had developed.[3] Endothelial cells may elaborate enzymes necessary for the digestion of Bruch's membrane,[6] leading to the hypothesis that endothelial cells may *produce* a break in Bruch's membrane, and then pro-

liferate as CNV rather than proliferating only through pre-existing breaks. A granulomatous inflammatory response to degenerated Bruch's membrane also has been suggested to contribute to the development of CNV. A chronic, low-grade inflammatory response has been associated with the development of CNV, although it is not known if this response is to existing degenerative changes within Bruch's membrane or is essential to the development of CNV.[7-9] In support of this hypothesis, experimentally produced subretinal neovascularization developing around intense retinal laser burns in the monkey eye may show macrophages at the site of the neovascularization.[10,11] The role of increased scleral rigidity in the formation of choroidal neovascular disease in AMD was suggested, with compromised blood flow in the vortex veins by progressively increased scleral rigidity as a possible explanation.[12]

Epidemiologic Studies

The Eye Disease Case-Control Study Group has suggested an association between increased dietary or serum levels of certain antioxidants and a decreased risk for neovascular AMD. In this study,[13,14] the increased risk of neovascular AMD was associated with cigarette smoking, higher levels of serum cholesterol, and parity greater than zero. This study also found that individuals with higher serum levels of various carotenoids or with greater dietary consumption of carotenoid-containing food sources were significantly less likely to have neo-

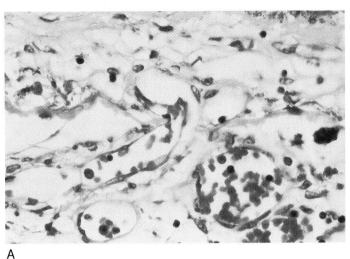

A

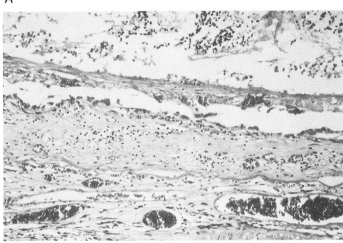

B

A, Early choroidal neovascularization in age-related macular degeneration. A capillary extends through a defect in Bruch's membrane and into a plane between RPE with basal laminar deposit and the remainder of Bruch's membrane. *B,* Age-related macular degeneration with a two-component scar—the thin subretinal and thicker intra–Bruch's membrane components are separated by residual retinal pigment epithelium and a layer of basal laminar deposit.

vascular AMD. High vitamin C consumption also was associated with a marginal reduction in disease risk. Serum levels of vitamin E, C, and dietary intake of vitamin E were not associated with the presence or absence of neovascular AMD.[13-15]

In a nested case-control study within the population-based cohort of the 4926 participants of the Beaver Dam Eye Study,[16] the average levels of individual carotenoids were similar in cases and controls. Patients with either soft drusen or geographic atrophy (GA) or CNV were less likely than controls to use supplements containing vitamin C, vitamin E, or zinc, although this finding was statistically significant only for vitamin C. Average levels of vitamin E (α-tocopherol) were significantly lower in cases than in controls. However, the difference was not statistically significant after controlling for levels of cholesterol in serum. Persons with levels of lycopene (the most abundant carotenoid in the serum), in the lowest quintile, were twice as likely to have AMD. Levels of carotenoids that compose macular pigment (lutein and zeaxanthin) in the serum were unrelated to AMD, and it was concluded that very low levels of only lycopene and not other dietary carotenoids or tocopherols were associated with AMD.

Thus, the pathogenesis of neovascular AMD is still not clarified and warrants much future research. Although several case-control studies have supported the theory that antioxidants may play a protective role against the development or progression of AMD, findings have been inconsistent and conflicting with respect to specific micronutrients. Until results of clinical trials prove that micronutrients are beneficial and clarify the risk of long-term potential toxicity, physicians probably should be reluctant to recommend micronutrients to prevent the development or progression of AMD. Further understanding of the pathogenesis is needed to determine the role of genetic and environmental factors in the development of AMD and the role of supplemental micronutrients in AMD prevention.

CLINICAL FEATURES

Regardless of the pathogenesis of CNV in AMD, clinicopathologic correlative studies[1,3,4] and natural history studies[17-21] have shown that CNV usually is accompanied by the ingrowth of fibrous scar tissue, eventually resulting in a disciform scar. This CNV–scar complex may have a variety of clinical and angiographic appearances.

Symptoms

The clinical symptoms of neovascular AMD vary from metamorphopsia, central or paracentral scotoma, to a sudden, nonspecific reduction in central vision.[22-24] CNV should be suspected and any pa-

tient with these symptoms should be evaluated for signs described below to determine if CNV is present, since treatment might be beneficial compared to no treatment in selected cases.

Signs

Not all patients with CNV will be symptomatic[25]; more specifically, some patients with CNV may not notice changes of metamorphopsia when testing for this symptom at home with an Amsler grid.[26] Therefore, the following clinical signs as well as angiographic features should be examined periodically in any patient over 50 years of age with non-neovascular features of AMD including large drusen (>63 μm in greatest linear dimension) and focal areas of hyperpigmentation. Furthermore, an ophthalmologist should scrutinize for these signs whenever a patient with large drusen or abnormalities of the RPE complains of metamorphopsia, new scotomas, or other sudden visual change. Signs of CNV may include a gray-green subretinal lesion that can be accompanied by subretinal fluid, subretinal hemorrhage or cystic retinal edema, elevation of the RPE, or visualization of the CNV itself. The presence of subretinal or sub-RPE blood may be so extensive as to obscure all other signs of the CNV. Often, however, this blood will be found along the periphery of the CNV. Most of the cases of CNV secondary to AMD have subretinal fluid. Accurate detection of subretinal fluid can be difficult but can be facilitated by biomicroscopy with a contact lens using a bright thin slit beam. The anterior portion of the beam will bow forward (convex to the surface of the RPE). An increased distance between the surface of the slit beam (which is visualized on the surface of the sensory retina) and the posterior portion of the beam (which is visualized on the surface of the RPE) is seen. As subretinal fluid is absorbed at the periphery of the CNV, subretinal lipid may precipitate in a circumferential pattern around the CNV. Another possible sign is elevation of the RPE, usually caused by the presence of fibrovascular tissue, which includes the CNV beneath the RPE.[1,27]

Differential Diagnosis

Similar clinical symptoms and signs of CNV due to AMD can be found in eyes with other causes of CNV, such as pathologic myopia, the ocular histoplasmosis syndrome (OHS), angioid streaks, and traumatic choroidal rupture. Subretinal blood in someone with AMD may not always be due to CNV, but could be seen, for example, in an eye with pathologic myopia with lacquer cracks or within areas of geographic atrophy when no CNV is seen on angiography and the blood is probably the result of disruption of the choriocapillaris at the periphery of the atrophy.[28] Occasionally, subretinal blood also may be seen in association with macro-aneurysms, a traumatic choroidal rupture, a posterior vitreous detachment, choroidal tumors, or any retinal vascular disease, such as branch vein occlusion, in which intraretinal hemorrhage dissects into the subretinal space. Although CNV almost always is associated with subretinal fluid, subretinal fluid also may be seen in eyes with central serous chorioretinopathy; inflammatory conditions such as Harada's disease or posterior scleritis; uveal effusion with evidence of shifting fluid; or in association with choroidal tumors such as nevi,

melanomas, cavernous hemangiomas, metastases, or osteomas. Fluorescein angiography is indicated to confirm the diagnosis of CNV secondary to AMD, to determine if treatment is indicated, and to serve as a guide for treatment when laser photocoagulation is indicated.

FLUORESCEIN ANGIOGRAPHY

A set of photographs to facilitate the identification of the variety of appearances of CNV secondary to

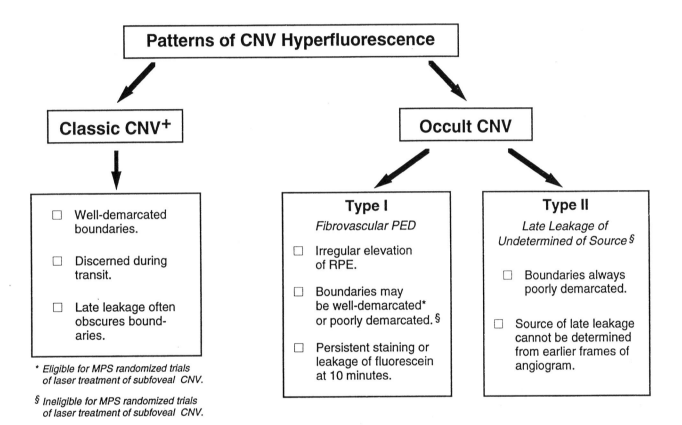

FIGURE 10–1   Angiographic characteristics of choroidal neovascular lesions. (From the Macular Photocoagulation Study Group: Subfoveal neovascular lesions in age-related macular degeneration. Guidelines for evaluation and treatment in the Macular Photocoagulation Study. Arch Ophthalmol 109:1242–1257, 1991. Copyright 1991, American Medical Association, with permission.)

AMD could include the following sequence of photographs obtained for documentation and management in the Macular Photocoagulation Study (MPS)[29]: (1) a black-and-white stereo pair of the macula obtained with a green monochromatic filter prior to dye injection; (2) rapid-sequence photographs of the macula taken during fluorescein dye transit, including at least one stereo pair; (3) stereo pairs of the macula taken at approximately 30, 40, 60, 90, 120, and 180 seconds after dye injection; (4) later stereoscopic pairs of the macula taken at 5 and 10 minutes after dye injection; and (5) stereoscopic color fundus photographs of the macula. Since CNV growth can be a continuous process,[30,31] the size of the CNV and the area of retina to be treated can change within a short time. Therefore, a fluorescein angiogram should be obtained ideally on the same day as any contemplated treatment and probably no more than 96 hours prior to treatment. Two basic angiographic patterns of CNV, reported by the MPS[32-36] and described by independent investigators,[1,19,24,37-39] include classic and occult CNV (Fig. 10-1).

Classic CNV

Classic CNV is an area of bright, well-demarcated fluorescence identified in the early phase of the angiogram with progressive pooling of dye in the overlying subsensory retinal space in the late phase of the angiogram (Fig. 10-2). Only occasionally will fluorescein angiography identify the actual capillary network of the CNV secondary to AMD.

Occult CNV

Occult CNV includes two fluorescent patterns. One, a fibrovascular pigment epithelial detachment (PED), consists of irregular elevation of the RPE consisting of stippled hyperfluorescence not as bright or discrete as classic CNV within 1 to 2 minutes after fluorescein injection, with persistence of staining or leakage of fluorescein dye within 10 minutes after injection (Fig. 10-3). Two, late leakage of undetermined source, consists of areas of leakage at the level of the RPE in the late phase of the angiogram not corresponding to an area of classic CNV or fibrovascular PED discernible in the early or middle phase of the angiogram to account for the leakage (Fig. 10-4).[36] Occasionally, the vessels of the fibrovascular tissue of which the occult CNV is composed can be visualized in the early phase of the angiogram.

Angiographic Features that Can Obscure CNV

These may be caused by one of the three following features: (1) blocked fluorescence due to visible blood contiguous with CNV (Fig. 10-5); (2) blocked fluorescence not due to visible blood (perhaps due

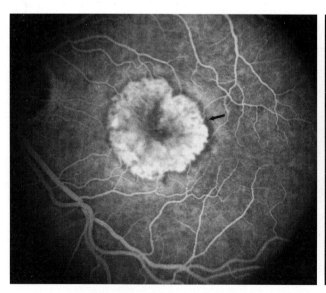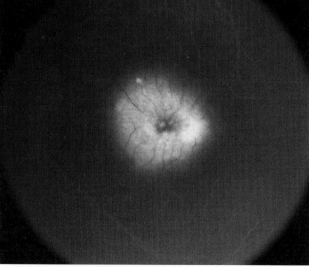

FIGURE 10-2   Classic choroidal neovascularization (CNV). *Left*, Early phase of angiogram shows fluorescein leakage from well-demarcated CNV surrounded by thin rim of blocked fluorescence (*arrow*); blocked fluorescence appeared flat on stereoscopic angiography. *Right*, Late phase of angiogram shows increased leakage from CNV. (From the Macular Photocoagulation Study Group: Subfoveal neovascular lesions in age-related macular degeneration. Guidelines for evaluation and treatment in the Macular Photocoagulation Study. Arch Ophthalmol 109:1242–1257, 1991. Copyright 1991, American Medical Association, with permission.)

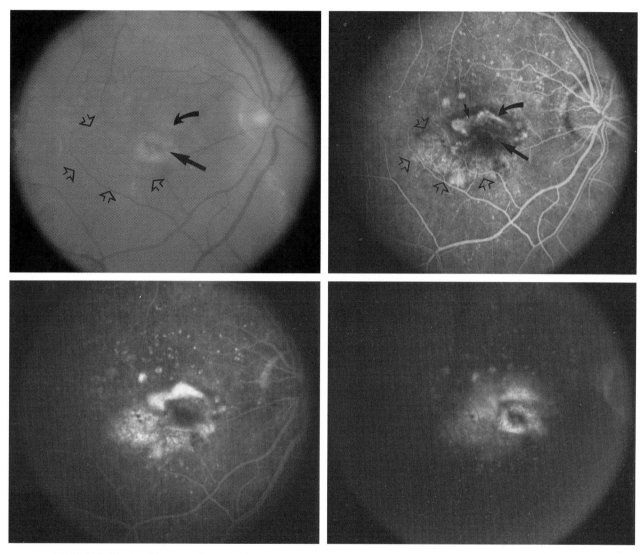

FIGURE 10–3   Classic and occult choroidal neovascularization (CNV) with well-demarcated borders. *Top left*, Color photograph shows scar from prior photocoagulation (*large arrow*) surrounded by subretinal hemorrhage, subretinal lipid, irregular elevation of retinal pigment epithelium (RPE) (*open arrows*), subretinal fibrosis (*curved arrow*), and overlying subretinal fluid. *Top right*, Early phase of fluorescein angiogram shows area of classic CNV (*small arrow*), scar from prior laser treatment (*large arrow*), and irregular elevation of RPE with stippled hyperfluorescence (*open arrows*) representing occult CNV (fibrovascular PED) inferior and temporal to scar. *Bottom left*, Midphase of fluorescein angiography showing leakage from classic CNV and increased intensity of stippled hyperfluorescence corresponding to fibrovascular PED. *Bottom right*, Late phase of angiogram (10 minutes) shows persistence of fluorescein staining and leakage within a sensory retinal detachment overlying lesion. (From the Macular Photocoagulation Study Group: Subfoveal neovascular lesions in age-related macular degeneration. Guidelines for evaluation and treatment in the Macular Photocoagulation Study. Arch Ophthalmol 109:1242–1257, 1991. Copyright 1991, American Medical Association, with permission.)

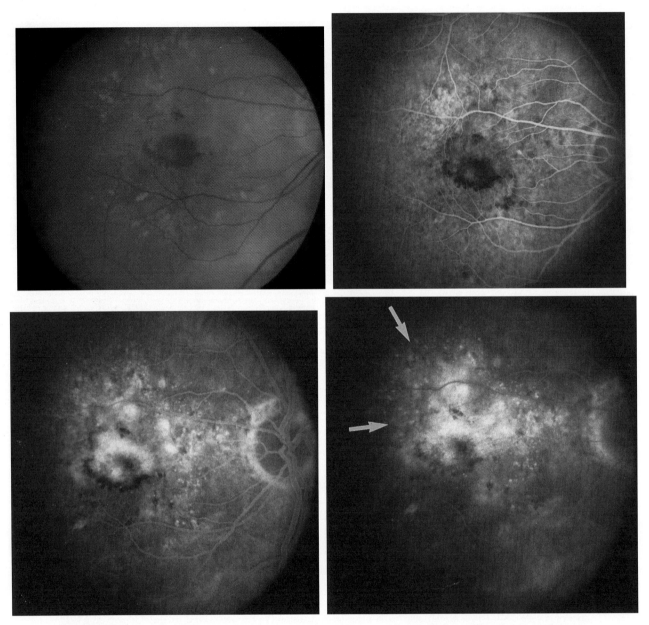

FIGURE 10–4   Occult choroidal neovascularization (CNV) causing late leakage of undetermined source. *Top left*, Color photograph showing subretinal hemorrhage, fluid, and drusen. *Top right*, Early phase of angiogram. *Bottom left*, Midphase of angiogram shows pinpoint areas of speckled hyperfluorescence and larger areas of hyperfluorescence, with accumulation of fluorescein leakage in overlying sensory retinal space in later phase of angiogram (*bottom right*). Source of late leakage in the late phase (*arrows*) does not correspond to classic CNV or an area of fibrovascular PED in either midphase (*bottom left*) or early phase (*top right*) of angiogram. (From the Macular Photocoagulation Study Group: Subfoveal neovascular lesions in age-related macular degeneration. Guidelines for evaluation and treatment in the Macular Photocoagulation Study. Arch Ophthalmol 109:1242–1257, 1991. Copyright 1991, American Medical Association, with permission.)

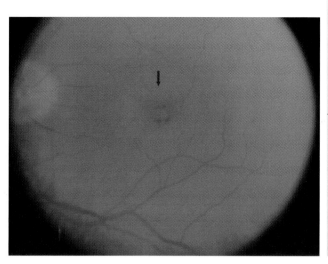

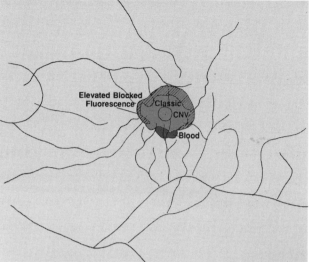

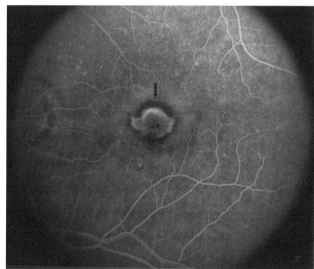

FIGURE 10–5 Elevated blocked fluorescence (EBF) and blood obscuring boundaries of choroidal neovascularization (CNV). *Top left*, Subfoveal CNV with contiguous blood inferior to CNV and hyperplastic pigment (*arrow*) along superior border. *Top right*, Composite drawing shows interpretation of angiogram. Boundaries of entire lesion are determined by peripheral boundaries of CNV, blocked fluorescence due to blood, and EBF. *Bottom*, Early phase of angiogram, shows hyperfluorescence of CNV, blocked fluorescence due to blood along inferior edge, and EBF presumably due to hyperplastic pigment, along superior edge (*arrow*). (From the Macular Photocoagulation Study Group. Subfoveal neovascular lesions in age-related macular degeneration. Guidelines for evaluation and treatment in the Macular Photocoagulation Study. Arch Ophthalmol 109: 1242–1257, 1991. Copyright 1991, American Medical Association, with permission.)

to blood that is not visible or hyperpigmentation or fibrin or fibrous tissue) (Fig. 10–5); or (3) hyperfluorescence from a serous PED (Fig. 10–6). As opposed to the first two features, which can obscure one's ability to detect CNV because of hypofluorescence, bright uniform early hyperfluorescence associated with a serous PED may obscure one's ability to detect hyperfluorescence from classic or occult CNV.

Numerous conditions in AMD may result in elevation or detachment of the RPE on stereoscopic biomicroscopy or angiographic evaluation. These various conditions all result in a "PED" in AMD, but can be differentiated by biomicroscopy and fluorescein angiography into the following types of PED: (1) a serous PED (Fig. 10–6); (2) a fibrovascular PED (Fig. 10–3); (3) a hemorrhagic PED in which blood from a CNV is noted at the level of the RPE (Fig. 10–7); and (4) a drusenoid PED, in which large areas of confluent, soft drusen are noted (Fig. 10–8).[40] A serous PED shows uniform, bright hyperfluorescence in the early transit phase with a smooth contour to the RPE; by the late phase, the bright hyperfluorescence shows no leakage into the overlying sensory retinal space; its boundaries are usually smooth and sharp. In a fibrovascular PED, the fluorescence is less fluorescent than in a serous PED, with a stippled appearance to the staining of the surface of the RPE, which may not be detected until the middle phase of the angiogram, with persistent staining or leakage of dye in the overlying subretinal space in the late phase. A hemorrhagic PED blocks choroidal fluorescence but is readily diagnosed by the dark appearance on biomicroscopy. A drusenoid PED fluoresces faintly during the transit phase, has no stippled appearance, usually does not have an irregularly elevated surface, and does not progress to bright hyperfluorescence or leakage in the late phase of the angiogram. It is usually quite small and shallow, very irregular in outline, and often has reticulated pigment clumping overlying it.

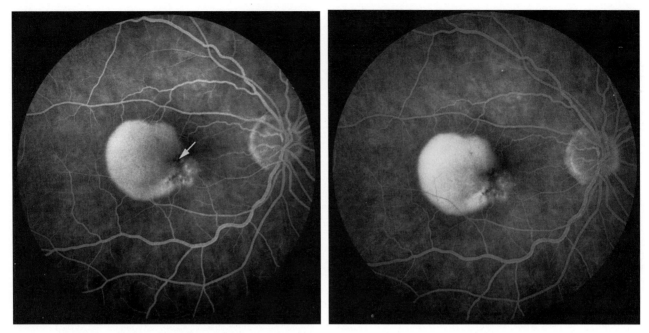

FIGURE 10–6   Serous pigment epithelial detachment (PED). *Left*, Early phase of fluorescein angiogram shows area of uniform, bright hyperfluorescence in the early transit phase with a smooth, sharp contour to the RPE; note the deformation of the otherwise round detachment by a notch in the hyperfluorescence (*arrow*). *Right*, Late phase showing no leakage at border of PED defined in early phase.

Other Clinical and Angiographic Features of CNV Secondary to AMD

Fading CNV

Fading CNV is a term defined by the MPS Group to describe CNV detected in the transit phase of the angiogram with staining or leakage in the late phase less than a minimum standard (Fig. 10–9),[33] and usually with no overlying subretinal fluid. It is probable that this angiographic pattern does represent CNV histologically, but without evidence of subretinal fluid or late staining or leakage, the MPS group chose not to include this finding as an area to receive treatment.

Feeder Vessels

Feeder vessels may be identified during the transit phase of the angiogram as vessels connected to leaking choroidal capillaries.[33] Feeder vessels have been described as extending from a laser-treated area to recurrent CNV across the perimeter of the laser-treated area (Fig. 10–10).[23,33,41] However, they also may be seen in untreated eyes, when peripheral untreated areas of CNV may be connected by feeder vessels to more central areas of CNV that are evolving toward natural scar formation[33] (Fig. 10–11).

Loculated Fluid

Loculated fluid consists of a well-demarcated area of hyperfluorescence, representing pooling of fluorescein in a compartmentalized space.[42] The loculated fluid may accumulate in a cystoid pattern or may pool within an area deep to the sensory retina in a shape that does not bear any resemblance to cystoid macular edema (Fig. 10–12).

RPE Tear or Rip of the RPE

These may occur spontaneously or during laser photocoagulation of CNV.[43-45] Upon its occurrence, visual acuity may fall abruptly. When not associated with CNV, RPE tears, even through the fovea, may be associated with preservation of good central visual acuity, provided that the torn area and not the scrolled-up RPE underlies the foveal center.[46] Angiography demonstrates early, bright, sharply demarcated hyperfluorescence within the torn region, with blocked fluorescence corresponding to heaped-up RPE at one side of the bright area (Fig. 10–13). The bright hyperfluorescence corresponds to fluorescein within the choriocapillaris that quickly leaks into the choroidal and scleral tissues, not blocked in this situation by the RPE that would normally overly these tissues. There may not be a sensory retinal detachment over an RPE tear, perhaps because the higher osmotic pressure of the choroid (compared with the subretinal space) allows fluid to be removed from the subretinal space at a rapid rate when the RPE cells with their tight junctions are absent and therefore unable to prevent free movement of fluid.[47]

Disciform Scar

The MPS group used the term "CNV/scar" to describe fibrous tissue in association with CNV in

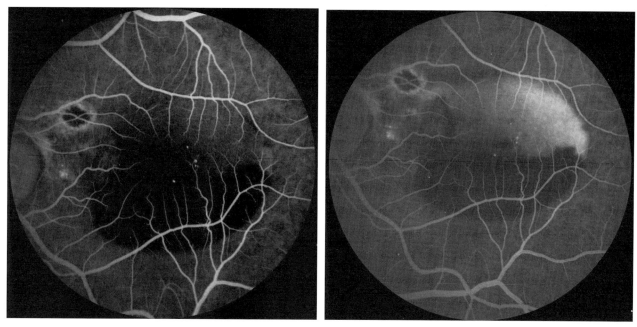

FIGURE 10–7 *Left,* Early phase of fluorescein angiography shows hypofluorescence along the inferior portion of the macula. *Right,* Midphase shows staining of pigment epithelial detachment (PED) along superior aspect of macula with persistent hypofluorescence from hemorrhage within PED.

which the fibrous tissue comprises more than 25% of the lesion. When no leakage is seen at the periphery of the lesion, the term "scar" is used by the MPS group. The term "disciform" is used to imply that the scar is circular in shape. The scar may contain brown or black pigment. It may have a variety of appearances depending on its location, the de-

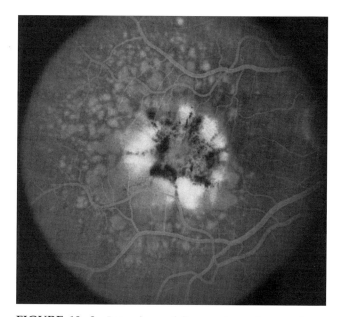

FIGURE 10–8 Late phase of fluorescein angiogram showing fainter staining of drusen centrally with hyperfluorescence of drusen peripherally in a drusenoid pigment epithelial detachment. No progression to bright hyperfluorescence or leakage is noted at the peripheral portion of the drusenoid pigment epithelial detachment.

gree of associated CNV, the presence of a retinal anastomosis into the scar, and the amount of RPE atrophy (Fig. 10–14).

Hemorrhage

Hemorrhage from CNV may collect in the subretinal pigment epithelial space, in the subneurosensory retinal space, or within the retina or vitreous. When a hemorrhage from a CNV lesion extends into the vitreous space, then on ultrasound, a relatively flat and broad-based lesion may be detected, with a fairly homogeneous pattern and without signs of choroidal excavation.[48,49] In 75% of patients, the vitreous hemorrhage clears spontaneously. If not, vitrectomy, which usually will restore the peripheral vision, should be considered.

INDOCYANINE GREEN ANGIOGRAPHY

One of the newest fields of imaging research in AMD is indocyanine green (ICG) angiography (see Chapter 4). Infrared angiography using ICG dye was introduced 20 years ago,[50,51] but was easier to evaluate due to advanced techniques and improved picture resolution in the last 5 years. Compared to fluorescein angiography, ICG angiography has two basic differences, namely, the use of near-infrared light (that is less absorbed than visible light by the pigment epithelium and the macular xanthophyll) and the use of a blood-protein-bound dye, ICG,

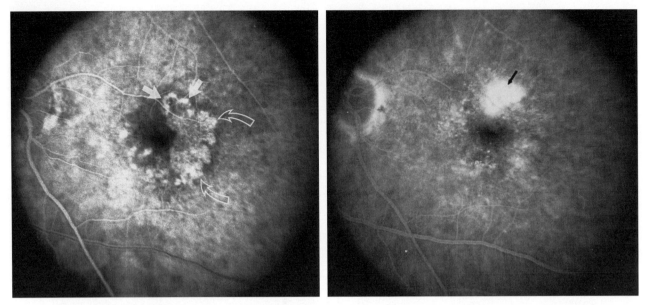

FIGURE 10–9   Fading fluorescence of occult choroidal neovascularization (CNV) contiguous with classic CNV. *Left*, Early phase of angiogram shows classic CNV (*closed arrows*) with contiguous areas of slightly elevated hyperfluorescent retinal pigment epithelium (RPE) (*open arrows*), presumably fibrovascular pigment epithelial detachment, another less well-demarcated area of hyperfluorescence nasal to fovea. *Right*, Later phase of angiogram shows fluorescein leakage from classic CNV (*arrow*). However, areas of elevated hyperfluorescent RPE on early phase of angiogram (*left*) begin to fade. Faded area is not considered lesion component to be treated because hyperfluorescence does not meet minimal leakage/staining standard for occult CNV. (From the Macular Photocoagulation Study Group: Subfoveal neovascular lesions in age-related macular degeneration. Guidelines for evaluation and treatment in the Macular Photocoagulation Study. Arch Ophthalmol 109:1242–1257, 1991. Copyright 1991, American Medical Association, with permission.)

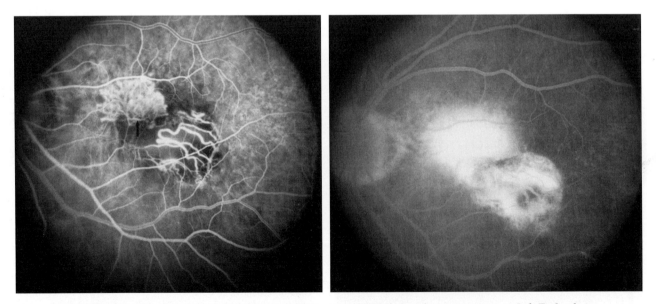

FIGURE 10–10   Recurrent choroidal neovascularization (CNV) that underwent treatment. *Left*, Early phase of angiogram shows recurrent lesion with classic CNV and feeder vessel (*arrow*). Larger choroidal vessels are seen within central portion of scar from previous laser treatment. *Right*, Late phase of angiogram shows fluorescein leakage of classic CNV. (From the Macular Photocoagulation Study Group: Subfoveal neovascular lesions in age-related macular degeneration. Guidelines for evaluation and treatment in the Macular Photocoagulation Study. Arch Ophthalmol 109:1242–1257, 1991. Copyright 1991, American Medical Association, with permission.)

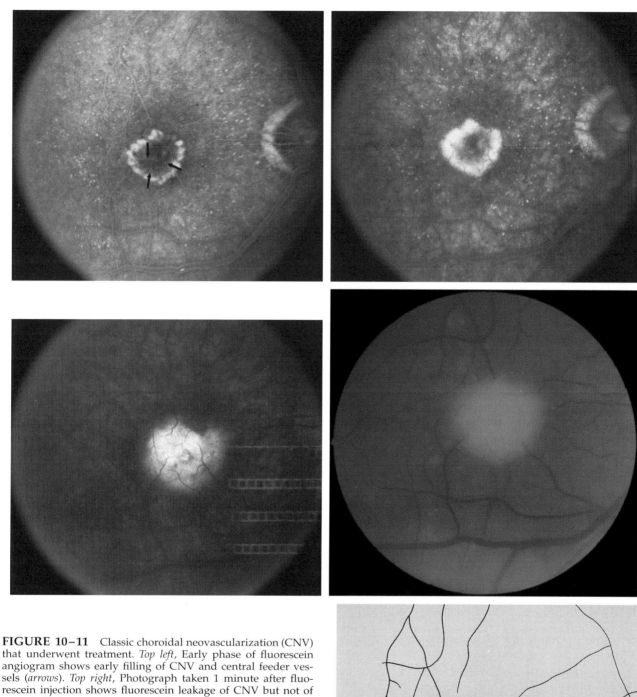

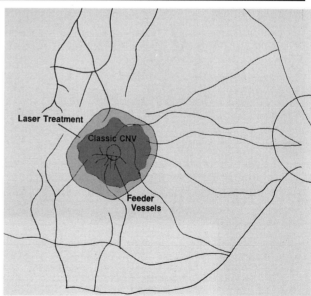

FIGURE 10–11   Classic choroidal neovascularization (CNV) that underwent treatment. *Top left,* Early phase of fluorescein angiogram shows early filling of CNV and central feeder vessels (*arrows*). *Top right,* Photograph taken 1 minute after fluorescein injection shows fluorescein leakage of CNV but not of central feeder vessels. *Center left,* Later phase of angiogram shows pooling of dye in subsensory retinal space, obscuring boundaries of CNV demarcated in early phase of angiogram (*top left*). *Center right,* Photography taken 12 to 48 hours after laser treatment. Note uniform whitening of retina. *Bottom,* Composite drawing using pretreatment fluorescein angiogram (*top left*) and posttreatment color photograph (*center right*) shows feeder vessels within CNV (green) and extent of treatment (orange). (From the Macular Photocoagulation Study Group: Subfoveal neovascular lesions in age-related macular degeneration. Guidelines for evaluation and treatment in the Macular Photocoagulation Study. Arch Ophthalmol 109:1242–1257, 1991. Copyright 1991, American Medical Association, with permission.)

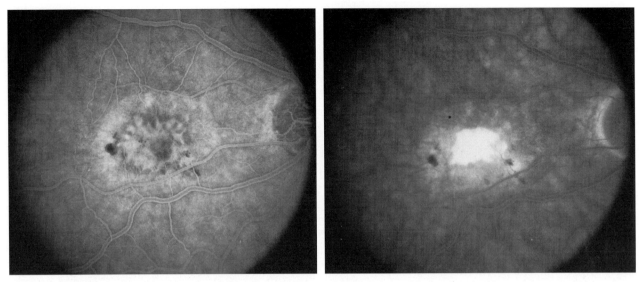

FIGURE 10–12   Loculated fluid. *Left,* Early frame of fluorescein angiography demonstrating hyperfluorescence from choroidal neovascularization (CNV) extending throughout the foveal center. *Right,* Late-phase frame demonstrating hyperfluorescent leakage as well as a distinct area of a well-defined, extremely bright, sharply demarcated collection of fluorescein dye corresponding to the loculated fluid. (From Bressler NM, Bressler SB, Alexander J, et al: Loculated fluid. A previously undescribed fluorescein angiographic finding in choroidal neovascularization associated with macular degeneration. Arch Ophthalmol 109:211–215, 1991. Copyright 1991, American Medical Association, with permission.)

which does not leak from the choriocapillaris, permitting more accurate visualization of choroidal vessels. The main disadvantage of ICG is its low fluorescence, which is only 4% of that of sodium fluorescein. One of the main areas in which ICG angiography theoretically might have a therapeutic role is in the study of CNV, particularly when it is only occult or has poorly defined borders, and thus not amenable to laser photocoagulation according to guidelines suggested by the MPS Group. The largest clinical series on ICG angiography published to date reported on 79 eyes in which rela-

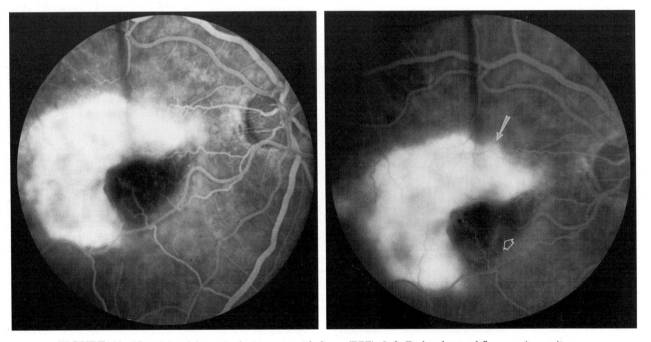

FIGURE 10–13   Tear of the retinal pigment epithelium (RPE). *Left,* Early phase of fluorescein angiogram of a tear of the pigment epithelium in which marked hyperfluorescence can be seen due to the absence of the normal RPE (*arrow*). Hypofluorescence can be seen in the area where the RPE has retracted and rolled upon itself (*open arrow*). *Right,* Late phase of a fluorescein angiogram in which staining, but no leakage, is seen in the area of the rip. (From Bressler NM, Bressler SB, Fine SL: Age-related macular degeneration. Surv Ophthalmol 32:375–413, 1988. Copyright 1988, American Medical Association, with permission.)

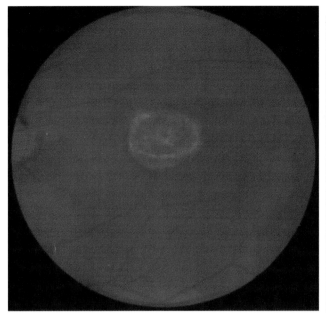

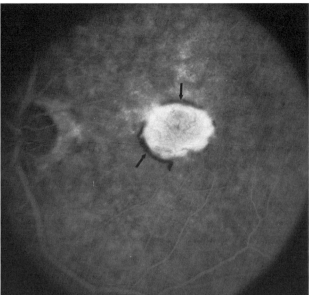

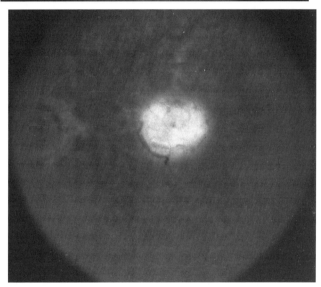

FIGURE 10–14   *Top left,* Subfoveal choroidal neovascularization (CNV) accompanied by fibrous tissue. *Top right,* Midphase of angiogram shows CNV in foveal center, with well-demarcated hyperfluorescence of CNV and/or fibrous tissue. Note areas of blocked fluorescence corresponding to blood (*arrows*). *Bottom,* Midphase of angiogram shows leakage from area of well-demarcated hyperfluorescence seen in early frame (*top right*). (From the Macular Photocoagulation Study Group: Subfoveal neovascular lesions in age-related macular degeneration. Guidelines for evaluation and treatment in the Macular Photocoagulation Study. Arch Ophthalmol 109:1242–1257, 1991. Copyright 1991, American Medical Association, with permission.)

tively small, well-delineated areas of hyperfluorescence (termed "focal spots") within the macula were demonstrated. In this series, these lesions were used to guide focal laser treatment with the assumption that these focal areas of hyperfluorescence represented an area of CNV for which photocoagulation might prove beneficial. Improvement of visual acuity (2 or more lines of Snellen acuity) was noted in 10 (13%) of these 79 eyes, and stabilization of vision occurred in an additional 42 eyes (53%) after a median follow-up time of 23 weeks.[52] In another study, which included 23 eyes, laser treatment was applied to focal spots of ICG hyperfluorescence at the edge of a plaque of ICG hyperfluorescence. Of the 15 eyes (70%) that had follow-up examinations at 1 year after treatment, 2 eyes (12.5%) improved by 2 or more lines and an additional 7 eyes (44%) had stabilization of visual acuity.[53] It should be noted that the information available from these studies for evaluating the beneficial or harmful effects of ICG-guided laser treatment on visual acuity in the absence of a randomized clinical trial comparing this treatment to no treatment does not necessarily suggest that the outcome is different from the natural course of untreated cases. Moreover, the short duration of follow-up and unavailability for follow-up in many cases could influence the conclusions of these studies.[54] Until randomized clinical trials demonstrate that ICG angiography can help preserve the vision in AMD, ophthalmologists should recognize that routine recommendation to obtain ICG angiography to guide laser treatment to preserve the patient's vision is not supported by available information.[53,54]

MANAGEMENT

The MPS trials, a series of large multicenter, randomized clinical trials, gave detailed information about the indications for laser treatment in CNV related to AMD (Table 10–1). The immediate goal of treatment in all MPS clinical trials that addressed this issue was to photocoagulate the entire area of CNV. To achieve this goal, the ophthalmologist needs to be able to identify the entire boundary of the CNV. It should also be remembered that the benefits of laser treatment have not been proven for a lesion with evidence of occult neovascularization in the absence of classic CNV, lesions with poorly demarcated boundaries, and lesions that are predominantly blocked fluorescence from blood or fibrous tissue.

Treatment Techniques

The principle of photocoagulation is that laser light is absorbed by pigment in the RPE and choroid and then is converted into heat, which dissipates into the adjacent tissues. If CNV is adjacent to an area of photocoagulation, it may be ablated by coagulation necrosis. Clinicopathologic correlative studies[55] suggest that the CNV may not be ablated completely by the laser. Rather, the neovascular lesion may become enveloped by multiple layers of RPE fibrous tissue and that this laser-induced scar limits continued growth of the neovascular lesion and therefore limits the extent of the retina that otherwise would be destroyed by the natural course of the neovascular lesion. Laboratory evidence suggests that proliferation of the RPE following laser treatment may play a role in treating CNV by enveloping the CNV and absorbing the fluid that separates the neovascularization from the overlying sensory retina.[56–58]

When preparing for laser treatment of CNV, a recent angiogram (preferably no more than 96 hours before treatment) should be obtained to reduce the possibility that the CNV has grown larger than that shown on the angiogram used to guide the boundaries of the treatment. Ideally, the angiogram is obtained on the same day of treatment. The greatest contrast and resolution to facilitate identifying the entire extent of the CNV lesion will

TABLE 10–1 Treatment Specifications of Laser Photocoagulation Protocol for CNV Followed by the MPS Group

Study	Lesion location	Laser technique
AMD, extrafoveal	Foveal edge of CNV (and blockage by pigment or blood if present) 200–2500 μm from FAZ center	Cover CNV, contiguous blockage, and 100 μm beyond CNV
AMD, juxtafoveal	Foveal edge of CNV (or blockage by pigment or blood if present) 1–199 μm from FAZ center or foveal edge of CNV >199 μm from FAZ center with contiguous blood or blocked fluorescence within 200 μm from FAZ center	*Nonfoveal side*: Cover CNV, contiguous blockage, and 100 μm beyond *Foveal side*: cover CNV; if CNV >100 μm from FAZ center and contiguous blood is present, also cover contiguous blood up to 100 μm beyond CNV
AMD, subfoveal, new*	CNV under FAZ center	Cover CNV, contiguous blockage, and 100 μm beyond
AMD, subfoveal, recurrent	Recurrent CNV under FAZ center	Cover CNV, contiguous blockage, and 100 μm beyond†

* At least some CNV must be classic; CNV must underlie foveal center; entire new lesion must be ≤3.5 MPS disc areas and have well-demarcated boundaries; entire recurrent lesion (including area of prior laser treatment) must be ≤6.0 MPS disc areas and have well demarcated boundaries; features that obscure boundaries of CNV must be smaller in area than CNV.

† At interface between recurrence and prior laser, extend treatment spots 300 μm into prior laser scar; cover feeder vessels 100 μm beyond lateral border and 300 μm radially beyond base (origin) of feeder vessel.

MPS, Macular Photocoagulation Study; CNV, choroidal neovascularization; FAZ, foveal avascular zone.

be obtained using 35-mm film when compared to videoangiography. It is unknown if the decreased contrast and resolution on videoangiography affects the management of these lesions. When considering where to treat, a representative frame of the angiogram that highlights the entire extent of the CNV lesion with respect to the retinal vasculature and other fundus landmarks should be projected onto a screen to allow for rapid and repeated extrapolations from the fluorescein landmarks as compared to the patient's fundus landmarks. Retrobulbar anesthesia may be used whenever necessary to ensure that neither ocular motility nor patient discomfort will compromise the success of treatment by preventing the ophthalmologist from delivering laser of sufficient intensity and duration of exposure to produce a uniform white treatment burn. This is especially true when treating near to or within the foveal avascular zone (FAZ), when there is a natural reluctance to treat on the foveal side of the lesion[59] and when small amounts of undertreatment may allow persistence of neovascularization or small amounts of overtreatment might obliterate foveal structures and result in unnecessary visual loss.[60] The initial laser burns are placed along the boundary of the CNV using a 200-μm spot size and 0.2- to 0.5-second duration. The long duration lowers the risk for a sudden break in Bruch's membrane, and the relatively large spot size minimizes the frequency of bleeding when adjusting from lower to higher milliwatts of power. Usually, photocoagulation is applied first to the foveal side of the planned treatment area in juxtafoveal or extrafoveal lesions. The desired end point for the intensity of the laser lesion was the creation of a uniformly white lesion. Specific treatment parameters are summarized in Table 10–1. Since this treatment approach was proven to be effective in randomized clinical trials, we employ this approach when treating similar lesions in our practice.

Wavelength Selection

A wide range of laser wavelengths is available for photocoagulation of CNV. The absorption spectrum of each wavelength dictates specific theoretical advantages and disadvantages for its use. When the MPS began in 1978, the argon blue-green laser was the one most commercially available to investigators. This laser no longer is recommended for treatment within the macular region because macular xanthophyll pigment directly absorbs the blue light of the argon blue-green laser, thereby inducing thermal damage to the inner retina.[61] In addition, the risk of inducing internal limiting membrane wrinkling, although rarely of clinical significance, is probably greatest with the argon blue-green laser.[62] Subsequent trials in the MPS for juxtafoveal lesions employed the krypton red laser because of

its theoretical advantage of penetrating through xanthophyll and passing through thin layers of red hemorrhage, allowing the uptake of the laser to be concentrated within the RPE and melanocytes of the inner choroid. When the MPS trials for subfoveal lesions were designed, eyes randomized to the treatment group also were randomized to either the argon green or the krypton red wavelength for treatment. Small trends in visual acuity outcomes favored argon green laser over krypton red laser for treatment of subfoveal CNV (new or recurrent), but only change in reading speed from baseline for the treatment of recurrent CNV attained statistical significance. Although argon laser–treated eyes lost fewer words per minute on reading speed tests as compared with krypton laser–treated eyes, reading speed remained markedly abnormal in each group. The average level of visual acuity was essentially the same for argon-treated and krypton-treated eyes. Likewise, the average change in visual acuity from baseline was essentially the same for both argon-treated and krypton-treated eyes. In both the new and recurrent CNV trials, argon-treated eyes had a small improvement in contrast sensitivity function, whereas krypton-treated eyes deteriorated further in this regard. Overall, however, there were no clinically significant differences in any of the visual outcome measures between the two laser wavelength groups.[33,34,63,64] Small differences in convenience of achieving the end point of a uniform white burn might be seen with red or yellow wavelengths when penetrating through the increased nuclear yellow lens in the older age group afflicted with CNV secondary to AMD, but any significant differences of clinical importance have not been shown. Rates of persistent or recurrent CNV were similar in each laser wavelength group and approached 50% within 3 years. However, argon-treated patients were more likely to demonstrate complete coverage of the entire neovascular lesion with heavy laser burns (which can reduce the likelihood of recurrence) as compared with krypton-treated patients. Clinically relevant complications of laser treatment were identified rarely, although iatrogenic rupture of Bruch's membrane and the creation of a retinal hole did occasionally occur with either wavelength. The only condition associated with treatment that was different between the two laser groups was focal narrowing of the retinal vessels in the region of photocoagulation. This occurred more often in argon-treated eyes than in krypton-treated eyes but was not shown to be of any clinical significance. Thus, no visible wavelength appears to have a significant advantage over other wavelengths. The treating ophthalmologist, therefore, should choose whatever wavelength will facilitate penetration of the ocular media and provide homogeneous and intense photocoagulation to the entire choroidal neovascular lesion, particularly since these aspects of treatment (intense burns and coverage of the entire lesion) have been shown to affect the final visual outcome.

Special Considerations

When overlying a major retinal vessel, the treatment burns should straddle the vessel, the reduce the possibility of causing hemorrhage or damaging the vessels by thermal vasculitis. There is no evidence to suggest that this technique compromises the effectiveness of the treatment.

When treating CNV that is contiguous with the optic nerve, treatment within 100 to 200 μm of the optic nerve should not be performed, to lower the chance of thermal necrosis of disc tissue and nerve fiber bundle defects.[65] In the treatment of peripapillary CNV, treatment was considered and proven to be effective only when at least 1.5 clock hours of the papillomacular bundle on the temporal side of the disc was spared of photocoagulation because there was no CNV in this area. However, most ophthalmologists will consider treatment of lesions contiguous with the optic nerve that spare even less than 1.5 clock hours. Treatment in this region can cause damage to the optic nerve. However, laser treatment to these lesions never caused severe visual loss unless a recurrence through the fovea subsequently developed.[66,67]

When treating recurrences, the treatment should extend 300 μm into the area of prior treatment at the interface of the prior treatment and the recurrent neovascular lesion. If a feeder vessel is present, the treatment should extend 100 μm beyond the lateral borders of the recurrent vessel and 300 μm radially beyond the base of the feeder vessel.

Risks and Benefits of Treatment of Extrafoveal CNV (Posterior Boundary of CNV Between 200 and 2500 μm from Geometric Center of FAZ)

The MPS group reported that laser treatment was beneficial at decreasing the risk of severe visual loss in eyes with extrafoveal CNV secondary to AMD when compared with no treatment (Table 10–2).[68] The proportion of eyes with severe visual loss (6 lines or more) 1 year after presenting with extrafoveal CNV was 41% in the eyes assigned to no treatment and 24% in the eyes assigned to laser treatment. By 3 years, 63% of the eyes assigned to no treatment and 45% of the eyes assigned to treatment had severe visual loss. The treatment benefit was maintained 5 years after treatment, at which time 64% of the eyes assigned to no treatment as opposed to 46% of eyes assigned to treatment had severe visual loss.[68] The relative risk of losing 6 lines or more of visual acuity from baseline among untreated eyes compared with laser-treated eyes was 1.5 from 6 months through 5 years after enrollment ($p = .001$). After 5 years, untreated eyes had lost a mean of 7.1 lines of visual acuity, whereas laser-treated eyes had lost a mean of 5.2

lines. Recurrent CNV was observed in 54% of laser-treated eyes by the end of the 5-year follow-up period. About 75% of these recurrences occurred by the end of the first year after treatment. An additional 17% occurred between 1 and 2 years of follow-up. The remaining 7% occurred between the end of the second year and the fifth year of follow-up. The effect of recurrence on visual acuity was devastating. Only 10% of the treated eyes with no recurrence had severe visual loss, compared with 80% of the treated eyes with recurrence. At the end of the third year of follow-up after treatment, the average visual acuity of the treated eyes with no recurrence was 20/50 and that of the treated eyes with recurrence was 20/250. This treatment benefit has been confirmed by two other similar randomized trials.[69,70] It should be emphasized that any recurrent CNV within 200 μm of the center of the FAZ was not treated in this trial; retreatment of these recurrences may have resulted in an even larger treatment benefit.

Risks and Benefits of Treatment to Juxtafoveal CNV (Posterior Boundary of CNV Between 1 and 199 μm from Geometric Center of FAZ)

In the Krypton Photocoagulation Study of lesions with AMD, lesions were included in which the posterior edge of the CNV was between 1 and 199 μm from the center of the FAZ, or lesions in which the posterior edge of the CNV was between 200 and 2500 μm from the center of the FAZ associated with blood or blocked fluorescence which extended within 200 μm of the FAZ center.[71] This study also showed that treatment was beneficial when compared with no treatment (Table 10–2). Forty per cent of the eyes assigned to no treatment, compared to 31% of the eyes treated, had severe visual loss by 1 year. The treatment benefit diminished by 3 years, but persisted even after 5 years; 25% of the treated eyes compared to 15% of the untreated eyes at least maintained their baseline visual acuity at this time. By 5 years after entry into the study, the mean visual acuity of laser-treated eyes was 20/200 compared to 20/250 in the untreated eyes; in addition, there were more than twice as many treated patients who retained visual acuity of 20/40 or better. Furthermore, only 25% of laser-treated eyes had a visual acuity of 20/400 or worse, whereas 40% of untreated eyes had this outcome.[72] Although untreated eyes with juxtafoveal CNV lost more visual acuity than treated eyes, both groups continued to lose vision throughout the study. Rates of severe visual loss (≥6 lines) rose to 52% among laser-treated eyes, and 61% among untreated eyes 5 years after enrollment. The disappointing long-term visual function among treated eyes was due to the great frequency of persistence or recurrence.

TABLE 10–2 Outcome of Treatment of CNV according to the MPS

Study	1 Year*		3 Years*		5 Years*		Risk of Persistent/ Recurrent CNV
	Treated Eyes	Untreated Eyes	Treated Eyes	Untreated Eyes	Treated Eyes	Untreated Eyes	
AMD, extrafoveal	24%	41%	45%	63%	46%	64%	54%
AMD, juxtafoveal	31%	40%	44%	63%	49%	58%	45%
juxtafoveal, classic, CNV only			48%	70%			
AMD, subfoveal, new	18%	23%	2 years 20%	37%	4 years 22%	47%	51%
AMD, subfoveal, recurrent	8%	19%	2 years 9%	28%	3 years 23%	44%	48%

* Risk of severe visual loss.

MPS, Macular Photocoagulation Study; CNV, choroidal neovascularization; FAZ, foveal avascular zone.

Thirty-two per cent of the treated eyes had evidence of leakage at the periphery of the laser-treated area within 6 weeks following treatment (termed a "persistence" of CNV). An additional 22% had evidence of leakage at the periphery of the laser-treated area that was not noted until sometime after the 6-week posttreatment visit. As with extrafoveal lesions, both persistence and recurrence had an adverse effect on visual acuity; the visual acuity in eyes with persistent or recurrent CNV after initial treatment was, on average, 3 to 4 lines worse than in eyes without peripheral leakage.[71,73] It is unknown whether an attempt to treat a more extensive area of treatment, as was done for the extrafoveal lesions (in which treatment was to extend for 100 μm beyond the entire boundary of the CNV) would have resulted in a better or worse treatment benefit. Although it was noted in this study that patients who were normotensive had a marked treatment benefit and patients with hypertension (manifested by elevated systolic or diastolic blood pressures or by the use of antihypertensive medications) had no treatment benefit, this finding was not noted consistently in other MPS trials and should not discourage an ophthalmologist from considering recommending treatment of a juxtafoveal lesion in a hypertensive patient.

At the time of enrollment of patients for the Krypton Photocoagulation Study, from April 1, 1981 through December 31, 1987, the study ophthalmologists and MPS Fundus Photographic Reading Center staff based their identification of CNV from stereoscopic fluorescein angiograms as fluorescein dye leakage at the level of the outer retina. At that time, CNV was not classified as classic or occult. During the 1980s, angiographic interpretation of CNV by the ophthalmologic community was refined, and by the end of 1988, the MPS in-

vestigators concluded that the standard interpretations of fluorescein angiograms that had been used in the MPS AMD Study for juxtafoveal lesions did not provide an adequate description of neovascular lesions. Therefore, the MPS Fundus Photograph Reading Center staff revised its interpretations of fluorescein angiograms to differentiate classic from occult CNV, guidelines which were critical to interpreting and applying the results of the subfoveal trials, which were published in 1991.[34] When the angiograms of patients who were enrolled in the MPS AMD Study for juxtafoveal lesions from 1981 to 1987 were re-evaluated[36] using the guidelines for interpretation of fluorescein angiograms adopted in 1988, it was noted that the number of eyes with classic CNV but no occult CNV (n = 237), classic and occult CNV (n = 158), and occult CNV but no classic CNV (n = 61) was almost identical for the eyes assigned randomly to treatment or observation. Classic CNV almost always was covered completely with intense laser treatment; nevertheless, recurrent CNV developed in more than half of these eyes within 1 year after initial laser treatment. In contrast, in more than half of the eyes with occult CNV, more than 50% of the occult CNV was not covered with heavy laser treatment. Laser treatment of eyes in which all of the CNV was classic was of greater benefit than for the entire group with juxtafoveal CNV. At 3 years after study entry, in the subgroup with classic CNV but no occult CNV, severe visual acuity loss occurred in 70% of the untreated eyes compared to 48% of the treated eyes. Subfoveal recurrent CNV was not retreated. However, had the treatment benefit for selected cases of subfoveal recurrent CNV been known and applied to these treated lesions that developed recurrence, severe visual acuity loss might have occurred in only 41% of the treated eyes, a marked treatment benefit compared to observation. For the eyes with classic and occult CNV, in which treatment usually covered all of classic CNV but less than 50% of the occult CNV, treatment was not beneficial.

Risks and Benefits of Treatment to Subfoveal CNV (CNV Lies Under Geometric Center of FAZ)

In 1986, the MPS group initiated two randomized clinical trials of laser treatment for subfoveal CNV secondary to AMD. One trial was initiated for *new* subfoveal CNV in eyes with no previous photocoagulation in the macula, and the other was initiated for *recurrent* subfoveal CNV that developed following laser treatment of an extrafoveal or juxtafoveal lesion. The subfoveal lesions had to have evidence of classic CNV (although occult CNV could be present with classic CNV). The entire boundary of the lesion had to be well-demarcated. The entire lesion size had to be less than or equal to 3.5 MPS disc areas (a circle whose radius is equal to approximately 1500 μm assuming a magnification of 3 on a Zeiss 30-degree photograph). In eyes with new subfoveal AMD,[33] laser was beneficial with respect to visual acuity, reading speed, and contrast sensitivity compared with no treatment, although there was an immediate decrease in visual acuity following treatment. Three months after randomization, 20% of the laser-treated eyes compared with 11% of the untreated eyes had lost 6 lines or more of visual acuity from the level at study entry. However, 24 months after enrollment, the percentage of eyes that lost 6 lines or more of visual acuity remained 20% in the laser-treated eyes, but had increased to 37% in the untreated eyes. Additional follow-up of eyes in the subfoveal new CNV study confirmed the benefits of laser photocoagulation that had been realized by 2 years after treatment and demonstrated that the treatment benefit lasted for at least 4 years. Few eyes, whether treated or not, had a visual acuity better than 20/200 at the 48-month examination. However, even though both treated and untreated eyes lost visual acuity, at 4 years after study entry the majority of treated eyes maintained visual acuity better than 20/400, whereas the majority of untreated eyes had a final visual acuity of 20/400 or worse. In the laser-treated group, more eyes had little or no change from their baseline level of visual acuity than in the untreated group, and more untreated eyes lost 6 or more lines of visual acuity from baseline than treated eyes by the 4 year follow-up examination.[74]

At the 4-year follow-up examination, laser treatment for new subfoveal CNV also was found to be beneficial when compared to untreated eyes with respect to two additional measures of visual outcome, reading speed and contrast sensitivity. At follow-up, eyes assigned to observation averaged fewer words per minute when reading compared

to eyes assigned to treatment. Half of the untreated study eyes could not read any words of enlarged text (Snellen equivalent of approximately 20/1500). Furthermore, laser-treated eyes retained pre-treatment levels of contrast threshold, whereas a larger and larger proportion of untreated eyes required more contrast to read large letters (Snellen equivalent of approximately 20/750) as follow-up continued.

The updated report on the benefit of laser treatment for new subfoveal CNV also demonstrated that specific vision or lesion features which had been shown to affect the outcome in the original report remained influential in affecting long-term results. Specifically, the treatment benefit diminished with increasing size of neovascular lesion at baseline, and the average visual acuity loss was greatest for those treated eyes with relatively good visual acuity (20/100 or better) at baseline. Further analysis was performed to determine the treatment benefit for eyes stratified according to the initial size of the lesion and the initial visual acuity.[75] This subgroup analysis suggested that treatment was not likely to be beneficial for lesions in the study that were larger than 2 MPS disc areas in size unless the visual acuity was 20/200 or worse (Figs. 10–15 and 10–16).

For small lesions (≤1 MPS disc area) and visual acuity of 20/125 or worse, or for medium sized lesions (>1 but ≤2 MPS disc areas) with a visual acuity of 20/200 or worse, treated eyes were less likely to have severe visual loss than untreated eyes at every examination during follow-up. Treatment for this situation should be considered strongly.

Study participants with large lesions and a visual acuity of 20/160 or better were more likely to have severe visual loss with treatment than with observation for up to 2 years with no appreciable treatment benefit through 4 years of follow-up. Hence, this situation is not likely to benefit from laser treatment. Close follow-up is recommended, since additional loss of vision, to 20/200 or worse, with absence of lesion growth beyond 3.5 MPS disc areas, might result in a situation that would benefit from laser treatment compared to observation.

Study participants with small lesions (≤1 MPS disc areas) and visual acuity of 20/100 or better, or medium-sized lesions (>1 but ≤2 MPS disc areas) and a visual acuity of 20/160 or better, tended to have a higher proportion developing severe visual loss compared with untreated eyes until 12 months after study entry. However, by 12 months after study entry and for at least 3 additional years thereafter, fewer treated eyes had severe visual loss compared to untreated eyes. Thus, these eyes are good candidates for laser treatment, but the patient must understand that the immediate visual loss that will occur after laser treatment likely will confine visual damage to a greater extent over several years than if treatment is not given. Although some ophthalmologists and patients, when confronted with this situation, may prefer careful follow-up at short

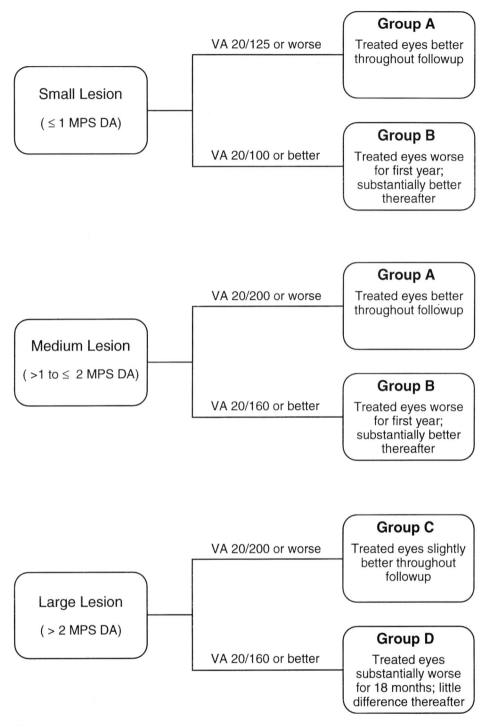

FIGURE 10–15 Schematic aid for determining the pattern of visual acuity loss in Macular Photocoagulation Study (MPS) eyes with new subfoveal choroidal neovascularization. DA, disc areas; VA, visual acuity. (From the Macular Photocoagulation Study Group: Visual outcome after laser photocoagulation for subfoveal choroidal neovascularization secondary to age-related macular degeneration: the influence of initial lesion size and initial visual acuity. Arch Ophthalmol 112:480–488, 1994. Copyright 1994, American Medical Association, with permission.)

time intervals instead of immediate laser treatment, so that treatment may be employed only if the visual acuity deteriorates, they must understand that there is considerable risk in deferring the treatment. In most cases, the lesion will enlarge to more than 3.5 MPS disc areas within 3 months such that laser treatment may no longer be an option and the opportunity to improve on the natural course of visual loss may be irretrievably lost. Thus if treatment of eyes with these features is deferred, follow-up certainly should be considered sooner than at 3 months, probably within 2 to 3 weeks, and oph-

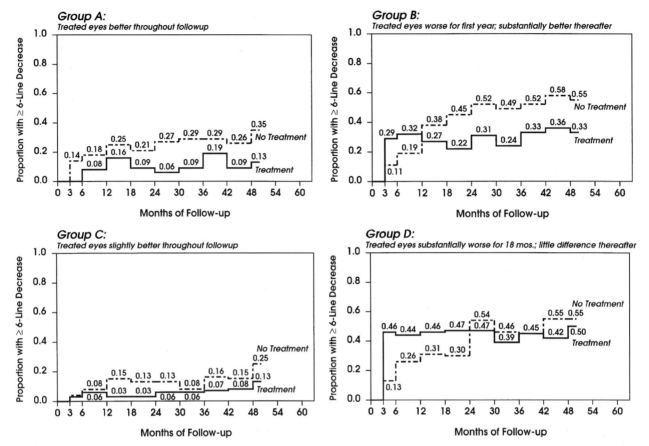

FIGURE 10–16 Proportion of eyes with decreases in visual acuity of 6 or more lines from baseline at each specified time in the various groups of the Macular Photocoagulation New Subfoveal CNV Study based on treatment benefit by initial size and initial visual acuity. *Solid line* indicates the treatment group; *broken line* indicates the no-treatment group. *Top,* Pattern A, treated eyes fared better throughout follow-up. *Upper center,* Pattern B, treated eyes fared better beginning 1 year after study entry. *Lower center,* Pattern C, treated eyes fared slightly better throughout follow-up. *Bottom,* Pattern D, treated eyes were substantially worse for first 18 months after study entry with little difference thereafter. (From the Macular Photocoagulation Study Group: Visual outcome after laser photocoagulation for subfoveal choroidal neovascularization secondary to age-related macular degeneration: the influence of initial lesion size and initial visual acuity. Arch Ophthalmol 112:480–488, 1994. Copyright 1994, American Medical Association, with permission.)

thalmologists should consider recommending treatment if the lesion grows within a few weeks, since waiting until vision deteriorates may not occur until the lesion first grows more than 3.5 MPS disc areas, a situation in which treatment is not likely to be beneficial.

The MPS group also reported on the incidence of recurrent CNV and its impact on visual outcome in eyes following initial laser therapy for new subfoveal CNV.[76] After initial treatment of new subfoveal CNV, 13% of treated eyes demonstrated persistent leakage for CNV within 6 weeks following treatment, while an additional 31% developed recurrent leakage from CNV within 2 years. In addition, a new, independent area of CNV developed in 3% of treated eyes over 3 years. Contrary to what had been observed in the extrafoveal and juxtafoveal trials, the development of persistent and recurrent CNV following treatment of new subfoveal

CNV had little effect on visual function. The mean visual acuity at 3 years following treatment was 20/400 for treated eyes with persistent CNV, 20/250 for treated eyes with recurrent CNV, and 20/320 for treated eyes with no peripheral leakage. Although persistent and recurrent CNV were common occurrences after initial treatment of new subfoveal CNV, it remains unknown whether additional treatment to these areas of posttreatment leakage protects the eye from further significant visual loss or leads to additional visual acuity loss from the retreatment itself. In the MPS new subfoveal CNV trial, half of the eyes with persistent or recurrent CNV were considered suitable for retreatment; that is, they had well-demarcated borders, properly applied treatment still would leave untreated some portion of the retina within 1500 μm of the center of the FAZ, and the old and newly treated areas together would not exceed 6 MPS disc areas. Although approximately half of all treated eyes were retreated, the number of eyes in the various subgroups based on suitability for retreatment and actual retreatment was too small to provide recommendation about the advisability of treatment of eyes that already had laser treatment for subfoveal CNV lesions. Nonetheless, it probably is justified to consider retreatment to areas of persistent or recurrent CNV that are detected when the recurrent lesion and area of prior subfoveal laser treatment is relatively small (<6 MPS disc areas), with the aim of minimizing further extensive visual acuity loss by confining the area of macular pathology. As in earlier MPS reports, patients with CNV or disciform scarring in the fellow eye at enrollment were at greater risk of having persistent or recurrent CNV in the study eye of the subfoveal trials as compared to individuals in whom the study eye was the first eye affected with CNV.[34,59,72]

Postoperative Management

Evaluating Extent of Laser Treatment

Since ophthalmologists might be reluctant to treat lesions that are very close to the fovea on the foveal side, and lack of adequate treatment in this area was shown to increase the chance for persistence at least threefold,[77] it is necessary to ensure complete coverage of the entire CNV lesion. When the CNV is not very close to the foveal center, it usually is not difficult for an ophthalmologist who is experienced at treating CNV to extend laser treatment over the entire extent of the CNV.[64,66] In such a situation, slight extension of the laser-treated area likely will have little effect on the visual acuity. However, when one is treating a juxtafoveal lesion, even the most experienced ophthalmologist may be reluctant to treat the foveal perimeter of the CNV too extensively.[59,77] Failure to cover the CNV in its entirety could lead to an increased risk of persistence within 6 weeks following treatment. In an attempt to minimize inadequate coverage, it is possible to compare the area of the laser treatment from a posttreatment photograph (e.g., using a 35-mm Polaroid transparency) to the area of the lesion from the pretreatment angiogram. The extent and location of the CNV with respect to the inner retinal vascular landmarks can be traced on a piece of plain white paper that is taped to the screen of a microfilm reader or projector upon which the pretreatment angiogram is projected. After treatment, a posttreatment 35-mm Polaroid transparency is taken. This transparency then is projected, and the area of heavy treatment and the same landmark vessels are outlined on a separate piece of plain white paper. The treatment drawing is placed on a light box, and the pretreatment drawing is placed over this, superimposing the landmark vessels. The area of heavy treatment then can be traced onto the pretreatment drawing to determine whether the

treatment has covered the CNV entirely. Any areas not treated adequately can be treated at the time that the inadequate treatment is identified.[23,29,78] The MPS group proved the usefulness of this method using 1-day posttreatment stereoscopic color photographs to identify areas of inadequate treatment; eyes with inadequate coverage did indeed have a higher rate of persistent CNV in the juxtafoveal trials.[59,77] It is likely that immediate posttreatment Polaroid photographs or videotape image evaluations are comparable to the 1-day posttreatment stereoscopic color photographs used in the MPS trials.

Follow-up Evaluations

The risk of recurrent CNV after treatment of an extrafoveal or juxtafoveal lesion is extremely high and treatment of these recurrences, even when extending through the foveal center, may be beneficial (Table 10–2) compared to no additional treatment. Recurrent CNV also may develop following treatment to a subfoveal lesion, and retreatment of these recurrences also may be beneficial. In order to identify these recurrences when additional treatment may be beneficial, follow-up evaluations are necessary. About 50% of treated eyes will develop recurrences within the first 1 to 2 years after treatment (especially within the first few months after treatment). Therefore, frequent follow-up evaluations are obtained during this time so that any recurrence that develops can be identified promptly while it is relatively small, when retreatment may cause the least amount of damage. At the first follow-up, approximately 2 to 3 weeks following treatment, an angiogram should be scrutinized for the presence of leakage at the periphery of the laser-treated area to identify the presence of persistent or recurrent CNV. Simultaneous projection of the fluorescein angiogram during biomicroscopic examination may help differentiate areas of atrophy, which stain, from areas of recurrent leakage. If no residual CNV is noted at this time, this evaluation, including fluorescein angiography, is repeated 3 to 4 weeks later. At that time the patient can begin to monitor the central vision of the treated eye for changes in distance and near vision, distortion, or increase in scotoma, which might indicate leakage from persistent or recurrent CNV. Ophthalmologists should be aware that these patients may need prompt re-evaluation if such symptoms develop so that recurrences can be identified when they are still amenable to treatment. This evaluation again is repeated at 3 to 4 months posttreatment and then every 3 to 4 months during the first year. Since it has been reported that in 12% of follow-up visits after laser photocoagulation, definite or questionable recurrent CNV that was not suspected clinically was identified subsequently on fluorescein angiogram,[79] clinical examination alone probably cannot replace fluorescein angiography in detecting all recurrent CNV within the first year after laser treatment. During the second year and thereafter, semiannual evaluation may be adequate. After 2 years, recurrences are unusual; follow-up every 6 months without angiography (unless signs or symptoms suggest a recurrence) probably is warranted.

Treatment of Recurrent CNV

The MPS group reported the results of a trial conducted among patients who had received laser treatment for an extrafoveal or a juxtafoveal neovascular lesion who subsequently developed recurrent CNV through the geometric center of the foveal avascular zone. These eyes were assigned randomly to additional laser treatment or to observation. Updated results of this trial were published in 1993, when the median period of follow-up was 3 years.[74] At 3 years after study entry, laser-treated eyes had better visual acuity than untreated eyes, although both groups had limited distance visual acuity (Table 10–2). Treated or not, most eyes suffered an additional loss of at least 2 lines of visual acuity by this time after study entry. However, twice as many treated eyes as compared with untreated eyes had visual acuity better than 20/200 at the 3-year examination, and fewer than half as many treated eyes as compared with untreated eyes had visual acuity of 20/400 or worse. The median reading speed among laser-treated eyes was more than twice that of untreated eyes. Likewise, contrast sensitivity thresholds were better among laser-treated eyes than among untreated eyes.

Unlike new subfoveal lesions with no prior laser treatment, the beneficial effects of laser treatment for recurrent lesions persisted for all subgroups stratified by initial lesion size or initial visual acuity. In each subgroup based on initial lesion size, the risk of severe visual loss was twice as high among untreated eyes as among treated eyes. In each subgroup based on initial visual acuity, treatment of recurrent subfoveal CNV was beneficial compared to no treatment. Treatment was beneficial even when the baseline visual acuity ranged from 20/40 to 20/100 inclusive; however, these eyes also were at greatest risk for vision loss with or without treatment.

Again, it should be emphasized that these MPS results of recurrent subfoveal lesions may be applicable only to eyes with CNV associated with AMD that meet the eligibility criteria used for study entry. These criteria specified that the lesion had to be a well-demarcated recurrent CNV lesion in which neovascularization was under the foveal center. Some component of the lesion had to be classic CNV; the size of the recurrent lesion plus the prior area of laser treatment was to be 6 MPS disc areas or less. Furthermore, lesions were eligible only if, after applying protocol treatment, some retina uninvolved by the CNV lesion within 1500 μm of the foveal center remained untreated. The treatment protocol was similar to that described previously for new subfoveal lesions, with the additional requirement that laser treatment extend 300 μm into the area of prior laser treatment at the interface of the recurrent CNV and the original area of photocoagulation. If a feeder vessel was present, treatment was to extend 100 μm beyond the lateral borders of the recurrent vessel, and 300 μm radially beyond the base of the feeder vessel.

Predicting Recurrences

As already mentioned, the risk of recurrence was greater if the lesion was not covered entirely by photocoagulation at least as intense as a minimum treatment intensity standard photograph (Fig. 10–17). The risk of recurrence in the treated eye also was increased if the fellow eye already had neovascular AMD at the time of treatment. Other factors that might increase the rate of recurrence include cigarette smoking,[32] hypertension,[32] and CNV that is very lightly pigmented[41]; the latter factor may reflect the difficulty in obtaining a uniform white confluent treatment in such cases, resulting in an increased risk of persistent CNV.

RISK OF FELLOW EYE DEVELOPING CNV

It is important to have the patient monitor the vision in the fellow eye if that macula did not already have CNV. The MPS group has shown that if a patient presents with extrafoveal CNV in one eye and no evidence of CNV or scarring in the fellow eye, about one third will develop CNV in the fellow eye within 5 years.[68] The risk of CNV developing in the fellow eye within 5 years after presenting with extrafoveal CNV in the first eye was 10% for eyes with small drusen only, 30% in eyes presenting with either large drusen or focal clumps of RPE hyperpigmentation, and approximately 60% for eyes presenting with both large drusen and focal clumps of RPE hyperpigmentation within 1500 μm of the foveal center.

This information was confirmed recently in a follow-up study of fellow eyes of 670 patients enrolled in the MPS randomized trials for new juxtafoveal CNV, new subfoveal CNV, or recurrent subfoveal CNV secondary to AMD. This study found that the 5-year incidence rate of CNV in the fellow eye ranged from 7% in fellow eyes with no risk factors to 87% in eyes with four independently identified risk factors (five or more drusen, focal hyperpigmentation, one or more large drusen, and definite systemic hypertension).[80]

Visual acuity changes in the fellow eye of the argon AMD extrafoveal trial paralleled the development of CNV in the fellow eye. For fellow eyes that developed CNV within 5 years, the average visual acuity loss was 8 lines of vision. For fellow eyes that had no evidence of CNV or scarring at baseline and did not have CNV develop within 5

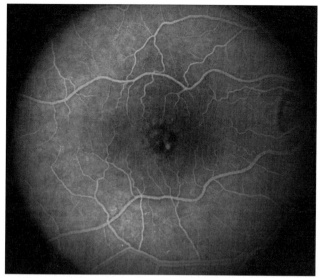

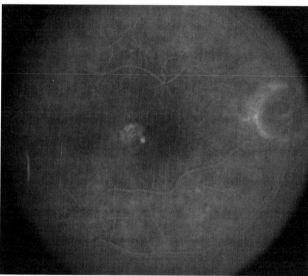

FIGURE 10–17 Minimal staining standard for occult choroidal neovascularization (CNV). *Top*, Early phase of angiogram shows fibrovascular pigment epithelial detachment with contiguous, flat, blocked fluorescence. *Bottom*, Late phase of angiogram shows fluorescein staining of occult CNV. If late staining was less apparent than minimal amount of staining noted in bottom section, area of presumed occult CNV was not considered to be lesion component. (From the Macular Photocoagulation Study Group: Visual outcome after laser photocoagulation for subfoveal choroidal neovascularization secondary to age-related macular degeneration: the influence of initial lesion size and initial visual acuity. Arch Ophthalmol 112:480–488, 1994. Copyright 1994, American Medical Association, with permission.)

years, the average visual acuity loss was only 0.4 lines.[68] Overall, 49% of participants in the argon AMD MPS trial were legally blind (visual acuity of 20/200 or less in both eyes) within 5 years of follow-up when the fellow eye initially had CNV or scarring, whereas only 12% of participants were legally blind within 5 years of follow-up when the fellow eye had no evidence of CNV or scarring initially.[68]

CONCLUSIONS AND FUTURE RESEARCH

Currently, the only treatment that has been shown to be beneficial for AMD based on large randomized clinical trials is photocoagulation. Unfortunately, this treatment is effective only for a small subgroup of patients with small, well-demarcated lesions that include a component of classic CNV. Furthermore, laser treatment has been shown to be beneficial at reducing the likelihood of developing additional severe visual acuity deterioration but usually causes an immediate decrease in visual acuity.

The majority of patients with neovascular AMD do not meet criteria to make laser treatment beneficial at reducing the risk of severe visual loss because the lesion is too large, or poorly demarcated, or does not include classic CNV at the time the patient presents to an ophthalmologist.[22,81] Thus, the search continues for therapies other than laser photocoagulation that may apply to more patients or may be less likely to cause damage to vision or may cause improvement in vision. New treatment strategies are aimed at limiting the degree and extent of destruction of retina overlying the CNV as well as applicability to a majority of patients in whom CNV develops, even those with large or poorly demarcated subfoveal lesions. Some of these new treatment strategies and their current status are detailed below.

Submacular Surgery

Theoretically, removal of CNV surgically may arrest the enlargement of the visual defect, limit central vision loss, and allow photoreceptors adjacent to the area of retina damaged by the neovascular lesion to function normally, as may be seen after selected cases of laser treatment. Additionally, surgical treatment may have the potential to preserve some of the neurosensory retina overlying the CNV with the expectation that some of macular photoreceptors will retain function. Surgery also may facilitate the management of CNV associated with large subfoveal hemorrhages.[82,83] During surgery, the submacular hemorrhage may be evacuated first and then the neovascular tissue removed or subsequently treated with laser, avoiding laser treatment that might have been too extensive if performed under the assumption that some or all of the hemorrhage was obscuring the boundaries of the CNV. Prompt surgical evacuation of blood in these eyes may limit toxic reactions to the overlying photoreceptors as well. Preliminary evidence on surgical treatment for CNV suggests that surgery may apply to a wide range of lesions and may be beneficial.[84–88] However, the available evidence suffers from limited follow-up of relatively few cases, nonstandardized methods of assessing visual outcomes, and lack of concurrent controls for comparison of outcomes. For cases reported to have stable or improved visual acuity following surgery, follow-up often has been of short duration (6 months or less). Case series have detailed the surgical technique but have not had concurrent controls or long follow-up. In contemplating this issue, the risks of submacular surgery should be considered, including acceleration of cataract, development of retinal tears, as well as retinal and choroidal detachments. Recurrence of CNV following surgical removal also has been reported.[84] Furthermore, relatively healthy RPE can be inadvertently removed.[89] The Submacular Surgery Trials Pilot Study, with support from the National Eye Institute of the National Institutes of Health, currently is assessing the benefits of submacular surgery in four trials including: (1) comparing surgery to observation for new subfoveal CNV secondary to AMD not currently amenable to laser treatment; (2) comparing surgery to photocoagulation for recurrent subfoveal CNV lesions secondary to AMD; (3) comparing surgery to observation for hemorrhagic subfoveal CNV lesion secondary to AMD in which more than 50% of the entire lesion is occupied by hemorrhage; and (4) comparing surgery to observation for new or recurrent subfoveal CNV lesions secondary to ocular histoplasmosis or idiopathic causes. The primary outcomes are stabilization of the presenting level of visual acuity or development of additional severe visual acuity loss, changes in contrast sensitivity, lens opacification, as well as quality of life, surgical complications, and costs. Expansion of one or more of these trials to a full-phase investigation to determine definitive benefits and risks of submacular surgery in an adequate number of participants followed for up to 4 years after study entry is anticipated in 1997.

Photodynamic Therapy

Selective destruction of CNV with preservation of the overlying neurosensory retina is the goal of photodynamic therapy (PDT) that relies on low-intensity light exposure of tissues treated with photosensitizers to produce photochemical effects.[90] In this technique, a photosensitizing dye is injected intravenously, followed by irradiation of the tissue at the absorbency maximum of the dye. The activated dye in its triplet state presumably interacts with oxygen and other compounds to form reactive intermediates, such as singlet oxygen, which then may cause disruption of cellular structures. Photodynamic therapy has been tried previously using hematoporphyrin derivative or rose bengal and has been limited by the weak photosensitizing ability or by prolonged cutaneous photosensitivity.[91] Newer photosensitizing agents have been designed to overcome these difficulties, with potentially improved clinical efficacy. One of these is benzopor-

phyrin derivative–monoacid (BPD-MA). Following intravenous injection of BPD-MA complexed with low-density lipoprotein to monkey eyes with subretinal neovascularization experimentally produced by intense laser lesions, eyes were irradiated with 692-nm light at a fluence of 50 to 150 J/cm^2 and irradiance of 150 to 600 mW/cm^2. The subretinal neovascularization was occluded on histopathology with minimal damage to the subjacent RPE, photoreceptors, and choriocapillaris. A randomized clinical trial is underway (the Treatment of Age-Related Macular Degeneration with Photodynamic Therapy [TAP] investigation) to evaluate the potential benefits of photodynamic therapy for CNV due to AMD.[90]

Radiation Therapy

It has been proposed that ionizing radiation may prevent the proliferation of endothelial cells of newly formed subretinal capillaries and may induce obliteration of the aberrant new vessels in CNV. Investigators of pilot studies evaluating the effect of radiation therapy on subfoveal CNV concluded that the results were promising, although lesions were generally large with poor vision, poorly demarcated boundaries, and may not always have had a component of classic CNV, all of which may have had an impact on results that suggested a favorable outcome compared to cases observed in the MPS trials.[92–95]

Pharmacologic Intervention

The possibility of using pharmacologic intervention, with the advantages of avoiding laser-induced retinal damage, treating poorly defined lesions or lesions with occult CNV but no classic CNV, lowering the recurrence rate following laser photocoagulation, and preventing eyes with nonneovascular AMD from progressing to the neovascular form of the disease, has been intriguing for many years. The rationale for the use of interferon alfa-2a as a potential antiangiogenic agent to treat CNV was based on work from basic science, studies on experimental neovascularization in monkeys, and the known effectiveness of the drug in the treatment of other angiogenic disorders in humans.[96,97] Conflicting results of various pilot studies have been published regarding its efficacy in AMD.[98–100] All of these studies had small sample sizes, and most of them were not designed such that cases were randomized to treatment or observation. Recently, a multicenter, randomized clinical trial that had enrolled patients with subfoveal CNV evaluated patients who were randomized into four groups receiving 1.5, 3, or 6 million international units or placebo treatment given 3 times a week for 12 months; 479 eyes were enrolled in 53 centers. At 12 months following study entry, treatment was not shown to be beneficial, and possibly was harmful.[101] These results serve to highlight the variable natural course of CNV in AMD, especially within 1 year of presentation. This variable course can lead to erroneous conclusions that a potential treatment is beneficial when such cases have no significant deterioration after a short follow-up; such cases might have had the same outcome without treatment. Nevertheless, given the public health impact of vision loss due to AMD, studies continue in animals and humans to investigate the potential effectiveness of other potential pharmacologic agents such as inhibitors of vascular endothelial growth factor, thalidomide, matrix metalloproteinase inhibitors, and angiotaxic steroids for the treatment of AMD.

Acknowledgment: We would like to thank Judith Alexander and the Wilmer Photograph Reading Center for assisting in the preparation and review of the figures.

REFERENCES

1. Bressler SB, Bressler NM, Alexander J, Green WR: Clinicopathologic correlation of occult choroidal neovascularization in age-related macular degeneration. Arch Ophthalmol 110:827–832, 1992.
2. Gass DM: Drusen and disciform macular detachment and degeneration. Arch Ophthalmol 90:201–217, 1973.
3. Green WR, Key SN: Pathologic features of senile macular degeneration. Ophthalmology 92:615–627, 1985.
4. Sarks SH: Aging and degeneration in the macular region: a clinicopathologic study. Br J Ophthalmol 60:324–341, 1976.
5. Smiddy WE, Fine SL: Prognosis of patients with bilateral macular drusen. Ophthalmology 91:271–284, 1984.
6. Herriot WJ, Henkind P, Bellhorn RW, Burns MS: Choroidal neovascularization can digest Bruch's membrane: a prior break is not essential. Ophthalmology 91:1603–1608, 1984.
7. Penfold PL, Provis JM, Billson FA: Age-related macular degeneration: ultrastructural studies of the relationship of leukocytes to angiogenesis. Graef Arch Clin Exp Ophthalmol 225:70–76, 1987.
8. Penfold PL, Killingsworth MS, Sarks SH: Senile macular degeneration: the involvement of immunocomponent cells. Graef Arch Clin Exp Ophthalmol 223:69–76, 1987.
9. Loeffler KU, Lee R: Basal linear deposit in the human macula. Graef Arch Clin Exp Ophthalmol 224:493–501, 1986.
10. Ryan SJ: Development of an experimental model of subretinal neovascularization in disciform macular degeneration. Trans Am Ophthalmol Soc 77:707–745, 1979.
11. Ryan SJ: Subretinal neovascularization: natural history of an experimental model. Arch Ophthalmol 100:1804–1809, 1982.
12. Friedman E, Ivry M, Ebert E, et al: Increased sclera rigidity and age-related macular degeneration. Ophthalmology 96:104–108, 1980.
13. Eye Disease Case-Control Study Group: Risk factors for neovascular age-related macular degeneration. Arch Ophthalmol 110:1701–1708, 1991.
14. Eye Disease Case-Control Study Group: Antioxidant status and neovascular age-related macular degeneration. Arch Ophthalmol 111:104–109, 1993.
15. Seddon JJ, Ajani UA, Sperduto RD, et al: Dietary carotenoids, vitamins A, C and E, and advanced age-related macular degeneration. JAMA 272:1413–1420, 1994.
16. Mares-Perlman JA, Brady WE, Klein R, et al: Serum antioxidants and age-related macular degeneration in a population-based case-control study. Arch Ophthalmol 113:1518–1523, 1995.
17. Bressler SB, Bressler, NM, Fine SL, et al: Natural course of choroidal neovascular membranes within the foveal avascular zone in senile macular degeneration. Am J Ophthalmol 93:157–163, 1982.
18. Bird AC: Macular disciform response and laser treatment. Trans Ophthalmol Soc UK 97:490–493, 1977.
19. Bressler NM, Frost LA, Bressler SB, et al: Natural course of poorly defined choroidal neovascularization associated with macular degeneration. Arch Ophthalmol 106:1537–1542, 1988.
20. Chandra SR, Gragoudas ES, Friedman E, et al: Natural history of disciform degeneration of the macula. Am J Ophthalmol 8:579–582, 1974.
21. Gragoudas ES, Chandra SR, Friedman E, et al: Disciform degeneration of the macula. II. Pathogenesis. Arch Ophthalmol 94:755–757, 1976.
22. Bressler NM, Bressler SB, Gragoudas ES: Clinical characteristics of choroidal neovascular membranes. Arch Ophthalmol 105:209–213, 1987.
23. Bressler NM, Bressler SB, Fine SL: Age-related macular degeneration. Surv Ophthalmol 32:375–413, 1988.
24. Boldt C, Bressler NM, Fine SL: Age-related macular degeneration. Curr Opin Ophthalmol 1:247–257, 1990.
25. Moisseiev J, Bressler NM: Asymptomatic neovascular membranes in the second eye of patients with visual loss from age-related macular degeneration. Invest Ophthalmol Vis Sci 31(s):462, 1990.
26. Fine AM, Elman MJ, Albert JE, et al: Earliest symptoms caused by neovascular membranes in the macula. Arch Ophthalmol 104:513–514, 1986.
27. Small ML, Green WR, Alpar JJ, et al: Senile macular degeneration: clinicopathologic correlation of two cases with neovascularization beneath the retinal pigment epithelium. Arch Ophthalmol 94:601–607, 1976.
28. Nasrallah F, Jalkh AE, Trempe CL, et al: Subretinal hemorrhage in atrophic age-related macular degeneration. Am J Ophthalmol 107:38–41, 1989.
29. Chamberlin JA, Bressler NM, Bressler SB, et al: The use of fundus photographs and fluorescein angiograms in the identification and treatment of choroidal neovascularization in the Macular Photocoagulation Study. Ophthalmology 96:1526–1534, 1989.
30. Klein ML, Zorizzo PA, Watzke RC: Growth features of choroidal neovascular membranes in age-related macular degeneration. Ophthalmology 96:1416–1421, 1989.
31. Vander JF, Morgan CV, Schatz H: Growth rate of subretinal neovascularization in age-related macular degeneration. Ophthalmology 96:1422–1429, 1989.
32. Macular Photocoagulation Study Group: Recurrent choroidal neovascularization after argon laser photocoagulation for neovascular lesions of neovascular maculopathy. Results of a randomized clinical trial. Arch Ophthalmol 104:503–512, 1986.
33. Macular Photocoagulation Study Group: Subfoveal neovascular lesions in age-related macular degeneration: guidelines for evaluation and treatment in the Macular Photocoagulation Study. Arch Ophthalmol 109:1242–1257, 1991.
34. Macular Photocoagulation Study Group: Laser photocoagulation of subfoveal neovascular lesions in age-related macular degeneration. Results of a randomized clinical trial. Arch Ophthalmol 109:1220–1231, 1991.
35. Macular Photocoagulation Study Group: Laser photocoagulation of subfoveal recurrent neovascular lesions in age-related macular degeneration. Results of a randomized clinical trial. Arch Ophthalmol 109:1232–1241, 1991.
36. Macular Photocoagulation Study Group: Occult choroidal neovascularization. Influence on visual outcome in patients with age-related macular degeneration. Arch Ophthalmol 114:400–412, 1996.

37. Soubrane G, Coscas G, Francis C, Loenig F: Occult sub-retinal new vessels in age-related macular degeneration. Ophthalmology 97:649–657, 1990.
38. Jalkh AE, Nasrallah FP, Marinelli I, Van de Velde F: Inactive subretinal neovascularization in age-related macular degeneration. Ophthalmology 97:1614–1619, 1990.
39. Schatz H, McDonald HR, Johnson RN: Retinal pigment epithelial folds associated with retinal pigment epithelial detachments in macular degeneration. Ophthalmology 97:658–665, 1990.
40. Casswell AG, Kohern D, Bird AC: Retinal pigment epithelial detachment in the elderly: classification and outcome. Br J Ophthalmol 69:397–403, 1985.
41. Sorenson JA, Yannuzzi LA, Shakin JL: Recurrent subretinal neovascularization. Ophthalmology 92:1059–1075, 1985.
42. Bressler NM, Bressler SB, Alexander J, et al: Loculated fluid. A previously undescribed fluorescein angiographic finding in choroidal neovascularization associated with macular degeneration. Arch Ophthalmol 109:211–215, 1991.
43. Gass JDM: Pathogenesis of tears of the retinal pigment epithelium. Br J Ophthalmol 68:514–519, 1984.
44. Decker WL, Sanborn GE, Ridley M, et al: Retinal pigment epithelial tears. Ophthalmology 90:507–512, 1983.
45. Cantrill HL, Ramsay RC, Knobloch WH: Rips in the pigment epithelium. Arch Ophthalmol 101:1074–1079, 1983.
46. Bressler NM, Finkelstein D, Sunness JS, et al: Retinal pigment epithelial tears through the fovea with preservation of good visual acuity. Arch Ophthalmol 108:1694–1697, 1990.
47. Marmor MF: Mechanisms of normal retinal adhesion. In Ryan S (ed): Retina. St Louis, CV Mosby Co, 1989, p 76.
48. Kreiger AE, Sterling JH: Vitreous hemorrhage in senile macular generation. Retina 3:318–321, 1983.
49. Tani M, Buettner H, Robertson DM: Massive vitreous hemorrhage and senile macular and choroidal degeneration. Am J Ophthalmol 90:525–533, 1980.
50. Flower R, Hochheimer BF: Clinical infrared absorption angiography of the choroid. Am J Ophthalmol 73:458–459, 1972.
51. Bischoff P, Flower RW: Ten years experience with choroidal angiography using indocyanine green dye. A new routine examination or an epilogue. Doc Ophthalmol 6:235–291, 1985.
52. Slakter JS, Yannuzzi LA, Sorenson JA, et al: A pilot study of indocyanine green videoangiography-guided laser photocoagulation of occult choroidal neovascularization in age-related macular degeneration. Arch Ophthalmol 112:465–472, 1994.
53. Guyer DR, Yannuzzi LA, Ladas I, et al: Indocyanine green-guided laser photocoagulation of focal spots at the edge of plaques of choroidal neovascularization. Arch Ophthalmol 114:693–697, 1996.
54. Bressler NM, Bressler SB: Indocyanine green angiography. Can it help preserve the vision of our patients? Arch Ophthalmol 114:747–749, 1996.
55. Green WR: Clinicopathologic studies of treated choroidal neovascular membranes. A review and report of two cases. Retina 11:328–356, 1991.
56. Miller H, Miller B, Ryan SJ: Correlation of choroidal subretinal neovascularization with fluorescein angiography. Am J Ophthalmol 99:263–271, 1985.
57. Miller H, Miller B, Ryan SH: Newly-formed subretinal vessels. Fine structure and fluorescein leakage. Invest Ophthalmol Vis Sci 27:204–213, 1986.
58. Miller H, Miller B, Ryan SJ: The role of the retinal pigment epithelium in the involution of subretinal neovascularization. Invest Ophthalmol Vis Sci 27:1644–1652, 1986.
59. Macular Photocoagulation Study Group: Persistent and recurrent neovascularization after krypton laser photocoagulation for neovascular lesions of age-related macular degeneration. Arch Ophthalmol 108:825–831, 1990.
60. Macular Photocoagulation Study Group: The influence of treatment extent on the visual acuity of eyes treated with krypton laser for juxtafoveal choroidal neovascularization. Arch Ophthalmol 113:190–194, 1995.
61. Smiddy WE, Fine SL, Quigley HA, et al: Comparison of krypton and argon laser photocoagulation in simulated clinical treatment of primate retina. Arch Ophthalmol 102:1086–1092, 1984.
62. Han DP, Folk JC: Internal limiting membrane wrinkling after argon and krypton laser photocoagulation of choroidal neovascularization. Retina 6:215–219, 1986.
63. Macular Photocoagulation Study Group: Evaluation of argon green versus krypton red laser for photocoagulation of subfoveal choroidal neovascularization in the Macular Photocoagulation Study. Arch Ophthalmol 112:1176–1184, 1994.
64. Macular Photocoagulation Study Group: Argon laser photocoagulation of neovascular lesions of age-related macular degeneration. Results of a randomized clinical trial. Arch Ophthalmol 100:912–918, 1982.
65. Goldberg MF, Herbst RW: Acute complications of argon laser photocoagulation. Arch Ophthalmol 89:311–318, 1973.
66. Macular Photocoagulation Study Group: Argon laser photocoagulation of neovascular lesions of ocular histoplasmosis. Results of a randomized clinical trial. Arch Ophthalmol 101:1347–1357, 1983.
67. Macular Photocoagulation Study Group: Laser photocoagulation for neovascular lesions nasal to the fovea. Results from clinical trials for lesions secondary to ocular histoplasmosis or idiopathic causes. Arch Ophthalmol 113:56–61, 1995.
68. Macular Photocoagulation Study Group: Argon laser photocoagulation for neovascular maculopathy: five-year results from randomized clinical trials. Arch Ophthalmol 109:1109–1114, 1991.
69. Coscas G, Soubrane G: Photocoagulation des neovaisseaux sous-retiniens dans la degenerescence macularie senile par laser a argon. Resultats de l'etude randomisee de 60 cas. Bull Mem Soc Fr Ophthalmol 94:149–154, 1982.
70. Moorfields Macular Study Group: Treatment of senile disciform macular degeneration: a single-blind randomized trial by argon laser photocoagulation. Br J Ophthalmol 66:745–753, 1982.
71. Macular Photocoagulation Study Group: Krypton laser photocoagulation for neovascular lesions of age-related macular degeneration. Results of a randomized clinical trial. Arch Ophthalmol 108:816–824, 1990.
72. Macular Photocoagulation Study Group: Laser photocoagulation for juxtafoveal choroidal neovascularization: five year results from randomized clinical trials. Arch Ophthalmol 112:500–509, 1994.
73. Macular Photocoagulation Study Group: Persistent and recurrent neovascularization after krypton laser photocoagulation for neovascular lesions of age-related macular degeneration. Arch Ophthalmol 108:825–831, 1990.
74. Macular Photocoagulation Study Group: Laser photocoagulation of subfoveal neovascular lesions of age-related macular degeneration: updated findings from two clinical trials. Arch Ophthalmol 111:1200–1209, 1993.
75. Macular Photocoagulation Study Group: Visual outcome after laser photocoagulation for subfoveal choroidal neovascularization secondary to age-related macular degeneration: the influence of initial lesion size and initial visual acuity. Arch Ophthalmol 112:480–488, 1994.
76. Macular Photocoagulation Study Group: Persistent and recurrent neovascularization after laser photocoagulation for subfoveal choroidal neovascularization of age-related macular degeneration. Arch Ophthalmol 112:489–499, 1994.
77. Macular Photocoagulation Study Group: Persistent and recurrent neovascularization after krypton laser photocoagulation for neovascular lesions of ocular histoplasmosis. Arch Ophthalmol 107:344–352, 1989.
78. Bressler NM, Bressler SB: Laser treatment in macular degeneration and histoplasmosis. Ophthalmol Clin North Am 4:565–581, 1989.

79. Sykes SO, Bressler NM, Maguire MG, et al: Detecting recurrent choroidal neovascularization. Comparison of clinical examination with and without fluorescein angiography. Arch Ophthalmol 112:1561–1566, 1994.
80. Macular Photocoagulation Study Group: Risk factors for choroidal neovascularization in the second eye of patients with juxtafoveal or subfoveal choroidal neovascularization secondary to age-related macular degeneration. Arch Ophthalmol (in press) 1998.
81. Freund KB, Yannuzzi LA, Sorenson JA: Age-related macular degeneration and choroidal neovascularization. Am J Ophthalmol 115:786–791, 1993.
82. Vander JF, Federman JL, Greven C, et al: Surgical removal of massive subretinal hemorrhage associated with age-related macular degeneration. Ophthalmology 98:23–27, 1991.
83. Lewis H: Intraoperative fibrinolysis of submacular hemorrhage with tissue plasminogen activator and surgical drainage. Am J Ophthalmol 118:559–568, 1994.
84. Thomas MA, Grand MG, Williams DF, et al: Surgical management of subfoveal choroidal neovascularization. Ophthalmology 99:952–968, 1992.
85. Berger AS, Kaplan HJ: Clinical experience with the surgical removal of subfoveal neovascular membranes. Ophthalmology 99:969–976, 1992.
86. Lambert HM, Capone A, Aaberg TM, et al: Surgical excision of subfoveal neovascular membranes in age-related macular degeneration. Am J Ophthalmol 114:241–242, 1992.
87. Ormerod LD, Puklin JE, Frank RN: Long-term outcomes after the surgical removal of advanced subfoveal neovascular membranes in age-related macular degeneration. Ophthalmology 101:1201–1210, 1994.
88. Hawkins BS, for the Submacular Surgery Trials Planning Group: Visual acuity outcomes following submacular surgery, laser photocoagulation, or observation of subfoveal choroidal neovascularization. Invest Ophthalmol Vis Sci 36(s):9, 1995.
89. Bynoe LA, Chang TS, Funata M, et al: Histologic examination of vascular patterns in subfoveal neovascular membranes. Ophthalmology 101:1112–1117, 1994.
90. Miller JW, Walsh AW, Kramer M, et al: Photodynamic therapy of experimental choroidal neovascularization using lipoprotein-delivered benzoporphyrin. Arch Ophthalmol 113:810–818, 1995.
91. Miller H, Miller B: Photodynamic therapy of subretinal neovascularization in the monkey eye. Arch Ophthalmol 111:5855–5860, 1993.
92. Bergink GJ, Deutman AF, van den Broek JE, et al: Radiation therapy for subfoveal choroidal neovascular membranes in age-related macular degeneration. A pilot study. Doc Ophthalmol 90:67–74, 1995.
93. Finger PT, Berson A, Sherr D, et al: Radiation therapy for subretinal neovascularization. Ophthalmology 103:878–889, 1996.
94. Frierichsen EJ, Redlands CA, Alater JD: Proton beam irradiation of subfoveal choroidal neovascularization in age-related macular degeneration. Invest Ophthalmol Vis Sci 34(s):171, 1995.
95. Mandai M, Ogura Y, Tanigumichi T: The effect of radiation therapy on subfoveal choroidal neovascular membrane in patients with ARMD. Invest Ophthalmol Vis Sci 34(s):146, 1995.
96. Miller JW, Stinson WG, Folkman J: Regression of experimental iris neovascularization with systemic alpha-interferon. Ophthalmology 100:9–14, 1993.
97. Ezekowitz RAB, Mulliken JB, Folkman J: Interferon alpha-2a for life threatening hemangiomas of infancy. N Engl J Med 326:1459–1463, 1992.
98. Guyer DR, Adamis AP, Gragoudas ES, et al: Systemic antiangiogenic therapy for choroidal neovascularization. What is the role of interferon alpha? Arch Ophthalmol 110:1383–1384, 1992.
99. Fung WE: Interferon alpha-2a for treatment of age-related macular degeneration. Am J Ophthalmol 112:349–350, 1992.
100. Engler CB, Sander B, Doefoed P, et al: Interferon alfa-2a treatment of patients with subfoveal neovascular macular degeneration. A pilot investigation. Acta Ophthalmol 71:27–31, 1993.
101. Thomas MA, Ibanez HE: Interferon alpha-2a in the treatment of subfoveal choroidal neovascularization. Am J Ophthalmol 115:563–568, 1993.
102. Guyer DR, Adamis AP, Yannuzzi LA, et al: Interferon alfa-2A is ineffective for patients with choroidal neovascularization secondary to age-related macular degeneration: results of a prospective randomized placebo-controlled clinical trial. Arch Ophthalmol (in press).

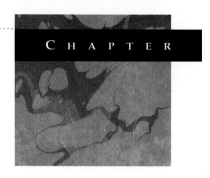

CHAPTER

11

Antiangiogenic Therapy

Anthony P. Adamis, M.D.

Age-related macular degeneration (AMD) is the leading cause of irreversible blindness in elderly Americans.[1] The etiology of the disorder remains unknown. Although the "dry" nonneovascular form of the disease is more prevalent, the "wet" neovascular form causes the majority of sudden and severe vision loss.[2] In the United States, $7^1/_2$ million cases of AMD are predicted by the year 2030.[2] Laser photocoagulation of choroidal neovascular membranes has shown some efficacy in stabilizing vision loss; however, the large majority of choroidal neovascular membranes are not treated because of their subfoveal location or incomplete visualization on angiography.[3] Antiangiogenesis, the pharmacologic inhibition of new blood vessel growth, represents a new therapeutic strategy that may see application in AMD and other neovascular disorders of the eye.

ANGIOGENESIS AND ANTIANGIOGENESIS

The endothelial cells lining the blood vessels of the normal adult eye rarely proliferate and possess a mitotic rate measured in years.[4] Angiogenesis, the process of new capillary growth from pre-existing vessels, occurs exclusively in disease and frequently leads to blindness. Angiogenesis characterizes the leading causes of blindness in the developed world including retinopathy of prematurity, diabetic retinopathy, neovascular glaucoma, and neovascular AMD. New vessels grow into normally avascular spaces of the eye and destroy the delicate ocular tissues. The orderly branching of normal blood vessels is replaced by a tangled web of capillaries that produce tissue edema and hemorrhage.

In the fully developed adult, angiogenesis is tightly controlled and occurs briefly during ovulation, menstruation, placental maturation, and wound healing.[5] Exclusive of these processes, growth in the vascular system is static. Specifically targeting growing vessels with systemic antiangiogenic therapy holds the promise of treating ocular diseases with few side effects.[5,6]

BIOLOGY OF ANGIOGENESIS

Inhibiting the growth of new vessels requires knowledge of the cell and molecular biology of angiogenesis. Much of the original work characterizing new blood vessel growth was done in models of tumor and corneal angiogenesis.[7,8] Angiogenesis proceeds through a series of defined but overlapping steps. They include:

1. Vessel dilation.
2. Basement membrane degradation of the parent venule.
3. Migration of the endothelial cell away from the parent venule.
4. Endothelial cell mitosis.
5. Alignment along an axis.
6. Formation of a lumen.
7. Fusion of adjacent capillary sprout tips.
8. Establishment of a circulation.
9. Remodeling of the primary capillary network to form venules and arterioles.
10. Selective capillary regression.

The presence and growth of vessels in normal and neoplastic tissues is regulated, in part, through a balance of angiogenic stimulators and inhibitors. Such a system is operative for both tumors[9,10] and the eye.[11,12] For example, the avascular cornea constitutively synthesizes both the angiogenic peptide basic fibroblast growth factor (bFGF)[11,12] and a potent nonprotein cornea angiogenesis inhibitor (CAI). Alterations in this angiogenic balance may lead to neovascularization. Regulation is tight and

122

multiple mechanisms control the production, post-transcriptional modification, cellular export, post-translational modification, and elimination of angiogenic molecules, permitting rapid and controlled bursts of angiogenesis.

MECHANISMS OF CHOROIDAL NEOVASCULARIZATION

The mechanisms of choroidal neovascularization are not well understood. However, the mechanisms of tumor, iris, and retinal neovascularization have been recently discovered and are largely conserved. Therefore, they may apply to choroidal neovascularization. In these systems, hypoxic ischemia increases the expression of the vascular endothelial growth factor (VEGF) gene,[13,14] a potent endothelial cell mitogen in vitro and vascular permeability and angiogenesis factor in vivo.[15,16] VEGF mRNA and protein levels are spatially and temporally correlated with ocular neovascularization in animal models[14,17] and in humans with diabetic retinopathy.[18-20] The specific inhibition of VEGF prevents neovascularization[21,22] and its introduction into normal primate eyes is able to produce pathologic neovascularization of the iris and retina.[23] Thus, VEGF is necessary and sufficient for retinal ischemia-associated neovascularization.

Recent preliminary studies have demonstrated high VEGF expression levels in the tissues surrounding choroidal neovascular membranes.[24,25] It is not known if ischemia precedes choroidal neovascularization, as it does for iris and retinal neovascularization. At first glance, this would seem unlikely, as the choriocapillaris is a very dense network of vessels with a high rate of blood flow. However, careful histopathologic and rheologic studies have shown a decreased density of capillaries in AMD[26] and a decreased rate of blood flow.[27] In the context of the extremely high metabolic rate for the outer retina, it is conceivable that relative outer retinal ischemia precedes choroidal neovascularization in AMD. The biochemical alterations in Bruch's membrane may also impede the diffusion of oxygen and metabolites from the choriocapillaris to the outer retina,[28] further provoking an up-regulation in VEGF by the retinal pigment epithelium. The latter has been demonstrated to occur in vitro in response to hypoxia.[29,30] Conversely, stimuli other than hypoxia may serve to increase VEGF levels. It is known that different cytokines, growth factors, as well as reactive oxygen intermediates, have this capacity.[31-33] The inflammatory cells associated with choroidal neovascularization may release these molecules and promote angiogenesis in an indirect fashion.[34]

Other known angiogenic factors may also be involved, including basic fibroblast growth factor (bFGF)[35] and interleukin-8 (IL-8).[36] Both are known to be synthesized by the retinal pigment epithelium.[37,38] Additionally, soluble stimulators and inhibitors may be retained in an insoluble state bound to glycosaminoglycans in Bruch's membrane and released locally upon its degeneration in AMD. Such a mechanism is operative in the cornea.[11,12] Choroidal neovascularization may also follow the concurrent down-regulation of an endogenous angiogenesis inhibitor. In support of this possibility, investigators have partially purified an inhibitor of endothelial cell proliferation from the conditioned media of cultured retinal pigment epithelial cells.[39]

ANGIOGENESIS INHIBITION IN CHOROIDAL NEOVASCULARIZATION

Although the exact mechanisms of choroidal neovascularization are not known, clinical trials with angiogenesis inhibitors have begun. Effective angiogenesis inhibitors for other conditions have been extrapolated for use in neovascular AMD. The first to be examined, interferon alfa, inhibits vascular endothelial cell proliferation and migration,[40] and prevents angiogenesis in rodents.[41] Interferon alfa is a molecule with multiple biologic actions on many different cell types. It is approved for use in hairy cell leukemia, viral warts, Kaposi's sarcoma, and other conditions. Notably, Kaposi's sarcoma is a tumor of vascular endothelial progenitor cells. Based in part on these data, interferon alfa was first used in 1989 to successfully treat a life-threatening infantile hemangioma.[42] Subsequent clinical trials confirmed its safety and efficacy for this condition.[43,44] Experiments in primates demonstrated efficacy at regressing iris neovascularization associated with retinal ischemia.[45] In 1991, a small series of patients with choroidal neovascular membranes secondary to AMD were treated with interferon alfa with apparent success.[46] Subsequent limited trials yielded conflicting data regarding its usefulness in AMD[47-49]; however, off-label use of the drug for AMD was common. Its safety and efficacy were definitively evaluated in a 500-patient, randomized, placebo-controlled clinical trial.[50] In spite of a high degree of statistical power and the use of the maximally tolerated dose, interferon alfa was found to be ineffective at preventing vision loss.

Several important conclusions from the interferon story can be drawn about antiangiogenic drug therapy. First, not all vascular beds behave similarly. There is a well known phenotypic heterogeneity to the vasculature that also extends to its biologic modulation.[51] Although interferon inhibits neovascularization in some vascular beds, it does not mean it can inhibit choroidal neovascularization. In support of this, Fidler and co-workers have shown that interferon is specifically effective at inhibiting only bFGF-induced angiogenesis.[52] Thus, it is best to test a potential antiangiogenic substance in relevant animal models prior to clinical trial. Models of choroidal neovascularization have been characterized in the primate and other species.[53,54] Although the neovascularization in these models is not part of a degenerative process, the models share many features with choroidal neovascularization secondary to AMD. Second, assessing the antiangiogenic efficacy of a compound in AMD requires at least 1 year of treatment in a large number of patients to achieve statistical significance. The disease is slow in its progression and highly variable in the short term. Except for exceptionally effective drugs, only large numbers of patients and the utilization of a control group will yield meaningful data. Third, in lieu of a highly specific antiangiogenic agent, pleotropic antiangiogenic molecules like interferon alfa are probably best delivered locally to the posterior segment in order to limit their side effects. Interferon alfa, like other nonspecific antiangiogenic agents, has many systemic side effects. Development of sustained drug delivery technologies for the posterior segment is needed to maximize the chances for success with these agents.

THE FUTURE

Recent discoveries of highly specific stimulators and inhibitors of angiogenesis hold promise for the safe and effective treatment of choroidal neovascularization secondary to AMD. New endogenous and physiologically relevant molecules have been discovered that are fundamentally important. They include the endothelial specific receptors Tie-1 and Tie-2, whose disruption results in lethal incomplete angiogenesis during development,[55] and angiostatin, a naturally cleaved fragment of plasminogen that is a highly specific inhibitor of endothelial cells in vitro and in vivo.[56] These molecules may play equally important roles in choroidal neovascularization, and along with VEGF, may serve as future therapeutic targets for the treatment of choroidal neovascularization.

REFERENCES

1. Ferris FL III: Senile macular degeneration: review of epidemiologic features. Am J Epidemiol 118:132–151, 1983.
2. Hyman LG, Lilienfeld AM, Ferris FL III, Fine SL: Senile macular degeneration: a case-control study. Am J Epidemiol 118:213–227, 1983.
3. Moisseiev J, Alhalel A, Masuri R, Treister G: The impact of the macular photocoagulation study results on the treatment of exudative age-related macular degeneration. Arch Ophthalmol 113:185–189, 1985.
4. Engerman RL, Pfaffenbach D, Davis MD: Cell turnover of capillaries. Lab Invest 17:738–743, 1967.
5. Folkman J, Klagsburn M: Angiogenic factors. Science 235:442–447, 1987.
6. Folkman J: Tumor angiogenesis: therapeutic implications. N Engl J Med 285:1182–1186, 1971.
7. Ausprunk DH, Folkman J: Migration and proliferation of endothelial cells in preformed and newly formed blood vessels during tumor angiogenesis. Microvasc Res 14:53–65, 1977.
8. Folkman J, Haudenschild C: Angiogenesis in vitro. Nature 288:551–556, 1980.
9. Kandel J, Bossy Wetzel E, Radvanyi F, et al: Neovascularization is associated with a switch to the export of bFGF in the multistep development of fibrosarcoma. Cell 66:1095–1104, 1991.
10. Good DJ, Polverini PJ, Rastinejad F, et al: A tumor suppressor-dependent inhibitor of angiogenesis is immunologically and functionally indistinguishable from a fragment of thrombospondin. Proc Natl Acad Sci U S A 87:6624–6627, 1990.
11. Folkman J, Klagsbrun M, Sasse J, et al: A heparin-binding angiogenic protein—basic fibroblast growth factor—is stored within basement membrane. Am J Pathol 130:393–400, 1988.
12. Adamis AP, Meklir B, Joyce NC: In situ injury-induced release of basic-fibroblast growth factor from corneal epithelial cells. Am J Pathol 139:961–967, 1991.
13. Shweiki D, Itin A, Soffer D, Keshet E: Vascular endothelial growth factor induced by hypoxia may mediate hypoxia-initiated angiogenesis. Nature 359:843–845, 1992.
14. Miller J, Adamis AP, Shima DT, et al: Vascular endothelial growth factor/vascular permeability factor is temporally and spatially correlated with ocular angiogenesis in a primate model. Am J Pathol 145:574–584, 1994.
15. Leung DW, Cachianes G, Kuang WJ, et al: Vascular endothelial growth factor is a secreted angiogenic mitogen. Science 246:1306–1309, 1989.
16. Keck PJ, Hauser SD, Krivi G, et al: Vascular permeability factor, an endothelial cell mitogen related to PDGF. Science 246:1309–1312, 1989.
17. Pierce EA, Avery RL, Foley ED, et al: Vascular endothelial growth factor/vascular permeability factor expression in a mouse model of retinal neovascularization. Proc Natl Acad Sci U S A 92:905–909, 1995.
18. Adamis AP, Miller J, Bernal M, et al: Increased vascular endothelial growth factor levels in the vitreous of eyes with proliferative diabetic retinopathy. Am J Ophthalmol 118:445–450, 1994.
19. Aiello LP, Avery RL, Arrigg PG, et al: Vascular endothelial growth factor in ocular fluid of patients wth diabetic retinopathy and other retinal disorders. N Engl J Med 331:1480–1487, 1994.
20. Malecaze F, Clamens S, Simorre-Pinatel V, et al: Detection of vascular endothelial growth factor messanger RNA and vascular endothelial growth factor-like activity in proliferative diabetic retinopathy. Arch Ophthalmol 112:1476–1482, 1994.
21. Adamis AP, Shima DT, Tolentino M, et al: Inhibition of VEGF prevents retinal ischemia-associated iris neovascularization in a primate. Arch Ophthalmol 114:66–71, 1995.
22. Aiello LP, Pierce EA, Foley ED, et al: Suppression of retinal neovascularian-suppression in vivo by inhibition of vascular endothelial growth factor (VEGF) using soluble VEGF-receptor chimeric proteins. Proc Natl Acad Sci USA 92:10457–10461, 1995.
23. Tolentino MT, Miller JW, Gragoudas ES, et al: Vascular endothelial growth factor is sufficient to produce iris neovascularization and neovascular glaucoma in a nonhuman primate. Arch Ophthalmol 114:964–970, 1996.
24. Dastgheib K, Li Q, Chan C, et al: Vascular endothelial growth factor (VEGF) in neovascular age-related macular degeneration (Abstract). Invest Ophthalmol Vis Sci 36:494, 1995.
25. Kliffen M, Sharma HS, Mooy CM, et al: Increased expression of angiogenic growth factors in age-related maculopathy (Abstract). Invest Ophthalmol Vis Sci 37:944, 1996.
26. Sarks SH: Ageing and degeneration in the macular region: a clinicopathological study. Br J Ophthalmol 60:324–341, 1976.
27. Friedman E, Krupsky S, Lane AM, et al: Ocular blood flow velocity in age-related macular degeneration. Ophthalmology 102:640–646, 1995.

28. Hewitt TA, Nakazawa K, Newsome DA: Analysis of newly synthesized Bruch's membrane proteoglycans. Invest Ophthlamol Vis Sci 30:478–486, 1985.
29. Adamis AP, Shima DT, Yeo KT, et al: Synthesis and secretion of vascular permeability factor/vascular endothelial growth factor by human retinal pigment epithelial cells. Biochem Biophys Res Commun 193:631–638, 1993.
30. Shima D, Adamis AP, Ferrara N, et al: Hypoxic induction of endothelial cell growth factors in retinal cells: identification and characterization of vascular endothelial growth factor (VEGF) as the sole mitogen. Mol Med 2:182–193, 1995.
31. Goldman CK, Kim J, Wong W, et al: Epidermal growth factor stimulates vascular endothelial growth factor production by human malignant glioma cells: a model of glioblastoma multiforme pathophysiology. Mol Biol Cell 4:121–133, 1993.
32. Harada S, Nagy JA, Sullivan KA, et al: Induction of vascular endothelial growth factor expression by prostaglandin E1 and E2 in osteoblasts. J Clin Invest 93:2490–2493, 1994.
33. Kuroki M, Voest E, Amano S, et al: Reactive oxygen intermediates increase vascular endothelial growth factor expression in vitro and in vivo. J Clin Invest 98:1667–1675, 1996.
34. Killingsworth MC, Sarks JP, Sarks SH: Macrophages related to Bruch's membrane in age-related macular degeneration. Eye 4:613–621, 1990.
35. Shing Y, Folkman J, Sullivan R, et al: Heparin affinity: purification of a tumor-derived capillary endothelial cell growth factor. Science 223:1296–1299, 1994.
36. Koch AE, Polverini PJ, Kunkel SL, et al: Interleukin-8 as a macrophage-derived mediator of angiogenesis. Science 258:1798–1801, 1992.
37. Schweigerer L, Malerstein B, Neufeld G, Gospodarowicz D: Basic fibroblast growth factor is synthesized in cultured retinal pigment epithelial cells. Biochem Biophys Res Commun 143:934–940, 1987.
38. Elner VM, Strieter RM, Elner SG, et al: Neutrophil chemotactic factor (IL-8) gene expression by cytokine-treated retinal pigment epithelial cells. Am J Pathol 136:745–750, 1990.
39. Glaser BM, Campochiaro PA, Davis JL Jr, Sato M: Retinal pigment epithelial cells release an inhibitor of neovascularization. Birth Defects 24:121–127, 1988.
40. Brouty-Boye D, Zetter BR: Inhibition of cell motility by interferon. Science 208:516–518, 1980.
41. Sidkey YA, Borden EC: Inhibition of angiogenesis by interferons: effects on tumor- and lymphocyte-induced vascular responses. Cancer Res 47:5155–5161, 1987.
42. White CW, Sondheimer HM, Crouch EC, et al: Treatment of pulmonary hemangiomatosis with recombinant interferon alfa-2a. N Engl J Med 320:1197–1200, 1989.
43. Ezekowitz RA, Mulliken JB, Folkman J: Interferon alfa-2a therapy for life-threatening hemangiomas of infancy. N Engl J Med 326:1456–1463, 1992.
44. White CW, Wolf SJ, Korones DN, et al: Treatment of childhood angiomatous diseases with recombinant interferon alfa-2a. J Pediatr 118:59–66, 1991.
45. Miller JW, Stinson WG, Folkman J: Regression of experimental iris neovascularization with systemic alpha-interferon. Ophthalmology 100:9–14, 1993.
46. Fung WE: Interferon alpha 2a for treatment of age-related macular degeneration (Letter). Am J Ophthalmol 112:349–350, 1991.
47. Lewis ML, Davis J, Chuang E: Interferon alfa-2a in the treatment of exudative age-related macular degneration. Graefes Arch Clin Exp Ophthalmol 231:615–618, 1993.
48. Gillies MC, Sarks JP, Beaumont PE, et al: Treatment of choroidal neovascularization in age-related macular degeneration with interferon alfa-2a and alfa-2b. Br J Ophthalmol 77:759–765, 1993.
49. Engler CB, Sander B, Koefoed P, et al: Interferon alpha-2a treatment of patients with subfoveal neovascular macular degeneration. A pilot investigation. Acta Ophthalmol 71:27–31, 1993.
50. Pharmacologic therapy for macular degeneration study group. Report #1. Interferon alfa-2a is ineffective for patients with choroidal neovascularization secondary to age-related macular degeneration. Results of a perspective randomized placebo-controlled clinical trial. Arch Ophthalmol 115:865–872, 1997.
51. Gumkowski F, Kaminska G, Kaminska M, et al: Heterogeneity of mouse vascular endothelium: in vitro studies of lymphatic, large blood vessel and microvascular endothelial cells. Blood Vessels 24:11–23, 1987.
52. Singh RK, Gutman M, Bucana CD, et al: Interferons alpha and beta down-regulate the expression of basic fibroblast growth factor in human carcinomas. Proc Natl Acad Sci U S A 92:4562–4566, 1995.
53. Ohkuma H, Ryan SJ: Experimental subretinal neovascularization in the monkey. Permeability of new vessels. Arch Ophthlamol 101:1102–1110, 1983.
54. Kimura H, Sakamoto T, Hinton DR, et al: A new model of subretinal neovascularization in the rabbit. Invest Ophthalmol Vis Sci 36:2110–2119, 1995.
55. Sato TN, Tozawa YD, Deutsch U, et al: Distinct roles of the receptor tyrosine kinases Tie-1 and Tie-2 in blood vessel formation. Nature 376:70–74, 1995.
56. O'Reilly MS, Holmgren L, Shing Y, et al: Angiostatin: a novel angiogenesis inhibitor that mediates the suppression of metastasis by a Lewis lung carcinoma. Cell 79:315–328, 1994.

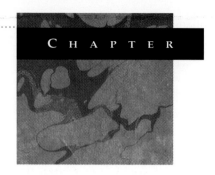

CHAPTER 12

Age-Related Macular Degeneration: Radiation Therapy for Choroidal Neovascularization

Mary E. Mendelsohn, M.D.
David H. Abramson, M.D.

Radiation has been used for years to treat benign and malignant ocular conditions. Recently, interest has arisen in using ionizing radiation to treat choroidal neovascularization in patients with macular degeneration. In this chapter, we discuss the theory, methods, results, and concerns of radiation therapy for macular degeneration. A brief review of radiation terminology and methodology is included, as many ophthalmologists are unfamiliar with this treatment modality.

Age-related macular degeneration (AMD) affects 10% of people over age 65 in the United States, and 30% of people over 75 years old.[1] The disease accounts for 16,000 new cases of blindness each year. Choroidal neovascularization (CNV), also called the "wet" form of macular degeneration, accounts for 90% of the patients with severe visual loss (20/200 or worse). The natural history of choroidal neovascularization is poor.[1-4] CNV destroys vision rapidly due to the leaking, bleeding, and fibrosing tendencies associated with the abnormal neovascular growth. Untreated, CNV tends to decrease vision to less than 20/400, often to the finger-counting range. One study of the natural history of subfoveal exudative macular degeneration showed that 75% of patients with subfoveal lesions for 2 years or more will lose four Snellen lines of visual acuity.[3]

CNV secondary to macular degeneration has proven difficult to treat. Only a small percentage of these patients meet the criteria for laser treatment published by the Macular Photocoagulation Study Group. Laser treatment is limited by the size of the membrane, whether the borders are clearly defined, the necessity for destruction of overlying retina (causing immediate worsening of vision if the net is subfoveal), visual field defects in paracentral nets, and spreading of scars following treatment into the foveal area.[5,6] There is a great need for vision-sparing treatment methods for this condition.

THEORY

There is basic science and clinical evidence to support the hypothesis that radiation delivered to the macula could prevent proliferation and/or cause regression of choroidal neovascularization. Radiation therapy is known to inhibit angiogenesis in two ways. It inhibits the growth of vascular endothelial cells; this has been seen in vitro in human cell culture.[7] Ocular wounds in rabbits were observed to have less neovascularization during healing after radiation treatment with iodine-125 plaque, using a 950-cGy dose.[8] As CNV is composed partly of growing vessels lined with endothelium, its proliferation may be prevented by radiation. Radiation therapy also causes sclerosing or obliteration of small vessels. Vaso-occlusive changes and ischemia follow high-dose radiation to the retina.[9] Radiation has been used therapeutically to cause regression of choroidal hemangiomas with 1200 to 2000 cGy photons.[10,11] Thus, the scientific rationale for using radiation for CNV seems sound.

RADIATION CHARACTERISTICS

Radiation treatment involves directing ionizing electromagnetic radiation to a site of pathology. Radiation damages proliferating tissue while causing minimal disruption to surrounding normal tissues. Ionizing radiation generates free radicals and reactive oxygen intermediates that damage cell components including DNA. The presence of oxygen acts as a radiosensitizer, reacting with the free radicals to enhance cell death. Hypoxic tissues are more resistant to photon beam irradiation. If the normal tissue's ability to sustain and repair radiation damage is not exceeded, it will tolerate the treatment well.[12] Choroidal neovascularization is a proliferating tissue, while the surrounding retina and optic nerve are not, so the eye should tolerate radiation to the posterior pole well. Dosage to dividing eye structures such as the lens and conjunctiva should be minimized.

Radiation has a variety of sources. Radioactive isotopes are one source, producing alpha or beta particles or gamma rays. Other sources for radiation are machines such as the linear accelerator or betatron, which produce X-rays, high-energy electromagnetic radiation. X-rays and gamma rays have identical physical properties and biologic effects; the term "photon" is often used interchangeably. Linear accelerators can also produce electron beams, which have rapid dose fall-off over distance and are useful for treating superficial lesions. Particle beams such as neutrons or protons are also used in radiation treatment; they are thought to be better for hypoxic tissue, and possibly offer affected cells less opportunity to repair induced damage. Brachytherapy, an alternative to external beam delivery, refers to the placing of a radioactive isotope within or near the target tissue for a specified time of constant exposure. The unit of measure of radiation is the centigray (1 cGy = 1 rad); it is the measure of the dose absorbed from ionizing radiation equivalent to 0.01 joule of energy per kilogram of tissue.

Radiation penetrates tissue to different extents depending on the energy of the radiation beam and the type of ionizing radiation used. The higher the energy, the more penetration is obtained in tissue. A 6-MV (megavolt) photon beam has less energy and so less penetration than a 10-MV photon beam. Alpha and beta particles are less penetrating than gamma rays; electrons are also less penetrating than photons. Electrons can be delivered with high energy to a surface location, but they lose that energy quickly as they enter tissue. For treatment of

choroidal neovascularization, studies to date have used photon radiation delivered by external beam or brachytherapy, proton beam, or beta emitters such as strontium-90 brachytherapy.

Radiation spreads from the source in a wave-like pattern through treated tissue. The dose of radiation delivered to a point will decrease with increasing distance away from the source. Isodose charts designed for patient treatment show the dose of radiation received by the target tissue, and dose to all surrounding structures (Figs. 12–1 and 12–2). Points on a single curve on an isodose chart represent equal doses; isodose curves are drawn until the dose drops to 10% of the treatment dose. For choroidal neovascularization, the macula is the target tissue. The isodose curves for a lateral and superior oblique approach with photon beam for a choroidal neovascularization patient are shown in Figures 12–1 and 12–2. Note that the opposite eye receives more radiation with the lateral approach, as it is in the exit path of the beam. The opposite retina receives 70% of the total dose with a lateral approach, while with the oblique approach, retina exposure is negligible. The lens receives some exposure with either technique; this is minimized by the use of blocks and beam splitting. The retina posterior to the equator receives 100% of the total dose.

When treating with external beam, the total dose is divided into smaller fractions that are delivered at intervals (i.e., daily) until the total dose is reached. A typical daily fraction is 200 cGy. Fractionation is an important concept; it allows normal tissue to repair any induced radiation damage (thought to take about 6 hours for most cells) before the next dose of radiation is given. Proliferating tissue such as cancer or neovascularization is more sensitive to damage from radiation and will be lethally affected. With fractionation, a tissue can tolerate a much higher total dose.[13]

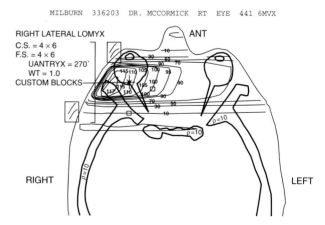

FIGURE 12–1 Isodose curves for lateral approach, photon beam treatment. Blocks in place to protect lens, posterior orbit, and brain. Exit through contralateral eye.

CUSTOM BLOCKS

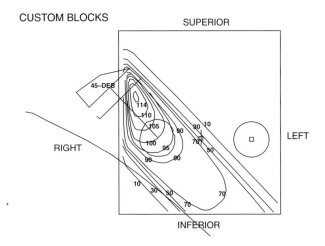

FIGURE 12-2 Isodose curves for oblique approach, photon beam treatment. Wedge in place to even distribution of radiation. Exit through nasal sinus, palate.

METHODS

Pretreatment and posttreatment evaluation at most centers includes visual acuity, ophthalmic examination, fluorescein angiography, and indocyanine green angiography in a manner similar to other CNV patients. No special posttreatment care is required. Radiation treatment techniques are used as described below.

External Beam Photon Radiotherapy

Simulation is done to accurately localize the target tissue and nearby radiosensitive structures in the path of the treatment beam. The patient lies on the treatment table. A mold of the patient's head is made of Aquaplast (a malleable plastic that hardens to the shape of the head), or other method of head fixation is employed. This ensures identical patient positioning with each treatment fraction. The eyes are positioned with laser beams that show the path of the treatment beam. A roentgenogram is taken of the treatment field to verify laser and patient alignment. Magnetic resonance imaging (MRI) or computed tomography (CT) images can be used if needed to aid in treatment planning. To further restrict the focus of external beam radiation, the portal through which the beam is delivered can be shaped (a D-shaped portal is commonly used when treating ocular pathology to decrease exposure to posterior structures like the brain). Shielding blocks that prevent passage of radiation can be placed to protect structures near the target tissue, such as the lens and conjunctiva. Wedge filters can be placed in the beam; they will progressively decrease the beam intensity across the field of radiation, to even out absorption to structures that are irregularly shaped yet where equal isodose exposure is desired.

The total dose is chosen and divided into daily fractions for treatment. Each treatment takes seconds to minutes and is painless. Most centers are using 800 to 2400 cGy total dose to treat choroidal neovascularization, in fractions of 144 to 800 cGy. As the dose per fraction increases, the risk for side effects also increases.

With photon beam irradiation, the entire retina posterior to the equator receives significant radiation, as does the anterior optic nerve. The lens receives much less radiation; as it is the most radiosensitive structure in the eye, the photon beam is angled to minimize lens exposure. The opposite eye receives more radiation when a lateral approach is used, as it is in the exit path of the beam. A superior oblique approach gives negligible exposure to the opposite eye, exiting through the maxillary sinus and palate.

Brachytherapy

Plaques surgically applied to the sclera just outside the macula have been used to locally deliver radiation. Isotopes used for CNV include the gamma emitter palladium-103, placed for 24 to 43 hours, and the beta emitter strontium-90, placed for 55 minutes.[16,19]

RESULTS

External photon beam was used as the treatment modality in several pilot studies. In Belfast, 19 patients were treated with 1000 or 1500 cGy (6-MV, 200-cGy fractions): 63% of treated patients had stabilization or improvement of visual acuity at 1 year, and regression of the CNV, while six of seven nontreated nonrandomized controls showed deterioration of the vision and enlargement of the neovascular net.[14] In the Netherlands, four groups of ten patients each were treated with 800-, 1200-, 1800-, and 2400-cGy doses (16-MV, 600-cGy fractions): 80% of the highest dose group had stable vision and neovascularization at 1 year; however, at 1½ years the next two highest dose groups showed just 50% stable vision.[15] In New York, one study treated 75 patients with 1440 cGy (6 MV, eight to ten fractions) and found overall 75% had stable vision after mean follow-up of 9 months.[16] Another New York study has treated over 100 patients to date with 1000 cGy (6-MV, 200-cGy fractions); preliminary results show 75% had stable vision at 6 months.[17]

Proton beam is being used by a group in California; they report a majority of eyes show regression at 6 months using a single dose of 800 to 1400 cGy in 21 patients.[18]

Brachytherapy is being investigated in New York using palladium-103 plaques, to a dose of 1500 cGy.[16] A strontium-90 plaque is used in Helsinki, to a dose of 1500 cGy, with three of three patients

TABLE 12–1 Acute and Late Radiation Effects for Eye Structures

Eye	Acute Radiation Effects	Dose* in cGy	Late Radiation Effects (Months to Years Later)	Dose* in cGy
Conjunctiva	Conjunctivitis, chemosis 1–3 wks after RT	Single dose >500	Telangiectasia, keratinization, metaplasia, symblepharon	>5000
Cornea	Epithelial defects, hyposensitivity, transient keratitis	>1000 >5000	Epithelial desquamation, neovascularization Ulceration	>2000 >4000
Sclera	Transient injection 2–4 wks after RT	NS	Tolerates high doses with plaques melt	>90,000
Lens	Edema (myopia) several wks after RT	NS	Cataract	200–500[†]
Iris	Iritis	6000 2000[†]	Rubeosis iridis, postsynechiae, iris atrophy	7000–17,000
Retina	Transient edema months after RT	3500–5000	Neovascularization, telangiectasias, vessel permeability, occlusion	2500–6000
Optic nerve	None		Optic nerve edema, optic neuropathy	5500–12,000[‡]
Lacrimal gland	None		Atrophy >6 months after RT	5000
Skin	Erythema, loss of lashes Dry dermatitis after 1 wk	>250 >1000	Blisters, moist dermatitis After 4 weeks telangiectasia, hyperpigmentation	>4000

* Total dose delivered; implies fractionated delivery unless otherwise stated. Doses are minimums at which side effect is seen; tissue may also tolerate listed dose without ill effect.

† Delivered as single fraction.

‡ Common with fractions >300 cGy.

RT, radiation therapy; NS, not specified.

showing some regression of CNV by 3 months, but with slight decrease in vision.[19]

In the months following treatment by any modality, most centers report clearing of subretinal hemorrhage and decreased edema associated with the CNV. Some centers have seen regression of the neovascular net; others report only lack of progression.

All of these pilot studies have low patient numbers and short-term follow-up to date, with no randomized control group. Further follow-up is required to evaluate whether any initial promising response is a lasting one. Controlled studies are required to show a difference from natural history of the disease.

CONCERNS

The tolerance of various eye structures to radiation must be remembered with any radiotherapy treat-ment. Side effects can occur if doses are high enough. Table 12–1 lists acute and late radiation effects to various parts of the eye, and the doses at which these have been seen.[20–23] As can be seen from the table, the retina and optic nerve are relatively resistant to radiation damage. The conjunctiva is more sensitive; any side effects from radiation should be treated with the usual modalities as they occur (lubricants, steroids). The most radiosensitive structure in the eye is the lens, because of the mitotic activity and the inability of the lens to clear damaged cells. After radiation, the pre-equatorial germinative zone cells divide rapidly but produce abnormal cells. These cells, known as Wedl cells, form layers at the posterior pole, eventually becoming a cataract. The higher the dose of radiation, the shorter the latency for the appearance of cataracts.

With external beam photon therapy in 200-cGy fractions, we have seen no side effects after 2 years of follow-up. With higher treatment fractions, skin erythema, conjunctival irritation, and other side effects become more common. Years after radiation therapy, increased incidence of cancer has occurred when patients were treated for benign conditions. Patients treated for ankylosing spondylitis had an increased incidence of leukemia, and patients treated for postpartum mastitis had an increased incidence of breast cancer.[24] An increased risk of cancer would be unlikely, given the small total doses delivered, but long-term follow-up is necessary to determine this.

It is necessary to exclude from treatment patients who have a history of radiation therapy to the head, as total exposure would be difficult to determine and treatment might exceed safe limits for surrounding structures. It is wise to exclude patients on chemotherapy, as certain agents can potentiate the effect of radiation. Diabetics are known to have their retinopathy worsen when treated with radioactive plaques, so they are best excluded from this treatment. CNV has much nonproliferating tissue associated with it—fibroblasts, macrophages, fibrous scaffold tissue, and glial cells. These may not be affected by radiation and may account for regrowth of CNV or uneven response to radiation.

Radiation treatment for choroidal neovascularization has a good theoretical foundation, and small pilot studies have had promising results. Several centers are now involved in prospective, randomized, controlled clinical trials with various doses and fractionation schedules. Future directions for this therapy include defining the best delivery method for radiation therapy (brachytherapy vs. external beam), the optimum total dose and fractions, and the optimum treatment schedule to cause regression of choroidal neovascularization. Treatment of choroidal neovascularization due to other conditions (pathologic myopia, choroidal rupture, angioid streaks) should also be considered. If successful, radiation will provide a much-needed vision-sparing treatment for this aggressive disease.

REFERENCES

1. Bressler NM, Bressler SB, Fine SL: Age-related macular degeneration. Surv Ophthalmol 32:375–412, 1988.
2. Bressler NM, Frost LA, Bressler SB, et al: Natural course of poorly defined choroidal neovascularization associated with macular degeneration. Arch Ophthalmol 106:1537–1542, 1988.
3. Guyer DR, Fine SL, Maguire MG, et al: Subfoveal choroidal neovascular membranes in age-related macular degeneration. Visual prognosis in eyes with relatively good visual acuity. Arch Ophthalmol 104:702–705, 1986.
4. Bressler SB, Bressler NM, Fine SL, et al: Natural course of choroidal neovascular membranes within the foveal avascular zone in senile macular degeneration. Am J Ophthalmol 93:157–163, 1982.
5. Macular Photocoagulation Study Group: Laser photoco-
agulation of subfoveal neovascular lesions in age-related macular degeneration. Arch Ophthalmol 109:1220–1231, 1991.
6. Macular Photocoagulation Study Group. Subfoveal neovascular lesions in age-related macular degeneration: guidelines for evaluation and treatment in the macular photocoagulation study. Arch Ophthalmol 109:1242–1257, 1991.
7. DeGowin RL, Lewis JL, Hoak JC, et al: Radiosensitivity of human endothelial cells in culture. J Lab Clin Med 84:42–48, 1974.
8. Chakravarthy U, Biggart JH, Gardiner TA, et al: Focal irradiation of perforating eye injuries: minimum effective dose and optimum time of irradiation. Curr Eye Res 8:1241–1250, 1989.
9. Sagerman RH, Chung CT, Alberti WE: Radiosensitivity of ocular and orbital structures. In Alberti WE, Sagerman RH (eds): Radiotherapy of Intraocular and Orbital Tumors. Berlin, Springer-Verlag, 1993.
10. Scott TA, Augsberger JJ, Brady LW, et al: Low-dose ocular irradiation for diffuse choroidal hemangiomas associated with bullous nonrhegmatogenous retinal detachment. Retina 11:389–393, 1988.
11. Plowman PN, Harnett AN: Radiotherapy in benign orbital disease. I. Complicated ocular angiomas. Br J Ophthalmol 72:286–288, 1986.
12. Haik BG, Jereb B, Abramson DH, Ellsworth RM. Ophthalmic radiotherapy. In Iliff NT (ed): Complications in Ophthalmic Surgery. New York, Churchill Livingstone, 1983, pp 449–483.
13. Perez CA, Brady LW: Principles and Practice of Radiation Oncology, 2nd edition. Philadelphia, JB Lippincott Co, 1992.
14. Chakravarthy U, Houston RF, Archer DB: Treatment of age-related subfoveal neovascular membranes by teletherapy: a pilot study. Br J Ophthalmol 77:265–273, 1993.
15. Bergink GJ, Deutman AF, van der Broek JE, et al: Radiation therapy for age-related subfoveal choroidal neovascular membranes: a pilot study. Doc Ophthalmol 90:67–74, 1995.
16. Finger PT, Berson A, Sherr D, et al: Radiation therapy for subretinal neovascularization. Ophthalmology 103:878–889, 1996.
17. Mendelsohn ME, Spaide RF, Abramson DH, Yannuzzi L: Radiation therapy for choroidal neovascularization from age related macular degeneration. American Academy of Ophthalmology paper presentation, 1995.
18. Friedrichsen EJ, Slater JD, Loredo LN, et al: Proton beam irradiation of subfoveal choroidal neovascularization in age related macular degeneration. Invest Ophthalmol Vis Sci 36:S224, 1995.
19. Immonen I, Jaakkola A, Heikkonen J: Treatment of subfoveal choroidal neovascular membranes using Strontium 90 plaque irradiation. Invest Ophthalmol Vis Sci 36:S224, 1995.
20. Brady LW, Shields J, Augsburger J, et al: Complications from radiation therapy to the eye. Front Radiat Ther Oncol 23:238–250, 1989.
21. Heyn R, Ragab A, Raney B, et al: Late effects of therapy in orbital rhabdomyosarcoma in children. A report from the Intergroup Rhabdomyosarcoma Study. Cancer 57:1738–1743, 1986.
22. Servodidio C, Abramson DH: Acute and long-term effects of radiation therapy to the eye in children. Cancer Nursing 16(5):371–381, 1993.
23. Brown GC, Shields JA, Sanborn G, et al: Radiation retinopathy. Ophthalmology 89:1494–1501, 1982.
24. U.S. Department of Health, Education and Welfare. A review of the use of ionizing radiation for the treatment of benign diseases. Washington, DC, HEW publication (FDA) 78-8043, September, 1977.

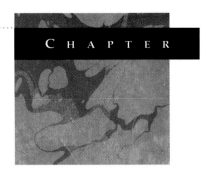

CHAPTER 13

Subretinal Surgery

Nancy M. Holekamp, M.D.
Matthew A. Thomas, M.D.

Removal of blood and scar tissue that interferes with retinal function is a mainstay of vitreous surgery. Until recently, most surgical manipulation has been performed in the preretinal vitreous cavity. Advances in vitreoretinal techniques now allow surgeons to approach a variety of clinical problems beneath the surface of the retina: choroidal neovascular membranes, thick subretinal hemorrhage, subretinal strands in proliferative vitreoretinopathy, subretinal fibrosis after inflammatory conditions, the rare infectious agent, and growths or deposits of malignant cells. This chapter presents current concepts regarding the use of vitreoretinal techniques to gain access to and operate in the subretinal space.

EARLY SUBRETINAL EXPERIENCE

In 1987, Hanscom and Diddie were the first to report using modern vitrectomy techniques, internal retinotomy, endodrainage of blood, and air-fluid exchange in the management of submacular hemorrhage.[1] One patient with age-related macular degeneration (AMD) and a large clot improved to an acuity of 20/400 from count fingers, and a second patient with subretinal hemorrhage from a retinal macroarterial aneurysm regained 20/80 visual acuity from hand motions following this intervention.

Shortly afterward in 1988, DeJuan and Machemer described vitreous surgery for hemorrhagic and fibrous complications of AMD.[2] Large retinotomies were created to gain access to the subretinal space and remove blood and disciform scars. Although the visual results in all four patients were disappointing, several seminal observations were made: surgery in the subretinal space could be

safely executed, the minimal bleeding that occurred stopped spontaneously, large retinotomies predisposed to recurrent detachment and proliferative vitreoretinopathy, and eyes with disciform scars had limited postoperative visual potential. In the time since that report, these conclusions have not changed.

In 1991, Blinder and associates also performed large flap retinotomies in treating eyes with extensive subfoveal neovascular scars.[3] Presumably to limit the risk of subsequent retinal detachment, they performed preoperative barrier laser photocoagulation around the area of proposed retinotomy. Although anatomically successful, visual outcome was disappointing. Understanding the importance of subfoveal retinal pigment epithelium (RPE) integrity following subretinal scar removal, they combined their technique with autologous RPE flaps and homologous RPE grafts with limited success.[4] These authors were the first to realize the importance of subfoveal RPE for postoperative visual acuity and to pursue the transplantation of RPE cells into the subfoveal space. These are still key issues in subretinal surgery.

SMALL RETINOTOMY TECHNIQUE

In 1991, Thomas and Kaplan reported an alternative approach to the subretinal space.[5] In removing subfoveal neovascular membranes in two patients with the presumed ocular histoplasmosis syndrome, they emphasized making a small retinotomy away from the center of the fovea. Through a small retinal hole rather than a large flap retinotomy, instruments were introduced into the subretinal space, abnormal tissue was dislodged, grasped with forceps, and extracted. The visual results were excellent, with acuity improving from 20/400 to 20/20 in one patient and from 20/400 to 20/40 in the second patient. Thomas and Kaplan made several important observations: there was little or no bleeding when active neovascular membranes were disconnected from their choroidal origin; large neovascular complexes could be removed through small retinotomies; and, most importantly, patients could regain visual function after surgical manipulation in the subfoveal space.

SURGICAL APPROACH

Subsequent to this early experience, subretinal surgery experienced a virtual revolution as numerous investigators applied the knowledge and techniques to a wider variety of cases.[6-9] The current surgical techniques and instruments[10-13] evolved over time from many innovative surgeons. Although largely designed to approach subfoveal choroidal neovascularization, the techniques with slight modification can address other subretinal pathology. Subretinal hemorrhage, subretinal fibrosis, and subretinal bands are all best approached through small retinotomies by angled, smaller gauge instruments. The evolution toward small retinotomies and smaller gauge instrumentation is not surprising given the movement toward small-incision cataract surgery, and minimally invasive dacryocystorhinostomy and filtering procedures using lasers and small-incision surgical innovations from other fields (orthopedics, abdominal surgery, etc.).

General Approach to the Subretinal Space

A standard three-port vitrectomy is used. The placement of sclerotomies is critical. The surgeon should decide preoperatively how the subretinal pathology is to be approached and place the sclerotomies accordingly. For example, in a right eye for a right-handed surgeon, a straight temporal retinotomy may minimize damage to major retinal vessels and provide adequate access to the subretinal pathology. Therefore, the superotemporal sclerotomy should be made near the horizontal meridian. In a left eye for a right-handed surgeon, much of the subretinal manipulation may be best handled with the dominant hand from a slightly superior position. Therefore, the superonasal sclerotomy should be made near the 9:30 meridian.

After a core vitrectomy is carried out, if the posterior hyaloid is not already detached, every effort is made to separate it from the retina, particularly in the region of the planned retinotomy. This can be accomplished using a silicone-tipped extrusion needle to aspirate over the attached cortical vitreous near the optic disc as described by Mein and

Flynn.[13] Often a Weiss ring is produced, confirming posterior vitreous separation. In younger patients with a tightly adherent cortical vitreous, a bent microvitreoretinal (MVR) blade or the angled 36-gauge subretinal pick can be used to engage the hyaloid at the optic nerve and manually elevate a Weiss ring, stripping the posterior hyaloid out to the equator. Often an expanding circumferential "wave" of posterior vitreous separation can be seen. The vitrector is reintroduced and the vitrectomy is completed.

The placement of the retinotomy takes into account (1) the location, size, and extent of the subretinal pathology; (2) surrounding major retinal vessels; (3) other retinal pathology (previous laser scars, retinochoroidal anastomoses); and (4) the dimensions of the subretinal instruments (specifically the length of the angled instrument tips so that the abnormal tissue can be reached without excessive stretching or tearing of the retinotomy). Rarely, more than one retinotomy may be needed. Because diathermized retinotomies easily tear and untreated retinotomies simply stretch during subretinal manipulation, a macular retinotomy location is not diathermized.[8]

The retinotomy should be made as small as possible for two reasons: (1) a small retinotomy appears to cause no significant damage to the nerve fiber layer. Consequently, small retinotomies can be made safely, even close to the papillomacular bundle, without fear of visual field defect, and (2) large subretinal complexes can be removed through relatively small retinotomies with little enlargement of the retinal hole. (The elastic properties of the retina allow it to stretch around tissues being delivered from the subretinal space much as the birth canal stretches around a crowning newborn.)

A 36-gauge angled pick, a 33-gauge angled infusion cannula, or an MVR blade can be used to perforate undiathermized retina. The 36-gauge angled pick seems superior to other instruments because of its smaller tip and the ease with which it creates an oblique perforation through neurosensory retina without damaging underlying RPE (Fig. 13–1). Care must be taken to not scrape underlying tissues, as choroidal bleeding or postoperative choroidal neovascularization can occur. Occasional slight retinal capillary hemorrhage can be controlled by transiently increasing the intraocular pressure. Careful attention must be paid to identify the precise location of the retinotomy so that other instruments can subsequently be introduced through the same hole.

If a neurosensory detachment does not accompany the subretinal pathology, then one is created with a subretinal infusion of a small amount of balanced salt solution. Theoretically, this allows for subretinal manipulation without damaging overlying photoreceptors. Generally, a 130-degree angled 33-gauge cannula with a 3-mm beveled tip is used[11] (Fig. 13–2). A controlled infusion is necessary to prevent retinal tears at points of retinal-

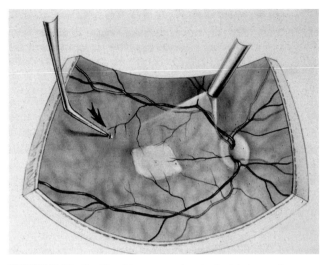

FIGURE 13–1 The 36-gauge subretinal pick is used to perforate nondiathermized neurosensory retina adjacent to the subfoveal neovascular complex.

subretinal adhesion, macular hole formation at the fovea, and extensive retinal detachment. This can be accomplished by a skilled assistant or a pediatric intravenous microinfusion pump. The infusion line (syringe, tubing, cannula) must be free of air to avoid infusing small bubbles into the subretinal space.

Approach to Subretinal Choroidal Neovascularization

If a subretinal choroidal neovascular membrane is to be removed, it is critical that all attachments to overlying neurosensory retina be cleaved (e.g., thinned retina from underlying laser scar adjacent to recurrent membrane). During the subretinal infusion of balanced salt solution, points of adhesion can be identified as fluid tracks. Separation can be

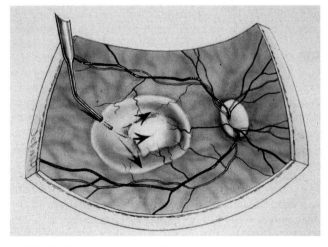

FIGURE 13–2 An angled 33-gauge infusion needle is used to fuse balanced salt solution beneath the neurosensory retina.

achieved with either additional hydrodissection[9] or with careful blunt dissection with an angled 36-gauge subretinal pick.[8] Care is taken to swing the pick in a pivoting or rotating manner over the surface of the membrane in attempt to break adhesions. This requires attention and concentration predominantly at the site of action at the membrane but also some attention to the instrument shaft in the retinotomy. If pressure from the pick fails to break the connections, horizontal subretinal scissors are necessary to cut firm adhesions. These scissors have a 130-degree bend and blades approximately 3 mm in length to allow manipulation through the retinotomy.[11] Adhesions are cut close to the membrane's surface. Retinochoroidal anastomoses sever with minimal petechial hemorrhages, which stop with temporarily elevated intraocular pressure. Occasionally it is advantageous to inject additional balanced salt solution to create more working space between the membrane and the overlying retina.

The membrane is dislodged by manipulations initially with the subretinal pick. The pick tip is gently pushed against the edge of the neovascular complex. Care is taken not to dig posteriorly behind the RPE but to use a stroking sideways motion against the top or edge of the complex, allowing it to peel up (with the intent of not disturbing underlying RPE). A plane of separation can often be identified, and the pick is slipped behind the complex to complete the separation (Fig. 13–3). Although it is well documented that extracted choroidal neovascular membranes are actually larger than the angiographic appearance,[14] often a larger rim of reactive fibrin can be seen to lift off the RPE with the edge of the membrane. Ideally, the neovascular tissue will separate easily from underlying subfoveal RPE, but if the membrane is in a sub-RPE location, then dislodging it will undoubtedly disrupt RPE. Other potential attachments are the edge of a laser scar (in recurrent cases) or the point of choroidal vascular ingrowth.

Once the pick has been used to free the membrane as fully as possible, it is necessary to extract the tissue with subretinal forceps. Positive-action horizontal forceps that are angled 130 degrees and have a 2.4-mm tip are introduced (closed) through the retinotomy, which has usually slightly enlarged during pick manipulation.[11] The blades are placed around the elevated edge of neovascular tissue or, if possible, around the ingrowth stalk. Gentle traction with the blades held closed breaks any remaining connections and allows the tissue to be delivered from the subretinal space (Fig. 13–3). This step is performed slowly and carefully. If traction on the neurosensory retina is seen, the membrane is released and further dissection is carried out. If excessive tugging and displacement of the surrounding RPE is seen, subretinal scissors can be used to sever remaining connections rather than breaking them with the forceps.

When the vascular connection to the choroid is

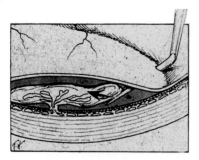

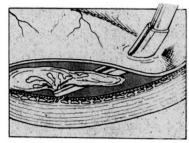

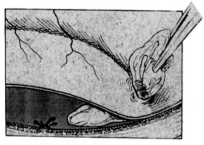

FIGURE 13–3 Subretinal pick manipulation of the neovascular complex followed by forceps removal through the retinotomy, which usually stretches slightly.

about to be severed, the intraocular pressure is raised to approximately 80 mm Hg. Despite high pressure, minimal subretinal hemorrhage may occur. To prevent massive bleeding, the membrane is patiently held in the middle of the vitreous cavity as the pressure remains elevated for at least 1 minute and then is slowly lowered. If more oozing hemorrhage occurs, the pressure is raised again. A thin accumulation of subretinal hemorrhage at the site of the extracted membrane is inconsequential, and is usually resorbed early in the postoperative period.

Once hemostasis is achieved, the membrane is removed from the eye through a sclerotomy or is cut and aspirated with the vitrectomy probe. Large membranes cannot be removed through a standard size sclerotomy. The specimen may be divided with intraocular scissors rather than enlarging the sclerotomy. Plugs are placed and scleral depression is performed 360 degrees to verify that no peripheral retinal tears have occurred.

A complete air-fluid exchange is performed using standard extrusion needles or silicone-tipped needles for the exchange with aspiration over the optic nerve. Care is taken to avoid optic nerve touch, as permanent peripheral visual field loss has been seen in a few cases.[15] Aspiration is not per-

formed over the retinotomy for fear of tearing or enlarging it. If the retinotomy is large, the straight 33-gauge extension needle may be used to aspirate through the retinotomy without engaging the edges of the neurosensory retina. Once the retina is flat, the retinotomy is inspected. In each case, the posterior hyaloid has been meticulously removed. No laser photocoagulation is used. If the retinotomy is small or moderate in size, the eye is gently refilled with fluid to leave a 10% air fill, and the patient is kept in a strict face-down position overnight. The retinotomy will usually be sealed on the first postoperative day. If the retinotomy is large or the patient cannot maintain a strict face-down position for one night, the eye is left with a 100% air fill. In the majority of cases, the retinotomy becomes invisible during the first postoperative month.[16]

Approach to Subretinal Hemorrhage

If a subretinal hemorrhage is to be removed, the surgeon must decide if tissue plasminogen activator (t-PA), manual clot extraction, or both are to be used. Although t-PA has certain theoretic advantages related to lysing fibrin-photoreceptor interdigitations and liquefying solid clots,[17–19] no randomized comparison proving the superiority of t-PA to manual extraction in the management of subretinal hemorrhage has been made. In fact, a consecutive series of 47 cases showed no apparent difference in visual outcome whether or not t-PA was used.[20] It is generally accepted that the fibrin within blood becomes cross-linked within days of the subretinal hemorrhage. Tissue plasminogen activator cannot dissolve this form of enmeshed molecules and thus cannot achieve lysis of clots present for more than 5 to 7 days.

t-PA Assisted Clot Extraction

If t-PA is used, a 130-degree angled 33-gauge cannula (connected to a syringe of 6 to 12 μg/0.1 ml of t-PA held by the surgical assistant) is gently inserted through an avascular extramacular portion of elevated retina into the subfoveal space. A small aliquot of t-PA is injected by the assistant into the clot in a controlled fashion. If the clot is large, another retinotomy with t-PA injection may be indicated. As studies in a rabbit model demonstrated no toxicity at 25 to 50 μg/0.1 ml,[19] the total amount of t-PA used safely should not exceed 25 to 50 total μg. Scleral plugs are then placed, and the eye is left undisturbed for 20 to 40 minutes.

Liquefied subretinal hemorrhage can be drained from the subretinal space in several ways: with a soft-tipped extrusion cannula held over the retinotomy; with a single 30-gauge angled subretinal extrusion cannula through the retinotomy; or with a Lewis double-lumen subretinal irrigator-aspirator through the retinotomy. Care is taken to avoid tearing the retinotomy site or damaging underlying RPE and choriocapillaris. Although bleeding can be tamponaded by raising the intraocular pressure, adequate clot formation is difficult to achieve in the presence of t-PA.

Several methods may be employed to maximize liquified clot removal from the subretinal space. A small bubble of perfluorocarbon liquid may be used to squeeze blood from the subretinal space.[21,22] A lavage of balanced salt solution, either through the same retinotomy or through a separate retinotomy with simultaneous aspiration through the first retinotomy, can clear the subretinal space of blood. Finally, an air-fluid exchange can generally increase the amount of subretinal blood removed. (In a phakic eye, this is the last step, as visibility may be lost if the eye is refilled with fluid.)

It is visually important to remove thick hemorrhage from the subfoveal space.[23] Remaining subretinal hemorrhage in extrafoveal and extramacular locations need not be aggressively removed. A complete air-fluid exchange is performed, aspirating over the retinotomy. The retinotomy should be free of clot and/or hemorrhage and lie flat. Depending upon its location, the retinotomy may or may not be lased. If the retinotomy is small, the eye may be left with a full air fill. If there is more than one retinotomy or a single retinotomy has enlarged, the surgeon may wish to infuse a nonexpansile concentration of long-acting gas. Patients are positioned face-down postoperatively.

Mechanical Clot Extraction

Thick, clot-like subretinal hemorrhages can be quickly and easily removed with manual extraction. If an associated choroidal neovascular membrane is also to be removed, then the surgeon may prefer a forceps extraction to subretinal infusion of t-PA.

A retinotomy site is created adjacent to the clot. Neurosensory retina is elevated from the blood by gentle infusion of balanced salt solution through a bent 33-gauge cannula. A silicone-tipped extrusion cannula or an angled 30-gauge subretinal cannula is placed through the retinotomy to aspirate any liquified blood. The clot is then engaged with the tip of the aspirating instrument and, at high suction, extraction is attempted. If unsuccessful, horizontal subretinal forceps can be placed through the retinotomy and used to mechanically extract the clot from the subretinal space in a slow, controlled manner. Often, associated neovascular tissue is simultaneously removed in one large hemorrhagic complex. To diminish the chances of additional subretinal bleeding, the intraocular pressure is increased during clot removal. The intraocular pressure is then gradually decreased while any new bleeding is sought. The clot is generally cut and aspirated with the vitrectomy probe rather than removed from the eye via sclerotomy.

Residual liquid subretinal blood is aspirated, and

a fluid-air exchange is performed to flatten the retinotomy. The retinotomy site may be lasered, especially if it is large and/or remote from the fovea, and either air or a nonexpansile concentration of long-acting gas is left in the eye. Patients are positioned face-down postoperatively.

Removal of Large Subretinal Hemorrhage

The intraoperative and postoperative complication rate for the removal of subretinal hemorrhage is generally higher than for other vitreous surgeries.[20–22,24,25] Larger subretinal hemorrhages, particularly those greater than 16 disc areas in size, are at higher risk for more complications. Intraoperative complications include enlarged retinotomies, inadvertent retinectomy, retinal incarceration in sclerotomies, unplanned lensectomy, retinal tear, limited suprachoroidal hemorrhage, and uncontrolled subretinal hemorrhage. Postoperative complications include retinal detachment with or without proliferative vitreoretinopathy (PVR), recurrent subretinal hemorrhage, massive subretinal fibrosis, recurrent neovascularization, postoperative RPE tears, and cataract. When approaching the removal of large subretinal hemorrhages, both surgeon and patient should be prepared for prolonged postoperative care, slow visual rehabilitation, and potentially disappointing results.

The randomized, prospective Submacular Surgery Trial will compare surgery versus observation in eyes with AMD and a lesion beneath the fovea, more than 50% of which is blood. This trial should establish whether surgery should be undertaken in such cases.

Approach to Subretinal Strands in Proliferative Vitreoretinopathy

Although subretinal bands may be encountered in up to 47% of eyes undergoing vitreous surgery for rhegmatogenous retinal detachment complicated by PVR,[26] one must decide (ideally preoperatively) if it is necessary to remove such bands to achieve retinal flattening. Successful reattachment of the retina is possible in 70 to 95% of eyes without removal of subretinal strands.[26,27] In general, subretinal bands in the posterior pole or those creating a "napkin ring" configuration require removal.

Access to a subretinal band in PVR is best obtained through a pre-existing retinal break. If this is not possible, intraocular diathermy is used to create a small retinotomy in extramacular retina in the vicinity of the subretinal band. This retinotomy may be used for drainage of subretinal fluid at the end of the case. Several retinotomies may be necessary depending on the vectors of subretinal traction and the configuration of the retinal detachment. To engage the subretinal band in a controlled fashion, subretinal forceps are preferred to a vitreoretinal pick. Using gentle tangential traction, the band is peeled off the outer surface of the retina and/or RPE. Complications at this point in the procedure include retinal or RPE tears, enlargement of the retinotomy, bullous retinal detachment, and subretinal hemorrhage. If firm adhesion to the overlying neurosensory retina or RPE precludes safe removal of the subretinal band, retroretinal traction can be relieved by segmentation with subretinal horizontal or vertical scissors in one or multiple places.

Once all anatomically significant subretinal bands have been removed, an air-fluid exchange is carried out through one of the existing retinotomies. Successful intraoperative flattening of the retina is possible in 95% of eyes requiring subretinal strand removal.[26] Given the nature of retinal detachments complicated by PVR, the retinotomy or retinotomies are treated with endolaser photocoagulation, and a nonexpansile, long-acting intraocular gas is left in the eye. The patient is positioned face-down postoperatively.

Approach to Other Subretinal Pathology

The surgical techniques outlines in this chapter can be modified to approach other subretinal pathology. The basic principles of small retinotomy—a small neurosensory retinal detachment to create working space under the retina; careful subretinal manipulation with small-gauge, angled instruments; and air tamponade with or without laser photocoagulation of most retinotomies—should be followed.

REFERENCES

1. Hanscom TA, Diddie KR: Early surgical drainage of macular subretinal hemorrhage. Arch Ophthalmol 105:1722–1723, 1987.
2. DeJuan E, Machemer R: Vitreous surgery for hemorrhagic and fibrous complications of age-related macular degeneration. Am J Ophthalmol 105:25–29, 1988.
3. Blinder KJ, Peyman GA, Paris CL, Gremillion CM Jr: Submacular scar excision in age-related macular degeneration. Int Ophthalmol 15:215–222, 1991.
4. Peyman GA, Blinder KJ, Paris CL, et al: A technique for retinal pigment epithelial transplantation for age-related macular degeneration secondary to extensive subfoveal scarring. Ophthalmic Surg 22:102–108, 1991.
5. Thomas MA, Kaplan HJ: Surgical removal of subfoveal neovascularization in the presumed ocular histoplasmosis syndrome. Am J Ophthalmol 111:107, 1991.
6. Berger AS, Kaplan HJ: Clinical experience with the surgical removal of subfoveal neovascularization membranes. Short term postoperative results. Ophthalmology 99:969–976, 1992.
7. Thomas MA, Grand MG, Williams DF, et al: Surgical management of subfoveal choroidal neovascularization. Ophthalmology 99:952–968, 1992.
8. Thomas MA, Dickinson JD, Melberg MS, et al: Visual results after surgical removal of subfoveal choroidal neovascular membranes. Ophthalmology 101:1384–1396, 1994.
9. Lamberg HM, Capone A, Aaberg TM, et al: Surgical excision of subfoveal neovascular membranes in age-related macular degeneration. Am J Ophthalmol 113:257–262, 1992.
10. Thomas MA, Lee CM, Pesin S, Lowe M: New instruments for submacular surgery. Am J Ophthalmol 112:733–734, 1991.
11. Thomas MA, Ibanez HE: Instruments for submacular surgery. Retina 14:84–87, 1994.
12. Wallace RT, Vander JF: A simple technique for controlled subretinal injections. Retina 13:260–261, 1993.
13. Mein CE, Flynn HW Jr: Recognition and removal of the posterior cortical vitreous during vitreoretinal surgery for impending macular hole. Am J Ophthalmol 112:611–615, 1991.
14. Bynoe LA, Chang TS, Funata M, et al: Histopathologic examination of vascular patterns in subfoveal membranes. Ophthalmology 101:1112–1117, 1994.
15. Melberg NS, Thomas MA: Visual field loss after pars plana vitrectomy with air/fluid exchange. Am J Ophthalmol 120:386–388, 1995.
16. Dickinson JD, Aguilar HE, Thomas MA: Retinotomy in subfoveal surgery: neither laser nor long acting gas tamponade is required. Presented at American Academy of Ophthalmology Meeting, 1994.
17. Toth CA, Mrose LS, Hjelmeland LM, Landres MB: Fibrin directs early retinal damage after experimental subretinal hemorrhage. Arch Ophthalmol 109:723–729, 1991.
18. Lewis H, Resnick SC, Flannery JG, Straatsma BR: Tissue plasminogen activator treatment of experimental subretinal hemorrhage. Am J Ophthalmol 111:197–204, 1991.
19. Lewis H: Intraoperative fibrinolysis of submacular hemorrhage with tissue plasminogen activator and surgical drainage. Am J Ophthalmol 118:559–568, 1994.
20. Ibanez HE, Williams DF, Thomas MA, et al: Surgical management of submacular hemorrhage. A series of 47 consecutive cases. Arch Ophthalmol 113:62–69, 1995.
21. Linn JI, Drews-Botch C, Sternberg P, et al: Submacular hemorrhage removal. Ophthalmology 102:1393–1399, 1995.
22. Kamei M, Tano Y, Maeno T, et al: Surgical removal of submacular hemorrhage using tissue plasminogen activator and perfluorocarbon liquid. Am J Ophthalmol 121:267–275, 1996.
23. Bennett SR, Folk JC, Blodi CF, Klugman M: Factors prognostic of visual outcome in patients with subretinal hemorrhage. Am J Ophthalmol 109:33–37, 1990.
24. Vander JF, Federman JL, Greven C, et al: Surgical removal of massive subretinal hemorrhage associated with age-related macular degeneration. Ophthalmology 98:23–26, 1991.
25. Wade EC, Flynn JW, Olsen KR, et al: Subretinal hemorrhage management by pars plana vitrectomy and internal drainage. Arch Ophthalmol 108:973–978, 1990.
26. Lewis H, Aaberg TM, Abrams GW, et al: Subretinal membranes in proliferative vitreoretinopathy. Ophthalmology 96:1403–1415, 1989.
27. Wallyn RH, Hilton GF: Subretinal fibrosis in retinal detachment. Arch Ophthalmol 97:2128–2135, 1979.

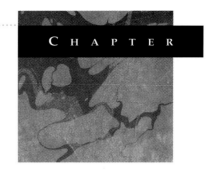

CHAPTER 14

Other Causes of Choroidal Neovascular Membranes

John H. Niffenegger, M.D.
Lawrence J. Singerman, M.D.

Choroidal neovascularization (CNV) has been observed in many macular diseases other than age-related macular degeneration (AMD). This chapter will review the clinical characteristics and treatment of these important diseases. They are much less common than AMD. Therefore, our knowledge of the pathology, natural history, and response to treatment is incomplete. In many situations, our management of these disorders is influenced by extrapolation from the results of the Macular Photocoagulation Study (MPS).[1] In ocular histoplasmosis syndrome and idiopathic choroidal neovascularization, the MPS directly studied the effectiveness of laser therapy.

Almost any pathologic process that disturbs the pigment epithelium and Bruch's membrane can be associated with choroidal neovascularization. Ocular histoplasmosis syndrome, idiopathic choroidal neovascularization, pathologic myopia, angioid streaks, multifocal choroiditis, serpiginous choroidopathy, choroidal osteoma, choroidal rupture, hereditary dystrophies, and many other conditions have been reported.

Pathologic investigation has not been possible for all of these diseases. The basic mechanisms of choroidal neovascularization have been derived from histopathologic studies of AMD.[2] These studies have been elaborated in earlier chapters. The common histopathologic feature appears to be a break in Bruch's membrane and capillary-like extension of new vessels from the choroid through the defect in Bruch's membrane. Because of the common characteristics of a break in Bruch's membrane in the early stages of CNV and the common occurrence of a disciform lesion late in the process, it is hypothesized that the pathogenesis of CNV has

important similarities regardless of the specific associated disease.

CNV has been divided histopathologically into two types according to the location of the new vessels.[3] In type I CNV, the initial growth of these new vessels appears to be between the inner and outer aspects of Bruch's membrane. Extension occurs within the subpigment epithelial space. This is the typical situation in AMD. In type II CNV, the growth pattern of CNV in young patients tends to be in the subsensory retinal space. This suggests that the removal of CNV in conditions where growth is anterior to the retinal pigment epithelium (RPE) has some chance of restoring useful visual function in these patients. Removal of CNV in AMD typically results in the removal of native RPE reducing the likelihood of useful central vision after subretinal surgery.[4]

The two treatments most commonly employed for CNV are laser photocoagulation and surgical removal of the neovascular membrane. Prognosis is largely dependent on the location of the CNV (Fig. 14–1). The MPS proved the efficacy of argon laser photocoagulation for extrafoveal CNV secondary to AMD, ocular histoplasmosis, and idiopathic CNV.[5–7] Krypton laser photocoagulation has been shown to be efficacious in juxtafoveal CNV.[8] The benefit of photocoagulation of subfoveal CNV has recently been demonstrated in select cases of AMD.[9–11] A pilot randomized study by several MPS investigators of photocoagulation for the treatment of subfoveal CNV secondary to ocular histoplasmosis did not demonstrate either a benefit or a detriment from laser treatment in 25 patients enrolled over a 2-year period.[12] The value of photocoagulation in less common causes of CNV has not been

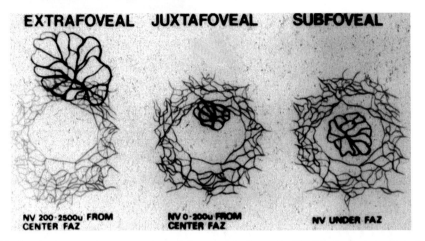

FIGURE 14-1   An important prognostic and therapeutic factor in CNV is its location in relation to the center of the foveal avascular zone. Proper assessment of location requires high-quality fluorescein angiography. (From Singerman LJ: Important points in the management of patients with choroidal neovascularization. Ophthalmology 92:610–614, 1985. Courtesy of Ophthalmology, with permission.)

studied thoroughly, and the results of the MPS must be cautiously considered. Differences as well as similarities between these disorders and those specifically studied in the MPS must be examined.

In some cases not eligible for photocoagulation, submacular surgery may offer the possibility of improved outcome. To date, no prospective randomized clinical trials have been completed comparing submacular surgery with either laser treatment or natural history. Uncontrolled series of subfoveal surgery for histoplasmosis CNV suggest impressive improvement in visual acuity is possible.[13,14] Currently, an arm of the Submacular Surgery Trial (a pilot prospective randomized controlled multicenter trial) is evaluating submacular surgery compared with natural history in subfoveal idiopathic and histoplasmic CNV. Other arms of this trial are evaluating submacular surgery for subfoveal CNV in AMD. Little is known regarding the response to surgery of less common forms of CNV.

OCULAR HISTOPLASMOSIS SYNDROME

Ocular histoplasmosis syndrome (OHS) is one of the more common causes of CNV not associated with AMD. It is endemic in the Ohio and Mississippi river valleys, where a relatively high proportion of young lifelong residents react positively to histoplasmin skin testing.[15] Positive reactions to skin testing are more common in patients with disciform lesions.[16-18] Reactivation of apparently inactive lesions has been reported with skin testing.[18-21] It is thought that most patients suffer a subclinical infection or mild flu-like illness.[22] Epidemic infection, however, has been reported to be associated with cleaning chicken coops,[23] demolition of old buildings,[24] or exposure to sites inhabited by bats.[25,26] Similar disease outside of endemic

areas such as in Europe has been reported and the etiology of this disorder is presumed in most cases.

The fundus findings in ocular histoplasmosis are described as a triad of macular scar or hemorrhage associated with peripapillary chorioretinal atrophy and punched-out peripheral chorioretinal lesions ("histo spots").[27] CNV may arise at a chorioretinal scar and cause loss of central vision.[28] End-stage lesions appear similar to the disciform scars found in AMD. CNV in ocular histoplasmosis syndrome, however, is not associated with drusen.[2] Some investigators suggest the CNV associated with ocular histoplasmosis tends to be subretinal, anterior to the plane of the RPE, more frequently than in CNV associated with AMD.[3]

It is hypothesized that focal choroiditis damages Bruch's membrane, retinal pigment epithelium, and choriocapillaris, causing an exudative detachment of the retina or subretinal hemorrhage. Resolution of the choroiditis leaves a focal area of atrophy. Choroidal vessels associated with the chorioretinal atrophy may decompensate, causing serous exudation, choroidal neovascularization, and transient serous detachment of the retina. A hemorrhagic detachment may occur that later resolves to form a disciform scar. Analysis of five choroidal neovascular membranes from patients with OHS showed growth in the subretinal space. The vessels tended to be engulfed by a monolayer of proliferating pigment epithelial cells. Surgical excision theoretically allows reapproximation of the retinal photoreceptors with the native RPE. Surgical removal may be associated with a significant improvement in vision.[4]

Differentiation of inactive scars from active CNV is essential in the management of patients with ocular histoplasmosis. Fluorescein angiography of chorioretinal scars demonstrates hyperfluorescence beginning first in the periphery, adjacent to normal choroid, with later spread to the center of the scar. In neovascularization, hyperfluorescence begins in the area of CNV and then spreads more peripherally. The late phase will show hyperfluorescence of the entire lesion in either case. The scar will show staining. The lesion with active CNV will have hyperfluorescence of the overlying serous subretinal detachment (Fig. 14–2). Recurrence must be recognized and treated promptly to reduce the risk of vision loss from foveal involvement.

The pathophysiology of recurrence is not well understood. Histopathology of subfoveal membranes suggests a nonuniform distribution of blood vessels and large areas of avascular membrane that would not likely be imaged adequately by angiography. This could contribute to incomplete treatment and thus to recurrence.[29]

Natural history studies have demonstrated a significant risk of vision loss from CNV, but at a rate lower than that seen in AMD, with a substantial number of eyes maintaining good vision.[30] Spontaneous improvement has been observed.[31,32] The MPS evaluated the efficacy of laser photocoagulation in extrafoveal and juxtafoveal CNV. Argon la-

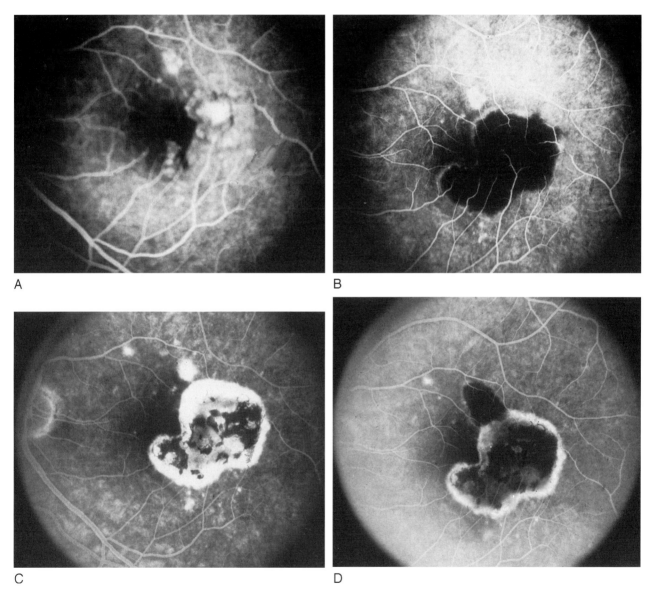

A

B

C

D

FIGURE 14–2   Laser photocoagulation of CNV in presumed ocular histoplasmosis syndrome (POHS). *A*, Angiogram shows two areas of CNV, one superotemporal and one inferior to the fovea. Hypofluorescence corresponded to subretinal hemorrhage, with secondary visual loss (20/80). A small area of hyperfluorescence superiorly corresponded to an inactive chorioretinal scar. *B*, Five days after laser treatment, the CNV is obliterated. *C*, One year later, there is increased hyperfluorescence at the superonasal margin of the previous treatment, contiguous with the previously inactive scar. Clinical examination revealed a small serous/hemorrhagic retinal detachment in this area (note the hypofluorescence corresponding to hemorrhage inferonasal to the upper lesion, highlighting probable CNV). *D*, One week following the second laser treatment to the area of reactivation, there is resolution of the detachment with no residual hyperfluorescence. Acuity improved to 20/30. (From Singerman LJ, Novak MA: Subretinal neovascularization. In Yannuzzi LA [ed]: Laser photocoagulation of the retina. Philadelphia, JB Lippincott, 1989, pp 27–46, with permission.)

ser photocoagulation has been shown to reduce the risk of severe visual loss in eyes with extrafoveal choroidal neovascular membranes.[6] Krypton laser has been found to be beneficial in juxtafoveal CNV associated with ocular histoplasmosis.[8]

In the argon study of extrafoveal CNV, 48% of eyes in the observation group, compared with 9% in the laser treatment group, lost six or more lines of visual acuity after 3 years of follow-up.[33] Visual acuity was worse than 20/200 in 39% of the untreated eyes, compared with 5% of treated eyes. In the treated group, 66% of treated eyes had a visual acuity of 20/40 or better, compared with 38% in the untreated group.

In the krypton study for juxtafoveal CNV, after 3 years of follow-up, 25% of eyes in the observation group versus 5% in the treatment group lost six or more lines of vision. The argon study for extrafoveal CNV and the krypton study for juxtafoveal CNV had similar treatment protocols. The MPS called for photocoagulation of the entire area of hyperfluorescence in an effort to completely obliterate the CNV.[5-8]

The treatment of subfoveal CNV associated with histoplasmosis was not specifically addressed by the MPS. The natural history is guarded, with more than 75% of patients developing 20/200 or worse visual acuity over a 2- to 3-year period.[34,35] A pilot randomized trial of photocoagulation of subfoveal CNV by some of the MPS investigators did not yield a definitive recommendation.[12]

Favorable results from subfoveal surgery have encouraged some investigators. Twenty eyes with subfoveal histoplasmic CNV were included in a report by Thomas and associates.[36] Significant improvement in visual acuity was obtained in six eyes. The mean follow-up was 6.5 months, and the rate of recurrence was 29%. Recently, Thomas and associates have reported on 67 eyes with an average follow-up of 10.5 months.[37] Final visual acuity improved in 83%. Over 30% had a final visual acuity of 20/40 or better.

IDIOPATHIC NEOVASCULARIZATION

Choroidal neovascularization in the absence of atrophic retinal scars, drusen, or other retinal abnormality is termed idiopathic. The MPS argon study of the treatment of extrafoveal CNV found a substantial reduction in the risk of losing six or more lines of visual acuity in the treated group (16%) compared with the group randomized to no treatment (34%).[7,34] The natural history of idiopathic subfoveal CNV has been retrospectively evaluated in 19 consecutive patients with idiopathic CNV.[38] The prognosis appears to be significantly better than in AMD and some other causes of CNV. Over a median follow-up of 87 months, 95% of the patients had a stable or improved visual acuity; 5%

had a significant loss in visual acuity. Initial lesions one disc area or smaller were more likely to have a final vision of 20/60 or better and less likely to have a final visual acuity of 20/200 or worse. This relatively favorable natural history must be considered when considering treatment of subfoveal lesions. Four eyes with idiopathic CNV were included in a report of 17 eyes treated with subfoveal surgery for CNV not associated with AMD or histoplasmosis.[39] Two eyes had visual acuity improved by two or more lines after surgery. In two eyes, visual acuities remained unchanged. Two eyes had recurrences during the follow-up period (range, 6 to 29 months). In a series of eight eyes undergoing surgery for idiopathic subfoveal CNV, a mean improvement of three Snellen lines and final acuity of 20/40 or better in two eyes was obtained.[37] Recurrence occurred in 50% (four of eight eyes).

PATHOLOGIC MYOPIA

Subretinal neovascularization occurs in between 5 and 10% of myopes and is more common in myopes with more than 5 diopters of myopia. Bilateral involvement is not uncommon.[40,41] Fuchs' spot is the term commonly used to describe a dark macular lesion from hemorrhage or RPE hyperplasia thought to represent changes secondary to or associated with the development of CNV in myopic patients.[42] Lacquer cracks, or linear breaks in Bruch's membrane, may develop in association with choroidal thinning and atrophy accompanying elongation of the globe in pathologic myopia. CNV may extend through these breaks, causing hemorrhage and disciform scarring.[2,28] Subretinal hemorrhage not associated with CNV is more common in younger patients and tends to resolve spontaneously in a few months. Vision usually remains stable or improves over several months in these cases.[43]

Choroidal neovascular membranes associated with myopia often appear as grayish circumscribed lesions occurring near the fovea. Subretinal fluid tends to be minimal, hemorrhage is limited, and subretinal exudation is not common. Hyperfluorescence on fluorescein angiography occurs early but does not leak profusely (Fig. 14–3). Hyperfluorescence may be confined to the borders of the choroidal neovascular membrane. Choroidal neovascularization may occur at the border of atrophic areas of RPE, which cause window defect, requiring careful attention to the angiogram to find any areas of discrete leakage. CNV may arise in the fovea in a large proportion of eyes with pathologic high myopia.[44,45]

The natural history of CNV in pathologic myopia is variable and complicates recommendations for laser treatment. Some authors report a poor prognosis. Hotchkiss and Fine found that 14 of 27 eyes lost two or more lines of visual acuity during

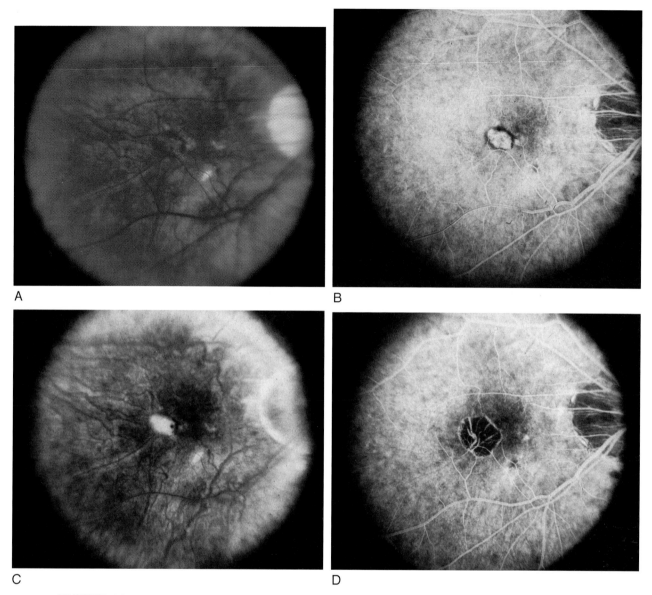

FIGURE 14–3   CNV secondary to pathologic myopia. *A,* Color photograph of a 33-year-old high myope complaining of sudden decrease in vision and metamorphopsia (acuity 20/400). Note the subretinal hemorrhage, and myopic chorioretinal atrophy. *B,* Fluorescein angiogram shows a circumscribed lacy CNV inferior to the fovea. *C,* The CNV stains in the late phase of the angiogram. *D,* Two months after photocoagulation the CNV is quiescent and acuity has improved to 20/200.

2 years of follow-up.[40] Twelve patients became legally blind. Other studies report a less severe prognosis. Two thirds of patients followed by Fried and co-workers had stable or improved vision without treatment, although in 50% the CNV involved the fovea during a 5-year follow-up period.[41]

Soubrane and Pisan randomized 38 eyes to photocoagulation and 28 eyes to observation.[46] The eyes not receiving treatment generally had a marked decline in vision, with 80% having a final visual acuity of less than 20/100. Treated eyes were remarkably stable but did not have any statistical improvement in vision compared with untreated eyes. The authors concluded that laser therapy for CNV in degenerative myopia probably is efficacious, although difficult and associated with significant risks and potential for complications. Progressive enlargement of atrophic laser scars has been reported.[47,48] Even if the atrophic laser scars extend to the fovea, however, they usually are not associated with serious vision loss.

Laser treatment in patients with subfoveal CNV associated with pathologic myopia may offer no improvement over its natural course. Surgical removal of the choroidal neovascular membrane has been performed in these cases. Information regarding outcomes remains preliminary, but there is hope that improvement over the natural history may be possible. Five eyes with CNV associated with pathologic myopia (>6 diopters of myopia and stigmata of myopic degeneration) were included in a report of subfoveal surgery.[39] Age ranged from 36 to 51 years. Four of the eyes had previous laser photocoagulation. Subfoveal CNV was present in the fellow eye of four patients. Visual acuity improved two lines or more in two eyes, and was stable or declined less than two lines in three eyes. There was one recurrence during the follow-up period of 6 to 15 months. In a series of ten myopic eyes undergoing surgical removal by Thomas et al, mean visual acuity declined by one line and recurrent CNV developed in two eyes.[37]

ANGIOID STREAKS

Angioid streaks are irregular radiating lines that appear similar to blood vessels in size and color, thus the term "angioid." Histopathologic examination reveals that these lines actually are calcified breaks in Bruch's membrane. A number of systemic disorders have been associated with angioid streaks including pseudoxanthoma elasticum, Paget's disease of bone, Ehlers-Danlos syndrome, sickle cell disease, thalassemia, and other blood dyscrasias (Figs. 14–4 and 14–5).[2,28,49–52] In a series of 50 patients, Clarkson and Altman found that 50% had an identifiable systemic diagnosis.[53] Skin biopsy specimens have exhibited changes suggestive of pseudoxanthoma elasticum in some patients with angioid streaks who did not have clinically evident skin changes.[54]

CNV may grow through the breaks in Bruch's membrane, causing serous or hemorrhage detachment of the RPE. Minor injury can cause traumatic

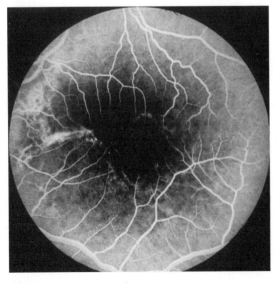

FIGURE 14–4 Angioid streaks in sickle cell anemia. Angiogram reveals a streak extending toward the fovea without evidence of CNV. (From Singerman LJ, Novak MA: Subretinal neovascularization. In Yannuzzi LA [ed]: Laser photocoagulation of the retina. Philadelphia, JB Lippincott, 1989, pp 27–46, with permission.)

rupture of the fragile, calcified Bruch's membrane, resulting in sudden loss of central vision.[28] Deterioration in visual acuity may occur in the absence of CNV by subtle, progressive atrophic degeneration. Visual acuity can drop to the 20/200 level, often in the absence of marked atrophy of the retinal pigment epithelium.

Most CNV associated with angioid streaks occurs in the papillomacular bundle, nasal to the fovea. Laser treatment in this region may cause visual field defects. In addition, there is a risk of damaging major vessels when treating near the optic disc. In Paget's disease, CNV may be large, increasing the difficulty of treatment. Prompt laser treatment may be considered in selected cases, as it has been found to reduce the rate of visual loss.

The visual prognosis in eyes with angioid streaks and CNV is poor. Typically, the CNV progresses to cause severe vision loss. Frequently, CNV occurs in the fellow eye. CNV has been treated with both argon and krypton laser.[52,55,56] Although untreated eyes cannot be considered adequate controls in these studies, treated eyes had better visual outcome than untreated eyes. Gelisken et al. reported long-term follow-up of patients treated with photocoagulation.[57] Patients were followed 2 months to 16 years with a mean follow-up of 3.4 years. The authors concluded that laser treatment was beneficial and allowed eyes to maintain useful vision longer than untreated eyes.

Five eyes with subfoveal CNV associated with angioid streaks were included in a report of subretinal surgery.[39] One patient had improvement from 20/300 to 20/50. Visual acuity was stable in three eyes and declined in one. There were no recurrences during the follow-up period, which ranged from 6.5 to 32 months. Thomas et al reported results in four patients undergoing subfoveal removal of choroidal neovascular membranes. Final visual acuity was 20/200 or worse in all eyes.[37]

MULTIFOCAL CHOROIDITIS

A number of investigators have reported multifocal choroiditis not related to ocular histoplasmosis syndrome but with end-stage findings similar to those found in histoplasmosis syndrome.[58–67] Unlike eyes with ocular histoplasmosis, these eyes often have evidence of vitreous inflammation, although this is a variable finding.[68] Anterior segment inflammation occurs in about 50% of eyes. Acute lesions appear as yellow or gray choroidal lesions that may initially block and later stain with fluorescein.[28] Inactive lesions typically are smaller than those seen in ocular histoplasmosis syndrome. Most patients are from areas where ocular histoplasmosis syndrome is not endemic. In 25% of unilateral cases, severe inflammation may occur in the second eye months or years later. Females and young patients (30s and

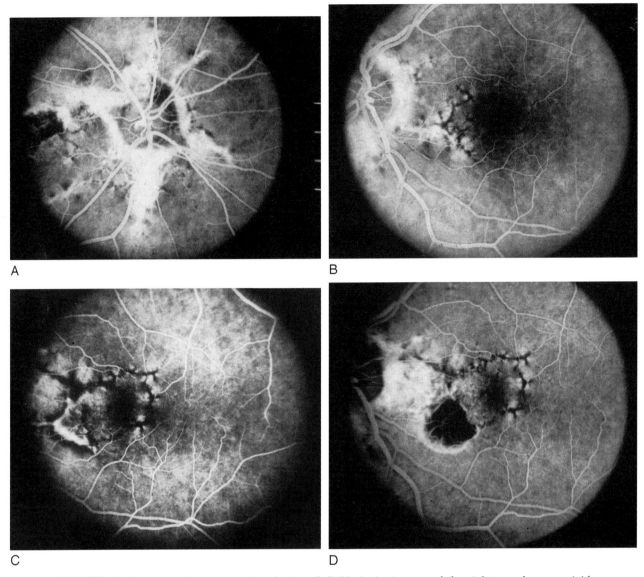

FIGURE 14–5 Angioid streaks and evolution of CNV. *A*, Angiogram of the right eye shows angioid streaks nasal to the fovea and surrounding the disc. A CNV treated nasal to the macula is quiescent. A medical evaluation and skin biopsy yielded a diagnosis of pseudoxanthoma elasticum. Visual acuity was 20/60. *B*, Angiogram of the left eye shows an angioid streak nasal to the macula (visual acuity is 20/25). *C*, Three years later the left eye developed sudden decrease in vision and metamorphopsia (visual acuity is 20/30-) associated with CNV. *D*, Three months after photocoagulation the CNV is quiescent and visual acuity has improved to 20/20-.

40s) are more commonly affected. The disorder has been reported in children. Multifocal choroiditis and choroidal neovascularization have been associated with multiple evanescent white dot and acute idiopathic blind spot enlargement syndrome in one series.[68]

CNV similar to that seen in ocular histoplasmosis syndrome often develops (Fig. 14–6). The final scar appears similar to scars seen in ocular histoplasmosis syndrome but the acute and subacute lesions in multifocal choroiditis appear quite different. Acute and subacute lesions have been observed to occur in ocular histoplasmosis syndrome but are rare. These lesions are more commonly observed in multifocal choroiditis and panuveitis. Chronic, subacute, and acute lesions may be present in the same eye. Subretinal fibrosis and scarring may become extensive and confluent.

Inflammatory lesions, and some CNV, may respond to steroid therapy[66] (Fig. 14–7). Photocoagulation may also be effective for CNV[66,69] (Fig. 14–6). In our experience, recurrent as well as new CNV may occur more commonly in multifocal choroiditis than in other causes of CNV. We recommend oral corticosteroid therapy for any active inflammation threatening the macula or optic nerve. Laser treatment is recommended for any CNV not under the center of the fovea. Active inflammation often

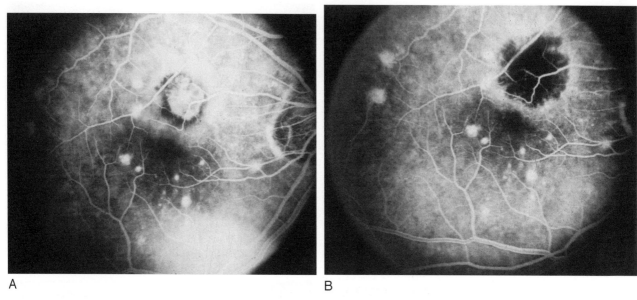

A   B

FIGURE 14–6   Multifocal choroiditis and CNV. *A*, Angiogram reveals well-defined hyperfluorescence superior to the fovea representing CNV. Scattered round hyperfluorescent lesions correspond to areas of choroiditis. *B*, Two weeks following photocoagulation the CNV is quiescent and the areas of choroiditis are stable.

accompanies CNV so concurrent steroid therapy and laser treatment are often required. Subfoveal CNV might be considered for surgical removal, but to date there is no proof of the benefits of this approach in this disease or in other diseases.

SERPIGINOUS CHOROIDITIS

Serpiginous choroiditis is a chronic, recurring inflammation of the RPE and choroid of unknown etiology. Lesions typically begin in the peripapillary region, extending in a radial or curvilinear pattern.[70] Patchy lesions may begin in the macula or periphery. Serpiginous choroiditis usually affects otherwise healthy young or middle-aged patients. The disease typically begins in one eye, eventually becoming bilateral, months or years later.[71] Recurrent attacks can occur weeks or years after the initial onset, involving larger areas of the fundus.[72] Visual field defects correspond to the affected fundus lesions and can be followed by Amsler grid. Often, the asymptomatic eye will have an area of chorioretinal scarring near the optic nerve.

The onset of paracentral and central scotoma tends to be sudden. Within weeks of the onset of symptoms, during the active phase of inflammation, examination reveals discrete grayish white discoloration of the RPE and inner choroid (Fig. 14–8). Anterior chamber reaction occasionally is present.[73] After a few weeks, the grayish lesions pale and later atrophy. A fibrous scar may be present in older lesions. Hyperplasia of the RPE often borders the atrophic areas.[74] In addition to inflammation of the RPE and choriocapillaris, retinal vasculitis and

branch vein occlusion have been associated with serpiginous choroiditis.[75] RPE detachment and neovascularization of the disc and retina have been reported.[76] Approximately 25% develop CNV near the border of atrophic scars.[28]

Clinicopathologic findings include a diffuse and focal infiltrate of lymphocytes in the choroid, with larger aggregations of lymphocytes at the margin of serpiginous lesions.[76] Lesions are characterized by a loss of RPE and photoreceptors, and variable amounts of RPE hyperplasia. Breaks in Bruch's membrane through which fibroglial scar tissue extends from the choroid are present in areas of CNV.

Patients may become symptomatic with recurrent inflammation at the margin of previous chorioretinal scarring.[78] In fluorescein angiography, hyperfluorescence from recurrent inflammation must be distinguished from leakage associated with CNV. Inflammatory lesions tend to have subtle hyperfluorescence and leakage late in the angiogram (Fig. 14–8). Blocked fluorescence is seen on indocyanine green angiography (ICG). CNV have earlier and more dramatic leakage. Subretinal hemorrhage or lipid indicates CNV (Fig. 14–9).

Treatment with oral or periocular steroids should be considered when inflammation threatens the fovea.[71,74,79] Hooper and Kaplan have advocated combination therapy of azathioprine, cyclosporine, and prednisone for patients unresponsive to steroids alone.[80] It is advisable to prescribe a systemic steroid for the patient to keep and use for the first day or two after symptoms recur, until a complete eye examination and fluorescein angiogram can be performed. Laser photocoagulation can be beneficial in treating CNV in selected patients and should be considered in patients with active CNV.

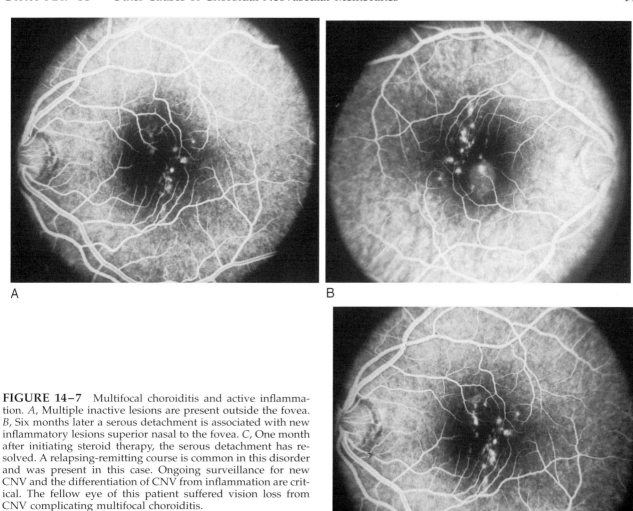

FIGURE 14–7   Multifocal choroiditis and active inflammation. *A,* Multiple inactive lesions are present outside the fovea. *B,* Six months later a serous detachment is associated with new inflammatory lesions superior nasal to the fovea. *C,* One month after initiating steroid therapy, the serous detachment has resolved. A relapsing-remitting course is common in this disorder and was present in this case. Ongoing surveillance for new CNV and the differentiation of CNV from inflammation are critical. The fellow eye of this patient suffered vision loss from CNV complicating multifocal choroiditis.

CHOROIDAL RUPTURE

Choroidal rupture is a fairly common complication of blunt ocular trauma. Direct choroidal ruptures are uncommon and tend to occur anterior to the equator where direct contusion of the globe occurred. Indirect choroidal rupture is more common and in one series was found to occur in 5 to 10% of blunt trauma cases.[81] In indirect choroidal rupture, breaks in the choriocapillaris, RPE, and Bruch's membrane occur posterior to the equator and tend to be concentric to the disc. Hemorrhage in the choroid, subretinal space, and retina often accompany choroidal rupture. CNV may develop, usually at the foveal margin of the choroidal rupture (Fig. 14–10). Visual loss resulting from serous exudation or hemorrhage from CNV can occur months or years after the original trauma. Laser photocoagulation may be helpful in cases of CNV.[82]

Neovascularization may involute without treatment.[83,84]

CHOROIDAL OSTEOMA

Choroidal osteoma was first described in detail by Gass and associates in 1978.[85] Most patients with this rare, benign tumor of cancellous bone are Caucasian women. In 10 to 25% of patients the osteoma is bilateral.[86,87] Lesions typically occur in the juxtapapillary region and macula. The majority of eyes maintain good visual acuity of 20/30 or better.[88] Osteoblasts grow in the choroid and may organize haversian systems. Slow growth of the tumor occurs in approximately half of patients. Choroidal vasculature may intermix with the compact bone of the osteoma, forming vascular tufts distinct from CNV.[89]

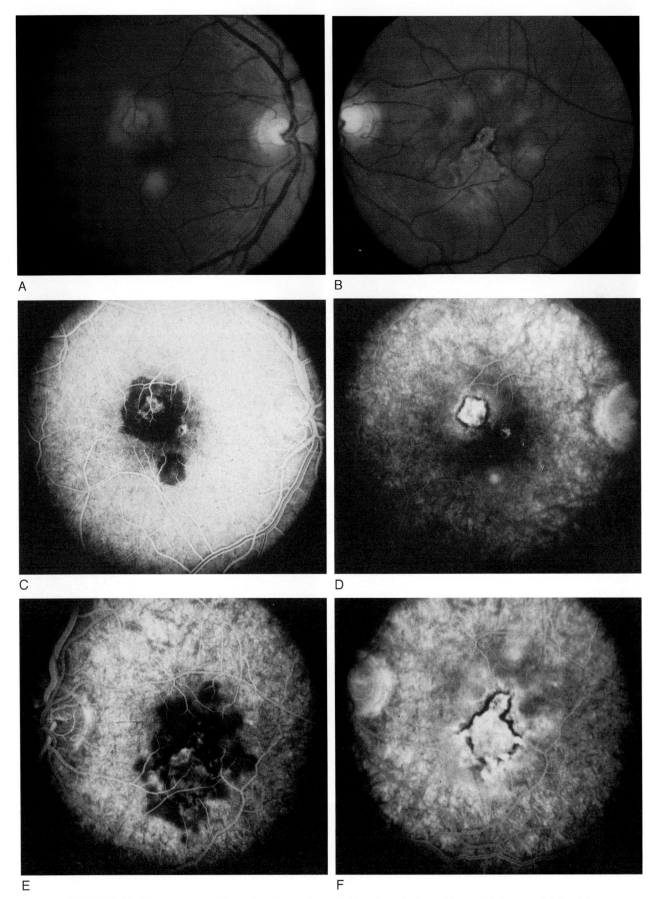

FIGURE 14–8 Serpiginous choroidopathy without CNV and resolution with steroid therapy. *A*, The right eye has whitening at the level of the RPE in the superior temporal fovea with a dense central area sharply demarcated with a pigmented border. Whitening at the level of the RPE is also present inferior to the fovea. Visual acuity is 20/40. *B*, The left eye has a much larger irregular, central sharply delineated lesion (visual acuity is 20/200). *C*, Fluorescein angiogram of the right eye demonstrates initial blocking in areas of choroidopathy surrounding a hyperfluorescence central area. *Illustration continued on opposite page*

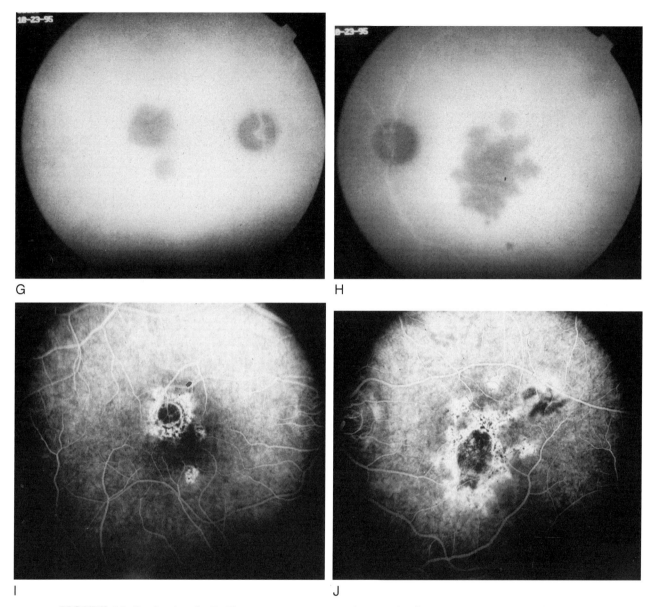

FIGURE 14–8 *Continued   D,* There is intense staining later in the fluorescein angiogram (right eye). *E,* The left eye has a similar pattern of hyperfluorescence and blocking early in the angiogram. *F,* Later in the angiogram there is intense staining (left eye). *G* and *H,* ICG demonstrates blocking in the areas of choroidopathy and lack of leakage, suggesting an absence of CNV (right eye, *G* and left eye *H*). *I* and *J,* The lesions became quiescent after systemic prednisone therapy. Five months after treatment the lesions remained stable. Fluorescein angiogram shows blocking from pigment hyperplasia, and shows window defects. *I,* Visual acuity in the right eye was 20/20. *J,* Visual acuity in the left was 20/100.

It is estimated that up to one third of patients with choroidal osteoma develop CNV.[89] Symptoms are associated with CNV and serous or hemorrhagic detachment of the macula. There has been little experience with the treatment of CNV in these tumors (Fig. 14–11).[90–93] Several treatments may be necessary to obliterate the CNV, but useful vision can be salvaged (Fig. 14–12).[94]

INFECTIOUS CHOROIDITIS

Infectious diseases have been associated with CNV. Focal choroiditis may play a role in the pathogen-esis. CNV has been reported in endocarditis with metastatic choroidal abscess[95,96] and in miliary choroidal tuberculosis.[97] Subretinal neovascularization with disciform scar formation is an uncommon but reported complication of rubella retinopathy.[98–101]

HEREDITARY DYSTROPHIES

There are several hereditary dystrophies that may be associated with CNV. Best's vitelliform dystrophy is an autosomal dominant disease that usually has its onset in children 3 to 10 years of age. Un-

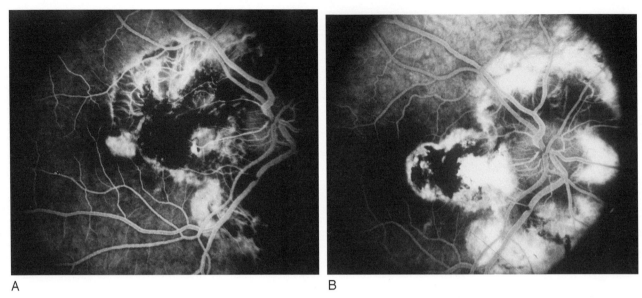

A   B

FIGURE 14–9   Serpiginous choroidopathy complicated by CNV and treated with laser. *A*, Active neovascularization is present nasal to the fovea adjacent to an area of previous inflammation and photocoagulation. Note the rim of blocked fluorescence corresponding to subretinal hemorrhage surrounding the CNV (visual acuity is 20/50). *B*, Three years after photocoagulation there is an inactive scar (visual acuity is 20/300). Recurrent CNV is common in this disorder. (From Singerman LJ, Novak MA: Subretinal neovascularization. In Yannuzzi LA [ed]: Laser photocoagulation of the retina. Philadelphia, JB Lippincott, 1989, pp 27–46, with permission.)

commonly, affected patients develop CNV and macular detachment with subsequent disciform scarring and loss of vision to 20/100 or worse.[28,102]

Fundus flavimaculatus is characterized by yellowish flecks that resemble drusen but are more irregular and, on fluorescein angiography, either do not fluoresce or fluoresce irregularly.[28] Patients with this disease generally begin losing central vision in childhood or early adulthood. CNV and disciform macular detachment occur uncommonly.[103,104]

Choroideremia is an X-linked recessive chorioretinal degenerative disease. It is characterized by progressive atrophy of the choroid and retinal pigment epithelium. Until recently, it was believed that vision was unaffected until the macula became involved late in the course of the disease. However, CNV may rarely develop in association with choroideremia.[105] Increased awareness by ophthalmologists of this complication may reveal more cases of neovascularization in choroideremia and other hereditary dystrophies, and some cases, if diagnosed early enough, may be treatable.

Patients with autosomal dominant Sorsby's fundus dystrophy are at a high risk for CNV and severe vision loss. In a retrospective study, ten eyes with well-defined extrafoveal CNV were treated with laser. All ten developed recurrent CNV and severe vision loss due to recurrent or persistent CNV occurring on the foveal side of the laser scar.[106]

IDIOPATHIC POLYPOID CHOROIDAL VASCULOPATHY

In 1985, several investigators reported a newly recognized, unusual hemorrhagic disorder of the posterior pole in middle-aged African-American women.[107] In 1990, three additional series describing similar cases were reported.[108–110] Terms used to describe these cases vary but include "idiopathic polypoid choroidal vasculopathy" and "posterior uveal bleeding syndrome." The majority of affected patients are African-American and women. Clinical findings include irregularly round serous and hemorrhagic detachments of the retinal pigment epithelium apparently derived from large vascular channels. The lesions cluster around the optic nerve, and drusen and macular RPE changes are conspicuously absent (Fig. 14–13). Digital pressure on the globe will not collapse these lesions. Vitreous hemorrhage occurs commonly and is a significant cause of visual loss. In a minority of cases, fluorescein angiography discloses CNV. In the majority, however, the lesions appear smaller angiographically and do not leak. Spontaneous regression typically leaves subretinal scarring, however. The disorder follows a remitting-relapsing course. Laser photocoagulation to the polypoidal "feeding" vessels has led to resolution. In many cases, vitrectomy is required to clear the media and recover vision.

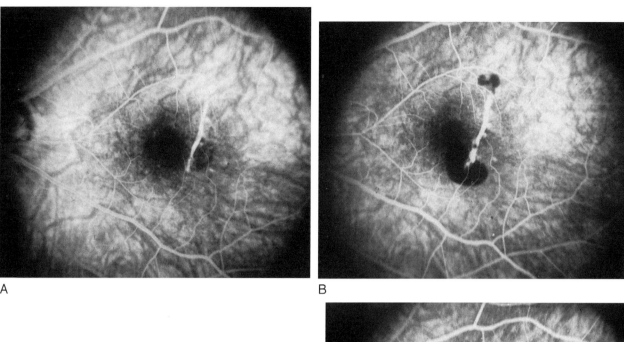

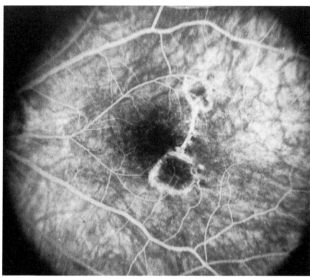

FIGURE 14–10 Choroidal rupture and CNV. *A*, Angiogram of an asymptomatic 34-year-old man (acuity 20/20) reveals crescentic hyperfluorescence temporal to the fovea corresponding to staining of inactive fibrovascular tissue. *B*, Angiogram of the same patient after acute visual loss (acuity 20/80). Examination revealed serous hemorrhagic detachment of the temporal macula. Active CNV is obscured by hemorrhage at each end of the choroidal rupture. *C*, Two months after treatment, the macular detachment and hemorrhage have resolved, and there is no active leakage. Acuity has returned to 20/25. (From Singerman LJ, Novak MA: Subretinal neovascularization. In Yannuzzi LA [ed]: Laser photocoagulation of the retina. Philadelphia, JB Lippincott, 1989, pp 27–46, with permission.)

IDIOPATHIC JUXTAFOVEAL TELANGIECTASIS

Irregular dilation and beading of the parafoveal capillary bed not associated with known predisposing conditions is termed idiopathic juxtafoveal telangiectasis. A number of subgroups have been described.[111–116] Type 1A is unilateral, most commonly affecting middle-aged men. Type 1B is unilateral as well, but occurs in older men with typically less edema and visual loss. Type 2 is bilateral and also affects women, involving small areas of the inferior temporal parafoveal capillaries. Multiple, yellow refractile opacities may be present near the inner retinal surface. Black pigment may be present in the retina temporal to the fovea. In type 3, there is bilateral cystic atrophy and foveal capillary nonperfusion.

The dilated capillaries may become incompetent, resulting in edema, exudate, and RPE changes accounting for mild to moderate visual loss. Because the disease may be self-limited, observation is probably warranted. Moderate grid laser photocoagulation for persistent or progressive visual loss can be performed in an effort to reduce macular edema.[117] CNV is uncommon but is a well-recognized cause for more severe vision loss. Subretinal exudation or hemorrhage should prompt angiography to search for CNV. The ophthalmologist should consider photocoagulaton if the CNV is outside the foveal avascular zone (FAZ) (Fig. 14–14).

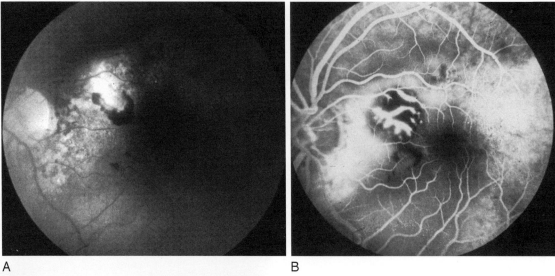

A

B

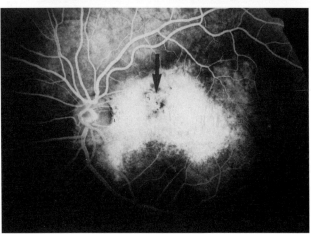

C

FIGURE 14–11   Choroidal osteoma and CNV. *A,* Angiogram from a 24-year-old woman with a choroidal osteoma. Superonasal to the fovea is a focus of intense hyperfluorescence surrounded by hemorrhage (acuity is 20/30). *B,* Two days after treatment (with blue-green laser in 1975), all new vessels have been obliterated; however, there is hyperfluorescence from thermal vasculitis. *C,* Eleven years later, a wide-angle angiogram shows further contraction and chorioretinal pucker at the treatment site (*arrow*), probably due to excessive absorption of blue wavelengths. (From Singerman LJ, Novak MA: Subretinal neovascularization. In Yannuzzi LA [ed]: Laser photocoagulation of the retina. Philadelphia, JB Lippincott, 1989, pp 27–46, with permission.)

MISCELLANEOUS DISORDERS

Probably any disease that affects the retinal pigment epithelium may eventually be associated with CNV. The list of diseases that have been reported to be associated with CNV is constantly growing.[28] These include toxocara canis,[28] ocular toxoplasmosis,[118] sarcoidosis,[28] Harada's disease,[119,120] central serous chorioretinopathy,[121] choroidal melanocytic nevus,[122] demarcation lines caused by rhegmatogenous retinal detachment,[28] chorioretinal folds,[123] photocoagulation,[124] focal treatment of diabetic maculopathy,[125] optic nerve drusen,[126] chronic papilledema,[127] and many, many more.

INDOCYANINE GREEN ANGIOGRAPHY

ICG is a tricarbocyanine dye with a peak absorbence (805 nm) and fluorescence (835 nm) in the near-infrared range. Light in the near infrared range penetrates media opacity better than shorter wavelength light.[128] The molecular weight is higher than that of fluorescein and ICG is highly protein bound. ICG tends to accumulate in the neovascular membrane and tends not to leak progressively as in fluorescein angiography.[129] These properties make ICG angiography a useful imaging technique in CNV that are not well defined by fluorescein angiography or in lesions that are obscured by hemorrhage or turbid fluid. A clinicopathologic correlation of choroidal neovascularization has demonstrated fibrovascular choroidal neovascular membrane corresponding to ICG imaging of occult CNV not well defined by fluorescein angiography.[130]

ICG angiography can add clinically useful information by identifying well-defined areas of hyperfluorescence in CNV poorly defined by fluorescein angiography, in eyes with pigment epithelial detachments, and in recurrent occult CNV.[131–133] The angiographic appearance of CNV well defined by fluorescein angiography may be variable, in some

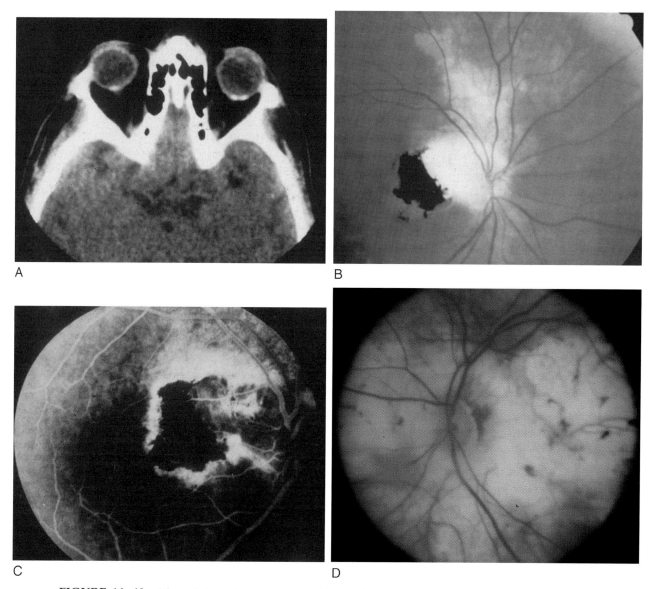

FIGURE 14–12   Bilateral choroidal osteoma in a 34-year-old man. *A*, Computed tomography of the head reveals bilateral calcification of the posterior pole. *B*, Fundus photograph from the same patient 18 years after photocoagulation in the superior papillomacular bundle. The hyperpigmentation at the temporal edge of the treated area is due to heavy blue-green absorption administered in 1974. The hypopigmentation superior to the superotemporal arcade is residual osteoma and overlying RPE change. *C*, Fluorescein angiogram of the treated area shows staining of its borders with no active leakage. Visual acuity is 20/20. *D*, Left eye of the same patient. Note the severe macular changes from a larger untreated tumor. Visual acuity is counting fingers. (From Singerman LJ, Lamkin JC, Addiego R, Zegarra H: Laser treatment of choroidal neovascularization. In Karlin DB [ed]: Lasers in Ophthalmic Surgery. Cambridge, MA, Blackwell Science, 1995, pp 112–139, with permission.)

instances showing only poorly demarcated leakage on ICG, in others showing well-demarcated leakage in areas defined as occult by fluorescein angiography.[134] ICG is also helpful to image disorders that disturb the RPE, Bruch's membrane, and choriocapillaris such as in angioid streaks.[135]

LASER TREATMENT TECHNIQUE

Fundamental aspects of the evaluation, laser treatment, and follow-up of patients with CNV have been described.[136] Prompt identification of CNV and timely treatment are essential to the optimal management of these patients. When CNV is suspected, referral to an experienced laser surgeon is preferable to obtaining a fluorescein angiogram that may take days or weeks to be developed and interpreted. Even a short delay in treatment may allow an extrafoveal lesion to progress into the fovea or require a larger treatment area, increasing scotoma size.[137,138] Optimally treatable lesions are more likely in patients who have good visual acuity, examined within a month of the onset of symptoms.[139] Patients with symptoms for several months

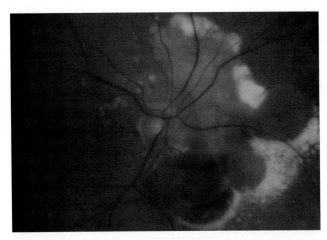

FIGURE 14–13 Idiopathic polypoidal choroidal vasculopathy. Note the several irregular and indistinct areas of serosanguinous RPE elevation with exudate at their margins. A polypoid vascular channel can be seen under the superior papillomacular bundle. (From Singerman LJ, Lamkin JC, Addiego R, Zegarra H: Laser treatment of choroidal neovascularization. In Karlin DB [ed]: Lasers in Ophthalmic Surgery. Cambridge, MA, Blackwell Science, 1995, pp 112–139, with permission.)

or a poor visual acuity on presentation have a lower probability of having an extrafoveal or juxtafoveal lesion treatable with laser, with potential for good central vision. Some subfoveal lesions may benefit from laser treatment, as recommended by the MPS foveal photocoagulation study, but not with the expectation of good central vision.

Optimal treatment is dependent on adequate patient education, recent angiography illustrating the area requiring treatment, proper laser technique, and rigorous follow-up. Once the decision to treat the CNV has been made, the patient should be informed that the goal of therapy is to reduce the risk of future vision loss, not to regain vision already lost. The high risk of recurrence and importance of daily monitoring of the Amsler grid should be emphasized. Office staff and receptionists must be trained to recognize symptoms of recurrence reported by the patient and to arrange prompt reexamination.

A recent, high quality, readily visible angiogram is used to guide precise localization and treatment of the CNV.[140] In certain cases, ICG angiography may provide information supplemental to fluorescein angiography. Because of the potential for rapid growth of the CNV, the angiogram should be less than 72 hours old. Prior to laser, retrobulbar anesthesia can be used for analgesia and akinesia, reducing the chance of inadvertent laser damage of the fovea or macula not involved by the CNV. Topical anesthetic may be adequate in cooperative patients.

Laser wavelength can be selected to improve the ease of treatment and may theoretically improve the efficacy of treatment. Commonly employed laser sources include argon green, krypton red, and dye yellow or red. Diode laser sources are less commonly used. Blue-green wavelengths should be avoided because of their greater absorbence by foveal xanthophyll (Fig. 14–15). Red sources have the advantage of greater transmission through corneal and lens opacities, turbid subretinal fluid, or hemorrhage. Less lenticular scatter and lower absorbence by hemoglobin allow more precise laser placement with red wavelengths. Yellow laser is better absorbed by hemoglobin, which may provide better absorption of laser directly in the CNV. This can be particularly useful in areas of atrophic RPE, which have poor absorption of the red wavelengths.

In the MPS subfoveal photocoagulation study, no consistent clinically or statistically significant difference between argon green or krypton red laser was found.[141] Focal retinal vascular narrowing was more common in eyes treated with green laser. In a Canadian study of extrafoveal CNV secondary to histoplasmosis, krypton red was no better than argon green.[142] The important point is for the laser surgeon to obtain an adequately intense burn to reliably destroy the CNV.

The initial stage of laser treatment involves outlining the CNV and blocked fluorescence with light, noncontiguous, 100- to 200-μm, 0.1- to 0.2-second burns placed 100 μm outside its margins (Fig. 14–16A). More intense burns are then placed contiguously on the perimeter closest to the fovea using 200-μm spots of 0.2- to 0.5-second duration (Fig. 14–16B). The power is adjusted to obtain a uniform white burn. The remainder of the perimeter is treated when appropriate burn intensity is reached (Fig. 14–16C). Finally, the internal portion of the membrane is treated with overlapping 200-μm, 0.5- to 1.0-second burns (Fig. 14–16D). Complete treatment requires dense whitening of the entire CNV plus a 100-μm margin beyond the angiographically evident lesion (except blood).

During photocoagulation, care is taken to avoid retinal vessels. Feeder vessels are treated directly, 100 μm beyond their lateral borders and 300 μm radially beyond their visible base. Thermal papillitis and nerve fiber layer defect field loss are potential complications of treatment of peripapillary CNV and large lesions nasal to the fovea.[143,144] Treatment of peripapillary lesions should spare 1.5 to 2 hours of the papillomacular bundle and not extend within 100 μm of the disc margin. Recurrent areas of CNV should have a treatment margin extending 300 μm into previously treated areas. The MPS has studied the effect of treatment of peripapillary and large lesions nasal to the fovea and found beneficial results consistent with those observed in the entire study group (nasal and nonnasal lesions).[148]

The need for accuracy in treatment of juxtafoveal CNV has recently been emphasized by an MPS report.[146] In the histoplasmosis group of CNV within 200 μm of the fovea, only 5% of eyes with adequate laser treatment covering the foveal side of the CNV had severe visual acuity loss compared to 25% of eyes with either some of the foveal side left un-

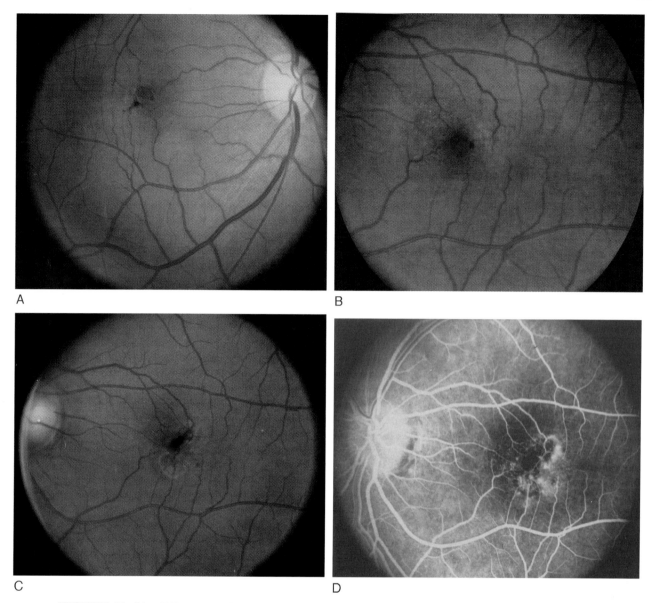

FIGURE 14–14   CNV in juxtafoveal telangiectasis. Fifty-three-year-old man with gradually progressive visual blurring in both eyes. Visual acuity is 20/50 OU. *A*, Right eye. Note the retinal vascular irregularity along with mild intraretinal edema and discoloration temporal to the fovea. There is a stellate RPE figure temporal to the fovea. *B*, Left eye. A smaller pigment figure is present temporally, along with crystalline deposits nasally. These findings are consistent with the diagnosis of juxtafoveal telangiectasis, type 2. *C*, Two years later, the visual acuity has decreased to 20/100 in the left eye. There is subretinal hemorrhage inferotemporal to the fovea, as well as a dirty gray area of retinal elevation inferior to the fovea. *D*, Fluorescein angiogram reveals an area of lacy early hyperfluorescence inferior to the fovea. Early hyperfluorescence superiorly corresponded to areas of RPE atrophy. *Illustration continued on following page*

treated or a wide border of treatment on the foveal side.

The objective of photocoagulation is to destroy the CNV while preserving as much of the fovea as possible. The MPS has established argon and krypton laser as standard methods of treatment. Sequential treatment of the CNV with red and yellow wavelengths with the dye laser offers theoretical advantages and may allow improved results (Fig. 14–17).[147] Whitening behind the CNV is accom-

plished first with red wavelength (630 to 647 nm), which penetrates the deep choroid (Fig. 14–17A). The vessels of the CNV may then be visible against the white background (Fig. 14–17B). Closure of these vessels may be enhanced by changing to yellow (577 nm), which is highly absorbed by hemoglobin (Fig. 14–17C). Although the exact mechanisms of efficacious photocoagulation are not well understood, it seems reasonable that optimal uptake of laser energy in the CNV may increase the

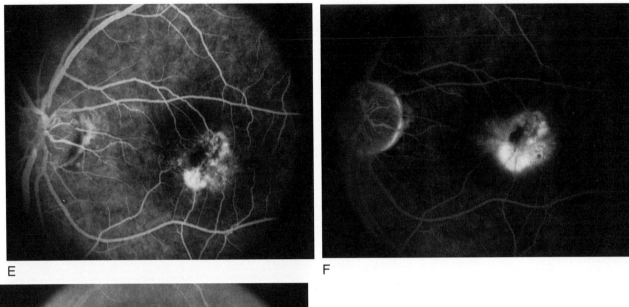

E

F

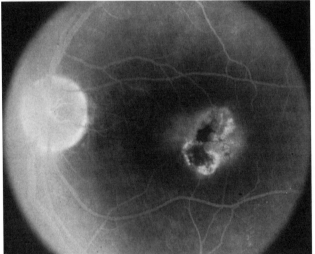

G

FIGURE 14–14 *Continued E,* The area of hyperfluorescence inferiorly has increased in intensity as dye transit continues. *F,* Late views reveal considerable leakage inferior to the fovea, consistent with CNV complicating juxtafoveal telangiectasis. The window defects superiorly have faded. *G,* Fluorescein angiogram of left macula shortly after sequential red-yellow photocoagulation for CNV. (From Singerman LJ, Addiego R, Lamkin JC, Zegarra, H: Laser treatment of less common macular diseases. In Karlin DB [ed]: Lasers in Ophthalmic Surgery. Cambridge, MA, Blackwell Science, 1995, pp 152–178, with permission.)

ability to obliterate the new vessels. Areas where the CNV is covered by hemorrhage are treated with red wavelengths. Areas of atrophic retinal pigment epithelium and visibly red membranes and feeder vessels are treated with yellow wavelength. If a dye or multiwavelength laser is not available, krypton can be used for the red wavelength and argon green substituted for the yellow dye laser.[148,149]

At the completion of the laser session, posttreatment fundus photography should be taken to document the area of treatment allowing comparison with pretreatment photographs and the appearance at follow-up visits.[150] It is very useful to immediately compare posttreatment red-free photographs, developed while the patient is still at the clinic, to allow retreatment of missed areas before he or she leaves.[151] If retrobulbar anesthesia was used, the eye is patched. The patient is reinstructed in the importance of daily monitoring of the Amsler grid and prompt re-examination if change in vision occurs (Fig. 14–18).

Exacting follow-up is required to promptly de-

tect and treat persistent or recurrent neovascularization. Fluorescein angiography is routinely repeated during the first several visits. The laser surgeon refers to the projected angiogram while examining the fundus with contact lens biomicroscopy. Fluorescein angiography of an adequately treated CNV should show an evenly hyperfluorescent rim of staining adjacent to the area of treatment. Areas of persistence will appear as a focal leak, usually at the margin of the treated area. Central leakage of a treatment scar that has a broad rim of surrounding hypofluorescence usually does not signify persistence and tends to resolve spontaneously. Retreatment is avoided unless enlargement of the hyperfluorescent area is seen on follow-up angiography.

At 1 to 2 weeks after treatment, residual edema and retinal vasculitis may prevent visualization of persistent CNV. During this period, only a positive angiogram is helpful to inform decisions regarding the possible need for additional treatment. A follow-up angiogram must be obtained by 1 month

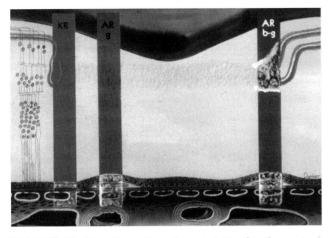

FIGURE 14–15 Absorption characteristics for the various laser modalities commonly used in the treatment of CNV must be kept in mind. Argon blue-green was the laser used in the early MPS studies but is rarely used for macular treatment due to absorption by foveal xanthophyll. Argon green and dye yellow are minimally absorbed by xanthophyll and are more commonly used for these treatments. Krypton or dye red sources penetrate media opacities and blood far more effectively than argon green. (From Singerman LJ: Important points in the management of patients with choroidal neovascularization. Ophthalmology 92:610–614, 1985. Courtesy of Ophthalmology, with permission.)

following treatment even if one has been obtained 1 to 2 weeks following treatment. An acceptable follow-up schedule between laser treatment and follow-up visits might be as follows:[1]

> 1 to 2 weeks (optional)
> 3 to 4 weeks (mandatory)
> 2 months
> 4 months
> 6 to 7 months
> 9 to 12 months
> Every 4 to 6 months in the second post-treatment year
> Every 6 to 12 months indefinitely

Follow-up is continued indefinitely because recurrence has been known to occur years after treatment. Any sign of recurrence should be evaluated with prompt angiography and treated unless the extent of treatment would exceed that suggested by the MPS protocol. In cases that do not meet MPS criteria, treatment must be considered on an individual basis. Visual acuity generally remains stable within 6 months of successful treatment. Late loss of acuity should prompt an evaluation to rule out recurrence but may be secondary to gradual en-

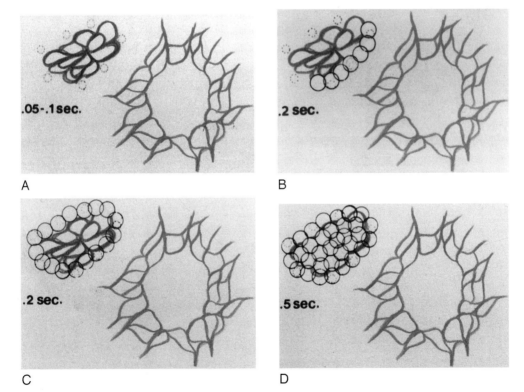

FIGURE 14–16 Laser treatment technique for extrafoveal and juxtafoveal CNV. *A*, The perimeter of the lesion is first lightly marked with noncontiguous 100-μm burns, 100 to 150 μm beyond its angiographically evident border. *B*, Next, the foveal side of the lesion's perimeter is covered with contiguous 200-μm burns. *C*, Next, the remainder of the lesion's perimeter is similarly treated. *D*, Finally, the center of the membrane is covered with 200- to 500-μm burns of longer duration (0.5 to 1.0 second). (From Singerman LJ: Important points in the management of patients with choroidal neovascularization. Ophthalmology 92:610–614, 1985. Courtesy of Ophthalmology, with permission.)

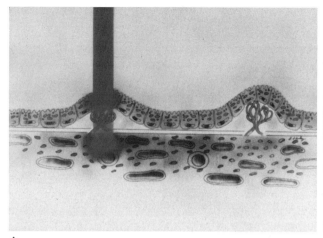

A

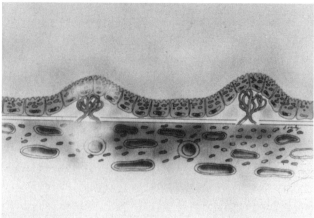

B

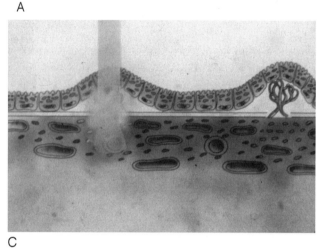

C

FIGURE 14–17   Sequential red-yellow treatment of CNV. *A,* Red wavelengths (dye or krypton) are used to treat the membrane deeply, lightly whitening its background and highlighting its extent. *B,* Appearance at the conclusion of red treatment. The entire extent of the membrane has been lightly whitened due to choroidal, RPE, and, possibly, outer retinal uptake. *C,* Intense yellow wavelength is then used to blanket the previously treated area. Enhanced uptake of yellow light by the new blood vessels may be helpful for effective treatment. (From Singerman LJ, Kalski RS: Tunable dye laser for choroidal neovascularization complicating age-related macular degeneration. Retina 9: 247–257, 1989, with permission.)

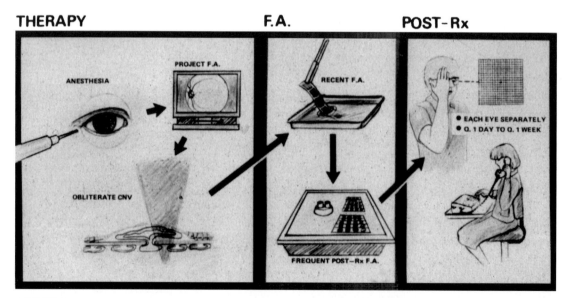

FIGURE 14–18   Critical points in the management of CNV include recent high-quality angiography magnified and projected in the treatment room, retrobulbar anesthesia for some juxtafoveal and subfoveal lesions, depending on patient cooperation as well as CNV location, and close posttreatment surveillance for recurrence including prompt examination if the patient notes new symptoms. (From Singerman LJ: Important points in the management of patients with choroidal neovascularization. Ophthalmology 92:610–614, 1985. Courtesy of Ophthalmology, with permission.)

largement of atrophy related to the area of treatment.[152,153]

Complications of laser treatment are uncommon. The most serious complication is inadvertent foveal treatment. Projection of a recent high-quality magnified angiogram is essential to reduce the risk of this complication. Retrobulbar anesthesia may also be helpful. The risk of choroidal hemorrhage can be reduced by employing durations 0.2 second or longer and by avoiding spot sizes smaller than 200 μm. Thermal vasculitis (Fig. 14–11B) and macular pucker (Fig. 14–11C) more commonly occur after blue-green laser treatment. Now that blue-green wavelengths are avoided, macular pucker is less frequent and tends not to be visually significant.

SUBFOVEAL SURGERY

Recent series of subfoveal surgery have suggested that CNV associated with focal conditions such as ocular histoplasmosis, idiopathic cause, multifocal choroiditis, punctate inner choroidopathy, and traumatic choroidal rupture may be responsive to subretinal surgery. In addition, pathologic myopia CNV may be a diffuse disorder treatable with this approach, although this surgery may be more difficult in high myopes. In many cases, patients tend to be younger than patients with AMD and may be more likely to have CNV in the subretinal space (type II CNV). Visual outcomes tend to be better than those seen in surgery for CNV in AMD. Candidates for subretinal surgery tend to have subfoveal lesions not eligible for photocoagulation according to MPS guidelines, significant thick subretinal hemorrhage, or characteristics preventing extrapolation of the MPS results. The natural history of the disorder must be considered.

Refinements in the surgical techniques have reduced the incidence of complications and simplified the procedure. A standard three-port vitrectomy is employed.[37] The posterior hyaloid is removed in most cases. A small retinotomy is made with a 36-gauge bent sharp spatula. Retinal vessels are avoided. A 33-gauge cannula is then used to inject balanced salt solution into the subretinal space to develop a working space around the CNV. Tissue plasminogen activator (t-PA) has recently been found to be useful in the evacuation of submacular hemorrhage.[154] Intraocular pressure is transiently elevated and subretinal forceps are used to grasp the CNV.

The retinotomy site is elastic and will allow a surprisingly large complex to be extracted. Care must be taken to ensure that all recognizable CNV is removed. Fragmentation and incomplete initial removal of the CNV is not uncommon. Several minutes after completing the extraction of the CNV, the intraocular pressure is normalized. Laser to the retinotomy site is avoided in uncomplicated cases. Partial fluid-air exchange is performed and the eye

is left with an air tamponade in uncomplicated cases.

Intraoperative complications include retinal holes near the macula. These tend to be more common in patients with extensive prior photocoagulation and in AMD. Choroidal hemorrhage is not uncommon but is usually controlled by transiently elevated intraocular pressure. The usual risks of vitrectomy surgery such as retinal breaks, retinal detachment, endophthalmitis, and cataract apply to these patients. The most common postoperative complication, as in laser surgery, is recurrence, which occurs in approximately 30 to 50% of cases.[36,37] Final visual outcomes are limited by recurrences, loss of photoreceptors and subfoveal RPE, and damage to the choriocapillaris.

INVESTIGATIONAL THERAPIES

A number of new therapies are being investigated in an effort to improve outcomes and to offer treatment to patients with CNV not eligible for photocoagulation or surgery. Pharmacologic approaches to the treatment of CNV are currently under investigation. The results of the Interferon Study have not yet been reported. A multi-center prospective randomized trial of interferon alfa-2a and a smaller uncontrolled trial of interferon alfa-2a for AMD did not find the therapy effective.[155,156] We are participating in the age-related macular degeneration and thalidomide study (AMDATS), which is a masked, randomized placebo controlled trial. Patients with small, well-demarcated subfoveal lesions and good vision are randomized to treatment or placebo. A recurrence prevention group randomizes patients with CNV to laser or thalidomide or laser and placebo.

Ionizing radiation may prevent endothelial cell proliferation in newly forming vessels in choroidal neovascular membranes. A number of small studies have investigated radiation therapy in AMD.[157,158] Treated eyes appear to have less progression. Results are preliminary and a prospective randomized trial would be helpful to determine the efficacy of this approach.

Photodynamic therapy offers the hope of improving the selectivity and effectiveness of laser therapy by using photochemically active dyes to produce localized tissue damage. Experimental generators of singlet oxygen[159] and lipoprotein-delivered benzoporphyrin[160] have the ability to selectively close choroidal new vessels and may be a promising, selective therapy for CNV. The treatment of AMD with photodynamic therapy (TAP) study is a randomized, controlled clinical trial in which we are participating. Patients with subfoveal lesions and moderate vision loss may be considered for possible eligibility.[161]

Techniques for subretinal surgery are improving, but damage to the RPE appears to be a limiting factor in visual recovery. Transplantation of RPE cells may allow improved function by repopulating the areas affected by RPE atrophy or damage. This technology remains in its early stages but has been applied to a limited group of patients.[162] Further evaluation will be required before this technique can be considered for wider application.

The Submacular Surgery Trial (SST) is a pilot randomized controlled clinical trial chaired by Neil Bressler in which we are participating. AMD is being studied in groups 1A to 3. OHS and idiopathic membranes are being studied in group 4. All groups have subfoveal involvement.

Eligibility criteria include the following: Lesions with evidence of classic CNV reducing vision to the 20/100 to 20/800 range are included in groups 1A, 1B, and 2. Patients assigned to group 1A and group 1B have not had prior laser treatment and have lesions with less than 50% of the affected area involved by hemorrhage. In group 1A, new subfoveal lesions with well-demarcated boundaries and moderate size (>2.0 to 3.5 disc areas) are randomized to surgery or laser. Group 1B includes poorly demarcated lesions, or well-demarcated CNV larger than allowed in group 1A. In group 1B, new subfoveal lesions with evidence of classic CNV but poorly demarcated boundaries, less than or equal to 9.0 disc areas in size, are randomized to surgery or observation. Well-demarcated lesions with evidence of classic CNV larger than those included in group 1A (>3.5 to 9.0 disc areas) are also included in group 1B and randomized to surgery or observation.

Recurrent lesions with prior laser treatment, evidence of classic CNV, less than or equal to 9.0 disc areas are eligible for group 2 and are randomized to surgery or laser. New or recurrent larger lesions (CNV ≤ 9.0 disc areas) with greater than 50% hemorrhage, CNV plus hemorrhage area greater than 3.5 disc areas, with greater than or equal to 75% of the hemorrhage in the posterior pole, are eligible for group 3 and are randomized to surgery or observation. Visual acuities may range from 20/100 to light perception (LP).

Patients with OHS or idiopathic CNV are included in group 4 and, if eligible, are randomized to surgery or observation. Lesions may be new or recurrent. Scars in OHS with an associated sensory detachment may also be eligible. The lesion must be less than or equal to 9.0 disc areas in size. Visual acuity must be in the range of 20/50 to 20/800.

No results are available from this trial to date. Thus far, the investigators have successfully recruited approximately 250 patients.[163] Plans are in progress to pursue National Institutes of Health (NIH) funding of the full-fledged clinical trial with the pilot study demonstrating the feasibility, it is hoped, in convincing fashion.

CONCLUSION

Even with the significant advances in subfoveal surgery, laser treatment probably is our best tool currently for treating CNV. Ultimately, prevention of CNV will be the best approach. Randomized clinical trials of laser treatment have been possible for common diseases associated with CNV, and the basis of modern laser therapy has been derived from these important studies. For less common diseases, such as angioid streaks, randomized trials would require many years and clinical centers to enroll sufficient patients to render a significant result. The rarity of some disorders precludes the development of such trials. In an effort to manage less common disorders associated with CNV we are compelled to extrapolate from the proven benefit described for more common diseases. Each of these has its own unique clinical setting. Technical advances in surgical management make subretinal surgery a therapeutic consideration in selected cases. A prospective pilot trial is underway that will expand our understanding of this modality in subfoveal AMD and ocular histoplasmosis. Advances in nonsurgical therapies raise hopes of improved outcomes.

Many factors need to be considered, including the patient's age, visual needs, coexistent vision-limiting ocular conditions, and adverse effects of treatment. Each disorder has its own pattern of these factors that must be considered to manage optimally patients with CNV.

REFERENCES

1. Singerman LJ, Lamkin JC, Addiego R, Zegarra H: Laser treatment of choroidal neovascularization. In Karlin DB (ed): Lasers in Opthalmic Surgery. Cambridge, MA, Blackwell Science, 1995, pp 112–139.
2. Green WR: Retina. In Spencer WH (ed): Ophthalmic Pathology. An Atlas and Textbook. Philadelphia, WB Saunders Co, 1985.
3. Gass JDM: Biomicroscopic and histopathologic considerations regarding the feasibility of surgical excision of subfoveal neovascular membranes. Trans Am Ophthalmol Soc 92:91–111, 1994.
4. Gass JDM: Biomicroscopic and histopathologic considerations regarding the feasibility of surgical excision of subfoveal neovascular membranes. Am J Ophthalmol 118:285–298, 1994.
5. Macular Photocoagulation Study Group: Argon laser photocoagulation for senile macular degeneration. Results of a randomized clinical trial. Arch Ophthalmol 100:912–918, 1983.
6. Macular Photocoagulation Study Group: Argon laser for ocular histoplasmosis. Results of a randomized clinical trial. Arch Ophthalmol 101:1347–1357, 1983.
7. Macular Photocoagulation Study Group: Argon laser for idiopathic neovascularization. Results of a randomized trial. Arch Ophthalmol 101:1358–1361, 1983.
8. Macular Photocoagulation Study Group: Krypton laser photocoagulation for neovascular lesions of ocular histoplasmosis. Results of a clinical trial. Arch Ophthalmol 105:1499–1507, 1987.
9. Macular Photocoagulation Study Group: Laser photocoagulation of subfoveal neovascular lesions in age-related macular degeneration. Results of a randomized clinical trial. Arch Ophthalmol 109:1220–1231, 1991.
10. Macular Photocoagulation Study Group: Subfoveal neovascular lesions in age-related macular degeneration. Guidelines for evaluation and treatment in the Macular

Photocoagulation Study. Arch Ophthalmol 109:1242–1257, 1991.

11. Macular Photocoagulation Study Group: Laser photocoagulation of subfoveal recurrent neovascular lesions in age-related macular degeneration. Results of a randomized clinical trial. Arch Ophthalmol 109:1232–1241, 1991.

12. Fine SL, Wood WJ, Isernhagen RD, et al: Laser treatment for subfoveal neovascular membranes in ocular histoplasmosis syndrome—results of a pilot randomized clinical trial. Arch Ophthalmol 111:19–20, 1993.

13. Thomas MA, Kaplan H: Surgical removal of subfoveal neovascularization in the presumed ocular histoplasmosis syndrome. Am J Ophthalmol 111:1–7, 1991.

14. Thomas MA, Grand G, Williams DF, et al: Surgical management of subfoveal choroidal neovascularization. Ophthalmology 99:952–968, 1992.

15. Edwards LB, Acquaviva FA, Livesay VT, et al: An atlas of sensitivity to tuberculin, PPD-B, and histoplasmin in the United States. Am Rev Respir Dis 99(4 pt 2):1–32, 1969.

16. Asbury T: The status of presumed ocular histoplasmosis: including a report of a survey. Trans Am Ophthalmol Soc 64:371–400, 1966.

17. Ganley JP: Epidemiologic characteristics of presumed ocular histoplasmosis. Acta Ophthalmol Suppl (Copenh) 119:1–63, 1973.

18. Schlaegel TF, Weber JC, Helveston E, Kenney D: Presumed histoplasmic choroiditis. Am J Ophthalmol 63(5 pt 1):919–925, 1967.

19. Krause AC, Hopkins WG: Ocular manifestations of histoplasmosis. Am J Ophthalmol 39:564–566, 1951.

20. McCulloch C: Histoplasmosis. Trans Can Ophthalmol Soc 26:107–125, 1963.

21. Woods AC, Wahlen HE: The probable role of benign histoplasmosis in the etiology of granulomatous uveitis. Trans Am Ophthalmol Soc 57:318–343, 1959.

22. Goodwin RA, Shapiro JL, Thurman GH, et al: Disseminated histoplasmosis: Clinical and pathologic correlations. Medicine (Baltimore) 59:1–33, 1980.

23. Loosli CG, Grayston JT, Alexander ER, Tanzi F: Epidemiological studies of pulmonary histoplasmosis in a farm family. Am J Hyg 55:392–401, 1952.

24. Wilcox KR, Waisbren BA, Martin J: The Walworth, Wisconsin, epidemic of histoplasmosis. Ann Intern Med 49:388–418, 1958.

25. Sorely DL, Levin ML, Warren JW, et al: Bat-associated histoplasmosis in Maryland bridge workers. Am J Med 67:623–626, 1979.

26. Johnson JE, Kabler JD, Gourley MF, et al: Cave associated histoplasmosis—Costa Rica. MMWR 37:312–313, 1988.

27. Woods AC, Wahlen HE: The probable role of benign histoplasmosis in the etiology of granulomatous uveitis. Trans Ophthalmol Soc 57:318–343, 1959.

28. Gass JDM: Stereoscopic Atlas of Macular Diseases. St. Louis, CV Mosby Co, 1987.

29. Bynoe LA, Chang TS, Funata M, et al: Histopathologic examination of vascular patterns in subfoveal neovascular membranes. Ophthalmology 101:1112–1117, 1994.

30. Schlaegel TF: Histoplasmic choroiditis. Ann Ophthalmol 6:237–252, 1974.

31. Singerman LG, Wong B, Ai E, Smith S: Spontaneous improvement in the first affected eye of patients with bilateral disciform scars. Retina 5:135–143, 1985.

32. Orlando RG, Davidorf FH: Spontaneous recovery phenomenon in the presumed ocular histoplasmosis syndrome. Int Ophthalmol Clin 23:137–149, 1983.

33. Macular Photocoagulation Study Group: Argon laser photocoagulation for neovascular maculopathy: three year results from randomized clinical trials. Arch Ophthalmol 104:694–701, 1986.

34. Kleiner RC, Ratner CM, Enger C, Fine SL: Subfoveal neovascularization in the ocular histoplasmosis syndrome: a natural history study. Retina 8:225, 1988.

35. Olk RJ, Burgess DB, McCormick PA: Subfoveal and juxtafoveal subretinal neovascularization in the presumed

36. Thomas MA, Grand MA, Williams DF, et al: Surgical management of subfoveal choroidal neovascularization. Ophthalmology 99:952–968, 1992.

37. Thomas MA, Dickinson JD, Melberg NS, et al: Visual results after surgical removal of subfoveal choroidal neovascular membranes. Ophthalmology 101:1384–1396, 1994.

38. Ho AC, Yannuzzi LA, Pisicano K, DeRosa J: The natural history of idiopathic subfoveal choroidal neovascularization. Ophthalmology 102:782–789, 1995.

39. Adelberg DA, Del Priore LV, Kaplan HJ: Surgery for subfoveal membranes in myopia, angioid streaks, and other disorders. Retina 15:198–205, 1995.

40. Hotchkiss ML, Fine SL: Pathologic myopia and choroidal neovascularization. Am J Ophthalmol 91:177–183, 1981.

41. Fried M, Siebert A, Meyer-Schwickerath G, Wessing A: Natural history of Fuch's spot: a long-term follow-up study. Doc Ophthalmol Proc Ser 28:215–221, 1981.

42. Gass JDM: Pathogenesis of disciform detachment of the neuroepithelium. VI. Disciform detachment secondary to heredodegenerative, neoplastic and traumatic lesions of the choroid. Am J Ophthalmol 63:689–711, 1967.

43. Hayasaka S, Uchida M, Setogawa T: Subretinal hemorrhages with or without choroidal neovascularization in the maculas of patients with pathologic myopia. Graefes Arch Clin Exp Ophthalmol 228:277–280, 1990.

44. Hampton GR, Kohen D, Bird AC: Visual prognosis of disciform degeneration in myopia. Ophthalmology 90:923–926, 1983.

45. Soubrane G, Pison J, Bornert P, et al: Neovaisseaux sous-retiniens de la myopie degenerative: resultats de la photocoagulation. Bull Soc Ophtalmol Fr 86:269–272, 1986.

46. Soubrane G, Pisan J: Myopie degenerative: resultats de la photocoagulation des neovaisseaux sous-Retiniens. In Coscas G, Sourane G (eds): Neovaisseaux Sous-retiniens Maculaires et Laser. Paris, Doin Editeurs, 1987, pp 180–184.

47. Brancato R, Menchini U, Pece A, et al: Dye laser photocoagulation of macular subretinal neovascularisation in pathological myopia. Int Ophthalmol 11:235–238, 1988.

48. Brancato R, Pece A, Avanza P, Radrizzani E: Photocoagulation scar expansion after laser therapy for choroidal neovascularization in degenerative myopia. Retina 10:239–243, 1990.

49. Gass JDM, Clarkson JG: Angioid streaks and disciform macular detachment in Paget's disease (osteitis deformans). Am J Ophthalmol 75:576–586, 1983.

50. Green WR, Friedman-Kien A, Banfield WG: Angioid streaks in Ehlers-Danlos syndrome. Arch Ophthalmol 76:197, 1976.

51. Singerman LJ: Angioid streaks in thalassemia major (Letter). Br J Ophthalmol 67:558, 1983.

52. Singerman LJ, Hatem G: Laser treatment of choroidal neovascular membranes in angioid streaks. Retina 1:75–83, 1981.

53. Clarkson JG, Altman RD: Angioid streaks. Surv Ophthalmol 26:235–246, 1982.

54. Lebwohl M, Phelps RG, Yannuzzi L, et al: Diagnosis of pseudoxanthoma elasticum by scar biopsy in patients without characteristic skin lesions. N Engl J Med 317:347–350, 1987.

55. Singerman LJ, Rice TA, Novak MA, Passoff RW: Red krypton and/or green and/or blue-green argon laser photocoagulation in treatment of angioid streaks. Invest Ophthalmol Vis Sci 25(Suppl):89, 1984.

56. Singerman LJ: Stries angioides: traitment par le laser a argon et le laser a krypton. In Coscas G, Soubrane GG (eds): Neovaisseaux Sous-Retiniens Maculaires et Laser. Paris, Doin Editeurs, 1987, pp 221–223.

57. Gelisken O, Hendrikse F, Deutman AF: A long-term follow-up study of laser coagulation of neovascular membrane in angioid streaks. Am J Ophthalmol 105:299–303, 1988.

58. Nozik RA, Dorsch W: A new chorioretinopathy associated with anterior uveitis. Am J Ophthalmol 76:758–762, 1973.

59. Dreyer RF, Gass JDM: Multifocal choroiditis and panuveitis: a syndrome that mimics ocular histoplasmosis. Arch Ophthalmol 102:1776–1784, 1984.

60. Watzke RC, Packer AJ, Folk JC, et al: Punctate inner choroidopathy. Am J Ophthalmol 98:572–584, 1984.

61. Palestine AG, Nussenblatt RB, Parver LM, Knox DL: Progressive subretinal fibrosis and uveitis syndrome. Br J Ophthalmol 68:667–673, 1984.

62. Palestine AG, Nussenblatt RB, Hooks JJ, et al: Histopathology of the subretinal fibrosis and uveitis syndrome. Ophthalmology 92:838–844, 1985.

63. Cantrill HL, Folk JC: Multifocal choroiditis associated with progressive subretinal fibrosis. Am J Ophthalmol 101:170–180, 1986.

64. Doran RML, Hamilton AM: Disciform macular degeneration in young adults. Trans Ophthalmol Soc UK 102:471–480, 1982.

65. Morgan CM, Schatz H: Recurrent multifocal choroiditis. Ophthalmology 93:1138–1143, 1986.

66. Yannuzzi LA, Sorenson J, Shakin J, Malch F: Acute disseminated chorioretinal spots: the New York experience. Presented at the Eighth Annual Meeting of the Macula Society, 1985.

67. Singerman LJ: In discussion, Morgan CM, Schatz H: Recurrent multifocal choroiditis. Ophthalmology 93:1143–1147, 1986.

68. Callanan D, Gass JDM: Multifocal choroiditis and choroidal neovascularization associated with the multiple evanescent white dot and acute idiopathic blind spot enlargement syndrome. Ophthalmology 99:1678–1685, 1992.

69. Coscas G, Soubrane G, Delayre T, Ramahefasolo C: Treatment of subretinal neovessels in idiopathic recurrent multifocal choroiditis. Bull Soc Ophtalmol Fr 89:1275–1279, 1989.

70. Laatikainen L, Erkkila H: A follow-up study on serpiginous choroiditis. Acta Ophthalmol (Copenh) 59:707–718, 1981.

71. Mansour AM, Jampol LM, Packo KH, Hrisomalos NF: Macular serpiginous choroiditis. Retina 8:125–131, 1988.

72. Hardy RA, Schatz H: Macular geographic helicoid choroidopathy. Arch Ophthalmol 105:1237–1242, 1987.

73. Masi RJ, O'Connor GR, Kimura SJ: Anterior uveitis in geographic or serpiginous choroiditis. Am J Ophthalmol 86:228–232, 1978.

74. Chisholm IH, Gass JDM, Hutton WL: The late stage of serpiginous (geographic) choroiditis. Am J Ophthalmol 82:343–351, 1976.

75. Friberg TR: Serpiginous choroiditis with branch vein occlusion and bilateral periphlebitis. Arch Ophthalmol 106:585–586, 1988.

76. Wojno T, Meredith TA: Unusual findings in serpiginous choroiditis. Am J Ophthalmol 94:650–655, 1982.

77. Wu JS, Lewis H, Fine SL, et al: Clinicopathologic findings in a patient with serpiginous choroiditis and treated choroidal neovascularization. Retina 9:292–301, 1989.

78. Jampol LM, Orth D, Daily MJ, Rabb MF: Subretinal neovascularization with geographic (serpiginous) choroiditis. Am J Ophthalmol 88:683–689, 1979.

79. Schatz H, Maumenee AE, Patz A: Geographic helicoid peripapillary choroidopathy: clinical presentation and fluorescein angiographic findings. Trans Am Acad Ophthalmol Otolaryngol 78:747–761, 1974.

80. Hooper PL, Kaplan HJ: Triple agent immunosuppression in serpiginous choroiditis. Ophthalmology 98:944–951, 1991.

81. Eagling EM: Ocular damage after blunt trauma to the eye. Br J Ophthalmol 58:126–140, 1974.

82. Fuller B, Gitter KA: Traumatic choroidal rupture with late serous detachment of the macula: report of successful argon laser treatment. Arch Ophthalmol 89:354–355, 1973.

83. Smith RE, Kelley JS: Late macular complications of choroidal ruptures. Am J Ophthalmol 77:650–658, 1974.

84. Hart JCD, Natsikos VE, Riastrick ER, Doran RML: Indirect choroidal tears at the posterior pole: a fluorescein angiographic and perimetric approach. Br J Ophthalmol 64:59–67, 1980.

85. Gass JDM, Guerry RK, Jack RL, Harris G: Choroidal osteoma. Arch Ophthalmol 96:428–435, 1978.

86. Grand MG, Burgess DB, Singerman LJ, Ransey J: Choroidal osteoma: treatment of associated subretinal neovascular membranes. Retina 4:84–89, 1984.

87. Shields CL, Shields JA, Augsburger JJ: Choroidal osteoma. Surv Ophthalmol 33:17–27, 1988.

88. Teich SA, Walsh JB: Choroidal osteoma. Ophthalmology 88:696–698, 1981.

89. Gass JDM: New observations concerning choroidal osteomas. Int Ophthalmol 1:71–84, 1979.

90. Burke JF, Brockhurst RJ: Argon laser photocoagulation of subretinal neovascular membrane associated with osteoma of the choroid. Retina 3:304–307, 1983.

91. Avila MP, El-Markabi H, Azzolini C, et al: Bilateral choroidal osteoma with subretinal neovascularization. Ann Ophthalmol 16:381–385, 1984.

92. Morrison DL, Magargal LE, Ehrlich DR, et al: Review of choroidal osteoma: successful krypton red laser photocoagulation of an associated subretinal neovascular membrane in involving the fovea. Ophthalmic Surg 18:299–303, 1987.

93. Rose SJ, Burke JF, Brockhurst RJ: Argon laser photoablation of a choroidal osteoma. Retina 11:224–228, 1991.

94. Grand MG, Burgess DB, Singerman LJ, Ramsey J: Choroidal osteoma. Treatment of associated subretinal neovascular membranes. Retina 4:84–89, 1984.

95. Munier F, Othenin-Girard P: Subretinal neovascularization secondary to choroidal septic metastasis from acute bacterial endocarditis. Retina 12:108–112, 1992.

96. Coll GE, Lewis H: Metastatic choroidal abscess and choroidal neovascular membrane associated with *Staphylococcus aureus* endocarditis in a heroin user. Retina 14:256–259, 1994.

97. Chung YM Yeh TS, Sheu SJ, Liu JH: Macular subretinal neovascularization in choroidal tuberculosis. Ann Ophthalmol 21:225–229, 1989.

98. Deutman AF, Grizzard WS: Rubella retinopathy and subretinal neovascularization. Am J Ophthalmol 85:82–87, 1987.

99. Slusher MM, Tyler ME: Rubella retinopathy and subretinal neovascularization. Ann Ophthalmol 14:292–294, 1982.

100. Orth DH, Fishman GA, Segall M, et al: Rubella maculopathy. Br J Ophthalmol 64:201–205, 1980.

101. Franke KE, Purnell EW: Subretinal neovascularization following rubella retinopathy. Am J Ophthalmol 86:462–466, 1978.

102. Miller SA, Bresnick GH, Chandra SR: Choroidal neovascular membrane in Best's vitelliform macular dystrophy. Am J Ophthalmol 82:252, 1976.

103. Klein R, Lewis RA, Meyers SM, Myers FL: Subretinal neovascularization associated with fundus flavimaculatus. Arch Ophthalmol 96:2054, 1978.

104. Leveille AS, Morse PH, Burch JV: Fundus flavimaculatus and subretinal neovascularization. Ann Ophthalmol 14:331, 1982.

105. Robinson D, Tiedeman J: Choroideremia associated with a subretinal neovascular membrane: a case report. Retina 7:70–74, 1987.

106. Holz FG, Haimovici R, Wagner DG, Bird AC: Recurrent choroidal neovasularization after laser photocoagulation in Sorsby's fundus dystrophy. Retina 14:329–334, 1994.

107. Stern RM, Zakov ZN, Zegarra HZ, Gutman FA: Multiple recurrent serosanguinous retinal pigment epithelial detachments in black women. Am J Ophthalmol 100:560–569, 1985.

108. Yannuzzi LA, Sorenson J, Spaide RF, Lipson B: Idiopathic polypoidal choroidal vasculopathy (IPCV). Retina 10:1–8, 1990.

109. Kleiner RC, Brucker AJ, Johnston RL: The posterior uveal bleeding syndrome. Retina 10:9–17, 1990.

110. Perkovich BT, Zakov ZN, Berlin LA, et al: An update on mutiple recurrent serosanguinous retinal pigment epithelial detachments in black women. Retina 10:18–26, 1990.
111. Chopdar S: Retinal telangiectasis in adults: fluorescein angiographic findings and treatment by argon laser. Br J Ophthalmol 62:243–250, 1978.
112. Hutton WL, Snyder WB, Fuller D, Vaiser A: Focal parafoveal retinal telangiectasis. Arch Ophthalmol 96:1362–1367, 1978.
113. Gass JDM: Idiopathic juxtafoveal telangiectasia. Arch Ophthalmol 100:769–780, 1982.
114. Millay RH, Klein ML, Handelman IL, Watzke RC: Abnormal glucose metabolism and parafoveal telangiectasia. Am J Ophthalmol 102:363–370, 1986.
115. Chew EY, Murphy RP, Newsome DA, Fine SL: Parafoveal telangiectasis and diabetic retinopathy. Arch Ophthalmol 104:71–75, 1986.
116. Casswell AG, Chaine G, Rush P, Bird AC: Paramacular telangiectasis. Trans Ophthalmol Soc UK 105:683–692, 1986.
117. Singerman LJ, Addiego R, Lamkin JC, Zegarra H: Laser treatment of less common macular diseases. In Karlin DB (ed): Lasers in Ophthalmic Surgery. Cambridge, MA, Blackwell Science, 1995, pp 152–178.
118. Gilbert HD: Unusual complications of ocular toxoplasmosis. In Fine SL, Owens SL (eds): Management of Retinal Vascular and Macular Disorders. Baltimore, Williams & Wilkins, 1983, pp 153–155.
119. Carlson MR, Kerman BM: Hemorrhagic macular detachment in Vogt-Koyanagi-Harada syndrome. Am J Ophthalmol 84:632, 1977.
120. Snyder DA, Tessler HH: Vogt-Koyanagi-Harada syndrome. Am J Ophthalmol 90:69–75, 1980.
121. Gomolin JE: Choroidal neovascularization and central serous chorioretinopathy. Can J Ophthalmol 24:20–23, 1989.
122. Waltmann DD, Gitter KA, Yannuzzi LA, Schatz H: Choroidal neovascularization associated with choroidal nevi. Am J Ophthalmol 85:704–710, 1978.
123. Friberg TR, Grove AS Jr: Subfoveal neovascularization of choroidal folds. Ann Ophthalmol 12:245–250, 1980.
124. Benson WE, Townsend RE, Pheasant TR: Choriovitreal and subretinal proliferation: Complications of photocoagulation. Ophthalmology. 86:283–289, 1979.
125. Varley M, Frank E, Purnell EW: Subretinal neovascularization after focal argon laser for macular edema. Ophthalmology 95:567–573, 1988.
126. Harris MJ, Fine SL, Owens SL: Hemorrhagic complications of optic nerve drusen. Am J Ophthalmol 92:70–76, 1981.
127. Jaimison RR: Subretinal neovascularization and papilledema associated with pseudotumor cerebri. Am J Ophthalmol 85:78–81, 1978.
128. Geeraets WJ, Berry ER: Ocular and spectral characteristics as related to hazards from laser and other sources. Am J Ophthalmol 66:15–20, 1968.
129. Bischoff PM, Flower RW: Ten years' experience with choroidal angiography using indocyanine green dye: a new routine examination or an epilogue? Doc Ophthalmol 60:235–291, 1985.
130. Chang TS, Freund KB, de la Cruz Z, et al: Clinicopathologic correlation of choroidal neovascularization demonstrated by indocyanine green angiography in a patient with retention of good visual acuity for almost four years. Retina, 14:114–124, 1994.
131. Lim JI, Sternberg P Jr, Capone A, et al: Selective use of indocyanine green angiography for occult choroidal neovascularization. Am J Ophthalmol 120:75–82, 1995.
132. Guyer DR, Yannuzzi LA, Slakter JS, et al: Digital indocyanine green videoangiography of occult choroidal neovascularization. Ophthalmology 101:1727–1735, 1994.
133. Sorenson JA, Yannuzzi LA, Slakter JS, et al: A pilot study of digital indocyanine green videoangiography for recurrent occult choroidal neovascularization in age-related macular degeneration. Arch Ophthalmol 112:473–479, 1994.
134. Avvad FK, Duker JS, Reichel E, et al: The digital indocyanine green videoangiography characteristics of defined neovascularization. Ophthalmology 102:401–405, 1995.
135. Quaranta M, Cohen SY, Krott R, et al: Indocyanine green videoangiography of angioid streaks. Am J Ophthalmol 119:136–142, 1995.
136. Singerman LJ: Important points in the management of patients with choroidal neovascularization. Ophthalmology 92:610–614, 1985.
137. Vander J, Morgan C, Schatz H: Growth rate of subretinal neovascularization in age-related macular degeneration. Ophthalmology 96:1422–1426, 1989.
138. Singerman LJ, Hionis R: In Discussion, Vander J, Morgan C, Schatz H: Growth rate of subretinal neovascularization in age-related macular degeneration. Ophthalmology 96:1426–1469, 1989.
139. Moorfields Macular Study Group: Treatment of senile disciform macular degeneration: a single-blind randomised trial by argon laser photocoagulation. Br J Ophthalmol 66:745–753, 1982.
140. Singerman LJ: Fluorescein angiography: practical role in the office management of macular diseases. Ophthalmology 93:1209–1215, 1986.
141. Macular Photocoagulation Study Group: Evaluation of argon green vs krypton red laser for photocoagulation of subfoveal choroidal neovascularization in the macular photocoagulation study. Macular photocoagulation study group (MPS) Group. Arch Ophthalmol 112:1176–1184, 1994.
142. The Canadian Ophthalmology Study Group: Argon green vs krypton red laser photocoagulation for extrafoveal choroidal neovascularization. One-year results in ocular histoplasmosis. Arch Ophthalmol 112:1166–1173, 1994.
143. Bloom SM: Thermal papillitis after dye red photocoagulation of a peripapillary choroidal neovascular membrane. Retina 10:261–264, 1990.
144. Turcotte P, Maguire MG, Fine SL: Visual results after laser treatment for peripapillary choroidal neovascular membranes. Retina 11:295–300, 1991.
145. Macular Photocoagulation Study Group: Laser photocoagulation for neovascular lesions nasal to the fovea. Results from clinical trials for lesions secondary to ocular histoplasmosis or idiopathic causes. Arch Ophthalmol 113:56–61, 1995.
146. Macular Photocoagulation Study Group: The influence of treatment extent on the visual acuity of eyes treated with krypton laser for juxtafoveal choroidal neovascularization. Arch Ophthalmol 113:190–194, 1995.
147. Singerman LJ, Kalski RS: Tunable dye laser for choroidal neovascularization complicating age-related macular degeneration. Retina 9:247–257, 1989.
148. Yannuzzi LA, Shakin JL: Krypton red photocoagulation of the ocular fundus. Retina 2:1–14, 1982.
149. Singerman LJ: Red krypton laser therapy of macular and retinal diseases. Retina 2:15–28, 1982.
150. Chamberlain JA, Bressler NM, Bressler SB, et al: The use of fundus photographs and fluorescein angiograms in the identification and treatment of choroidal neovascularization in the Macular Photocoagulation Study. Ophthalmology 96:1526–1534, 1989.
151. Monahan PM, Gitter KA, Eichler JD, Cohen G: Evaluation of persistence of subretinal membranes using digitized angiographic analysis. Retina 13:196–201, 1993.
152. Elman MJ, Fine SL, Murphy RP, et al: The natural history of serous retinal pigment epithelium detachment in patients with age-related macular degeneration. Ophthalmology 93:224–230, 1986.
153. Rice TA, Murphy RP, Fine SL, Patz A: Stability of argon laser photocoagulation scars in ocular histoplasmosis. In Fine SL, Owens SL (eds): Management of Retinal Vascular and Macular Disorders. Baltimore, Williams & Wilkins, 1983, pp 187–190.
154. Lewis H: Intraoperative fibrinolysis of submacular hem-

orrhage with tissue plasminogen activator and surgical drainage. Am J Ophthalmol 118:559–568, 1994.

155. Jaakkola A, Anttila PM, Immonen I: Interferon alpha-2a in the treatment of exudative senile macular degeneration. Acta Ophthalmol (Copenh) 72:545–549, 1994.

156. Pharmacological therapy for macular degeneration study group: interferon alfa-2a is ineffective for patients with choroidal neovascularization secondary to age related macular degeneration. Results of prospective randomized placebo controlled clinical trial. Arch Ophthalmol 115: 865–872, 1997.

157. Bergink GJ, Deutman AF, van den Broek JF, et al: Radiation therapy for subfoveal choroidal neovascular membranes in age-related macular degeneration. A pilot study. Graefes Arch Clin Exp Ophthalmol 232:591–598, 1994.

158. Hart PM, Archer DB, Chakravarty U: Asymmetry of disciform scarring in bilateral disease when one eye is treated with radiotherapy. Br J Ophthalmol 79:562–568, 1995.

159. Kliman GH, Puliafito CA, Stern SD, et al: Phthalocyanine photodynamic therapy: new strategy for closure of choroidal neovascularization. Lasers Surg Med 15:2–10, 1994.

160. Miller JW, Walsh AW, Kramer M, et al: Photodynamic therapy of experimental choroidal neovascularization using lipoprotein-delivered benzoporphyrin. Arch Ophthalmol 113:810–818, 1995.

161. Treatment of AMD with photodynamic therapy: The TAP study, 520 W. 6th Avenue, Vancouver, BC, Canada. Andrew Strong, Clinical Director (in progress).

162. Algvere PV, Berglin L, Gouras P, Sheng Y: Transplantation of fetal retinal pigment epithelium in age-related macular degeneration with subfoveal neovascularization. Graefes Arch Clin Exp Ophthalmol 232:707–716, 1994.

163. Submacular Surgery Trial: Operations manual.

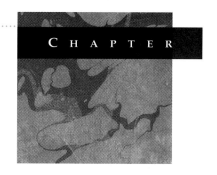

CHAPTER 15

Angioid Streaks

Gabriel Coscas, M.D.
Gisèle Soubrane, M.D., Ph.D.
Maddalena Quaranta, M.D.

Angioid streaks have been described first by Doyne during the meeting of the Ophthalmologic Society of United Kingdom, in 1889. The worsening of visual acuity after an ocular trauma was due to a hemorrhage, defined as choroidal. After reabsorption, fundus examination disclosed irregular zigzagging dark lines in the peripapillary region, extending to the periphery. Three years later Knapp[1] described streaks as an unusual complication of retinal hemorrhage and called them angioid streaks. Kofler[2] first thought that angioid streaks were at the level of Bruch's membrane, far beyond retinal vessels, and histologic studies confirming this hypothesis were done by Böck in 1938 and Hagedoorn in 1939.[3,4] The latter connected the ruptures of Bruch's membrane to the degeneration of the elastic layer and to an accumulation of calcium and iron in a patient with pseudoxanthoma elasticum (PXE).

A number of systemic diseases are associated with angioid streaks. Angioid streaks and PXE have been associated in Stockholm by an ophthalmologist, Grönblad, and by a dermatologist, Strandberg.[5] Thus, the disease was named Grönblad-Strandberg syndrome. Osteitis deformans was first described by Paget in 1876[6] in a patient who lost his vision in both eyes due to macular hemorrhages. Despite this observation, angioid streaks and Paget's disease were only linked by Rowland, in 1933.[7] The association between angioid streaks and sickle cell disease has been even more recently described by Lieb, in 1959.

HISTOPATHOLOGY

Angioid streaks represent visible cracks in Bruch's membrane. Histopathologic studies performed on eyes of patients affected with PXE[3,4,8–11] disclosed an accumulation of calcium in Bruch's membrane which presents multiple cracks with well-defined borders. In PXE, the elementary alteration is a degeneration of the elastic fibers of the whole body and the calcium accumulation seems to be a secondary phenomenon[12] of unknown origin. At the level of angioid streaks, the elastic layer of Bruch's membrane is primarily altered. Studies with high-resolution electron microscopy have identified an abundant granulofilamentous material, related to an abnormal elastic layer, suggesting an abnormal elastogenesis in PXE, instead of normal elastic units.[13] The elastic fibers are charged with calcium. This accumulation of calcium weakens and hardens the elastic fibers.

In Paget's disease this accumulation is better explained. In fact, the remodeling of the bone in this disease produces a large mobilization of calcium that is susceptible to bind to elastic fibers.

In sickle cell disease, iron deposition has been for a long time incriminated in the formation of angioid streaks. However, in other hemolytic diseases and hemochromatosis, in which iron levels are also elevated, angioid streaks are not observed. Moreover, histochemical and light electron microscopic studies of two eyes of a patient with homozygous sickle cell disease and angioid streaks demonstrated heavy calcification, suggesting that calcification is responsible for the brittleness of membrane in these patients.[14] Calcium could be mobilized during the medullar phenomena of compensation due to anemia.[12]

Other histologic abnormalities have been described in angioid streaks independent of the associated systemic disease, such as absence or rupture of the choriocapillaris beneath the streaks.[15] Retinal pigment epithelium, contiguous to the borders of streaks, can be hypopigmented or thinned.

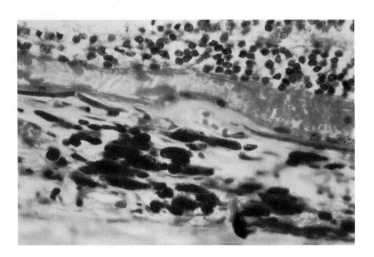

Angioid streak with defect in Bruch's membrane and early choroidal neovascularization. (From Dreyer R, Green WR: Pathology of angioid streaks. Trans Penn Acad Ophthalmol Otolaryngol 31:158–167, 1978, with permission.)

CLINICAL SIGNS

Symptoms

Angioid streaks are asymptomatic. Macular symptoms due to progression of streaks towards the fovea (Fig. 15–1) or to proliferation of choroidal neovascularization appear usually after the third decade of life. The relatively late appearance of symptoms can explain the late discovery of the disease, especially in the nonfamilial forms.

Fundus Examination

Angioid streaks are usually bilateral and asymmetric. In the early phases of the disease, diagnosis can be difficult, when only an atrophic crescent localized nasally to the optic disc, associated with scarce and tiny streaks, is visible. Angiographies can then help in the diagnosis.

In more advanced cases, angioid streaks appear like irregular, radiating, zigzagging, tapering lines that extend from the peripapillary area towards the peripheral fundus (Fig. 15–2).[4,16–20] Near the optic disc, they are often interconnected by circular breaks. The size of streaks is variable (50 to 500 μm).[21]

The color of streaks varies from reddish orange to dark red or brown, depending on the pigmentary characteristics of the choroid that becomes visible through the thinned retinal pigment epithelium overlying the streaks. In some cases, streaks are dark and abundantly interconnected to each other, giving the fundus the appearance of a "spider's web."

With aging, angioid streaks become darker and the surrounding pigment epithelium appears de-

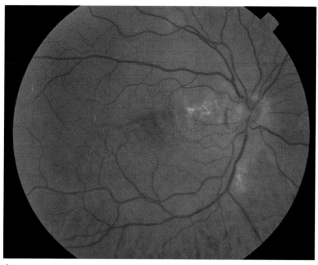

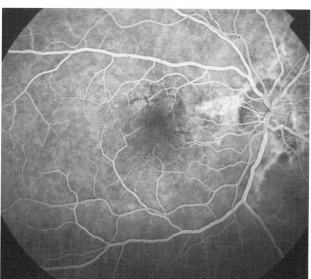

A   B

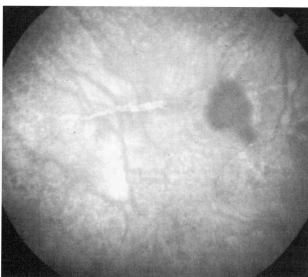

FIGURE 15–1   Angioid streak crossing the foveal region. Visual acuity was reduced at 20/200. *A*, Color fundus picture visualizes better than *B*, fluorescein angiography of the streak crossing the foveal region. *C*, ICG angiography perfectly visualizes the foveal streak.

C

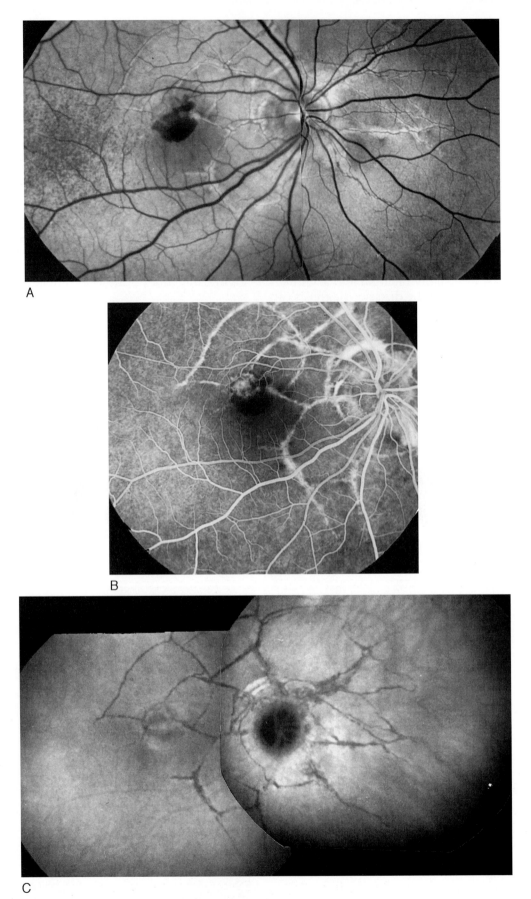

FIGURE 15–2 *A*, Red-free picture showing typical angioid streaks surrounding the optic disc. A subretinal hemorrhage is visible in the macular region, and peau d'orange appearance of the posterior pole, more evident temporally, is visualized. *B*, Fluorescein angiography discloses well-defined choroidal new vessels, partly masked by the hemorrhage. *C*, Composite of late-phase indocyanine green pictures shows hypofluorescent streaks, probably marking the relatively recent onset of the streaks, and in the upper inner macula, a hyperfluorescent zone corresponding with the choroidal new vessels.

pigmented. Sometimes, a whitish irregular reflex, due to the presence of fibrous tissue,[22] covers the streaks, blurring them. On the contrary, in other cases, streaks appear black due to pigmentary proliferation along their course.[23]

The topography of the streaks seems related to the lines of forces within the eye, resulting from the pull of intrinsic and extrinsic muscles on the relative fixed site of the optic disc.[24] Such forces, acting on a brittle Bruch's membrane, surely account for the configuration of angioid streaks.

Fluorescein Angiography

Frames of the fundus shot before dye injection can be useful to detect the autofluorescence of the optic disc with drusen frequently associated with angioid streaks (see below).

Usually, angioid streaks become hyperfluorescent in the retinal arterial phase and their fluorescence persists after the dye has disappeared from the retinal vessel (Fig. 15–2). These findings indicate atrophic retinal pigment epithelium at the site of the streaks. In the absence of neovascular complications, angioid streaks do not leak fluorescein dye, even on late frames.

Angiographic features are inconstant, and sometimes streaks perfectly visible on fundus examination are barely visible on fluorescein angiography and vice versa (Figs. 15–1 and 15–3). Variability of the angiographic behavior of streaks[15] depends on multiple factors: (1) blockage due to the presence of pigment; (2) hypofluorescence due to atrophy of the choriocapillaris; or (3) hyperfluorescence due to transmission of the choroidal fluorescence, which can appear early (window defect) or late during the sequence, due to staining of streaks by the dye arising from the surrounding normal choriocapillaris.

Indocyanine Green Angiography

Indocyanine green (ICG) angiography must be retained for cases of angioid streaks in which the other diagnostic tools have failed to detect precisely the nature of the disease: either pigmentary disturbances, frequently associated with the most advanced cases, and can interfere with the identification of the hyperfluorescence of streaks; or hemorrhages, which can mask the fluorescence of streaks or of their neovascular complications.

During the sequence, angioid streaks appear like hyperfluorescent lines with some more hyperfluorescent pinpoints along and inside their course.[25] This angiographic feature does not depend on the degree of pigmentation of streaks, or of atrophy of the choriocapillaris (Fig. 15–4).

Recent streaks, on the contrary, appear like hypofluorescent lines around the disc (Fig. 15–2) or in the midperiphery of the fundus even when they remain undetected with fundus examination and fluorescein angiography. This latter characteristic can be useful in early diagnosis of angioid streaks, in young patients.

SYSTEMIC DISEASES ASSOCIATED WITH ANGIOID STREAKS

Angioid streaks have been reported to be associated with a large number of systemic diseases (Table 15–1). Some associations are probably due to chance, but some others, such as pseudoxanthoma elasticum and sickle cell disease, are well known.

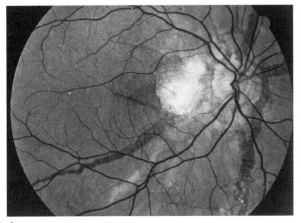
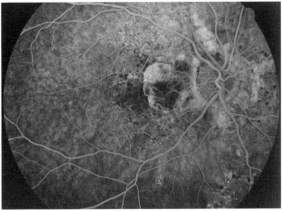

A   B

FIGURE 15–3   A, Red-free picture and (B) fluorescein angiography of typical angioid streaks. Note the presence, in the inferopapillary region, of crystalline bodies.

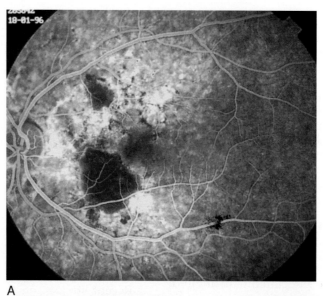

A

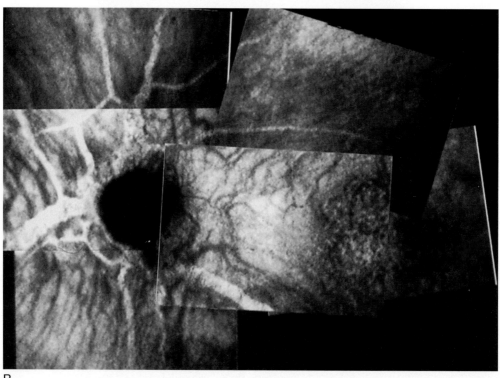

B

FIGURE 15–4   *A,* Fluorescein angiography and (*B*) ICG angiography of angioid streaks. Angioid streaks are in both angiographies visualized as hyperfluorescent lines. Note that angioid streaks seem to be longer and better individualized on ICG than on fluorescein angiography.

Pseudoxanthoma Elasticum (PXE, Grönblad-Strandberg Syndrome)

PXE is a systemic disease whose prevalence is estimated to be 1 per 100,000.[23] PXE is autosomal recessive,[23] although some authors suggest the possibility of an autosomal dominant form as well.[26–28] The disease is normally present at an early age, but the time of the first diagnosis is variable.

Systemic Manifestations

SKIN. The typical lesions of PXE are yellowish confluent papules, localized in areas of wear and tear (such as the face; neck; axillary, cubital, and inguinal folds; and in the periumbilical region) that give to the skin a "plucked chicken" appearance (Fig. 15–5). The biopsy performed on scar tissue or on flexural folds differentiate PXE lesions from those

TABLE 15–1 Systemic Diseases Associated with Angioid Streaks

Disease	Systemic Manifestations

Pseudoxanthoma elasticum	Usually autosomal recessive[23,26–28]
	Skin:
	  Yellowish, confluent papules on the flexural folds[17,27,29]
	Cardiovascular system:
	  Peripheral, cardiac, or cerebral arterial occlusion[17]
	  Systemic hypertension
	  Mitralic valve prolapse[30]
	  Digestive hemorrhage[31]
	  Uterine hemorrhage and risk of abortion[32]
	Ocular manifestations :
	  Angioid streaks[17,20,23,33–35]
	  Peau d'orange pigmentary change[19,36–39]
	  Focal atrophic lesion of RPE[16,17,20,36,40]
	  Crystalline bodies[18,20,41]
	  Optic disc drusen[16,17,20,40]

Ehlers-Danlos disease	Hereditary disease
	Ligament and skin hyperelasticity
	Ocular manifestations:
	  Strabismus
	  Blue sclera
	  Myopia
	  Keratoconus
	  Lens ectopia
	  Hypertelorism
	  Angioid streaks[42–44]

Osteitis deformans or Paget's disease of the bone	Chronic, progressive, sometimes hereditary thickening and deformity of bones associated with pain Hearing loss Coronary insufficiency Hyperparathyroidism Arteritis and calcium accumulation in midcaliber arteries Angioid streaks (rare)[18,23,34,45,46]

Sickle cell disease	Abnormal S or C hemoglobin (SS or SC sickle cell disease)
	Hemolysis and reduction of red cells deformability
	Acute bone ache
	Peripheral and visceral arterial occlusions
	Ocular manifestations:
	  Sickle cell retinopathy and associated signs
	  Angioid streaks[18,20,47,48,50–53]

Thalassemia	Autosomal dominant β Chain of hemoglobin non- or poorly synthesized (homozygous form or β thalassemia major; heterozygous or β thalassemia minor) Hemolytic anemia Hemochromatosis Recurrent infections Ocular manifestations: angioid streaks[54–58]
Hereditary spherocytosis	Autosomal dominant Hemolytic anemia Red cell membrane abnormalities Icterus or subicterus Splenomegaly Ocular manifestations: angioid streaks[59,60]

Table continued on following page

TABLE 15–1   *Continued*

Disease	Systemic Manifestations
Abetalipoproteinemia	Autosomal recessive β-Apolipoprotein nonsynthetized Acanthocytosis Peripheral neuropathy Deficit in lipid absorption Congestive cardiopathy Ocular manifestations: Rod degeneration (retinitis pigmentosa) Nystagmus Ophthalmoplegia Ptosis Cataract Anisocoria Angioid streaks[61–63]

of senile elastosis, and of work-related exposure to calcium salts (colliers or road workers). This method of biopsy allows diagnosis of PXE even in patients without evident skin lesions.[64] Sometimes the interpretation of skin biopsy is difficult, especially in skin regions normally exposed to sun.[27,29]

Histologic and ultrastructural analysis of these lesions discloses deposits of salts of calcium and calcium phosphates in the deep and reticular derma.

CARDIOVASCULAR SYSTEM. Calcification of elastic fibers in the mid- and large-caliber arteries has been found. The risk of peripheral, cardiac, or cerebral vascular occlusion in PXE has been estimated to be 26%.[23] Systemic hypertension is frequent (about 20%) and appears after the fourth decade. Arterial involvement in the extremities is also frequent (about 30%) and particularly affects the femoral artery.

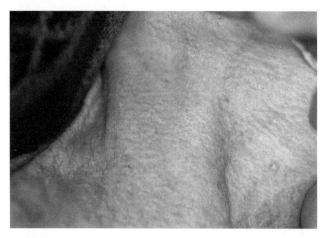

FIGURE 15–5   Typical lesions on the skin of neck in a 53-year-old patient suffering from pseudoxanthoma elasticum.

The most frequent cardiac manifestation of PXE is angor (15%), which can occur even early in life. Mitral valve prolapse has been found in 70% of PXE patients systematically examined by ultrasound cardiac examination.[30]

Gastrointestinal hemorrhages are frequent (14% according to Connor[23]), and sometimes very severe.[30] Hemorrhages occur in young people, often during pregnancy, and are due to diffuse bleeding of the gastric mucosa. Alterations of blood vessels in PXE are localized in the lamina media of blood vessels, contrary to the lesions of arteriosclerosis, which are localized mainly in the intima.[65]

GYNECOLOGIC AND OBSTETRIC MANIFESTATIONS. The risk of abortion during the first 3 months of pregnancy is high (22%).[32] Uterine hemorrhages have been reported.

Ocular Manifestations

PXE represents the main cause of angioid streaks in 34 to 83% of patients affected with PXE.[17,20,23,25,34,35] The differences may be due to the difficult interpretation of the skin biopsy. They have been described even in childhood.

TABLE 15–2   Frequency of Systemic Diseases in Patients with Angioid Streaks

Disease	Frequency
Idiopathic forms	20–65.6%
Pseudoxanthoma elasticum	34–59%
Paget's disease of the bone	1.4–15%
Sickle cell hemoglobinopathies	1–6%
Other systemic diseases	Rare

PEAU D'ORANGE PIGMENTARY CHANGE. Description of the "peau d'orange" lesion is attributed to Smith et al,[36] although this feature had already been described by previous authors.[37,38] It consists of a widespread pattern of yellow-brown, sometimes confluent spots, in patients affected with PXE, with or without angioid streaks. This feature is usually more evident in the midperipheral fundus, particularly on the temporal side (Fig. 15–2). This feature is characteristic of PXE, but it is not pathognomonic. It can exist before the occurrence of the streaks,[37,39] and could represent a marker of the heterozygous recessive form.[39]

The fluorescein angiographic behavior is an irregular and sudden masking effect, visible since the choroidal phase of the sequence and fading later on (Fig. 15–6).[19,39]

Indocyanine green angiography identified that peau d'orange pigmentary change is a diffuse alteration of the fundus, only more prominent on the temporal side. A pattern of hypofluorescent spots, corresponding to the pigmentary changes of peau d'orange, appears in the midphase and persists until the late phases of the ICG sequence.[25]

The site of the alteration is unknown. According to Krill's theory, it could correspond to a localized alteration of elastic tissue of Bruch's membrane.[30]

FOCAL ATROPHIC LESIONS OF RETINAL PIGMENT EPITHELIUM. Small chorioretinal atrophic lesions

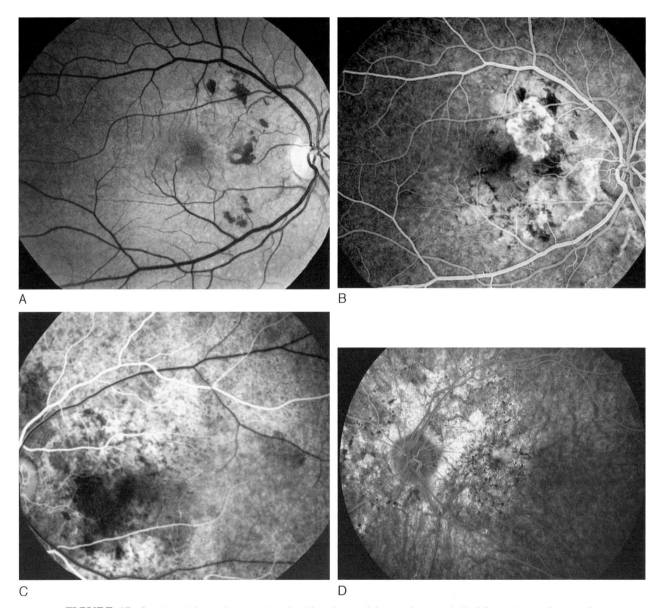

A   B   C   D

FIGURE 15–6 Angioid streaks associated with subretinal hemorrhages. *A*, Red-free picture shows subretinal hemorrhages. *B* and *C*, Fluorescein angiography discloses reticular alterations of retinal pigment epithelium at the posterior pole and two foci of choroidal well-defined new vessels. Note the nonhomogenous fluorescence of the temporal side of the posterior pole due to the presence of peau d'orange. *D*, Fluorescein angiography 3 months after photocoagulation shows the presence of laser scars.

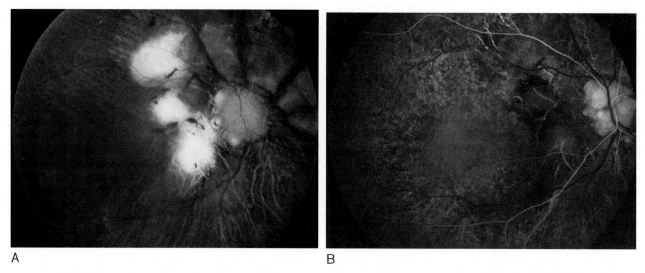

A   B

FIGURE 15–7   *A*, Red-free picture and (*B*) early-phase fluorescein angiography of drusen of the optic disc in a patient affected with pseudoxanthoma elasticum.

have been observed in the peripheral fundus in PXE patients. These lesions have been referred to by several different names: salmon spots,[20,30,36] punched-out lesions,[26] and focal lesions.[16,19,20] These white scars present with varying amounts of surrounding pigment, similar to those observed in the presumed ocular histoplasmosis syndrome. They can be present before appearance of the streaks,[30] and have been reported in 44% of PXE patients.[16]

CRYSTALLINE BODIES. Crystalline bodies consist of small, yellow, round subretinal lesions, localized in the midperiphery, especially in the inferior juxtapapillary region and midperiphery (Fig. 15–3). They can be encircled by a pigment epithelium hyperplasia and, in some cases, be contiguous to a

"tail" of pigment epithelium thinning that gives them the appearance of a comet.[20] In patients with PXE, crystalline bodies occur in 75% of patients.[41] They could represent focal ruptures in Bruch's membrane.[18]

OPTIC DISC DRUSEN. Optic disc drusen have been frequently reported in patients affected with PXE.[16,17,20,30] They are usually visible on fundus examination as discrete, multiple, amorphous, calcified structures in the prelaminar portion of the optic nerve (Figs. 15–7 and 15–8). In a small number of patients, they can be buried in a normal-appearing optic disc. In such cases, autofluorescence fundus photographs and ultrasound examination can help in the diagnosis. Their pathogenesis is unknown.

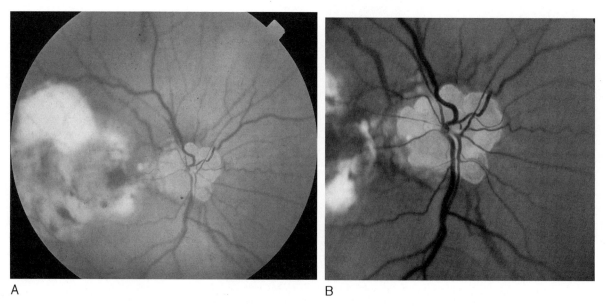

A   B

FIGURE 15–8   *A*, Fundus and (*B*) red-free photographs of drusen of the optic disc in a patient with pseudoxanthoma elasticum.

They could be due to localized axoplasmic transport alterations secondary to calcium accumulation in the lamina cribrosa of optic disc.[66] The lesion can be responsible for an optic neuropathy.[20]

Paget's Disease of the Bone (Osteitis Deformans)

Systemic Manifestations

Paget's disease of the bone is a chronic, progressive, and sometimes hereditary disease in which abnormal osteoclastic and osteoblastic phenomena cause thickening, calcification, and deformity of spongeous bones, confined to some bones or generalized. Patients develop, usually after the age of 40 years, enlargement of the skull, deformity of the long bones, and kyphoscoliosis. Bone deformations are associated with pain. Other complications of this disease are hearing loss, coronary failure, hyperparathyroidism, arteritis, and calcium deposition in the midcaliber arteries.

The diagnosis of the disease is based on clinical and radiologic signs associated with elevation of serum alkaline phosphatase and elevation of urine peptide hydroxyproline.

Ocular Manifestations

Prevalence of angioid streaks in Paget's disease has been evaluated as varying from 8 to 15%.[17,18,34,45] Considering the frequency of Paget's disease (3% >40 years old, and 9% >80 years old), angioid streaks should be found in thousands of patients with osteitis deformans, but this is not the case. Dabbs and Skjodt published a series of 70 randomly selected patients with Paget's disease of bones and found only one patient to have angioid streaks.[46]

Sickle Cell Disease

Sickle cell disease is a hemoglobinopathy affecting preferentially black people. Substitution of one or several normal beta-hemoglobin by an abnormal S or C hemoglobin leads to a characteristic deformation of red cells, associated with a reduction of their deformability. Ocular complications of sickle cell disease are broadly described, and in particular include retinopathy. Angioid streaks were first described by Lieb et al in 2 of 65 patients with SS sickle cell disease.[47] Nowadays, angioid streaks are classically associated with this hematologic disease.[20,48] The prevalence varies from 1 to 2%,[18,20,50] but higher values have been found.[67]

Streaks in these patients rarely occur before the age of 25 years,[51,52] but frequency increases dramatically after this age to reach 22% in those over the age of 40 years.[50,53] Central visual loss due to cho-

roidal neovascularization occurs infrequently in sickle cell patients with angioid streaks.[20]

EVOLUTION AND PROGNOSIS

Evolutional Stages of Angioid Streaks

Natural history of angioid streaks, except for their complications, is scarcely documented. Size and length increase are considered normal in angioid streaks, but there is no publication concerning their rate of progression.

With aging, angioid streaks become less pigmented, losing their typical red-brown color.[20]

Complications

Posttraumatic Bruch's Membrane Ruptures

The extreme brittleness of Bruch's membrane can explain the high risk of extensive choroidal ruptures from relatively mild contusion of the eye.[20] According to a retrospective study on angioid streaks, 15% of patients experience sudden visual loss following ocular trauma.[68]

These ruptures are usually associated with large subretinal hemorrhages, which can be misdiagnosed as complications of choroidal neovascularization (CNV) (Fig. 15–9).[35,70–72] Hemorrhages are usually in proximity to streaks, but can frequently involve the macular region.

Choroidal Neovascularization

CNV modifies dramatically the prognosis of angioid streaks. Patients become symptomatic usually because of central visual decrease and metamorphopsia.

Fundus examination usually discloses a serous retinal detachment, frequently surrounded by subretinal hemorrhages (Figs. 15–2 and 15–6). These are mainly localized to the macular or interpapillomacular region and the immediate proximity of streaks. Rarely the neovascular lesion is superior or nasal to the optic disc.

Fluorescein angiography confirms the presence of CNV[73] and enables localization of it on the border or inside the streaks. Choroidal neovascularization has the typical angiographic features of well-defined new vessels, with leakage in the late phases (Fig. 15–10). The limits of CNV are sometimes difficult to ascertain, because of the pigmentary changes that frequently are associated with angioid streaks, and because of hemorrhages (Fig. 15–8). In these cases, ICG angiography can be useful (see above).[25]

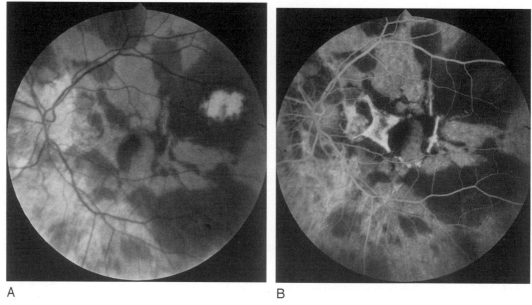

A   B

FIGURE 15-9   Posttraumatic subretinal hemorrhages in a young patient suffering from angioid streaks and pseudoxanthoma elasticum. Hemorrhage from posttraumatic streaks occurred after relatively mild trauma.

Risk Factors and Natural History

The risk of occurrence of CNV increases with age.[20,74] Additional risk factors in the development of CNV are density, length, and localization of streaks at less than one disc diameter from the center of the macula.[75]

Angioid streaks are frequently complicated by CNV if associated with PXE,[74] while CNV is rare in association with sickle cell disease.[18,35,48,53,76] Bilateralization occurs in 42 to 60% of cases, with an interlapsing time of about 18 months.[68,75]

Natural prognosis of CNV complicating angioid streaks is poor, evolving almost always towards macular involvement and central visual loss.[77] Legal blindness secondary to CNV has been noted in more than 50% of patients.[68,74,79] The frequency of this complication varies among studies from 72 to 86%.[16,33,34,68]

Management and Treatment

Several studies have reported the results of laser photocoagulation for CNV complicating angioid streaks.

Investigators, initially disappointed with the results, postulated that the poor outcome may have been caused by incomplete treatment of CNV or laser-induced stimulation of CNV.[18,80] Hilton stated that laser treatment encouraged development and further growth of CNV.[81]

Thereafter, other isolated case reports described successful laser treatment.[82-85] Four case series[68,86-89]

comprising ten or more eyes with CNV secondary to angioid streaks treated with laser have been reported.

Piro, Scheraga, and Fine[68] described the treatment results in 21 eyes. Although over 80% of them had an initial visual acuity of 20/40 or better, visual acuity progressed to legal blindness in more than 70%, 55% of which decreased to this level within 6 months of treatment.

Brancato and associates[86] found that visual prognosis was better in the 13 eyes in which CNV was amenable to laser treatment (whose final visual acuity was 25/200), in comparison to 10 eyes in which CNV was not amenable to laser photocoagulation, whose final visual acuity was 20/300. Follow-up ranged from 10 to 72 months. In this study, 10 of the 13 treated eyes developed recurrences within 3 months of treatment.

Gelisken, Hendrikse, and Deutman[87] described retrospectively 30 treated eyes of 24 patients. Visual acuity was stabilized or improved in 16 eyes (53%). Twelve of the remaining 14 treated eyes (46%) maintained a visual acuity better than 20/200. Eleven of 16 fellow eyes had untreated CNV, and central visual acuity was lost. Ten treated eyes did not recur, but the mean follow-up period of these eyes was only 1.3 years, while eyes with recurrences had a follow-up of 3.4 years.

A retrospective study conducted in France by Esente et al[88] on 23 eyes found an improvement or a stabilization of visual acuity in 13 eyes, over a period of 33 months. The final visual acuity depended on the distance of CNV from the foveola, being better in CNV at more than 400 μm. This study also demonstrated the high rate of neovas-

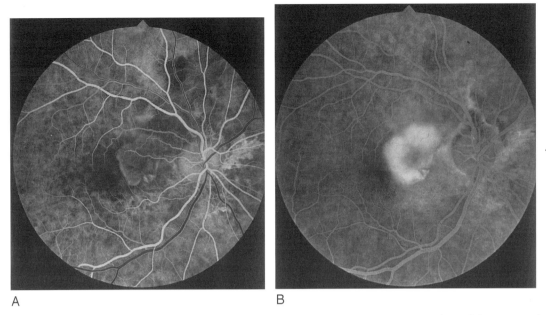

A   B

FIGURE 15–10   *A*, Early- and (*B*) late-phase fluorescein angiography of visible choroidal new vessels complicating angioid streaks.

cular recurrences: 17 eyes (74%) presented one or more recurrences. In 70% of eyes, recurrences were on the foveal border of the scar.[88]

A recent case series by Lim et al[89] followed 24 treated eyes of 20 patients, for 3 months to 9 years (mean, 3.5 years). In this study, 18 of 24 eyes (75%) maintained visual acuity better than 20/200. Visual deterioration and the rates of recurrence and persistence were more marked if the fellow eye presented with scar, CNV, or both.

All these case series concluded that laser pho-

tocoagulation of nonsubfoveal neovascular lesions must be considered. Laser treatment may slow down the rate of visual loss and may result in a less severe final visual acuity decrease than natural scarring (Fig. 15–6). The necessity of long-term follow-up after treatment is emphasized by the high rate of recurrence (Fig. 15–11).

In the absence of prospective randomized studies, laser photocoagulation of CNV secondary to angioid streaks can be only suggested. The utility of laser treatment is, however, strongly supported

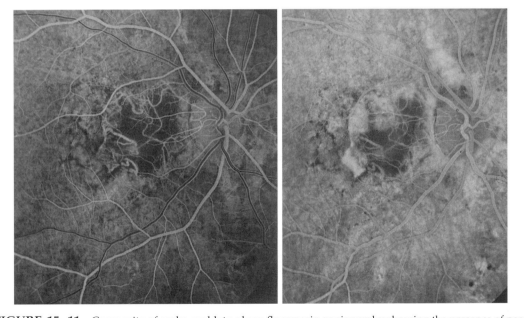

FIGURE 15–11   Composite of early- and late-phase fluorescein angiography showing the presence of neovascular recurrence on the foveal border of the laser scar. The recurrence occurred 2 months after laser photocoagulation.

by the above-mentioned studies. The early diagnosis and treatment of CNV, before involvement of the foveal center, remains a crucial point, underscored by each study.

REFERENCES

1. Knapp H: On the formation of dark angioid streaks as unusual metamorphosis of retinal hemorrhage. Arch Ophthalmol 26:289–292, 1892.
2. Kofler A: Beitrage zur Kenntnis der angioid Streaks (Knapp). Klin Augenheilkd 82:134–149, 1917.
3. Böck J: Zur Klinik und Anatomie der gefässähnlichen Streifen im Augenhintergrund. Z Augenheilkd 95:1–50, 1938.
4. Hagedoorn A: Angioid streaks. Arch Ophthalmol 21:746–774 and 935–965, 1939.
5. Groenblad E: Angioid streaks. Acta Ophthalmol 7:328, 1929.
6. Paget J: Royal medical and surgical society report: on a form of chronic inflammation of bone (osteitis deformans). Lancet 2:714–716, 1876.
7. Rowland WD: Bilateral caerulean cataract. N Engl Ophthalmol Soc 16:61, 1932.
8. Gass JD, Clarkson JG: Angioid streaks and disciform macular detachment in Paget's disease (osteitis deformans). Am J Ophthalmol 75:576–686, 1973.
9. Klien BA: Angioid streaks: a clinical and histopathologic study. Am J Ophthalmol 30:955–968, 1947.
10. McWilliam RJ: On the histology of angioid streaks. Trans Ophthalmol Soc UK 71:243–249, 1951.
11. Verhoeff FH: Histological findings in case of angioid streaks. Br J Ophthalmol 32:531–544, 1948.
12. Dhermy P: Histopathologie des stries angioides. In Coscas G, Soubrane G (eds): Neovaisseaux sous-retiniens et laser. Paris, Doin, 1987, pp 210–211.
13. Huang SN, Steele HD, Kumar G, Parker JO: Ultrastructural changes of elastic fibers in pseudoxanthoma elasticum: a study of histogenesis. Arch Pathol 83:108–113, 1967.
14. Jampol LM, Acheson R, Eagle RC Jr, et al: Calcification of Bruch's membrane in angioid streaks with homozygous sickle cell disease. Arch Ophthalmol 105:93–98, 1987.
15. Federman JL, Shields JA, Tomer TL, Annesley WH: Angioid streaks. In Yannuzzi LA, Gitter KA, Schatz H (eds): The macula. A Comprehensive Text and Atlas. Baltimore, Williams & Wilkins, 1978, pp 218–231.
16. Shields JA, Federman JL, Tomer TL, Annesley WH Jr: Angioid streaks I. Ophthalmoscopic variations and diagnostic problems. Br J Ophthalmol 59:257–266, 1975.
17. Walker ER, Frederick RG, Mayes MD: The mineralization of elastic fibers and alterations of extracellular matrix in pseudoxanthoma elasticum. Arch Dermatol 125:70–76, 1989.
18. Clarkson JG, Altman RD: Angioid streaks. Surv Ophthalmol 26:235–246, 1982.
19. Federman JL, Shields JA, Tomer TL: Angioid streaks II. Fluorescein angiographic features. Arch Ophthalmol 93:951–926, 1975.
20. Gass JD: Stereoscopic Atlas of Macular Diseases, 3rd edition. St Louis, CV Mosby Co, 1987, pp 102–109.
21. Donaldson EJ: Angioid streaks. Aust J Ophthalmol 11:55–58, 1983.
22. Newsome DA: Angioid streaks and Bruch's membrane degeneration. In Newsome DA (ed): Retinal dystrophies and degenerations. New York, Raven Press, 1988, pp 271–283.
23. Neldner KH: Pseudoxanthoma elasticum. Clin Dermatol 6: 1–159, 1988.
24. Adelung JC: Zur Genese der angioid Streaks. Klin Monatsbl Augenheilkd 119:241–250, 1951.
25. Quaranta M, Cohen SY, Krott R, et al: Indocyanine green videoangiography of angioid streaks. Am J Ophthalmol 119:136–142, 1995.
26. McKusik, VA: Heritable Disorders of Connective Tissue, 4th edition. St Louis, CV Mosby Co, 1992, pp 474–520.
27. Pope FM: Two types of autosomal recessive pseudoxanthoma elasticum. Arch Dermatol 110:209–212, 1974.
28. Stutz SB, Schnyder UW, Vogel A: Clinical and genetic criteria in pseudoxanthoma elasticum (PXE). Hautarzt 36: 265–268, 1985.
29. Paton D: The Relation of Angioid Streaks to Systemic Disease. Springfield, IL, Charles C Thomas, 1972, pp 20–41.
30. Lebwohl M, Stefano D, Prioleau P, Uman M: Pseudoxanthoma elasticum and mitral valve prolapse. N Engl J Med 307:228–231, 1982.
31. Eddy DD, Farber EM: Pseudoxanthoma elasticum. Internal manifestations: a report of cases and statistical review of the literature. Arch Dermatol 86:729–732, 1962.
32. Voljoen DL, Beatty S, Beighton P: The obstetric and gynaecological implications of pseudoxanthoma elasticum. Br J Obstet Gynaecol 94: 884–888, 1987.
33. Connor PH, Juergens JL, Perry HO, et al: Pseudoxanthoma elasticum and angioid streaks: a review of 106 cases. Am J Med 30:537–543, 1961.
34. Scholz RO: Angioid streaks. Arch Ophthalmol 26:677–695, 1941.
35. Archer DB, Logan WC: Angioid streaks. In Krill AE (ed): Hereditary Retinal and Choroidal Diseases. Clinical Characteristics. Hagerstown, MD, Harper & Row, 1976, pp 851–909.
36. Smith JL, Gass JDM, Justice JJ: Fluorescein fundus photography of angioid streaks. Br J Ophthalmol 48:517–521, 1964.
37. Bischler V: Le fond d'oeil moucheté multicolore: manifestation fruste de la maladie de Groenblad et Strandberg. Bull Mem Soc Fr Ophtalmol 68: 287–291, 1955.
38. Shimizu K: Mottled fundus in association with pseudoxanthoma elasticum. Jpn J Ophthalmol 5:1–13, 1961.
39. Gills JP, Paton D: Mottled fundus oculi in pseudoxanthoma elasticum. Arch Ophthalmol 73:792–795, 1965.
40. Krill AE, Klien BA, Archer DB: Precursor of angioid streaks. Am J Ophthalmol 76:875–879, 1973.
41. Meislik J, Neldner K, Reeve EB, Ellis PP: Atypical drusen in pseudoxanthoma elasticum. Ann Ophthalmol 11:653–656, 1979.
42. Cottini GB: Association des syndromes de Groenblad-Strandberg et d'Ehler-Danlos dans le même sujet. Acta Derm Venereol 28:544–549, 1959.
43. Pelbois F, Rollier M: Association d'un syndrome d'Ehler-Danlos et d'un syndrome de Groenblad-Strandberg. Bull Soc Fr Derm Syph 59:141–143, 1952.
44. Green WR, Friedman-Kien A, Banfield WG: Angioid streaks in Ehler-Danlos syndrome. Arch Ophthalmol 76: 197–204, 1966.
45. Terry TT: Angioid streaks and osteitis deformans. Trans Am Ophthalmol Soc 32:555–573, 1934.
46. Dabbs TR, Skjodt K: Prevalence of angioid streaks and other ocular complications of Paget's disease of bone. Br J Ophthalmol 74:579–582, 1990.
47. Lieb VA, Geeraets WJ, Guerry D III: Sickle cell retinopathy: ocular and systemic manifestations of sickle cell disease. Acta Ophthalmol 58:1–45, 1959.
48. Paton D: Angioid streaks and sickle cell anemia. Arch Ophthalmol 62:852–858, 1959.
49. Paton D: The significance of angioid streaks. Middle East Med J 1:301–336, 1963.
50. Nagpal KC, Asdourian G, Goldbaum M, et al: Angioid streaks and sickle haemoglobinopathies. Br J Ophthalmol 60:313–334, 1976.
51. Condon PI, Serjeant GR: Ocular findings in homozygous sickle cell anemia in Jamaica. Am J Ophthalmol 74:1105–1109, 1972.
52. Majecodunmi SA, Akinyanju OO: Ocular findings in homozygous sickle cell disease in Nigeria. Can J Ophthalmol 12:160–162, 1978.
53. Condon PI, Serjeant GR: Ocular findings in elderly cases of homozygous sickle cell disease in Jamaica. Br J Ophthalmol 60:361–364, 1976.

54. Gibson JM, Raichaudhuri P, Rosenthal AR: Angioid streaks in a case of beta thalassemia major. Br J Ophthalmol 667:29–31, 1983.
55. Theodossiadis G, Ladas I, Koutsandrea C, et al: Thalassemia et neovaisseaux sous-retiniens maculaires. J Fr Ophtalmol 7:115–118, 1984.
56. Kinsella FP, Mooney DJ: Angioid streaks in beta thalassaemia minor. Br J Ophthalmol 72:303–304, 1988.
57. Singerman LJ: Angioid streaks in thalassaemia major. Br J Ophthalmol 67:558, 1983.
58. Daneshmend TK: Ocular findings in case of haemoglobine H disease. Br J Ophthalmol 63:842–844, 1979.
59. McLane NJ, Grizzard WS, Kousseff BG, et al: Angioid streaks associated with hereditary spherocytosis. Am J Ophthalmol 97:444–449, 1984.
60. Singerman LJ: Angioid streaks associated with hereditary spherocytosis. Am J Ophthalmol 98:647–648, 1984.
61. Duker JS, Belmont J, Bosley TM: Angioid streaks associated with abetalipoproteinemia. Arch Ophthalmol 105:1173–1174, 1987.
62. Runge P, Muller PR, McAllister J: Oral vitamin E supplements can prevent the retinopathy of abetalipoproteinemia. Br J Ophthalmol 70:166–173, 1986.
63. Yatzkan DN: Angioid streaks of the fundus in association with post-hemorrhagic amaurosis. Am J Ophthalmol 43:219–222, 1957.
64. Lebwohl M, Phelps RG, Yannuzzi LA, et al: Diagnosis of pseudoxanthoma elasticum by scar biopsy in patients without characteristic skin lesions. N Engl J Med 317:347–350, 1987.
65. Goodman RM, Smith EW, Paton D: Pseudoxanthoma elasticum: a clinical and histopathological study. Medicine 42:297–334, 1963.
66. Coleman K, Ross MH, McCabe M, et al: Disk drusen and angioid streaks in pseudoxanthoma elasticum. Am J Ophthalmol 112:166–170, 1991.
67. Geeraets WJ, Guerry D III: Angioid streaks and sickle cell disease. Am J Ophthalmol 49:450–470, 1960.
68. Piro PA, Scheraga D, Fine SL: Angioid streaks: natural history and visual prognosis. In Fine SL, Owens SL (eds): Management of Retinal Vascular and Macular Disorders. Baltimore, Williams & Wilkins, 1983, pp 136–139.
69. Britten MJ: Unusual traumatic retinal haemorrhages associated with angioid streaks. Br J Ophthalmol 50:540–542, 1965.
70. Howard GM: Angioid streaks in acromegaly. Am J Ophthalmol 56:137–139, 1963.
71. Hagedoorn A: Angioid streaks and traumatic ruptures of Bruch's membrane. Br J Ophthalmol 59:267, 1975.
72. Turut P, Malthieu D, Courtin J: Membrane neovasculaire choroidienne et rupture choroidienne traumatique sur stries angioides. Bull Soc Ophtalmol Fr 82:591–594, 1982.
73. Gass JD: Pathogenesis of disciform detachment of the neuroepithelium VI. Disciform detachment secondary to heredodegenerative, neoplastic and traumatic lesions of the choroid. Am J Ophthalmol 63:689–711, 1967.
74. Shilling GS, Blach RK: Prognosis and therapy of angioid streaks. Trans Ophthalmol Soc UK 95:301–305, 1975.
75. Mansour AM, Shields JA, Annesley WH, et al: Macular degeneration in angioid streaks. Ophthalmologica 197:36–41, 1988.
76. Hamilton AM, Pope FM, Condon PL: Angioid streaks in Jamaican patients with homozygous sickle cell disease. Br J Ophthalmol 65:341–347, 1981.
77. Hochart G, Turut P, Francois P: Evolution spontanée des néovaisseaux sous-rétiniens dans les stries angioides. Bull Soc Ophtalmol Fr 87:289–290, 1987.
78. Wise GN, Dollery CT, Hendkind P: Macular degeneration in angioid streaks. In The Retinal Circulation. London, Harper & Row, 1971, pp 491–492.
79. Groenblad E: Color photographs of angioid streaks in the late stages. Acta Ophthalmol 36:472–474, 1958.
80. Wilkinson CP: Stimulation of subretinal neovascularization. Am J Ophthalmol 81:104–106, 1976.
81. Hilton GF: Late serosanguineous detachment of the macula after traumatic choroidal rupture. Am J Ophthalmol 79:997–1000, 1975.
82. Peabody R, Warren H: Angioid streaks in macular diseases. In L'Esperance FA (ed): Current Diagnosis and Management of Chorioretinal Diseases. St Louis, CV Mosby Co, 1977, pp 527–539.
83. Fine SL: Angioid streaks. Int Ophthalmol Clin 17:173–182, 1979.
84. Deutman AF, Kovacs B: Argon laser treatment in complications of angioid streaks. Am J Ophthalmol 88:12–17, 1979.
85. Meislik J, Neldner KH, Reeve EB, Ellis PP: Laser treatment in maculopathy of pseudoxanthoma elasticum. Can J Ophthalmol 13:210–212, 1978.
86. Brancato R, Menchini U, Pece A, et al: Laser treatment of macular subretinal neovascularizations in angioid streaks. Ophthalmologica 195:84–87, 1987.
87. Gelisken O, Hendrikse F, Deutman AF: A long-term follow-up study of laser coagulation of neovascular membranes in angioid streaks. Am J Ophthalmol 105:299–303, 1988.
88. Esente S, Francais C, Soubrane G, Coscas G: Stries angioides et néovaisseaux sous-rétiniens: étude rétrospective des résultats de la photocoagulation au laser au krypton et au laser à argon vert. Bull Soc Ophtalmol Fr 87:293–296, 1987.
89. Lim JI, Bressler NM, Marsh MJ, Bressler SB: Laser treatment of choroidal neovascularization in patients with angioid streaks. Am J Ophthalmol 116:414–423, 1993.

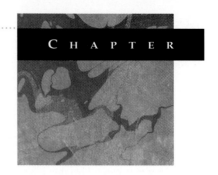

CHAPTER 16

Ocular Histoplasmosis

Eric S. Mann, M.D., Ph.D.
Travis A. Meredith, M.D.

The presumed ocular histoplasmosis syndrome (POHS), or simply ocular histoplasmosis syndrome (OHS), describes a choroidopathy that afflicts healthy young adults and may cause severe visual loss. The syndrome is most prevalent in areas of the United States where the fungus *Histoplasma capsulatum* is endemic. The primary cause of visual loss in ocular histoplasmosis is the sequelae of choroidal neovascularization (CNV) in the macula, which results in exudation and subsequent scarring causing permanent reduction in visual acuity. Current treatment to prevent visual loss includes laser photocoagulation to ablate neovascular membranes that spare the center of the fovea and submacular surgery to remove these membranes once they become subfoveal. Other less common types of ocular involvement by *H. capsulatum* not reviewed here include histoplasmic endophthalmitis and solitary histoplasmic chorioretinal granulomas often found in immunocompromised individuals. Herein, we describe the pathogenesis, natural history, and clinical features of the ocular histoplasmosis syndrome and review its current management and treatment.

HISTORICAL BACKGROUND

Woods and Whalen in 1959 were the first to describe an ocular syndrome of disciform macular detachment associated with peripheral chorioretinal scars in healthy young adults.[1] Schlaegel and Kenney in 1966 later added peripapillary atrophy to form the classic triad of the presumed ocular histoplasmosis syndrome.[2]

Activation of these atrophic chorioretinal lesions with histoplasmin skin testing[1,3,4] along with positive reactions to histoplasmin antigen in many of the patients with this ocular syndrome[1] led many investigators to conclude that the fungus *H. capsulatum* may be the cause of such a choroiditis without inflammation in the vitreous.

POHS and *H. capsulatum*

The clinical entity ocular histoplasmosis is often termed POHS because Koch's postulates have not proven the dimorphic fungus *H. capsulatum* to be the causative agent of this ocular disease.[5,6] The *H. capsulatum* organism has never been cultured from an individual with POHS or isolated from an eye with any of the classic lesions of POHS. Other reports of histopathologic identification of *H. capsulatum* in ocular tissue have either been contested[7] or occurred in patients with disseminated histoplasmosis.[8–10]

Instead, epidemiologic evidence has been used to implicate this fungus as the etiologic agent of POHS. The etiologic relationship between *H. capsulatum* and POHS is based on both the similar geographic distribution of POHS and *H. capsulatum* infection in the United States (i.e., areas endemic to histoplasmosis) and on results of histoplasmin skin testing in patients with POHS. The highest prevalence of POHS occurs in areas endemic for histoplasmosis and is rare outside these areas.[11] In addition, almost all patients with POHS have lived in or visited an endemic area.[12,13] Finally, more than 90% of patients with POHS demonstrate a positive histoplasmin skin test,[14–16] and such skin testing has reportedly activated previously quiescent chorioretinal lesions in POHS.[1,3,4] Histoplasmin skin testing is therefore not recommended for the clinical diagnosis of POHS because of the possibility of activation of old choroidal lesions.

178

HISTOPATHOLOGICAL FEATURES

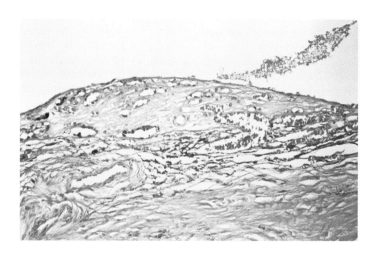

Mound-shaped macular scar, covered by retinal pigment epithelium, composed of fibrovascular tissue, hyperplastic retinal pigment epithelium, and blood vessel from the choroid is from a patient with the ocular histoplasmosis syndrome. (From Meredith TA, Green WR, Kay SN III, et al: Ocular histoplasmosis: clinicopathologic correlation of three cases. Surv Ophthalmol 22:189–205, 1977, with permission.)

GEOGRAPHIC DISTRIBUTION

The similar geographic distribution of POHS and infection with histoplasmosis (as determined by positive histoplasmin skin testing) is suggestive evidence of the etiological role of *H. capsulatum* in this ocular condition. Endemic areas of histoplasmosis include most of the Ohio and Mississippi river valleys encompassing Indiana, Ohio, Illinois, Kentucky, Tennessee, and Mississippi. This region of the United States places approximately 80 million people at risk for ocular involvement with this condition. The organism is also encountered in the Southeast and Middle Atlantic states within the United States as well as other areas of the world. Ocular findings that are clinically indistinguishable from POHS in patients from Europe and Great Britain who have negative skin tests[17] and have never visited or lived in an endemic area may result from infection with an organism that produces an ocular syndrome which is a phenocopy of POHS.[18] Infection with *H. capsulatum* is localized to endemic areas where infection is documented by positive skin tests to histoplasmin in over 60% of the population.[16] Ocular disease, though, remains uncommon among patients with a positive histoplasmin skin test. For example, in Maryland (an endemic state for histoplasmosis) approximately 4% of those infected with histoplasmosis demonstrate clinical evidence of POHS.[16] Residing in an endemic area for at least 2 weeks (Nozik, personal communication) incurs a risk of infection with histoplasmosis.

CLINICAL FEATURES

The diagnosis of POHS is suggested by the characteristic clinical features which include the observation of small atrophic "punched-out" chorioretinal scars ("histo spots") in the midperiphery or posterior pole and peripapillary chorioretinal scarring, with and without active choroidal neovascularization or disciform scarring in the macula (Fig. 16–1). These discrete focal lesions occur frequently in both eyes without anterior or vitreous inflammation. Linear streaks of atrophic scars in a curvilinear row may be found about the equator in 5% of patients.[18,19] Visual loss occurs as a sequela of macular CNV formation. Choroidal neovascularization grows through defects in Bruch's membrane. Typically, a gray-green lesion is seen beneath the retina. There may be some blood, fluid, or lipid associated with this (Fig. 16–2). The fluorescein angiography in these lesions usually shows early hyperfluorescence of a cartwheel lesion with sharply defined margins. As the angiogram goes forward, there is leakage of dye into the subretinal space, usually leading to a fuzzy area of hyperfluorescence in the late phases.

PREVALENCE

POHS afflicts young adults between the second and fifth decades of life[20,21] without preference for gender. Population-based studies of ocular histoplasmosis in the United States show that peripheral atrophic lesions are more common than the macular disciform scar; atrophic scars occur in 1.6 to 2.5% of people living in an endemic area[16,22,23] but in 4.4% of positive responders to the histoplasmin skin test.[16] The prevalence rate of disciform scarring in an endemic population is estimated to be 1.2 per 1000 or 0.1%.[16] Prevalence rates of ocular histoplasmosis with regard to race reveal blacks rarely manifest disciform macular lesions[15,24] despite the prevalence of peripheral atrophic scars and positive histoplasmin skin tests being equal among black and whites.[15,22,15]

INCIDENCE AND NATURAL HISTORY

The natural history of atrophic scars in the various regions of the fundus reveals evolution in a significant percentage of eyes.[26,27] Long-term follow-up of eyes with ocular histoplasmosis demonstrate both new atrophic scars and changes in old scars.[28] Old scars in the macula may disappear and reappear in the same spot or in new areas as choroiditis develops elsewhere in the macula. Changes in atrophic scarring manifested by increased size or formation of new scars in the macula, peripapillary region, or retinal periphery occurred in 57% of eyes studied in one report.[27] In other studies new macular scars not present on the baseline fluorescein angiogram developed in 17 to 19% of eyes followed on average 8.5 to 10 years.[23,29] Fluorescein angiography often reveals defects in the retinal pigment epithelium (RPE) that may not be visible in color photographs. The incidence of new scars found in the retinal periphery by color photographs is similar to that observed in the macular area.[27]

Incidence of Fellow Eye Involvement

The risk to the second eye is of great concern to the patient who has lost vision in one eye from POHS. The fellow eye of a patient with a disciform lesion in the contralateral eye must be observed carefully by the ophthalmologist and self-monitored by the patient with the daily use of an Amsler grid. The average interval between the onset of symptoms in the first eye and the second eye is 4 years.[27]

The risk of developing CNV in the fellow eye with visual loss depends on the initial ocular findings in the second eye. The presence of macular and peripapillary scars are significant risk factors for CNV formation and subsequent visual loss in the

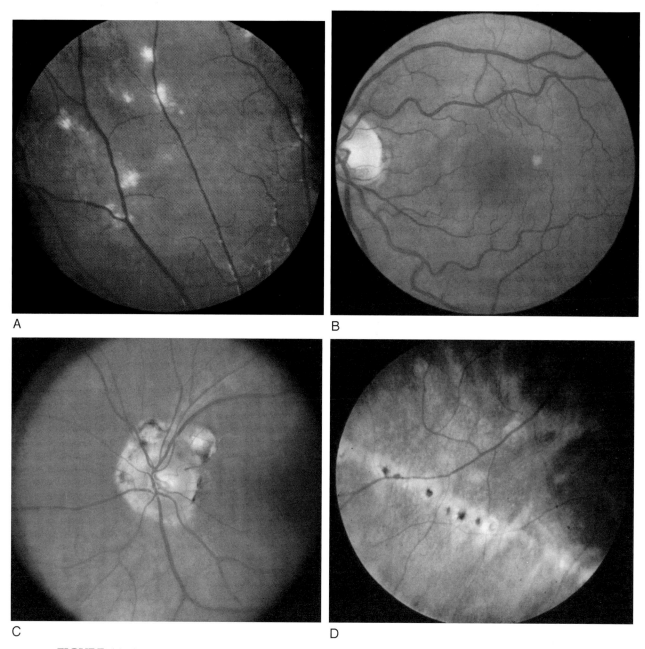

FIGURE 16–1   Clinical features of ocular histoplasmosis. *A,* Peripheral "histo spots." *B,* Macular histo spots. *C,* Peripapillary atrophy. *D,* "Linear streaks."

fellow eye.[15,20] Most CNV occurs at the sites of previous "histo scars." The risk of developing symptomatic choroidal neovascularization within the macula in the second eye with macular scars is estimated to be approximately 20 to 24%,[15,23,27,31,32] whereas the risk of a peripapillary membrane in eyes with peripapillary scarring is approximately 4%[23] over 8 years' average follow-up. In the Macular Photocoagulation Study (MPS) the incidence of development of choroidal neovascularization in 394 fellow eyes was a nearly constant rate of about 2% per year for the 5 years of follow-up. Notably, one study found only an 8% incidence of CNV in asymptomatic fellow eyes with atrophic spots during an average follow-up of 39 months.[39]

The risk of developing symptomatic lesions in the second eye is not influenced by the age of onset of visual symptoms in the primary eye or by the distribution, severity, and changes (size and number) in atrophic macular scars in the fellow eye. Because the chance of macular involvement with CNV depends primarily on the presence of histo spots within the macula,[23] eyes without atrophic macular scars have a much better prognosis, al-

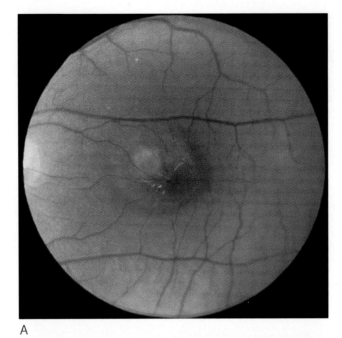

A

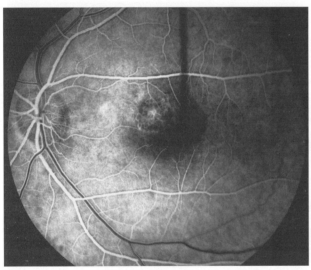

B1

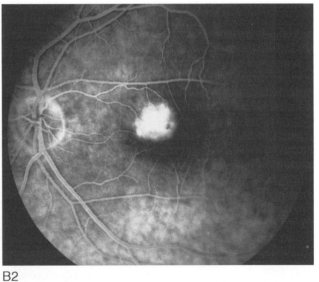

B2

FIGURE 16–2   Choroidal neovascularization (CNV) of ocular histoplasmosis. *A,* Fundus photograph. The photograph shows a classic gray-green lesion beneath the retina. These membranes are often anterior to the pigment epithelium. *B,* Fluorescein angiogram. (1) Early phase of fluorescein angiogram shows early hyperfluorescence of CNV. (2) Late phase of fluorescein angiogram shows late leakage of fluorescein dye from the CNV.

though de novo subretinal neovascularization can occur.[34,35] In the absence of macular scars, the risk of a symptomatic lesion in the fellow eye is less than 1% per year of follow-up.[23,36] In the MPS, macular histo spots of any kind tripled the risk of later development of subretinal new vessels compared to eyes with no spots.

VISUAL PROGNOSIS, RECOVERY, AND EXACERBATION

Exudative maculopathy due to new vessel membranes and subsequent disciform scarring accounts for most of the visual loss observed in POHS. Atrophic scars alone usually do not affect visual function. Approximately 1 adult in 1000 of the population in an endemic area will have disciform maculopathy in one eye from POHS.[16,37] It has also been estimated that one affected patient in ten will have involvement in both macula.[37] Since over 50% of patients with untreated disciform maculopathy within the foveal avascular zone ultimately end up with 20/200 or worse vision in the involved eye,[15,27,31,33,38–40] approximately 1 adult in 40,000 will become legally blind without treatment.[20] POHS remains an uncommon cause of blindness with an annual incidence of 2.8% and prevalence of 0.5% in the blind population of Tennessee.[20]

Spontaneous visual recovery after visual loss may follow active exudation[41–44] or occur after disciform macular scarring secondary to CNV.[33,45,46] Spontaneous involution of subfoveal neovascularization has been observed in POHS as well as in response to corticosteroid therapy.[37,47] The phenomenon of improvement in Snellen acuity in an affected eye after loss of vision in the fellow eye has been described and is not unique to POHS. When patients experience visual loss in the fellow eye, spontaneous visual recovery may occasionally occur with eccentric fixation[48] or by reversal of an organic amblyopia with disappearance of the central scotoma.[49]

PATHOGENESIS

The pathogenesis of POHS is believed to begin with an initial benign systemic infection with *H. capsulatum*. The overwhelming majority of histoplasmosis infections are benign and asymptomatic; upper respiratory symptoms are the most common symptomatic presentation. Ocular histoplasmosis, however, does not become apparent until some 10 to 30 years later.[13] POHS rarely follows disseminated infection with *H. capsulatum* or chronic pulmonary histoplasmosis.

Histoplasmosis infection is acquired early in life, probably during adolescence, through inhalation of mycelial spores. Transformation to the yeast phase of the organism occurs within the lung. Subsequent hematogenous dissemination of this yeast phase results in the finding of multiple foci of dead or latent *Histoplasma* in numerous organs at autopsy.[26] These foci may become sources themselves of subsequent asymptomatic transient episodes of *Histoplasma* fungemia. Such episodes of fungemia may eventually seed the choroid to produce a multifocal granulomatous chorioretinitis that heals as atrophic scars as the host response rapidly destroys the organism.[50–53] Such a model explains why organisms are not identified by histopathology or culture. Hematogenous dissemination of *H. capsulatum* to the eye also explains the frequent bilaterality, the number and random distribution of histo spots throughout the fundus,[15,21] and the evolution of changing patterns of peripheral atrophic histo spots over many years.[26,27,30,54]

When the focus of chorioretinitis involves the macula, injury to Bruch's membrane, RPE, or choriocapillaris may result in an atrophic scar, choroidal neovascular membrane, or exudative retinal detachment. Subretinal hemorrhage, from either choroidal neovascularization or direct damage to the RPE or choriocapillaris, may heal as a fibrovascular scar. The clinical observation of disciform maculopathy contiguous to atrophic scars in individuals with POHS[15,50] supports such a pathophysiologic model.

The cause of abnormal growth of blood vessels is unknown. Choroidal neovascularization may be a wound-healing response particular to the unique anatomic properties of the macula. Genetic predisposition to form atrophic scars and disciform lesions at these histo spots within the macula is suggested from histocompatibility data. Ophthalmoscopic findings at the time of initial systemic infection with histoplasmosis are rarely seen probably because of the asymptomatic nature and small subclinical size of the funduscopic lesions. Reactivation of these lesions with re-exposure to the histoplasmin antigen years later may explain why the choroidal vasculature surrounding an atrophic scar proliferates as a neovascular membrane.[15]

HUMAN LEUKOCYTE ANTIGEN ASSOCIATIONS

Why do some patients infected with *H. capsulatum* develop POHS whereas most do not? Hereditary differences in infected patients marked by histocompatibility antigens may predispose some to ocular disease. The prevalence of histocompatibility antigens among cases of POHS suggests a genetic predisposition for the development of peripheral atrophic spots and disciform macular scarring. Human leukocyte antigen (HLA) analysis in POHS patients reveals both HLA-B7[55,56] and HLA-DRw2[57] to be more common among patients with disciform lesions than control populations. POHS patients with only peripheral atrophic scars demonstrate an increased frequency of the HLA-DRw2 but not the HLA-B7 allele.[58] Perhaps expression of both the B7 and DRw2 alleles predispose patients to exudative maculopathy. Interestingly, POHS in black patients with disciform lesions shows no HLA-B7 association but a strong correlation with DRw2 compared with control populations.[24]

TREATMENT

Multiple treatment modalities have been advocated for patients with POHS and exudative maculopathy that typically end in visual loss from disciform macular scars. Only laser ablation of CNV has been demonstrated to reduce the risk of visual loss from CNV in the macula.[41–43] Treatment paradigms of choroidal neovascularization in eyes with POHS to prevent visual loss are governed by the location of the CNV with respect to the center of the foveal avascular zone. Laser photocoagulation of well-defined extrafoveal or juxtafoveal neovascular membranes (Table 16–1) has been demonstrated by the MPS studies to be unequivocally effective in reducing the risk of visual loss when compared to the natural history of the disease.[41–43] A recent report from the MPS study also recommends treatment of peripapillary CNV lesions.[59] Prophylactic treatment of inactive macular scars to prevent the development of exudative neovascular membranes is not recommended.[60,61]

TABLE 16–1   Macular Photocoagulation Study: Distribution of Laser-Treated and Untreated Eyes by Specific Visual Acuity 5 Years After Enrollment for Extrafoveal CNV*

Visual Acuity (Snellen Fraction)†	OHS, Laser-Treatment Group‡ No. (%)	OHS, No-Treatment Group§ No. (%)
20/20 or better	45 (39)	34 (29)
20/25 to 20/40	34 (29)	16 (14)
20/50 to 20/80	18 (16)	14 (12)
20/100 to 20/160	9 (8)	10 (9)
20/200 to 20/320	9 (8)	28 (24)
20/400 to 20/640	1 (1)	10 (9)
20/800 or worse	0	4 (3)
Total	116 (100)	116 (100)

* Macular Photocoagulation Study Group: Argon laser photocoagulation for neovascular maculopathy. Five-year results from randomized clinical trials. Arch Ophthalmol 109:1109–1114, 1991. Copyright 1991, American Medical Association, with permission.

† Wilcoxon rank sum, $p < .001$.

‡ Mean visual acuity, 20/40.

§ Mean visual acuity, 20/80.

Laser Photocoagulation: Macular Photocoagulation Study

Early reports of the benefit of photocoagulation using xenon or argon treatment of CNV provided no clarification as to the role of photocoagulation in the treatment of POHS.[15,27] The MPS was a multicenter, randomized clinical trial supported by the National Eye Institute which assessed the role of argon (blue-green) laser photocoagulation as a treatment for symptomatic choroidal neovascular membranes that do not involve the center of the fovea.

In 1983, the MPS group demonstrated the effectiveness of argon laser photocoagulation of active, well-defined extrafoveal CNV (i.e., CNV >200 μm from the center of the foveal avascular zone) secondary to POHS in reducing the risk of severe visual loss.[41] In the MPS studies, severe visual loss corresponds to a loss of six lines of Snellen acuity equivalent to quadrupling the minimum angle of resolution. The 5-year results reported in 1991 by the MPS group for eyes treated for extrafoveal CNV secondary to POHS upheld earlier recommendations of the MPS. Untreated eyes had 3.6 times the risk of severe visual loss of laser-treated eyes with 42% of untreated eyes as compared to only 12% of laser-treated eyes, demonstrating a decrease in visual acuity of six lines or more from baseline.[43] Table 16–1 demonstrates the distribution of laser-treated and untreated eyes at each specific level of visual acuity five years after enrollment and randomization.

The proportion of eyes at each follow-up examination that had lost six or more lines of visual acuity from the baseline examination to each follow-up exam for both treated and untreated eyes is demonstrated in Figure 16–3. Patients are advised to undergo prompt treatment of extrafoveal CNV with laser photocoagulation.

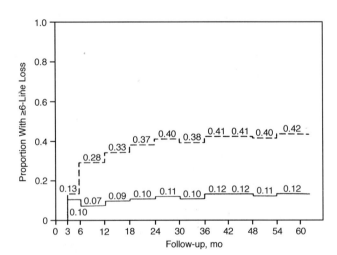

FIGURE 16–3   MPS: Proportion of eyes with severe visual loss (six or more lines of visual acuity loss from baseline level) at each follow-up examination for laser-treated (*solid line*) and untreated eyes (*dashed line*) with extrafoveal CNV. (From Macular Photocoagulation Study Group: Argon laser photocoagulation for neovascular maculopathy. Five-year results from randomized clinical trials. Arch Ophthalmol 109:1109–1114, 1991. Copyright 1991, American Medical Association, with permission.)

Krypton laser photocoagulation for juxtafoveal CNV (i.e., CNV 1 to 199 μm from the center of the foveal avascular zone or 200 μm or more from the center of the foveal avascular zone with blood and/or blocked fluorescence within 200 μm of the foveal avascular zone center) secondary to POHS was demonstrated in 1987 by the MPS to prevent severe visual loss.[42] The visual results after laser photocoagulation of CNV reveal that after 5 years of follow-up, 28% of untreated eyes in contrast to 12% of treated eyes had lost six or more lines of visual acuity.[62] Figure 16−4 demonstrates the distribution of laser-treated and untreated eyes at each specific level of visual acuity. The proportion of eyes at each follow-up examination that had lost six or more lines of visual acuity from the baseline examination for both treated and untreated eyes is demonstrated in Figure 16−5. Accurate and complete krypton laser treatment of juxtafoveal CNV, particularly on the foveal side, lessens persistent CNV[63] and is required to avoid further severe visual loss.[64] In a retrospective, nonrandomized analysis, the long-term visual results of laser-treated extrafoveal and juxtafoveal CNV in eyes with POHS demonstrated the long-term benefit of photocoagulation proposed by the MPS over an average follow-up of 9.6 years.[65]

Persistent and recurrent CNV are a significant concern in laser-treated CNV and a cause of severe visual loss after laser treatment. In defining recurrent CNV, the MPS included CNV occurring at 6 weeks or later from the time of laser treatment. Persistent CNV occurs within 6 weeks of laser treatment. Persistent or recurrent CNV may occur contiguous with the border or within the laser treatment scar (frequently on the foveal side). New independent neovascular complexes not contiguous or within the photocoagulation scar were not classified as recurrent CNV. The MPS Group re-

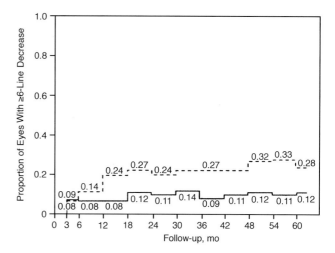

FIGURE 16−5   MPS: Proportion of eyes with severe visual loss (six or more lines of visual acuity loss from baseline level) at each follow-up examination for laser-treated (*solid line*) and untreated eyes (*dashed line*) with juxtafoveal CNV. (From Macular Photocoagulation Study Group: Laser photocoagulation for juxtafoveal choroidal neovascularization. Arch Ophthalmol 112: 500−509, 1994. Copyright 1994, American Medical Association, with permission.)

ported a 5-year incidence of recurrence of 26% with treated extrafoveal CNV.[43] New areas of CNV not contiguous with the laser scar developed in another 7% of laser-treated eyes.[43] Krypton-treated juxtafoveal CNV in eyes with POHS demonstrated an incidence of persistent or recurrent CNV of 33% and new independent CNV in noncontiguous laser-treated areas in an additional 2% of eyes.[62] Thus, recommendations for high-risk patients (i.e., those with atrophic macular scars, recently treated with laser, or who have lost vision in the fellow eye) include self-monitoring with an Amsler grid and urgent fundus examination if symptoms occur.

Visual loss may also occur due to CNV origination from a peripapillary scar.[66−68] Although the natural history of POHS-related peripapillary CNV is not well known, it is believed to be better than macular CNV, due to the greater distance from the foveal avascular zone. The MPS has recently evaluated whether laser photocoagulation of peripapillary CNV mitigates severe visual loss when compared to no treatment. Among eyes with peripapillary lesions, no statistically significant effect of treatment was observed, although 12% more untreated eyes lost six lines or more of visual acuity than did treated eyes. The difference between laser-treated and untreated eyes was more marked when the change in visual acuity from baseline to the 3-year examination was considered (Table 16−2). Therefore, the MPS group recommended laser treatment of peripapillary CNV.[59] Severe visual loss and extensive visual field defects occur rarely after photocoagulation of peripapillary CNV from thermal damage to the optic disc or retinal nerve fiber layer.[59,66,69] The risks of laser treatment of peripapillary CNV appear to be outweighed by the loss of

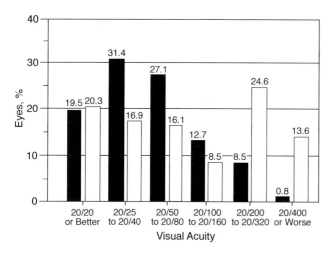

FIGURE 16−4   MPS: Percent distribution of laser-treated and untreated eyes by specific visual acuity 5 years after enrollment for juxtafoveal CNV. (From Macular Photocoagulation Study Group: Laser photocoagulation for juxtafoveal choroidal neovascularization. Arch Ophthalmol 112:500−509, 1994. Copyright 1994, American Medical Association, with permission.)

TABLE 16–2   Macular Photocoagulation Study: Distribution by Specific Visual Acuity and Change from Baseline for Laser-Treated and Untreated Eyes 3 Years After Enrollment for Peripapillary CNV*

	Peripapillary, No. (%)		Nasal, No. (%)		All, No. (%)	
	Treatment	Observation	Treatment	Observation	Treatment	Observation
Visual acuity						
20/20 or better	3 (14)	3 (13)	9 (28)	3 (11)	12 (22)	6 (12)
20/25 to 20/40	8 (36)	7 (30)	5 (16)	5 (18)	13 (24)	12 (24)
20/50 to 20/100	3 (14)	4 (17)	11 (34)	6 (21)	14 (26)	10 (20)
20/125 to 20/200	4 (18)	2 (9)	4 (13)	5 (18)	8 (15)	7 (14)
20/250 to 20/400	2 (9)	2 (9)	2 (6)	7 (25)	4 (7)	9 (18)
20/500 or worse	2 (9)	5 (22)	1 (3)	2 (7)	3 (6)	7 (14)
Total	22	23	32	28	54	51
_p_†	.54		.02		.03	
Visual acuity change						
≥2 lines increase	3 (14)	5 (22)	8 (25)	4 (14)	11 (20)	9 (18)
No change	10 (45)	4 (17)	14 (44)	5 (18)	24 (44)	9 (18)
2–3 lines decrease	4 (18)	4 (17)	5 (16)	2 (7)	9 (17)	6 (12)
4–5 lines decrease	2 (9)	4 (17)	2 (6)	2 (7)	4 (7)	6 (12)
≥6 lines decrease	3 (14)	6 (26)	3 (9)	15 (54)	6 (11)	21 (43)
Total	22	23	32	28	54	51
_p_†	.29		<.001		<.001	

* From Macular Photocoagulation Study Group: Laser photocoagulation for neovascular lesions nasal to the fovea (results from clinical trials for lesions secondary to ocular histoplasmosis or idiopathic causes). Arch Ophthalmol 113:56–61, 1995. Copyright 1995, American Medical Association, with permission.

† _p_ value for exact trend test with quantitatively ordered classes.

vision caused by the growth of CNV with involvement of the fovea.[59]

Although photocoagulation remains our current therapeutic tool in the treatment of CNV that spares the center of the fovea in eyes with POHS, subfoveal CNV demonstrates no clear benefit from laser treatment.[70] Patients with POHS complicated by subfoveal CNV have a poor visual prognosis.[15,27,31,33,38–40] A pilot, randomized trial produced no conclusive evidence in an effort to determine whether laser treatment of subfoveal CNV in POHS was effective.[70] Nevertheless, most experts feel that laser photocoagulation of subfoveal CNV in patients with POHS offers little benefit over the natural history without treatment. Laser treatment must justify sacrificing the 14 to 23% of eyes with POHS complicated by subfoveal CNV that retain a visual acuity of 20/40 or better[33,40,65] in order to reduce the severity of visual loss in the majority of eyes destined to develop 20/200 or less. A treatment algorithm of subfoveal choroidal neovascularization may include systemic or periocular steroids for several weeks in an attempt to elicit resolution or inactivation of small subretinal neovascular complexes. Oral prednisone at a daily dose of 60 to 100 mg for several weeks has been

anecdotally reported to cause inactivation of CNV in POHS. However, no controlled trial has ever demonstrated treatment with systemic or periocular corticosteroids to result in better visual results than the natural course without treatment.[33] Nevertheless, subfoveal CNV in POHS usually leads to significant and permanent loss of central vision. Ninety per cent of eyes with visual acuity of 20/200 or less from subfoveal CNV will remain with severely reduced vision after 3 years.[33] Given the poor natural history and limited therapeutic value of laser photocoagulation, surgical alternatives have recently been explored.

Submacular Surgery

Surgical removal of subfoveal CNV is potentially less damaging to the neurosensory retina than laser treatment. Submacular surgery for subfoveal CNV in POHS appears to improve visual function compared with either the natural history of the disease or with laser photocoagulation. In a nonrandomized, uncontrolled, retrospective report, 31% of 67 eyes with POHS that underwent surgery for subfoveal CNV achieved a visual acuity of 20/40 or better with an average follow-up of 10.5 months.[71] Eyes with better preoperative vision (>20/100) had a significantly better final visual acuity than eyes with poor preoperative vision (<20/200).[71] Recurrence of CNV did not affect the final visual acuity because many of these recurrences were treated successfully with laser photocoagulation. Further data will allow appropriate case selection and surgical timing of intervention to maximize visual benefit from submacular surgery.

Thus, surgical removal of CNV is technically feasible and usually can be accomplished without serious complications.[71-73] The surgical instrumentation and techniques have been refined[74,75] and allow the surgical management of CNV of many different etiologies. CNV in eyes with POHS often arise from focal defects in Bruch's membrane and proliferate anterior to the RPE.[76] This type of membrane may be removed with preservation of the underlying RPE and choriocapillaris requisite to restoring visual function. Submacular surgery, though, has specific operative risks in addition to the inherent risks of all vitrectomy surgery, which include severe ocular and systemic morbidity. Retinal detachment, retinal tears without detachment, endophthalmitis, subretinal hemorrhage, progressive cataract, and premacular fibrosis may all be encountered.

A randomized, controlled, prospective, multicenter clinical trial to further evaluate subfoveal surgery has been organized. The Submacular Surgery Trial (SST) will evaluate subfoveal surgery as compared to observation for the treatment of eyes with POHS and subfoveal CNV. Further research is needed to better understand the pathophysiologic process that results in choroidal neovascularization and to develop animal models to explore potential antiangiogenic drugs to intervene in that process.

REFERENCES

1. Woods AC, Whalen HE: The probable role of benign histoplasmosis in the etiology of granulomatous uveitis. Trans Am Ophthalmol Soc 57:318–343, 1959.
2. Schlaegel TF, Kenney D: Changes around the optic nerve head in presumed ocular histoplasmosis. Am J Ophthalmol 62:454–458, 1966.
3. Krause AC, Hopkins WG: Ocular manifestation of histoplasmosis. Am J Ophthalmol 39:564–566, 1951.
4. Schlaegel TF: Granulomatous uveitis: an etiologic survey of 100 cases. Trans Am Acad Ophthalmol Otolaryngol 62:813–825, 1958.
5. Wong VG, Kwong-Chung KJ, Hill WB: Koch's postulates and experimental ocular histoplasmosis. Int Ophthalmol Clin 15:139–145, 1975.
6. Schlaegel TF, Weber JC, Helveston E, Kenney D: Presumed histoplasmic choroiditis. Am J Ophthalmol 63:919–925, 1967.
7. Gass JD, Zimmerman LE: Histopathologic demonstration of Histoplasma capsulatum. Am J Ophthalmol 85:725, 1978.
8. Craig EL, Suie T: Histoplasma capsulatum in human ocular tissue. Arch Ophthalmol 91:285–289, 1974.
9. Klintworth GK, Hollingsworth AS, Lusman PA, Bradford WD: Granulomatous choroiditis in a case of disseminated histoplasmosis. Arch Ophthalmol 92:45–48, 1973.
10. Goldstein BG, Buettner H: Histoplasmic endophthalmitis. A clinicopathologic correlation. Arch Ophthalmol 101:774–777, 1983.
11. Ellis FD, Schlaegel TF: The geographic localization of presumed histoplasmic choroiditis. Am J Ophthalmol 75:953–956, 1973.
12. Van Metre TE, Maumence AE: Specific ocular uveal lesions in patients with evidence of histoplasmosis. Arch Ophthalmol 71:314–324, 1964.
13. Ganley JP: Epidemiologic characteristics of presumed ocular histoplasmosis. Acta Ophthalmol Suppl 119:1–63, 1973.
14. Check IJ, Diddie KR, Jay WM: Lymphocyte stimulation by yeast phase Histoplasma capsulatum in presumed ocular histoplasmosis syndrome. Am J Ophthalmol 87:311, 1979.
15. Gass JDM, Wilkinson CP: Follow-up study of presumed ocular histoplasmosis. Trans Am Acad Ophthalmol Otolaryngol 76:672–694, 1972.
16. Smith RE, Ganley JP: An epidemiological study of presumed ocular histoplasmosis. Trans Am Ophthalmol Otolaryngol 75:994–1005, 1971.
17. Braunstein RA, Rosen DA, Bird AC: Ocular histoplasmosis syndrome in the United Kingdom. Br J Ophthalmol 58:893–898, 1974.
18. Bottoni FG, Deutman AF, Aandekerk AL: Presumed ocular histoplasmosis syndrome and linear streak lesions. Br J Ophthalmol 73:528–535, 1989.
19. Fountain JA, Schlaegel TFJ: Linear streaks of the equator in presumed ocular histoplasmosis syndrome. Arch Ophthalmol 99:246, 1981.
20. Feman SS, Podgorski SF, Penn MK: Blindness from presumed ocular histoplasmosis in Tennessee. Ophthalmology 89:1295–1298, 1982.
21. Smith RE, Ganley JP, Knox DL: Presumed ocular histoplasmosis. II. Patterns of peripheral and peripapillary scarring in persons with nonmacular disease. Arch Ophthalmol 87:251–257, 1972.
22. Asbury T: The status of presumed ocular histoplasmosis; including a report of a survey. Trans Am Ophthalmol Soc 64:371–400, 1966.
23. Lewis ML, Schiffman JC: Long-term follow-up of the second eye in ocular histoplasmosis. Int Ophthalmol Clin 23:281–285, 1983.
24. Baskin MA, Jampol LM, Huamonte FU, et al: Macular lesions in blacks with the presumed ocular histoplasmosis syndrome. Am J Ophthalmol 89:77–83, 1980.
25. Edwards PQ, Palmer CE: Sensitivity to histoplasmin among negro and white residents of different communities in the USA. Bull WHO 30:575–585, 1964.
26. Schlaegel TF: The natural history of histo spots in the disc and macular area. Int Ophthalmol Clin 15:19, 1975.
27. Lewis ML, Van Newkirk MR, Gass JD: Follow-up study of presumed ocular histoplasmosis syndrome. Ophthalmology 87:390, 1980.
28. Watzke RC, Claussen RW: The long-term course of multifocal choroiditis (presumed ocular histoplasmosis). Am J Ophthalmol 91:750–760, 1981.
29. Watzke RC, Claussen R: The long term course of multifocal choroiditis (presumed ocular histoplasmosis). Am J Ophthalmol 91:750, 1981.
30. Krill AE, Christi MI, Klein BA: Multifocal choroiditis. Trans Am Acad Ophthalmol Otolaryngol 73:222–245, 1969.
31. Elliot JH, Jackson DJ: Presumed histoplasmic maculopathy: clinical course and prognosis in nonphotocoagulated eyes. Int Ophthalmol Clin 15:29, 1975.
32. Sawelson H, Goldberg RE, Annesley WH, Tomer TL: Presumed ocular histoplasmosis syndrome. The fellow eye. Arch Ophthalmol 94:221–224, 1976.
33. Olk RJ, Burgess DB, McCormick PA: Subfoveal and juxtafoveal subretinal neovascularization in the presumed ocular histoplasmosis syndrome. Visual prognosis. Ophthalmology 91:1592–1602, 1984.
34. Miller SA, Stevens TS, DeVenecia G: De novo lesions in presumed ocular histoplasmosis-like syndrome. Br J Ophthalmol 60:700–712, 1976.

35. Ryan SJ Jr: De novo subretinal neovascularization in the histoplasmosis syndrome. Arch Ophthalmol 94:321–327, 1976.

36. Schlaegel TF: In discussion of Gass JDM and Wilkinson CP: Follow-up study of presumed ocular histoplasmosis. Trans Am Acad Ophthalmol Otolaryngol 76:695, 1972.

37. Schlaegel TF: Treatment of the POHS. In Schlaegel TF (ed): Ocular Histoplasmosis New York, Raven Press, 1977, pp. 209–259.

38. Klein ML, Fine SL, Patz A: Follow-up study in eyes with choroidal neovascularization caused by presumed ocular histoplasmosis. Am J Ophthalmol 83:830–835, 1977.

39. Gutman FA: The natural course of active choroidal lesions in the presumed ocular histoplasmosis syndrome. Trans Am Ophthalmol Soc 77:515–541, 1979.

40. Kleiner RC, Ratner C, Enger C: Subfoveal neovascularization in the ocular histoplasmosis syndrome. Retina 8:225, 1988.

41. Macular Photocoagulation Study Group: Argon laser photocoagulation for histoplasmosis: results of a randomized clinical trial. Arch Ophthalmol 101:1347–1357, 1983.

42. Macular Photocoagulation Study Group: Krypton laser photocoagulation for neovascular lesions of ocular histoplasmosis: results of a randomized clinical trial. Arch Ophthalmol 105:1499–1507, 1987.

43. Macular Photocoagulation Study Group: Argon laser photocoagulation for neovascular maculopathy. Five-year results from randomized clinical trials. Arch Ophthalmol 109:1109–1114, 1991.

44. Campochiaro PA, Morgan KM, Conway BP, Stathos J: Spontaneous involution of subfoveal neovascularization. Am J Ophthalmol 109:668–675, 1990.

45. Orlando RG, Davidorf EH: Spontaneous recovery phenomenon in the presumed ocular histoplasmosis syndrome. Int Ophthalmol Clin 23:137–149, 1983.

46. Singerman LJ, Wong BA, Smith S: Spontaneous visual improvement in the first affected eye of patients with bilateral disciform scars. Retina 5:135, 1985.

47. Gass JDM: Stereoscopic Atlas of Macular Diseases: Diagnosis and Treatment. 3rd edition. St Louis, CV Mosby Co, 1987, pp 112–128.

48. Harris MJ, Robbins D, Dieter JM: Eccentric visual acuity in patients with macular disease. Ophthalmology 92:1550, 1985.

49. Jost BF, Olk RJ, Burgess DB: Factors related to spontaneous visual recovery in the ocular histoplasmosis syndrome. Retina 7:1–8, 1987.

50. Smith RE, O'Connor GR, Halde CJ, et al: Clinical course in rabbits after experimental induction of ocular histoplasmosis. Am J Ophthalmol 76:284, 1973.

51. Smith RE, Scalarone M, O'Connor GR, et al: Detection of *Histoplasma capsulatum* by fluorescent antibody techniques in experimental ocular histoplasmosis. Am J Ophthalmol 76:375, 1973.

52. Smith RE, Dunn S, Jester JV: Natural history of experimental choroiditis in the primates. Am J Ophthalmol 76:284, 1984.

53. Smith RE, Dunn S, Jester JV: Natural history of experimental histoplasmic choroiditis in the primate. II. Histopathologic features. Invest Ophthalmol Vis Sci 25:810, 1984.

54. Tewari RP, Sharma DK, Mathur A: Significance of thymus-derived lymphocytes in immunity elicited by immunization with ribosomes or live yeast cells of *Histoplasma capsulatum*. J Infect Dis 138:605–613, 1978.

55. Braley RE, Meredith TA, Aaberg TM, et al: The prevalence of HLA-B7 in presumed ocular histoplasmosis. Am J Ophthalmol 85:859–861, 1978.

56. Godfery WA, Sabates R, Cross DE: Association of presumed ocular histoplasmosis with HLA-B7. Am J Ophthalmol 85:854–858, 1978.

57. Meredith TA, Smith RE, Duquesnoy RJ: Association of HLA-DRW2 antigen with presumed ocular histoplasmosis. Am J Ophthalmol 89:70–76, 1980.

58. Meredith TA, Smith RE, Braley RE, et al: The prevalence of HLA-B7 in presumed ocular histoplasmosis in patients with peripheral atrophic scars. Am J Ophthalmol 86:325–328, 1978.

59. Macular Photocoagulation Study Group: Laser photocoagulation for neovascular lesions nasal to the fovea (results from clinical trials for lesions secondary to ocular histoplasmosis or idiopathic causes). Arch Ophthalmol 113:56–61, 1995.

60. Gitter C, Cohen G: Photocoagulation of active and inactive lesions of presumed ocular histoplasmosis. Am J Ophthalmol 79:428–436, 1975.

61. Fine SL, Patz A, Orth DH, et al: Subretinal neovascularization developing after prophylactic laser photocoagulation of atrophic macular scars. Am J Ophthalmol 82:352, 1976.

62. Macular Photocoagulation Study Group: Laser photocoagulation for juxtafoveal choroidal neovascularization. Arch Ophthalmol 112:500–509, 1994.

63. Macular Photocoagulation Study Group: Persistent and recurrent neovascularization after krypton laser photocoagulation for neovascular lesion of ocular histoplasmosis. Arch Ophthalmol 107:344–352, 1989.

64. Macular Photocoagulation Study Group: The influence of treatment extent on the visual acuity of eyes treated with krypton laser for juxtafoveal choroidal neovascularization. Arch Ophthalmol 113:190–194, 1995.

65. Cummings HL, Rehmar AJ, Wood WJ, Iserhagen RD: Long-term results of laser treatment in the ocular histoplasmosis syndrome. Arch Ophthalmol 113:465–468, 1995.

66. Meredith TA, Aaberg TM: Hemorrhagic peripapillary lesion in presumed ocular histoplasmosis. Am J Ophthalmol 84:160–168, 1977.

67. Cantrill HL, Burgess D: Peripapillary neovascular membranes in presumed ocular histoplasmosis. Am J Ophthalmol 89:192–203, 1980.

68. Lopez PF, Green WR: Peripapillary subretinal neovascularization. A review. Retina 12:147–171, 1992.

69. Turcotte P, Maguire MG, Fine SL: Visual results after laser treatment for peripapillary choroidal neovascular membranes. Retina 11:295–300, 1991.

70. Fine SL, Wood WJ, Isernhagen RD, et al: Laser treatment for subfoveal neovascular membranes in ocular histoplasmosis syndrome—results of a pilot randomized clinical trial. Arch Ophthalmol 111:19–20, 1993.

71. Thomas MA, Dickerson JC, Melberg NS, et al: Visual results after surgical removal of subfoveal choroidal neovascular membranes. Ophthalmology 101:1384–1396, 1994.

72. Thomas MA, Grand MG, Williams DF: Surgical management of subfoveal choroidal neovascularization. Ophthalmology 99:952–968, 1992.

73. Thomas MA, Kaplan HJ: Surgical removal of subfoveal neovascularization in the presumed ocular histoplasmosis syndrome. Am J Ophthalmol 111:1–7, 1991.

74. Thomas MA, Ibanez HE: Instruments for submacular surgery. Retina (in press) 1994.

75. Thomas MA: The use of vitreoretinal surgical techniques in subfoveal choroidal neovascularization. Curr Opin Ophthalmol 3:349–356, 1992.

76. Gass JDM: Biomicroscopic and histopathologic consideration regarding the feasibility of surgical excision of subfoveal neovascular membranes. Am J Ophthalmol 118:285–298, 1994.

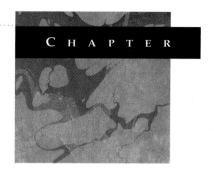

CHAPTER 17

Myopia

Gisèle Soubrane, M.D., Ph.D.

Gabriel Coscas, M.D.

Dagmar Kuhn, M.D.

Myopia is the most common ocular abnormality. *Physiologic myopia* is a normal chance variation in the refractive power. It may also result from excessive convergent power caused by the cornea or the lens. *Degenerative myopia* is characterized by a refractive error of at least −6.00 diopters with an axial length of the globe of more than 26 mm. Progressive choroidal degeneration is then usually associated in the posterior pole.

The *prevalence* of myopia varies from 11 to 36%,[1,2] being least in blacks and greatest in Asians. Degenerative myopia has been reported to range from 0.2 to 9.6%,[3,4] also influenced by ethnicity.[5] Higher prevalence rates were found in females, in higher socioeconomic classes, and in those with greater academic training.

The precise *pathophysiology* in the determination of the development of degenerative myopia has not been elucidated. Degenerative myopia is thought to be the result of a combination of both genetic and environmental factors. It is also one of the manifestations of a wide variety of genetic disorders such as Marfan's, Ehler-Danlos, Down's, and Stickler's syndromes. No animal model reproduces faithfully the human condition of degenerative myopia.

Visual disabilities due to degenerative myopia are numerous and their incidence is related to the degree of myopia. The global expansion of the globe with scleral thinning results in the hallmark ectasia of degenerative myopia: the posterior staphyloma. Progressive axial elongation appears directly involved in the occurrence of the posterior vitreous detachment, of peripheral breaks, and of posterior pole degeneration. Central visual impairment can be due to lacquer cracks, atrophic areas, choroidal new vessels, or macular hole with posterior retinal detachment.[86]

MYOPIC FUNDUS

The posterior staphyloma is pathognomonic of degenerative myopia. The slowly progressive chorioretinal stretching results in the posterior pole abnormalities typical for the disease: optic disc crescent, retinal and choroidal abnormalities, ruptures of Bruch's membrane (lacquer cracks), and atrophic chorioretinal areas associated with vitreous disturbances. Histologically, changes occur in the sclera, the choroid and the retinal pigment epithelium (RPE). The collagen fibrils are reduced in diameter and their organization is disturbed.[7] The generalized thinning of the choroid which progresses to loss of the choriocapillaris, leads toward absence of the choroid, especially at the base of the staphyloma.[8] The RPE cells are flatter and larger than usual before degeneration.[6] Bruch's membrane undergoes a variety of changes, including thinning, splitting, and rupturing. The severity of the changes is more pronounced in the area of the staphyloma.

The clinical features of the myopic fundus have been well studied by means of indirect ophthalmoscopy, color and red-free photographs, fluorescein angiography, and more recently indocyanine green (ICG) angiography.

Posterior Staphyloma

This localized ectasia involves the sclera, the choroid, and the pigment epithelium. Its prevalence increases with axial length. Posterior pole staphyloma is present in early life and increases gradually with age.[9]

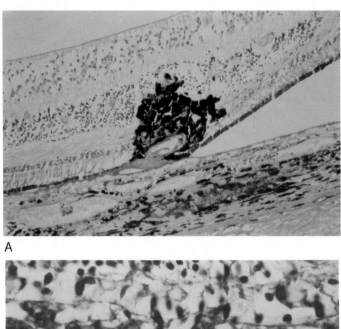

A

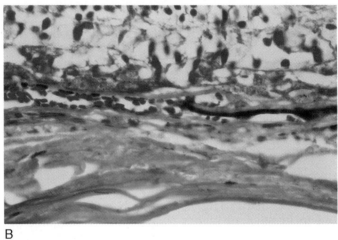

B

A, Fuchs' spot with intraretinal neovascular tuft of blood vessels from the choroid surrounded by hyperplastic retinal pigment epithelium. *B*, One margin of a lacquer crack where choroidal neovascularization extends under the retinal pigment epithelium. (From Grossniklaus HE, Green WR: Pathologic findings in pathologic myopia. Retina 12:127–133, 1992, with permission.)

On biomicroscopic examination and stereoscopic color fundus photographs, the area of the staphyloma is pale and reveals the deep choroidal vessels (Fig. 17–1A). The location, depth, and size of posterior staphyloma are best assessed with stereopsis and ultrasound examination. Some pigment epithelium alterations sometimes underline the limit of the staphyloma.

The atrophy of choriocapillaris and choroid as well as the abnormal distribution of choroidal vessels in the ectasic area are disclosed on fluorescein angiography (Fig. 17–1B), and are even more obvious on ICG angiography. In the latter examination, choroidal arteries seem to originate mainly at the borders of the staphyloma. In the late phase, a circular reflex underlines the borders of the staphyloma in some eyes. Furthermore, retrobulbar vessels are visualized, demonstrating the scleral thinning.[10] Staphyloma involving the macula is commonly associated with decreased vision,[11] but it also causes cumulative damage that can be blind-

ing: 53.3% of eyes with staphyloma are legally blind after the age of 60 years.[9]

Optic Disc Abnormalities

The typical myopic disc is oval with a vertical axis. The disc may appear tilted with an oblique insertion (Fig. 17–1B).

The earliest sign of tissue traction is seen at the temporal margin of the optic disc. Dragging of the pigment epithelium and choroid from the nerve produces a concentric area of depigmentation, the so-called temporal crescent, in which bright white sclera can be visualized through the transparent neurosensory retina (Fig. 17–1). The myopic crescent usually appears as a sharply defined area. Some crescents are underlined with pigment clumps. This change can be extensive and can surround the disc according to the location of the

FIGURE 17–1   Posterior staphyloma. *A*, Fundus photography. The area inferior to the disc is pale and discretely out of focus. A large choroidal vessel is visible within this staphylomatous area. The myopic crescent surrounds the temporal border of the disc. *B*, Fluorescein angiography. The posterior staphyloma is difficult to identify (*arrowheads*). The large choroidal vessels image in negative on the late frame only in that area. Choroidal vessels are also visible in the myopic crescent (*arrows*). The foveal avascular zone is difficult to delimit precisely (*white arrows*).

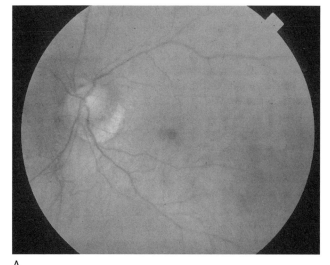

A

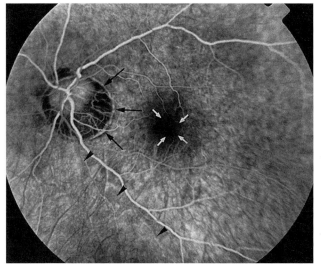

B

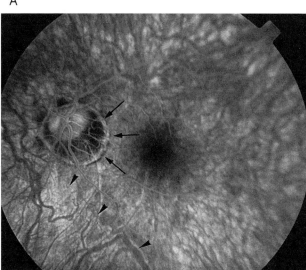

staphyloma. The choroidal layer usually extends closer to the temporal edge of the disc and is visualized on angiography. Histopathologically, RPE and Bruch's membrane stop at some distance from the disc margin, leaving a variable amount of choroid uncovered. Usually, the choroid itself terminates short of the disc edge, leaving the underlying sclera exposed. In constrast, the nasal side frequently has a raised edge, called supertraction, due to the coverage of a portion of the optic foramen.[12]

Vitreous Abnormalities

Spontaneous posterior detachment of the vitreous gel from the inner limiting membrane is premature in degenerative myopia. Biochemical analysis of the vitreous discloses that about 99% of the gel is water and 0.1% consists of soluble proteins and hyaluronic acid. Rare cells, mainly hyalocytes, are located in the cortical area. Its structural or fibrillar component is composed of type II collagen[13] concentrated in the cortical area. The collagen fibers attach to the retinal cells after penetration through the inner limiting membrane in a perpendicular fashion at the vitreous base, resulting in a firm attachment. A relatively firm attachment is located at the foveal and parafoveal areas, at the margin of the optic nerve head and along the major retinal vessels in a more tangential fashion. Acquired attachments more firm occur at points of degeneration of the inner limiting membrane, at areas of lattice degeneration, at some chorioretinal scars, and at the optic nerve head as the result of glial cell proliferation. The hydrated hyaluronic acid polymers maintain a certain spatial relationship with the dipolar water molecules. The spatial integrity of the vitreous is lost by elimination of the polymer hyaluronic acid with introduction of positively charged molecules which results in liquefaction with collapse and condensation of the collagen framework. The vitreous syneresis of irregular fluid-filled cavities within the gel substance occurs with aging. The fluid within the syneretic cavities then enters the potential subhyaloid space and dissects the rest of the cortex away from the retina.

In myopic eyes, the resulting posterior vitreous detachment (PVD) occurs earlier, is more extensive,[14] and its incidence increases with the degree of myopia.

If acute in onset, PVD may be accompanied by photopsia resulting from vitreoretinal traction and migratory small scotomata, or "floaters."[15] Kinetic contact B-scan ultrasonography[16] is an important adjunct to Goldmann contact lens[17] and El Bayadi-Kajiura lens examination in determining the status of the vitreous-retinal interface. Acute PVD might occasionally result in avulsion of a retinal vessel or in formation of full-thickness retinal tear, especially along the margin of vitreous adhesion to a peripheral strip of lattice degeneration. These findings present an increased risk for recurrent vitreous hemorrhage and retinal detachment, particularly if located in the superior half of the fundus. Laser photocoagulation or cryocoagulation of retinal breaks and all other areas of retinal degeneration are recommended preventive measures. Retinal detachment requires scleral buckling for definitive management.

Retinal and Choroidal Abnormalities

The thinning of the retinal pigment epithelium and of the choriocapillaris, referred to as "tigroid" or "tessellated" fundus, is often localized inferior to the disc in the lower fundus. Degeneration may involve the whole fundus (Fig. 17–2A).

The stretching of the neurosensory retina in the macular staphyloma results in a straightening of the retinal vessels and a decreased identification of the luteal pigment.

The large choroidal vessels, arteries, and veins become clearly visible. The anatomic distribution of the major choroidal veins is abnormal in degenerative myopia. Vortex-like choroidal veins may cross the macular area or surround the optic disc. On ICG angiography, the choroidal arteries are scarce and of small caliber.

The thinning and loss of the choriocapillaris is confirmed. The islands of remaining choriocapillaris are demonstrated by a patchy filling of irregular grayish hyperfluorescent zones contrasting with the hypofluorescence of reduced or absent choriocapillaris. The choroidal venous system is also attenuated.[18]

Atrophic Areas

As the myopic staphyloma progresses in association with RPE and choriocapillaris atrophy, areas of focal atrophy may be clinically identified (Fig. 17–3). *On biomicroscopic examination*, these areas may be round or irregular in shape, small or extensive, isolated or multiple, and yellowish white. A variable amount of pigment clumping may exist within these areas or sometimes on their margins. With progressive atrophy, yellowish or whitish choroidal vessels, previously described as choroidal sclerosis, appear in the atrophic areas and seem sheathed. As these vessels are perfused with fluorescein, their whitish appearance may be due to changes in the overlying RPE cells.

On *fluorescein* and *ICG angiography*, the large choroidal vessels crossing the hypofluorescent atrophic areas fill early. With fluorescein, the atrophic areas stain progressively, whereas with ICG they remain hypofluorescent. Their limits remain sharp, as there is no leakage with either dye. Depending on its density, pigment clumping masks the underlying fluorescence.

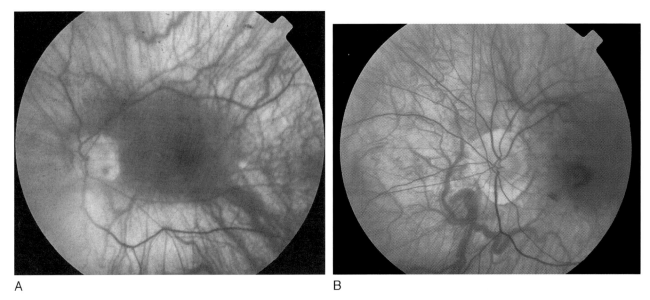

A   B

FIGURE 17–2   Retinal and choroidal abnormalities. *A*, The posterior pole presents a nearly normal red color contrasting with the surrounding pale fundus in which choroidal vessels are easily visible. *B*, Choroidal vessels are obvious around the optic disc. A prominent large choroidal vein is located next to the inferior crescent.

Increase of the number of atrophic areas and their progressive enlargement and coalescence result in large lesions (Fig 17–3). When the fovea is involved, central vision can be markedly decreased. Beyond the sixth decade, myopic eyes with posterior staphyloma have a high incidence of chorioretinal atrophy.[6]

Lacquer Cracks

Ruptures of Bruch's membrane are more prevalent in myopic eyes with an anatomically distorted posterior pole. Lacquer cracks involve 4.3% of eyes with an axial length greater than 26.5 mm,[19] although their number and extent do not directly correlate to it. Their presence is associated with visual decrease, especially when involving the fovea.[20]

On biomicroscopy, lacquer cracks are linear or stellate (Figs. 17–4 and 17–5). The lines are fine, irregular in caliber, yellowish white, usually horizontally oriented, single (Fig. 17–4) or multiple (Fig. 17–5), and often branching with crisscrossing. When cracks are numerous, a reticular or fishnet pattern predominates.[21] Most cracks occur in the macular region within the base of the staphyloma; some are connected with the temporal peripapillary crescent. They are located in the deepest layers of the retina. On their borders, a fine pigmentary mottling is often noted. When the lacquer cracks are large, choroidal vessels may traverse the lesion posteriorly. The inner layers of the retina are undisturbed. With time, lacquer cracks may widen and coalesce with adjacent atrophic areas. Finally, the cracks become lost in a large area of myopic chorioretinal degeneration.

Fluorescein angiography helps to detect lacquer cracks that may be subtle and missed or incompletely identified on routine examination. In the early phase, the crack is an irregular and discretely hyperfluorescent line produced by abnormal transmission from a partially atrophic choriocapillaris (Fig. 17–6C). The fluorescence increases moderately during transit. In the late phase, the linear lesion is only faintly hyperfluorescent (Fig. 17–5C), probably as a consequence of some scleral staining. The hyperfluorescence does not extend into the width of the crack. No intraretinal or subretinal leakage of dye has been noted in uncomplicated lacquer cracks.

ICG angiography discloses even more numerous and longer lacquer cracks in the macular area. In addition, thin lacquer cracks radiate from the optic disc. They appear as hypofluorescent streaks, first discernible during the mid phases and more evident during the late phase.[18]

The acute occurrence or extension of a lacquer crack can be accompanied by a subjective light flash followed by metamorphopsia and a positive scotoma caused by a *macular subretinal hemorrhage* from the choriocapillaris or go unnoticed if they are not near the visual axis. The subretinal hemorrhage is focal, dense, of variable size, and round. They may be multiple and sequential. The crack underlying the subretinal hemorrhage is usually difficult to identify on biomicroscopic examination. Fluorescein angiography provides clues, especially on the border of the hemorrhage due to the decrease of thickness of the blood layer. ICG angiography may show the lacquer crack that underlies the hemorrhage and help to rule out choroidal new vessels. The prognosis for the retention of central vision is good after the resolution of the hemorrhage in 80

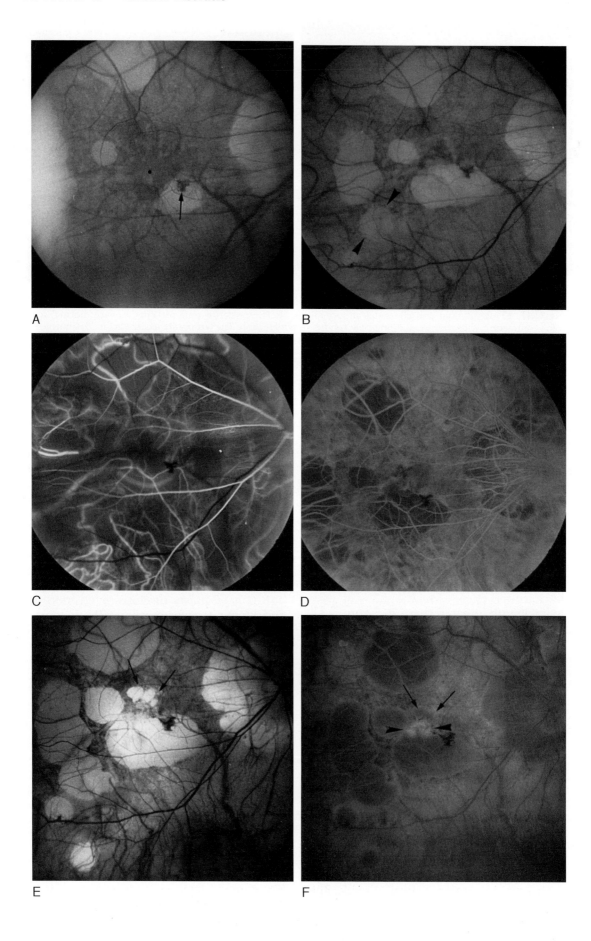

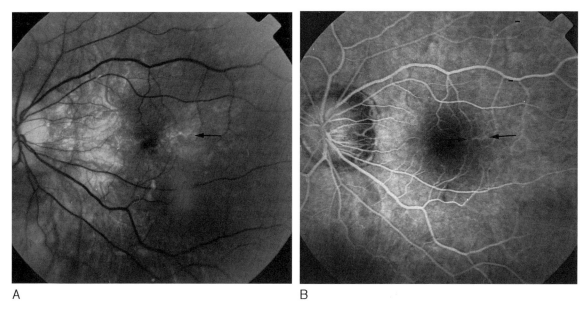

A   B

FIGURE 17–4   Isolated lacquer cracks. *A,* Red-free photograph. The temporal macular area of this myopic fundus presents RPE disturbances. A linear aspect can be suspected (*arrows*). *B,* Early frame of fluorescein angiography discloses a linear window defect due to a single crack (*arrows*).

to 90% of cases unless a lacquer crack has involved the fovea.[20,22]

Lacquer cracks carry a guarded prognosis because of their frequent association with choroidal neovascularization and with focal degenerative lesions involving the macula along their course.[23]

COMPLICATIONS OF DEGENERATIVE MYOPIA

With time, the development of macular abnormalities may jeopardize the visual prognosis. The most devastating macular lesions of degenerative myopia are progressive: macular chorioretinal atrophy resulting from the spontaneous increase of the atrophic areas, posterior retinal detachment secondary to a macular hole, and/or neovascularization.

Posterior Retinal Detachment

A foveal break induces a relatively shallow posterior retinal detachment confined within the temporal vascular arcades (Fig. 17–6). The detachment may spread peripherally, raising the suspicion of an additional peripheral break. Usually, the posterior detachment remains stable in size. A cystoid degeneration occurs in the detached retina.

Surgical repair is still controversial but, when considered, is internal than external. Internal surgery consists of a vitreous fluid-gas exchange with filtered air, C3F8 or SF6, and postoperative prone positioning of the head for internal tamponade or an injection of silicone oil. The internal tamponade may be performed either after aspiration of the liquefied vitreous[24,25] or after a pars plana vitrectomy.[26,27] Some surgeons apply endolaser treatment to the gas-occluded break. If the internal approach fails, or if the surgeon is confronted by an extreme posterior staphyloma with advanced atrophy of the retina, pigment epithelium, and choroid, the external method can be successful. Small convex solid silicone rubber button explant may close the break. If the break remains elevated, a careful posterior sclerotomy is performed. The resulting hypotony is reversed with a controlled pars plana injection of filtered air or systemic gas.

←

FIGURE 17–3   Natural progression of atrophic areas. *A,* In 1986, a few atrophic areas are observed in this right eye. Pigment clumping is present in the nasal patch (*arrow*). A large crescent surrounds the temporal part of the disc. *B,* Two years later, the pre-existing atrophic areas have enlarged even on this smaller magnification. A new atrophic patch developed (*arrowheads*). *C,* The corresponding fluorescein angiography shows the early filling of the choroidal vessels due to RPE and choriocapillaris atrophy. The retinal vessels are linear. *D,* Later during the sequence of fluorescein angiography, the hypofluorescent atrophic areas are well delineated. *E,* Four years later, the progression of atrophy results in confluence of the previous areas and development of new patches superior to the macula (*arrows*). *F,* On the corresponding late fluorescein, these new patches are less prominent (*arrows*). Only a small central area in hyperfluorescent (*arrowheads*).

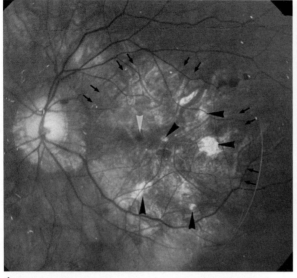

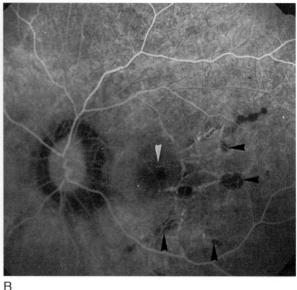

A

B

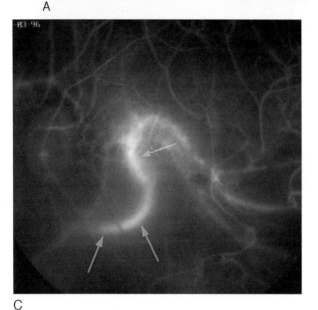

C

FIGURE 17–5   Multiple lacquer cracks. *A,* Red-free photograph. The posterior pole demonstrates atrophic areas (*black arrowheads*) and a small central hemorrhage (*white arrowhead*) within the staphyloma (*arrows*). A patch of pigmentation is located inferior to the macula. The global but irregular thinning does not permit the precise identification of the lacquer cracks. Note a hemorrhage along the superior temporal vessels. *B,* Mid phase of fluorescein angiography. The multiple temporal lacquer cracks have a fishnet pattern. Superior to the hemorrage (*white arrowhead*) a faint hyperfluorescent line can be suspected. The atrophic areas are mainly dark (*black arrowheads*). *C,* Early frame of ICG angiography. A large artery (*white arrows*) shows a fluorescent hyperfluorescence at the arterial choroidal phase. The dark area corresponds to the RPE hyperplasia.

Choroidal Neovascularization

Myopia is the second most common cause of choroidal new vessels (CNVs). The risk of CNVs increases with the degree of myopia.[28] The neovascular process is believed to affect 5 to 10% of the myopic population, especially in eyes with more than 6 diopters of myopia[29] or an axial length of 26.5 mm or more.[19]

Clinical Signs

Macular CNV ingrowth tends to occur suddenly and to induce a sudden painless decrease in vision, usually associated with metamorphopsia. The biomicroscopic features of CNVs in a degenerative myopic fundus include a shallow serous retinal detachment, often limited and difficult to detect even

in stereopsis, and thin and scarce hemorrhages. Hard exudates are uncommon. The neovascular lesion is usually small, light gray, and round or elliptic. A dark pigmented rim may underline the lesion (Fig. 17–7).

The development of CNVs may be related to pre-existing breaks in Bruch's membrane or atrophic areas (Fig. 17–8),[30] as suggested by several clinical studies.[11,31] However, the relation is not clear, as macular lacquer cracks are not always complicated by CNVs and as CNVs do not arise always from these ruptures. Nevertheless, ruptures in Bruch's membrane were found to be more numerous in myopic eyes with new vessels.[32] About one third of CNVs arise from a lacquer crack crossing the macular area in its portion next to the fovea (Fig. 17–8A). On the contrary, 18 to 43% of degenerative myopic eyes with a neovascular ingrowth have no detectable breaks (Fig. 17–7).[20,33] It has been suggested

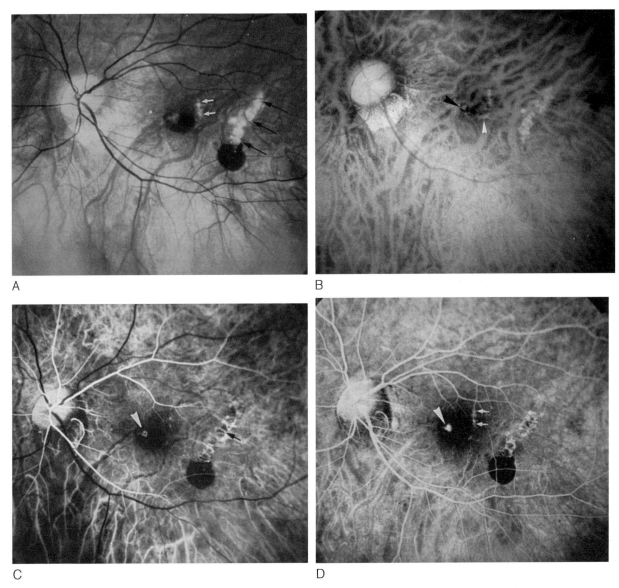

FIGURE 17–6   Lacquer cracks with hemorrhages. *A*, Red-free photograph. A large temporal lacquer crack (*black arrows*) presents at its inferior extremity with a round deep retinal hemorrhage. Another crack (*white arrows*) is visible temporal to a macular subretinal hemorrhage. *B*, Red light photograph. A third lacquer crack is identified inferior to the central area as a depigmented line (*black arrowhead*). A dark circle is obvious (*white arrowhead*). *C*, Early frame of fluorescein angiography. The deep choroidal arteries are perfused with dye within the larger rupture (*black arrow*). A small nasal round area is hyperfluorescent (*white arrowhead*). *D*, Late frame of fluorescein angiography. The large lacquer crack is less striking. The thin crack (*white arrows*) shows hyperfluorescence. The choroidal new vessels have increased in visibility (*white arrowhead*).

that CNVs might be preferentially located on the macular side of the staphyloma.[34]

Fluorescein Angiography

Fluorescein angiography discloses the neovascular component. In the early dye transit phase, CNVs appear usually as bright hyperfluorescent spots without a discernible vascular pattern in young myopes. Throughout the course of dye transit, the leakage, suggestive of the presence of CNVs, does not extend significantly.[35,44] The location of the neovascular tissue is a main concern at the time of pre-

sentation: 58[36] to 74%[37] directly involve the foveal zone on initial examination. Nearly all of the remaining membranes are located within 100 to 300 μm of the fovea. The initial size of the CNV is almost always less than 1/2 disc diameter.[38]

It is difficult to ascertain a neovascular ingrowth on the edge of a macular break in Bruch's membrane, as the new vessels usually do not present a lacy pattern and give rise to a very limited amount of leakage. The same difficulty exists when new vessels arise from atrophic patches.

In elderly patients, choroidal neovascularization exhibits more leakage, resulting in the exten-

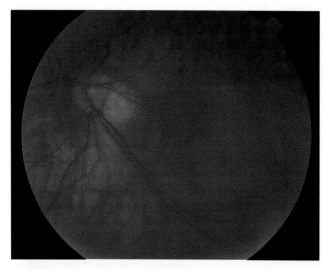

FIGURE 17–7 Macular hole. Color photograph. An obvious retinal detachment involves the macular area. The macular hole is at very low contrast.

sion of dye beyond the boundaries of the neovascular net that is delineated in the early dye transit. This increase in exudation may be due to associated age-related degenerative changes. The modification of the new vessels' behavior on the late phases of angiography with increasing age of the patient explains the description by some authors of two types of CNV.[33] Most studies include elderly patients (up to 96 years), which might confuse neovascular degeneration of degenerative myopia with age-related macular degeneration in myopic eyes.

ICG Angiography

Early frames of ICG angiography reveal either a hyperfluorescent net or a fluorescent area of intensity similar to that of the choroidal background (Fig. 17–8C). CNVs are then detectable by the presence of a surrounding hypofluorescent rim. CNV filling is concomitant with the choroidal arteries filling, increases during the choroidal venous phase, then fades with dye washout from the large choroidal vessels. In the late phases, the neovascular net remains mildly hyperfluorescent in eyes with clear media but does not leak ICG dye, which remains mainly in the vascular compartment.[10,18]

ICG angiography may be of crucial importance to diagnose a neovascular process on the border of a lacquer crack or of an atrophic area. These latter abnormalities remain hypofluorescent during the course of the examination. Thus, only CNVs will exhibit hyperfluorescence. Similarly, ICG angiography may reveal CNVs as hyperfluorescent areas in eyes with macular subretinal hemorrhages, allowing differentiation of them from ruptures of Bruch's membrane.

Natural History

The visual prognosis in degenerative myopia remains controversial. After the initial rapid decrease in visual acuity, a relative stabilization of vision probably reflects the reabsorption of the transudate and the hemorrhages, together with the establishment of an eccentric point of fixation.[36] The basis for the claimed benign visual prognosis of myopic CNVs may be related to a low acuity at inclusion,[33] to a limited follow-up period, and even to the lack of fluorescein angiographic diagnosis.[39] However, after 2 years of follow-up, deterioration of vision was observed in 43[36] and 51% of eyes.[32] With longer observation, a three-line decrease in visual acuity affects more eyes: 62% at 5 years,[37] 58% at 8 years, and 76% at 10 years.[38] Furthermore, the prevalence of legal blindness reaches at long term 34[9] to 47%,[38] as a consequence of the enlargement of the macular RPE atrophy.

As time passes, a typical Foerster-Fuchs spot[40,41] develops. It evolves into a round or oval, slightly elevated deep lesion. The fibrovascular scar presents varying degree of pigmentation. Histologically, the scar, containing hyperplastic RPE and basement membrane, extends into the retina. This fibrous tissue contains melanin, and waste products secondary to hemosiderin and xanthophyll degradation.[42]

With time, this scar remains the same size as the initially detected CNVs. However, an area of chorioretinal atrophy progressively surrounds the central lesion and progresses, involving at long term the whole posterior pole. The only evidence of previous existence of a Fuchs' spot may be a certain amount of macular clumped pigment within a large atrophic area. The increase of the halo of atrophy usually obliterates the previous eccentric fixation and necessitates the use of another area farther from the fovea.

In rare cases, recurrent subretinal hemorrhages occur. In elderly patients, the disciform scar might be extensive and induce exudation.

CNVs initially sparing fixation progress to involve the fovea.[38,39] Furthermore, a bilateral neovascular involvement occurs in 12[32] to 41%[39] of patients. Therefore, the presence of a Fuchs' spot indicates a guarded prognosis.

Treatment Approaches

As the poor functional outcome of myopic CNVs comes into prominence, treatment approaches are more often considered. Limited studies have been performed using photocoagulation for juxtafoveal CNVs[32,43,44]; rare surgical excisions have been performed for subfoveal myopic CNVs; antiangiogenic medical treatments have only been considered.

Laser photocoagulation may be performed when the new vessels spare the foveola (Fig. 17–10A and B) and reduce or threaten to reduce central vision. The main difficulty in the treatment is related to the localization of the foveola in relation to the CNVs. Xanthophyll pigment that is normally well delineated on blue-light frames is rarely visible in myopic eyes. The foveal avascular zone is rarely identifia-

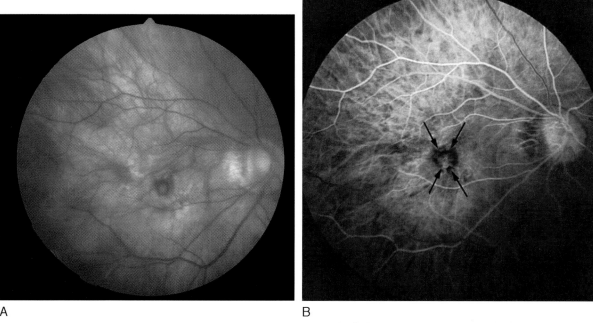

A   B

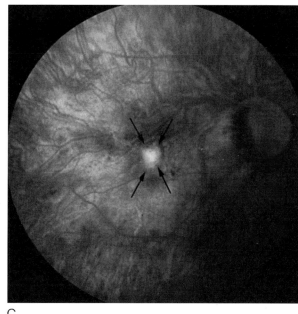

C

FIGURE 17–8   Choroidal new vessels. *A*, Color photograph. The posterior macular staphyloma is depigmented, allowing the visualization of the choroidal vessels. In the macular area, a pigmentated circle is disclosed. *B*, Early frame of fluorescein angiography. The fluorescence of the new vessels (*arrows*) is of the same intensity as that of the choroidal background. Their location is subfoveal. A hypofluorescent rim underlines the CNVs. *C*, Late frame of fluorescein angiography. The leakage of dye does not extend at distance of the CNVs (*arrows*). It is, however, manifest by the disappearance of the dark rim.

ble on early frames of fluorescein angiography in degenerative myopia (Fig 17–10*B*). Thus, a normal reading vision (despite metamorphopsia), the convergence of retinal vessels, and the use of the scanning laser ophthalmoscope and the 50-μm laser aiming beam at very low intensity might be of help in the determination of fixation.

Encouraging results of laser photocoagulation treatment (Fig. 17–11) have been published[35,47] despite a high rate of recurrences and of scar enlargement. A randomized controlled trial[37] has shown that krypton laser photocoagulation was useful in preventing visual loss in myopic eyes with evidence of recent CNVs outside the fovea. At 2 years, the 35 treated eyes did statistically better than the 35 untreated eyes with respect to the outcome of distance and reading vision ($p<.01$ and $p<.001$, respectively). After 5 years' follow-up, the difference between the two groups was no longer statistically significant.[48] Recently, a retrospective study on 100 consecutive eyes has confirmed the previous randomized study.[38] However, 42 and 63% of treated eyes reached legal blindness at 5 and 10 years of follow-up, respectively, compared to 68% in the natural history group.

Both studies identified a high recurrence rate (31.4 and 72%). About half of them were amenable to further photocoagulation, resulting in a better, although transient, visual preservation (Fig. 17–12). Most of the recurrences occur the first year follow-

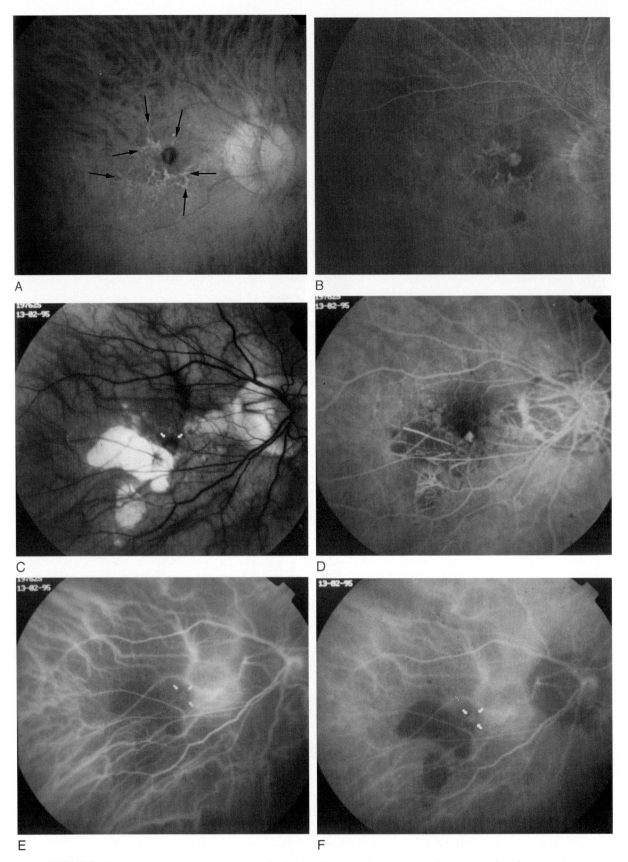

FIGURE 17-9 Choroidal new vessels. *A*, Red light photograph. Numerous lacquer cracks of various pigmentation and width (*arrows*) extend in the macula. A pigmented circle is located on their crossing. *B*, Late frame of fluorescein angiography. The lacquer cracks are discretely hyperfluorescent. The CNV do not leak heavily. *C*, Red-free photograph. A large atrophic area occupies the inferior temporal area of the posterior pole. A hemorrhage (*white arrows*) underlines its superior border. *D*, Middle phase of fluorescein angiography. The hyperfluorescent CNVs are located at the border of the atrophy in which the choroidal vessels are visible. *E*, Middle phase of ICG angiography. Choroidal arteries and veins are already perfused with the dye. The atrophic areas are less fluorescent than the rest of the fundus. A small neovascular tuft is discernible (*white arrows*). *F*, Late phase of ICG angiography. The hyperfluorescence of the CNVs (*arrows*) contrasts with the dark atrophic areas.

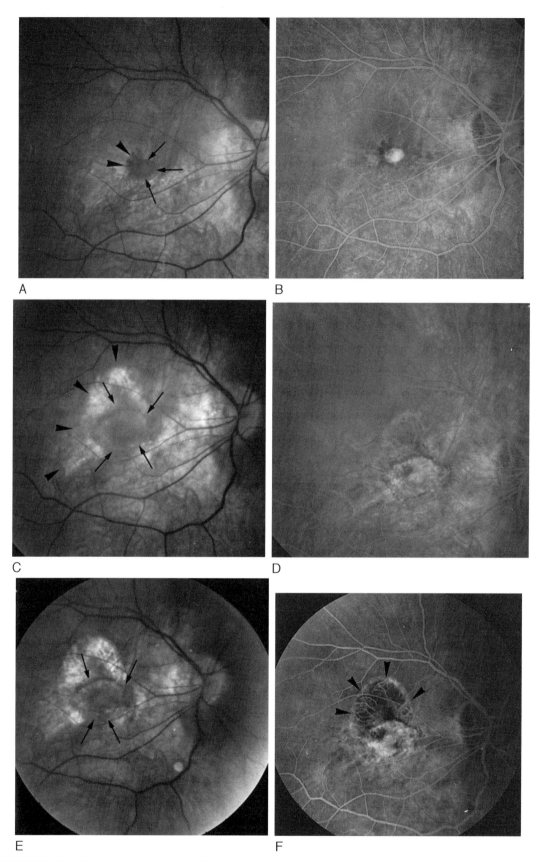

FIGURE 17–10 Natural history of CNVs. *A*, Red-free photograph. A submacular hemorrhage (*arrowheads*) extends on the temporal border around a pigmented area (*arrows*). *B*, Late frame of fluorescein angiography. Late staining of dye from CNVs located centrally in the macula. *C*, Two years later. Red-free photograph. Central fibrosis (*arrows*) surrounded by atrophy (*arrowheads*). *D*, Corresponding fluorescein angiography. The area of atrophy is not profound. *E*, Two years later. Red-free photograph. The glial tissue (*arrows*) has not extended. *F*, Corresponding fluorescein angiography. The area of atrophy (*arrowheads*) has increased, involving the superior posterior pole.

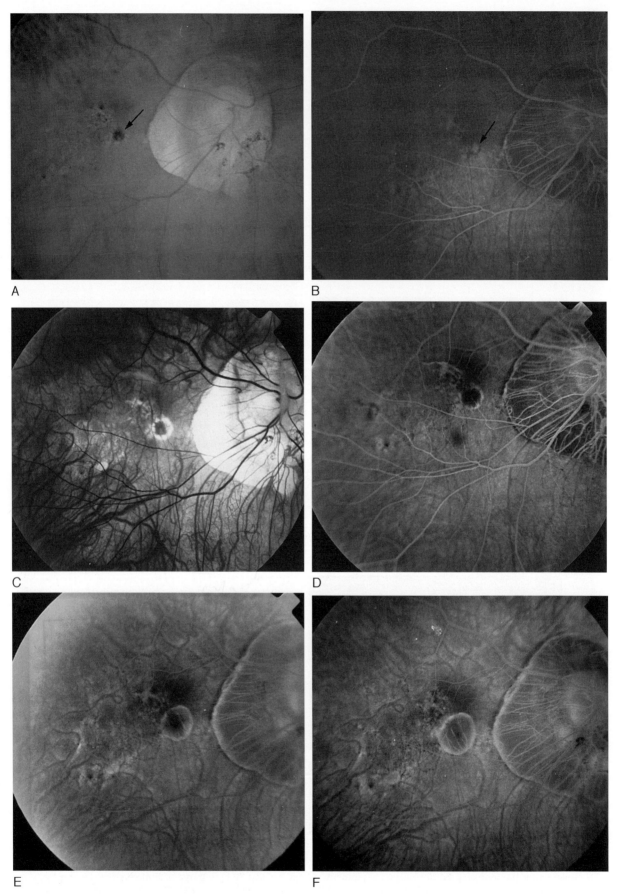

FIGURE 17–11 Photocoagulation of choroidal new vessels. *A*, Red photograph. The macular RPE presents multiple disturbances. A small pigmented ring is discernible (*arrow*). *B*, Late frame of fluorescein angiography. A moderate hyperfluorescence (*arrow*) is sparing the central macula as retinal vessels are visible. *C*, Red-free photograph of posttreatment control. The photocoagulation scar covers adequately the CNV area. *D*, Corresponding fluorescein. The treatment scar is hypofluorescent, surrounded by a uniform hyperfluorescent border. *E*, Three months later. The treatment scar has increased, although no recurrence has occurred. *F*, One year later. The size of the scar has further enlarged.

ing treatment on the foveal side of the photocoagulation scar. This high recurrence rate emphasizes the need of a close follow-up for early detection and treatment after performing laser photocoagulation.

Progressive enlargement of the treatment scar (Fig. 17–11C, E, and F) is seen in 92 to 100% of eyes despite use of different laser wavelengths.[44,49,50] It is greatest in the same direction as the maximal peripapillary crescent expansion.[47] This spontaneous enlargement does not result in a compulsory visual decrease. However, treatment strategies should take the traction lines into consideration.

Surgical Removal

Few attempts have been performed to excise subfoveal myopic CNVs. In the only series published,[51] the mean change in final visual acuity compared with preoperative vision was a decrease of one line.

In two out of ten eyes, recurrences developed, both within 2 months of surgery. Thus, myopic CNVs are not favorable for surgical excision (Fig. 17–12).

The macula of eyes with degenerative myopia is threatened by atrophy, by macular hole, and by neovascular process. In case of neovascular involvement, photocoagulation treatment is of only limited effect in delaying visual loss but may maintain useful central vision in some eyes. Even though the risk of large posttreatment scars may be less vision threatening than are the deleterious effects of CNVs, laser photocoagulation and surgical excision are not satisfactory therapies.

TREATMENT OF DEGENERATIVE MYOPIA

Treatment to prevent the development of degenerative myopia in children from families at risk has

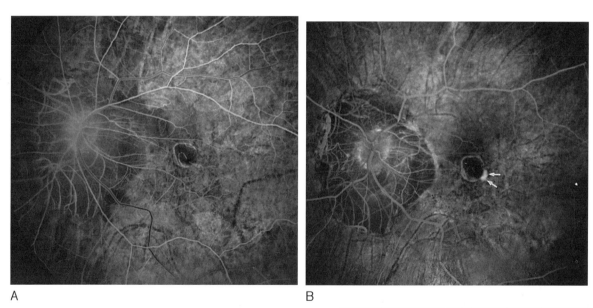

A   B

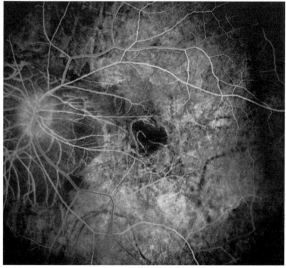

C

FIGURE 17–12 CNV recurrence. *A,* Early phase of fluorescein angiography. A deep choroidal vessel within the photocoagulation scar is perfused with dye. The temporal rim of the scar is interrupted. *B,* Early frame of fluorescein angiography. One month later, a recurrence (*arrows*) occurred on the foveal border of the scar. *C,* Early frame of fluorescein angiography. Two weeks after treatment of the recurrence, no further abnormality is identified.

been tested in limited studies. Neither dietary supplementation with vitamins or oligo elements[52] nor instillation of atropine[53,54] nor the wearing of bifocal glasses[53] has demonstrated any efficacy.

Patients with degenerative myopia, particularly those with lacquer cracks, should avoid abrupt elevation in intraocular pressure (rubbing of the eyes, blunt trauma). Lowering of intraocular pressure is important in individuals with open-angle glaucoma and is also advised for patients with low-tension or suspected glaucoma. Valsalva's maneuver and intense exercises are inadvisable. Chronic use of aspirin and other anticoagulants should be avoided.

The use of pharmacologically induced ocular hypotension in nonglaucomatous individuals to retard the progression of degenerative myopia has been suggested.[55] Chronic cycloplegia could be effective to some degree but its usefulness is outweighed by its adverse effects.[53,56] Refractive surgery, anterior chamber intraocular lens implantation, and extraction of a clear lens fail to address the basic problem of progressive scleral expansion and its deleterious effects.

Scleral reinforcement has been performed to arrest staphyloma progression.[57] A number of materials have been employed, including donor sclera,[58] autologous or animal fascia lata,[59] dura mater,[60] silicone rubber,[61] Dacron mesh, and polytetrafluoroethylene (Gore-Tex).[62] Although thousands of operations have been performed, the efficacy of the procedure is not yet proven. Scleral reinforcement would be recommended to prevent the development of posterior staphyloma before irreversible damage has occurred.

REFERENCES

1. Sorsby A, Sheridan M, Leary GA, Benjamin B: Vision, visual acuity and ocular refraction of young men. Br Med J 1:1394–1398, 1960.
2. Sperduto RD, Seigel D, Roberts J, Rowland M: Prevalence of myopia in the United States. Arch Ophthalmol 101: 405–470, 1983.
3. Michaels DD: Visual Optics and Refraction; A Clinical Approach, 2nd edition. St Louis, CV Mosby Co, 1980, p 513.
4. Stromberg E: Uber Refraktion und Achsenlange des menschlichen Auges. Acta Ophthalmol 14:281–293, 1981.
5. Fuchs AW, Soubrane G: Frequency of myopia gravis. Am J Ophthalmol 49:1418, 1960.
6. Green JL, Rabb MF: Degeneration of Bruch's membrane and retinal pigment epithelium. Int Ophthalmol Clin 21: 27–50, 1981.
7. Curtin BJ, Iwamoto T, Renaldo DP: Normal and staphylomatous of high myopia: an electron microscopic study. Arch Ophthalmol 97:912–915, 1979.
8. Okabe S, Nobuhiko M, Okamoto S, Kataoka H: Electron microscopic studies on retinochoroidal atrophy in the human eye. Acta Med Okayama 36:11–21, 1982.
9. Curtin BJ: The posterior staphyloma of pathologic myopia. Trans Am Ophthalmol Soc 75:67–86, 1977.
10. Coscas G, Soubrane G: ICG angiography in myopic degeneration. Second International Symposium on Indocyanine Green Angiography, Nara, July 4, 1996.
11. Noble KG, Carr RE: Pathologic myopia. Ophthalmology 89:1099–1100, 1982.
12. Grossniklaus HE, Green WE: Pathologic findings in pathologic myopia. Retina 12:127–132, 1992.
13. Snowden JM, Swann DA: Vitreous structure. V. The morphology and thermal stability of vitreous collagen fibers and comparison to articular cartilage (type II) collagen. Invest Ophthalmol Vis Sci 19:610–618, 1980.
14. Goldmann H: Senile changes of the lens and the vitreous. Am J Ophthalmol 57:1–13, 1964.
15. Murakami K, Jalkh AE, Avila MP, et al: Vitreous floaters. Ophthalmology 90:1271–1276, 1983.
16. Fisher YL, Slakter JS, Friedman RA, Yanuzzi LA: Kinetic ultrasound evaluation of the posterior vitreoretinal interface. Ophthalmology 98:1135–1138, 1991.
17. Buzney SM, Weiter JJ, Furukawa H, et al: Examination of the vitreous: a comparison of biomicroscopy using the Goldmann and El Bayadi-Kajiura lenses. Ophthalmology 92:1745–1748, 1985.
18. Quaranta M, Arnold J, Coscas G, et al: Indocyanine green angiographic features of pathologic myopia. Am J Ophthalmol 122:663–671, 1996.
19. Curtin BJ, Karlin DB: Axial length measurements and fundus changes of the myopic eye. Am J Ophthalmol 71:42–53, 1971.
20. Klein RM, Curtin BJ: Lacquer crack lesions in pathologic myopia. Am J Ophthalmol 79:386–392, 1975.
21. Pruett RC, Weiter JJ, Goldstein RB: Myopic cracks, angioid streaks, and traumatic tears in Bruch's membrane. Am J Ophthalmol 103:537–543, 1987.
22. Milch FA, Yannuzzi LA, Rudick AJ: Pathologic myopia and subretinal hemorrhage. Ophthalmology 94(Suppl):117, 1987.
23. Ohno-Matsui K, Tokoro T: The progression of the lacquer cracks in pathologic myopia. Retina 16:29–37, 1996.
24. Blankenship GW, Ibanez-Langlois S: Treatment of myopic macular hole and detachment. Intravitreal gas exchange. Ophthalmology 94:333–336, 1987.
25. Garcia-Arumi J, Correa CA, Corcostegui B: Comparative study of different techniques of intraocular gas tamponade in the treatment of retinal detachment due to macular hole. Ophthalmologica 201:83–91, 1990.
26. Binder S, Zugner M, Velikay M: Does vitrectomy followed by intraocular gas tamponade offer sufficiently effective treatment of retinal detachment due to holes in the posterior pole? Int Ophthalmol 11:25–30, 1987.
27. Lai YT: Treatment of macular hole retinal detachment. Br J Ophthalmol 74:201–202, 1990.
28. Balacco-Gabrieli C: Aetiopathogenesis of degenerative myopia: a hypothesis. Ophthalmologica 185:199–204, 1982.
29. Campos R: La tache de Fuchs. In Problemes Actuels D'Ophtalmologie. Basel, Karger, 1957, pp 363–364.
30. Gass JDM: Pathogenesis of disciform detachment of the neuroepithelium. VI. Disciform detachment secondary to heredodegenerative, neoplastic and traumatic lesions of the choroid. Am J Ophthalmol 63:689–711, 1967.
31. Rabb MF, Garron I, La Franco FP: Myopic macular degeneration. Int Ophthalmol Clin 21:51–69, 1981.
32. Hotchkiss ML, Fine SL: Pathologic myopia and choroidal neovascularization. Am J Ophthalmol 91:177–183, 1981.
33. Avila MP, Weiter JJ, Trempe CL, et al: Natural history of choroidal neovascularization in degenerative myopia. Ophthalmology 91:1573–1581, 1984.
34. Cohen SY, Quentel G, Guiberteau B, Delahaye C: Subretinal leakage in tilted disc syndrome. Am Acad Ophthalmol 102(Suppl):147, 1995.
35. Soubrane G, Pison J, Bornert P, et al: Néovaisseaux sous-rétiniens de la myopie dégénérative: résultats de la photocoagultaion. Bull Soc Ophtalmol Fr 86:26–272, 1986.
36. Hampton GR, Kohen D, Bird AC: Visual prognosis of disciform degeneration in myopia. Ophthalmology 90:923–926, 1983.
37. Soubrane G, Pison J, Bornert P, et al: Néovaisseaux sous-rétiniens de la myopie dégénérative: résultats de la photocoagulation. Bull Soc Ophtalmol Fr 86:269–272, 1986.
38. Secretan M, Kuhn D, Soubrane G, Coscas G: Long term follow-up of choroidal neovascularization in pathologic

myopia: natural history compared to evolution after laser treatment. Europ J Ophthalmol (accepted for publication).

39. Fried M, Siebert A, Meyer-Schwickerath G, Wessing A: Natural history of Fuchs' spot: a long term follow-up study. Doc Ophthalmol Proc Ser 28:215–221, 1981.

40. Foerster R: Ophthalmologische Beiträge. Berlin, Enslin, 1862, p 55.

41. Fuchs E: Der centrale schwarze Fleck bei Myopie. Z Augenheilkd 5:171–178, 1901.

42. Green WR: Retina. In Spencer WH (ed): Ophthalmic Pathology—An Atlas and Textbook, 3rd edition. Philadelphia, WB Saunders Co, 1985, pp 913–924.

43. Jalkh AE, Weiter JJ, Trempe CL, et al: Choroidal neovascularization in degenerative myopia: role of laser photocoagulation. Ophthalmic Surg 18:721–725, 1987.

44. Brancato R, Menchini U, Pece A, et al: Dye laser photocoagulation of macular subretinal neovascularisation in pathological myopia. Int Ophthalmol 11:235–238, 1988.

45. Pece A, Serini P, Avanza P, Brancato R: Myopie dégénérative: récidives de néovaisseaux sous-rétiniens après photocoagulation au laser. J Fr Ophtalmol 13:24–28, 1990.

46. Tanev V, Ilieva E: La tache de Fuchs chez le myope grave. Aspect angiofluorographiques et traitement au laser. Bull Soc Ophtalmol Fr 85:369–370, 1985.

47. Deutman AF, Hendrikse F: Traitement des néovaisseaux sous-rétiniens dans la myopie dégénérative. Ophtalmologie 3:299–301, 1989.

48. Fardeau C, Soubrane G, Coscas G: Photocoagulation des néovaisseaux sous-rétiniens compliquant la dégénérescence myopique. Bull Soc Fr Ophtalmol 92:239–242, 1992.

49. Brancato R, Pece A, Avanza P, Raddrizzani E: Photocoagulation scar expansion after laser therapy for choroidal neovascularization in degenerative myopia. Retina 10: 239–243, 1990.

50. Bressler SB, Pieramici D, Marsh MJ, et al: Laser scar expansion in pathologic myopia and ocular histoplasmosis following treatment of choroidal neovascularization. Invest Ophthalmol Vis Sci 33:1207, 1992.

51. Thomas MA, Dickinson JP, Melberg NS, et al: Visual results after surgical removal of subfoveal choroidal neovascular membranes. Ophthalmology 101:138–1396, 1994.

52. Silverstone BZ, Seelenfreud MH, Berson D: Zinc and copper metabolism in patients with high myopia and senile macular degeneration. Doc Ophthalmol Proc Series. Junk, The Hague, 1987, pp 215–217.

53. Brodstein RS, Brodstein DE, Olson RJ, et al: The treatment of myopia with atropine and bifocals. Ophthalmology 91: 1373, 1984.

54. Greene PR: Mechanical considerations in myopia: relative effects of accomodation, convergence, intraocular pressure and the extraocular muscles. Am J Optom Physiol Ophthalmol 57:902–914, 1980.

55. Jensen H: Timolol maleate in the control of myopia: a preliminary report. Acta Ophthalmol 185(Suppl) 66:128, 1988.

56. Brenner RL: Further observations on use of atropine in the treatment of myopia. Ann Ophthalmol 17:137, 1985.

57. Malbran J: Una neuva orientacion quirergica contra la miopia. Arch Soc Oftal Hisp Am 14:1167, 1954.

58. Borley WE, Miller WW: Surgical treatment of degenerative myopia. Trans Am Acad Ophthalmol Otolaryngol 62:791, 1958.

59. Vancea P: New concept in the treatment of progressive myopia. Ann Ophthalmol 3:1105–1108, 1971.

60. Miller WW: Surgical treatment of degerative myopia: scleral reinforcement. Trans Am Acad Ophthalmol Otolaryngol 78:896, 1974.

61. Snyder AA, Thompson FB: A simplified technique for surgical treatment of degenerative myopia. Am J Ophthalmol 74:273, 1972.

62. Thompson FB: Scleral reinforcement. In Thompson (ed): Myopia Surgery: Anterior and Posterior Segments. New York, MacMillan, 1990, pp 267–297.

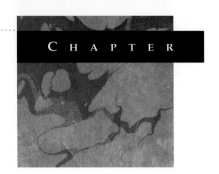

CHAPTER 18

Central Serous Chorioretinopathy

Lisabeth S. Hall, M.D.

David R. Guyer, M.D.

Lawrence A. Yannuzzi, M.D.

Central serous chorioretinopathy (CSC) is defined as an idiopathic serous detachment of the macula due to the accumulation of serous fluid at the posterior pole. Since 1866 when this disorder was first described by von Graefe[1] and called *recurrent central retinitis*, many clinicians have sought to describe and understand this disorder. There was great difficulty in defining this disorder due to a lack of understanding concerning the anatomic site responsible for the clinical findings. It was not until 100 years later, in the 1960s, that Maumenee[2] and Gass[3] contributed greatly to our understanding of CSC. By describing the unique patterns seen on fluorescein angiography in patients with this condition, in 1965 Maumenee[2] defined the source of subretinal fluid to be a leak through the retinal pigment epithelium (RPE). Two years later, Gass[3] added the classic description of the disease reporting angiographic findings on additional patients and coined the term "central serous chorioretinopathy."

Klein[4] further described the clinical characteristics of CSC and noted that in 95% of cases there is fluid accumulation confined to under the neurosensory retina (type I CSC), whereas 3% of cases have an isolated detachment of the RPE (type II) and 3% show detachment of both the neurosensory retina and the RPE (intermediate type CSC).

DEMOGRAPHICS

CSC typically occurs in young to middle-aged adults ranging from 20 to 45 years of age.[1,3,5-15] It affects males ten times more often than females.[5,15,16] Recently, CSC has been described more frequently than previously reported in individuals over 50 years of age. Women are more commonly affected as they get older,[15] with the male/female ratio approaching 2:1 past age 50.[17] It remains important to recognize CSC in this population and differentiate it from choroidal neovascularization. CSC is most common in Caucasians, Hispanics, and Asians, particularly those of Japanese origin. It is uncommon in blacks.[18-20]

CLINICAL HISTORY

The typical patient with CSC notes a unilateral decrease in central vision or a central scotoma. They may complain of metamorphopsia or microsomia in the involved eye. Rarely, the symptoms are preceded by a migraine-like headache.[3] CSC is not consistently reported in association with systemic disease. Cases of CSC are often reported in patients with a supercharged or "type-A" personality.[18] The vast majority of patients are emmetropes or mild hyperopes; CSC is not associated with high myopia.

CLINICAL EXAMINATION

In the acute stage of CSC, visual acuity can range from 20/20 to 20/200.[15] In one series, 52% of patients had acuity of 20/30 or better at presentation. With a small hyperopic correction, vision often im-

TABLE 18–1 Ophthalmic Findings

Serous retinal detachment
Serous detachment of the retinal pigment
  epithelium (RPE)
Subretinal precipitates
Extramacular RPE atrophic tracts
Multiple bullous serous retinal and RPE
  detachments
RPE atrophic changes

proves due to the anterior displacement of the neurosensory retina. Amsler grid testing often shows a small central scotoma or metamorphopsia. There is a delay in retinal recovery time after exposure to bright light.[21] Examination of the anterior segment, vitreous, optic nerve, and retinal vasculature are normal.

The following findings may be present on fundus examination (Table 18–1)[3,6,15]:

1. *Serous retinal detachment*: In the macula there is a round to oval, well-delineated shallow serous retinal detachment (Fig. 18–1). The detachment varies considerably from a small elevation at the fovea to a large detachment that may appear bullous with sloping margins.[22] The normal foveal reflex is absent. Instead, a mildly darkened area is surrounded by a halo of light reflex with an average size of 2 disc diameters.

2. *Pigment epithelial detachments (PEDs)*: One or more discrete round to oval, well-demarcated areas of detached RPE may be observed. These areas are often present under the superior half of the macular detachment and are infrequent in the fovea. They may also be found above the macular detachment. This is due to the effects of gravity forcing the subretinal fluid inferiorly.[3] The PEDs are yellow to yellow-gray and often have a yellow halo surrounding them representing the border between attached and detached RPE. These detachments are often less than $1/4$ of a disc diameter in size and are often difficult to visualize if shallow or obscured by turbid subretinal exudate.

3. *Subretinal precipitates*: At the level of the RPE, multiple, variably sized, yellow dot-like specks can be noticed that are thought to be proteinaceous precipitates. These are probably caused by turbidity of subretinal fluid.[3] Diffuse gray-white subretinal deposits are occasionally present, which may represent fibrin (Fig. 18–2).[6] A small, yellow, round spot may be seen in the fovea that may be caused by increased xanthophyll visibility.

4. *RPE atrophic changes*: RPE changes corresponding to previous CSC episodes may be present in either or both eyes. Atrophic changes in the fovea can also be explained by shifting of subretinal fluid while the patient is in the supine state during sleep and then upright during the day moving fluid inferiorly away from the fovea.

5. *Multiple bullous serous retinal and RPE detachments*: An atypical presentation of CSC is that of multiple serous retinal detachments (Fig. 18–3), usually seen in healthy middle-aged men.[6,11,23,24] These posterior pole or midperipheral detachments are often associated with subretinal fibrinous exudate and multiple serous RPE detachments with areas of shifting subretinal fluid.

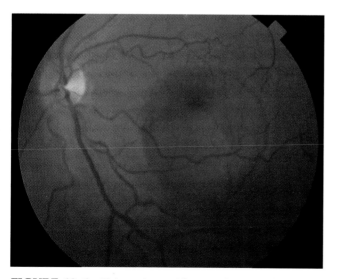

FIGURE 18–1 This patient with central serous chorioretinopathy has a serous macular detachment.

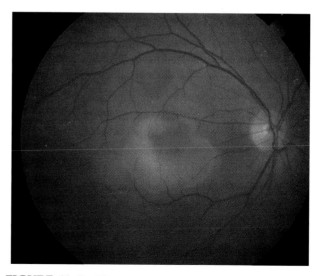

FIGURE 18–2 This patient with central serous chorioretinopathy has a serous macular detachment with fibrin deposition.

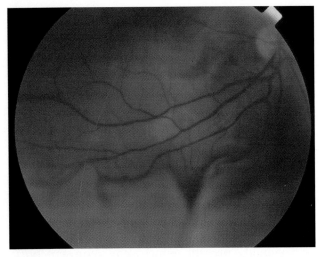

FIGURE 18–3 This patient developed a bullous retinal detachment with central serous chorioretinopathy.

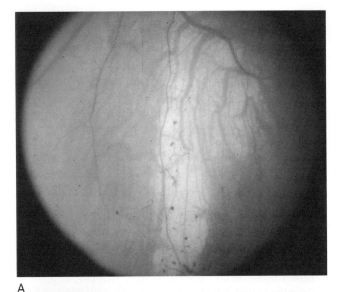

A

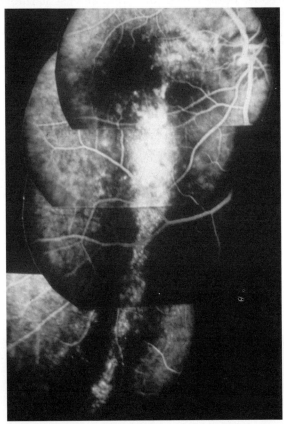

B

FIGURE 18–4 This patient with central serous chorioretinopathy has an inferior tract (*A*). These tracts can often be well delineated by fluorescein angiography (*B*).

6. *Extramacular RPE atrophic tracts*: Yannuzzi and co-workers[25] described 25 patients with extramacular inferior hemispheric RPE atrophic tracts related to an antecedent retinal detachment (Fig. 18–4). Five of these patients actually had a peripheral retinal detachment. Other findings that were reported in this subset of CSC patients included retinal capillary telangiectasia, retinal capillary leakage cystoid macular edema, lipid deposition, choriocapillaris atrophy, choroidal neovascularization, and disciform scar formation. This group tended to have unusually poor visual outcomes as expected. The underlying pigment epithelial changes or precipitates may serve as a guide to the full extent of the detachment and area of fluid leakage.[22]

Ie and associates[26] reported 11 patients with the diagnosis of CSC who were found to have subretinal exudation presumed to be fibrin. This finding has traditionally been suggestive of CNV due to age-related macular degeneration (AMD), which was not present in any of these patients. Exudates in cases of CSC were previously reported in association with pregnancy or in reported cases of large bullous detachments. Ie suggests that a significant alteration in the normal physiology must occur to allow fibrinogen, the necessary precursor of fibrin, to enter the subretinal space.

DIFFERENTIAL DIAGNOSIS

Several disease processes can cause a localized detachment of the macula and thus mimic CSC (Table 18–2). These disorders include presumed ocular histoplasmosis syndrome (POHS), AMD, multifocal choroiditis, metastatic cancer, Harada's disease, tumors, vascular disorders, Eales' disease, uveal effusion syndrome, segmental retinitis pigmentosa, retinoschisis, lymphoma, and optic nerve pit with serous macular detachment.

Patient history, clinical examination, and exami-

TABLE 18–2 Differential Diagnosis

Presumed ocular histoplasmosis syndrome
   (POHS)
Age-related macular degeneration (AMD)
Multifocal choroiditis
Metastatic cancer
Harada's disease
Tumors
Vascular disorders
Eales' disease
Uveal effusion syndrome
Segmental retinitis pigmentosa
Retinoschisis
Lymphoma
Optic nerve pit with serous macular detachment

nation with fluorescein angiography (FA) can usually distinguish CSC from the other disorders mentioned. It is especially important that in patients over age 50 choroidal neovascularization be ruled out. The findings of drusen in the macula may help to exclude CSC, but indocyanine green (ICG) angiography may be invaluable in differentiating the two entities.

NATURAL HISTORY/ CLINICAL COURSE

Idiopathic CSC is a self-limited disease, remaining mild in most patients, with the majority recovering excellent vision without medical intervention. Klein and associates prospectively studied 34 eyes with CSC and reported 100% resolution without treatment.[15] The average time for resolution is 3[15] to 4 months.[3] On follow-up examination (average, 23 months), 100% of eyes had 20/40 or better vision and 94% had 20/30 or better.[15] A 100% rate of recovery, without treatment, to 20/20 has been reported in another series.[27] Although the serous detachment is self-limited and visual acuity typically is excellent, patients may complain of minor visual disturbance including decreased contrast sensitivity, relative scotomas, decreased color vision, metamorphosis, and nyctalopia.[15,28,29] Patients may be reassured that improvement in vision may continue for more than 1 year following resolution of the detachment.[15] Despite spontaneous healing and return to good visual function, pigment epithelial scars can be observed around the original areas of leakage. They can be much larger than the previous area of leakage and no longer leak on FA.[30] After resolution of the detachment other findings can include focal yellow deposits, precipitates, and cystic changes.[3]

Recurrences

Recurrences of CSC are quite common. Clinical series report a 45[15] to 49%[15,27] chance of a recurrence after an episode of CSC; 10% of patients suffer three or more recurrences. Almost 50% of patients will experience a recurrence within 1 year of the first episode, although recurrences have been reported up to 10 years later.[30] Occasionally, a patient will present with a seemingly "first" attack of CSC, but careful history and examination will reveal that the patient had suffered a prior episode of CSC.

Complicated Cases

Despite an excellent visual prognosis in the majority of patients, a small subset of approximately 5% have a poor outcome. Reports of cystoid macular edema, peripheral atrophic tracks,[31] choroidal neovascularization,[32] and severe RPE degeneration are correlated with poor visual outcome.

Yannuzzi and co-workers[25] reported a subset of 32 eyes with CSC who demonstrated RPE atrophic tracks resulting in a final visual acuity of 20/200 or worse in 25% of patients. Diffuse RPE abnormalities may accompany one or recurrent episodes of CSC and lead to an unfavorable outcome. Levine and associates[33] studied 14 eyes by FA and found diffuse areas of RPE abnormalities within the previous detachments in 100% of cases and outside these areas in 43% of cases. They observed new RPE window defects in 42% of fellow eyes. The authors concluded that CSC may represent a diffuse, progressive disturbance of the RPE. They confirmed other reports that more severe forms of CSC are more common in patients of nonwhite heritage. In their series 23% of patients were black and the average age was older. Other reports have shown a poorer visual outcome in patients of Asian and Hispanic heritage. Gass reported severe and permanent visual loss resulting from subretinal fibrosis secondary to fibrin in the subretinal space.[34]

CSC in Older Adults

Traditionally, central serous choroidopathy has been a disease reported most often in young men, but more recent studies have identified many cases of CSC in adults over 50. Spaide has reported cases of CSC in patients over 50 and found a higher percentage of female patients (50%).[17] Schatz[35] reported 13 patients over 60 with 4 of 17 female, and a higher incidence of multiple small PEDs but no signs of AMD in any patients. Berger[36] studied 47 patients with CSC who were over 50 at presentation and found an increased risk of choroidal neovascularization especially in patients with multiple leaks on FA.

CSC in Women

Recent studies have looked at the characteristics of CSC in women[37] and have found that women tend to be older (average age, 53). This is consistent with earlier studies that found a higher percentage of women in the older population of patients with CSC.[38,39] CSC has been reported in association with pregnancy in several papers.[40-42] Some studies have suggested a nonwhite predominance of patients, and most studies report a much higher incidence of fibrinous subretinal exudates (up to 90%).[41,42] CSC tends to occur in the third trimester and resolves spontaneously by 1 to 2 months with an excellent prognosis despite subretinal exudates.

A chronic benign form of CSC was reported in 14 patients with juxtafoveal cystic lesions, good vision, and angiographic evidence of pigment epithelial detachments.[43]

FLUORESCEIN ANGIOGRAPHY

Fluorescein angiography provided unique insight into the understanding of CSC by demonstrating that the fluid accumulating under the neurosensory retina originated from a tiny leakage point in the RPE.[2,3] On FA in over 95% of patients with CSC there is at least one leakage point seen. In the early phase of the angiogram the leakage of dye from the choroid through the RPE is seen as a focal dot of hyperfluorescence.

Types of Leakage

Two types of leakage may then be observed (Figs. 18–5 and 18–6). Typically, the dye spreads sym-

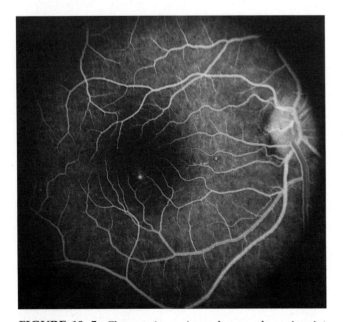

FIGURE 18–5 Fluorescein angiography reveals a pinpoint area of hyperfluorescence.

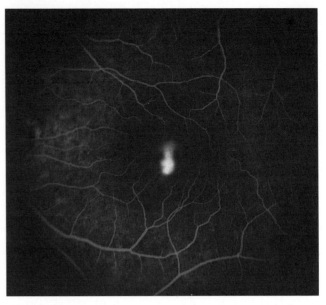

FIGURE 18–6 Fluorescein angiography of Figure 18–2 showing enlargement to a smokestack-like lesion.

metrically, staining the subretinal fluid under the detachment but never extends outside the borders of the detachment. In as many as 93% of patients a uniform type of filling is seen.[44] In 7[44]–20%[27,45,46] of cases the classic or smokestack type of leakage is observed where fluorescein first ascends and then flows laterally as it reaches the superior border of the detachment (Fig. 18–6). This pattern, described in 1971 by Shimizu and Tobari,[46] is felt to result from an osmotic pressure gradient generated by differences between the protein concentration of the subretinal fluid under the detachment and the fluorescein dye entering the detachment.

Location of Leakage Points

Spitznas and Huke[44] confirmed previous reports[46-48] concerning the location of the leakage points. Leakage points are most often found in the superior nasal quadrant (33.2%), followed by the inferior nasal (21.2%), superior temporal (19%), and inferior temporal (14.8%) in decreasing order of frequency. In 25.4% the leakage points were located in the papillomacular bundle. The majority of points are within a 1-mm zone around the fovea but less than 10% are found actually within the foveal area. In 11.8% of cases leakage points were found in an area more than 3 mm from the foveal center. In these cases they were most often found in the upper nasal quadrant.[44] These authors also studied the location points in patients with a recurrence of CSC and found 62% of the new leakage points to be within 0.5 mm[44] and 80%[27,44] within 1 mm of the old leakage points. Although several studies have confirmed an obvious anatomic predilection for RPE leakage, regional differences in the choriocapillary, RPE, neurosensory retina, or Bruch's membrane have failed to explain this.[30] The commonly observed movement of exudate into the fovea despite fewer than 10% of leakage points found there is curious. It is hypothesized to result from the decreased adhesion force between the RPE and neurosensory retina in the foveal region due to the paucity of rods there.[44]

Number of Leakage Points

Patients with CSC typically have one leakage point on FA but they may have multiple. In 430 eyes with CSC (without detachment of the RPE),[44] 71.6% of patients were found to have one leakage point and 17% had two and some patients had as many as seven leakage points observed simultaneously in the same eye.

Gilbert et al[27] reported long-term follow-up of CSC patients and noted several rare leakage patterns including persistent leakage at the site of a healed CSC scar and diffuse leakage without any discrete leakage point.

INDOCYANINE GREEN ANGIOGRAPHY

Abnormalities in the choroidal circulation have been hypothesized to be causative factors in the pathogenesis of CSC.[10,11,17] Fluorescein angiography has limited usefulness in defining choroidal effects in CSC. ICG dye (Fig. 18–7) is a larger molecular that is highly protein bound and therefore does not leak extensively through the fenestrations of the choriocapillaris. This allows less obscuration of the choroidal vasculature than with FA and for this reason has proven invaluable in studying CSC. In several studies, digital ICG videoangiograms (ICG-V)

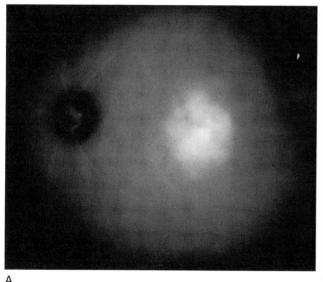

A

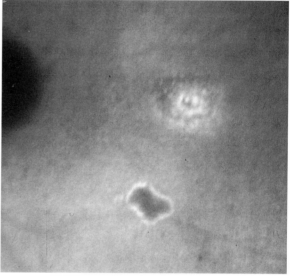

B

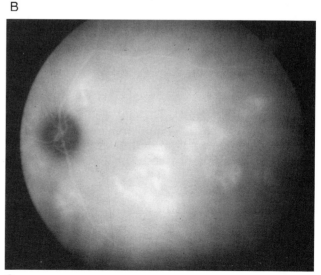

C

FIGURE 18–7 ICG angiography findings of central serous chorioretinopathy include a focal spot surrounded by an area of choroidal hyperpermeability (A), pigment epithelial detachments with hypofluorescent centers and hypofluorescent rims (B), and diffuse focal areas of choroidal hyperpermeability (C).

were used to study eyes with CSC previously evaluated by FA.[10,11,35,36] All investigators discovered choroidal abnormalities that were not previously identifiable on FA.

Active leakage points identified on FA were confirmed with ICG-V by Cardillo Piccolino[49] in 80% of patients and by Guyer[50] in 100%. In eyes with the classic "smokestack" on FA the pattern was not clearly seen on ICG.[22] No additional leakage points were identified and no areas of ischemia or decreased perfusion were evident.

ICG has been used by several investigators to study the unique characteristics of PEDs.[35] ICG studies revealed "occult" pigment epithelial detachments (PEDs) not identified on FA,[35] with unique characteristics of staining.[35,36] Guyer found that 75% of patients with acute CSC had PEDs, while 84% with chronic CSC demonstrated early staining and late hypofluorescence characteristics of PED in patients with CSC. In the late phase the dye pools at the margins of the PED, forming a distinct ring (Fig. 18–7). On the contrary, serous PEDs seen in AMD are not stained by ICG and remain hypofluorescent.[38] A specific staining pattern was noted, leading to the conclusion that choroidal hyperpermeability may underlay CSC. Guyer reported that 100% of patients had multiple bright areas of hyperfluorescence 0.3 to 3 disc areas around the areas of leakage and elsewhere. The boundaries were independent of the neurosurgery retinal detachment and clearly choroidal in origin. These areas of fluorescence were noted in eyes with inactive disease,[17] after resolution of disease, and preceding the appearance of leakage and clinical disease.[22] We have also studied ICG in patients over age 50 with CSC, and in over 30 patients 100% were noted to have bilateral multifocal choroidal vascular hyperpermeability (MCVH). In normal controls ICG was not found to exude in detectable quantities and late choroidal staining was not found in patients without CSC.[39]

OTHER MODALITIES OF DIAGNOSIS

Optical Coherence Tomography

Hee et al found optical coherence tomography (OCT) to be effective in detecting serous detachment undetected by slit lamp biomicroscopy,[51] making it a potentially useful tool in cases where noninvasive testing may be necessary.

Electrophysiologic Studies

Several investigators have investigated CSC with the use of electroretinography (ERG).[52–56] They found reduced b-wave (macular response) amplitudes in most patients with CSC. In one study[53] 18 patients were studied after resolution of CSC and were found to have recovery of the b-waves and shortened implicit times. The findings of oscillatory potentials that did not recover suggest a middle to inner retinal layer abnormality.

PATHOGENESIS

Many suggestions regarding the etiology of CSC have been made. They include vitreous traction,[57] hypotony,[58] infection,[1,59–61] malnutrition,[58] toxicity,[8,62] psychogenic behavior,[3,18,63–65] episcleritis,[66] familial causes,[6,7] and allergy. Reports of CSC in association with systemic disease, medication use, pregnancy, and emotional states are multiple. These include membranoproliferative glomerulonephritis type II,[67] cardiac and renal organ transplantation,[68] and dialysis.[69,70]

The primary tissue site affected and the cause of CSC remain controversial. Previously, Gass hypothesized that the choroid was the site of involvement. This has been recently substantiated with the introduction of ICG angiography. Through studies of patients with CSC, investigators have pointed to the choroidal vasculature as the primary site of involvement. In studying our patients using ICG angiography we found choroidal staining beneath leakage points previously identified on FA. The question still remains as to the specific physiologic mechanism causing a serous detachment of the retina, and the underlying disturbance of chorioretinal hemostasis.

Under normal circumstances, the retina remains apposed to the RPE and the RPE to Bruch's membrane. Although it remains poorly understood, there are several factors responsible. Under normal physiologic conditions, there is a net movement of fluid from the vitreous toward the choroid due to osmotic pressure differences and ionic differences. Specifically, three components of the retinal adhesion force must be overcome in order for subretinal fluid to accumulate: (1) hydrostatic pressure (related to intraocular pressure [IOP]), (2) high osmotic pressure in the choroid in comparison to the retina, and (3) active transport by the RPE pump from the subretinal space to the choroid.[71] Some authors point to the RPE as the site of disturbance.[72–74] The anatomic sequence of events remains controversial. Gass suggested that a detachment of the RPE preceded leakage, but in contrast, Wessing[47] concluded that a direct penetration through the RPE causing accumulation of subretinal fluid is the rule based upon his observations with FA. Cardillo Piccolino[71] suggested that in CSC a lesion induces permeability decreasing the influence of colloid osmotic pressures allowing flow from choriocapillaris to the subretinal space. Spitznas[74] proposed the possibility of reversed polarity of ion movement causing fluid to move from the

TABLE 18–3   Proposed Pathogenesis for Central
Serous Chorioretinopathy*

Choroidal hyperpermeability
⇓
Serous RPE detachment
⇓
Pressure on RPE
⇓
Mechanically induced leak or RPE decompensation
⇓
RPE leakage
⇓
Neurosensory retinal detachment

* From Guyer DR, Yannuzzi LA, Slakter JS: Digital
indocyanine green angiography of central serous
chorioretinopathy. Arch Ophthalmol 112:1057–1062,
1994. Copyright 1994, American Medical Association,
with permission.

choroid to the subretinal space. Guyer et al[50] proposed a model of the physiologic sequence of
events based upon recent work with ICG angiography (Table 18–3).

Several investigators have offered invaluable insight into the mechanisms involved in CSC. A hypothesis involving increased adrenergic stimulation
has been investigated based upon clinical observations of CSC in situations of high stress and type
A personalities. An animal model of CSC has been
created with the use of intravenous epinephrine in
rabbits[75–78] and monkeys.[79–81] Clinical observations
of CSC in pregnancy[79–81] and in Cushing's disease
(Bouzas EA 1993) also support a hormonal mechanism for disease. Most clinicians support the idea
that stress plays a role in the etiology of CSC based
upon their patients' histories. Yoshioka found that
experimental CSC induced in rabbits using intravenous adrenalin is completely suppressed by pretreatment with β-adrenergic receptor agents and
ganglionic blocking agents, supporting the strong
role of stress in this disease.[82]

Yannuzzi[18] suggests that the cause of CSC may
be multifactorial, consisting of genetic, environmental, and behavioral factors. Patients with CSC
were more likely to demonstrate a type A personality and increased levels of catecholamines in patients with type A personality traits have been demonstrated. It is not known precisely how the
adrenergic stimulation produces CSC. One possibility is that it causes damage to the choriocapillaris, thus inducing a hyperpermeable state.

HISTOPATHOLOGY

There is little information available concerning the
histopathology of CSC. Gass[6] reported histopathology on a 52-year-old male without a history of visual complaints. Postmortem examination revealed
a serous detachment of the RPE and retina with
normal choroid, choriocapillaris, and pigment epithelium. Three other histopathologic reports describe serous macular detachments with normal
RPE[83–85] but without prior documentation of CSC
clinically or by FA. De Venecia reported a case
where classic smokestack leakage was documented
on FA and evidence of fibrinous exudate in the subretinal and sub-RPE space with a normal choriocapillaris was noted on histopathologic examination.[86] Since patients with CSC have an excellent
visual prognosis and tend to be young, histopathologic examination is rare and therefore does not
contribute much to our understanding of the
pathogenesis.

TREATMENT

Medical treatment has not been shown to shorten
the course of the macular detachment or lead to a
better long-term prognosis. Systemic corticosteroids
have been shown to exacerbate CSC. Reports of
CSC in association with Cushing's syndrome suggest that in certain cases glucocorticoids may play
a role in the etiology of the disease. Treatment of
the psychogenic components of this disorder with
barbiturates or sedatives has been advocated but
not proven to be beneficial. Other suggested modes
of therapy including β-blockers and acetazolamide
have not been shown to be beneficial.

The use of laser photocoagulation to treat CSC
has been controversial. In the acute state, photocoagulation at the site of the angiographic pigment
epithelial leak can result in resolution of the serous
detachment within 3 to 4 weeks in most patients.
Spitznas[30] reported on a nonrandomized study of
139 untreated and 109 xenon arc–treated cases of
CSC. Either the leakage point was directly treated
or indirect treatment was applied to the edge of the
detachment. All three groups had identical final visual acuity (median, 20/25). The duration of the
detachment was 80 days in the untreated group
and 10 days in both treated groups. Klein and associates[15] studied 34 untreated patients prospectively and found that all cases resolved and 94% of
eyes had 20/30 or better acuity at follow-up. Studies have not shown that laser treatment results in a
better long-term prognosis, only a faster resorption
of serous fluid.[87] Because of the overall good visual
prognosis without therapy, and the potential risk
for iatrogenic choroidal neovascularization, photocoagulation for CSC is recommended only in special circumstances. We would recommend laser
treatment only for patients with occupational needs
for binocular vision (such as pilots or surgeons),
persistent serous fluid (>6 months), or those eyes
with chronic pigment epithelial changes.

REFERENCES

1. von Graefe A: Ueber centrale recidivierende Retinitis. Graefes Arch Clin Exp Ophthalmol 12:211–215, 1866.
2. Maumenee AE: Symposium: macular diseases, clinical manifestations. Trans Am Acad Ophthalmol Otolaryngol 69:605–613, 1965.
3. Gass JDM: Pathogenesis of disciform detachment of the neuroephithelium. II. Idiopathic central serous choroidopathy. Am J Ophthalmol 63:587–615, 1960.
4. Klein BA: Symposium: macular diseases: clinical manifestations. Central serous retinopathy and chorioretinopathy. Trans Am Acad Ophthalmol Otolaryngol 69:614–620, 1965.
5. Bennett G: Central serous retinopathy. Br J Ophthalmol 39:600–618, 1955.
6. Gass JDM: Stereoscopic Atlas of Macular Diseases. St Louis, CV Mosby Co, 1987, pp 46–59.
7. Gragoudas ES: Unpublished data.
8. Burton TC: Central serous retinopathy. In Blodi FC (ed): Current Concepts in Ophthalmology, Vol 3. St Louis, CV Mosby Co, 1972, pp 1–28.
9. Edwards TS, Priestley BS: Central angiospastic retinopathy. Am J Ophthalmol 57:988–996, 1964.
10. Gass JD, Norton EWD, Justice J: Serous detachment of the retinal pigment epithelium. Trans Am Acad Ophthalmol Otolaryngol 70:990–1015, 1966.
11. Gass JDM: Bullous retinal detachment: an unusual manifestation of idiopathic central serous choroidopathy. Am J Ophthalmol 75:819–821, 1973.
12. Klein BA: Symposium: macular diseases, clinical manifestations. I. Central serous retinopathy and chorioretinopathy. Trans Am Acad Ophthalmol Otolaryngol 69:614–620, 1968.
13. Mitsui Y, Sakanishi R: Central angiospastic retinopathy. Am J Ophthalmol 41:105–114, 1956.
14. Seraatsma BR, Allca RA, Pettit TH: Central serous retinopathy. Trans Pacific Coast Otolaryngol Ophthalmol Soc 47:107–127, 1966.
15. Klein ML, Van Buskirk EM, Friedman E, et al: Experience with nontreatment of central serous choroidopathy. Arch Ophthalmol 91:247–250, 1974.
16. Cohen D, Gaudric A, Coscas G, et al: Epitheliopathie retinienne diffuse ct chorioretinopathie sereuse centrale. J Fr Ophthalmol 6:339–349, 1983.
17. Spaide RF, Hall LS, Hass A, et al: Indocyanine green videoangiography of older patients with central serous chorioretinopathy. Retina 16:203–213, 1996.
18. Yannuzzi LA: Type A behavior and central serous chorioretinopathy. Trans Am Ophthalmol Soc 84:799–845, 1986.
19. Hirose I: Therapy of central serous retinopathy. Folia Ophthalmol Jpn 20:1003–1034, 1969.
20. Fukunaga K: Central chorioretinopathy with disharmony of the autonomic nervous system. Acta Soc Ophthalmol Jpn 73:1468–14n, 1969.
21. Lyons DE: Conservative management of central serous retinopathy. Trans Ophthalmol Soc U K 97:214, 1977.
22. Yannuzzi L, Schatz H, Gitter K: Central Serous Choroidopathy in the Macula. Baltimore, Williams & Wilkins, 1978, pp 145–165.
23. Mazzuca DE, Benson WE: Central serous retinopathy: variants. Surv Ophthalmol 31:173–174, 1986.
24. Benson WE, Shields JA, Annesley WH, Tasman W: Central serous chorioretinopathy with bullous retinal detachment. Ann Ophthalmol 12:920–924, 1980.
25. Yannuzzi LA, Shakin J, Fisher Y, et al: Peripheral retinal detachment and retinal pigment epithelial atrophic tracts secondary to central serous pigment epitheliopathy. Ophthalmology 91:1554, 1984.
26. Ie D, Yannuzzi LA, Spaide RF, et al: Subretinal exudative deposits in central serous chorioretinopathy. Br J Ophthalmol 77:349–353, 1993.
27. Gilbert CM, Owens SL, Smith PD, Fine SL: Long-term follow-up of central serous chorioretinopathy. Br J Ophthalmol 68:815–820, 1984.
28. Folk JC, Thompson HS, Han DP, Brown CK: Visual function abnormalities in central serous retinopathy. Arch Ophthalmol 102:1299–1302, 1984.
29. Tsuneoka H, Kabayama T, Fukada I, Narazaki S: Night visual acuity in patients with idiopathic central serous choroidopathy. Jpn J Ophthalmol 24:17–187, 1980.
30. Spitznas M: Central serous retinopathy. In Ryan SJ (ed): Retina. St Louis, CV Mosby Co, 1989, pp 217–227.
31. Yannuzzi LA, Shakin JL, Fisher YI, Altomonte MA: Peripheral retinal detachments and retinal pigment epithelial atrophic tracts secondary to central serous pigment epitheliopathy. Ophthalmology 91:1554–1572, 1984.
32. Schatz H, Yannuzzi LA, Gitter KA: Subretinal neovascular membrane following argon laser photocoagulation treatment for central serous choriodopathy: complication or misdiagnosis? Trans Am Acad Ophthalmol Otolaryngol 83:893–906, 1977.
33. Levine R, Brucker A, Robinson F: Long-term follow-up of idiopathic central serous chorioretinopathy by fluorescein angiography. Ophthalmology 96:854–859, 1989.
34. Gass JDM: Central serous chorioretinopathy and white subretinal exudation during pregnancy. Arch Ophthalmol 109:677–681, 1991.
35. Schatz H, Madeira D, Johnson RN, McDonald HR: Central serous chorioretinopathy occurring in patients 60 years of age or older. Ophthalmology 99:63–67, 1992.
36. Berger AR, Olk RJ, Burgess D: Central serous choriodopathy in patients over 50 years of age. Ophthalmic Surg 22:583–590, 1991.
37. Quillen DA, Gass DM: Central serous chorioretinopathy in women. Ophthalmology 103:72–79, 1996.
38. Yannuzzi LA, Slakter JS, Sorenson JA, et al: Digital indocyanine green videoangiography and choroidal neovascularization. Retina 12:191–223, 1992.
39. Scheider A, Volth A, Neuhauser L: Fluorescence characteristics of indocyanine green in the normal choroid and in subretinal neovascular membranes. Ger J Ophthalmol 1:7–11, 1992.
40. Fastenberg DM, Ober RR: Central serous choriodopathy in pregnancy. Arch Ophthalmol 101:1055, 1993.
41. Sunness JS, Haller JA, Fine SL: Central serous choriodopathy and pregnancy. Arch Ophthalmol 111:360, 1993.
42. Gass JDM: CSC and white subretinal exudation during preganancy. Arch Ophthalmol 109:677–681, 1991.
43. Lachapelle K, Ballantyne M, Cruess A: Chronic benign retinal pigment epithelial detachment: a subtype of central serous choriodopathy. Can J Ophthalmol 29(2):70–72, 1994.
44. Spitznas M, Huke J: Number, shape, and topography of leakage points in acute type I central serous retinopathy. Graefes Arch Clin Exp Ophthalmol 225:437–440, 1987.
45. Spitznas M: Central serous chorioretinopathy. Ophthalmology 87(8S):88, 1980.
46. Shimizu K, Tobari I: Central serous retinopathy dynamics of subretinal fluid. Mod Probl Ophthalmol 9:152–157, 1971.
47. Wessing A: Grundsatzliches zum diagnostoschen Fortschutt durch die Fluoreszenzangiographie. Ber Dtsch Ophthalmol Ges 73:560–568, 1973.
48. Bonamour G, Bonnet M, Grange ID, et al: Topographische Studien uber angiographisch beobachtete Lasionen bei Retinitis centralis serosa. Klin Monatsbl Augenheilkd 171:862–866, 1977.
49. Cardillo Piccolino F, Borgia L: Central serous chorioretinopathy and indocyanine green angiography. Retina 14:231–242, 1994.
50. Guyer DR, Yannuzzi LA, Slakter JS: Digital indocyanine green angiography of central serous chorioretinopathy. Arch Ophthalmol 112:1057–1062, 1994.
51. Hee MR, Puliafito CA, Wong C: Optical coherence tomography of central serous chorioretinopathy. Am J Ophthalmol 120(1):65–74, 1995.
52. Nagata M, Honda Y: Macular ERG in central serous retinopathy. Jpn J Ophthalmol 15:9–16, 1971.

53. Miyake Y, Shiroyama N, Ota I, Horiguchi M: Local macular electroretinographic responses in idiopathic central serous chorioretinopathy. Am J Ophthalmol 106:549–550, 1988.

54. van Meel GJ, Smith VC, Pokomy J, van Norren D: Foveal densitometry in central serous choroidopathy. Am J Ophthalmol 98:359–368, 1984.

55. Chuang EL, Sharp DM, Fitzke FW, et al: Retinal dysfunction in central serous retinopathy. Eye 1:120–125, 1987.

56. Tian N: A study of spectral electroretinogram of color vision defects due to macular diseases. Eye Sci 10(3):163–167, 1994.

57. Tolentinto EI, Freeman HM, Schepens CC: Vitreoretinal traction in serous and hemorrhagic macular retinopathy. Arch Ophthalmol 78:23–20, 1967.

58. Duke-Elder WS: System of Ophthalmology: Diseases of the Retina, Vol 10. St Louis, CV Mosby Co, 1967, pp 121–137.

59. Fuchs E: Ein Fall zentraler, Rezidivierender Syphilitischer Net zhautntzundung. Centralbl f Prakt Augenh 40:105–108, 1916.

60. Kitahara S: Ueber klinische Beobachtungen bei der in Japan haufig vorkommenden Chorioretinitis centralsi serosa. Klin Monatsbl Augenheilkd 97:345–362, 1936.

61. Sie-Boen-Lian: The etiologic agent of serous central chorioretinitis. Ophthalmologica 148:269–270, 1964.

62. Redman SI: A review of solar retinitis as it may pertain to macular lesions seen in persons of the armed forces. Am J Ophthalmol 28:1155–1165, 1945.

63. Gifford SR, Marquardt G: Central angiospastic retinopathy. Arch Ophthalmol 21:211–228, 1939.

64. Werry H, Arends C: Untersuchung zur Objektivierung von Personlichkeitsmerkmalen bei Patienten mit Retinopathia centralis serosa. Klin Monatsbl Augenheilkd 172:363–370, 1978.

65. Lipowski ZJ, Kiriakos RZ: Psychosomatic aspects of central serous retinopathy: a review and case report. Psychosomatics 12:398–401, 1971.

66. Fine SL, Owens SL: Central serous retinopathy in a 7-year-old girl. Am J Ophthalmol 90:871–873, 1985.

67. Ulbig MR, Riordan-Eva P, Holz FG: Membranoproliferative glomerulonephritis type II associated with central serous retinopathy. Am J Ophthalmol 116(4):410–413, 1993.

68. Friberg TR, Eller AW: Serous retinal detachment resembling central serous chorioretinopathy following organ transplantation. Grafes Archive Clin Exp Ophthalmol 228(4):305–309, 1990.

69. Friberg TR, Elter AW: Serous retinal detachment resembling central serous chorioretinopathy following organ transplantation. Graefes Arch Clin Exp Ophthalmol 228:305–309, 1990.

70. Gragoudas ES: Unpublished data.

71. Piccolino FC: Central serous retinopathy: some considerations on the pathogenesis. Ophthalmologica 182:204–210, 1981.

72. Marmor MF: Control of subretinal fluid: experimental and clinical studies. Eye 4:340–344, 1990.

73. Negi A, Marmor MF: Experimental serous retinal detachment and focal pigment epithelium damage. Arch Ophthalmol 102:440–449, 1984.

74. Spitznas M: Pathogenesis of central serous retinopathy: a new working hypothesis. Graefes Arch Clin Exp Ophthalmol 224:321–324, 1986.

75. Ikeda I, Komi T, Nakaji K, et al: Chorioretinitis central serous. Acta Soc Ophthalmol Jpn 60:1261–1266, 1956.

76. Nagayoski K: Experimental study of chorioretinopathy by intravenous injection of adrenaline. Acta Soc Ophthalmol Jpn 75:1720–1727, 1971.

77. Miki T, Sunada I, Higaki T: Studies on chorioretinitis induced in rabbits by stress (repeated administration of epinephrine). Acta Soc Ophthalmol Jpn 75:1037–1045, 1972.

78. Yasuzumi T, Miki T, Sugimoto K: Electron microscopic studies of epinephrine choroiditis in rabbits. I. Pigment

79. Chumbley LC, Frank RN: Central serous retinopathy and pregnancy. Am J Ophthalmol 77:158–160, 1974.

80. Cruysberg JRM, Deutman AF: Visual disturbances during pregnancy caused by central serous choroidopathy. Br J Ophthalmol 66:240–241, 1982.

81. Fastenberg DM, Ober RR: Central serous choroidopathy in pregnancy. Arch Ophthalmol 101:1055–1058, 1983.

82. Yoshioka H: The etiology of CSC (Japanese) Nippon Ganka Gakkai Zasshi. Acta Soc Ophthalmol Jpn 95(12):1181–1195, 1991.

83. Klien BA: Macular and extramacular serous chorioretinopathy. Am J Ophthalmol 51:231–242, 1961.

84. Fry WE, Spaeth EB: Subacute arcumscribed macular retinochoroiditis simulating intraocular tumor. Trans Am Acad Ophthalmol 59:346–355, 1955.

85. Ikui H: Histopathological examination of central serous retinopathy. Folia Ophthalmol Jpn 20:1035–1043, 1969.

86. de Venecia G: Fluorescein angiographic smoke stack. Case presentation at Verhoeff Society Meeting. Washington, DC, April 2 25, 1982.

87. Watzke RC, Burton TC, Leverton PE: Ruby laser photocoagulation therapy of central serous retinopathy. I. A controlled clinical trial. 11. Factors affecting prognosis. Trans Am Acad Ophthalmol Otolaryngol 78:205–211, 1974.

88. Horniker E: Su di una forma retinite centrale di origine vasoneurotica (retinite central capillaro-spastica). Ann Ottal 55:578–600, 1927.

89. Walsh FB, Sloan LL: Idiopathic flat detachment of the macula. Am J Ophthalmol 19:195–228, 1936.

90. Klien BA: Macular lesions of vascular origin. II. Functional vascular conditions leading to damage of the macula lutea. Am J Ophthalmol 36:1–13, 1953.

91. Maumenee AE: Serous and hemorrhagic disciform detachment of the macula. Trans Pacific Coast Oto-Ophthalmol Soc 40:139–16U, 1959.

92. Fine SL: Personal communication, 1989.

93. Gass IDM: Photocoagulation treatment of idiopathic central serous choroidopathy. Trans Am Acad Ophthalmol Otolaryngol 83:456–463, 1977.

94. Friberg TR, Campagna J: Central serous chorioretinopathy: an analysis of the clinical morphology using image-processing techniques. Graefes Arch Ophthalmol 227:201–205, 1989.

95. Nadel AJ, Turan MI, Coles RS: Central serous retinopathy: a generalized disease of the pigment epithelium. Mod Probl Ophthalmol 20:76–88, 1979.

96. Bettman JW: Allergic retinosis. Am J Ophthalmol 28:132:1323–1328, 1945.

97. Berens S, Sayad WY, Girard LJ: Symposium on ocular allergy. The uveal tract and retina: consideration of certain experimental and clinical concepts. Trans Am Acad Ophthalmol Otolaryngol 56:220–241, 1952.

98. Henry F: Angiospastic retinopathy. Am J Ophthalmol 35:1509–1510, 1952.

99. Yoshioka H, Sugita T, Nagayoski K: Fluorescein angiography findings in experimental retinopathy produced by intravenous adrenaline injection. Folia Ophthalmol Jpn 21:648–652, 1970.

100. Yoshioka H, Katsume Y, Akune H: Experimental central serous chorioretinopathy in monkey eyes. II. Fluorescein angiographic findings. Ophthalmologica 185:168–178, 1982.

101. Yoshioka H, Katsume Y: Experimental central serous chorioretinopathy. III. Ultrastructural findings. Jpn J Ophthalmol 26:397–409, 1982.

102. Kazuhiko H, Hasegawa Y, Tokoro T: Indocyanine green angiography of central serous chorioretinopathy. Int Ophthalmol 9:37–41, 1986.

103. Amber JS, Zagarra H, Myers SM: Chronic macular detachment following pneumatic retinopexy. Retina 10:125–130, 1990.

104. Cox SN, Hay E, Bird AC: Treatment of chronic macular edema with acetazolamide. Arch Ophthalmol 106:1190–1195, 1988.
105. Robertson DM, Ilstrup D: Direct, indirect, and sham laser photocoagulation in the management of central serous chorioretinopathy. Am J Ophthalmol 95:457–466, 1983.
106. Watzke RC, Burton TC, Woolson RF: Direct and indirect laser photocoagulation of central serous choroidopathy. Am J Ophthalmol 88:914–918, 1979.
107. Slusher MM: Krypton red laser photocoagulation in selected cases of central serous chorioretinopathy. Retina 6:81–84, 1986.
108. Robertson DM: Argon laser photocoagulation treatment in central serous chorioretinopathy. Ophthalmology 93:972–974, 1986.
109. Yazawa M, et al: Indocyanine green videoangiographic findings in detachment of the retinal pigment epithelium. Ophthalmology 102(4):622–629, 1995.
110. Matsunga H: Occurrence of CNV following photocoagulation treatment for CSC NGGZ. Acta Soc Ophthalmol Jpn 99(4):460–468, 1995.

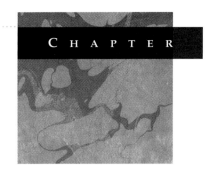

CHAPTER 19

Macular Hole

Allen C. Ho, M.D.

A macular hole is a full-thickness defect or tear of retinal tissue involving the anatomic fovea of the eye. Recently, there has been renewed interest in this previously untreatable condition with the refinement of vitreoretinal surgical techniques. Therapeutic approaches to macular hole surgery have ushered in new considerations of pharmacosurgical interventions in vitreoretinal surgery. Although significant progress has been made toward an understanding of macular hole lesions, significant controversy exists regarding the terminology, pathophysiology, diagnosis, natural history, and management of macular holes and precursor lesions.

The first macular hole descriptions were made in the second half of the 19th century and it was not until early in this century that macular holes were recognized as a clinical entity by most ophthalmologists. Early case descriptions of macular holes focused on young traumatized eyes, but it is now known that "idiopathic," age-related macular holes of the elderly comprise the vast majority of these lesions. In the beginning of the century traumatic macular holes were believed to account for half of all cases of macular holes; in a 1983 series, however, 83% were idiopathic and only 15% were due to accidental or surgical trauma.[1]

PATHOGENESIS: HISTORICAL, TRAUMATIC, AND CYSTOID DEGENERATION AND VASCULAR THEORIES

There are three basic historical theories on the pathogenesis of macular holes: the traumatic theory, the cystic degeneration and vascular theory, and the vitreous theory.[2] In 1869, Knapp made the first case description of a macular hole in a patient with ocular trauma and an initial diagnosis of a macular hemorrhage. He and most other early observers attributed macular holes to ocular trauma. Two years later Noyes provided the first accurate and detailed ophthalmoscopic description of a macular hole that was secondary to blunt trauma in a 13-year-old girl.[3] Noyes noted the difference in depth of focus from the retinal surface to the base of the lesion and probably was the first to recognize that the hallmark of the lesion was a full-thickness defect in retinal tissue within the center of the macula. Blunt ocular trauma could effect immediate macular hole formation from mechanical energy created by vitreous fluid waves and contrecoups macular necrosis or macular laceration.

The first histopathologic descriptions of full-thickness and lamellar macular holes were provided by Fuchs (1907) and Coats (1901), which supported a cystic degeneration theory of macular hole formation. Coats noted cystic intraretinal changes adjacent to the macular hole and surmised that these changes could be caused by trauma as well as other atraumatic mechanisms. Intraretinal cyst coalescence could then create a full-thickness macular hole. The major atraumatic theory of macular hole formation was the vascular theory of pathogenesis. Many believed that aging changes of the retinal vasculature led to cystoid retinal degeneration and subsequent macular hole formation. This vascular theory, sometimes characterized as ocular angiospasm, was the basis for a variety of interesting therapies including anxiolytics, vasodilators such as acetylcholine, nicotinic acid, calcium chloride, sodium and potassium iodide, retrobulbar atropine or prisicoline, vitamins, minerals, hormones, sedation, and recommendations of abstinence from tobacco.

HISTOPATHOLOGICAL FEATURES

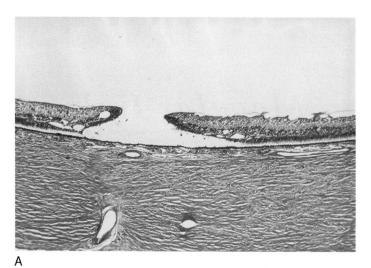

A

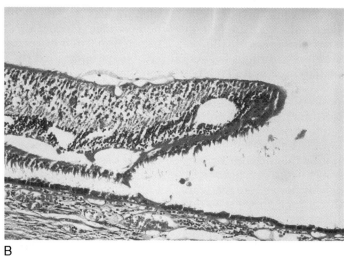

B

A, Idiopathic macular hole with rounded margins, cystoid macular edema, a thin layer of tapered cortical vitreous, and a small area of surrounding retinal detachment. *B,* Higher power view of rounded margin of idiopathic macular hole with tapered cortical vitreous, cystoid macular edema, and area of detachment with partial atrophy of the photoreceptor cell layer.

VITREOUS THEORIES AND CURRENT CONCEPTS OF MACULAR HOLE FORMATION

The vitreous theory of macular hole formation reflects both contemporary and historical perspectives on the pathogenesis of this condition. As early as 1912, the histopathology of overlying premacular vitreous condensation adjacent to foveal cystoid degeneration was recognized.[4] In 1924, Lister was the first of many to implicate anteroposterior vitreous forces in the pathogenesis of macular holes.[5] Several investigators, however, could not completely reconcile this theory of contracting vitreous bands with clinical observations of relatively clear vitreous, devoid of obvious vitreous traction bands.

Other proponents of a vitreous theory emphasized that the process of vitreous separation from the macula was the critical event in the pathogenesis of a macular hole. The problem with this hypothesis is that the incidence of posterior vitreous detachment and macular hole has been reported to be as variable as 12 to 100%. Data on the vitreous condition as it relates to macular hole formation are muddled by multiple problems including: the definition of vitreous separation (partial vs. complete, vitreofoveal separation vs. vitreomacular separation), the lack of uniform criteria used for vitreous separation (clinical: Weiss ring, posterior vitreous lacuna, posterior hyaloid; echographic: B scan ultrasonography; intraoperative: with endoilluminator and retinal pick or silicone-tipped cannula), and the timing of the observation of the vitreous (single vs. prospective observation; e.g., was vitreous attachment or separation noted before, after, or during the evolution of a macular hole?). Because posterior vitreous detachment is a common event in the age group of those at greatest risk for idiopathic macular hole formation, it is difficult to ascribe a causal relationship between these two events without a prospective evaluation of eyes correlating the status of the vitreous and the evolution of macular holes.

Morgan and Schatz proposed a mechanism of macular hole formation that they described as involutional macular thinning, which incorporates vitreous, vascular, and cystic degeneration theories.[6] In the first step of their proposed mechanism, the authors suggested that choroidal vascular changes could lead to altered submacular choroidal vascular perfusion leading to focal foveal, retinal, and pigment epithelial changes. In their view, these vascular changes then lead to cystic degeneration of the retina which then produce permanent structural changes in the fovea or in the retinal pigment epithelium, leading to involutional macular thinning. The final step in the pathogenesis of a macular hole in this theory is vitreous traction on now-susceptible, thinned foveal tissue.[6,7] These authors did not specify the nature of the vitreous traction

(anteroposterior forces vs. tangential traction) in their theory.

In 1988, Gass and Johnson described a classification scheme for idiopathic macular holes and their precursor lesions incorporating their ideas of the pathogenesis of these lesions.[8,9] From their clinical studies, these authors concluded that attached vitreous appears to move freely and without significant anteroposterior vitreous to macula traction forces. They also believed that an attached vitreous was critical to macular hole formation and that prior observations of macular holes developing despite posterior vitreous separation were incorrect because an optically empty area of a posterior vitreous lacuna may easily be misdiagnosed as a posterior vitreous detachment. Because each of the presumed stages of development of a macular hole caused loss of the normal foveal anatomic depression but no elevation of tissue above the parafoveal retina, they hypothesized that focal shrinkage of the prefoveolar vitreous cortex and tangential retinal traction are responsible for macular hole formation. Tangential vitreous contraction as a factor in the development of macular holes refocused attention on the vitreous and eyes deemed at risk for macular hole formation (premacular hole lesions). In their view, focal shrinkage of the prefoveal vitreous cortex causes anterior traction on the foveolar and then the foveal area, which creates an anterior traction detachment of the fovea.[8] This anterior traction is different from prior theories incorporating ideas on anteroposterior vitreous traction originating from the vitreous base and transmitted by shrinking transvitreal vitreous fibers.

GASS CLASSIFICATION OF PREMACULAR HOLE AND MACULAR HOLE LESIONS

Recently, Gass has updated his biomicroscopic classification and interpretation of macular hole formation.[10] (Fig. 19–1, Table 19–1). Spontaneous tangential traction of the external part of the prefoveolar cortical vitreous detaches foveolar retina thereby creating an intraretinal yellow spot approximately 100 to 200 μm in diameter (stage 1A).[8–10] The yellow color may result from intraretinal xanthophyll pigment. The foveal retina then elevates to the level of the surrounding perifoveal retina, elongating the foveal retina around the umbo. This transforms the yellow spot to a small donut-shaped yellow ring (stage 1B)[10] (Fig. 19–2).

Stage 1 lesions often demonstrate fine radiating retinal striae best observed with retroillumination. Vision is typically in the 20/25 to 20/70 range. Eventually the centrifugal displacement of the retinal receptors, xanthophyll, and radiating nerve fibers leads to a dehiscence of the deeper retinal receptor layer at the umbo[10] (Fig. 19–1, Table 19–1). The overlying internal limiting membrane, horizon-

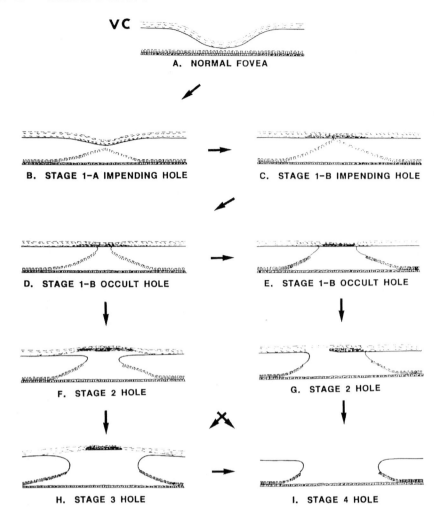

FIGURE 19–1   1995 Gass biomicroscopic classification of macular hole. (From Gass JD: Reappraisal of biomicroscopic classification of stages of development of a macular hole. Am J Ophthalmol 119(6):752–759, 1995. Ophthalmic Publishing Company, with permission.)

tally oriented Müller cell processes, and prefoveolar vitreous condensation may remain intact (stage 1B, occult macular hole) and thereby preclude biomicroscopic detection.[10] An *occult* macular hole is a new concept in Gass' revised classification scheme. The center of the yellow ring may often appear reddish in color and the yellow ring itself develops a serrated or irregular edge. Spontaneous vitreofoveal separation may then occur, creating a semitranslucent prefoveal opacity (pseudo-operculum) that is often larger than the underlying occult foveolar hole.[10] The yellow ring appears at the edge of the centrifugally displaced retinal receptors and disappears, presumably because of relief of prefoveolar vitreous traction on the edge of the expanding occult macular hole.[10] The *first biomicroscopically identifiable full-thickness retinal defect is a stage 2 hole* (*redefined as <400 μm in diameter*) and may be obscured by the overlying pseudo-operculum[10] (Fig. 19–3). Most macular hole "opercula" probably do not harbor retinal receptors; they are comprised of vitreous condensation and reactive glial proliferation.[10,11] These generally enlarge to stage 3 holes

(≥400 μm) (Fig. 19–4). Stage 3 holes (partial vitreomacular separation) may then evolve to stage 4 macular holes (complete separation of the vitreous from the entire macular surface and optic disc).[10] Vision usually varies between 20/70 and 20/400 in stage 3 or 4 lesions (Fig. 19–5). An overlying operculum may be observed and with time, fine radiating retinal striae (26%), drusen or yellow-white deposits (42%), and atrophy of the retinal pigment epithelium may appear in the base of the hole.[12] Epiretinal membranes, cystic degeneration of the retina, and underlying cuffs of subretinal fluid that effect shallow macular detachments are also observed.

DIFFERENTIAL DIAGNOSIS OF PREMACULAR HOLE AND MACULAR HOLE LESIONS

Macular holes and particularly premacular holes are often misdiagnosed. Careful examination with

TABLE 19–1 1995 Gass Biomicroscopic Classification of Age-Related Macular Hole*

Stage	Biomicroscopic Findings	Anatomic Interpretation	
		Old	New
1A (impending hole)	Central yellow spot, loss of foveolar depression, no vitreofoveolar separation	Early serous detachment of foveolar retina	Same
1B (impending or occult hole)	Yellow ring with bridging interface, loss of foveolar depression, no vitreofoveolar separation	Serous foveolar detachment with lateral displacement of xanthophyll	Same for small ring. For larger ring, central occult foveolar hole with centrifugal displacement of foveolar retina and xanthophyll, with bridging contracted prefoveolar vitreous cortex. Cannot detect transition from impending to occult hole
2	Eccentric oval, crescent, or horseshoe retinal defect inside edge of yellow ring	Hole (tear) in peripheral foveolar retina	Hole (tear) in contracted prefoveolar vitreous bridging round retinal hole, no loss of foveolar retina
	Central round retinal defect with rim of elevated retina		
	With prefoveolar opacity	Hole with operculum,† rim of retinal detachment	Hole with pseudo-operculum,‡ rim of retinal detachment
	Without prefoveolar opacity	Hole, no posterior vitreous detachment from optic disc and macula	Same
3	Central round ≥400 μm diameter retinal defect, no Weiss's ring, rim of elevated retina		
	With prefoveolar opacity	Hole with operculum, no posterior vitreous detachment from optic disc and macula	Hole with pseudo-operculum, no posterior vitreous detachment
	Without prefoveolar opacity	Hole, no posterior vitreous detachment from optic disc and macula	Same
4	Central round retinal defect, rim of elevated retina, Weiss's ring		
	With prefoveolar opacity§	Hole with operculum and posterior vitreous detachment from optic disc and macula	Hole with pseudo-operculum and posterior vitreous detachment from optic disc and macula
	Without prefoveolar opacity	Hole and posterior vitreous detachment from optic disc and macula	Same

* From Gass JD: Reappraisal of biomicroscopic classification of stages of development of a macular hole. Am J Ophthalmol 119(6):752–759, 1995, Ophthalmic Publishing Company, with permission.

† Operculum contains foveolar retina.

‡ Pseudo-operculum contains no retinal receptors.

§ Usually found near temporal border of Weiss's ring.

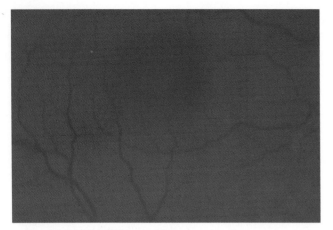

FIGURE 19–2 Stage 1B presumed occult macular hole. Note the serrated edges of the inner aspect of the yellow ring. Visual acuity is 20/30.

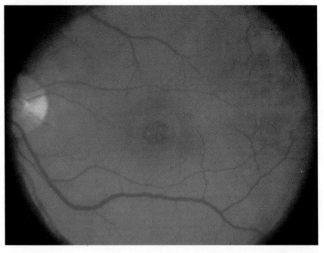

FIGURE 19–4 Stage 3 macular hole. This is a generally well-circumscribed 400-μm full-thickness retinal defect with an irregular inferotemporal border. Note the yellow clumps of presumed glial cells in the base of the macular hole and the surrounding cuff of subretinal fluid. The posterior hyaloid is attached at the optic nerve and the major temporal retinal arcades. Visual acuity is 20/100.

a contact lens is required to make an accurate diagnosis. In one series, only 1 of 18 subjects referred with the diagnosis of stage 1 macular hole was correctly diagnosed, while other cases were actually an aborted stage of macular hole formation (8 cases), stage 2 holes (4 cases), stage 3 holes (1 case), and unrelated lesions (4 cases).[13] Patients with age-related macular degeneration and a large central druse, central serous retinopathy and a foveal neurosensory detachment, cystoid macular edema, vitreomacular traction syndrome, or a foveal yellow lesion associated with solar retinopathy may all be misdiagnosed as having a stage 1 macular hole. In general, macular hole patients are older than most affected by central serous retinopathy and have intraretinal yellow changes rather than at the level of the retinal pigment epithelium. Careful contact lens examination of both eyes along with a medical history to rule out recent solar exposure is helpful. Subretinal fluid is not observed in premacular hole patients, although there is foveal elevation in stage 1 lesions. Patients with cystoid macular edema, vit-

reomacular traction syndrome, and stage 1B lesions all may have cystic intraretinal features; in patients with stage 1B macular holes, however, the foveola is not elevated above the level of the surrounding retina as observed in vitreomacular traction.

Full-thickness macular holes are also often misdiagnosed. Most commonly, an epiretinal membrane will create a central retinal depression that simulates a stage 3 macular hole (Fig. 19–6). These pseudoholes do not demonstrate a surrounding cuff of subretinal fluid or drusen-like yellow precipitates on the surface of bare retinal pigment epithelium. Careful contact lens examination should be directed to observe small eccentric retinal defects, the presence of an associated cuff of subretinal fluid, the status of the vitreoretinal interface,

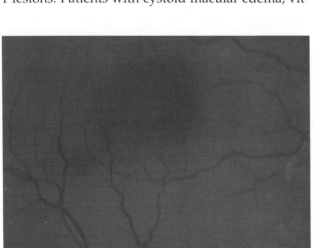

FIGURE 19–3 Stage 2 macular hole. There is a central foveolar retinal dehiscence less than 200-μm in greatest diameter and no detectable subretinal fluid. Visual acuity is 20/60.

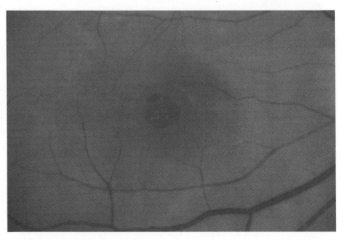

FIGURE 19–5 Stage 4 macular hole. The full-thickness retinal defect is surrounded by an epiretinal membrane and elevated by a large rim of subretinal fluid. Yellow deposits are noted in the base of the macular hole. Visual acuity is 20/300.

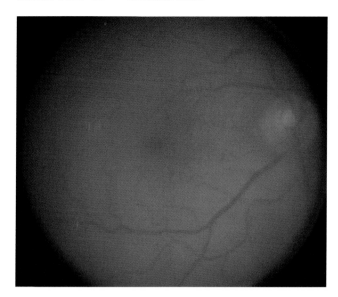

FIGURE 19-6 Pseudomacular hole. The most common misdiagnosis of a full-thickness macular hole is an epiretinal membrane that creates a circular central depression without any retinal defect. Note the tortuosity of the macular vessels and subtle retinal striae (pseudohole). The Watzke sign was negative and the visual acuity was 20/25.

whether the depression is lamellar or full-thickness, and the presence of any drusen-like precipitates on bare retinal pigment epithelium. A positive Watzke's sign and the laser aiming beam test (50-μm laser photocoagulator aiming beam is directed within and around the macular hole) are more specific than Amsler grid abnormalities for detecting macular holes.[14,15] Visual acuity is typically reduced to 20/60 or worse with macular holes, often at the level of 20/100 to 20/200, while macular pseudoholes fare better.

One condition that may be misdiagnosed as a true macular hole is a lamellar macular hole, which is a partial thickness defect of macular retina typically described as a red, petal-shaped depression in the inner retinal surface.[13] This is thought to represent a macular lesion created by spontaneous release of vitreous upon an impending macular hole lesion.[8,9] A pseudo-operculum may be observed overlying the lamellar macular hole, which contributes to misdiagnosis of the lesion as a true macular hole.[16] The pseudo-operculum may appear larger than the underlying defect and probably represents condensed cortical vitreous. Newer imaging modalities such as optical coherence tomography (OCT) or laser biomicroscopy may help to distinguish macular holes and precursor lesions from simulating lesions.[17,18]

Associated Conditions

The majority of macular holes are "idiopathic" in origin; however, many other associations have been previously reported. Full-thickness macular holes

have been described in association with a variety of conditions including proliferative diabetic retinopathy, optic disc coloboma, high myopia, choroidal neovascularization, Best's disease, adult vitelliform macular degeneration, retinal arteriovenous communication, scleral buckling for retinal reattachment, pneumatic retinopexy for retinal reattachment, trauma, and topical pilocarpine.

Lamellar macular holes (partial thickness retinal defect) have been described in association with topical pilocarpine, cystoid edema after cataract extraction, and idiopathic parafoveal telangiectasia.

HISTOPATHOLOGY

Full-Thickness Macular Hole

Two large histopathologic series have been reported on macular holes.[19,20] Histopathologic examination of full-thickness macular holes demonstrates round or oval retinal defects surrounded by rounded retinal edges and a cuff of detached neurosensory retina with subretinal fluid (Fig. 19-7A). In the most recent series, 79% demonstrated cystoid macular edema and 68% had epiretinal membranes. Photoreceptor atrophy was variable (200 to 750 μm; mean, 480 μm from the edge of the retinal margin) in this group of globes some of which had longstanding macular holes[19] (Fig. 19-7B). In some of the eyes, a thin tapered layer of cortical vitreous is noted that may effect traction on the edges of the macular hole. Two cases of probable resolved macular holes have also been reported.[19] In these specimens, there was no surrounding cuff of subretinal fluid and the photoreceptors were reapposed to Bruch's membrane. One eye demonstrated hyperplastic retinal pigment epithelium at the margin of the retinal defect that appeared to seal the macular hole.

Lamellar Macular Hole

Histopathology of lamellar macular holes has also been described.[19,20] Lamellar macular holes are characterized by a partial loss of neurosensory retina which looks like a sharply circumscribed round or petal-shaped red depression in the inner retinal surface. In half of these eyes, there was evidence of a thin layer of epicortical vitreous membrane causing tangential traction.[19]

Premacular Vitreous and Opercula

The histopathology of tissue removed during vitreous surgery for impending macular holes has been described.[22,23] In one study, the primary tissue specimen was a thin sheet of acellular premacular vitreous collagen, which is difficult to detect bio-

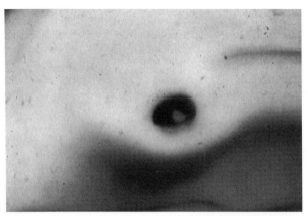

A

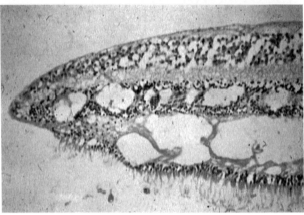

B

FIGURE 19–7 *A*, Gross examination of this autopsy eye demonstrates a full-thickness macular hole with an associated operculum. *B*, Histopathologic examination of this macular hole demonstrates rounded edges of retina, intraretinal cystoid macular edema, subretinal fluid and atrophy of photoreceptors particularly near the edge of the macular hole. (From Guyer DR, Green WR, de Bustrus S, Fine SL: Histopathologic features of idiopathic macular holes and cysts. Ophthalmology 97:1045–1051, 1990, with permission.)

microscopically and may be present even when there is an apparent posterior vitreous detachment.[22] The second report used immunocytochemical labeling of the premacular vitreous sheet and demonstrated cellular, potentially contractile glial and retinal pigment epithelial cells in the surgical specimens[23] consistent with prior studies on the vitreoretinal interface.[24]

A very interesting report on two surgically retrieved opercula overlying full-thickness macular holes reveals that opercula probably do not represent displaced neurosensory photoreceptors.[11] The opercula were comprised of a proliferation of dislodged, reparative fibrous astrocytes and Müller cells. This observation is consistent with Gass' revised theory on macular hole pathogenesis, which describes a dehiscence at the umbo with lateral displacement of photoreceptors; the operculum represents the overlying reparative tissue and not neurosensory retina.

There are two reports on the histopathology of surgically treated macular holes.[25,26] These clinico-pathologic studies demonstrated that macular holes can be sealed by fibrous astrocytes and Müller cells, without significant inflammation, disruption of the underlying retinal pigment epithelium, or cystoid macular edema. There is a closer reapproximation of retinal edges compared with spontaneously resolved macular holes,[19,25] suggesting that surgically treated holes may seal in different ways than spontaneously resolved macular holes. The same fibrous astrocytes and Müller cells that have been shown to help seal surgically treated macular holes may also contribute to epiretinal membrane formation and recurrent macular holes if the reparative process goes awry.[27]

NATURAL HISTORY

Premacular Hole Lesions, Stage 1A and 1B

The natural history of stage 1 lesions has been controversial. The best information currently available on the natural history of stage 1 lesions is derived from the Vitrectomy for Prevention of Macular Hole Study Group, which reported that 14 (40%) of 35 patients randomized to observation progressed to a full-thickness macular hole over a 2-year follow-up period.[28] Generally, a stage 1A lesion progresses to a stage 1B lesion within a few weeks to a few months.[28] Stage 1 lesions progressing to full-thickness lesions do so in an average time of 4.1 months (range 1 to 13 months) after diagnosis.[28] Prior reports estimated the progression rate of stage 1 or other premacular hole lesions to be 10 to 75%.[1,6,9,13,29–35] Several of these studies were limited by their retrospective nature.

In general, resolution of a stage 1 lesion is accompanied by vitreofoveal separation. Sixty per cent of stage 1 lesions abort macular hole formation. The resolved fovea may appear normal or may demonstrate the red-faceted, slightly depressed lesion characteristic of a lamellar macular hole. There may be an overlying pseudo-operculum suspended anterior to the fovea that may be confused with a stage 1 lesion itself.[13,16] Lamellar macular holes do not progress to macular holes.[10,13] Moreover, posterior vitreous detachment is generally believed to confer protection from macular hole evolution,[13,29,33,34,36,37] although one small series of five patients was believed to develop macular hole despite a complete posterior vitreous detachment.[38]

The visual acuity of stage 1 lesions ranges between 20/25 and 20/80. Initial visual acuity is believed to predict progression to full-thickness macular hole.[1,39] Recent data from the Vitrectomy for the Prevention of Macular Hole Study Group revealed that eyes with stage 1 macular holes and best-corrected visual acuity between 20/50 and 20/80 had a 66% (10 of 15 eyes) rate of progression to full-thickness macular hole, whereas eyes with best-corrected visual acuity between 20/25 and 20/40 had a 30% (6 of 20 eyes) risk of progression to full-thickness macular hole. The risk of progression to macular hole is significantly higher in eyes with stage 1 macular holes with best-corrected visual acuity of 20/50 or worse.[39]

Risk Factors for Full-Thickness Macular Hole

While the demographic features of age-related macular hole patients are generally widely accepted, risk factors for development of full-thickness lesions are more controversial. The Eye Disease Case-Control Study Group reported on the demographics and risk factors for "idiopathic" macular hole comparing 198 subjects with macular hole and 1023 matched controls. Seventy-two per cent of subjects with macular hole were female[40]; explanations for this female preponderance are speculative. Only 3% of subjects with idiopathic macular hole were less than 55 years of age. This study did not find an association of macular hole with hysterectomy, hypertension, or cardiovascular disease, in contradistinction to prior reports.[1,7] Interestingly, the most significant risk factor for macular hole formation was increased plasma fibrinogen (>2.95 g/liter) which more than doubled the risk for macular hole formation[40]; again, explanations are speculative. Estrogen users were at a reduced risk for hole formation.[40] The Eye Disease Case-Control Study Group did not examine two ocular characteristics that have been previously associated with macular hole formation: macular retinal pigment epithelial changes (involutional macular thinning) and macular vitreous attachment.

Stage 2 Lesions

According to the revised Gass classification, Stage 1B occult holes become manifest (stage 2 holes) either after early separation of the contracted prefoveolar vitreous cortex from the retina surrounding a small hole or as an eccentric can-opener-like tear in the contracted prefoveolar vitreous cortex at the edge of larger stage 2 holes.[10]

The majority of stage 2 holes demonstrate progression to stage 3 and 4 macular holes with subsequent loss of vision. The most optimistic study reported a 33% resolution rate with 67% progressing to larger stage 3 and 4 lesions.[35] Hikichi reported a 96% (n = 48 eyes) progression of stage 2 lesions to stage 3 or 4, while only 4% remained in stage 2, with no eyes demonstrating resolution during a median follow-up period of 4 years (range, 2 to 8 years).[41] Eighty-five per cent of stage 2 eyes enlarged their hole size to greater than 400 μm, 64% experienced vitreomacular separation, and visual acuity decreased two or more Snellen lines during

the follow-up period in 71% of 48 eyes. These authors concluded that even though vitreomacular separation may improve the prognosis of a macular hole, stage 2 lesions usually will develop an enlarged hole and decreased visual acuity.[29,41] Most stage 2 holes progress and enlarge to stage 3 or 4 within 6 months.

Stage 3 and 4 Macular Holes

Most full-thickness macular holes greater than 400 μm retain peripheral vision but suffer loss of central vision to the level of 20/100 and worse. Some stage 3 or 4 lesions will enlarge their hole size and a minority will undergo progressive loss of central visual acuity. Hikichi reported that 32 (55%) of 58 eyes with a stage 3 lesion, and 5 (16%) of 31 eyes with a stage 4 lesion, underwent macular hole enlargement during the median follow-up period of 3 years. Visual acuity decreased two or more lines of Snellen equivalent during the follow-up period in 17 (29%) eyes with a stage 3 lesion, and in four (13%) eyes with a stage 4 lesion.[29]

Visual deterioration may be related to increasing and chronic subretinal fluid, cystoid retinal changes, or photoreceptor atrophy. Less commonly, loss of central and then peripheral vision is related to a progressive retinal detachment. This is most commonly associated with myopia 6 diopters or greater.[42]

Uncommonly (5 to 12% of stage 3 or 4), spontaneous flattening and improvement in vision may occur.[1,7,35,43] The mechanism of spontaneous flattening is unclear, although two cases have been reported in association with epiretinal membrane formation and vision improving to the 20/20 to 20/30 level.[44,45] Because macular holes demonstrate absolute scotomata on microperimetry within the hole and probable relative scotomata in the surrounding neurosensory detachment,[46,47] spontaneously flattened macular holes may improve their visual function in ways similar to those who have experienced successful surgical repair.[48]

Fellow Eyes of Patients with Macular Holes

Patients with a unilateral macular hole are understandably concerned about the prognosis for their fellow eye. The vast majority of fellow eyes will not develop a macular hole. The risk of fellow eye involvement has been reported to be from 3 to 22%.[31,34] Normal fellow eyes have a very low incidence (0 to 2%) of macular hole formation, particularly if there is a pre-existant posterior vitreous detachment.[6,34–36,39] Fellow eyes with stage 1 lesions and vitreous attachment are probably at a similar risk for hole formation as previously described (about 40%).

Focal electroretinography (FERG) may further refine the prognosis of a fellow eye.[50] In an interesting prospective study, these authors found that foveal ERG amplitude was significantly related to subsequent macular hole formation, suggesting that this test can provide an objective measure of macular function to help identify eyes at risk for macular hole formation.[50]

MANAGEMENT OF MACULAR HOLE LESIONS

Because the majority of patients with macular hole suffer from unilateral loss of central vision with a preserved fellow eye, indications for intervention have been questioned.[51] Nevertheless, many vitreoretinal surgeons offer surgical intervention to afflicted patients because of refinements in surgical technique, better visual outcomes, and up to a 20% chance that the fellow eye will become affected. The first step in the management of a macular hole lesion is to reconfirm the diagnosis, since pseudomacular holes are commonly misdiagnosed as full-thickness macular holes. The management of premacular hole lesions has been guided by the Vitrectomy for Prevention of Macular Hole Study findings.[28]

Historically, therapy for macular holes has evolved from anxiolytics and vasodilator therapies to current-day strategies utilizing intraocular tamponade and vitrectomy surgery. Until recently, most surgeons focused their attention on retinal detachments that were associated with macular hole. Meyer-Schwickerath in 1961 proposed cerclage, subretinal fluid drainage, and light laser photocoagulation employing scleral buckling techniques to flatten a macular hole. Subsequent reports in the next two decades advocated variations on this theme including Y-shaped plombs, "armed" silicone implants, diathermy, laser photocoagulation, cryotherapy, silicone oil, and intravitreal gas—all without vitrectomy—to flatten the macula and associated retinal detachment. Not surprisingly, many of the subjects of these reports were greater than 6 diopters myopic.

Full-Thickness Macular Hole

In 1991, Kelly and Wendel reported on vitrectomy, removal of cortical vitreous and epiretinal membranes, and strict face-down gas tamponade to stabilize or improve vision in full-thickness idiopathic macular holes.[52] Their hypothesis was that by removing tangential vitreous and membrane forces, they could flatten the macular hole, and possibly reduce the adjacent cystic retinal changes and neurosensory macular detachment. The overall results were a 58% anatomic success rate and visual improvement of two or more lines in 42% of eyes (73%

of anatomically successful eyes). A critical surgical step in their technique is the induction of a complete posterior vitreous detachment with a soft-tipped silicone suction needle that is swept over the retinal surface near the major retinal vascular arcades and temporal to the macula; engagement of cortical vitreous results in the "fish strike" sign, which is then removed to the posterior equatorial zone (Fig. 19–8). Because surface cortical vitreous can be difficult to identify, one report advocates the use of autologous blood to stain this tissue.[53] In addition, fine and often friable epiretinal membranes are removed with a microbarbed microvitreoretinal (MVR) blade and tissue forceps stripping, which often causes small retinal hemorrhages near the macular hole. The peripheral retina is inspected carefully for iatrogenic retinal tears. A total air-fluid gas exchange is performed to desiccate the vitreous cavity and accumulated posterior retinal fluid followed by a nonexpansive concentration of long-acting gas. Strict face-down positioning to position the gas bubble against the macular hole for at least 1 week is as important as the technical components of the procedure. Surgical complications include cataract, retinal detachment, retinal trauma, macular light toxicity, and postoperative intraocular pressure rises.

More recently, Kelly and Wendel improved their overall results to 73% anatomic success and 55% of patients improving two or more lines of visual acuity.[54] This group and other investigators have noted that macular hole surgery is more successful in patients with macular holes of less than 6 months' duration compared with those up to 2 years or longer. In a small series, one group noted that surgery on longstanding stage 3 macular holes (1 year

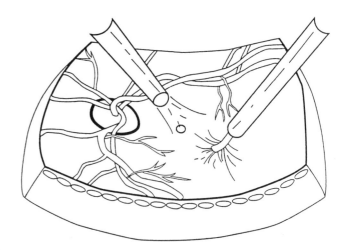

FIGURE 19–8 Identification, engagement, and removal of the vitreous posterior hyaloid and cortical vitreous is important to successful macular hole surgery. The "fish strike" sign occurs when a silicone-tipped extrusion needle with active suction is swept over the retinal surface and engages cortical vitreous. (From Kelly NE, Wendel RT: Vitreous surgery for idiopathic macular holes. Results of a pilot study [see comments]. Arch Ophthalmol 109:654–659, 1991. Copyright 1991, American Medical Association, with permission.)

duration) or longer can result in 58% anatomic success rate with improvement in central visual acuity, although recovery of central vision may be delayed for 6 months or longer.[55] An uncontrolled series of surgery for stage 2 macular holes demonstrated that 61% improved visual acuity, 27% remained stable, and 12% progressed to a stage 3 macular hole with worse vision[56]; 61% of these eyes had a final visual acuity of 20/50 or better. These results compare favorably to prior reports on the natural history progression rates of stage 2 macular holes (67 to 96%).

Glaser and co-workers first reported on the novel use of intravitreal bovine transforming growth factor β_2 (TGF-β_2), pars plana vitrectomy, fluid–gas exchange for full-thickness macular hole with anatomic success rates of about 90%.[57–59] In contradistinction to the surgical technique by Kelly and Wendel, these investigators did not strip surrounding epiretinal membranes in some cases.[59] Longer acting gas tamponade with 16% perfluoropropane gas improved their surgical success rate compared with air but was associated with significant nuclear sclerotic cataract formation (76% requiring cataract extraction with follow-up $\geq$24 months).[12,60] Unfortunately, production recombinant TGF-β_2 (non–bovine derived) did not yield similarly successful surgical results as bovine TGF-β_2.

What then are the indications for treatment of a full-thickness macular hole? Controversy exists, since the majority of these subjects will not develop a macular hole in their fellow eye and one group has noted that with careful refraction many eyes with full-thickness macular hole may enjoy better visual acuity than previously believed.[61] On the other hand, refinements in surgical techniques have clearly made recovery of central acuity possible in this group of patients, and currently the Vitrectomy for Macular Hole Study is gathering prospective and controlled clinical data on this issue.

Preliminary results from this multicenter study reveal that some visual benefit of vitrectomy surgery for macular hole exists (reading speed and potential acuity vision), however, visual acuity benefit as measured by the early treatment diabetic retinopathy study chart was modest. These results may be due to surgical complications such as cataract. Long-term study of this subject is necessary.

The ideal surgical candidate has recent-onset, bilateral, small, full-thickness macular holes and will have no problems maintaining a face-down postoperative position. Perhaps preoperative diagnostic testing, such as laser interferometry, will help select candidates with postoperative visual potential.[62] Potential surgical candidates need to be informed about nuclear cataract progression as well as a host of other posterior segment complications including but not limited to retinal tears, rhegmatogenous retinal detachment, and retinal pigment epithelial alterations.[63–66] Some patients who have anatomically unsuccessful surgery may undergo another vitrectomy with successful flattening of the macular

hole and visual improvement.[67] Others have suggested macular laser photocoagulation with or without intraocular gas tamponade for primary[68] or recurrent macular hole.[69]

Premacular Hole Lesions

Because tangential vitreous traction is believed to play a role in the formation of macular holes, removal of cortical vitreous should reduce the rate of progression of stage 1A and 1B premacular hole lesions to full-thickness macular holes. Smiddy and then Jost reported small, uncontrolled pilot series on the technical feasability of vitrectomy surgery for impending macular holes.[58,70] In another small, uncontrolled series Chan has described intravitreal injection of an expansile gas bubble without vitrectomy surgery to induce a posterior vitreous detachment with resolution of stage 1A (seven of seven) and 1B (three of four) premacular hole lesions.[71]

The Vitrectomy for Prevention of Macular Hole Study subsequently reported multicenter, prospective, randomized data on vitrectomy surgery and careful peeling of the cortical vitreous for presumed stage 1A and 1B lesions.[28] A full-thickness macular hole developed in 10 (37%) of 27 patients in the vitrectomy group compared with 14 (40%) of 35 patients randomized to observation ($p = .81$). This study could not demonstrate a significant benefit of vitrectomy surgery for stage 1A and 1B lesions, and the study was terminated because of low recruitment. At this time, I do not recommend vitrectomy surgery for these premacular hole lesions but rather suggest careful follow-up, since a significant proportion will go on to full-thickness macular holes within a year.

Other surgeons question the role of tangential vitreous traction in the pathogenesis of macular hole, since surgical peeling of cortical vitreous did not reduce the rate of full-thickness macular hole formation in the Vitrectomy for Prevention of Macular Hole Study.[72] It may be that some premacular hole stage 1 lesions were actually ''occult'' macular holes as noted intraoperatively by Jost and co-workers or that the intervention may have been too late in the disease process.[70,73] On the other hand, it may be that tangential traction may only be part of the pathogenesis of this condition and other retinal, retinal pigment epithelial, or choroidal factors may also be important.[6,73]

REFERENCES

1. McDonnell PJ, Fine SL, Hillis AI: Clinical features of idiopathic macular cysts and holes. Am J Ophthalmol 93:777–786, 1982.
2. Aaberg TM: Macular Holes: A Review. Surv Ophthalmol 15(3):139–162, 1970.
3. Noyes HD: Detachment of the retina, with laceration at the macula lutea. Trans Am Ophthalmol Soc 1:128–129, 1871.

4. Zeeman WPC: Uber Loch-und cystenbildung der fovea Centralis. Graefe Arch Ophthalmol 80:259–269, 1912.

5. Lister W: Holes in the retina and their clinical significance. Br J Ophthalmol 8:1–20, 1924.

6. Morgan CM, Schatz H: Involutional macular thinning. A pre-macular hole condition. Ophthalmology 93(2):153–161, 1986.

7. Morgan CM, Schatz H: Idiopathic macular holes. Am J Ophthalmol 99:437–444, 1985.

8. Gass JD: Idiopathic senile macular hole. Its early stages and pathogenesis. Arch Ophthalmol 106(5):629–639, 1988.

9. Johnson RN, Gass JD: Idiopathic macular holes. Observations, stages of formation, and implications for surgical intervention. Ophthalmology 95(7):917–924, 1988.

10. Gass JD: Reappraisal of biomicroscopic classification of stages of development of a macular hole. Am J Ophthalmol 119(6):752–759, 1995.

11. Madreperla SA, McCuen BWN, Hickingbotham D, Green WR: Clinicopathologic correlation of surgically removed macular hole opercula. Am J Ophthalmol 120(2):197–207, 1995.

12. Thompson JT, Hiner CJ, Glaser BM, et al: Fluorescein angiographic characteristics of macular holes before and after vitrectomy with transforming growth factor beta-2. Am J Ophthalmol 117(3):291–301, 1994.

13. Gass JD, Joondeph BC: Observations concerning patients with suspected impending macular holes. Am J Ophthalmol 109(6):638–646, 1990.

14. Watzke RC, Allen L: Subjective slitbeam sign for macular disease. Am J Ophthalmol 68:449–453, 1969.

15. Martinez J, Smiddy WE, Kim J, Gass JD: Differentiating macular holes from macular pseudoholes. Am J Ophthalmol 117(6):762–767, 1994.

16. Gass JD, Van NM: Xanthic scotoma and yellow foveolar shadow caused by a pseudo-operculum after vitreofoveal separation. Retina 12(3):242–244, 1992.

17. Kiryu J, Shahidi M, Ogura Y, et al: Illustration of the stages of idiopathic macular holes by laser biomicroscopy. Arch Ophthalmol 113(9):1156–1160, 1995.

18. Puliafito C, Hee M, Lin C, et al: Imaging of macular diseases with optical coherence tomography. Ophthalmology 102:217–229, 1995.

19. Guyer DR, Green WR, de Bustrus S, Fine SL: Histopathologic features of idiopathic macular holes and cysts. Ophthalmology 97:1045–1051, 1990.

20. Frangieh GT, Green WR, Engel HM: A histopathologic study of macular cysts and holes. Retina 1:311–336, 1981.

21. Gass JD: Lamellar macular hole: a complication of cystoid macular edema after cataract extraction. Arch Ophthalmol 94(5):793–800, 1976.

22. Smiddy WE, Michels RG, de Bustros S, et al: Histopathology of tissue removed during vitrectomy for impending idiopathic macular holes. Am J Ophthalmol 108(4):360–364, 1989.

23. Campochiaro PA, Van NE, Vinores SA: Immunocytochemical labeling of cells in cortical vitreous from patients with premacular hole lesions [see comments]. Arch Ophthalmol 110(3):371–377, 1992.

24. Foos RY: Vitreoretinal junction; topographical variations. Invest Ophthalmol 11:801–808, 1972.

25. Madreperla SA, Geiger GL, Funata M, et al: Clinicopathologic correlation of a macular hole treated by cortical vitreous peeling and gas tamponade. Ophthalmology 101(4):682–686, 1994.

26. Funata M, Wendel RT, de la Cruz Z, Green WR: Clinicopathologic study of bilateral macular holes treated with pars plana vitrectomy and gas tamponade. Retina 12:289–298, 1992.

27. Fekrat S, Wendel RT, de la Cruz Z, Green WR: Clinicopathologic correlation of an epiretinal membrane associated with a recurrent macular hole. Retina 15(1):53–57, 1995.

28. de Bustros S: Vitrectomy for prevention of macular holes. Results of a randomized multicenter clinical trial. Vitrectomy for Prevention of Macular Hole Study Group. Ophthalmology 101(6):1055–1059, 1994.

29. Hikichi T, Yoshida A, Akiba J, Trempe CL: Natural outcomes of stage 1, 2, 3, and 4 idiopathic macular holes [see comments]. Br J Ophthalmol 79(6):517–520, 1995.

30. Gass JD: Risk of developing macular hole [letter; see comments]. Arch Ophthalmol 109(5):610–612, 1991.

31. Bronstein MA, Trempe CL, Freeman HM: Fellow eyes with macular holes. Am J Ophthalmol 92:757–761, 1981.

32. Atmaca LS: Follow-up of macular holes. Ann Ophthalmol 16(11):1064–1065, 1984.

33. Akiba J, Yoshida A, Trempe CL: Risk of developing a macular hole [see comments]. Arch Ophthalmol 108(8):1088–1090, 1990.

34. Akiba J, Kakehashi A, Arzabe CW, Trempe CL: Fellow eyes in idiopathic macular hole cases. Ophthalmic Surg 23(9):594–597, 1992.

35. Guyer DR, de Bustros S, Diener WM, Fine SL: Observations on patients with idiopathic macular holes and cysts. Arch Ophthalmol 110(9):1264–1268, 1992.

36. Fisher YL, Slakter JS, Yannuzzi LA, Guyer DR: A prospective natural history study and kinetic ultrasound evaluation of idiopathic macular holes. Ophthalmology 101(1):5–11, 1994.

37. Wiznia RA: Reversibility of the early stages of idiopathic macular holes. Am J Ophthalmol 107(3):241–245, 1989.

38. Gordon LW, Glaser BM, Ie D, et al: Full-thickness macular hole formation with a pre-existing complete posterior vitreous detachment. Ophthalmology 102:1702–1705, 1995.

39. Kokame GT, de Bustros S: Visual acuity as a prognostic indicator in stage I macular holes. The Vitrectomy for Prevention of Macular Hole Study Group. Am J Ophthalmol 120(1):112–114, 1995.

40. Eye Disease Case Control Study Group: Risk factors for idiopathic macular holes. Am J Ophthalmol 118:754–761, 1994.

41. Hikichi T, Yoshida A, Akiba J, et al: Prognosis of stage 2 macular holes. Am J Ophthalmol 119(5):571–575, 1995.

42. Aaberg TM: Macular holes. Am J Ophthalmol 69:555–562, 1970.

43. Yuzawa M, Watanabe A, Takahashi Y, Matsui M: Observation of idiopathic full-thickness macular holes: follow-up observation. Arch Ophthalmol 112:1051–1056, 1994.

44. Bidwell AE, Jampol LM: Macular holes and excellent visual acuity. Arch Ophthalmol 106:1350, 1988.

45. Lewis H, Cowan GM, Straatsma BR: Apparent disappearance of a macular hole associated with development of an epiretinal membrane. Am J Ophthalmol 102(2):172–175, 1986.

46. Sjaarda RN, Frank DA, Glaser BM, et al: Assessment of vision in idiopathic macular holes with macular microperimetry using the scanning laser ophthalmoscope. Ophthalmology 100(10):1513–1518, 1993.

47. Acosta F, Lashkari K, Reynaud X, et al: Characterization of functional changes in macular holes and cysts. Ophthalmology 98:1820–1823, 1991.

48. Sjaarda RN, Frank DA, Glaser BM, et al: Resolution of an absolute scotoma and improvement of relative scotomata after successful macular hole surgery. Am J Ophthalmol 116(2):129–139, 1993.

49. Trempe CL, Weiter JJ, Furukawa H: Fellow eyes in cases of macular hole. Biomicroscopic study of the vitreous. Arch Ophthalmol 104(1):93–95, 1986.

50. Birch DG, Jost BF, Fish GE: The focal electroretinogram in fellow eyes of patients with idiopathic macular holes. Arch Ophthalmol 106(11):1558–1563, 1988.

51. Fine SL: Vitreous surgery for macular hole in perspective. Is there an indication? [editorial; comment]. Arch Ophthalmol 109(5):635–636, 1991.

52. Kelly NE, Wendel RT: Vitreous surgery for idiopathic macular holes. Results of a pilot study [see comments]. Arch Ophthalmol 109(5):654–659, 1991.

53. Ryan EA, Lee S, Chern S: Use of intravitreal autologous blood to identify posterior cortical vitreous in macular hole surgery. Arch Ophthalmol 113(6):822–823, 1995.

54. Wendel RT, Patel AC, Kelly NE, et al: Vitreous surgery for macular holes [see comments]. Ophthalmology 100(11):1671–1676, 1993.

55. Orellana J, Lieberman RM: Stage III macular hole surgery. Br J Ophthalmol 77(9):555–558, 1993.
56. Ruby AJ, Williams DF, Grand MG, et al: Pars plana vitrectomy for treatment of stage 2 macular holes. Arch Ophthalmol 112(3):359–364, 1994.
57. Glaser BM, Michels RG, Kuppermann BD, et al: Transforming growth factor-beta 2 for the treatment of full-thickness macular holes. A prospective randomized study. Ophthalmology 99(7):1162–1172, 1992.
58. Smiddy WE, Michels RG, Glaser BM, de Bustros S: Vitrectomy for impending idiopathic macular holes. Am J Ophthalmol 105(4):371–376, 1988.
59. Lansing MB, Glaser BM, Liss H, et al: The effect of pars plana vitrectomy and transforming growth factor-beta 2 without epiretinal membrane peeling on full-thickness macular holes. Ophthalmology 100(6):868–871, 1993.
60. Thompson JT, Glaser BM, Sjaarda RN, Murphy RP: Progression of nuclear sclerosis and long-term visual results of vitrectomy with transforming growth factor beta-2 for macular holes. Am J Ophthalmol 119(1):48–54, 1995.
61. Freeman WR: Vitrectomy surgery for full-thickness macular holes. Am J Ophthalmol 2:233–235, 1992.
62. Smiddy WE, Thomley ML, Knighton RW, Feuer WJ: Use of the potential acuity meter and laser interferometer to predict visual acuity after macular hole surgery. Retina 14: 305–309, 1994.
63. Park SS, Marcus DM, Duker JS, et al: Posterior segment complications after vitrectomy for macular hole. Ophthalmology 102(5):775–781, 1995.
64. Duker JS: Retinal pigment epitheliopathy after macular hole surgery [letter; comment]. Ophthalmology 100(11): 1604–1605, 1993.
65. Poliner LS, Tornambe PE: Retinal pigment epitheliopathy after macular hole surgery [see comments]. Ophthalmology 99(11):1671–1677, 1992.
66. Charles S: Retinal pigment epithelial abnormalities after macular hole surgery (letter). Retina 13:176, 1993.
67. Ie D, Glaser BM, Thompson JT, et al: Retreatment of full-thickness macular holes persisting after prior vitrectomy: a pilot study. Ophthalmology 100:1787–1793, 1993.
68. Schocket SS, Lakhanpal V, Xiaoping M, et al: Laser treatment of macular holes. Ophthalmology 95:574, 1988.
69. Del Priore LV, Kaplan HJ, Bonham RD: Laser photocoagulation and fluid-gas exchange for recurrent macular hole. Retina 14(4):381–382, 1994.
70. Jost BF, Hutton WL, Fuller DG, et al: Vitrectomy in eyes at risk for macular hole formation. Ophthalmology 97(7): 843–847, 1990.
71. Chan CK, Wessels IF, Friedrichsen EJ: Treatment of idiopathic macular holes by induced posterior vitreous detachment. Ophthalmology 102(5):757–767, 1995.
72. Melberg NS, Williams DF: More on macular holes. Ophthalmology 101(11):1764–1765, 1994.
73. de Bustros S: Author's reply. Ophthalmology 101(11):1765, 1994.

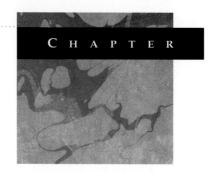

CHAPTER 20

Epimacular Membranes

Steve Charles, M.D.

Membranes on the macular surface can result from several pathogenic mechanisms,[1-4] with the common theme of tissue damage and subsequent repair. Epimacular membranes (EMMs) are hypocellular, largely collagen structures. Epimacular membranes are also called macular puckers, cellophane maculopathy, surface wrinkling retinopathy, epiretinal membranes, preretinal membranes, premacular fibroplasia, and premacular fibrosis. Each of these names has certain deficiencies; hence, the currently accepted name—epimacular membranes.

PATHOGENESIS

The so-called idiopathic type of epimacular membrane has been shown to be caused by glial proliferation through a defect in the internal limiting lamina, usually created by a posterior vitreous separation.[5-7] Retinal breaks, retinopexy, photocoagulation, inflammation, and vascular disease[8] can lead to glial proliferation[9-13] on the retinal surface. Retinal pigment epithelium (RPE) cells[14,15] can migrate through a retinal break and proliferate on the retinal surface, just as in the case of proliferative vitreoretinopathy (PVR). Epimacular membranes can be thought of as localized glial or RPE-induced proliferative vitreoretinopathy.

ETIOLOGY OF VISUAL LOSS

Hypocellular contraction of the epimacular membrane causes nonrhegmatogenous elevation of the macula, thought by the author to be responsible for a major fraction of the associated visual loss, with retinal distortion a minor factor. Reversible macular edema secondary to macular separation from the fluid-pumping mechanism of the RPE contributes to visual loss as well. Although the terms "macular

pucker" and "surface wrinkling retinopathy" emphasize retinal distortion, some patients have marked improvement in postoperative vision in spite of persistent retinal distortion and metamorphopsia.

HISTORY

The typical epimacular membrane patient experiences a relatively rapid loss of vision accompanied by metamorphopsia over a period of several weeks, followed by relative stabilization of the visual function. In spite of this typical history, it is common practice for doctors to advise a patient with a recent history of visual loss to, for example, the 20/50 level, that they should wait until the vision is reduced to 20/80 or worse before considering surgery. In fact, the vision will usually stabilize at a visual level at or near that noted on initial presentation. Because improved visual outcomes are associated with higher preoperative vision and shorter duration, it is a better practice to make a decision on surgical intervention at the first visit.

CASE SELECTION

As with all surgical procedures, the decision to operate is a multifactorial process based on symptoms, extent of visual loss, visual needs, status of the other eye, age, duration, medical status, and the presence of other ocular diseases. There is no substitute for ethical, sound clinical judgment in making the decision to operate. The author's visual acuity threshold for surgery has moved from 20/200 to 20/40 in selected cases, as the methodology has improved. The author operates on patients with preoperative vision at the 20/40 level, or better, if the patient is significantly symptomatic from dis-

HISTOPATHOLOGICAL FEATURES

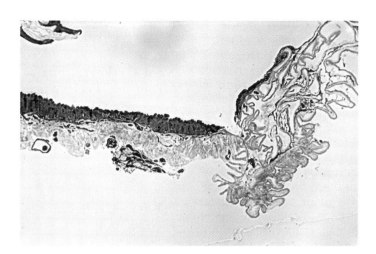

Surgically removed idiopathic epiretinal membrane that is composed of a thin layer of fibrous tissue with a blood vessel. It is lined internally by a monolayer of tall retinal pigment epithelium. A large gathered aggregate of internal limiting lamina of the retina is attached (*to the right*). (From Michels RG: A clinical and histopathologic study of epiretinal membranes affecting the macula and removed by vitreous surgery. Trans Am Ophthalmol Soc 80: 580–656, 1982, with permission.)

abling metamorphopsia, is in good health, is relatively young, and understands the issues. Duration is a relative rather than absolute criteria because cases of 10 years' duration have had significant visual improvement following surgery. This remarkable visual improvement is presumably because the minimal amount of subretinal fluid present in these cases leads to minimal irreversible photoreceptor degeneration, just as is the case in central serous retinopathy. Macular edema concurrent with EMMs, except in the vascular disease subgroup, is probably secondary to macular elevation, typically reversible, and not a contraindication to vitreoretinal surgery. Knowledge that the patient had significantly poor vision before the membrane occurred is an absolute contraindication to surgery. The slow recovery of vision after retinal reattachment surgery coupled with the typical 1-month onset of EMMs makes it difficult to make a surgical decision in this situation.[16,17] Patients with severe hereditary photoreceptor degeneration or a previous central retinal artery occlusion frequently have wrinkling of the retinal surface without an epiretinal membrane because of marked decrease in retinal thickness. Surgery is contraindicated in this situation.

SURGICAL SEQUENCE AND TECHNIQUES

Vitreomacular Traction

The posterior vitreous cortex is rarely adherent to typical epimacular membranes. On occasion, patients present with macular elevation secondary to hypocellular contraction of the posterior vitreous cortex with marked adherence of the vitreous to the macula. When operating on these cases, care must be taken to avoid tearing the fovea by imbricating the vitreous into the port of the vitreous cutter. Horizontal scissors should be used to delaminate the posterior vitreous cortex from the fovea prior to any removal of the vitreous (Fig. 20–1).

Nonrhegmatogenous Proliferative Vitreoretinopathy

Some patients have multiple star folds from PVR in addition to the epimacular component. Removing these additional epiretinal membranes is a stimulus for recurrent PVR and is unnecessary unless it is causing macular elevation or distortion.

Need for Vitrectomy at the Time of Membrane Peeling

The need to remove the vitreous at the time of epiretinal membrane surgery has not been established. If vitrectomy is performed, however, it will prevent late complications from hypocellular gel contraction and patients will not complain of floaters. Vitrectomy can lead to postoperative rhegmatogenous retinal detachment because of intraoperative suction forces, cutter-movement-induced traction, and vitreous incarceration in the sclerotomies. If the vitreous has been removed, a postoperative retinal detachment can be managed by in-office, two-needle, fluid-gas exchange and laser retinopexy (Fig. 20–2). Anterior vitreous cortex removal is correlated with an increased incidence of posterior subcapsular cataract, possibly caused by fluid turbulence. Avoiding the anterior vitreous cortex may reduce postoperative posterior subcapsular cataract and rhegmatogenous retinal detachment.

Epiretinal Membrane Removal

Machemer developed the concept of membrane peeling in 1972, soon after his introduction of vitrectomy. Originally, peeling was performed with a bent needle.[18] O'Malley subsequently developed the concept of using a rounded, angulated instrument he called a pic to perform the peeling. This method was popularized by the author and the late Ron Michels.[3,19] Bent needles and pics require the presence of a visible outer margin of the EMM, frequently called an "edge."[20] The author subsequently developed the concept of inside-out mem-

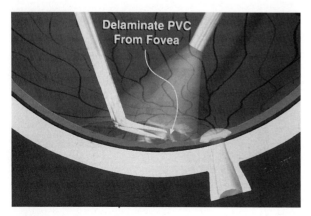

FIGURE 20–1 Delaminate the posterior vitreous cortex from the fovea before removal of the vitreous.

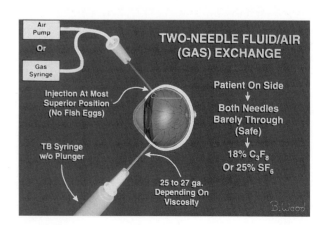

FIGURE 20–2 Two-needle fluid-air (gas) exchange.

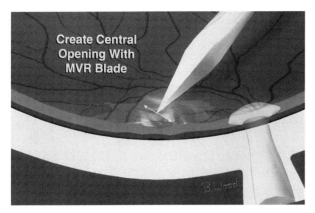

FIGURE 20–3   Make central slit using the MVR blade.

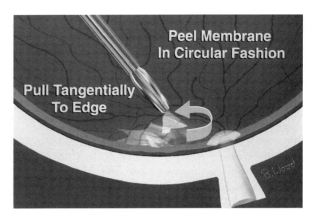

FIGURE 20–5   Move forceps tangentially along the surface of the retina.

brane peeling because of the difficulty of finding an "edge" in certain cases.[21] In contrast to Machemer's outside-in membrane peeling method, inside-out peeling is initiated by making a slit in the apparent center of the epimacular membrane using the microvitreoretinal (MVR) blade (Fig. 20–3). The MVR blade is the same one used to make the sclerotomies. The MVR blade should not be bent, as there is no intent to place it between the membrane and the retina. The center of the membrane can be identified by noting the orientation of radial striae, the most elevated retinal region, the most opaque region of the membrane, and relative movement of the membrane with respect to the retina induced by lateral movement of the MVR blade tip. After a slit is made in the apparent center of the membrane, diamond-coated, microforceps are utilized to grasp the edge of the slit. These end-opening forceps were developed by the author and Hans Grieshaber for end grasping and must have precise alignment of the tips of the blades (Fig. 20–4). The peeling should be accomplished by moving the forceps tangentially along the surface of the retina (Fig. 20–5). This motion should be continued in a circular fashion, similar to capsulorrhexis. If the membrane tears, it can be regrasped without removing any membrane from the forceps because the diamonds penetrate numerous layers of membrane and facilitate removal of the membrane through the pars plana as well. The surgeon should always observe the fovea during the peeling process, rather than focusing on the end of the forceps,

in order to prevent tearing the fovea. Areas of stronger adherence to the ILL can be detected by noting fine fibers being lifted from the retinal surface during the peeling process. Scissors delamination rather than peeling is utilized if strong adherence to the fovea, vessels, or any region of the retina is noted during the peeling process (Fig. 20–6). Right-angle 20-gauge scissors (Charles modification of the Grieshaber Sutherland scissors) with the blades parallel to the retinal surface can delaminate the glial attachment points without trauma to the ILL. If there are marked folds, the blunt, polished end of the vitrectomy instrument can be used to gently push the retinal folds into better position. Moderately sized peeled or delaminated membrane should be removed through the pars plana with the diamond-coated forceps. If the membrane is very large or dense it should be removed with the vitrectomy probe.

Management of Retinal Breaks

No posterior retinal breaks occurred in the author's series of 841 consecutive cases, but other series re-

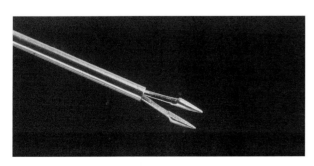

FIGURE 20–4   Diamond-coated microforceps.

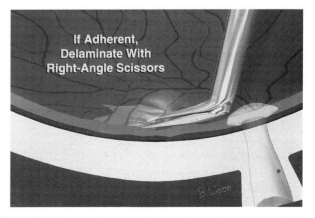

FIGURE 20–6   Scissors delamination rather than peeling is used if strong adherence to the fovea, vessels, or any region of the retina is noted during peeling.

port a 1 to 15% incidence of posterior retinal breaks.[23-25] All series, including the author's, report a 5 to 6% incidence of peripheral retinal breaks. The peripheral retina should be inspected at the end of the case, and all retinal breaks with associated subretinal fluid (SRF) should be managed with fluid-air exchange, internal drainage of subretinal fluid, air-gas exchange with 25% sulfur hexafluoride (SF_6), and laser endophotocoagulation around the break.[26] Scleral buckling is not indicated in these cases. Retinal breaks without SRF can be treated with endolaser retinopexy.

MANAGEMENT OF COEXISTENT CATARACT

Some surgeons recommend that cataract surgery be performed prior to vitreous surgery if visually significant cataract is present. This approach increases costs and subjects the patient to double the anesthesia and operative risk. Epimacular membrane surgery requires excellent visualization and should not be attempted if greater than 2+ nuclear sclerosis or a posterior subcapsular cataract is present. The fact that vitreous surgery causes relatively rapid progression of preexisting nuclear sclerotic cataract in a significant number of cases should be taken into account when considering whether to remove the lens.[27,28]

Cataract surgery can be combined with vitreous surgery using many different approaches. Some recommend that the cataract surgeon or the vitreoretinal surgeon perform phakoemulsification and intraocular lens insertion before initiating vitreous surgery. This is not an ideal approach because pigment released from the iris, blood, viscoelastics, miosis, and corneal changes frequently cause the view for membrane peeling to be adversely affected. The author recommends use of pars plana lensectomy with preservation of the anterior lens capsule before the vitreous surgery, as first reported by Blankenship.[29] A posterior chamber intraocular lens is inserted in the ciliary sulcus through a scleral tunnel incision after the vitrectomy and membrane peeling. The author has modified Blankenship's technique by performing a circular posterior capsulorrhexis rather than entering the lens through the equatorial capsule. A bent, 20-gauge titanium fragmentor (Alcon) is then used to remove the nucleus and epinucleus while carefully avoiding the anterior lens capsule (Fig. 20–7). Aspiration is used to clean all cortex off the lens capsule. Any lens material that falls posteriorly can be removed with the fragmentor after vitreous removal is accomplished. The lens fragments should be picked up with suction alone and moved to the anterior vitreous space before engaging fragmentation with the foot pedal. A small, 20-gauge, sandblasted or diamond-dusted capsule polisher is utilized to remove material from the anterior lens capsule (Fig.

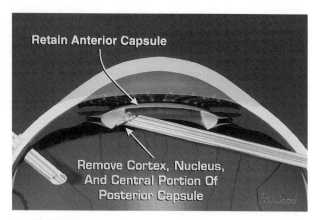

FIGURE 20–7   After performing a circular posterior capsulorrhexis, a bent 20-gauge titanium fragmentor is used to remove the nucleus and epinucleus.

20–8). Careful capsule polishing obviates the need for primary anterior capsulotomy. The author currently uses acrylic (Acrysof by Alcon), foldable lenses through a 3.1-mm keratome, scleral tunnel incision (Fig. 20–9).

VISUAL RESULTS

Approximately 40% of the patients in the author's series of 841 cases had their vision improved to 20/40 or better, and approximately 56% improved to 20/80 or better. Over 52.7% of the patients improved 2 lines or greater in visual acuity, with an average of 3.9 lines of visual improvement. As expected, those with the worst preoperative visual acuity tended to get the most number of lines of visual improvement postoperatively. Among patients with a preoperative visual acuity in the 20/800 to light perception (LP) range, almost 74% improved, with an average number of 3.5 lines of improvement. Among patients with preoperative vision in the 20/50 to 20/400 range, 66.3% improved, with an average of 2.5 lines of improve-

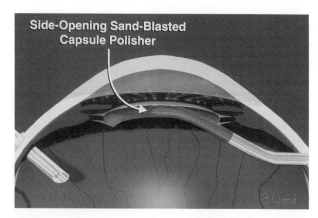

FIGURE 20–8   A small 20-gauge, sandblasted or diamond-dusted capsule polisher is used to polish the anterior lens capsule.

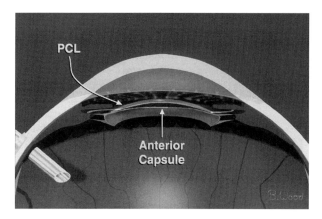

FIGURE 20–9   Acrylic (Acrysof by Alcon), foldable lenses through a 3.1-mm keratome, scleral tunnel incision are used.

ment. Among patients with preoperative vision in the 20/20 to 20/40 range, 48.8% had an average of 1.9 lines of visual improvement. Many of these patients in the latter group achieved dramatic symptomatic reduction of metamorphopsia, despite the fact that their vision could only improve a few lines at best.

COMPLICATIONS

Retinal Breaks

No posterior retinal breaks were caused in the author's series of 841 consecutive vitrectomies for EMMs. Other authors[23–25, 30–33] have reported an incidence of 0 to 15%. Although the author's series was not randomized to outside-in versus inside-in peeling, this marked difference probably indicates that inside-out, forceps membrane peeling is a safer method than using pics and outside-in peeling.

Rhegmatogenous Retinal Detachment

The author's series had a similar incidence of postoperative retinal detachment to that reported by other authors (6%). This complication is related to inadvertent force on the vitreous base during vitreous removal, instrument introduction forces, and incarceration of vitreous in the sclerotomies. This complication can be decreased by using high-quality cutters, low suction force (<80 mm Hg), and highest possible cutting rates, and by avoiding pulling the cutter away when cutting is activated. The retinal periphery should be inspected with the indirect ophthalmoscope at the end of the case and any retinal breaks treated with laser or cryoretinopexy. If subretinal fluid is present, retinal breaks can be managed with a fluid-gas exchange utilizing 25% SF_6.

Proliferative Vitreoretinopathy Recurrence

If PVR was successfully repaired prior to the development of a membrane, it can be stimulated to recur by epimacular membrane surgery. Usually, the PVR-induced redetachment can be successfully repaired with repeat vitrectomy and silicone oil, but little improvement in pre-EMM surgery vision is then obtained.

Endophthalmitis

The author's series of 841 cases had no cases of postoperative endophthalmitis, while the literature reports an average incidence of 0.7%. The author uses a one-piece surgical drape that is folded over the lid margins, and a microscope drape in all cases. Subconjunctival Nebcin and Rocephin are injected at the end of the case. High-quality infusion fluid (Alcon BSS Plus) is used in all cases. Absorbable sclerotomy sutures are not used.

Recurrence of Epimacular Proliferation

Approximately 3% of treated EMM cases in published series are followed by a recurrence of EMM.[23,25,27,30,31,34,35] Approximately 1.6% of treated EMM cases resulted in clinically significant recurrent epimacular membranes in the author's series of 841 cases. Successful reoperation can usually be performed with sustained visual improvement. The recurrence rate emphasizes the reparative nature of the process due to the damage to the retinal surface associated with membrane peeling. All patients probably have some repair of the retinal surface after membrane peeling. The criteria for defining a recurrence has not been established in the literature. In some patients, the folds disappear completely and a recurrence can easily be determined to be present if folds recur. In some patients, the folds never completely resolve, although vision can return to normal levels with resolution of metamorphopsia. In other patients, the recurrent membrane causes macular elevation with minimal striae, and the membrane is more difficult to visualize. Decreased visual function is usually the best indicator of clinically significant recurrences if the patient had initially experienced gradual visual improvement. Visually significant cataract must be ruled out before the visual loss can be attributed to the macula.

Retinal Whitening

Immediate postoperative retinal whitening occurs at the removal site in a significant percentage of cases. This disappears spontaneously in several days and does not seem to affect the visual outcome. It is probable that this phenomenon represents ganglion cell axoplasmic flow disruption. Michels noted that retinal whitening can be present preoperatively in a significant number of cases.

Cataract

Posterior subcapsular cataracts after vitrectomy are largely avoidable. Posterior subcapsular cataracts can be caused by instrument contact with the lens, or by using low-quality infusion fluids (such as lactated Ringer's solution) rather than glutathione bicarbonate Ringer's (Alcon BSS Plus).

The observed increase in the incidence of nuclear sclerosis associated with EMM surgery is thought by the author to result from ultraviolet (UV) irradiance and heating from infrared (IR) light exposure from the microscope light source and/or the endoilluminator. The author's series of 841 cases resulted in 7% of the patients requiring cataract surgery from progression of nuclear sclerosis after vitrectomy. The incidence of progression of nuclear sclerosis has been reported to range from 7% to over 50%.[23–25,27,30,36,37] This wide variation could be accounted for by many factors, including follow-up period, definition of clinical significance, postoperative refraction, operating time, intraoperative cataract surgery, light source UV and IR content, and unknown factors. The author has used cooling of the infusion fluid for the past 10 years in an attempt to reduce heating of the nucleus secondary to infrared irradiation. Cooling lessens the effect of the ultraviolet as well. Heating and ultraviolet exposure are thought by many cataract researchers to be factors in the development of nuclear sclerosis.

Acknowledgments: The author would like to thank Joseph C. Schwartz, M.D. for his help in compiling the references, and Byron Wood for the illustrations.

REFERENCES

1. de Juan E Jr, Lambert HM, Machemer R: Recurrent proliferations in macular pucker, diabetic retinopathy and retrolental fibroplasialike disease after vitrectomy. Graefes Arch Ophthalmol 223:174–183, 1985.
2. Green WR: Clinicopathologic correlation of pigmented epiretinal membranes. Am J Ophthalmol 106:536–545, 1988.
3. Smiddy WE, Michels RG, Green WR: Morphology, pathology, and surgery of idiopathic vitreoretinal macular disorders, a review. Retina 10:288–296, 1990.
4. Smiddy WE, Michels RG, Gilbert HD, Green WR: Clinicopathologic study of idiopathic macular pucker in children and young adults. Retina 12:232–236, 1992.
5. Roth AM, Foos RY: Surface wrinkling retinopathy in eyes enucleated at autopsy. Trans Am Acad Ophthalmol Otolaryngol 75:1047–1058, 1971.
6. Hirokawa H, Jalkh AE, Takahashi M, et al: Role of the vitreous in idiopathic pre-retinal macular fibrosis. Am J Ophthalmol 106:536–545, 1988.
7. Kishi S, Shimizu K: Oval defect in detached posterior hyaloid membrane in idiopathic preretinal fibrosis. Am J Ophthalmol 118:451–456, 1994.
8. Wise GN: Clinical features of idiopathic preretinal macular fibrosis. Am J Ophthalmol 79:349, 1975.
9. Kenyon KR, Michels RG: Ultrastructure of epiretinal membrane removed by pars plana vitreoretinal surgery. Am J Ophthalmol 83(6):815, 1977.
10. Clarkson SG, Green WR, Massof D: A histopathologic review of 168 cases of preretinal membrane. Am J Ophthalmol 84:1, 1977.
11. Green WR, Kenyon KR, Michels RG, et al: Ultrastructure of epiretinal membranes causing macular pucker following retinal reattachment. Trans Ophthalmol Soc UK 99:63, 1979.
12. Kampik A, Green WR, Michels RG, Nase PK: Ultrastructural features of idiopathic progressive epiretinal membrane removed by vitreous surgery. Am J Ophthalmol 90:797, 1981.
13. Michels RG: A clinical and histopathological study of epiretinal membranes affecting the macula and removed by vitreous surgery. Trans Am Ophthalmol Soc 80:580, 1982.
14. Laqua H: Pigmented macular pucker. Am J Ophthalmol 86(1):56, 1978.
15. Lindsey PS, Michels RG, Luckenbach M, Green WR: Ultrastructure of epiretinal membrane causing retinal starfold. Ophthalmology 90:578, 1983.
16. de Bustros S, Rice TA, Michels RG, et al: Vitrectomy for macular pucker, use after treatment of retinal tears or detachment. Arch Ophthalmol 106: 758–761, 1988.
17. Shea M: The surgical management of macular pucker in rhegmatogenous retinal detachment. Ophthalmology 87(1):70–75, 1980.
18. Machemer R: A new concept for vitreous surgery: two instrument techniques in pars plana vitrectomy. Arch Ophthalmol 92:407–412, 1974.
19. Michels RG, Wilkinson CP, Rice TA: Retinal Detachment. St Louis, CV Mosby Co, 1990, 850–857.
20. Shea M: The surgical management of macular pucker. Can J Ophthalmol 2:110–113, 1979.
21. Charles S: Vitreous Microsurgery. Baltimore, Williams & Wilkins, 1987, 153–157.
22. Rice TA, de Bustros S, Michels RG, et al: Prognostic factors in vitrectomy for epiretinal membranes of the macula. Ophthalmology 93:602–610, 1986.
23. McDonald HR, Verre WP, Aaberg TM: Surgical management of idiopathic epiretinal membranes. Ophthalmology 93:978–983, 1986.
24. Pilkerton AR, Gilbert WS, Perraut LE Sr, et al: Idiopathic preretinal fibrosis: a review of 237 cases. Ophthalmol Surg 23(2):113–116, 1992.
25. Pesin SR, Olk RJ, Grand MG, et al: Vitrectomy for premacular fibroplasia. Ophthalmology 98:1109–1114, 1991.
26. Charles S: Vitreous Microsurgery. Baltimore, Williams & Wilkins, 1987, p 98.
27. Michels RG: Vitreous surgery for macular pucker. Am J Ophthalmol 92:628, 1981.
28. Margherio RR: Discussion of Michels RG: Vitrectomy for macular pucker. Ophthalmology 91: 1387–1388, 1984.
29. Blankenship GW, Flynn HW Jr, Kokame GT: Posterior chamber intraocular lens insertion during pars plana lensectomy and vitrectomy for complications of proliferative diabetic retinopathy. Am J Ophthalmol 108(1):1–5, 1989.
30. Margherio RR, Cox MS, Trese MT, et al: Removal of epimacular membranes. Ophthalmology 92:1075–1083, 1985.
31. Michels RG: Vitrectomy for macular pucker. Ophthalmology 91:1384, 1984.
32. de Bustros S, Thompson JT, Michels G, et al: Vitrectomy for idiopathic epiretinal membranes causing macular pucker. Br J Ophthalmol 72:692–695, 1988.
33. Poliner LS, Olk RJ, Grand MG, et al: Surgical management of premacular fibrosis. Arch Ophthalmol 106:761–764, 1988.

34. Michels RG: Surgery of macular pucker. In Fine SL, Owens SL (eds): Management of Retinal Vascular and Macular Disorders. Baltimore, Williams & Wilkins, 1983, 120–130.
35. Wilkinson CP: Recurrent macular pucker. Am J Ophthalmol 88(6):1029, 1979.
36. de Bustros S, Thompson JT, Michels RG, et al: Nuclear sclerosis after vitrectomy for idiopathic epiretinal membranes. Am J Ophthalmol 105:160–164, 1988.
37. Cherfan GM, Michels RG, de Bustros S, et al: Nuclear sclerotic cataract after vitrectomy for idiopathic epiretinal membranes causing macular pucker. Am J Ophthalmol 111:434–438, 1991.

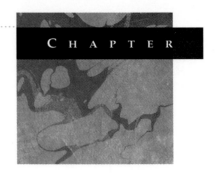

CHAPTER 21

Postsurgical Cystoid Macular Edema

Andrew A. Chang, M.B.B.S.
Richard F. Spaide, M.D.
Lawrence A. Yannuzzi, M.D.

Cystoid macular edema (CME) represents one of the most common causes of unexpected poor visual acuity after cataract surgery. Although postsurgical CME occurs most frequently after cataract extraction,[1-15] it may also occur following almost any other ocular surgery including neodymium: yttrium-aluminum-garnet (Nd:YAG) capsulotomy,[16-24] penetrating keratoplasty,[25] scleral buckling,[26] and filtering procedures.[1-27] CME develops following uneventful cataract surgery in about 60% of patients with intracapsular[1] and 20 to 30% of patients with extracapsular surgery.[2] Generally, visual loss tends to be self-limiting; however, chronic CME with permanent visual loss occurs in approximately 1% of patients undergoing extracapsular cataract extraction. The precise pathogenesis of CME continues to perplex ophthalmologists. As yet there are a number of different therapies that have been proposed based on theories of pathogenesis. However, no definitive treatment regimen exists. The goal of treatment of chronic CME is to reduce the edema and improve the visual acuity.[28]

HISTORICAL PERSPECTIVE

In 1953 Irvine described a syndrome following intracapsular cataract surgery with late rupture of the anterior vitreous face with vitreous prolapse into the anterior chamber incarceration in the cataract wound. Decreased vision was felt due to vitreous opacities or macular changes.[8] Gass and Norton subsequently (1966) described cystoid macular edema occurring in aphakic eyes with intraretinal

fluorescein angiographic cystoid spaces and optic nerve head staining.[10]

The syndrome of CME following cataract surgery has therefore been termed the *Irvine-Gass syndrome.*

CLASSIFICATION

Angiographic Macula Edema

This term is used when there is leakage of fluorescein detected on angiography that may or may not be accompanied by decreased visual acuity. Many of these cases have subtle biomicroscopic changes.

Clinically Significant Macular Edema

Clinically significant macular edema is associated with a *reduction in visual acuity*. The exact relationship that angiographic CME has to clinically significant CME is uncertain. It is possible that patients with clinically significant CME may have a chronic form of "angiographic" CME. On the other hand, clinically significant CME may be a separate condition on a histologic or pathophysiologic level that initially is unable to be differentiated from angiographic CME using conventional fluorescein angiography. Patients with clinically significant CME as a group are more likely to have undergone complicated surgery with vitreous loss or implantation of an anterior chamber intraocular lens (IOL).[5,7,29]

The overwhelming majority of patients have

HISTOPATHOLOGICAL FEATURES

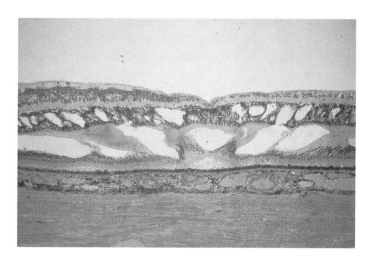

Marked cystoid macular edema with cystic spaces in the outer plexiform layer and, to a lesser degree, in the inner nuclear layer.

spontaneous resolution of their CME in the months following surgery. In a subset of patients, when macular edema persists for longer than 6 months it is less likely to resolve spontaneously. These patients are said to have *chronic macular edema*.

CLINICAL PRESENTATION

Symptoms

The majority of patient with aphakic and pseudophakic CME have undergone uncomplicated cataract surgery. In the angiographic type of CME, patients are often asymptomatic. The usual onset of clinically significant CME occurs 4 to 12 weeks after uncomplicated surgery, peaking at about 4 to 6 weeks. The typical presentation is with poor postoperative central visual acuity followed by a fluctuation in visual symptoms. Some patients may also report low-grade eye redness, photophobia, and eye irritability.

Clinical Examination

CME is best visualized by careful slit lamp biomicroscopic examination using a contact lens. There is loss of the foveal depression. The perifoveal area may take on a yellow xanthophyllic color (Fig. 21–1A). Using a thin, angled slit beam, the macula appears thickened with translucent intraretinal cystoid spaces (Fig. 21–1B). These cystoid spaces are larger in the perifoveal region and become progressively smaller away from the center of the macula. Small splinter hemorrhages may be seen within the retina,[3] and blood may accumulate within the cystoid spaces. In some patients, the underlying choroidal details may be obscured either from severe edema or a concomitant shallow serous detachment of the macula.

Epiretinal membranes are seen in about 10% of patients.[4,5] They have the appearance of a translucent, grayish membrane with a glinting reflex from the inner surface of the retina as the light beam is swept across the macula. The epiretinal membrane

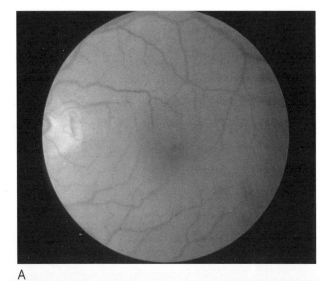

A

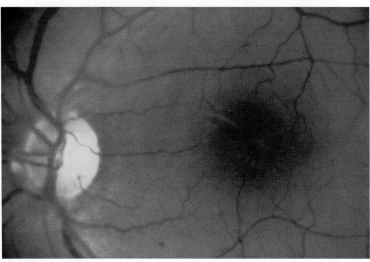

B

FIGURE 21–1   *A,* Loss of the foveal reflex with prominent foveal xanthophyll pigment. *B,* Magnified view of the macula showing fusiform cystoid spaces.

may limit potential for visual recovery upon resolution of the CME.

In chronic edema the intraretinal cystoid spaces may coalesce, producing what is referred to as a foveal cyst, which is actually a foveal schisis cavity. Patients with foveal cysts generally have poorer vision and may be less likely to have satisfactory visual recovery. Unroofing of the foveal cyst with the formation of an inner lamellar macular hole may occur.[3,30] This has the appearance of a sharp step from the perifoveal cystoid spaces to a circular or oval indented area in the foveal area. This usually results in permanent loss of visual acuity.

Patients with chronic CME may develop mottling of the retinal pigment epithelium (RPE), which may relate to the presence of chronic subretinal serous fluid. The granular clumping of the pigment remains unchanged with resolution of the CME.

Some degree of optic nerve head swelling is almost always present. This may be only detected on comparison with the fellow optic nerve. The optic nerve head has an erythematous appearance with slight thickening and elevation of the rim and decrease in the cup size. The relative contribution of the nerve head swelling to decreased visual function is unknown.

Signs of low-grade intraocular inflammation may be present as indicated by a ciliary injection of the globe and anterior chamber flare and cells. Vitreous syneresis and detachment is commonly seen.

Concomitant ocular abnormalities from complications of cataract surgery such as iris or vitreous incarceration in the wound, posterior capsular rupture, iridovitreal synechiae, corneal edema, anterior vitreous strands and incarceration, and IOL pupillary capture (retention of large amounts of lens cortex) may be visible.

FLUORESCEIN ANGIOGRAPHY

Fluorescein angiography is very useful in making the definitive diagnosis of cystoid macular edema. Early in the fluorescein angiographic study, capillary dilation and leakage are conspicuous. The fluorescein leakage occurs from small points in the midsection of each capillary segment. Later pooling in the outer plexiform layer (Henle's layer) gives rise to the classic petaloid staining pattern in the perifoveal region (Fig. 21–2). The fusiform spaces may be arranged in a radial pattern. There is often patchy hyperfluorescence extending outside the cystic spaces, implying more widespread capillary leakage.

In more severe cases of CME, the cystoid spaces may form within the macula located outside of the immediate perifoveal region. In these areas the outer plexiform layer is oriented vertically and cys-

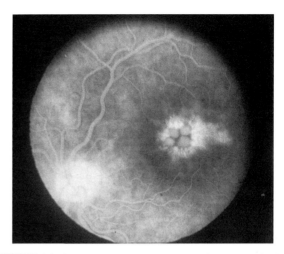

FIGURE 21–2 Fluorescein angiogram. Fluorescein leakage from perifoveal capillaries with the classic petalloid appearance. Note that the cysts appear less hyperfluorescent.

toid spaces that form have a honeycomb appearance.

Late staining of the optic nerve due to leakage of the capillaries in the optic nerve head is almost always seen. Improvement in the CME is accompanied by a parallel decrease in optic nerve staining. This suggests that factors causing macular capillary leakage also cause leakage from capillaries within the optic nerve head.

In certain eyes, particularly those with pseudophakic bullous keratopathy, significant capsular opacities, or small pupils, fluorescein angiography may be technically difficult, resulting in a dark or indistinct study. In these patients, details in the early and mid phases of the angiogram may be barely visible, while an area of hyperfluorescence frequently can be seen in the later phases of the angiogram. It may be extremely difficult to distinguish CME from other conditions such as choroidal neovascularization based on the angiographic findings alone in these eyes.

The area of dye leakage seen during angiography correlates poorly with visual acuity.[5,29] There are several possible explanations for this disparity. First, the actual amount of foveal thickening is one of the most important predictors of visual acuity.[29] The poor correlation between the angiographic findings and visual acuity suggests that the two-dimensional area of fluorescein leakage seen during angiography is not strictly related to the amount of macular or foveal thickening, which is in the third dimension. Second, the cystoid spaces seen during fluorescein angiography lie in the outer plexiform layer and loss of visual acuity may depend on accumulation of fluid in other regions, such as within or under the photoreceptor layer. Finally, there may be pathologic factors occurring in the retina besides the simple accumulation of fluid, that may contribute to the degradation of visual function without causing additional changes in the fluorescein angiogram.

HISTOPATHOLOGY

Histopathologic examination of eyes with CME demonstrate cystoid spaces predominantly in the outer plexiform layer of the fovea (Henle's fiber layer)[31-38] (Fig. 21–3). These cystoid spaces may also be seen in the inner nuclear, ganglion, and nerve fiber layers. There is some debate regarding the histopathologic mechanism of development of the cystoid spaces. Some authors have stated that these spaces represent extracellular collection of fluid,[31] while others considered the possibility of Müller cell swelling and necrosis coupled with vascular decompensation leading to the formation of the cystoid spaces.[36,38] The inner and outer segments of the photoreceptors may appear shortened with swelling and loss of Müller cells. Subretinal fluid may be present. Atrophy, vacuolization, and proliferation of the RPE may also occur.[37]

Cystoid spaces tend to form in the perifoveal region as opposed to the macula outside of this area. This may relate to the unique retinal anatomy and the peculiar capillary arrangement in the foveal and perifoveal area. Fluid transport from the retina occurs at the RPE and at the retinal vessels.[39] Fluid leaks out from retinal capillaries and is then resorbed by the retinal vessels and RPE. Inflammation may increase the fluid flux through the retina. In addition, the macular region has an unusual vascular arrangement—an avascular area is bounded on all sides by a highly vascularized region. Fluid produced in the perifoveal region may spill into the avascular portions of the fovea where resorption may be limited.

Correlations between histopathologic findings and CME have been made.[33] The presence of iridovitreal synechiae, cyclitis and vitritis were associated with CME, whereas the presence of phlebitis and iritis were not.[33] A posterior vitreous detachment was always present with no discernable persistent vitreomacular adhesions. One study demonstrated that only 6 of 31 eyes with vitreous incarceration in the wound had CME.[34] It is possible that other eyes in that study previously had CME that resolved. All eyes had a posterior vitreous detachment. Of the six eyes with CME, six had iridovitreal synechiae, five had periphlebitis, and in those who did not have diabetes as an additional risk factor for macular edema, all four had pars plicata distortion.[34]

Eyes with CME appear to have a global blood-ocular barrier breakdown. Iris angiography and anterior chamber fluorophotometry have shown leakage from the iris.[40,41] Fluorophotometric studies have shown diffuse fluorescein leakage into the vitreous cavity.[42,43]

ELECTROPHYSIOLOGY

On electrophysiologic evaluation, abnormalities may be seen on focal and pattern electroretinograms with normal visual evoked potentials.[44,45]

DIFFERENTIAL DIAGNOSIS

A number of ocular and systemic diseases may mimic postsurgical cystoid macular edema. In addition, cystoid macula edema may be secondary to other ocular pathology. Table 21–1 lists some other conditions associated with CME.

Branch Retinal Vein Occlusion

Branch vein occlusions acutely produce a sector-shaped area of intraretinal hemorrhage and edema corresponding to the distribution of the draining vein. With time the hemorrhages may clear, leaving an area of retinal edema. Capillary telangiectasis and dilatation of the affected segments of the occluded vein may be seen. However, macular tributary vein occlusions may not result in obvious

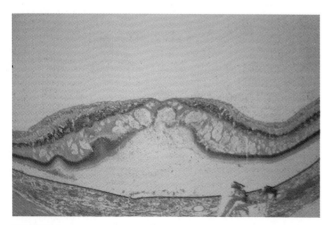

FIGURE 21–3 Histopathologic section through macula illustrating aphakic cystoid macular edema. Extensive deposits of serous exudate in outer plexiform and inner nuclear layers.

TABLE 21–1 Other Conditions Associated with Cystoid Macular Edema

Diabetes
Vascular occlusions
Hypertensive retinopathy
Epiretinal membrane
Intraocular tumors (e.g., melanoma, choroidal hemangioma)
Intraocular inflammation (e.g., pars planitis)
Macroaneurysm
Retinitis pigmentosa
Drugs: epinephrine in aphakia
Choroidal neovascularization
Radiation retinopathy

vessel dilatation as would be seen in larger vessel occlusions. Flecks of intraretinal lipid may develop, which does not occur in CME following cataract surgery. Fluorescein angiography demonstrates asymmetric venous filling. Small patches of capillary nonperfusion may be seen. In the later phases of the angiogram, intraretinal hyperfluorescence accumulates and is centered in the area of the branch retinal vein occlusion.

Diabetic Macular Edema

Postsurgical CME must be differentiated from focal or diffuse diabetic maculopathy, as the treatment is different for each condition. In a study of patients sent to a referral practice for CME, approximately 8% were diabetic.[5] Patients with pre-existing macular edema frequently have a severe exacerbation of their macular edema following cataract surgery.[46,47] In diabetic patients the relative contribution of diabetic retinopathy and postsurgical CME may be difficult to estimate. In diabetic macular edema there may be lipid deposition and intraretinal hemorrhages. During fluorescein angiography, diabetic macular edema has diffuse leakage that may not be localized to the foveal area. Absence of disc leakage may be a helpful distinguishing feature. Absence of disc leakage in diabetic maculopathy may be helpful in distinguishing this from postsurgical macular edema. In a diabetic patient with macular edema, the presence of optic nerve staining implies the macular edema is, at least in some part, related to the surgical process.

Choroidal Neovascularization

Cataract and age-related macular degeneration are often coexistent in this age group. Choroidal neovascularization (CNV), the hallmark of exudative age-related macular degeneration, is manifested by a grayish green membrane associated with overlying neurosensory detachment, RPE detachments, flecks of subretinal lipid, and sub-RPE and subretinal hemorrhage. These findings are not seen in postsurgical CME. Occult neovascularization is a slower growing variant of CNV and may be more difficult to recognize. Occult CNV may cause CME and thus may be confused with postsurgical CME. Patients with occult CNV have thickening at the level of the RPE, a shallow overlying neurosensory detachment, and may have flecks of subretinal lipid, but may not necessarily have sub-RPE or subretinal hemorrhage. The fluorescein angiographic findings of occult choroidal neovascularization include ill-defined hyperfluorescence at the level of the RPE, pinpoint leakage (ooze) from the RPE, and "thumbprints," which are small irregular folds of the RPE.[48-50] In occult CNV the new vessels themselves are not visible during fluorescein angiog-

raphy. There is no late staining of the optic nerve head in occult CNV.

Retinal Detachment

Shallow retinal detachments that clinically are difficult to detect can extend into the macula, causing poor visual acuity.[51] These detachments may cause folds in the macula that give the appearance of CME. These patients may have angiographic evidence of CME, which may be related to either the previous cataract surgery or the retinal detachment. In one study of patients seen in a referral practice for CME, 9 of 150 (6%) actually had retinal detachments.[5] Patients with CME usually complain of blurring of vision with some slight distortion. Patients with retinal detachment may notice that their vision changes with head position and that their visual acuity is better in the morning than in the evening. There may be retinal folds in the macular region, which does not occur in CME. Subretinal fluid may gravitate inferiorly in retinal detachments. Contact B-scan ultrasonography can aid in confirming the diagnosis.

Endophthalmitis

Acute postoperative endophthalmitis usually presents with a sudden onset of pain, loss of vision, and severe uveitis. Endophthalmitis from less virulent organisms such as *Propionibacterium acnes* or *Candida parapsilosis* may produce an indolent intraocular inflammation resulting in a less conspicuous clinical presentation.[52] Infection with *P. acnes* most commonly occurs following extracapsular cataract surgery,[52,53] although it has been reported following intracapsular surgery.[54] This anaerobic bacterium becomes sequestered within the lens capsule or between the lens capsule and the intraocular lens, causing a chronic uveitis. A white plaque may be seen in the posterior lens capsule. Vitrectomy, capsulectomy, culture, and intraocular antibiotic administration are indicated if this diagnosis is suspected.[52]

Photic Maculopathy

These patients usually present on the first or second postoperative day with a paracentral scotoma. Clinically, an irregularly shaped, oval, yellow-white lesion may be seen close to the fovea. Fluorescein angiography reveals an area of fluorescein staining. This is later replaced by fine mottling of the retinal pigment epithelium.

Hypotonous Retinopathy

Intraocular hypotony may be caused by a wound leak or cyclodialysis cleft. Broad irregular choroidal folds are seen initially. The choroid may be swollen around the peripapillary area and may simulate papilledema. Retinal vessels are tortuous and may be engorged. Vision loss is secondary to folding of the choroid, RPE, and retina. Cystoid macular edema is not commonly seen.

Impending Macular Hole

An impending macular hole may appear as a yellowish spot in the fovea. A full-thickness macular hole may be mistaken for a large cystic space.

PREVALENCE

The prevalence of CME following cataract surgery has declined with improvement in surgical technique. However, it continues to be a significant disappointment for both the patient and the ophthalmologist. Following intracapsular cataract extraction (ICCE) about 1 to 2% of patients will have clinically significant CME. Iris-fixated IOLs implanted after ICCE were associated with a prevalence of clinically significant CME of 2% to more than 5% depending on the IOL geometry and how the IOL was manufactured.[55–57] There has been a shift in surgical technique from intracapsular techniques to preserving the posterior capsule through extracapsular cataract extraction (ECCE) and phacoemulsification. Concurrently with this change, posterior chamber IOLs became more popular. With these advances, the prevalence of clinically significant CME decreased to approximately 1%.[2,58,59,60]

Complicated cataract extraction is associated with an increased risk of CME. Cystoid macular edema is more commonly seen when some complication of cataract surgery occurs such as disruption of the anterior vitreous hyaloid, vitreous loss, retention of lens cortex, vitreous strands to the wound, if the IOL is unstable or poorly positioned, inadequate wound closure, and chronic inflammation.[5,7] A study of 141 patients with visual loss from chronic CME revealed that iris incarceration, rather than vitreous incarceration in the wound, was the most important predictor of poor vision.[5] If primary capsulotomy or vitreous loss occurs, the incidence of clinically significant CME increases to 5 to 8%.[1,2,10,11] In a retrospective cohort study of 46 cases of vitreous loss during ECCE salvaged by anterior vitrectomy and anterior chamber IOLs, there was a significantly higher incidence of clinically significant CME of 20% compared to 1% in the control group.[60]

Following ECCE or phacoemulsification many patients require Nd:YAG capsulotomy when they develop capsular opacities that limit visual acuity. This second surgical procedure is associated with the development of CME in a small proportion of patients. The prevalence of CME after Nd:YAG capsulotomy varies widely among different series,[16–24] with an average of 1.5%. Many of these studies used higher energy levels than what are commonly used today; thus, the actual prevalence using current techniques may be somewhat lower.

THEORIES OF PATHOGENESIS

Vitreous Traction on the Macula

Since the syndrome of postcataract surgery CME was first described, investigators have proposed that vitreous traction on the macula is important in the pathogenesis of CME.[8] Schepens[62] demonstrated attachments of the vitreous to the macula and suggested a role for the vitreous in the production of macular changes. Reese and coworkers[63] as well as Tolentino and Schepens[6] further developed the hypothesis and proposed that vitreous changes brought about by cataract surgery may lead to traction on the macula with formation of CME. Some investigators have proposed that the pattern of fluorescein leakage in the cystoid spaces of the macula with late staining of the nerve head is due to "invisible" strands of vitreous inserting into the optic nerve and macula.[64,65] Vitreoretinal traction on the internal limiting membrane and Müller cells may affect distant or adjacent retinal blood vessels with release of inflammatory mediators.[64]

Gass and Norton first discounted the theory of vitreous traction as the sole cause of CME, as many of their patients had no demonstrable vitreomacular attachment.[11] This finding has been supported by other investigators. In a prospective vitrectomy study of 136 eyes with aphakic CME, only 5 (3.6%) had a demonstrable vitreous strand to the macula.[66] In a histopathologic study of eyes with CME,[35] and in eyes with CME and vitreous incarceration in the wound,[36] no attachment of the vitreous to the macula could be found.

In the vitreomacular traction syndrome vitreous traction does cause CME.[67–69] This condition is caused by an incomplete posterior vitreous detachment where the vitreous remains attached to the macula and, usually, the optic nerve. Vitreomacular traction syndrome may occur in patients who never had ocular surgery. Since cataract extraction frequently precipitates posterior vitreous separation, it is possible that cataract extraction is associated with a higher prevalence of vitreomacular traction syndrome.

Vitreous Incarceration in the Wound

Vitreous incarceration in the wound has been shown to be associated with CME.[11,12] In one study of patients with clinically significant CME, many of whom had complicated cataract surgery, 35% had vitreous incarceration in the wound.[5] CME takes much longer to resolve in eyes with vitreous incarceration when compared to eyes without vitreous incarceration.[11,12] With continuing developments in cataract surgery, including improved wound suturing, extracapsular surgery and phacoemulsification, posterior chamber IOLs, and improvements in handling operative complications, vitreous incarceration in the wound has become less common.

Vitreous-Uveal Traction

Iridovitreal adhesions and vitreal distortion of the pars plicata have been correlated with the presence of CME. After cataract extraction complicated by vitreous loss, iridovitreal adhesions may form. It is possible for vitreous adhesions with the posterior iris, pars plicata, or both to form in eyes with or without vitreous loss. Pars plana vitrectomy can be used to relieve these adhesions. Removing the vitreous traction from the uveal structures may affect the prognosis of CME in several different ways. Vitreous traction may chronically stimulate the involved uveal tract to release inflammatory mediators. Vitreous traction on the pars plicata can alter aqueous humor dynamics and intraocular pressure, factors that may participate in the formation of CME.[70] Transport of prostaglandins from the eye occurs in the area of the ciliary body.[71] It is possible that chronic traction in this area may change the dynamics of inflammatory mediator transport within the eye, leading to CME.

Inflammation

Irvine considered inflammation as one of the causes of decreased vision in patients with spontaneous rupture of the vitreous face and macular changes.[8] In 1954, Chandler described macular edema causing "cystic degeneration" occurring after cataract surgery, and considered prolonged postoperative inflammation as a predisposing cause.[13]

Eyes with CME often have signs of intraocular inflammation. Eyes with CME have evidence of blood-ocular barrier breakdown during fluorophotometry. On histopathologic examination chronic inflammatory cells in the iris, ciliary body, and retina blood vessels may be seen.

The iris is a metabolically active tissue able to release a number of different inflammatory mediators.[72] Incarceration of iris in the wound may cause the production and release of these mediators, resulting in CME, which may represent a possible distal effect. Iris clip lenses and rigid anterior chamber intraocular lenses have chronic iris stimulation as the common element in CME. The only factors found to be associated with a chronic breakdown of the blood-aqueous barrier in a study of patients

after cataract surgery and posterior chamber lens implantation were abnormal pupil shape and posterior synechiae, both implying iris involvement.[73] Entrapment of the peripheral iris in the wound might cause chronic irritation of the ciliary body leading to cyclitis, which has been strongly associated with chronic CME.[34]

Inflammatory Mediators That May Be Involved in CME

A number of inflammatory mediators have been implicated in the formation of CME. Worst[74] suggested that during cataract extraction, potentially toxic substances including prostaglandins normally contained in the anterior segment may diffuse posteriorly to the macula. Prostaglandins were among the first inflammatory mediators to be implicated in the pathophysiology of CME.[74,75]

Prostaglandins are synthesized from arachidonic acid, a 20-carbon acid derived from dietary linoleic acid. Arachidonic acid is released from cell membranes by the action of phospholipase A_2 in response to trauma, ischemia, and neuronal or hormonal stimuli. Cyclo-oxygenase converts arachidonic acid to cyclic endoperoxide intermediates that are then converted to prostaglandins.[76–78] Light exposure to the retina also has been suggested as a factor that may increase the production of prostaglandins mediated through the generation of free radicals.[79] Corticosteroids can indirectly block the action of phospholipase A_2, thus preventing the release of arachidonic acid. Nonsteroidal anti-inflammatory drugs (NSAIDs) such as aspirin, indomethacin, or ketorolac block the synthesis of prostaglandins from arachidonic acid by inhibiting cyclo-oxygenase.[76–78]

Inflammation may arise from traction on the iris by vitreous or by immunologic reaction to antigens (IOL) in the anterior segment. This causes breakdown of the blood-aqueous barrier by disrupting the tight junctions of the iris and ciliary body with increased vascular permeability and leakage of protein into the aqueous.

Inflammatory mediators[80] diffuse posteriorly into the vitreous cavity, as no significant diffusion barrier exists for the vitreous[81] where they result in disruption of the blood retinal barrier. Immunohistochemical localization of the blood-retinal barrier breakdown sites has shown that the barrier breakdown occurs primarily at the inner blood-retinal barrier (retinal vessels) but also at the outer barrier (RPE).[82] Vitreous fluorophotometry in aphakic CME suggests that backward diffusion may play a significant role in the development of CME.[42]

The causal link between prostaglandins and CME, though appealing, has been difficult to confirm. CME has not been induced in animal eyes through the injection of prostaglandins. Topical application of prostaglandins is being used as an antiglaucoma medication in humans, and use of prostaglandins has not been associated with CME.[83,84]

Arachidonic acid may be metabolized by enzymes such as 5-lipoxygenase,[77] to produce leukotrienes and peptidoleukotrienes. Additional mediators, not produced from arachidonic acid, such as neuropeptides, cytokines, bradykinin, histamine, tumor necrosis factor, and platelet-activating factor, have been shown to have roles in inflammation. During an inflammatory response a spectrum of these inflammatory mediators are produced. Some of these inflammatory mediators involved in ocular inflammation are listed in Table 21–2.[76–91]

Inflammatory mediators ordinarily interact in an integrated manner to effect the proper response. For example, neuropeptides can cause prostaglandin release in the eye. Prostaglandins require intact innervation in the eye, though, to produce inflammatory effects.[85] Denervation reduces the sensitivity of the eye to the inflammatory effects of prostaglandins.[85] Effects of platelet-activating factor are mediated through peptidoleukotrienes.[86] Platelet-activating factor may increase the release of arachidonic acid and the production of prostaglandins.[87] Prostaglandins and leukotrienes interact to increase vascular permeability. Tumor necrosis factor increases aqueous prostaglandin and leukotriene concentrations.[88] Tumor necrosis factor can also induce interleukin-1 (IL-1), which is a potent agent causing vascular leakage, and IL-1 can in turn induce prostaglandins.[89]

There are a number of mediators that promote inflammation and others, such as transforming growth factor-β (TGF-β), that are immunosuppressive[92] (Table 21–2).[92–94] These immunosuppressive mediators, which appear in the eye, participate in the maintenance of an altered immune response in the eye termed anterior chamber associated immune deviation (ACAID). TGF-β helps establish ACAID through a secondary mediator, prostaglandin E_2.[92] Thus, prostaglandins appear to both promote and suppress certain aspects of intraocular inflammation. Ocular use of immunosuppressive cytokines, or analogues of these cytokines, may be one avenue to treat CME, and uveitis, in the future.

Light Damage

Chromophores in the cataractous lens reduce the transmission of shorter wavelength light. Following cataract extraction, the retina is exposed to large amounts of light, and increased proportion of shorter wavelength light. Exposure to UV light may generate free radicals that increase prostaglandin release. It has been theorized that this excess light causes or potentiates the tendency to form CME, possibly through increased formation of prostaglandins.[79]

Phototoxicity from the operating microscope has been proposed as a possible contributory factor in the pathogenesis of CME. Blocking UV light from the microscope has not been shown to have a statistically significant effect on the prevalence of CME.[95] Pupillary light occluders used during cataract surgery have not been found to have an effect on the prevalence of CME.[96] In one randomized study, UV-absorbing IOLs have been shown to reduce the incidence of angiographically detected CME, but no effect on the visual acuity was found.[97] In two other smaller studies no effect on the prevalence of CME was found in patients receiving UV-absorbing IOLs.[98,99]

Patients who were either scheduled for enucleation or who had a blind eye were exposed to the light of an operating microscope to investigate the phototoxic effects on the retina.[100–102] Extensive RPE necrosis and disruption of the outer lamellae of the photoreceptors was demonstrated.[102] Photic injury from the microscope could be produced with both infrared and UV filters in use.[101] In these studies, no patient developed CME despite the intentional photic damage.[100–102]

TABLE 21–2 Mediators of Ocular Inflammation

Promoters of Ocular Inflammation	Inhibitors of Ocular Inflammation
Cytochrome P-450 products	α-Melanocyte–stimulating hormone
Histamine	Endogenous glucocorticoids
Interferon-γ	Prostaglandins
Interleukins (esp. 1, 2, 6, and 8)	Transforming growth factor-β
Leukotrienes	Vasoactive intestinal peptide
Neuropeptides	
Platelet-activating factor	
Prostaglandins	
Serotonin	
Tumor necrosis factor	

TREATMENT OF POSTSURGICAL CME

The aim of CME treatment is to improve visual acuity by decreasing macular edema once it forms. This theoretically would reduce the risk of subsequent pathologic events such as foveal cysts and inner lamellar holes. Effective and rational treatment hinges on an understanding of the pathophysiology of the disease process. Most treatment strategies for CME have concentrated on either vitreous traction or inflammation as the primary etiology. Other additional treatments have been proposed to reduce the edema without directly treating the cause for the edema formation. These methods include use of carbonic anhydrase inhibitors, grid laser photocoagulation to the macula, and hyperoxic therapy. Therapeutic agents used in the medical treatment of CME are listed in Table 21–3.

Corticosteroids

Corticosteroids are known to improve uveitis-related CME such as pars planitis. Steroids block the release of arachidonic acid from cell membranes. Although they were among the first medications used to treat CME following cataract surgery, corticosteroids have never been the subject of a randomized double-blind study for the treatment of CME.

TABLE 21–3   Therapeutic Agents in the Medical Treatment of CME

Corticosteroids
Topical
Prednisolone acetate 1% four times daily
Prednisolone sodium phosphate 1% four times daily
Dexamethasone 0.1% four times daily
Peribulbar
Triamcinolone 20 mg (0.5 ml) every 3–6 weeks
Methylprednisolone (Depo-Medrol) 20 mg every 3–6 weeks
Oral
Prednisone 1–1/5 mg/kg daily

Cyclo-oxygenase Inhibitors
Topical
Diclofenac sodium 0.1% (Voltaren) four times daily
Flurbiprofen sodium 0.03% (Ocufen) four times daily
Ketorolac tromethamine 0.5% (Acular) four times daily

Carbonic Anhydrase Inhibitors
Acetazolamide (Diamox) 500 mg daily

Topical, subtenon and systemic steroids have all been investigated in several series, which have demonstrated a visual improvement occurring in 60 to 100% of cases. However, this improvement was not long-lasting, with a tendency of CME to return after cessation of therapy.[55,103–105]

Stern and colleagues[55] studied 50 patients who had chronic CME associated with iris-fixated lenses. Of the 50 patients, 49 were treated with varying combinations of oral, subtenon, and topical corticosteroids. Eleven patients responded quickly with corticosteroids and had no recurrence of CME, although some of these patients were continued on a lower dose schedule. Thirty patients had recurrences after corticosteroids were tapered; with resumption of corticosteroids, 16 of these improved to 20/40 or better, while 14 had a final visual acuity between 20/40 and 20/80. Nine patients did not seem to respond to corticosteroids.

Gehring[103] treated 17 patients with macular edema detected by contact lens examination. After treatment using 20 to 40 mg of systemically administered prednisone per day for varying periods, 13 patients (76%) improved to 20/30 and 15 patients (88%) improved by two or more lines of visual acuity. Several patients had recurrences of CME with discontinuance of prednisone, and these cases improved with resumption of prednisone. Although these results appear impressive, many of the cases in this series were of relatively recent onset, and may have spontaneously resolved without treatment.

Corticosteroids have many adverse ocular and systemic side effects, particularly in older patients. Topical steroids are known to cause cataracts, worsen herpes keratitis, and impair wound healing. The most common ocular complication in patients treated for CME with corticosteroids is elevated intraocular pressure. McEntyre[106] suggested that ocular hypertension induced by corticosteroid administration altered hydrostatic dynamics in the macula. He treated patients with enough corticosteroids to induce ocular hypertension and found these patients had a decrease in their cystoid macular edema. A complete account of the intraocular pressures for these patients was not reported. Most patients apparently had a pressure rise of 5 to 10 mm Hg, but some had intraocular pressures as high as 38 mm Hg. Melberg and Olk[107] compared the success rate of treatment for two groups of patients with postsurgical CME: one group that did have an elevation of intraocular pressure with treatment and a control group that did not. All 16 patients without vitreous attachment to anterior chamber structures who developed increased intraocular pressure had improvement of their CME. In contrast, only 4 of 14 control patients without an increase in intraocular pressure had improvement in their CME.[107]

Corticosteroid-induced ocular hypertension may influence the fluid flux from leaking macular capillaries by increasing the hydrostatic tissue fluid pressure. Other possible explanations for the observed effect were that the corticosteroid responders differed genetically, had different corticosteroid receptors, or had better drug penetration than the nonresponders. Another possibility suggested was that inflammation causes decreased intraocular pressure, and patients having the best response to anti-inflammatory therapy would be expected to have a greater restoration of intraocular pressure than those who did not.[108]

NSAIDs, such as the cyclo-oxygenase inhibitors (COIs), decrease intraocular inflammation without causing elevated intraocular pressure.[109] As will be discussed subsequently, more recent studies have shown an improvement in CME in patients treated with COIs. With COIs there appears to be a dissociation between increased intraocular pressure and improvement of CME. This may suggest that the increased intraocular pressure found in corticosteroid-treated patients may not be the sole mechanism causing improvement in CME.

Increased intraocular pressure induced by corticosteroids may be treated with additional medications, but lowering intraocular pressure may alter the therapeutic efficacy. Withdrawal of the corticosteroids may be the most prudent approach for patients with markedly elevated intraocular pressure.

Systemic steroids offer the most sustained systemic levels of steroid. However, there are potentially serious side effects especially in elderly patients with prolonged use limiting their use. Systemic complications associated with corticosteroids in patients being treated for CME include hyperglycemia, hypertension, and neuropsychiatric problems.

Periocular steroids potentially allow higher concentration of steroid delivery to the macula. However, there are potential complications of risk of ocular perforation and elevation of intraocular pressure. Subtenon injection of corticosteroids reduces the potential for systemic complications. There is no proof of any long-term improvement or alteration of the natural course of CME after dissipation of the corticosteroids. It is possible, though, that some severe sequelae such as the formation of foveal cysts or inner lamellar holes may be avoided with the reduction of edema.

Nonsteroidal Anti-inflammatory Drugs

COIs block the cyclo-oxygenase and the synthesis and release of prostaglandins during surgery. Based on this premise, NSAIDs have been investigated in the prophylaxis and therapy of CME. Numerous studies have been conducted to examine the efficacy of systemic and topical COIs both in the prophylaxis and treatment of established CME.[110–126]

Topical administration has higher ocular penetration as compared with systemic administration.[110] Side effects are relatively few with topical

administration. Some ocular burning and irritation is common and superficial punctate keratopathy may occur.

Prophylaxis of Postsurgical CME

Oral indomethacin and piroxicam have been effective in prophylactically reducing the incidence of angiographic CME. However, no difference in visual outcome between treated or untreated groups was demonstrated.[111,112] In one study, systemic aspirin did not appear to have an effect on visual acuity from postsurgical CME.[113]

Miyake administered topical indomethacin to prevent angiographic CME after cataract surgery.[114–116] In a long-term follow-up study[116] they found that patients treated with topical indomethacin prophylactically had improvement in visual acuity early after surgery. However, this effect did not persist. Other investigators found that patients treated prophylactically with topical indomethacin had a decreased incidence of angiographically demonstrable CME by approximately one half, but no improvement in visual acuity was found.[60,117]

The prophylactic use of topical diclofenac[118] and ketorolac[119] has been shown to also decrease the incidence of angiographic CME, but with no effect on clinical CME and no sustained improvement in CME.

A randomized, double-blind clinical trial showed that treatment with flurbiprofen or indomethacin preoperatively and continued 3 months postoperatively reduces the incidence of angiographic and clinical CME and severity of CME in the earlier postoperative period. The flurbiprofen-treated patients had good visual acuity (20/40 or better) sooner than vehicle-treated patients. By days 121 to 240 there was no significant difference between groups in clinical CME.[120]

Most of these studies included the concurrent use of corticosteroids in the postoperative period. Corticosteroids inhibit the generation of prostaglandins, raising the possibility of synergy.[110] Many of the studies investigating indomethacin employed concurrent corticosteroid treatment.[110] This may obscure the true treatment benefit from indomethacin.

A well-controlled, paired comparison study by Flach and associates showed[119] that ketorolac tromethamine used without corticosteroids was effective in reducing the incidence of angiographic CME. Since no study has been done to evaluate the effectiveness of topical corticosteroids in reducing the incidence of angiographic CME, the practical benefit of this finding is difficult to quantify. The visual acuity of the patients was not mentioned in the results of this study.[119]

Treatment of Clinically Significant CME

A more pragmatic approach would be to treat patients with clinically significant CME.[121–126] Neither oral indomethacin[121] nor topical fenoprofen[122] caused a statistically significant improvement in visual acuity. Yannuzzi[123] treated 40 consecutive patients with CME using indomethacin and corticosteroids and found 80% improved by two or more Snellen lines. There were no control patients. In several patients the visual acuity declined with cessation of treatment, and then improved with resumption of therapy. In another study by Peterson and associates,[124] use of topical indomethacin was associated with an improvement of three Snellen lines or more in 80% of patients treated. This particular study only included patients who could tolerate the medication for 8 weeks, and the study had no controls. Of the patients who initially responded, 53% displayed an "on-off" phenomenon when treatment was started and stopped.[124]

However, two double-blind, prospective, randomized studies have suggested that topical ketorolac tromethamine 0.5% is effective for the treatment of visually significant chronic CME.[125,126] In the second multicenter study, aphakic and pseudophakic CME had been present for at least 4 months. The randomized, prospective, double-blind, placebo-controlled trial demonstrated an improvement in vision of at least two Snellen lines and angiographic CME in 19 of 56 treated eyes after 1 month of treatment and 22 eyes after 3 months of treatment. This was significantly better than the 10 of 57 control subjects during the same interval. This statistical difference remained for at least 1 month after cessation of therapy.[126] The limitations of this study were that there was no comparison made with topical corticosteroids and that follow-up was limited to 120 days.

There may be several explanations for why COIs have not further improved vision in CME. Chronic edema may produce profound structural alterations in the fovea, causing permanent damage. Inflammation itself may damage the fovea. Müller cell abnormalities, the possibility of ischemic damage, and RPE changes may contribute to the long-term visual loss.

The optimal effective dose of COIs is not known with certainty. Oral COIs penetrate into the eye poorly[112] and topical COIs penetrate to varying degrees. Because of the large number of different classes of mediators released in inflammation, blocking prostaglandin synthesis alone may not be sufficient. A nonsteroidal drug that blocks production or dampens the effect of more than one type of inflammatory mediator might be more efficacious in treating CME. It may be possible to inhibit inflammation and its sequelae without experiencing the side effects of corticosteroids.

Carbonic Anhydrase Inhibition

Carbonic anhydrase inhibitors may work by improving the ability of the retinal pigment epithelium to pump out edema fluid within the retina.[127] Carbonic anhydrase inhibitors, such as acetazolamide, have been shown in nonrandomized studies to decrease CME and improve visual acuity in patients after cataract surgery[128,129] and scleral buckling.[130] Patients displayed an on-off effect with initiation and cessation of treatment. This drug has been effective in only a minority of patients, some of these patients experience tachyphylaxis, and the effect of the medication lasts only as long as the patients use the drug.

Methazolamide has been tried in the treatment of macular edema in retinitis pigmentosa. It was effective in relatively few patients and rebound was noted with continued use.[131,132]

Long-term carbonic anhydrase inhibitor use is associated with many adverse effects, particularly in older patients. Serious but rare side effects include bone marrow depression, aplastic anemia, and Stevens-Johnson syndrome.

Grid Laser Photocoagulation

Grid laser was described as a method of treatment of postsurgical CME using ruby and argon laser photocoagulation. Zweng and associates treated 17 patients using a ruby laser.[133] Of the five patients who improved, three attained 20/30 or better visual acuity. Schepens suggested using argon laser for grid photocoagulation to treat CME.[134] However, he did not report the results of this treatment. Two pilot studies investigating argon laser for chronic CME unresponsive to medical therapy found that approximately one half of the treated patients showed improvement in their visual acuity.[135,136]

Grid laser treatment has not been investigated in the context of a controlled clinical trial, and so there is no information available concerning its efficacy or safety. It is possible that grid laser treatment, particularly in elderly patients, may induce or accelerate RPE atrophy in the macular region, which is an unacceptable trade-off causing detriment over time to the central vision.

Hyperoxic Therapy

One study of five patients with chronic CME after cataract extraction or secondary IOL implantation were treated with intermittent hyperbaric oxygen for 21 days and had an improvement in visual acuity.[137] The fluorescein angiography results did not improve after the conclusion of treatment in two patients and showed minimal change in a third patient. The visual acuity improvement did not seem to be correlated to the change in the fluorescein angiography result. The authors suggested that constriction of perifoveal capillaries by hyperbaric oxygen may facilitate the reformation of damaged junctional complexes in the capillary wall.[137] Although this explanation may be true, it does not adequately explain the rapid improvement in visual acuity without a parallel change in the amount of macular edema. The hyperbaric oxygen may also affect the anterior segment of the eye, or it may alter ischemia of the macula.

In another study, high concentrations of oxygen were administered to three eyes with chronic aphakic CME through the use of modified swimmer's goggles.[138] All three patients had an improvement in visual acuity. It was suggested that the locally administered oxygen increased the partial pressure of oxygen (PO_2) of the inner retina.[138] Transcorneal delivery of oxygen has been shown to increase the PO_2 of the anterior segment,[139] but whether or not this also increases retinal oxygenation is speculative. It is also possible that the local increase of the PO_2 in the anterior segment altered the production or metabolism of inflammatory mediators produced.

Nd:YAG Vitreolysis

CME complicated with vitreous incarceration in the wound resolves more slowly than CME without vitreous incarceration. Therefore, removing or cutting the offending vitreous might shorten the time for resolution of the associated CME.

Nd:YAG vitreolysis has been reported to cause improvement in vision and associated resolution of CME in some post–cataract surgery patients.[140–142] At the present time, the precise benefit of this treatment cannot be evaulated with certainty for several reasons. First, these studies had no controls. Second, the patients were treated with corticosteroids after Nd:YAG vitreolysis, which may have a separate, beneficial, effect on CME. Third, many of the patients had CME for a very short period of time,[140,141] and may have spontaneously improved. Vitreous fibers that are chronically incarcerated in the wound become much more difficult to lyse. The corneal endothelium migrates over the vitreous strands and lays down basement membrane, making the strands more tenacious.

Nd:YAG vitreolysis is performed using a contact lens with an auxiliary button dioptric element (such as the Abraham lens). Patients who have corneal opacities or peripheral corneal edema require the use of a mirrored gonioscopy lens. The strands are always larger and broader than they first appear even on gonioscopy. Repeated sessions may be required with higher risk of local complications such as bleeding from the iris and increased inflammation. Iridovitreal synechiae posterior to the iris cannot be reliably lysed with an Nd:YAG laser. In one series of 12 patients, 1 developed a retinal detachment and another developed IOP rise after laser.[142]

Vitrectomy

Vitrectomy has been investigated as a therapeutic intervention for CME. It would allow removal of vitreous adhesions. In addition, vitrectomy would theoretically be effective by removing the inflammatory mediators in the vitreous as well as allowing greater access of topical steroids to the posterior segment. Several series have yielded encouraging results for vitrectomy.

Following favorable results of nonrandomized vitrectomy studies in aphakic eyes,[143,144] a national multicenter randomized, prospective clinical trial[66,145] demonstrated a visual benefit of vitrectomy for *aphakic* chronic macular edema with vitreous incarceration in the wound; however, the treatment effect was not large. The patients in the vitrectomy group were treated with topical atropine and corticosteroids, but the patients in the control group were not, which might have favorably affected the vitrectomy group. The investigators[66] recommended that vitrectomy be delayed until CME was stable for at least 2 to 3 months. Vitrectomy was considered if vision was 20/80 or worse and before the visual acuity was 20/80 for 2 years. Vitrectomy was performed via a pars plana or combined pars plana and limbal approach.

Dugel and co-workers[146] performed vitrectomy on 11 eyes of nine patients with chronic macular edema unresponsive to topical, subtenon and systemic steroids. Five eyes improved vision to better than 20/40. Seven eyes had visual improvement of four lines or more. Angiographic CME improved in nine eyes.

A review of 24 patients with chronic *pseudophakic* CME[147] revealed that vitrectomy for CME unresponsive to medical therapy with vitreous adhesions to anterior segment structures or iris capture of the IOL resulted in improvement in vision of all patients with a mean of 4.7 Snellen lines. There was no significant difference for anterior or posterior chamber IOLs. The length of time from cataract surgery to vitrectomy had no correlation with the postoperative vision.

Because of changes in cataract surgery as well as the improvement in anterior vitrectomy techniques, most patients with CME do not have vitreous incarceration. In addition, almost every patient undergoing cataract surgery has an intraocular lens implantation, and consequently is not aphakic. There are few data concerning vitrectomy for pseudophakic patients with CME who do not have vitreous incarceration.

Intraocular Lens Removal and Replacement

Intraocular lenses have been associated with CME by several mechanisms. Certain earlier IOLs, through the method of packaging, poor quality of the finish, or impurities in the plastic, were associated with CME.[56] These problems have largely been eliminated with modern manufacturing techniques. Some IOLs, such as the iris clip and rigid closed loop anterior chamber IOLs, appear to have chronically stimulated the iris and caused CME.[56,57,148,149] These IOLs are no longer being used.[57] CME may be more frequent in eyes with iris tuck by an IOL haptic or capture of the iris by the lens.[150]

Many patients with IOL-related CME also have concurrent problems such as pseudophakic bullous keratopathy, glaucoma, hyphema, and chronic inflammation. These patients ultimately may require surgery with explanation or exchange of their IOLs as a part of a larger effort to salvage the eye.

In one study examining the effect of lens removal in IOL-related CME, five of ten eyes attained a visual acuity of 20/50 or better.[151] In another study, six eyes had lens exchange, and four of the eyes had visual acuity improvement of two Snellen lines or more.[152] Many eyes with pseudophakic bullous keratopathy have concurrent CME, but the exact prevalence is difficult to determine due to the difficulty in performing fluorescein angiography. However, one study showed resolution of angiographic CME in 18 of 25 patients treated with penetrating keratoplasty, anterior chamber IOL removal, and replacement with a posterior chamber IOL.[153]

CME Treatment Strategy

The management of the patient with CME should begin with a careful examination to exclude and rule out an occult infectious process, intraocular derangement such as entrapment of the iris or vitreous in the wound, or a contributory factor such as primary uveitis or diabetic retinopathy.

The best course of action for a patient with CME for only a few months after cataract surgery is to wait, as most of these patients will spontaneously resolve. In cases where pharmacologic therapy is indicated, what is the drug of choice and how should it be delivered? The lack of randomized therapeutic trials limits the objective information available to base definitive recommendations for the treatment of CME. Given the imperfect nature of current knowledge, recommendations for treatment are formed from consolidating information from past therapeutic studies and considerations of the pathophysiology of CME.[154]

There may be pressure to treat these patients with a number of medications simultaneously to try to improve the vision by any means possible. However, treatment in a graded manner represents a rational approach. A stepwise strategy is shown in Table 21–4. Each step is continued without change for 6 to 8 weeks. If no progress is made at the end of this time then the next therapeutic step is taken without discontinuing the previous step. If at any point a response is noted, the medications can be tapered slowly. If the vision deteriorates, then the medication is increased to the previous level.

Corticosteroids are probably the most commonly used medications in the treatment for CME, but have not been the subject of a randomized, controlled trial. COIs offer the possibility of less adverse systemic and ocular side effects. Oral COIs do not appear to penetrate the eye very well, and have not been shown to be efficacious.

As corticosteroids and COIs act synergistically to suppress the production of prostaglandins,[110] it is rational to commence these two agents concomitantly from the outset. Topical steroid and COI are commenced at four times daily for 6 to 8 weeks. If a response is noted, then the frequency of administration is gradually decreased. Studies using both corticosteroids and COIs together suggest that

TABLE 21–4 Stepwise Therapeutic Approach to CME

Step 1	Topical corticosteroid Topical COI
Step 2	Sub–Tenon's capsule orbital corticosteroid injection
Step 3	Acetazolamide Oral corticosteroid

Step 4	*Surgery*
	   Laser Nd:YAG laser vitreolysis
	   Vitrectomy

Other therapeutic options	Diamox Hyperoxic therapy Grid laser photocoagulation

COI, cyclo-oxygenase inhibitor; Nd:YAG, neodymium:yttrium-aluminum-garnet.

some patients may respond to a short course of therapy without recurrence of CME. The withdrawal of corticosteroids and COIs, though, has been associated with the recurrence of CME in a number of patients. This suggests that some patients may have a chronic inflammatory condition that may require chronic treatment. The use of corticosteroids and COIs together may reduce the amount of corticosteroid necessary to achieve a desired amount of anti-inflammatory effect.

If there is no improvement on this regimen, periocular steroid injections can be considered. A total of three or four injections may be given. Ocular hypertension following subtenon corticosteroid injection appears to be relatively less common unless the medication dissects forward under the conjunctiva. If no effect is seen following this, it is not advisable to give further injections.

In patients who either have had no response to or could not receive subtenon corticosteroids, oral corticosteroids or a carbonic anhydrase inhibitor such as acetazolamide can be prescribed. Only a minority of patients have a satisfactory response to this medication.

Lack of response to any medication suggests the need for evaluation of alternate approaches. Some patients may require IOL replacement or removal as indicated by careful examination of the anterior segment. Rarely, other methods of treatment such as grid laser photocoagulation or hyperoxic therapy should be considered.

Patients with chronic CME who have vitreous incarceration in the surgical wound usually merit a course of pharmacologic treatment before any attempt of surgical repair for the vitreous incarceration. Nd:YAG vitreolysis may be convenient for the physician and the patient but has distinct technical limitations. In addition, there is little knowledge of the efficacy of Nd:YAG vitreolysis in more chronic cases of CME. Vitrectomy, either through an anterior or posterior approach, has the potential to effect a better repair of vitreous adhesions to the wound or iris, especially in more chronic cases. Iris incarceration may be repaired during the same procedure.

SUMMARY

CME following cataract surgery represents a disappointment for both patient and ophthalmologist alike. Improved surgical technique already has reduced the incidence of CME following cataract surgery, and further refinements in cataract surgery will undoubtedly continue this trend. However, despite improvements in surgical technique and newer IOL materials, a certain proportion of patients will probably develop clinically significant CME because of surgical trauma. The effective prevention and treatment of CME requires clarification of the basic mechanisms responsible for CME. Evaluation of newer therapeutic agents, as well as re-evaluation of older drugs such as corticosteroids, requires randomized, double-blind clinical trials to determine their efficacy. Although vitrectomy may be useful for aphakic CME and pseudophakic CME, to define the role of vitrectomy further prospective studies are required.

REFERENCES

1. Hitchings RA, Chisholm IH, Bird AC: Aphakic macular edema: incidence and pathogenesis. Invest Ophthalmol 14:68, 1975.
2. Wright PL, Wilkinson CP, Balyeat HD, et al: Angiographic cystoid macular edema after posterior chamber lens implantation. Arch Ophthalmol 106:740, 1988.
3. Bovino JA, Kelly TJ, Marcus DF: Intraretinal hemorrhages in cystoid macular edema. Arch Ophthalmol 102:1151, 1984.
4. Gass JDM: Stereoscopic Atlas of Macular Diseases. St. Louis, CV Mosby Co, 1987, pp 368–380.
5. Spaide RF, Yannuzzi LA, Sisco LJ: Chronic cystoid macular edema and predictors of visual acuity. Ophthalmic Surg 24:262, 1993.
6. Tolentino FI, Schepens CL: Edema of the posterior pole after cataract extraction. A biomicroscopic study. Arch Ophthalmol 74:781, 1965.
7. Ruiz RS, Saatchi OA: Visual outcome in pseudophakic eyes with clinical cystoid macular edema. Ophthalmic Surg 22:190, 1991.
8. Irvine SR: A newly defined vitreous syndrome following cataract surgery. Interpreted according to recent concepts of the structure of the vitreous. Am J Ophthalmol 36:599, 1953.
9. Reese AB, Jones IS, Cooper WC: Macular changes secondary to vitreous traction. Trans Am Ophthalmol Soc 64:123, 1966.
10. Gass JDM, Norton EWD: Cystoid macular edema and papilledema following cataract extraction: a fluorescein fundoscopic and angiograpic study. Arch Ophthalmol 76:646, 1966.
11. Gass JDM, Norton EWD: Follow-up study of cystoid macular edema following cataract extraction. Trans Am Acad Ophthalmol Otolaryngol 73:665, 1969.
12. Wilkinson CP: A long-term follow-up study of cystoid macular edema in aphakic and pseudophakic eyes. Trans Am Ophthalmol Soc 79:810, 1981.
13. Chandler PA: Complications after cataract surgery: clinical aspects. Trans Am Acad Ophthalmol Otolaryngol 58:382, 1954.
14. Hoyt CS, Nickel D: Aphakic cystoid macular edema. Occurrence in infants and children after transpupillary lensectomy and anterior vitrectomy. Arch Ophthalmol 100:746, 1982.
15. Nicholls JVV: Macular edema in association with cataract extraction. Am J Ophthalmol 37:665, 1954.
16. Keates RH, Steinert RF, Puliafito CA, Maxwell SK: Long-term follow-up of Nd:YAG laser posterior capsulotomy. Am J Intraocular Implant Soc 10:164, 1984.
17. Johnson S, Kratz R, Olson P: Clinical experience with the Nd:YAG laser. Am J Intraocular Implant Soc 10:452, 1984.
18. Chambless WS: Neodymium YAG laser posterior capsulotomy results and complications. Am J Intraocular Implant Soc 11:31, 1985.
19. Winslow RL, Taylor BC: Retinal complications following YAG capsulotomy. Ophthalmology 92:785, 1985.
20. Stark WJ, Worthen D, Holladay JT, Murray G: Neodymium: YAG lasers. An FDA report. Ophthalmology 92:209, 1985.
21. Liesegang TJ, Bourne WM, Ilstrup DM: Secondary surgical and neodymium-YAG laser discissions. Am J Ophthalmol 100:510, 1985.

22. Shah GR, Gills JP, Durham DG, Asmus WH: Three thousand YAG lasers in posterior capsulotomies. An analysis of complications and comparison to polishing and surgical discission. Ophthalmic Surg 17:473, 1986.

23. Bath PE, Frankhauser F: Long-term results of Nd:YAG laser posterior capsulotomy with the Swiss laser. J Cataract Refract Surg 12:150, 1986.

24. Steinert RF, Puliafito CA, Kumar SR, et al: Cystoid macular edema, retinal detachment and glaucoma after Nd: YAG laser posterior capsulotomy. Am J Ophthalmol 112: 373, 1991.

25. Kramer SG: Cystoid macular edema after aphakic penetrating keratoplasty. Ophthalmology 88:782, 1981.

26. Miyake K, Miyake Y, Maekubo K, et al: Incidence of cystoid macular edema afer retinal detachment surgery and the use of topical indomethacin. Am J Ophthalmol 95:451, 1983.

27. Choplin NT, Bene CH: Cystoid macular edema following laser iridotomy. Ann Ophthalmol 15:172, 1983.

28. Spaide RF, Yannuzzi LA: Post-cataract surgery cystoid macular edema. In Schwartz B (ed): Clinical Signs in Ophthalmology. St. Louis, Mosby-Year Book, 1992, pp 2–16.

29. Gass JDM: Lamellar macular hole: a complication of cystoid macular edema after cataract extraction: a clinicopathologic case report. Trans Am Ophthalmol Soc 73:231, 1975.

30. Nussenblatt RB, Kaufman SC, Palestine AG, et al: Macular thickening and visual acuity. Measurement in patients with cystoid macular edema. Ophthalmology 94: 1134, 1987.

31. Gass JDM, Anderson DR, Davis EB: A clinical, fluorescein angiographic, and electron microscopic correlation of cystoid macular edema. Am J Ophthalmol 100:82, 1985.

32. Yanoff M, Fine BS, Brucker AJ, Eagle RC Jr: Pathology of human cystoid macular edema. Surv Ophthalmol 28:205, 1984.

33. Martin NF, Green WR, Martin LW: Retinal phlebitis in the Irvine-Gass syndrome. Am J Ophthalmol 83:377, 1977.

34. McDonnell PJ, de la Cruz ZC, Green WR: Vitreous incarceration complicating cataract surgery. A light and electron microscopic study. Ophthalmology 93:247, 1986.

35. Norton AL, Brown WJ, Carlson M, Pilger IS: Pathogenesis of aphakic macular edema. Am J Ophthalmol 80:96, 1975.

36. Fine BS, Brucker AJ: Macular edema and cystoid macular edema. Am J Ophthalmol 92:466, 1981.

37. Tso MOM: Pathology of cystoid macular edema. Ophthalmology 89:902, 1982.

38. Streeten B: Discussion of Tso MOM: Pathology of cystoid macular edema. Ophthalmology 89:914, 1982.

39. Mutra JN, Cunha-Vaz JG, Sabo CA, et al: Microperfusion studies on the permeability of retinal vessels. Invest Ophthalmol Vis Sci 31:471, 1990.

40. Kottow M, Hendrickson P: Iris angiography in cystoid macular edema after cataract extraction. Arch Ophthalmol 93:487, 1975.

41. Easty D, Dallas N, O'Malley R: Aphakic macular oedema following prosthetic lens implantation. Br J Ophthalmol 61:321, 1977.

42. Cunha-Vaz JG, Travassos A: Breakdown of the blood retinal barriers and cystoid macular edema. Surv Ophthalmol 28(Suppl):485, 1984.

43. Blair NP, Elman MJ, Rusin MM: Vitreous fluorophotometry in patients with cataract surgery. Graefes Arch Clin Exp Ophthalmol 223:441, 1987.

44. Salzman J, Seiple W, Carr R, et al: Electrophysiological assessment of aphakic cystoid macular oedema. Br J Ophthalmol 70:819, 1986.

45. Miyake Y, Miyake K, Shiroyama N: Classification of aphakic cystoid macular edema with focal electroretinograms. Am J Ophthalmol 116:576–583, 1993.

46. Jaffee GJ, Burton TC, Kuhn E, et al: Progression of nonproliferative diabetic retinopathy and visual outcome after extracapsular cataract extraction and intraocular lens implantation. Am J Ophthalmol 114:448, 1992.

47. Pollack A, Leiba H, Bukelman A, Oliver M: Cystoid macular edema following cataract extraction in patients with diabetes. Br J Ophthalmol 76:221, 1992.

48. Boldt HC, Folk JC: Slow leakage from the retinal pigment epithelium (ooze) in age-related macular degeneration. Retina 10:244, 1990.

49. Frederick AR Jr, Morely MG, Topping TM, et al: The appearance of stippled retinal pigment epithelial detachments. A sign of occult choroidal neovascularization in age-related macular degeneration. Retina 13:3, 1993.

50. Schatz H, McDonald HR, Johnson RN: Retinal pigment epithelial folds associated with retinal pigment epithelial detachment in macular degeneration. Ophthalmology 97: 658, 1990.

51. Lakhanpal V, Schocket SS: Pseudophakic and aphakic retinal detachment mimicking cystoid macular edema. Ophthalmology 94:785, 1987.

52. Fox GM, Joondeph BC, Flynn HW Jr, et al: Delayed-onset pseudophakic endophthalmitis. Am J Ophthalmol 111: 163, 1991.

53. Meisler DM, Palestine AG, Vastine DW, et al: Chronic propionibacterium endophthalmitis after extracapsular cataract extraction and intraocular lens implantation. Am J Ophthalmol 102:733, 1986.

54. Chien AM, Raber IM, Fischer DH, et al: *Propionibacterium acnes* endophthalmitis after intracapsular cataract extraction. Ophthalmology 99:487, 1992.

55. Stern AL, Taylor DM, Dalburg LA, Cosentino RT: Pseudophakic cystoid maculopathy: a study of 50 cases. Ophthalmology 88:942, 1981.

56. Apple DJ, Mamalis N, Loftfeld K: Complications of intraocular lenses: a historical and histopathological review. Surv Ophthalmol 29:1, 1984.

57. Stark WJ, Worthen DM, Holladay JT, et al: The FDA report on intraocular lenses. Ophthalmology 90:311, 1983.

58. Powe NR, Schein OD, Gieser SC, et al: Synthesis of the literature on visual acuity and complications following cataract extraction with intraocular lens implantation. Arch Ophthalmol 112:239–252, 1994.

59. Colin J, Bonnet P: Comparaison de la phaco-emulsification et de l'extraction extracapsulaire manuelle du cristallin. Ophthalmologie 3:233,1989.

60. Kraff MC, Sanders DR, Jampol LM, et al: Prophylaxis of pseudophakic cystoid macular edema with topical indomethacin. Ophthalmology 89:885, 1982.

61. Frost NA, Sparrow JM, Strong NP, Rosenthal AR: Vitreous loss in planned extracapsular cataract extraction does lead to a poorer visual outcome. Eye 9:446, 1995.

62. Schepens CL: Fundus changes caused by alterations of the vitreous body. Am J Ophthalmol 39:631, 1955.

63. Reese AB, Jones IS, Cooper WC: Macular changes secondary to vitreous traction. Am J Ophthalmol 64:544, 1967.

64. Schubert HD: Cystoid macular edema: the apparent role of mechanical factors. In Bito LZ, Stjernschantz J (eds): The Ocular Effects of Prostaglandins and Other Eicosanoids. New York: Alan R Liss, 1989, pp 277–291.

65. Jaffe NS: Vitreous traction at the posterior pole of the fundus due to alterations in the vitreous posterior. Trans Am Acad Ophthalmol Otolaryngol 71:642, 1967.

66. Fung WE, Vitrectomy-ACME Study Group: Vitrectomy for chronic aphakic cystoid macular edema: results of a national, collaborative, prospective, randomized investigation. Ophthalmology 92:1102, 1985.

67. Smiddy WE, Michels RG, Green WR: Morphology, pathology and surgery of idiopathic vitreoretinal macular disorders. Retina 10:288, 1990.

68. Smiddy WE, Green WR, Michels RG: Vitreomacular traction syndrome—ultrastructural characteristics. Am J Ophthalmol 107:177, 1989.

69. Margherio RR, Trese MT, Margherio AR, Cartwright K: Surgical management of vitreomacular traction syndromes. Ophthalmology 96:1437, 1989.

70. Zarbin MA, Michels RG, Green WR: Dissection of epiciliary tissue to treat chronic hypotony after surgery for ret-

inal detachment with proliferative vitreoretinopathy. Retina 11:208–213, 1991.

71. Bito LZ, Salvador EV: Intraocular fluid dynamics. III. The site and mechanism of prostaglandin transfer across the blood intraocular fluid barriers. Exp Eye Res 14:233, 1972.

72. Bhattacherjee P, Kulkarni PS, Eakins KE: Metabolism of arachidonic acid in rabbit ocular tissues. Invest Ophthalmol Vis Sci 18:172, 1979.

73. Ferguson VMG, Spalton DJ: Continued breakdown of the blood aqueous barrier following cataract surgery. Br J Ophthalmol 76:453, 1992.

74. Worst JGF: Bioxizitat des Kammerwassers. Eine vereinheitlichende pathologische Theorie, begrundel auf hypothetische biotoxische Kammerwasserfaktoren. Klin Monatsbl Augenheilkd 167:376, 1975.

75. Mishima H, Masuda K, Miyake K: The putative role of prostaglandins in cystoid macular edema. Prog Clin Biol Res 312:251, 1989.

76. Bazan NG, de Abreu MT, Bazan HE, Blfort R Jr: Arachidonic acid cascade and platelet-activating factor in the network of eye inflammatory mediators: therapeutic implications in uveitis. Int Ophthalmol 14:335, 1990.

77. Williams KI, Higgs GA: Eicosanoids and inflammation. J Pathol 156:101, 1988.

78. Smith WL: The eicosanoids and their biochemical mechanisms of action. Biochem J 259:315, 1989.

79. Jampol LM: Aphakic cystoid macular edema. A hypothesis. Arch Ophthalmol 103:1134, 1985.

80. Miyake K, Mibu H, Horiguchi M, et al. Inflammatory mediators in post-operative aphakic and pseudophakic baboon eyes. Arch Ophthalmol 108:1764, 1990.

81. Cunha-Vaz J: The blood-ocular barriers. Surv Ophthalmol 23:279, 1979.

82. Vinores SA, Amin A, Derevjanik NL, et al: Immunohistochemical localization of blood-retinal barrier breakdown sites associated with post-surgical macular oedema. Histochem J 26:655–665, 1994.

83. Stjernschantz J, Bito LZ: The ocular effects of eicosanoids and other autocoids: historic background and the need for a broader perspective. In Bito LZ, Stjernschantz J (eds): The Ocular Effects of Prostaglandins and Other Eicosanoids. New York, Alan R Liss, 1989, pp 1–13.

84. Bito LZ, Camras CB, Gum GG, Resul B: The ocular hypotensive effects and side effects of prostaglandins on the eyes of experimental animals. In Bito LZ, Stjernschantz J (eds): The Ocular Effects of Prostaglandins and Other Eicosanoids. New York, Alan R Liss, 1989, pp 349–368.

85. Butler JM, Hammond BR: The effects of sensory denervation on the responses of the rabbit eye to prostaglandin E_2, bradykinin, and substance P. Br J Pharmacol 69:495, 1980.

86. Muller A, Meynier F, Bonne C: PAF-induced conjunctivitis in the rabbit is mediated by peptido-leukotrienes. J Ocul Pharmacol. 6:227–232, 1990.

87. Snyder F: Platelet-activating factor and related acetylated lipids as potent biologically active cellular mediators. Am J Physiol 259 (Cell Physiol) 28:C697, 1990.

88. Fleisher LN, Ferrell JB, Smith MG, McGahan MC: Lipid mediators of tumor necrosis factor-alpha-induced uveitis. Invest Ophthalmol Vis Sci 32:2393, 1991.

89. De Vos AF, Hoekzema R, Kijlstra A: Cytokines and uveitis. Curr Eye Res 11:581, 1992.

90. Franks WA, Limb GA, Stanford MR, et al: Cytokines in human intraocular inflammation. Curr Eye Res 11(Suppl): 187, 1992.

91. Murray PI, Hoekzema R, van Haren MA, et al: Aqueous humor interleukin-6 levels in uveitis. Invest Ophthalmol Vis Sci 31:917, 1990.

92. Streilein JW, Wilbanks GA, Taylor A, Cousins S: Eye-derived cytokines and the immunosuppressive intraocular microenvironment: a review. Curr Eye Res 11(Suppl): 41, 1992.

93. Lipton JM, Macaluso A, Hiltz ME, Catania A: Central administration of the peptide alpha-MSH inhibits inflammation in the skin. Peptides 12:795, 1991.

94. Catania A, Arnold J, Macaluso A, et al: Inhibition of acute inflammation in the periphery by central action of salicylates. Proc Natl Acad Sci USA 88:8544, 1991.

95. Jampol LM, Kraff MC, Sanders DR, et al: Near-UV radiation from the operating microscope and pseudophakic cystoid macular edema. Arch Ophthalmol 103:28, 1985.

96. Kraff MC, Lieberman HL, Jampol LM, Sanders DR: Effect of a pupillary light occluder on cystoid macular edema. J Cataract Refract Surg 15:658, 1989.

97. Kraff MC, Sanders DR, Jampol LM, Lieberman HL: Effect of an ultraviolet-filtering intraocular lens on cystoid macular edema. Ophthalmology 92:366, 1985.

98. Komatsu M, Kanagami S, Shimizu K: Ultraviolet-absorbing intraocular lens versus non-UV-absorbing intraocular lens: comparison of angiographic cystoid macular edema. J Cataract Refract Surg 15:654, 1989.

99. Clarke MP, Yap M, Weatherill JR: Do intraocular lenses with ultraviolet absorbing chromophores protect against macular oedema? Acta Ophthalmol 67:593, 1989.

100. Robertson DM, Feldman RB: Photic retinopathy from the operating room microscope. Am J Ophthalmol 101: 561, 1986.

101. Robertson DM, McLaren JW: Photic retinopathy from the operating room microscope. Study with filters. Arch Ophthalmol 107:373, 1989.

102. Green WR, Robertson DM: Pathologic findings of photic retinopathy in the human eye. Am J Ophthalmol 112:520, 1991.

103. Gehring JR: Macular edema following cataract extraction. Arch Ophthalmol 80:626, 1968.

104. Suckling RD, Malsin KF: Pseudophakic cystoid macular oedema and its treatment with local steroids. Aust N Z J Ophthalmol 16:353–359, 1988.

105. McDonell PJ, Ryan SJ, Walkoner AF, Miller-Scholte A: Prediction of visual acuity recovery in cystoid macular edema. Opthalmic Surg 23:354–358, 1992.

106. McEntyre JM: A successful treatment for aphakic cystoid macular edema. Ann Ophthalmol 10:1219, 1978.

107. Melberg NS, Olk RJ: Corticosteroid-induced ocular hypertension in the treatment of aphakic or pseudophakic cystoid macular edema. Ophthalmology 100:164, 1993.

108. Jampol LM: Discussion of Melberg NS, Olk RJ: Corticosteroid-induced ocular hypertension in the treatment of aphakic or pseudophakic cystoid macular edema. Ophthalmology 100:167, 1993.

109. Gieser DK, Hodapp E, Goldberg I, et al: Flurbiprofen and intraocular pressure. Ann Ophthalmol 831, 1981.

110. Flach AJ: Cyclo-oxygenase inhibitors in ophthalmology. Surv Ophthalmol 36:259, 1992.

111. Klein RM, Katzin HM, Yannuzzi LA: The effect of indomethacin pretreatment on aphakic cystoid macular edema. Am J Ophthalmol 87:487, 1979.

112. Abelson MB, Smith LM, Ormerod LD: Prospective, randomized trial of oral piroxicam in the prophylaxis of postoperative cystoid macular edema. J Ocular Pharmacol 5:147, 1989.

113. Shammas HJ, Milkie CF: Does aspirin prevent postoperative cystoid macular edema? J Am Intraocul Implant Soc 5:337, 1979.

114. Miyake K: Prevention of cystoid macular edema after lens extraction by topical indomethicin. (I) A preliminary report. Albrecht von Graefes Arch Klin Exp Ophthalmol 203:81, 1977.

115. Miyake K: Prevention of cystoid macular edema after lens extraction by topical indomethicin. II A control study in bilateral extractions. Jpn J Ophthalmol 22:80, 1978.

116. Miyake K, Sakamura S, Miura H: Long-term follow-up study on the prevention of aphakic cystoid macular edema by topical indomethacin. Br J Ophthalmol 64:324, 1980.

117. Yannuzzi LA, Landau AN, Turtz AL: Incidence of aphakic cystoid macular edema with the use of topical indomethacin. Ophthalmology 88:947, 1981.

118. Quentin CD, Behrens-Baumann W, Gaus W: Prophylaxe des zystoiden Makulaodems mit Diclofenac-Augentrop-

fen bei i.c. Kataraktextraktion mit Choyce-Mark-IX-Vor der Kammerlinse. Fortschr Ophthalmol 86:546, 1989.

119. Flach AJ, Stegman RC, Graham J, Kruger LP: Prophylaxis of aphakic macular edema without corticosteroids. Ophthalmology 97:1253, 1990.

120. Solomon R: Efficacy of topical flurbiprofen and indomethacin in preventing pseudophakic cystoid macular edema. J Cataract Refract Surg 21:73–81, 1995.

121. Yannuzzi LA, Klein RM, Wallyn RH, et al: Ineffectiveness of indomethacin in the treatment of chronic cystoid macular edema. Am J Ophthalmol 84:517, 1977.

122. Burnett J, Tessler H, Isenberg S, Tso MOM: Double masked trial of fenoprofen sodium treatment of chronic aphakic cystoid macular edema. Ophthalmic Surg 14:150. 1983.

123. Yannuzzi LA: A perspective on the treatment of aphakic cystoid macular edema. Surv Ophthalmol 28(Suppl):540, 1984.

124. Peterson M, Yoshizumi MO, Hepler R, et al: Topical indomethacin in the treatment of chronic cystoid macular edema. Graefes Arch Clin Exp Ophthalmol 230:401, 1992.

125. Flach AJ, Dolan BJ, Irvine AR: Effectiveness of ketorolac 0.5% solution for chronic aphakic and pseudophakic cystoid macular edema. Am J Ophthalmol 103:479, 1987.

126. Flach AJ, Jampol LM, Weinberg D, et al: Improvement in visual acuity in chronic aphakic and pseudophakic cystoid macular edema after treatment with topical 0.5% ketorolac tromethamine. Am J Ophthalmol 112:514, 1991.

127. Marmor MF, Maack T: Enhancement of retinal adhesion and subretinal fluid absorption by acetazolamide. Invest Ophthalmol Vis Sci 23:121, 1982.

128. Cox SN, Hay E, Bird AC: Treatment of chronic macular edema with acetazolamide. Arch Ophthalmol 106:1190, 1988.

129. Tripathi RC, Fekrat S, Tripathi BJ, Ernest JT: A direct correlation of the resolution of pseudophakic cystoid macular edema with acetazolamide therapy. Ann Ophthalmol 23:127, 1991.

130. Weene LE: Cystoid macular edema after scleral buckling responsive to acetazolamide. Ann Ophthalmol 24:423, 1992.

131. Fishman GA, Gilbert LD, Anderson RJ, et al: Effect of methazolamide on chronic macular edema in patients with retinitis pigmentosa. Ophthalmology 101:687–693, 1994.

132. Fishman GA, Glenn AM, Gilbert LD: Rebound of macular edema with continued use of methazolamide in patients with retinitis pigmentosa. Arch Ophthalmol 111:1640–1646, 1993.

133. Zweng HC, Little HL, Peabody RR: Laser photocoagulation of macular lesions. Trans Am Acad Ophthalmol Otolaryngol 72:377, 1968.

134. Schepens CL: Retinal Detachment and Allied Diseases, Vol 2. Philadelphia, WB Saunders Co, 1983, p 1018.

135. Perez R, Provenzano J, Muoz D, Vzquez L: Argon laser for clinically significant pseudophakic foveal edema. Ophthalmology 98(Suppl):250, 1991.

136. Haller JA: Grid photocoagulation for chronic cystoid macular edema. Invest Ophthalmol Vis Sci 33(Suppl):1316, 1992.

137. Pfoff DS, Thom SR: Preliminary report on the effect of hyperbaric oxygen on cystoid macular edema. J Cataract Refract Surg 13:136, 1987.

138. Benner JD, Xiaoping M: Locally administered hyperoxic therapy for aphakic cystoid macular edema. Am J Ophthalmol 113:104, 1992.

139. Jampol LM, Orlin C, Cohen SB, et al: Hyperbaric and transcorneal delivery of oxygen to the rabbit and monkey anterior segment. Arch Ophthalmol 106:825, 1988.

140. Katzen LE, Fleischman JA, Trokel S: YAG laser treatment of cystoid macular edema. Am J Ophthalmol 95:589, 1983.

141. Steinert RF, Wasson PJ: Neodymium:YAG laser anterior vitreolysis for Irvine-Gass cystoid macular edema. J Cataract Refract Surg 15:304, 1989.

142. Tchah H, Rosenberg M, Larson RS, Lindstrom RL: Neodymium-YAG laser vitreolysis for treatment and prophylaxis of cystoid macular oedema. Aust N Z J Ophthalmol 17:179, 1989.

143. Federman JL, Annesley WH Jr, Sarin LK, Remer P: Vitrectomy and cystoid macular edema. Ophthalmology 87:622, 1980.

144. Fung WE: Anterior vitrectomy for aphakic cystoid macular edema. Ophthalmology 87:189, 1980.

145. Fung WE: The national, prospective, randomized vitrectomy study for chronic aphakic cystoid macular edema. Progress report and comparison between control and nonrandomized groups. Surv Ophthalmol 28(Suppl):569, 1984.

146. Dugel PU, Rao NA, Ozler S, et al: Pars plan vitrectomy for intraocular inflammation-related cystoid macular edema unresponsive to corticosteroids. Ophthalmology 99:1535, 1992.

147. Harbour JW, Smiddy WE, Rubsamen PE, et al: Pars plana vitrectomy for chronic pseudophakic cystoid macular edema. Am J Ophthalmol 120:302–307, 1995.

148. Apple DJ, Olson RJ: Closed-loop anterior chamber lenses. Arch Ophthalmol 105:52, 1987.

149. Smith PW, Wong SK, Stark WJ, et al: Complications of semiflexible, closed-loop intraocular lenses. Arch Ophthalmol 105:52, 1987.

150. Lindstrom RL, Nelson JD, Neist RL: Anterior chamber lens subluxation through a basal peripheral iridectomy. J Am Intraocul Implant Soc 9:53, 1983.

151. Smith SG: Intraocular lens removal for chronic cystoid macular edema. J Cataract Refract Surg 15:442, 1989.

152. Stark WJ, Gottsch JD, Goodman DF, et al: Posterior chamber intraocular lens implantation in the absence of capsular support. Arch Ophthalmol 107:1078, 1989.

153. Price FW, Whiston WE: Natural history of cystoid macular edema in pseudophakic bullous keratopathy. J Cataract Refract Surg 16:163, 1990.

154. Spaide RF, Yannuzzi LA: Cystoid macular edema after cataract surgery. Semin Ophthalmol 8:121, 1993.

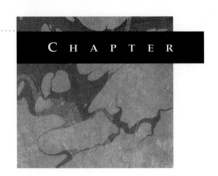

CHAPTER 22

Chorioretinal and Retinal Folds

David J. Weissgold, M.D.

Alexander J. Brucker, M.D.

Undulations of the choroid and the overlying retinal pigment epithelium (RPE) and neurosensory retina produce choroidal, or "chorioretinal", folds. On the other hand, ripples in the neurosensory retina alone are termed "retinal folds." The two conditions are distinct, and each may be seen in numerous clinical settings. We will discuss choroidal (we prefer the term "chorioretinal") and retinal folds separately, and will outline some of the more common and important conditions giving rise to each of them.

CHORIORETINAL FOLDS

Background

Since their original clinical description in 1884 by Nettleship[1] in a patient with optic atrophy following papilledema and their original histopathologic description in 1915 by Birch-Hirschfeld and Siegfried[2] in a patient with an orbital tumor, chorioretinal folds have been reported in many different clinical settings.

Clinical Evaluation

Chorioretinal folds may occur in patients of any age or race, and of either sex. They may be unilateral or bilateral. Acquired folds are usually symptomatic, with patients reporting distortion and/or blurring. In contrast, patients with longstanding folds are normally asymptomatic; these chorioretinal folds are most commonly of the idiopathic or hyperopic variety (see "Causes").

Ophthalmoscopically, chorioretinal folds normally are found posterior to the equator as narrow, alternating dark and light bands. They are rarely evident in the fundus periphery. In most cases, the bands are oriented horizontally and point, at their medial ends, towards the optic disc (Figs. 22–1*A* and *B*). However, vertically oriented chorioretinal folds (Fig. 22–1*D*) and irregular, reticular patterns (Figs. 22–1*E* and *F*) are not uncommon, the latter being especially frequent in cases of hypotony. Eccentrically located, radially arranged folds have also been described.[3] Slit lamp biomicroscopic examination is important for confirming that the folds are deep to the retina.

In contrast, retinal folds are translucent and superficial. They are frequently seen emanating from an identifiable area of other retinal pathology. However, clinical distinction between chorioretinal folds and retinal folds can be difficult at times. Fluorescein angiography is especially helpful in distinguishing between the two.

Fluorescein Angiography

The light and dark bands seen ophthalmoscopically in cases of chorioretinal folds have a specific appearance during fluorescein angiography. Alternating hyper- and hypofluorescent lines corresponding to the bands appear early in the angiogram and persist throughout all phases (Fig. 22–1*B*). Owing to thinning of the overlying RPE over the peaks of the folds and compression of the RPE in the valleys, or troughs, the hyperfluorescent lines seen on an-

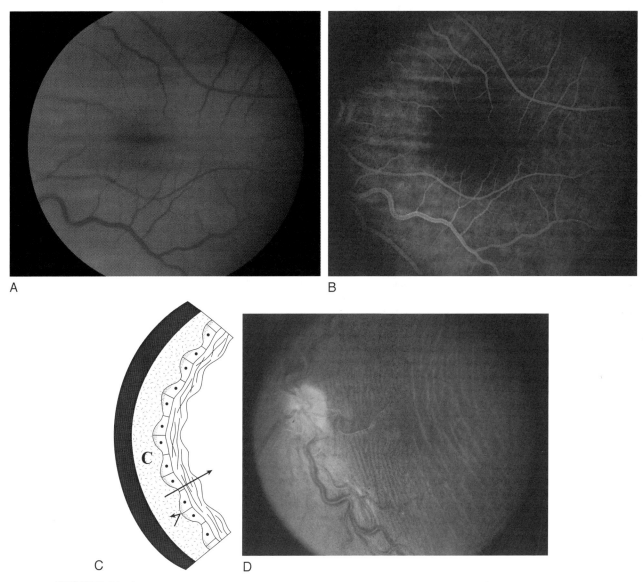

FIGURE 22–1   *A*, Horizontally oriented chorioretinal folds in the posterior pole. *B*, Fluorescein angiogram of the chorioretinal folds seen in *A*. *C*, Diagrammatic representation of cause for alternating bands of hyper- and hypofluorescence seen in *B*. Choroidal (C) fluorescence is blocked (*reflected arrow*) in areas where the concentration of the pigment granules in the overlying RPE cells is high. Choroidal fluorescence passes through the RPE and the overlying neurosensory retina (*straight arrow*) where the RPE cells are thinned and their pigment granules are widely dispersed. (Courtesy of Mr. Peter O. Branscombe.) *D*, Vertically oriented chorioretinal folds. *Illustration continued on following page*

giography correspond to the light bands seen ophthalmoscopically and the hypofluorescent lines correspond to the dark bands (Figs. 22–1*B* and *C*).[4–9] One report contradicts this, however, showing normal-appearing RPE at the peaks of the folds and attenuation of the RPE in the troughs[10]; the meaning of this difference is unclear. There is no late leakage of dye ascribed to chorioretinal folds themselves. If the underlying cause of the chorioretinal folds is treated and they largely disappear ophthalmoscopically, fluorescein angiography may still demonstrate faint lines of hypofluorescence where RPE cells are presumably still crowded.[11,12]

In much of the early literature written prior to the advent of fluorescein angiography there is con-

fusion about whether the ophthalmoscopically evident folds reported are full-thickness chorioretinal folds or more superficial retinal folds. Fluorescein angiography has been an important tool for use in making this distinction.

Ultrasound

Although fluorescein angiography remains the single most important test for demonstrating chorioretinal folds after clinical examination, a few investigators have attempted to show that ophthalmic ultrasound may play a role in their demonstration.

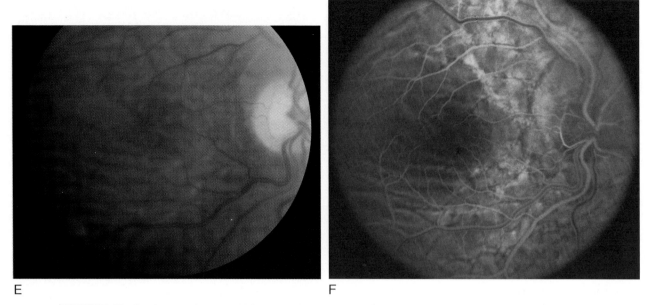

E   F

FIGURE 22–1   *Continued   E,* Irregular, reticular chorioretinal folds. (Courtesy of Dr. Donald L. Budenz.) *F,* Fluorescein angiogram of the chorioretinal folds seen in *E.* (Courtesy of Dr. Donald L. Budenz.)

Sonography can be useful in revealing underlying causes of chorioretinal folds but not in determining the presence or absence of the folds themselves.

The use of B-scan ophthalmic ultrasound for the evaluation of patients with chorioretinal folds was first reported by Cappaert and co-workers.[13] All of their cases demonstrated flattening of the posterior pole with thickening of the retinochoroidal and scleral layers at the posterior pole. None of their patients had identifiable orbital masses. Because two of their patients responded to oral prednisone with resolution of their folds and normalization of their B-scans, the authors proposed that scleral and/or retrobulbar inflammation, coupled with scleral thickening and subsequent scleral shrinkage, may play roles in the development of chorioretinal folds.

Later, Atta and Byrne[14] corroborated some of the previously described ultrasonographic findings in 31 eyes of 24 patients, also without orbital masses. Flattening of the posterior pole was the most common echographic finding (18 eyes), and was present more often in the horizontal plane than in the vertical plane. The authors propose that this is likely related to the usual horizontal orientation of chorioretinal folds in the posterior pole. Retinochoroidal layer thickening and shortened axial lengths were demonstrated by standardized A-scan. Atta and Byrne concluded that chorioretinal folds may be produced by (1) scleral shortening, as in cases of hyperopia; (2) choroidal thickening, as in cases of trauma, scleritis, or hypotony; or (3) enlargement of retrobulbar structures (e.g., optic nerve, extraocular muscles, Tenon's space). These conclusions are in agreement with those of other investigators (see "Mechanisms").

Singh and colleagues,[15] in a study of patients with posterior scleritis, and Leahy and co-workers,[16] in the largest series of cases of chorioretinal folds, both found a high incidence of retinochoroidal thickening using ultrasound, confirming Atta and Byrne's findings. However, in the study by Singh and colleagues, there were also a number of cases of posterior scleritis with retinochoroidal thickening in the absence of chorioretinal folds.

Mechanisms

Despite the length of time that has elapsed since the first report of chorioretinal folds by Nettleship,[1] controversy still exists regarding their exact cause. This is surely due, at least in part, to the myriad of clinical situations in which they are seen (see "Causes"). A few reports have appeared that have attempted to answer the questions of how and why chorioretinal folds form, and why they should do so secondary to so many different underlying ophthalmic disorders.

Bullock and Egbert,[17,18] working with human cadaver and live cat eyes, produced experimental chorioretinal folds by compressing and stretching strips of posterior eye wall, torquing optic nerve insertions, and creating hypotony via anterior chamber paracenteses. They were not able to generate folds by placing a mass in the retrobulbar space. From their experiments, review of the literature, and their own clinical experiences, the authors concluded that any force causing compression of Bruch's membrane, which is located between the RPE and the choriocapillaris, will result in folding of those adjacent layers as well. They invoked Laplace's law governing tension across the wall of a sphere as a function of the pressure gradient across that wall as a partial explanation for the existence of chorioretinal folds in cases of ocular hypotony. Bullock and Egbert also concluded that tension on the insertion site of the optic nerve into the back of the globe is a factor in producing chorioretinal folds, and may be particularly important in defining the direction and location of the folds.

In 1988, Friberg and Lace[19] elaborated on the theory of optic nerve tension as a force responsible for the generation of chorioretinal folds. Working with fresh cadaver globes, they measured the tensile strengths of choroid and sclera, individually. From these figures, they calculated the elasticity of each tissue. Friberg and Lace then determined that a compressive force exerted against the eye wall would have to be manyfold greater to buckle, or cause folds in, sclera than it would to buckle choroid. These authors postulated that minimal tension exerted at the optic nerve–posterior eye wall junction may be enough to cause folds in adjacent choroid without disrupting sclera.

Later, Friberg[20] carried this explanation one step further. He reasoned that buckling of the RPE and Bruch's membrane over the relatively inelastic choroid occurs when compressive forces within the RPE–Bruch's membrane–choroid complex exceed the normal tensile force generated in the choroid by intraocular pressure. Friberg concluded further that, in cases of hypotony, thickening of the choroid leads to a decreased internal surface area and, hence, buckling of the overlying Bruch's membrane–RPE complex. In cases of orbital tumors, Graves's ophthalmopathy, and scleral buckles used for the repair of retinal detachment, the author feels that folds are due to external compressive forces on the globe, changing its shape and thus the configurations of the various layers of the eye wall.

To date, no investigator has provided a single, unifying explanation for the appearance of chorioretinal folds in so many different clinical settings. Perhaps most or all of the above theories play roles. By analogy, myocardial fibrosis is seen following a multitude of different cardiac ailments; once injured, the myocardium has a limited repertoire for reaction. Perhaps chorioretinal folds are a common clinical end point generated by the coats of the eye wall reacting to external and/or intrinsic forces in the only way they are physically capable of reacting.

Causes

Chorioretinal folds have been reported in cases of orbital masses and orbital inflammatory processes, excessive hyperopia, optic nerve and disc swelling, choroidal neovascular membranes (CNVMs) in age-related macular degeneration (AMD), localized suprachoroidal hemorrhages, posterior scleritis, and choroidal tumors.[1–16,18,21–43] In addition, chorioretinal folds have been seen following ocular surgery in cases of ocular hypotony, especially after glaucoma filtration surgery; after posterior segment laser treatments; following scleral buckling for the repair of retinal detachments, and in other postsurgical situations.[18,44–54] Finally, in some cases the presence of chorioretinal folds defies explanation and the folds have been termed "idiopathic."

Recently, Leahey and colleagues reported the largest series of chorioretinal folds in the literature, and payed particular attention to laterality of the condition.[16] They found that most causes of retinal folds tend to produce them either unilaterally or bilaterally (Table 22–1). Furthermore, Leahey's group recommended that those patients with unilateral chorioretinal folds receive the most aggressive diagnostic evaluations, as they tended to have the most serious ocular causes and the highest incidence of orbital disease. It is important to perform complete clinical ophthalmologic examinations and histories on all patients with chorioretinal folds in an effort to identify any underlying causes of the folds.

What follows are descriptions of the more common and important causes of chorioretinal folds.

Orbital Masses and Inflammation

Many early reports of chorioretinal folds are from cases in which retrobulbar tumors or inflammation were evident.[2,5,7–9,23,24,28,30] This continues to be the case in the more modern literature as well.[4,6,10–12,14,16,18,21,22,25–27,29,31] The authors of many of these reports, as well as others,[17–20] have speculated about why orbital masses should cause chorioretinal folds. Unfortunately, the only investigators to attempt to produce chorioretinal folds experimentally in response to a mass introduced in the orbit were not able to do so.[17] It seems likely that distortion of the globe contour secondary to the mass effect, twisting of the optic nerve at its insertion into the globe, and retrobulbar/posterior eye wall inflammation with concomitant choroidal thickening, all play roles in the production of chorioretinal folds in cases of orbital disease.

Orbital masses discovered in patients with chorioretinal folds have been diverse: sphenoid meningioma,[5,21] invasive maxillary sinus carcinoma,[6] lacrimal gland tumors,[6,7,21,25] rhabdomyosarcoma,[9] hemangiopericytoma,[10] hemangioma,[11,12,18,21–23,25,28] mucocoele or mucopyocoele,[12,23,25,26] orbital hemorrhage following blunt trauma,[14] infectious abscess,[14] cholesteatoma,[23] metastatic carcinoma,[23–25] fibrous dysplasia of bone,[24] meningioma of the optic nerve,[25] dermoid cyst,[25] neurofibrosarcoma,[25] choristomatous cyst,[27] and osteosarcoma[28] have been reported. Less discrete orbital inflammatory diseases, such as Graves' ophthalmopathy, orbital pseudotumor, and orbital cellulitis have also been reported as causes of chorioretinal folds.[5,6,16,18,22,23,29–31]

As emphasized by Leahey and co-workers,[16] pa-

TABLE 22–1 Unilateral Versus Bilateral Chorioretinal Folds*

| | No. (%) of Eyes | | |
Cause	Unilateral Cases (n = 30)	Bilateral Cases (n = 48)	Total Cases (n = 78)
Macular degeneration	3 (10)	14 (29)	17 (22)
Hyperopia	1 (3)	12 (25)	13 (17)
Idiopathic	1 (3)	10 (21)	11 (14)
Hypotony	4 (13)	4 (8)	8 (10)
Scleritis	5 (17)	2 (4)	7 (9)
Vascular occlusion	4 (13)	—	4 (5)
Ocular tumor	4 (13)	—	4 (5)
Thyroid	—	2 (4)	2 (3)
Uveitis	—	2 (4)	2 (3)
Nerve edema	2 (7)	—	2 (3)
Retinal detachment	2 (7)	—	2 (3)
Choroiditis	—	2 (4)	2 (3)
Orbital tumor	1 (3)	—	1 (1)
Trauma	1 (3)	—	1 (1)
Optic atrophy	1 (3)	—	1 (1)
Bone	1 (3)	—	1 (1)

* From Leahey AB, Brucker AJ, Wyszynski RE, Shaman P: Chorioretinal folds: a comparison of unilateral and bilateral cases. Arch Ophthalmol 111:357–359, 1993, with permission. Copyright 1993, American Medical Association.

tients with chorioretinal folds secondary to orbital disease, especially in cases of tumors, usually have unilateral pathology and, hence, unilateral folds (Table 22–1). This is often not the case with folds secondary to orbital inflammatory diseases, however, such as Graves' ophthalmopathy and orbital pseudotumor. As these processes may involve both orbits, the chorioretinal folds produced are frequently bilateral.[14,16,18,23]

Most of the above-cited case descriptions do not comment on the persistence or regression of chorioretinal folds following medical or surgical treatment of the underlying causative disease. However, there are many descriptions of folds regressing after therapy just as there are numerous illustrations of instances in which the folds persist after treatment. There are a few papers that pay particular attention to this issue.[5,12,16,23] While it is often the case that chorioretinal folds may disappear and leave no ophthalmoscopic or fluorescein angiographic trace of their existence, in many cases of chronic folds and in some cases of resolved folds, telltale pigmentary changes occur in an interrupted linear fashion.[16,23]

Most investigators have not been able to demonstrate a relationship between the location of orbital masses and the orientation, or direction, of the chorioretinal folds they yield. However, in a detailed analysis of the locations of orbital masses and

the patterns and orientation of the chorioretinal folds they produce, Friberg and Grove were able to show that intra- and extraconal orbital tumors produce folds that appear different in their orientation with respect to the tumor location; intraconal tumors generated folds radiating from the disc, whereas extraconal masses yielded concentric folds with their convex sides directed toward the optic disc (Fig. 22–2).[25] Furthermore, in their series, far posterior tumors, such as those in the orbital apex, rarely gave rise to chorioretinal folds.

Hyperopia

There have been many reports of chorioretinal folds occurring in hyperopic eyes or myopic eyes with recent hyperopic shifts without other evident causes for the presence of folds.[6,8,14,16,21–23,25,32–35] The most excessive hyperopia reported in an eye with chorioretinal folds is +22.0 diopters, in an 11-year-old boy affected bilaterally with posterior microphthalmos.[35] Chorioretinal folds due to relative hyperopia may be observed in patients of all ages, but they are most common in middle-aged adults.[16,32–34] While they may occur unilaterally in such cases, most are seen bilaterally.[8,14,16,21–23] Mills and co-workers have written extensively on this subject.[32–34] They reported that visual prognosis is excellent in these patients, with very few patients

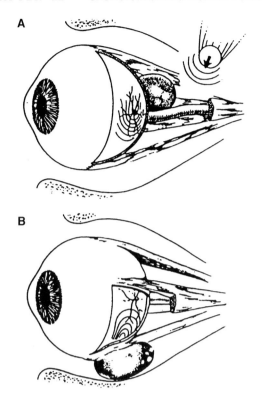

FIGURE 22-2 *A*, Intraconal tumors displace the optic nerve, compress the choroid in front of the nerve, and put the choroid under tensile stress on the opposite side. Folds are oriented in the direction of displacement as shown in the *inset. B*, Extraconal tumors tend to buckle the wall of the globe, thereby compressing the sclera and choroid forming folds, which trail off along the leading edge of the tumor. (From Friberg TR: The etiology of choroidal folds: a biomechanical explanation. Graefes Arch Ophthalmol 227:459–464, 1989, with permission.)

complaining of visual disturbances once hyperopic correction is worn and, of those few who do experience distortion, micropsia, or blurring, many resolve completely while only a few progress.

Some reports show a preponderance of males over females in populations with chorioretinal folds secondary to hyperopia.[32–34] The significance of this possible sex-biased distribution is not known and has not been reproduced in other studies.

Cangemi and colleagues emphasized the importance of ruling out orbital mass lesions in patients with unilateral folds in eyes with acquired hyperopia or hyperopic shifts.[22] Interestingly, Friberg and Grove demonstrated that intraconal orbital tumors are much more likely to produce these hyperopic shifts than extraconal tumors.[25]

Optic Disc Swelling

Optic disc swelling is commonly "part and parcel" of some clinical scenarios in which chorioretinal folds are observed, such as hypotonous maculopathy, posterior uveitis and scleritis, and orbital neoplasms and inflammatory disease. In addition, apparent disc engorgement—or pseudopapille-

dema—is often seen in excessive hyperopia in the abscence of other pathology. As we have already described, chorioretinal folds are frequently encountered in all of these settings. Although optic disc swelling does occur in the settings of hypotony and orbital disease, these entities are considered separately as causes of chorioretinal folds.

The earliest report of chorioretinal folds was in a patient with optic atrophy observed 18 months after an attack of "papillitis" likely secondary to tertiary syphilis.[1] Since that report, the literature has seen examples of chorioretinal folds in the setting of papilledema in cases of meningitis,[6] venous sinus thrombosis,[6] systemic hypertension,[6] pseudotumor cerebri,[12,36–40] intracranial tumors,[18,36] aqueductal stenosis,[36] and intracerebral hemorrhage.[36] Chorioretinal folds have also been observed in patients with optic disc edema, some bilateral, who had ultrasonographic and computed tomographic evidence of retrobulbar nerve sheath distention where no definitive diagnosis was made, despite extensive diagnostic evaluation.[14]

These reports have included both descriptions of chorioretinal folds observed concomitant with disc swelling and of folds recorded after abatement of the swelling, (i.e., in instances of optic atrophy). Just as is seen with chorioretinal folds due to other causes, those seen with disc swelling may be observed in patients of both sexes and all ages, they may resolve or persist, and they may be symptomatic or asymptomatic. While chorioretinal folds in disc edema may be unilateral or bilateral, most reported cases illustrate bilateral folds, as there are a large proportion of cases of true papilledema.

Obviously, it is of paramount importance to look closely at the disc for signs of acute or chronic edema when chorioretinal folds are noted. Furthermore, diagnostic evaluation, including orbital and/or cranial computed tomographic or magnetic resonance imaging and other tests, such as cerebrospinal fluid analysis and measurement of intracranial pressure via lumbar puncture, should be included in the evaluation of such patients where appropriate.

Choroidal Neovascular Membranes

There are a number of reports of chorioretinal folds occuring with CNVMs in AMD.[3,6,11,16,22,23] Combining the two largest series of chorioretinal folds reported to date, AMD was the underlying pathology in 25 of 137 (18%) eyes.[16,22] Although fluorescein angiography was performed in 86% of cases in Leahey's et al's series,[16] the authors do not mention whether CNVMs were seen in their cases at the time the folds were evident. Cangemi and coworkers made no mention of the presence or absence of neovascular membranes either.[22]

Two different theories regarding the natural history of chorioretinal folds and CNVMs in AMD have been proposed. Friberg and Grove feel that undulations in Bruch's membrane somehow weaken it, predisposing the eye to develop subretinal neovascular complexes.[11] Gass, on the other hand, has argued that contraction of CNVMs gives rise to surrounding folds that radiate from around the causative neovascular membrane.[3] However, no investigation published to date has aimed specifically at answering the question of why and how CNVMs and chorioretinal folds are sometimes related in eyes with AMD.

Posterior Scleritis

If one subscribes to the concept that congestion and thickening of the choroid, coupled with scleral shrinkage, is one etiologic factor in the development of chorioretinal folds, then it is not surprising that there are numerous reports of such folds in cases of posterior scleritis.[13–16,18,22,42,43] Many of these reports discuss the likelihood that choroidal thickening and congestion lead to a mismatch in the surface area covered by the inner and outer choroidal faces with subsequent folding at the inner choroidal surface.

Posterior scleritis can frequently be an elusive diagnosis, and the presence of chorioretinal folds has been observed to aide in making its diagnosis. Benson and co-workers reported a series of seven patients with posterior scleritis who were initially misdiagnosed as having such disorders as intraocular neoplasm, orbital mass, choroiditis, and idiopathic central serous chorioretinopathy.[42] They pointed to the presence of chorioretinal folds in five of their cases as one of a number of helpful clues to the true diagnosis. Interestingly, chorioretinal folds were not visible ophthalmoscopically in two of their patients due to the presence of overlying turbid subretinal fluid but were detected by the use of fluorescein angiography. Later, in a review of posterior scleritis, Benson reported that chorioretinal folds were present in 7 of 43 (16%) cases evaluated at Wills Eye Hospital in Philadelphia.[43] He pointed out that in mild cases of posterior scleritis, where clinical findings may be minimal, chorioretinal folds may be the only clue to the true diagnosis.

Patients suspected of having posterior scleritis should undergo thorough general medical evaluation and laboratory investigation in an attempt to discover an underlying cause.

Hypotony and Other Postoperative Scenarios

While many recent papers credit Gass with first describing the entity of hypotonous maculopathy, Gass himself[44] credited Dellaporta[45] with initially reporting the constellation of posterior pole findings seen in postoperative hypotonous eyes. Dellaporta described disc swelling, nasal subretinal linear pigment clumping, and macular changes that he ascribed to intraretinal macular edema in four

eyes of three patients who developed hypotony after intracapsular cataract extraction. Seventeen years later, Gass expanded and refined Dellaporta's triad of posterior segment changes seen in hypotony. He described the now well-known peripheral serous choroidal detachments and argued that what he had observed in his series of ten patients and what he believed Dellaporta had actually seen in the maculae of his three patients was not retinal edema but chorioretinal folds. Gass also emphasized the importance of fluorescein angiography in demonstrating the folds. Since the time of these reports, many other investigators have added cases of chorioretinal folds occurring in postoperative hypotony.[14,16,18,20–23,46–49]

As noted previously (see "Clinical Evaluation"), chorioretinal folds in hypotonous maculopathy are somewhat unique in that they are not linear or parallel, but rather assume an irregular, reticular pattern (Fig. 22–1E and F).

Most pathophysiologic explanations for the presence of chorioretinal folds in hypotonous eyes center around the concept of choroidal congestion and thickening, just as do the explanations for chorioretinal folds in the presence of posterior scleritis.[17,18,20] Since the sclera is inelastic relative to the choroid, decreasing the intraocular pressure (i.e., increasing the pressure differential across the eye wall) generates choroidal congestion and thickening. The choroid can only expand inward, toward the center of the globe, and thus the area covered by the internal choroidal face–Bruch's membrane complex decreases, leading to undulations of Bruch's membrane and its neighbors, the RPE and the choroid. Bullock and Egbert successfully produced chorioretinal folds in cats by creating hypotony through the use of anterior paracenteses.[17,18] Interestingly, once the cat eyes were made hypotonous and typical irregular, reticular chorioretinal folds were present, the folds could be made to line up parallel to one another by applying traction to the optic nerve. However, prior to the creation of hypotony, folds could not be generated by pulling on the nerve. Newell reported being able to experimentally induce chorioretinal folds in vivo in three normal human eyes by raising the intraocular pressure through the use of an ocular suction cup followed by abrupt release of the suction.[23] Once again, he explains the appearance of folds at the time of the release of suction upon choroidal congestion and thickening from relative hypotony.

Finally, chorioretinal folds have been reported following a variety of ophthalmic procedures that would not, by themselves, be expected to induce hypotony. Folds have been seen after scleral buckling for repair of retinal detachment,[8,18,22] in concert with an acute macular hole following craniofacial surgical repair of congenital bony anomalies,[50] following diode endolaser treatment for an iatrogenic retinal tear during vitrectomy for the correction of idiopathic macular hole,[51] after krypton red laser ablation of a CNVM,[52] in a case of photic maculopathy following cataract surgery,[53] and after ne-odymium:yttrium-aluminum-garnet (Nd:YAG) cy-clocryotherapy for the treatment of refractory glaucoma.[54]

Miscellaneous

Chorioretinal folds have also been reported in the setting of a variety of other ophthalmic and systemic disorders. There are numerous instances of both primary (benign nevi, melanomas) and metastatic (breast, rectal, and bronchogenic carcinomas) choroidal neoplasms giving rise to chorioretinal folds.[6,8,18] Other masses that may give rise to chorioretinal folds and which have been mistaken for intraocular neoplasms are localized suprachoroidal hematomas, as reported by Augsberger and colleagues.[41] There have also been a few reports of chorioretinal folds occurring in relation to retinal detachments, central serous chorioretinopathy, and retinal vascular occlusions.[5,6,16] One published case exists of chorioretinal folds occurring secondary to a dural cavernous sinus fistula; once again, the mechanism of choroidal congestion is invoked by the authors of this report as an etiologic explanation.[55]

Systemic diseases that have ocular manifestations may also produce chorioretinal folds. Alagille syndrome, or arteriohepatic dysplasia, is an autosomal dominant disorder producing multiple systemic problems: dysmorphic facies, intrahepatic cholestasis, skeletal anomalies, and peripheral pulmonic stenosis, among other less common features. The hepatic and cardiac involvement in Alagille syndrome yield significant morbidity, but the disease is rarely lethal. Some ocular features are also characteristic, such as posterior embryotoxon. Chorioretinal folds, strabismus, band keratopathy, anomalous optic discs, and ectopic pupils are all less common features.[4,56,57]

Whipple's disease, a multisystem inflammatory process due to a poorly characterized bacillus organism, has mostly neuro-ophthalmic manifestations from central nervous system involvement, such as motility disturbances. However, Avila and co-workers have described two patients with direct ocular involvement, primarily diffuse chorioretinal inflammation, one of whom had chorioretinal folds.[58]

In their description of a series of six patients with circulating antineutrophil cytoplasmic antibodies with ocular involvement, Pulido and colleagues included one case of a woman with bilateral chorioretinal folds. These antibodies are seen in cases of systemic vasculitis, especially in Wegener's granulomatosis.[59]

Lastly, chorioretinal folds were seen in 1 of 17 (6%) patients with scleromyxedema, a rare connective tissue disorder characterized by generalized dermal sclerosis and superficial lichenoid skin papules.[60] Other ophthalmic manifestations observed in a total of 4 of the 17 patients (24%) were corneal opacities, thickened brow or eyelid skin, ectropion, lagophthalmos, and papilledema.

RETINAL FOLDS

Background

Retinal folds (i.e., those that involve only the neurosensory retina) must be distinguished from chorioretinal folds. Large retinal folds occurring singly or in small groups that are associated with retinopathy of prematurity (ROP), familial exudative vitreoretinopathy (FEVR), and scleral buckles, for example, bear little resemblance to chorioretinal folds. However, smaller, multiple retinal folds, especially when located in the posterior pole, are easily confused with chorioretinal folds. While retinal and chorioretinal folds have some overlapping causes, there are numerous underlying disorders that uniquely cause retinal folds (Table 22–2). So, the distinction between the two can provide a useful clue as to their underlying cause.

Clinical Evaluation

In the proper setting, such as in cases of ROP, FEVR, proliferative vitreoretinopathy (PVR), and following scleral buckling surgery, and with the proper clinical appearance, retinal folds are easily diagnosed by ophthalmoscopy alone. Such folds are usually large and either single or in small numbers. Vitreoretinal traction may be evident, depending on the cause of the folds. Of course, other findings on examination in eyes with this sort of retinal fold will depend upon their underlying cause and other concomitant pathology.

Those retinal folds that are more easily confused with chorioretinal folds are generally fine, multiple, and linear. They commonly accompany epiretinal membranes and involve the inner retinal layers.[4] They frequently assume a radiating pattern (Fig. 22–3) as do those chorioretinal folds associated with CNVMs. They are often located in the posterior pole, another characteristic common to AMD-related chorioretinal folds. These fine retinal folds normally appear somewhat narrower and have less alterations of color than chorioretinal folds.[4,16] The fine, multiple retinal folds observed in bullous rhegmatogenous retinal detachments involve the outer retina and assume an irregular, reticular appearance not unlike that of chorioretinal folds in hypotonous eyes (Fig. 22–1E and F). Folds of the RPE have more coloration than those of the neurosensory retina, and are seen in patients with AMD who have RPE detachments associated with CNVMs.[61]

Again, additional biomicroscopic and ophthalmoscopic findings in eyes with fine retinal folds

TABLE 22–2 Causes of Chorioretinal and Retinal Folds

Chorioretinal Folds	Retinal Folds
Orbital masses	ROP
Orbital inflammatory processes	FEVR
Hyperopia	Congenital retinal fold
Optic disc swelling	Posterior microphthalmia
Localized suprachoroidal hemorrhage	PHPV
Posterior scleritis	Shaken baby syndrome
Choroidal tumors	Terson's syndrome
Postoperative hypotony	PVR
Following posterior segment laser	Epiretinal membrane
Alagille, Whipple's and other systemic disorders	Rhegmatogenous retinal detachment
	Following internal retinal tamponade
Idiopathic	Drug-induced myopia
CNVMs in AMD	CNVMs and AMD
Following scleral buckle surgery	Following scleral buckle surgery

ROP, retinopathy of prematurity; FEVR, familial exudative vitreoretinopathy; PHPV, persistent hyperplastic primary vitreous; PVR, proliferative vitreoretinopathy; CNVMs, choroidal neovascular membranes; AMD, age-related macular degeneration.

vary with their underlying causes and any other ophthalmic pathology present.

Fluorescein Angiography

As mentioned previously (see under "Chorioretinal Folds"), fluorescein angiography can be particularly useful in distinguishing between chorioretinal and fine retinal folds. While alternating relative hyper- and hypoflourescent lines are seen in cases of chorioretinal folds, there are no such lines or any

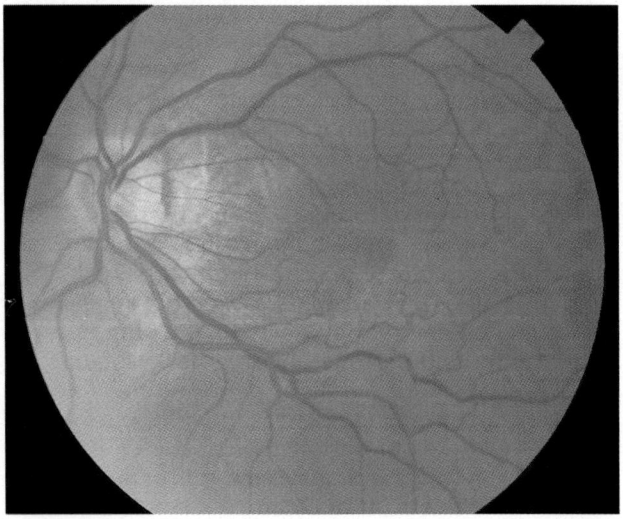

FIGURE 22–3 Multiple, fine retinal folds seen in the macula of an eye with an idiopathic epiretinal membrane. (Courtesy of Dr. Donald J. D'Amico.)

other specific fluorescein angiographic findings in cases of retinal folds. Abnormal fluorescein angiographic findings in instances where retinal folds are present relate to any underlying or coincident ocular pathology and not to the folds themselves. Tortuosity of the retinal vasculature around retinal folds is very common.

Mechanisms

There is little written regarding experimental work designed to study the exact biomechanical or other causes of retinal folds. If one considers the majority of causes (see "Causes") of retinal folds, though, it is apparent that they often arise secondary to tangential traction on the retina. In the case of epiretinal membranes, for example, the traction is applied at the inner retinal surface, whereas in the case of retinal folds from subretinal scars the pulling occurs at the outer retinal surface. Normally, there is no disturbance of the retinal circulation or the RPE–Bruch's membrane–choriocapillaris complex directly attributable to retinal folds themselves; hence the reason for the unremarkable fluorescein angiographic studies.

Causes

We will now describe the more common and important causes of retinal folds in more detail. What follows is not an exhaustive analysis of all reported instances in which retinal folds occur, but rather an outline.

Retinal Folds in Infants and Children

There are many reports of large, single or low-multiple retinal folds occurring in disorders primarily diagnosed in pediatric patients. These include ROP[62-66]; FEVR[67-74]; congenital retinal fold[75-76]; posterior microphthalmos[77-80]; persistent hyperplastic primary vitreous[81]; and an unusual syndrome of microcephaly, microphthalmia, falciform retinal folds, and blindness.[82] In many of these situations the folds themselves or collateral damage or deformities are a major detriment to the development of normal vision. The success of the surgical correction of deformities and amblyopia therapy depends on many factors, such as the degree and location of the abnormalities, the age of the child at the time of the initiation of therapy, the presence of concurrent central nervous system dysfunction, the preexisting visual capabilities, and others. There are reports of successful surgical flattening of such folds in children.[68,76,83-86]

Peculiar circinate, perimacular retinal folds have been observed in young children with shaken baby syndrome.[87-91] Massicotte and co-workers suggested that these folds arise from lateral vitreous traction induced by violent shaking of the head, but that direct head injury was not likely to play a role.[88] However, Keithan and colleagues called this theory into question with a report of two adult patients with Terson's syndrome following direct head trauma who had fine, perimacular retinal folds similar to those previously observed in cases of shaken baby syndrome.[92]

After Surgery

Peripheral, radially oriented folds are common following scleral buckling surgery for repair of retinal detachment.[93,94] They commonly appear immediately following drainage of subretinal fluid. However, while these are often referred to as retinal folds, they are really full-thickness folds of the entire eye wall: sclera, choroid, and retina.[94]

Recently, large, true retinal folds have been noted to complicate retinal reattachment surgeries in which internal tamponade is employed.[95-99] These have been observed both in cases where gas and oil were employed for tamponade. Unlike the radial folds discussed above that appear overlying scleral buckles just after drainage of subretinal fluid, these postoperative retinal folds are frequently single and tend to originate at one end of the scleral explant and course posteriorly.[95] Larrison and co-workers feel that air introduced during air-fluid exchange plays a role in the development of posterior retinal folds in vitrectomy cases where internal drainage of subretinal fluid is performed.[100] They propose that the small amount of subretinal fluid often left behind after drainage shifts posteriorly during prone positioning for air-fluid exchange, and that it then pools at the tethered junction of attached and detached retina, only to be pumped out later by the RPE, leaving behind a long posterior retinal fold.

Proliferative Vitreoretinopathy

Retinal folds are observed in moderate and severe cases of PVR.[101-104] In fact, they are an integral part of the disorder and are included in commonly used classification schemes of PVR.[101] When one considers the presence of fibroglial proliferation in the vitreous cavity and behind the retina in cases of PVR and posterior segment trauma, with all of the ensuing traction exerted on the retina, it is not surprising that the retina should become folded.

Epiretinal Membranes

Numerous different names are used to refer to epiretinal membranes, such as internal limiting membrane wrinkling, surface-wrinkling retinopathy, macular pucker, cellophane maculopathy, premacular fibrosis syndrome, and others. Macular epiretinal membranes, as seen in idopathic cases, in those following successful retinal reattachment surgery, and in a host of other ocular disorders, exert lateral traction on the retina and very often result in retinal folds. These folds may be course or fine, single or multiple. They are likely one of the most important reasons that patients with epiretinal membranes experience metamorphopsia and decreased visual acuity.

While many epiretinal membranes are not sufficiently troublesome to patients to warrant surgical correction, in some cases distortion and blurring are severe enough to justify intervention. Such membranes can be successfully removed from the retinal surface during vitrectomy surgery by using a combination of a fine pick and other microsurgical instruments. The underlying retinal folds frequently flatten intra- and postoperatively. Epiretinal membranes may also separate from the retinal surface spontaneously, although this is rare.[105]

Drug-Induced Myopia

In 1986, Ryan and Jampol reported a case of transient myopia with fine, radial, perimacular retinal folds believed to be secondary to an over-the-counter cold medication containing acetaminophen, chlorpheniramine, phenylpropanolamine, and dextromethorphan.[106] Interestingly, this was not the first report of drug-induced myopia with macular changes.[107-112] Previous authors had attributed the macular striae to edema. However, they had not performed fluorescein angiography. Ryan and Jampol demonstrated normal fluorescein angiography without evidence of macular edema in their patient and believe that the striae reported in the earlier cases were retinal folds, not some manifestation of retinal edema.

Summary

Chorioretinal and retinal folds each occur in a variety of clinical settings. Hence, single, unifying theories regarding the mechanisms of their production remain elusive. Fluorescein angiography is particularly useful in distinguishing between the two, and may yield clues as to causative reasons for the presence of folds, as well. In some cases, the underlying causes of chorioretinal and/or retinal folds may be quite serious. Thus, careful, complete ophthalmologic examinations are always necessary, and systemic medical evaluation is sometimes indicated, too.

REFERENCES

1. Nettleship E: Peculiar lines in the choroid in a case of post-papillitic atrophy. Trans Ophthalmol Soc U K 4: 167–171, 1884.
2. Birch-Hirschfeld A, Siegfried C: Zur Kenntnis der Veranderungen des Bulbus durch Druck eines Orbitaltumors. Graefes Arch Ophthalmol 90:404–412, 1915.
3. Gass JDM: Radial chorioretinal folds: a sign of choroidal neovascularization. Arch Ophthalmol 99:1016–1018, 1981.
4. Gass JDM: Stereoscopic Atlas of Macular Diseases: Diagnosis and Treatment, 3rd edition. St Louis, Mosby-Year Book, 1987.
5. Kroll AJ, Norton EWD: Regression of choroidal folds. Trans Am Acad Ophthalmol Otolaryngol 74:515–525, 1970.
6. Von Winning CHOM: Fluorography of choroidal folds. Doc Ophthalmol 31:209–249, 1972.
7. Francois J, De Laey JJ: Fluoro-angiographic aspects of acquired chorio-retinal folds. Mod Probl Ophthalmol 9: 129–135, 1970.
8. Norton EWD: A characteristic fluorescein angiographic pattern in choroidal folds. Proc R Soc Med 62:119–128, 1969.
9. Wolter JR: Parallel horizontal choroidal folds secondary to an orbital tumor. Am J Ophthalmol 77:669–673, 1974.
10. Shields JA, Shields CL, Rashid RC: Clinicopathologic correlation of chorioretinal folds: secondary to massive cranioorbital hemangiopericytoma. Ophthal Plast Reconstr Surg 8:62–68, 1992.
11. Friberg TR, Grove AS: Subretinal neovascularization and choroidal folds. Ann Ophthalmol 12:245–250, 1980.
12. Newell FW: Fundus changes in persistent and recurrent choroidal folds. Br J Ophthalmol 68:32–35, 1984.
13. Cappaert WE, Purnell EW, Frank KE: Use of B-sector scan ultrasound in the diagnosis of benign choroidal folds. Am J Ophthalmol 84:375–379, 1977.
14. Atta HR, Byrne SF: The findings of standardized echography for choroidal folds. Arch Ophthalmol 106:1234–1241, 1988.
15. Singh G, Guthoff R, Foster CS: Observations on long-term follow-up of posterior scleritis. Am J Ophthalmol 101: 570–575, 1986.
16. Leahey AB, Brucker AJ, Wyszynski RE, Shaman P: Chorioretinal folds: a comparison of unilateral and bilateral cases. Arch Ophthalmol 111:357–359, 1993.
17. Bullock JD, Egbert PR: Experimental choroidal folds. Am J Ophthalmol 78:618–623, 1974.
18. Bullock JD, Egbert PR: The origin of choroidal folds—a clinical, histopathological and experimental study. Doc Ophthalmol 2:261–263, 1974.
19. Friberg TR, Lace JW: A comparison of the elastic properties of human choroid and sclera. Exp Eye Res 47:429–436, 1988.
20. Friberg TR: The etiology of choroidal folds: a biomechanical explanation. Graefes Arch Ophthalmol 227:459–464, 1989.
21. Steuhl KP, Richard G, Weidle EG: Clinical observations concerning choroidal folds. Ophthalmologica 190:219–224, 1985.
22. Cangemi FE, Trempe CL, Walsh JB: Choroidal folds. Am J Ophthalmol 86:380–387, 1978.
23. Newell FW: Choroidal folds. The Seventh Harry Searls Gradle Memorial Lecture. Am J Ophthalmol 75:931–942, 1973.
24. Hedges TR Jr, Leopold IH: Parallel retinal folds: their significance in orbital space-taking lesions. Arch Ophthalmol 62:353–355, 1959.
25. Friberg TR, Grove AS Jr: Choroidal folds and refractive errors associated with orbital tumors: an analysis. Arch Ophthalmol 101:598–603, 1983.
26. Kaufman S: Orbital mucopyoceles: two cases and a review. Surv Ophthalmol 25:253–262, 1981.
27. Newton C, Dutton JJ, Klintworth GK: A respiratory epithelial choristomatous cyst of the orbit. Ophthalmology 92:1754–1757, 1985.
28. Wolter JR: Parallel horizontal retinal folding. Am J Ophthalmol 53:26–29, 1962.
29. Kowal L, Georgievski Z: Choroidal folds in Graves' ophthalmology (Letter). Aust N Z J Ophthalmol 22:216, 1994.
30. Hyvarinen L, Walsh FB: Benign chorioretinal folds. Am J Ophthalmol 70:14–15, 1970.
31. Takahashi T, Ikushima K, Arizawa T: Orbital myositis simulating infectious cellulitis: report of two cases. Jpn J Ophthalmol 27:626–630, 1983.
32. Kalina RE, Mills RP: Acquired hyperopia with choroidal folds. Ophthalmology 87:44–50, 1980.
33. Dailey RA, Mills RP, Stimac GK, et al: The natural history and CT appearance of acquired hyperopia with choroidal folds. Ophthalmology 93:1336–1342, 1986.
34. Stimac GK, Mills RP, Dailey RA, et al: CT of acquired hyperopia with choroidal folds. Am J Neuroradiol 8: 1107–1111, 1987.
35. Fried M, Meyer-Schwickerath G, Koch A: Excessive hypermetropia: review and case report documented by echography. Ann Ophthalmol 14:15–19, 1982.
36. Bird AC, Sanders MD: Choroidal folds in association with papilledema. Br J Ophthalmol 57:89–97, 1973.
37. Mitchell DJ, Steahly LP: Pseudotumor cerebri and macular disease. Retina 9:115–117, 1989.
38. Gittinger JW Jr, Asdourian GK: Macular abnormalities in papilledema from pseudotumor cerebri. Ophthalmology 96:192–194, 1989.
39. Corbett JJ, Savino PJ, Thompson HS, et al: Visual loss in pseudotumor cerebri: follow-up of 57 patients from five to 41 years and a profile of 14 patients with permanent severe visual loss. Arch Neurol 39:461–474, 1982.
40. Baker RS, Bundic JR: Sudden visual loss in pseudotumor cerebri due to central retinal artery occlusion. Arch Neurol 41:1274–1276, 1984.
41. Augsberger JJ, Coats TD, Lauritzen K: Localized suprachoroidal hemorrhages: ophthalmoscopic features, fluorescein angiography, and clinical course. Arch Ophthalmol 108:968–972, 1990.
42. Benson WE, Shields JA, Tasman WS, Crandall AS: Posterior scleritis. Arch Ophthalmol 97:1482–1486, 1979.
43. Benson WE: Posterior scleritis. Surv Ophthalmol 32:297–316, 1988.
44. Gass JDM: Hypotony maculopathy. In Bellows JG (ed): Contemporary Ophthalmology: Honoring Sir Stewart Duke-Elder. Baltimore, Williams & Wilkins, 1972, pp 343–366.
45. Dellaporta A: Fundus changes in postoperative hypotony. Am J Ophthalmol 40:781–785, 1955.
46. Newhouse RP, Beyrer C: Hypotony as a late complication of trabeculectomy. Ann Ophthalmol 14:685–686, 1982.
47. Stamper RL, McMenemy MG, Lieberman MF: Hypotonous maculopathy after trabeculectomy with subconjunctival 5-flourouracil. Am J Ophthalmol 114:544–553, 1992.

48. Altan T, Temel A, Bavbek T, Kazokoglu H: Hypotony maculopathy after trabeculectomy with postoperative use of 5-fluorouracil. Ophthalmologica 208:318–320, 1994.

49. Duker JS, Schuman JS: Successful surgical treatment of hypotony maculopathy following trabeculectomy with topical mitomycin C. Ophthal Surg 25:463–465, 1994.

50. Hertle RW, Leahey AB, Bloom S, et al: Chorioretinal folds and a macular hole secondary to craniofacial surgery. Ophthal Plast Reconstr Surg 6:278–282, 1990.

51. Diskin J, Maguire AM, Margherio RR: Choroidal folds induced with diode endolaser (Letter). Arch Ophthalmol 110:754, 1992.

52. Grabowski WM, Decker WL, Annesley WH Jr: Complications of krypton red laser photocoagulation to subretinal neovascular membranes. Ophthalmology 91:1587–1591, 1984.

53. Johnson RN, Schatz H, McDonald HR: Photic maculopathy: early angiographic and ophthalmoscopic findings and late development of choroidal folds. Arch Ophthalmol 105:1633–1634, 1987.

54. Lam S, Tessler HH, Lam BL, Wilensky JT: High incidence of sympathetic ophthalmia after contact and noncontact neodymium:YAG cyclotherapy. Ophthalmology 99:1818–1822, 1992.

55. Gonshor LG, Kline LB: Choroidal folds and dural cavernous sinus fistula (Letter). Arch Ophthalmol 109:1065–1066, 1991.

56. Wells, KK, Pulido JS, Judisch GF, et al: Ophthalmic features of Alagille syndrome (arteriohepatic dysplasia). J Pediatr Ophthalmol Strabismus 30:130–135, 1993.

57. Romanchuk KG, Judisch GF, LaBrecque DR: Ocular findings in arteriohepatic dysplasia (Alagille's syndrome). Can J Ophthalmol 16:94–98, 1981.

58. Avila MP, Jalkh AE, Feldman E, et al: Manifestations of Whipple's disease in the posterior segment of the eye. Arch Ophthalmol 102:384–390, 1984.

59. Pulido JS, Goeken JA, Nerad JA, et al: Ocular manifestations of patients with circulating antineutrophil cytoplasmic antibodies. Arch Ophthalmol 108:845–850, 1990.

60. Davis ML, Bartley GB, Gibson LE, Maguire LJ: Ophthalmic findings in scleromyxedema. Ophthalmology 101:252–255, 1994.

61. Schatz H, McDonald HR, Johnson RN: Retinal pigment epithelial folds associated with retinal pigment epithelial detachment in macular degeneration. Ophthalmology 97:658–665, 1990.

62. Kushner BJ, Gloeckner E: Retrolental fibroplasia in full-term infants without exposure to supplemental oxygen. Am J Ophthalmol 97:148–153, 1984.

63. Shapiro DR, Stone RD: Ultrasonic characteristics of retinopathy of prematurity presenting with leukocoria. Arch Ophthalmol 103:1690–1692, 1985.

64. Foos RY: Chronic retinopathy of prematurity. Ophthalmology 92:563–574, 1985.

65. Sternberg P Jr, Lopez PF, Capone A Jr, et al: Management of threshold retinopathy of prematurity. Retina 12:S60–S63, 1992.

66. Brockhurst RJ, Chishti MI: Cicatricial retrolental fibroplasia: its occurrence without oxygen administration and in full term infants. Albrecht Von Graefes Arch Klin Exp Ophthalmol 195:113–128, 1975.

67. Fullwood P, Jones J, Bundey S, et al: X linked exudative vitreoretinopathy: clinical features and genetic linkage analysis. Br J Ophthalmol 77:168–170, 1993.

68. van Nouhuys CE: Signs, complications, and platelet aggregation in familial exudative vitreoretinopathy. Am J Ophthalmol 111:34–41, 1991.

69. van Nouhuys CE: Dominant exudative vitreoretinopathy. Ophthalmic Paediatr Genet 5:31–38, 1985.

70. Nishimura M, Yamana T, Sugino M, et al: Falciform retinal fold as sign of familial exudative vitreoretinopathy. Jpn J Ophthalmol 27:40–53, 1983.

71. van Nouhuys CE: Congenital retinal fold as a sign of dominant exudative vitreoretinopathy. Albrecht Von Graefes Arch Klin Exp Ophthalmol 217:55–67, 1981.

72. Nicholson DH, Galvis V: Criswick-Schepens syndrome (familial exudative vitreoretinopathy). Study of a Columbian kindred. Arch Ophthalmol 102:1519–1522, 1984.

73. Feldman EL, Norris JL, Cleasby GW: Autosomal dominant exudative vitreoretinopathy. Arch Ophthalmol 101:1532–1535, 1983.

74. Dudgeon J: Familial exudative vitreo-retinopathy. Trans Ophthalmol Soc U K 99:45–49, 1979.

75. Theodore FH, Ziporkes J: Congenital retinal fold. Arch Ophthalmol 23:1188–1197, 1940.

76. Maguire AM, Trese MT: Visual results of lens-sparing vitreoretinal surgery in infants. J Pediatr Ophthalmol Strabismus 30:28–32, 1993.

77. Meire F, Leys M, Boghaert S, de Laey JJ: Posterior microphthalmos. Bull Soc Belge Ophthalmol 231:101–106, 1989.

78. Spitznas M, Gerke E, Bateman JB: Hereditary posterior microphthalmos with papillomacular fold and high hyperopia. Arch Ophthalmol 101:413–417, 1983.

79. Boynton JR, Purnell EW: Bilateral microphthalmos without microcornea associated with unusual papillomacular retinal folds and high hyperopia. Am J Ophthalmol 79:820–826, 1975.

80. Ryckewaert M, Zanlonghi X, Bertrand-Cuignet H, Constantinides G: High hyperopia with papillomacular fold. Ophthalmologica 204:49–53, 1993.

81. Pruett RC: The pleomorphism and complications of posterior hyperplastic primary vitreous. Am J Ophthalmol 80:625–629, 1975.

82. Jarmas AL, Weaver DD, Ellis FD, Davis A: Microcephaly, microphthalmia, falciform retinal folds, and blindness. A new syndrome. Am J Dis Child 135:930–933, 1981.

83. Snir M, Nissenkorn I, Wineberger D, et al: Surgical flattening of retinal fold of stage III cicatricial retrolental fibroplasia (RLF). Metab Pediatr Syst Ophthalmol 10:55–58, 1987.

84. Machemer R: Closed vitrectomy for severe retrolental fibroplasia in the infant. Ophthalmology 90:436–441, 1983.

85. Trese MT: Surgical results of stage V retrolental fibroplasia and timing of surgical repair. Ophthalmology 91:461–466, 1984.

86. Chong LP, Machemer R, de Juan E: Vitrectomy for advanced stages of retinopathy of prematurity. Am J Ophthalmol 102:710–716, 1986.

87. Gaynon MW, Koh K, Marmor MF, Frankel LR: Retinal folds in the shaken baby syndrome. Am J Ophthalmol 106:423–425, 1988.

88. Massicotte SJ, Folberg R, Torczynski E, et al: Vitreoretinal traction and perimacular retinal folds in the eyes of deliberately traumatized children. Ophthalmology 98:1124–1127, 1991.

89. Han DP, Wilkinson WS: Late ophthalmic manifestations of the shaken baby syndrome. J Pediatr Ophthalmol Strabismus 27:299–303, 1990.

90. Munger CE, Pfeiffer RL, Bouldin TW, et al: Ocular and associated neuropathologic observations in suspected whiplash shaken baby syndrome. A retrospective study of 12 cases. Am J Forensic Med Pathol 14:193–200, 1993.

91. Elner SG, Elner VM, Arnall M, Albert DM: Ocular and associated systemic findings in suspected child abuse. Arch Ophthalmol 108:1094–1101, 1990.

92. Keithahn MAZ, Bennett SR, Cameron D, Mieler WF: Retinal folds in Terson syndrome. Ophthalmology 100:1187–1190, 1993.

93. Michels RG, Wilkinson CP, Rice TA: Retinal Detachment, 1st edition. St Louis, CV Mosby Co, 1990.

94. Thompson JT: The effects and action of scleral buckles in the treatment of retinal detachment. In Ryan SJ, Glaser BM (eds): Retina, 2nd edition, Vol 3. St Louis, Mosby-Year Book, 1994, pp 2019–2033.

95. Twomey JM, Leaver PK: Retinal compression folds. Eye 2:283–287, 1988.

96. Pavan PR: Retinal fold in macula following intraocular gas. An avoidable complication of retinal detachment surgery. Arch Ophthalmol 102:83–84, 1984.

97. Pavan PR: Arcuate retinal folds after intraocular gas injection (Letter). Arch Ophthalmol 106:164–165, 1988.

98. Lewen RM, Lyon CE, Diamond JG: Scleral buckling with intraocular air injection complicated by arcuate retinal folds. Arch Ophthalmol 105:1212–1214, 1987.

99. van Meurs JC, Humalda D, Mertens DAE, Peperkamp E: Retinal folds through the macula. Doc Ophthalmol 78:335–340, 1991.

100. Larrison WI, Frederick AR Jr, Peterson TJ, Topping TM: Posterior retinal folds following vitreoretinal surgery. Arch Ophthalmol 111:621–625, 1993.

101. The Retina Society Terminology Committee: The classification of retinal detachment with proliferative vitreoretinopathy. Ophthalmology 90:121–125, 1983.

102. Mandai M, Takanashi T, Ogura Y, Honda Y: Proliferative vitreoretinopathy shows predilection for the inferior fundus. Graefes Arch Clin Exp Ophthalmol 228:335–337, 1990.

103. Lewis H, Aaberg TM: Causes of failure after repeat vitreoretinal surgery for recurrent proliferative vitreoretinopathy. Am J Ophthalmol 111:15–19, 1991.

104. Elner SG, Elner VM, Diaz-Rohena R, et al: Anterior proliferative vitroretinopathy. Clinicopathologic, light microscopic, and ultrastructural findings. Ophthalmology 95:1349–1357, 1988.

105. Sjaarda RN, Michels RG: Macular pucker. In Ryan SJ, Glaser BM (eds): Retina, 2nd edition, Vol 3. St Louis, Mosby-Year Book, 1994, pp 2301–2311.

106. Ryan EH Jr, Jampol LM: Drug-induced acute transient myopia with retinal folds. Retina 6:220–223, 1986.

107. Maddalena M: Transient myopia associated with acute glaucoma and retinal edema. Arch Ophthalmol 80:186–188, 1968.

108. Bovino J, Marcus D: The mechanism of transient myopia induced by sulfonamide therapy. Am J Ophthalmol 94:99–102, 1982.

109. Garland M, Sholk A, Guenter K: Acetazolamide induced myopia. Am J Obstet Gynecol 84:69–71, 1962.

110. Muirhead JF, Scheie HG: Transient myopia after acetazolamide. Arch Ophthalmol 63:315–318, 1960.

111. Beasley F: Transient myopia and retinal edema during hydrochlorothiazide (Hydrodiuril) therapy. Arch Ophthalmol 65:212–213, 1961.

112. Beasley F: Transient myopia and retinal edema during ethoxzolamide (Cardrase) therapy. Arch Ophthalmol 68:490–491, 1962.

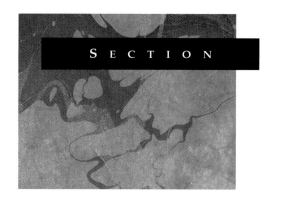

SECTION

III

*Retinal
Vascular
Diseases*

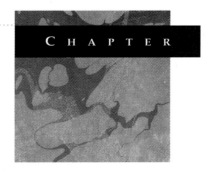

Retinal Arterial Occlusive Diseases

Gary C. Brown, M.D.

CENTRAL RETINAL ARTERY OBSTRUCTION

In 1859, von Graefe[1] described an embolic central retinal artery obstruction in a patient with endocarditis and multiple systemic emboli. Knapp,[2] however, mentions that several years earlier Virchow had suggested that an embolus might be seen directly in a retinal artery with the ophthalmoscope. Duke-Elder[3] nicely elaborates further history on the entity. Within 5 years after von Graefe's report, Sweiger described the histopathologic correlate of central retinal artery obstruction. In 1868 Mauthner suggested that spasmodic contractions could lead to retinal arterial obstruction, and in 1874 Loring implicated focal obstructive disease within the retinal vessels as a cause. By the turn of the 20th century, over two dozen reports of retinal arterial obstruction were present in the ophthalmic literature.

Background

Data concerning the incidence of central retinal artery obstruction (occlusion) are not readily available, but from information gathered at Wills Eye Hospital, it has been estimated to occur with a frequency of about 1 per 10,000 outpatient visits. The abnormality is most commonly encountered in older adults, but can also be seen in children.[4] The mean age at the time of presentation is the early sixties.[5-7] There appears to be no predilection for one eye over the other, and men are affected more frequently than women. In approximately 1 to 2% of cases there is bilateral involvement.[5] When both eyes are simultaneously affected by retinal artery

obstruction, the differential diagnosis should include cardiac valvular disease, giant cell arteritis, and other vascular inflammations.[6]

Clinical Features

Patients with acute central retinal artery obstruction usually relate a history of painless visual loss occurring over several seconds. In some instances, there is a preceeding history of amaurosis fugax.

The anterior segment examination is most often initially normal in eyes with acute central retinal artery obstruction. If rubeosis iridis is present at the time the obstruction occurs, the presence of concomitant carotid artery obstruction should be considered. Under these circumstances, increased intraocular pressure resulting from the rubeosis iridis induced by the carotid artery obstruction can exceed the perfusion pressure in the central retinal artery and predispose to central retinal artery obstruction.

An afferent pupillary defect usually develops within seconds after obstruction of the central retinal artery.[8] During the early phases of the obstruction the fundus appearance can be normal, but an afferent pupillary defect will still be present unless the obstruction has spontaneously resolved.

Acutely, the superficial retina in the posterior pole becomes opacified and assumes a yellow-white appearance, except in the region of the foveola, where a cherry-red spot is present (Fig. 23–1). Ischemic necrosis in the affected inner half of the retina corresponds to the whitening seen clinically. The size of the cherry-red spot is variable, depending upon the width of the foveola. A cherry-red spot develops because the retina in this region is

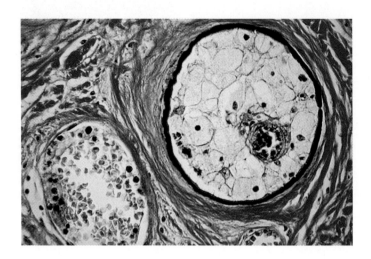

Near total occlusion of central retinal artery by an atheromatous
plaque (AFIP 868622).

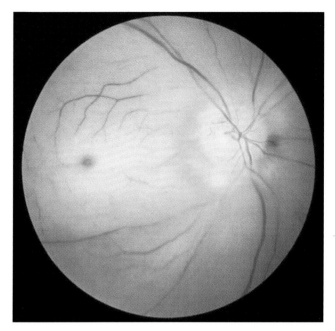

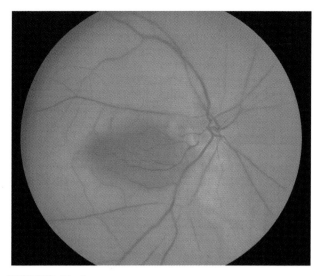

FIGURE 23-2   Central retinal artery obstruction with cilio-retinal sparing of the papillomacular bundle and the foveola. The visual acuity returned to 20/20.

FIGURE 23-1   Acute central retinal artery obstruction. The retinal arteries are narrowed, superficial retinal whitening is present, and a cherry-red spot can be seen in the foveola.

extremely thin, allowing a view of the underlying retinal pigment epithelium (RPE) and choroid. Additionally, the foveolar retina is probably nourished, to an extent, by the underlying choroid, therefore opacifying to a lesser degree. The retinal opacification diminishes rapidly once outside the macular area. The opacification can require hours to become apparent, although we have been able to induce it in the subhuman primate model following complete retinal arterial obstruction within 10 to 15 minutes. In most cases the retinal opacification resolves over a period of 4 to 6 weeks, usually leaving a pale optic disc, narrowed retinal vessels, and visible absence of the nerve fiber layer in the region of the optic disc. Resultant pigmentary changes are usually absent unless there is also involvement of the choroidal circulation. Acutely, the retinal arteries are most often thin, although the retinal veins can be thin, dilated, or even normal in appearance. In cases of severe obstruction, segmentation or "boxcarring" of the blood column can be seen in both the arteries and the veins.

At the time of initial examination, the visual acuity in eyes with central retinal artery obstruction ranges between counting fingers and light perception in 90% of eyes.[5] The presence of an embolus in the fundus is usually associated with poorer vision.[5] Absence of light perception is rarely encountered. In such instances, the clinician should suspect the presence of concomitant choroidal circulatory compromise of damage to the optic nerve.[5]

Approximately 25% of eyes with an acute central retinal artery obstruction have a patent cilioretinal artery that supplies part of all of the papillomacular

bundle.[9] If only a part of the papillomacular bundle is spared the resultant visual acuity is still usually no better than 20/100. In about 10% of eyes the cilioretinal artery spares the foveola (Figs. 23-2 and 23-3), in which case the visual acuity improves to 20/50 or better in 80% of eyes over a 2-week period. Only a small island of central vision may remain, but in some eyes a surprising amount of peripheral visual field returns.

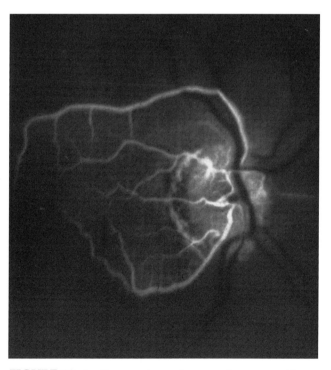

FIGURE 23-3   Fluorescein angiogram of an eye with an acute central retinal artery obstruction and sparing by two cilioretinal arteries (at the 7:30 and 10:30 positions) reveals a characteristic pattern of filling of the patent cilioretinal artery and the retinal vein that drains the area supplied by it.

Emboli are visible within the retinal arterial system in about 20% of eyes with central retinal artery obstruction.[5] The most common variant is the glistening, yellow cholesterol embolus (Hollenhorst plaque) (Fig. 23–4). This type of embolus is believed to most commonly arise from atherosclerotic deposits in the carotid arteries[6] but certainly can also originate from the aortic arch, ophthalmic artery, or even the more proximal central retinal artery. Cholesterol emboli are often small and may not totally obstruct retinal arteries. They frequently occur asymptomatically. In some eyes with central retinal artery obstruction, a large, nonglistening embolus is seen within the central retinal artery on the optic disc, while numerous small cholesterol emboli are present in the more peripheral retinal arteries. It is likely that the larger embolus on the disc is of the same origin, but appears different because it is surrounded by a fibrin-platelet thrombus. Calcific emboli (Fig. 23–5) are less common than cholesterol emboli, but tend to be larger and cause more severe obstructions. They usually originate from the cardiac valves.[6] Fibrin-platelet thrombi can be transient and cause amaurosis fugax, but can also be seen with central retinal artery obstruction without other types of emboli (Fig. 23–6).

The presence of a retinal arterial embolus, whether seen in conjunction with a retinal arterial obstruction or not, is associated with increased mortality. Savino and associates[10] found a mortality rate of 56% over 9 years in such patients, as compared to a rate of 27% during the same time in an age-matched control group without arterial emboli. Similar to what has been noted with the ocular ischemic syndrome,[11] the leading cause of death was cardiac disease.

The incidence of rubeosis iridis after acute central retinal artery obstruction was previously

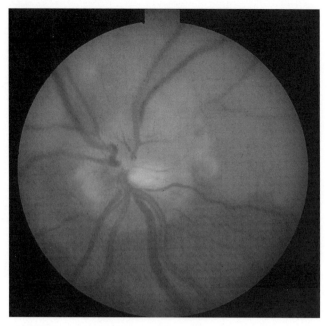

FIGURE 23–5 White calcific plaque from the aortic valve causing a superior papillary retinal artery obstruction.

thought to be in the 1 to 5% range.[12] More recent studies,[13–15] however, have shown that the figure approaches 20%, similar to that seen after central retinal vein obstruction.[16] In a prospective study on the subject, Duker and associates[15] found that 18.2% of eyes with acute central retinal artery obstruction progressed to develop rubeosis iridis. Unlike eyes with central retinal vein obstruction, in which the new iris vessels develop at a mean time of 5 months

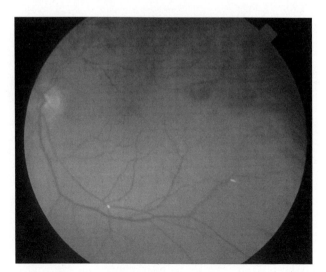

FIGURE 23–4 Two glistening cholesterol emboli (Hollenhorst plaques) in the inferotemporal vascular arcade, most probably arising from the ipsilateral carotid artery. The emboli did not cause an obstruction in this eye.

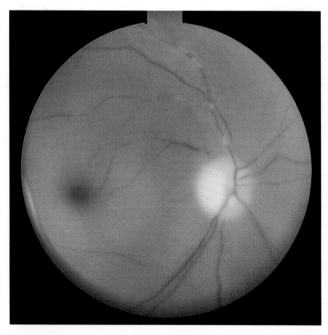

FIGURE 23–6 Fibrin-platelet thrombi in the superotemporal artery in an eye with an acute central retinal artery obstruction.

after the obstruction,[17] with central retinal artery obstruction they develop at a mean of 4 to 5 weeks after the event, with a range of 1 to 15 weeks.[14,15] Eyes in which the obstruction is severe and prolonged for a week or longer appear to be at greater risk for the development of rubeosis iridis than those in which the obstruction is reversed within the first few days after its occurrence. Laser panretinal photocoagulation is effective in causing regression of the new iris vessels in about 65% of eyes.[18] Neovascularization of the optic disc has also been noted to occur after acute central retinal artery obstruction, and develops in about 2 to 3% of eyes.[16,19]

Similar to the case with neovascularization of the iris, when neovascularization optic disc is already present in an eye at the time an acute central retinal artery obstruction develops, the clinician should suspect a cause other than the acute blockage. In particular, underlying carotid artery obstruction should be considered.[20]

Ancillary Studies

Intravenous fluorescein angiography (Fig. 23–7) may reveal a delay in retinal arterial filling, but the most commonly seen fluorescein angiographic sign with acute central retinal artery obstruction is a delay in retinal arteriovenous transit time (time elapsed from the appearance of dye within the arteries of the temporal vascular arcade until the corresponding veins are completely filled; normal is ≤11 seconds).[5] Late staining of the optic disc is variable, but staining of the retinal vessels is unusual. Complete lack of filling of the retinal arteries is distinctly unusual[21] and probably occurs in less than 2% of cases.[5]

The choroidal vascular bed in eyes with central retinal artery obstruction usually fills normally, although delays of 5 seconds or greater are seen in about 10% of cases.[5] In a normal eye the choroid generally begins to fill 1 to 2 seconds prior to filling of the retinal arteries, and is completely filled within 5 seconds of the first appearance of dye. A marked prolongation of choroidal filling in the presence of a cherry-red spot should arouse suspicion of an ophthalmic artery obstruction[22] (Fig. 23–8) or a concomitant carotid artery obstruction.[20] With an acute ophthalmic artery obstruction the cherry-red spot may be absent and the visual acuity is often no light perception.

The retinal circulation has a marked propensity to re-establish the circulation following an acute central retinal artery obstruction. Therefore, arterial narrowing and visual loss may persist, but the fluorescein angiogram can revert to normal at varying times after the insult.[6]

Electroretinography (Fig. 23–9) typically discloses a diminution in the amplitude of the b-wave (corresponding to the function of the Müller and/or bipolar cells) secondary to inner layer retinal ischemia. The a-wave, which corresponds to photoreceptor function, is generally unaffected. In some eyes the study is normal in the presence of decreased vision, possibly because of the re-establishment of retinal blood flow.

Visual field studies frequently demonstrate a remaining temporal island of vision, presumably because the choroid nourished the corresponding nasal retina. In the presence of a patent cilioretinal artery, small areas of central vision are preserved. Depending upon the degree and the extent of the obstruction, varied portions of the peripheral field may remain.[9]

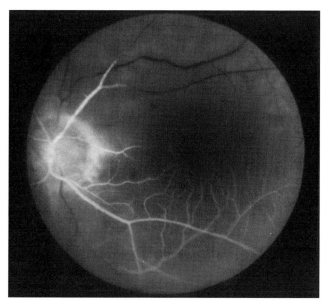

FIGURE 23–7 Fluorescein angiogram of an eye with an acute central retinal artery obstruction at 60 seconds after injection reveals delays in filling of the retinal arterial and venous systems.

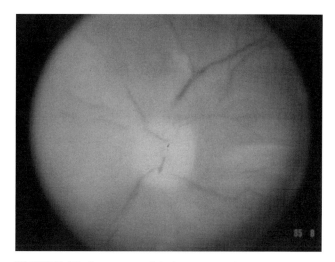

FIGURE 23–8 Acute ophthalmic artery obstruction secondary to mucormycosis. Intense opacification of the retina is present and a cherry-red spot is absent. The visual acuity was no light perception.

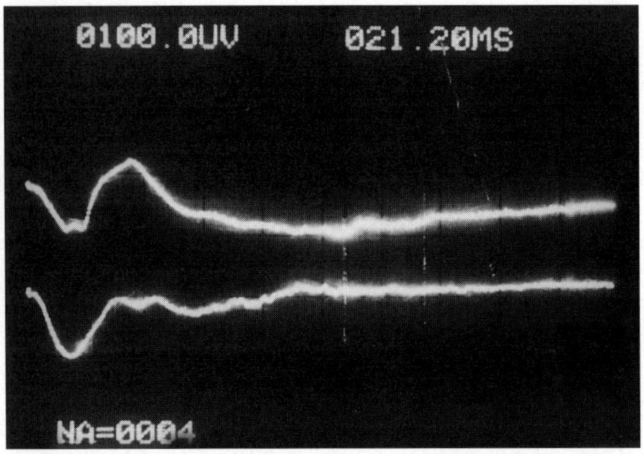

FIGURE 23–9 Electroretinographic tracing from an eye with a central retinal artery obstruction (*bottom tracing*) demonstrates diminished amplitude of the b-wave due to inner layer retinal ischemia. The amplitude of the a-wave is normal. The unaffected opposite eye (*top tracing*) shows a- and b-waves of normal amplitude.

Systemic Associations and Etiology

In many instances it is impossible to ascertain the exact pathophysiologic process responsible for a central retinal artery obstruction. Those that probably account for the majority of cases include the following:

Emboli[4–7,10,23]
Intraluminal thrombosis[12]
Hemorrhage under an atherosclerotic plaque[12,24]
Vasculitis[4,6,7,23]
Spasm[4,25–27]
Circulatory collapse[6]
Dissecting aneurysm[28]
Hypertensive arterial necrosis[29]

A consideration of the causes of central retinal artery obstruction is intimately related to the associated systemic abnormalities. Systemic arterial hypertension is found in about two thirds of patients with central retinal artery obstruction and diabetes mellitus is present in approximately one fourth.[5] Cardiac valvular disease is also present in about one fourth.[5,23] Carotid atherosclerosis, in the form of an ipsilateral plaque or stenosis, is seen in 45% of cases. In about 20% of cases the stenosis is 60% or greater.[30]

Systemic and ocular abnormalities that have been associated with retinal arterial obstruction are listed in Table 23–1. The site of the pathologic process determines whether the obstruction will be a central retinal artery obstruction, ophthalmic artery obstruction, branch retinal artery obstruction, cilioretinal artery obstruction, or cotton-wool spot. In some cases there is an overlap between the mechanisms and specific disease entities that cause the blockage. It should also be noted that the list is constantly enlarging as more associations are discovered.

TABLE 23–1 Systemic and Ocular Abnormalities Associated with Retinal Arterial Obstruction

Abnormalities contributing to embolus formation
  Systematic arterial hypertension (via atherosclerotic plaque formation) [5,6]
  Carotid atherosclerosis[23,30]
  Cardiac valvular disease
    Rheumatic[5,23,30]
    Mitral valve prolapse[31,32]
  Thrombus after myocardial infarction[33]
  Cardiac myxoma[34,35]
  Tumors[36]
  Intravenous drug abuse[4,37]
  Lipid emboli
    Pancreatitis[38]
    Purtscher's retinopathy (trauma)[39]
  Loiasis[40,41]
  Radiologic studies
    Carotid angiography[42]
    Lymphangiography[43]
    Hysterosalpingography[44]
  Head and neck corticosteroid injection[45]
  Retrobulbar corticosteroids[46]
  Deep vein thrombosis (via paradoxical embolus through cardiac wall defect) (Wills Eye Hospital Retina Vascular Unit files)
Trauma (via compression, spasm, or direct vessel damage)
  Retrobulbar injection[47–50]
  Orbital fracture repair[4,51,52]
  Anesthesia[53]
  Penetrating injury[54]
  Drug- and/or alcohol-induced stupor[22,23]
  Nasal surgery[55]
Coagulopathies
  Sickle cell disease[56,57]
  Homocystinuria[58]
  Oral contraceptives[4,59]
  Platelet and factor abnormalities[4]
  Pregnancy[4]
  Lupus anticoagulants[60]
  Protein S deficiency[61,62] (also consider protein C deficiency and antithrombin III deficiency)
Ocular conditions associated with the retinal arterial obstruction
  Prepapillary arterial loops[63,64]
  Optic disc drusen[4,65]
  Increased intraocular pressure (with sickling hemoglobinopathy)[4,56]
  Toxoplasmosis[66]
  Optic neuritis[67]
Collagen vascular diseases
  Systemic lupus erythematosus[4,68,69]
  Polyarteritis nodosa[6]
  Giant cell arteritis[70]
  Wegener's granulomatosis[71]
  Liebow's lymphoid granulomatosis[72]

Table continued on opposite page

TABLE 23–1 *Continued*

        Other vasculitides
           Orbital mucormycosis[22]
           Radiation retinopathy[73]
           Behçet's disease[74]
        Miscellaneous associations
           Ventriculography[75]
           Fabry's disease[76]
           Sydenham's chorea[77]
           Migraine[4,25–27]
           Hypotension[6]
           Fibromuscular hyperplasia*
           Nasal oxymethazolone use[78]
           Lyme disease[79]

 * F. Milch, personal communication, 1985.

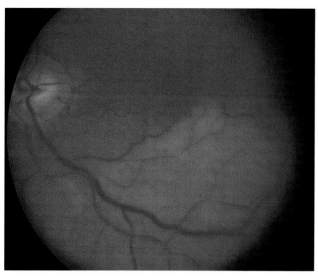

FIGURE 23–10   Branch retinal artery obstruction reveals superficial retinal whitening in the distribution of the obstructed inferotemporal branch artery.

The causes of retinal arterial obstruction in patients under the age of 30 years often differ from those found in older adults.[4] While carotid artery atherosclerosis can be seen in the thirties, it is very unusual for it to cause retinal arterial obstructive disease prior to this age. Disease entities that more commonly cause retinal arterial obstructive disease in the young include migraine, coagulation abnormalities, cardiac disorders, trauma, sickling hemoglobinopathies, and ocular abnormalities such as optic nerve drusen and prepapillary arterial loops[4] (Fig. 23–10).

The finding of a retinal arterial obstruction generally merits a complete systemic work-up to look for etiologic factors. Associated systemic abnormalities can be found in approximately 90% of affected patients.[4,5,80]

Long-term survival seems to be decreased in people with retinal arterial obstruction. Lorentzen[81] noted a survival time of 5.5 years in people with central retinal artery obstruction, as compared to an expected survival of 15.4 years in an age-matched population.

Treatment

At the same time that ocular therapy is administered, a systemic work-up should be undertaken. In particular, patients over the age of 55 years without emboli in the fundus should have an erythrocyte sedimentation rate (ESR) drawn on an urgent basis to screen for giant cell arteritis. On the Retina Vascular Unit at Wills Eye Hospital, giant cell arteritis accounts for approximately 1 to 2% of cases of retinal arterial obstruction. If the disease is suspected, aggressive treatment with systemic corticosteroids should be instituted without delay, since we have seen the second eye become involved

within hours. Unfortunately, this therapy rarely helps the vision in the affected eye.

Work in subhuman primates suggests that the retina sustains irreversible damage when the central retinal artery has been obstructed for 90 to 100 minutes.[82] While this may be the case in the experimental model, the central retinal artery is rarely completely obstructed in the human clinical situation. Additionally, in the animal model the obstruction was created at the point of entrance of the central retinal artery into the optic nerve; in the human the obstruction probably does not routinely occur at this location. Recovery of good vision has been noted to occur as long as 3 days after central retinal arterial obstruction.[83] For the above reasons, it has been recommended that ocular treatment be given if a patient with an acute central retinal artery obstruction is seen within 24 hours after the onset of visual loss.

Ocular massage can be attempted with an in-and-out movement with a Goldmann contact lens or via digital massage. In rare instances, this manipulation can dislodge an obstructing embolus. Repeated increased pressure for 10 to 15 seconds, followed by a sudden release, has been recommended.[84] The technique can produce retinal arterial dilation, theoretically improving retinal perfusion as well. Russell[85] demonstrated a 16% increase in retinal arterial diameter, probably secondary to autoregulation, when the intraocular pressure was raised to 60 mm Hg. When a sudden increase in intraocular presence was followed by a sudden decrease, ffytche and associates[86] demonstrated an 86% increase in volume of flow.

The use of an oxygen and carbon dioxide (95% oxygen, 5% carbon dioxide) mixture has been applied systemically in some cases.[87] Although higher oxygen concentrations can lead to retinal arterial vasoconstriction,[88,89] it has been shown that inspiration of 100% oxygen can, in the presence of acute central retinal artery obstruction, produce a normal PO_2 at the surface of the retina via diffusion from the choroid.[90] There is also clinical evidence to suggest that high-dose oxygen can improve visual function in eyes with central retinal artery obstruction.[91] Carbon dioxide, on the other hand, is a vasodilator and can produce increased retinal blood flow.[89] In the absence of a carbon dioxide mixture, rebreathing into a paper bag can be considered in the office.

Anterior chamber paracentesis has also been advocated for the treatment of acute central retinal artery obstruction. Augsburger and Magargal[87] found a three-gradation improvement in vision using the Snellen classification at 1 month after the acute event in eyes that initially underwent an anterior chamber paracentesis. Nevertheless, it is uncertain whether this treatment yields better vision than the natural course of the disease.[92] This maneuver causes a sudden decrease in intraocular pressure, with the hope that the perfusion pressure behind the obstruction will push on an obstructing embolus. The technique can be performed at the slit lamp using topical cocaine anesthesia with a 25-gauge or smaller needle. In general, 0.1 to 0.4 ml of aqueous is removed. Intravenous acetazolamide can also be used to induce a relatively rapid decrease in intraocular pressure.[84]

Treatment with antifibrinolytic agents has been reported.[93,94] Although data suggest that they may be of benefit in improving visual acuity, systemic complications, such as stroke, have been reported. The injection of fibrinolytic agents through the supraorbital artery has been reported to be of benefit in eyes with acute central retinal artery obstruction. Watson[95] noted improvement in about 50% of eyes treated in this fashion. The drug travels retrograde into the ophthalmic artery and allows doses in the central retinal artery that are over 100 times greater than those that would be achieved if a similar amount of drug was injected intravenously.

Other treatment modalities that have been described include a retrobulbar injection or systemic administration of vasodilators such as papaverine or tolazoline.[6] A possible pitfall with retrobulbar injection is the development of a retrobulbar hemorrhage, which could further compromise retinal arterial flow. Sublingual nitroglycerin, a potent vasodilating agent has been reported to re-establish flow in some cases.[96,97] Systemic anticoagulants have generally not been employed for the treatment of central retinal artery obstruction.[6]

BRANCH RETINAL ARTERY OBSTRUCTION

Funduscopically, a branch retinal vein obstruction appears as a localized region of superficial retinal whitening (Fig. 23–10). The whitening is most prominent in the posterior pole, along the distribution of the obstructed vessel. Areas of more intense whitening are often seen at the borders of the area of ischemia. These probably occur secondary blockage of axoplasmic flow in the nerve fiber layer as it reaches the hypoxic retina.

Among cases of acute retinal arterial obstruction, central retinal artery obstructions account for approximately 57%, branch retinal artery obstruction for 38%, and cilioretinal artery obstruction for 5%.[9] Over 90% of branch retinal artery obstructions involve the temporal retinal vessels.[9] It is unclear whether indeed the temporal arteries are more commonly affected, or whether nasal branch retinal artery obstructions are often asymptomatic.

The visual prognosis in eyes with symptomatic branch retinal artery obstruction is usually quite good unless the foveola is completely surrounded by retinal whitening. About 80% of eyes eventually improve to 20/40 or better,[4] although residual field defects generally remain.

Neovascularization of the iris occurring secondary to branch retinal artery obstruction is very rare. Occasionally, posterior segment neovascularization can arise after branch retinal artery obstruction particularly in patients with diabetes mellitus.[98,99] Artery-to-artery collateral vessels may develop in the retina and are pathognomonic for branch artery obstruction.

The causes of branch retinal arterial obstruction are similar to those seen with central retinal artery obstruction; thus, the systemic work-up is often the same. In cases in which the obstruction occurs at an arterial bifurcation, the cause is more likely to be embolic than when a vessel is obstructed elsewhere along its course.

Since the visual prognosis is substantially better with branch retinal artery obstruction than with central retinal artery obstruction, aggressive therapy is usually not undertaken unless all of the perifoveolar capillaries are involved. Laser therapy has been suggested as a mechanism of obliterating emboli,[100] but its clinical usefulness remains to be seen. Additionally, we have caused a retinal arterial embolus to move further peripherally via manipulation during a pars plana vitrectomy. Again, it is uncertain whether this technique will have clinical applicability.

COMBINED CENTRAL RETINAL ARTERY/VEIN OBSTRUCTION

Combined cental retinal artery/vein obstruction demonstrates clinical features that are common to both entities.[101,102] There is usually a history of sudden visual loss. The fundus examination (Figs. 23–11 and 23–12) discloses superficial retinal opacification with a cherry-red spot in the posterior pole, similar to that seen with acute central retinal artery obstruction. The signs suggestive of venous ob-

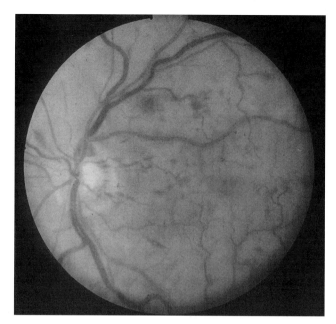

FIGURE 23–11 Combined central retinal artery/central retinal vein obstruction in the eye of a 61-year-old man. The retinal veins are dilated and tortuous, retinal hemorrhages are present, and retinal whitening with a cherry-red spot is evident in the macula.

struction often include dilated and tortuous retinal veins, retinal hemorrhages, a swollen optic disc, and marked thickening of the retina in the posterior pole.

Fluorescein angiography typically shows severe retinal capillary nonperfusion, as well as sudden termination of the midsized retinal vessels (Fig. 23–13). Despite the marked retinal thickening seen clinically in the posterior pole, there is often a minimal amount of leakage of dye into the macular area, probably because of shutdown of the retinal vessels.[102]

The visual prognosis is generally very poor in these eyes,[102] but occasionally spontaneous improvement can be seen.[103] The mean acuity is in the hand-motions range. Approximately 80% of these eyes will progress to develop rubeosis and neovascular glaucoma. This complication can develop as rapidly as 1 to 2 weeks or at greater than 1 year after the obstruction, with a median time of about 6 weeks.[102] Aggressive panretinal laser photocoagulation should be considered in an attempt to prevent neovascular glaucoma, although it can still develop after such treatment is administered.[102]

The causes of combined central retinal artery/central retinal vein obstruction are probably similar to those seen with central retinal artery obstruction. Richards[101] noted predominantly systemic diseases that cause vasculitis, although this was not the case in a larger series.[102] Retrobulbar injection can produce this entity, and probably accounts for about one fourth of cases.[102]

Although the entity has clinical features suggestive of both central retinal artery and central retinal vein obstruction, it is uncertain whether simultaneous obstructions of both vessels are necessary to induce this abnormality. A similar funduscopic appearance has been produced experimentally in the subhuman primate model by occluding both vessels at their point of entrance into and exit from the retrobulbar nerve.[104] Nonetheless, complete blockage of the central retinal vein on the optic nerve

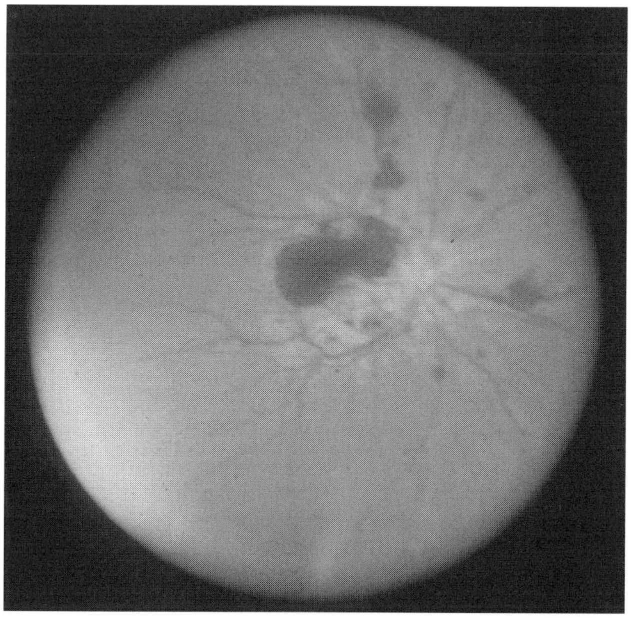

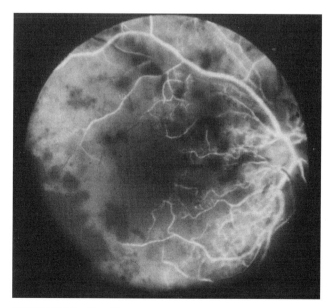

FIGURE 23–12 Equator-plus photograph showing a combined central retinal artery/central retinal vein obstruction at 1 day after cataract surgery performed with retrobulbar anesthesia.

FIGURE 23–13 Fluorescein angiogram of an eye with a combined central retinal artery/central retinal vein obstruction discloses marked retinal capillary nonperfusion and abrupt terminations of the midsized retinal vessels.

TABLE 23–2 Features Used for Distinguishing Combined Central Retinal Artery/Vein Obstruction from Aminoglycoside Toxicity

	Combined Obstruction	Aminoglycoside Toxicity
Electroretinogram	Reduced b-wave	Extinguished
Late serious retinal detachment	No	Sometimes
Retinal perforation from needle	No	Yes
Cataract formation	No	Yes

head in the same model has also reproduced this ophthalmoscopic picture.[105] At several months after the onset of visual loss, histopathologic features in the retina consistent with the hemorrhagic necrosis of central retinal vein obstruction and the inner retinal atrophy seen after central retinal artery obstruction have been demonstrated.[102]

Included in the differential diagnosis of central retinal artery/central retinal vein obstruction is the entity of aminoglycoside toxicity. This form of ischemic and hemorrhagic retinopathy was described by McDonald and associates[106] after intraocular gentamicin injection in 1986. It has since been reported in the subhuman primate model.[107] The two entities can be very difficult to differentiate clinically. Within the first day or so after ocular surgery, the fundus appearance from inadvertent aminoglycoside injection into the eye can mimic a central retinal artery obstruction; the hemorrhagic component may take longer to develop than the retinal whitening. Features that help to differentiate the two are shown in Table 23–2, above.[106,107]

CILIORETINAL ARTERY OBSTRUCTION

Cilioretinal arteries usually enter the retina from the temporal aspect of the optic disc, separate from the central retinal artery, and can been seen clinically in about 20% of eyes. Fluorescein angiographically, they are visible in approximately 32% of eyes.[108] In a normal fluorescein angiographic sequence the usually fill concomitantly with the choroidal circulation, about 1 to 2 seconds before filling of the retinal arteries.

Ophthalmoscopically, a cilioretinal artery obstruction appears as an area of superficial retinal whitening along with course of the vessel. Three clinical variants have been described[109]: (1) isolated cilioretinal artery obstruction, (2) cilioretinal artery obstruction associated with central retinal vein obstruction, and (3) cilioretinal artery obstruction associated with anterior ischemic optic neuropathy.

Isolated cilioretinal artery obstruction (Fig. 23–14) usually has good visual prognosis.[109] Ninety per cent of affected eyes improve to 20/40 or better vision, with 60% returning to 20/20. Even when the papillomacular bundle is severely damaged, the eye has potentially excellent vision, presumably due to intact superior and inferior nerve fiber layer bundles that course above and below to supply the fovea. This variant accounts for greater than 40% of eyes with cilioretinal artery obstruction.

Cilioretinal artery obstruction in conjunction with central retinal vein obstruction (Fig. 23–15) also comprises just greater than 40% of cases of cilioretinal artery obstruction.[109] The venous obstruction are generally nonischemic, and therefore do not usually lead to rubeosis iridis and neovascular glaucoma.[109,111] It is possible, however, that a cilioretinal artery obstruction is difficult to detect in the presence of an ischemic central retinal vein obstruction, causing the incidence of rubeosis iridis to be

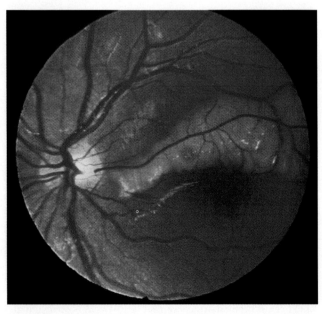

FIGURE 23–14 Isolated cilioretinal artery obstruction. The visual acuity returned to 20/20 in this eye.

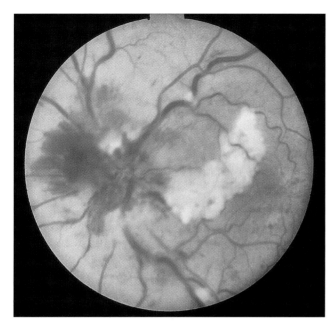

FIGURE 23–15 Cilioretinal artery obstruction in association with a central retinal vein obstruction.

falsely low in this subgroup with cilioretinal artery obstruction. Approximately 70% of eyes achieve 20/40 or better vision,[109] with the venous obstructive component probably accounting for the greatest degree of visual loss. From the venous point of view, Fong and associates[112] have noted that 5% of patients with central retinal vein obstruction also have a cilioretinal artery obstruction. The reasons for the association of cilioretinal artery obstruction with central retinal obstruction are unclear. Reduced hydrostatic pressure in the cilioretinal artery, as compared to the central retinal artery, may predispose the cilioretinal artery to stasis and thrombosis in the setting of increased hydrostatic pressure within the retinal venous system.[110,111] Additionally, swelling of the optic disc may compromise the cross-sectional area of the cilioretinal artery and lead to reduced flow. According to Poiseuille's law, the flow within a blood vessel is proportional to the fourth power of the radius of the vessel. Thus, flow within a vessel with twice the radius of a second vessel will be 16 times that within the smaller vessel.

In the group of eyes with cilioretinal artery obstruction in association with anterior ischemic optic neuropathy the visual prognosis is typically quite poor (20/400 to no light perception), primarily due to the optic nerve damage.[109] Hyperemic or pale swelling of the optic disc is seen in conjunction with superficial retinal whitening along the course of the obstructed cilioretinal artery. Acute pale swelling of the optic disc is suggestive of the giant cell arteritis as the underlying cause, and is usually associated with more severe visual loss than hyperemic swelling. It is not surprising that cilioretinal artery obstruction and anterior ischemic optic neuropathy occur together, since both appear to be

manifestations of posterior ciliary insufficiency.[113,114] This variant comprises approximately 15% of all cilioretinal artery obstructions.[109]

The systemic work-up for causes of cilioretinal artery obstruction is similar to that for central retinal artery obstruction. An extensive work-up for embolic sources is probably not indicated, however, for cases associated with central retinal vein obstruction. Ocular treatment is generally not given for isolated cilioretinal artery obstruction or cilioretinal artery obstruction associated with central retinal vein obstruction. For cases associated with anterior ischemic optic neuropathy, the possibility of underlying giant cell arthritis as a cause should be investigated.

COTTON-WOOL SPOTS

A cotton-wool spot, or soft exudate, is a yellow-white lesion in the superficial retina that usually occupies an area less than one fourth that of the optic disc. A cotton-wool spot can occur singly or in conjunction with many others (Figs. 23–16). Fluorescein angiographically, these lesions correspond to focal areas of retinal capillary nonperfusion (Fig. 23–17). In some cases they are bordered by microaneurysmal abnormalities.

A cotton-wool spot is believed to develop secondary to obstruction of a retinal arteriole and resultant ischemia.[115,116] The focal hypoxia leads to blockage of axoplasmic flow within the nerve fiber layer of the retina, with the subsequent deposition of intra-axonal organelles.[117] Light microscopy of a cotton-wool spot reveals cytoid bodies, cellular ap-

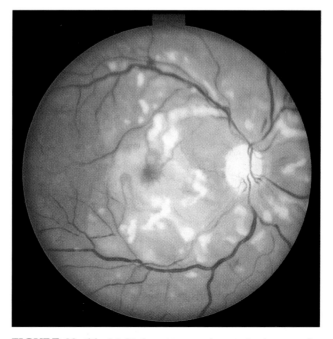

FIGURE 23–16 Multiple cotton-wool spots in the eye of a patient with systemic lupus erythematosus.

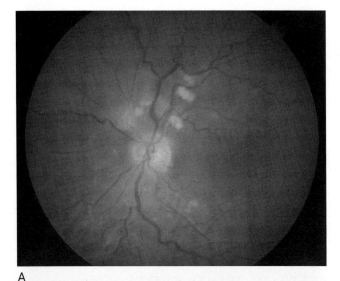

A

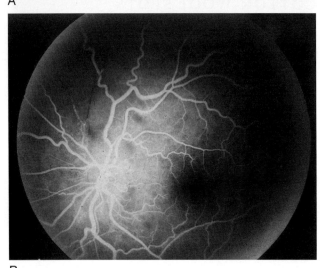

B

FIGURE 23–17   A, Multiple cotton-wool spots, as well as a superonasal retinal artery obstruction in the eye of a patient with metastatic carcinoma. B, Fluorescein angiogram corresponding to A reveals areas of hypofluorescence corresponding to the cotton-wool spots.

pearing bodies with a "pseudonucleus," within the nerve fiber layer. Transmission electron microscopy has shown that cytoid bodies are composed largely of mitochondria, and that they appear to have a major lipid component.[119]

Cotton-wool spots usually do not cause visual loss, but many patients relate a history of seeing "spots" in their visual field. Most resolve within 5 to 7 weeks,[119] although in diabetics they can remain for longer periods of time.[120]

Diabetes mellitus is the most common cause of cotton-wool spots. When known diabetics are excluded, the most common causes of a fundus appearance in which there is a predominance of cotton-wool spots or a single cotton-wool spot are undiscovered diabetic retinopathy (20% of cases) and systemic arterial hypertension (20% of cases).[119]

An increasing cause of cotton-wool spots is the

acquired immunodeficiency syndrome (AIDS). Clinically, cotton-wool spots have been observed in as many as 50% of AIDS patients.[121] In an autopsy group the figure was 71%,[122] suggesting that the true incidence may be higher than seen on clinical examination. The suggestion has been made that the deposition of immune complexes in retinal blood vessels are responsible for the formation of cotton-wool spots in AIDS patients.[123,124]

The finding of even one cotton-wool spot in a nondiabetic patient with an otherwise normal fundus examination necessitates a systemic work-up for possible etiologies. In approximately 95% of cases, a serious underlying systemic disorder can be found.[119] The blood pressure should be measured very soon after noting such a fundus finding, since cotton-wool spots rarely develop unless the diastolic pressure is at least 110 to 115 mm Hg.

In theory, almost any abnormality that can cause an obstruction of the central retinal artery or a branch retinal artery (see "Central Retinal Artery

TABLE 23–3   Abnormalities Associated with Cotton-Wool Spots in the Fundus

Diabetic retinopathy
Systemic arterial hypertension
Collagen vascular disease
   Systemic lupus erythematosus
   Dermatomyositis
   Polyarteritis nodosa
   Scleroderma
   Giant cell arteritis
Cardiac valvular disease
   Mitral valve prolapse
   Rheumatic heart disease
   Endocarditis
Acquired immunodeficiency syndrome (AIDS)
Central and branch retinal vein obstruction
Partial central retinal artery obstruction
Leukemia
Trauma
Radiation retinopathy
Metastatic carcinoma
Leptospirosis
Rocky Mountain spotted fever
High-altitude retinopathy
Severe anemia
Acute blood loss
Papilledema
Papillitis
Carotid artery atherosclerosis
Dysproteinemias
Septicemia
Aortic arch syndrome (pulseless disease)
Intravenous drug abuse
Acute pancreatitis
Onchocerciasis
Systemic interferon alfa administration

Obstruction'') could also cause a cotton-wool spot. A list of many of the abnormalities that have been associated with cotton-wool spots is shown in Table 23–3.

REFERENCES

1. Von Graefe A: Ueber Embolie der arteria centralis retinae als Urscahe plotzlicher Erblingdung. Arch Ophthalmol 5:136–157, 1859.
2. Knapp H: Embolism of a branch of the retinal artery with hemorrhage infraretus in the retina. Arch Ophthalmol 1:64–84, 1869.
3. Duke-Elder S, Dobree H: System of Ophthalmology, Vol 10. St Louis, CV Mosby Co, 1967, pp 66–97.
4. Brown GC, Magargal LE, Shields JA, et al: Retinal arterial obstruction in children and young adults. Ophthalmology 88:18–25, 1981.
5. Brown GC, Magargal LE: Central retinal artery obstruction and visual acuity. Ophthalmology 89:14–19, 1982.
6. Gold D: Retinal arterial occlusion. Trans Am Acad Ophthalmol Otolaryngol 83:392–408, 1977.
7. Karjalainen K: Occlusion of the central retinal artery and retinal branch arterioles. Acta Ophthalmol Suppl 109:5–96, 1971.
8. Brown GC, Shields JA: Amaurosis fugax secondary to presumed cavernous hemangioma of the orbit. Ann Ophthalmol 13:1205–1209, 1981.
9. Brown GC, Shields JA: Cilioretinal arteries and retinal arterial occlusion. Arch Ophthalmol 97:84–92, 1979.
10. Savino PJ, Glaser JS, Cassady J: Retinal stroke. Is the patient at risk? Arch Ophthalmol 95:1185–1189, 1977.
11. Sivalingam A, Brown GC, Magargal LE, Menduke H: The ocular ischemic syndrome II. Mortality and morbidity. Int Ophthalmol 13:187–191, 1989.
12. Perraut LE, Zimmerman LE: The occurrence of glaucoma following occlusion of the central retinal artery. A clinicopathologic report of six cases with a review of the literature. Arch Ophthalmol 61:845–865, 1959.
13. Hayreh SS, Podhajsky P: Ocular neovascularization with retinal vascular occlusion. II. Occurrence in central and branch retinal artery occlusion. Arch Ophthalmol 100:1585–1596, 1982.
14. Duker JS, Brown GC: Iris neovascularization associated with obstruction of the central retinal artery. Ophthalmology 95:1244–1249, 1988.
15. Duker JS, Sivalingam A, Brown GC, Reber R: A prospective study of acute central retinal artery obstruction. The incidence of secondary ocular neovascularization. Arch Ophthalmol 109:339–342, 1991.
16. Brown GC: Central retinal vein obstruction. Diagnosis and management. In Reinecke R (ed): Ophthalmology Review. Norwalk, CT, 1985, pp 65–97.
17. Magargal LE, Brown GC, Augsburger JJ, Parrish RK: Neovascular glaucoma following central retinal vein obstruction. Ophthalmology 88:1095–1011, 1981.
18. Duker JS, Brown GC: The efficacy of panretinal photocoagulation for neovascularization of the iris after central retinal artery obstruction. Ophthalmology 95:1244–1249, 1988.
19. Duker JS, Brown GC: Neovascularization of the optic disc associated with obstruction of the central retinal artery. Ophthalmology 96:87–91, 1989.
20. Brown GC, Magargal LE: The ocular ischemic syndrome. Clinical, fluorescein angiographic and carotid angiographic features. Int Ophthalmol 11:239–251, 1988.
21. David NJ, Norton EWD, Gass JD, Beauchamp J: Fluorescein angiography in central retinal artery occlusion. Arch Ophthalmol 77:619–629, 1967.
22. Brown GC, Magargal LE, Sergott R: Acute obstruction of the retinal and choroidal circulations. Ophthalmology 93:1373–1382, 1986.

23. Appen RE, Wray SH, Cogan DG: Central retinal artery occlusion. Am J Ophthalmol 79:374–381, 1975.
24. Dahrling BE: The histopathology of early central retinal artery occlusion. Arch Ophthalmol 78:506–510, 1965.
25. Graveson GS: Retinal arterial occlusion in migraine. Br Med J 2:838–840, 1949.
26. Carroll D: Retinal migraine. Headache 10:9–13, 1970.
27. Silberberg DH, Laties AM: Occlusive migraine. Trans Pa Acad Ophthalmol Otolaryngol 27:34–38, 1974.
28. Wolter JR, Hansen KD: Intimo-intimal intussusception of the central retinal artery. Am J Ophthalmol 92:486–491, 1981.
29. Leishman R: The eye in general vascular disease. Hypertension and arteriosclerosis. Br J Ophthalmol 41:641–701, 1957.
30. Shah HG, Brown GC, Goldberg RE: Digital subtraction carotid angiography and retinal arterial obstruction. Ophthalmology 92:68–732, 1985.
31. Woldoff HS, Gerber M, Desser KB, Benchimol A: Retinal vascular lesions in two patients with prolapsed mitral valve leaflets. Am J Ophthalmol 79:382–385, 1975.
32. Wilson LA, Keeling PWN, Malcolm AD, et al: Visual complications of mitral leaf prolapse. Br Med J 2:86–88, 1977.
33. Zimmerman LE: Embolism of central retinal artery secondary to myocardial infarction with mural thrombus. Arch Ophthalmol 73:822–826, 1965.
34. Jampol LM, Wong AS, Albert DM: Atrial myxoma and central retinal artery occlusion. Am J Ophthalmol 75:242–249, 1973.
35. Cogan DG, Wray SH: Vascular occlusions in the eye from cardiac myxomas. Am J Ophthalmol 80:396–403, 1975.
36. Tarkkanen A, Merenmies L, Makinen J: Embolism of the central retinal artery secondary to metastatic carcinoma. Acta Ophthalmol 51:25–33, 1973.
37. Atlee WE: Talc and cornstarch emboli in eyes of drug abusers. JAMA 219:49–51, 1972.
38. Inkeles DM, Walsh JB: Retinal fat emboli as a sequela to acute pancreatitis. Am J Ophthalmol 80:935–938, 1975.
39. Madsen PH: Traumatic retinal angiopathy (Purtscher). Ophthalmologica 1965:453–458, 1972.
40. Corrigan MJ, Hill DW: Retinal artery occlusion in loaisis. Br J Ophthalmol 52:477–470, 1968.
41. Toussaint M, David NJ: Retinopathy in generalized Loaloa filariasis. A clinicopathologic study. Arch Ophthalmol 74:470–476, 1965.
42. Carlson MR, Pilger IS, Rosenbaum AL: Central retinal artery occlusion after carotid angiography. Am J Ophthalmol 81:103–104, 1976.
43. Rasmussen KE: Retinal and cerebral fat emboli following lymphangiography with oily contrast media. Acta Radiol 10:199–202, 1970.
44. Charawanamuttu AM, Hughes-Nurse J, Hamlett JD: Retinal embolism after hysterosalpingography. Br J Ophthalmol 57:166–169, 1973.
45. Wilson RS, Havener WH, McGrew RN: Bilateral retinal artery and choriocapillaris occlusion following the injection of long acting corticosteroid suspensions in combination with other drugs. I. Clinical studies. Ophthalmology 85:967–974, 1978.
46. Ellis PP: Occlusion of the central retinal artery after retrobulbar corticosteroid injection. Am J Ophthalmol 85:352–356, 1978.
47. Klein ML, Jampol LM, Condon PI, et al: Central retinal artery occlusion without retrobulbar anesthesia. Am J Ophthalmol 93:573–577, 1981.
48. Kraushar MF, Seelenfeund MH, Freilich DB: Central retinal artery closure during orbital hemorrhage after retrobulbar injection. Trans Am Acad Ophthalmol Otolaryngol 78:65–70, 1974.
49. Sullivan KL, Brown GC, Forman AR, et al: Retrobulbar anesthesia and retinal vascular obstruction. Ophthalmology 90:373–377, 1983.
50. Roth SE, Magargal LE, Kimmel AS, et al: Central retinal artery occlusion in proliferative sickle-cell retinopathy after retrobulbar injection. Ann Ophthalmol 20:221–224, 1988.

51. Emery JM, Huff JD, Justice J Jr: Central retinal artery occlusion after blow-out fracture repair. Am J Ophthalmol 78:538–540, 1974.

52. Nicholson DH, Guzak SV Jr: Visual loss complicating repair of orbital floor fractures. Arch Ophthalmol 86:369–375, 1971.

53. Hollenhorst RW, Svien RJ, Benoit CF: Unilateral blindness occurring during anesthesia for neurosurgical operations. Arch Ophthalmol 52:819–830, 1954.

54. Brown GC, Magargal LE: Sudden occlusion of the retinal and posterior choroidal circulations in a youth. Am J Ophthalmol 88:690–693, 1979.

55. Rossazza C, Ployet MJ, Garant G, Reynaud J: Obstruction of the central retinal artery after resection-repositioning under the nasal septum mucosa. Rev Otoneuroophthalmol 49:161–162, 1977.

56. Michelson PE, Pfaffenbach D: Retinal arterial occlusion following ocular trauma in youths with sickle-trait hemoglobinopathy. Am J Ophthalmol 74:494–497, 1972.

57. Sorr EM, Goldberg RE: Traumatic central retinal artery occlusion with sickle cell trait. Am J Ophthalmol 80:648–652, 1975.

58. Wilson RS, Ruiz RS: Bilateral central retinal artery occlusion in homocystinuria. A case report. Arch Ophthalmol 82:267–268, 1969.

59. Friedman S, Golan A, Shoenfeld A, Goldman J: Acute ophthalmologic complications during the use of oral contraceptives. Contraception 10:685–692, 1974.

60. Kleiner R, Najarian LV, Schatten S, et al: Vaso-occlusive retinopathy associated with antiphospholipid antibodies (lupus anticoagulant retinopathy). Ophthalmology 96:896–904, 1989.

61. Greven CM, Weaver RG, Owen J, Slusher MM: Protein S deficiency and bilateral branch retinal artery occlusion. Ophthalmology 98:33–34, 1991.

62. Comp PC, Esmon CT: Recurrent venous thromboembolism in patients with a partial deficiency of protein S. N Engl J Med 311:1525–1528, 1984.

63. Brown GC, Magargal LE, Augsburger JJ, Shields JA: Preretinal arterial loops and retinal arterial occlusion. Am J Ophthalmol 87:646–651, 1979.

64. Degenhart W, Brown GC, Augsburger JJ, Magargal LE: Prepapillary vascular loops. Ophthalmology 88:1126–1131, 1981.

65. Purcell JJ Jr, Goldberg RE: Hyaline bodies of the optic papilla and bilateral acute vascular occlusions. Ann Ophthalmol 6:1069–1074, 1974.

66. Braunstein RA, Gass JD: Branch artery obstruction caused by acute toxoplasmosis. Arch Ophthalmol 98:512–513, 1980.

67. Brown GC, Tasman WS: Retinal arterial obstruction in association with presumed Toxocara canis neuroretinitis. Ann Ophthalmol 13:1385–1387, 1981.

68. Gold DH, Morris DA, Henkind P: Ocular findings in systemic lupus erythematosus. Br J Ophthalmol 56:800–804, 1972.

69. Wong K, Ai E, Jones JV, Young D: Visual loss as the initial symptom of systemic lupus erythematosus. Am J Ophthalmol 92:238–244, 1981.

70. Eagling EM, Sanders MD, Miller SJH: Ischaemic papillopathy. Clinical and fluorescein angiographic review of forth cases. Br J Ophthalmol 58:990–1008, 1974.

71. Artero Mora A, Serrano-Comino M, Melano A, Teus MA: Obstruction of the central artery of the retina in Wegener's granulomatosis. Med Clin (Barc) 87:736–737, 1986.

72. Saraux H, Krulik M, Laroche L: Retinal arteritis in Liebow's lymphomatoid granulomatosis. J Fr Ophthalmol 6:565–569, 1983.

73. Shulovsky LJ, Fletcher GH: Retinal and optic nerve complications in a high dose irradiation technique of ethmoid sinus and nasal cavity. Radiology 104:629–634, 1972.

74. Colvard DM, Robertson DM, O'Duffy D: The ocular manifestations of Behçet's disease. Arch Ophthalmol 95:1813–1817, 1977.

75. Keane JR: Sudden blindness after ventriculography. Bilateral retinal vascular occlusion superimposed on papilledema. Am J Ophthalmol 78:275–278, 1974.

76. Sher NA, Reiff W, Letson RD, Desnick RJ: Central retinal artery occlusion complicating Fabry's disease. Arch Ophthalmol 96:815–817, 1978.

77. Ling W, Oftedal G, Simon T: Central retinal artery occlusion in Sydenham's chorea. Am J Dis Child 118:525–527, 1969.

78. Magargal LE, Sanborn GE, Donoso LA, Gonder JR: Branch retinal artery occlusion after excessive use of nasal spray. Ann Ophthalmol 17:500–501, 1985.

79. Lightman DA, Brod RD: Branch retinal artery occlusion associated with lyme disease. Arch Ophthalmol 109:1198–1199, 1991.

80. Brown GC, Brown MM, Hiller T, et al: Cotton-wool spots. Retina 5:206–214, 1985.

81. Lorentzen SE: Occlusion of the central retinal artery. A followup. Acta Ophthalmol 47:690–703, 1969.

82. Hayreh SS, Kolder HE, Weingeist TA: Central retinal artery occlusion and retinal tolerance time. Ophthalmology 87:75–78, 1980.

83. Duker J, Brown GC: Recovery following acute obstruction of the retinal and choroidal circulations. A case history. Retina 8:257–260, 1988.

84. ffytche TJ: A rationalization of treatment of central retinal artery occlusion. Trans Ophthalmol Soc U K 94:468–479, 1974.

85. Russell RWR: Evidence for autoregulation in human retinal circulation. Lancet 2:1048–1050, 1973.

86. ffytche TJ, Bulpitt CJ, Kohner EM, et al: Effects of changes in intraocular pressure on the retinal microcirculation. Br J Ophthalmol 58:514–522, 1974.

87. Augsburger JJ, Magargal LE: Visual prognosis following treatment of acute central retinal artery obstruction. Br J Ophthalmol 64:913–917, 1980.

88. Eperon G, Johnson M, David NJ: The effect of arterial pO2 on relative retinal blood flow in monkeys. Invest Ophthalmol 13:342–352, 1975.

89. Frayser R, Hickham JB: Retinal vascular response to breathing increased carbon dioxide and oxygen concentrations. Invest Ophthalmol 3:427–431, 1964.

90. Landers MB III: Retinal oxygenation via the choroidal circulation. Trans Am Ophthalmol Soc 76:528–556, 1978.

91. Patz A: Oxygen inhalation in retinal arterial occlusion. A preliminary report. Am J Ophthalmol 40:789–795, 1955.

92. Atebara NH, Brown GC, Cater J: Efficacy of anterior chamber paracentesis and Carbogen in treating acute nonarteritic central retinal artery occlusion. Ophthalmology 102:2029–2034, 1995.

93. Leydhecker W, Krieglstein GK, Brunswig D: Indications and limitations of fibrinolytic therapy for central retinal artery occlusion. Klin Monatsbl Augenheilkd 172:43–46, 1978.

94. Schmidt D, Schumacher M, Wakhloo AK: Microcatheter urokinase infusion in central retinal artery occlusion. Am J Ophthalmol 113:429–434, 1992.

95. Watson PG: The treatment of acute central retinal artery occlusion. In Cant JS (ed): The Ocular Circulation in Health and Disease. St Louis, CV Mosby Co, 1969, pp 234–245.

96. Kuritzky S: Nitroglycerin to treat acute loss of vision. N Engl J Med 323:1428, 1990.

97. Charness ME, Liu GT: Central retinal artery occlusion in giant cell arteritis: treatment with nitroglycerin. Neurology 41:1698–1699, 1991.

98. Brown GC, Reber R: An unusual presentation of branch retinal artery obstruction in association with ocular neovascularization. Can J Ophthalmol 21:103–106, 1986.

99. Kraushar MF, Brown GC: Retinal neovascularization after branch retinal arterial obstruction. Am J Ophthalmol 104:294–296, 1987.

100. Dutton GN, Craig G: Treatment of a retinal embolus by photocoagulation. Br J Ophthalmol 73:580–581, 1989.

101. Richards RD: Simultaneous occlusion of the central retinal artery and vein. Trans Am Ophthalmol Soc 77:191–209, 1979.

102. Brown GC, Duker J, Lehman R, Eagle R Jr: Combined central retinal artery–central retinal vein obstruction. Int Ophthalmol 17:9–17, 1993.
103. Jorizzo PA, Klein ML, Shults WT, Linn ML: Visual recovery in combined central retinal artery and central retinal vein occlusion. Am J Ophthalmol 104:358–363, 1987.
104. Hayreh SS, van Heuven WAJ, Hayreh MS: Experimental retinal vascular occlusion. I. Pathogenesis of central retinal vein occlusion. Arch Ophthalmol 96:311–323, 1978.
105. Fujino T, Curtin VT, Norton EWD: Experimental central retinal vein occlusion. Arch Ophthalmol 81:395–406, 1969.
106. McDonald HR, Schatz H, Allen AW, et al: Retinal toxicity secondary to intraocular gentamicin injection. Ophthalmology 93:871–877, 1986.
107. Brown GC, Eagle RC Jr, Shakin E, et al: Retinal toxicity of intravitreal gentamicin. Arch Ophthalmol 108:1740–1744, 1990.
108. Justice J Jr, Lehmann RP: Cilioretinal arteries. A study based on review of stereo fundus photographs and fluorescein angiographic findings. Arch Ophthalmol 94:1355–1358, 1976.
109. Brown GC, Moffat K, Cruess A, et al: Cilioretinal artery obstruction. Retina 3:182–187, 1983.
110. McLeod D, Rig CP: Cilio-retinal infarction after retinal vein occlusion. Br J Ophthalmol 60:419–427, 1976.
111. Schatz H, Fong ACO, McDonald HR, et al: Cilioretinal artery occlusion in young adults with central retinal vein occlusion. Ophthalmology 98:594–601, 1991.
112. Fong ACO, Schatz H, McDonald HR, et al: Central retinal vein occlusion in young adults. Retina 12:3–11, 1992.
113. Hayreh SS: The cilio-retinal arteries. Br J Ophthalmol 47:71–89, 1963.
114. Henkind P, Charles NC, Pearson J: Histopathology of ischemic optic neuropathy. Am J Ophthalmol 69:78–90, 1970.
115. Ashton N, Henkind P: Experimental occlusion of retinal arterioles (using graded glass ballotini). Br J Ophthalmol 49:225–234, 1965.
116. Ashton N: Pathological and ultrastructural aspects of the cotton-wool spot. Proc R Soc Med 62:1271–1276, 1969.
117. McLeod D, Marshall J, Kohner EM, Bird AC: The role of axoplasmic transport in the pathogenesis of retinal cotton-wool spots. Br J Ophthalmol 61:177–191, 1977.
118. Ashton N: Pathophysiology of retinal cotton-wool spots. Br Med Bull 26:143–150, 1970.
119. Brown GC, Brown MM, Hiller T, et al: Cotton-wool spots. Retina 5:206–214, 1985.
120. Kohner EM, Dollery CT, Bulpitt CJ: Cotton-wool spots in diabetic retinopathy. Diabetes 18:691–704, 1969.
121. Freeman WR, Lerner CW, Mines JA, et al: A prospective study of the ophthalmologic findings in the acquired immune deficiency syndrome. Am J Ophthalmol 97:133–142, 1984.
122. Pepose JS, Holland GN, Nestro MS, et al: An analysis of retinal cotton-wool spots in the acquired immunodeficiency syndrome. Am J Ophthalmol 95:118–120, 1983.
123. Seilgmann M, Chess L, Fahey JL, et al: AIDS: an immunologic reevaluation. N Engl J Med 311:1286–1292, 1984.
124. Freeman WR, Helm M: Retinal and ophthalmologic manifestations of AIDS. In Ryan SJ (ed): Retina, Vol 2, Baltimore, CV Mosby Co, 1989, pp 597–615.

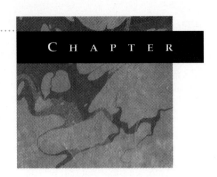

Central Retinal Vein Occlusion: A Primer and Review

Antonio P. Ciardella, M.D.

John G. Clarkson, M.D.

David R. Guyer, M.D.

Reem Z. Renno, M.D.

Lawrence A. Yannuzzi, M.D.

DEFINITION AND CLINICAL APPEARANCE

Central retinal vein occlusion (CVO) is a common retinal vascular disorder with potentially blinding complications. Following diabetic retinopathy, retinal venous occlusive disease (including both branch and central vein occlusion) is the most common retinal vascular disorder.[1] CVO is an easily diagnosed condition. Critical signs include diffuse retinal hemorrhages in all quadrants of the retina, and dilated and tortuous retinal veins. The clinical appearance varies from a few small scattered retinal hemorrhages and a few cotton-wool patches to a marked hemorrhagic appearance with both deep and superficial retinal hemorrhages, which occasionally may break through into the vitreous cavity.

The two major complications associated with CVO are persistent macular edema, and neovascular glaucoma secondary to iris neovascularization. Vitreomacular attachment may play an important role in the pathogenesis and chronicity of macular edema in CVO.[2] Macular hemorrhage or macular nonperfusion, or both, may also occur.[2] Severe visual loss may develop, including blindness, as a result of neovascular glaucoma.

PATIENT POPULATION

Most patients who develop central vein occlusion are over 50 years of age.[1] A cross-sectional study conducted at the Wilmer Ophthalmological Institute between 1980 and 1985 on 197 patients diagnosed with CVO revealed a significant increase in the prevalence of hypertension and diabetes mellitus in CVO cases, while the prevalence of cerebrovascular or cardiovascular disease was the same as in the normal population, as was overall mortality.[3] The Eye Disease Case-Control Study Group findings (1986–1990; 258 patients with CVO) reinforce the recommendations to diagnose and treat systemic hypertension and consider use of exogenous estrogens in postmenopausal women to prevent CVO.[4]

Most authors have concluded that successful treatment of these systemic conditions is not effective in the management of the ocular complications.[1] However, Trempe[5] reported that meticulous treatment of underlying medical conditions can prevent complications as well as the development of CVO in the fellow eye.

Hayreh et al analyzed data on 1108 patients (1229 eyes) and found a cumulative probability of developing a second episode of the same or a dif-

HISTOPATHOLOGICAL FEATURES

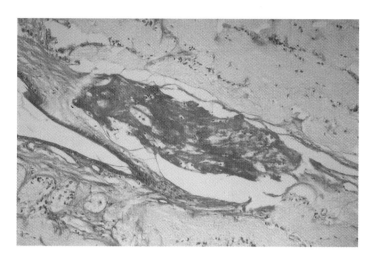

Thrombus of 24 hours' duration in the central retinal vein in the retrolaminar area of the optic nerve. (From Green WR, Chan CC, Hutchins GM, Terry JM: Central retinal vein occlusion: a prospective histopathologic study of 29 eyes in 28 cases. Retina 1:27–55, 1981, with permission.)

ferent type of retinal vein occlusion in the same eye to be 0.9% within 2 years and 2.5% within 4 years and in the fellow eye 7.7 and 11.9%, respectively.[6]

YOUNG PATIENT POPULATION

CVO can be seen in young adults and although it is occasionally associated with a systemic disease,[7] in the majority of cases it occurs in an otherwise healthy patient with no known systemic or ocular disorder. Inflammation of the central retinal vein has been proposed as a cause of the occlusion in young adults, and for that reason it has been called papillophlebitis.[8] A recent review of 17 patients aged 40 years or less with CVO[9] showed little evidence to support an inflammatory etiology or underlying vascular disease in most of the patients. An alternative explanation for the development of CVO in young patients might be congenital anomaly of the central retinal vein.

PREDISPOSING FACTORS, ETIOLOGY, DIFFERENTIAL, AND PATIENT POPULATION

Although some patients have factors predisposing them to CVO, such as glaucoma (open or narrow angle; most common associated ocular disease),[10] diabetes mellitus, hypertension, polycythemia, sickle cell trait, dysproteinemias, carotid artery insufficiency, carotid-cavernous sinus fistula, and use of oral contraceptives and diuretics, most patients have no recognizable cause for developing venous thrombosis.[11–18] Retinal venous obstruction occasionally may also occur following retrobulbar anesthesia,[19] and lung–heart transplantation.[20] CVO has also been seen in patients with ischemic optic neuropathy,[21] bilaterally as an initial manifestation of pseudotumor cerebri[22]; associated with meningeal carcinomatosis,[23] congenital anomalies of the optic disc including tilted disc,[24] and drusen of the optic nerve head[25]; in pregnancy[26]; following hepatitis B vaccination[27]; as a first manifestation of Crohn's disease[28]; and in iron deficiency anemia.[29] Other factors incriminated in venous thrombosis include hypercoagulable states such as multiple myeloma[30]; hyperhomocysteinemia[31]; factor XII deficiency[32]; antiphospholipid antibodies syndrome[33]; high lipoprotein A level[34]; and inherited plasminogen deficiency,[35] acquired protein S deficiency,[36] protein C deficiency,[37] resistance to activated protein C,[38] and essential thrombocythemia.[39] It may also be associated with systemic vasculitis diseases such as syphilis[40] and human immunodeficiency syndrome (HIV) infection.[41,42] Furthermore CVO is also associated with primary empty-sella syndrome[43] and with anorexia nervosa.[44] The Central Retinal Vein Occlusion Study Group followed 725

TABLE 24–1   Baseline Characteristics of CVOS Patients and Eyes

	No. of Patients	Percentage
Patient Characteristics (n = 711)		
Male	375	53
Age >65	406	57
White	665	94
Hypertension (on medication and/or elevated pressure)	435	61
Diabetes	52	7
Current smoker	90	13
Former smoker	277	39
Bilateral CVO at entry	3	0.4
Prior CVO nonstudy eye	38	5
Any prior vascular occlusion, nonstudy eye (CVO, BVO, BAO)	62	9
Characteristics of the Study Eye (n = 714)		
Hypertensive retinopathy	12	2
Controlled glaucoma	77	11
Myopia (2+ diopters)	71	10
Hyperopia (2+ diopters)	205	29
Visual acuity better than 20/50	209	29
Visual acuity worse than 20/200	201	28

patients with CVO for a 3-year period. Risk factors for CVO in their patient population are shown in Table 24–1.

CLINICAL TYPES

The fundus appearance in CVO reflects the degree of obstruction of all of the venous outflow from the retina (central retinal vein plus collateral vessels and not just the central retinal vein alone). In fact a patient may have complete anatomic obstruction of the central retinal vein at the level of the lamina cribrosa, with well-developed collateral venous channels and manifest only minimal funduscopic changes of venous occlusion.

CVO is of two types: ischemic/nonperfused (hemorrhagic retinopathy) and nonischemic/perfused (venous stasis retinopathy).

Ischemic CVO

Ophthalmoscopy shows the following:

1. Marked tortuosity and engorgement of the retinal vessels.
2. Extensive retinal hemorrhage involving both the peripheral retina and posterior pole and widespread capillary nonperfusion on fluorescein angiogram.
3. Multiple cotton-wool spots.
4. Severe optic disc edema and hyperemia. Often, a relative afferent pupillary defect (RAPD) is present and visual acuity at presentation is 20/200 or worse (the RAPD is helpful in differentiating the ischemic type from the

nonischemic type in both the early and the late stage of the disease).
5. Macula covered by hemorrhages, possibly showing cystoid changes (Figs. 24–1 through 24–7).

Nonischemic CVO

Nonischemic CVO is the most common type, accounting for about 75% of all cases. These are mild fundus changes, and no afferent pupillary defect is present; often, visual acuity is better than 20/200 (Figs. 24–8 through 24–11).

Patients initially exhibiting one of the lesser degrees of obstruction may subsequently progress into a more severe form. The reviewed records of 160 patients with CVO between 1980 and 1985 at the Wilmer Ophthalmological Institute showed that 9% of initial nonischemic CVO converted to the ischemic variant.[45]

Hayreh et al[46] investigated prospectively 128 patients (140 eyes) to determine the role of six routine clinical tests in the differentiation of ischemic CVO from nonischemic CVO during its early phase. There were four functional tests (visual acuity, visual fields, RAPD, and electroretinography [ERG]) and two morphologic tests (ophthalmoscopy and fluorescein fundus angiography). It was found that none of the six tests had 100% sensitivity and specificity in such a differentiation during the early acute phase, so that no one test can be considered a "gold standard." However, combined information from all six is almost always reliable. Overall, the four functional tests proved far superior to the two morphologic tests in differentiating ischemic from nonischemic CVO: RAPD was the most reliable in monocular CVO (with a normal fellow eye) followed closely by ERG; combined information

Text continued on page 296

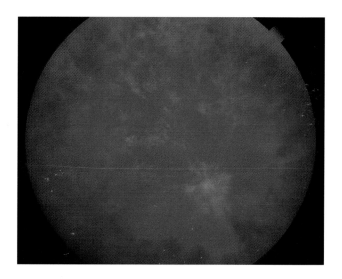

FIGURE 24–1   Clinical photograph of the right eye of a patient who experienced a CVO. Note the presence of massive intraretinal hemorrhages and optic disc swelling. This occlusion was classified in group I (indefinite). Subsequently, it evolved to a nonperfused CVO. (From Yannuzzi LA, Guyer DR, Green WR: The Retina Atlas. Philadelphia, Mosby-Year Book Inc, 1995, pp 380–387, with permission.)

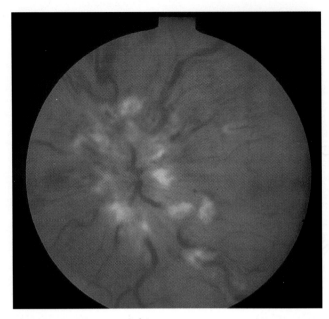

FIGURE 24–2   Clinical photograph of a nonperfused CVO. Note the presence of a swollen optic disc and multiple peripapillary cotton-wool spots, in addition to retinal hemorrhages. (From Yannuzzi LA, Guyer DR, Green WR: The Retina Atlas. Philadelphia, Mosby-Year Book Inc, 1995, pp 380–387, with permission.)

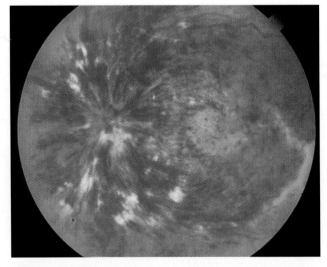

FIGURE 24–3   Clinical photograph of a patient who developed a nonperfused CVO. There are widespread hemorrhages and axoplasmic debris as well as macular edema. Note the arcuate feature of the superficial retinal hemorrhages, which follow the course of the arcuate nerve fiber layer. (From Yannuzzi LA, Guyer DR, Green WR: The Retina Atlas. Philadelphia, Mosby-Year Book Inc, 1995, pp 380–387, with permission.)

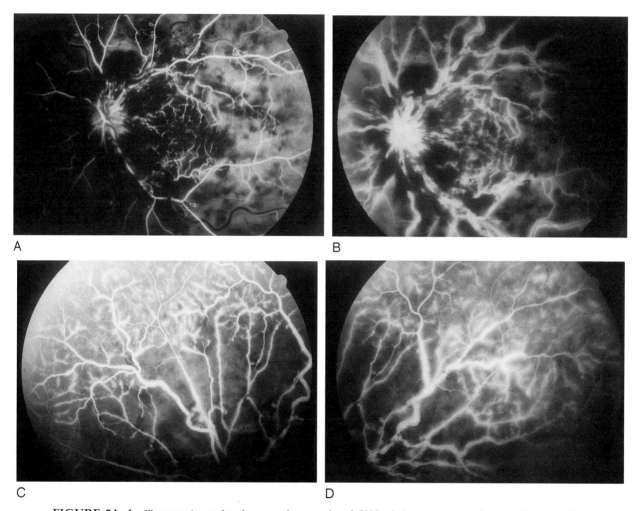

FIGURE 24–4   Fluorescein study of a case of nonperfused CVO. *A*, Arteriovenous-phase angiogram of the posterior pole showing blockage of underlying choroidal fluorescence by intraretinal hemorrhages. Note the presence of retinal vessel tortuosity and capillary nonperfusion. *B*, Late-phase angiogram of the posterior pole showing staining of the optic nerve head and of the walls of the retinal vessels. *C* and *D*, Fluorescein study of the superonasal (*C*) and superotemporal (*D*) periphery better demonstrates the presence of extensive retinal nonperfusion.

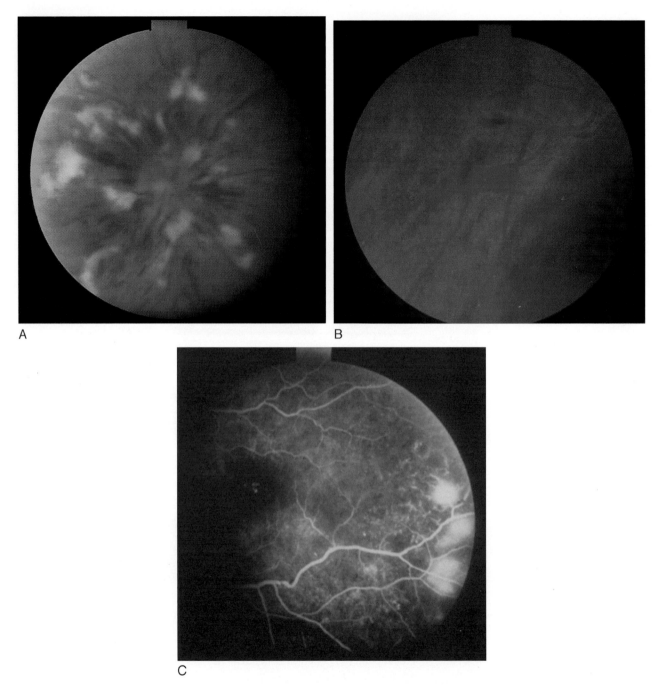

A

B

C

FIGURE 24–5   This patient had a nonperfused CVO complicated by neovascularization elsewhere (NVE) and vitreous hemorrhage. *A,* Clinical photograph of the left eye showing tortuous retinal vessels, blurred optic disc margins, flame-shaped intraretinal hemorrhages, and cotton-wool patches. *B,* Ophthalmoscopic examination a few weeks later revealed the presence of epiretinal neovascularization along the inferior temporal arcade. *C,* Fluorescein angiography confirmed the presence of retinal neovascularization. (From Yannuzzi LA, Guyer DR, Green WR: The Retina Atlas. Philadelphia, Mosby-Year Book Inc, 1995, pp 380–387, with permission.)

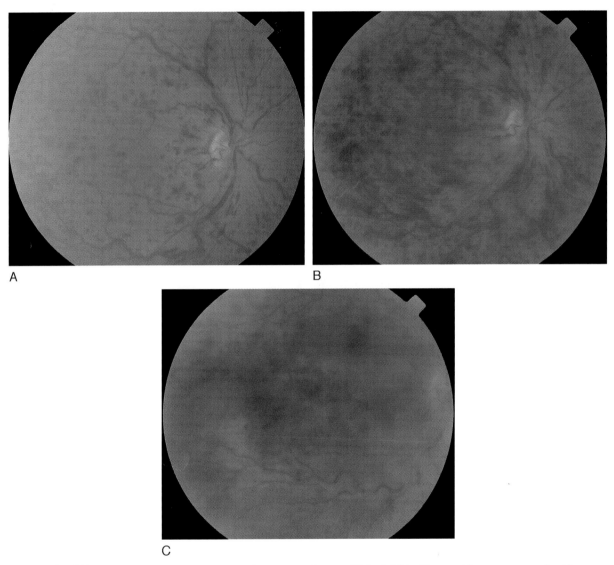

FIGURE 24–6 Progression from nonischemic to ischemic CVO. *A*, This 66-year-old man presented with nonischemic CVO in the right eye. Visual acuity was 20/50 and fundus examination revealed the presence of a CVO with mild macular edema and a few scattered hemorrhages at the posterior pole. *B*, Three weeks later, the patient complained of further decrease of vision in his right eye to the level of 20/200. There was progression of the CVO to the ischemic type. Note the presence of more diffuse intraretinal hemorrhages. *C*, The patient refused laser treatment. Eleven months later, he presented with a vitreous hemorrhage.

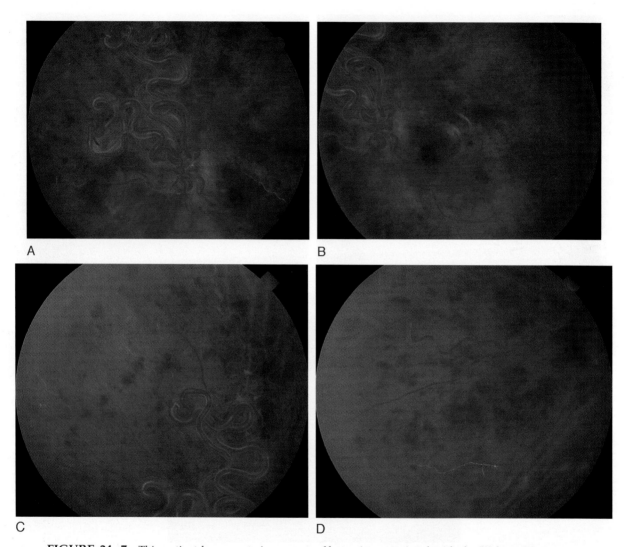

A

B

C

D

FIGURE 24–7   This patient has an arteriovenous malformation associated with the Wyburn-Mason syndrome and developed a central retinal vein occlusion. *A–D*, Clinical photographs of the left eye show a markedly dilated superonasal vein and artery. There is optic disc swelling and diffuse intraretinal hemorrhages at the posterior pole and the periphery. *E–J*, Fluorescein angiography study of the same eye reveals the presence of telangiectatic vessels in the macular region. There is also blockage secondary to the blood and capillary nonperfusion in the periphery. (From Yannuzzi LA, Guyer DR, Green WR: The Retina Atlas. Philadelphia, Mosby-Year Book Inc, 1995, pp 380–387, with permission.)

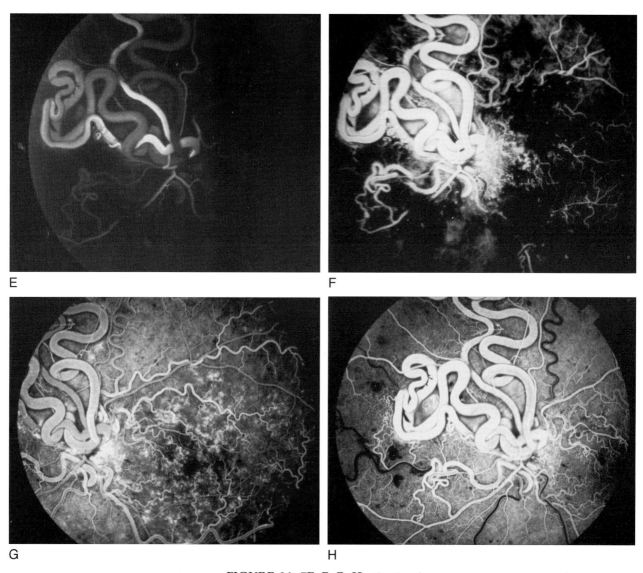

FIGURE 24–7E, F, G, H   *Continued*

Illustration continued on following page

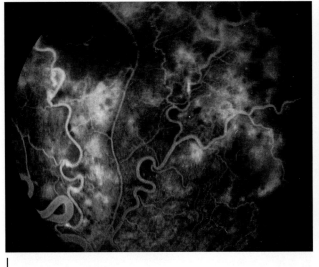
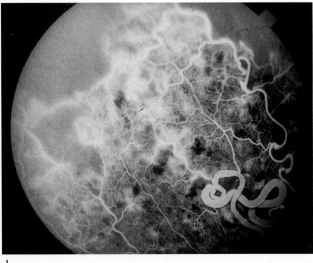

I   J

FIGURE 24–7I, J   *Continued*

from RAPD and ERG differentiated 97% of cases; perimetry was the next most reliable followed by visual acuity. The two morphologic tests performed worst; fluorescein angiography provided no information at all on retinal capillary nonperfusion (in at least one third of the eyes during the early acute phase) because of the masking effect caused by retinal hemorrhages. Ophthalmoscopic appearance is the least reliable, most misleading parameter.

HISTOLOGY AND PATHOPHYSIOLOGY

Coats was the first to suggest that almost all cases of occlusion of the central vein are caused by thrombosis.[47–49] Leber's conclusion was similar to that of Coats.[50] Both investigators agreed that the preferred site for obstruction of the central vein is in the region of the lamina cribrosa. In 1923, Scheerer[51,52] made a thorough study of the histologic changes leading to the obstruction of the central vein, and also investigated the normal condition in the region of the lamina cribrosa. He found that both the central retinal artery and vein have their own and distinct tunic of connective tissue in the optic nerve, whereas both vessels share the same connective sheath in the lamina cribrosa. Normally, in this area there is no connective tissue between the vessels, and the walls of the vessels touch one another. Here the lumen of each vessel may be round or the vein may be flattened against the artery. Behind the lamina cribrosa the vessels are more independent of one another and the lumen of each vessel is round. He found the thickness of the walls of the vessels in the region of the lamina on the average to be not more than 20 to 26 μm for

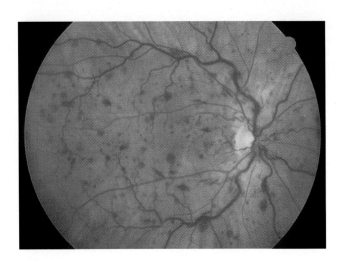

FIGURE 24–8   Clinical photograph of the right eye of a patient with perfused CVO. Note the presence of dilated and tortuous retinal veins and intraretinal hemorrhages. (From Yannuzzi LA, Guyer DR, Green WR: The Retina Atlas. Philadelphia, Mosby-Year Book Inc, 1995, pp 380–387, with permission.)

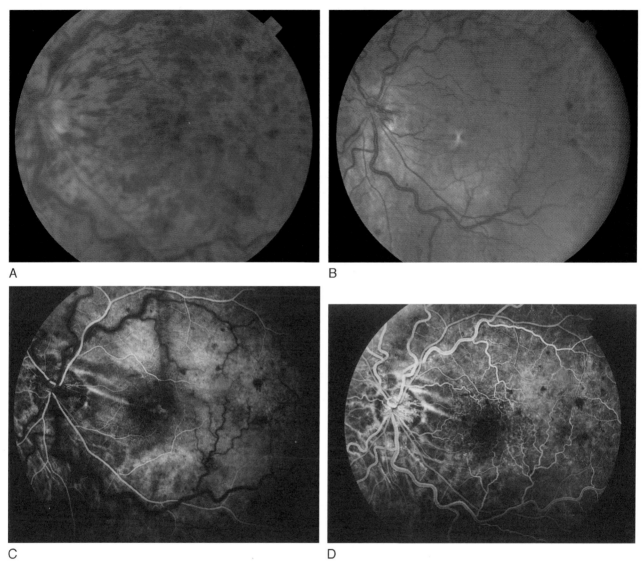

FIGURE 24–9 Natural course of a perfused CVO. *A*, Clinical photograph of an acute CVO. Note the presence of dilated retinal veins and intraretinal hemorrhages. Visual acuity at that time was 20/50 in the left eye. *B*, Clinical photograph of the same eye 16 months later. There was almost complete resolution of retinal hemorrhages and persistence of dilated retinal veins. Note also the presence of retinochoroidal anastomosis at the disc. A light reflex is present over the macula. Visual acuity was improved to the level of 20/ 30. *C*, Early-phase fluorescein study reveals the presence of chorioretinal folds around the disc. Note the lack of filling of the retinochoroidal collaterals at this time of the study. *D*, Late-phase fluorescein angiogram shows presence of telangiectatic capillaries temporally. The anastomotic capillaries at the disc are now filled with dye. Differently from neovascularization of the disc (NVD), they do not leak dye.

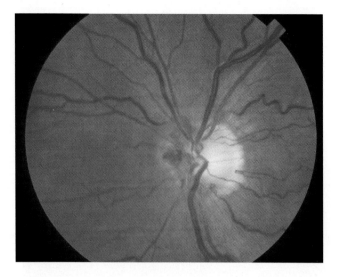

FIGURE 24–10   Clinical photograph of a patient who developed compensatory retinochoroidal anastomosis at the disc following a CVO. Note the similarity of the anastomotic capillaries with NVD. On fluorescein angiography these compensatory vessels perfuse slowly, and do not leak. (From Yannuzzi LA, Guyer DR, Green WR: The Retina Atlas. Philadelphia, Mosby-Year Book Inc, 1995, pp 380–387, with permission.)

the artery and 10 to 13 μm for the vein. He came to the conclusion that in arteriosclerotic disease sclerotic changes occur in the walls of the central vessels in the lamina cribrosa—they cause the artery to be hard and unyielding and the connective tissue surrounding the vessels to increase in thickness. The space occupied by the vein becomes less and less and the vein is compressed until the endothelial layers come in contact with one another. At this point the turbulent flow in the constricted central retinal vein may cause the formation of a thrombus.

Green and co-workers[53] studied 29 eyes with CVO and documented thrombosis of the central retinal vein in the area of the lamina cribrosa as a constant pathologic finding (Fig. 24–12).

In the end-artery system of the retina, venous occlusion causes an elevation of venous and capillary pressure and stagnation of the blood flow. This stagnation results in hypoxia of the retina drained by the obstructed vein. The hypoxia, in turn, results in damage to the capillary endothelial cells leading to extravasation of blood constituents into the extracellular space. The extracellular pressure is consequently increased, causing further stagnation of the circulation and hypoxia leading to a vicious circle.

The visual defects and retinal damage produced

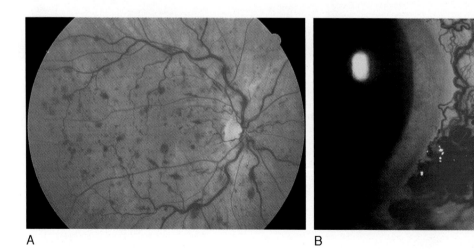

A   B

FIGURE 24–11   *A,* This patient has intraretinal hemorrhages and tortuous vessels. *B,* The same patient also has dilated conjunctival vessels due to a carotid cavernous fistula. Carotid cavernous fistula should be considered in the differential diagnosis of central retinal vein occlusion. (Courtesy of Robert Hammond. From Yananuzzi LA, Guyer DR, Green WR: The Retina Atlas. Philadelphia, Mosby-Year Book Inc, 1995, pp 380–387, with permission.)

by venous obstruction depend primarily on the rapidity of its development, the degree of obstruction, and the availability of collateral pathways of venous outflow. If the degree of obstruction is mild, capillary endothelial damage is minimal and leakage of serous exudation and extravasation of erythrocytes into the retina may be unassociated with significant ischemic damage to the retina. Complete resolution of the fundus changes and return of the retinal function may occur following venous recanalization and the establishment of collateral venous channels. Opticociliary venous collateral vessels at the optic disc indicate that blood is being shunted from the retinal circulation to the lower pressure choroidal circulation to leave the eye by the vortex veins. Opticociliary shunts are derived from dilation of normal vascular channels on the optic disc and their appearance indicates that obstruction has probably been present for some time.[54,55]

With moderate venous obstruction, the degree of retinal hemorrhage, exudation, and ischemia is greater. Following restoration of normal venous pressure, the retina may remain edematous secondary to prolonged or permanent damage to the retinal capillary endothelium. If the degree of venous obstruction is greater, hemorrhagic infarction of the retina causes extensive loss of the retinal capillary bed and postischemic cystoid degenerative and atrophic changes that remain after restoration of the normal venous pressure. Exudative neurosensory detachment has been described as a potential complication of CVO.[56]

Permanent macular changes include chronic macular edema (CME) with or without evidence of cystic degeneration, an inner lamellar macular hole, a full-thickness macular hole, retinal pigment epithelium (RPE) atrophy and proliferation caused by dissection of blood beneath the retina during the acute phase of the disease, epiretinal membrane formation, and traction detachment of the macula. For uncertain reasons, proliferative retinopathy occurs less frequently after central than after branch retinal vein occlusion.[57-59]

Complete posterior vitreous detachment (PVD) may protect against retinal or optic disc neovascularization in eyes with severe CVO. Vitreomacular attachment may cause persistent macular edema in eyes with mild CVO.[60,61] The result of a retrospective study of the relationship between the vitreous condition and the development of retinal or optic

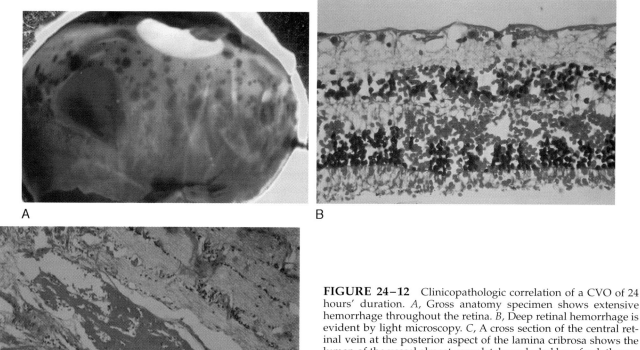

A

B

C

FIGURE 24–12 Clinicopathologic correlation of a CVO of 24 hours' duration. *A,* Gross anatomy specimen shows extensive hemorrhage throughout the retina. *B,* Deep retinal hemorrhage is evident by light microscopy. *C,* A cross section of the central retinal vein at the posterior aspect of the lamina cribrosa shows the lumen of the vessel almost completely occluded by a fresh thrombus. (From Green WR, Chan CC, Hutchins GM, Terry JM: Central retinal vein occlusion: a prospective histopathologic study of 29 eyes in 28 cases. Retina 1:27–55, 1981, with permission.)

disc neovascularization in 60 eyes with CVO associated with extensive retinal ischemia suggests that CVO may induce the development of PVD, and that PVD may play a role in protecting eyes with CVO from posterior segment neovascularization.[62]

Vascular endothelial growth factor (VEGF) plays a major part in mediating active intraocular neovascularization in patients with ischemic retinal disease, including CVO.[63,64] Also, the increase in insulin-like growth factor I (IGH-I) in the vitreous may play an important role in the development and pathogenesis of proliferative retinal disease.[65]

The role of associated arterial disease in CVO pathogenesis remains controversial, but as the central retinal artery and vein share a common sheath within the optic nerve, thickening and hypertrophy of the artery is likely to compromise the venous diameter, leading to obstruction.[66]

A combination of CVO and cilioretinal artery obstruction has been reported by several investigations.[67-72] Since the perfusion pressure in the choroidal circulation (and consequently in the cilioretinal artery) is inferior to the perfusion pressure in the retinal artery, an increase in the resistance to the outflow in the capillary bed caused by vein occlusion may result in blood flow stasis and occlusion of the cilioretinal artery.

CVO can also complicate carotid-cavernous sinus fistulas,[73,74] and congenital retinal arteriovenous (AV) fistula.[75,76] It has been proposed that turbulent flow, high intravascular volume, and arteriolar pressure in the venous side of the retinal arteriovenous malformation may lead to vessel wall damage, thrombosis, and occlusion. It was suggested that compression of the central retinal vein by the mass effect of the AV malformation on the optic nerve further leads to turbulence and thrombosis.

SYMPTOMS

Patients usually present with abrupt painless loss of vision, usually unilateral, ranging from transient episodes of blurring of vision to severe loss of visual acuity that is usually less than 20/200 and frequently reduced to counting fingers or worse, along with a marked Marcus Gunn pupil (relative afferent pupillary conduction defect).

Less frequently, patients may present with a history of transient obstruction of vision, lasting a few seconds to minutes, with complete recovery to normal.

These symptoms may recur over several days to weeks followed by a decrease in vision, or by a complete recovery of normal vision without recurrent symptoms. Invariably, funduscopic evaluation typically shows scattered retinal hemorrhages in all retinal quadrants, with varying degrees of severity, usually accompanied by some dilation of the venous system. Some patients will present with redness and photophobia of the involved eye. On examination, these patients manifest ciliary injection and some dilation of normal iris vessels. This occurs usually within the first days to a few weeks after the onset of visual disturbance. It is important to recognize these changes as a manifestation of the acute process and to differentiate dilation of normal iris vessels from frank iris neovascularization (INV).

Unfortunately, some patients present with pain and evidence of iris neovascularization and neovascular glaucoma at the time of their initial examination. This usually follows a loss of vision, roughly 3 to 4 months before the onset of the pain. This clinical presentation has been called "90-day glaucoma." These eyes typically have corneal edema, high intraocular pressure, and extensive iris neovascularization.

Initial Assessment

Initial patient's evaluation should include:

1. Assessing *visual acuity* (VA).
2. Looking for *afferent pupillary defect* (RAPD).
3. High-magnification *slit lamp examination* of the iris with *undilated* pupil to detect the presence of INV, and gonioscopy to detect the presence of angle neovascularization (ANV) are recommended at the first visit and at every follow-up visit.
4. Measurement of *intraocular pressure* should be obtained because of the reported association with open angle glaucoma.
5. *Ophthalmoscopy.*

Further Assessment

Fluorescein Angiography

Wide-angle fluorescein angiography using a 60-degree fundus camera is helpful in evaluating retinal circulation and in documenting the degree of retinal nonperfusion.[1] It is important to include images of the midperipheral fundus and the posterior pole, since capillary nonperfusion is most likely to occur in these areas. In the presence of widespread confluent hemorrhages, it may not be possible to determine angiographically the extent of capillary closure.

Electroretinography

Although high-quality fluorescein angiography is useful in determining the perfusion characteristics of the retinal vasculature and the extent of retinal nonperfusion, the fluorescein angiogram cannot distinguish between ischemic viable retina and nonviable infarcted retina. The ERG is a record of the electrical activity of the retina in response to a high stimulus; it is a test of retinal function that can be used to determine the functional consequences of retinal circulatory disturbance. In diabetic retinopathy, abnormalities in the ERG have been shown to relate to the severity of retinopathy and in identifying those at high risk for development of proliferative retinopathy.[77,78] The b-wave arises in the inner nuclear layer of the retina, probably in the Müller cells, whereas the a-wave arises in the photoreceptors. Since the inner nuclear layer receives its blood supply from the inner retinal circulation, it might be expected that eyes with CVO would more likely show an effect of the b-wave than of the a-wave, which is produced by the photoreceptors that receive their blood supply from the choroid. Based upon this rationale, the b/a ratio has been measured and found to be reduced in CVO. However, loss of b-wave amplitude is not necessarily associated with irreversible loss of inner retinal functions.[79-84]

NATURAL COURSE AND PROGNOSIS

The natural course of this disorder is variable: a patient may end with a complete recovery of the vision or marked reduction of vision caused by persistent macular edema, or neovascular glaucoma leading to frank blindness.[85-92] The prognosis is related directly to the type of CVO present. There are many gradations between the perfused and nonperfused types.

Retinal microaneurisms usually develop after a CVO. Anastomotic connections between the choroidal circulation and the retinal veins, which appear as tortuous vessels at the edge of the optic disc, develop in about 50% of cases. They can be differentiated by disc neovascularization because of their larger caliber and lack of leakage on fluorescein angiography.[93]

Massive lipid exudation is rare in CVO, and when it is present it may indicate the presence of hypertriglyceridemia.[94]

Development of Iris Neovascularization, Angle Neovascularization, and Neovascular Glaucoma

The Central Vein Occlusion Study Group[45a,95-99] followed 725 patients with CVO for a 3-year period. In the first 4 months of follow-up, 81 (15%) of the 547 perfused (group P) eyes converted to nonperfused (group N). Over the next 32 months of follow-up an additional 19% of eyes were found to have converted to ischemia for a total of 34% after 3 years (Table 24–2). The development of nonperfusion or ischemia was most rapid in the first 4 months and progressed continuously throughout the entire duration of follow-up (Table 24–3 and Fig. 24–13).

INV/ANV developed in 117 (16%) of the 714 eyes. Sixty-one of the 117 eyes that developed INV/ABV were initially categorized as nonperfused (group N) or intermediate (group I), and 56 of the 117 eyes were initially categorized as perfused (group P). The strongest predictors of INV/ANV

TABLE 24–2　Central Vein Occlusion Study Eligibility and Exclusion Criteria

Eligibility Criteria
Confirmed presence of central vein occlusion (CVO)
Intraocular pressure of <30 mm Hg
Ability to obtain good-quality fundus photographs and fluorescein angiography
Willingness to sign consent form
Visual acuity light perception or better
Duration of CVO of <1 year with intraretinal hemorrhage present in all four quadrants
Study eye retina, iris, and angle free of any neovascularization

Exclusion Criteria
Previous photocoagulation for retinal vascular disease of study eye
Intercurrent eye disease that is likely to affect visual acuity over study period
Presence of any diabetic retinopathy in either eye, new or old branch arterial and/or vein occlusion in study eye, retinal neovascularization in study eye, other retinal vascular disease in study eye, or vitreous hemorrhage other than breakthrough in study eye
Presence of peripheral anterior synechia in the study eye
Patient cannot stop receiving heparin sodium and/or warfarin sodium (Coumadin) for duration of study

TABLE 24–3 Number and Proportion of Eyes Developing INV/ANV

	All Eyes	
Status	N	Number and Proportion that Developed INV/ANV
Visual acuity 20/40 or better		
No perfusion or <10 DA	200	9 (0.05)*
10 to <30	8	1
30+	0	0
Indeterminate	1	1
Visual acuity 20/50–20/200		
No perfusion or <10 DA	259	32 (0.12)
10 to <30	25	5 (0.25)
30+	7	2
Indeterminate	13	6
Visual acuity worse than 20/200		
No perfusion or <10 DA	79	15 (0.19)
10 to <30	36	9 (0.25)
30+	50	25 (0.50)
Indeterminate	36	13 (0.36)

* Proportions shown only for groups with denominators of 20 or more.

INV/ANV, iris neovascularization of at least 2 clock hours and/or angle neovascularization; DA, disc areas.

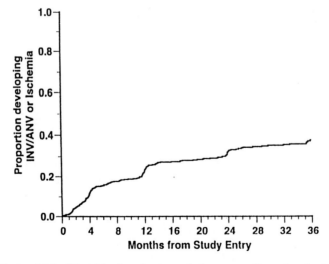

FIGURE 24–13 Kaplan-Meier life table showing cumulative proportion of patients who had developed INV/ANV by study month.

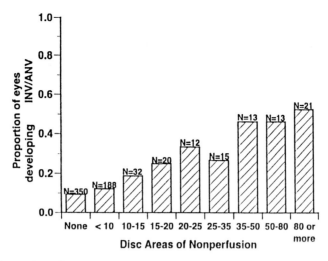

FIGURE 24–14   Proportion of patients developing INV/ANV (2 clock hours of iris neovascularization or any angle neovascularization) during study period by number of disc areas of nonperfusion measured at baseline.

were the amount of nonperfusion by fluorescein angiogram ($p < .001$) (Fig. 24–14) and the initial visual acuity ($p = .0001$) (Fig. 24–15).

MANAGEMENT FOLLOW-UP AND TREATMENT

To date there is no miracle solution to CVO, nor is there a protocol in managing patients and following them. It is widely agreed upon that laser treatment is the mainstay in managing patients with CVO. When to use laser, what groups or subgroups of CVO patients will benefit from it, when to do it,

and what type of laser are questions to be addressed by the proceedings of the CRVO study.

Recently, McAllister and Constable[100] have described the creation of laser-induced chorioretinal venous anastomosis for treatment of nonischemic CVO. In their pilot study, 24 patients with nonischemic CVO and progressive visual loss were treated, and a successful chorioretinal venous anastomosis was created in 33% of cases, with improvement in visual acuity and resolution of the funduscopic appearance of venous occlusion. Their technique consisted of creating the anastomosis with a blue-green or green argon laser, with a 50-μm spot size of 0.1-second duration and with a power level of 1.5 to 2.5 W. Several spots on the

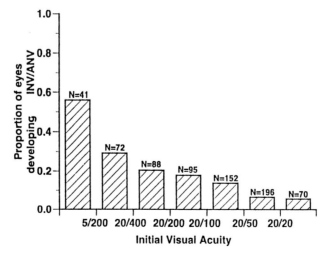

FIGURE 24–15   Proportion of patients developing INV/ANV (2 clock hours of iris neovascularization or any angle neovascularization) during study period by Snellen visual acuity measurement at baseline.

edge of the tributary vein were usually necessary to disrupt the wall of the vein and to rupture the underlying Bruch's membrane. The procedure can be complicated by total occlusion of the venous tributary, intraocular hemorrhage, and subretinal and intravitreal neovascularization.

Further study is necessary to assess the real value of this technique in CVO, and imaging of choroidal circulation may be helpful in choosing the site of treatment.

MEDICAL TREATMENT

Conventional medical treatment for vascular disease, such as anticoagulants and aspirin, has unfortunately not proven effective in treating or preventing CRVO.[101-103] Moreover, anticoagulant therapy can be associated with systemic complications and can increase the severity of intraretinal hemorrhage during the first weeks of the disease.[104] Thrombolytic agents such as streptokinase, urokinase, and more recently tissue plasminogen activator are associated with a high risk of systemic hemorrhage complications, and the beneficial effect on retinal blood flow and visual acuity may be only temporary.[105,106] There is increasing interest in substances that might decrease blood viscosity and improve microcirculatory blood flow. Among these substances, pentoxifylline[107-109] and troxerutin[110-112] have been proposed as rheologic treatments for CVO. Pentoxifylline increases erythrocyte deformability and has been reported to clinically increase the final visual acuity in patients with CVO. Troxerutin is a hemisynthetic, flavonoid derivative of rutin which, when administrated in high doses, has been shown to inhibit platelet and blood cell aggregation and increase red blood cell deformability, thereby reducing blood viscosity and improving microcirculatory flow.

Other experimental medical treatments for CVO include nasaruplase,[113] prostaglandin E$_1$, stellate ganglion block and warfarin potassium,[114] plasmapheresis,[115] hemodilution,[116-119] heparin-induced extracorporeal LDL precipitation (HELP),[120] cervicothoracic continuous epidural block,[121,122] ticlid,[123] hyperbaric oxygen treatment,[124] central retinal vein decompression surgery,[125] and Fundus-III (a composite herbal recipe for Huoxoue-Huayu or invigoration of blood circulation).[126]

However, further studies are necessary to assess the efficacy of these drugs in CVO and their effectiveness in improving the final visual acuity.

REFERENCES

1. Clarkson JG: Central retinal vein occlusion. In Ryan SJ (ed): Retina, Vol 2, Medical Retina. St Louis, CV Mosby Co, 1989.
2. Kado MI, Jalkh AE, Toshida A, et al: Vitreous changes and macular edema in the central retinal vein occlusion. Ophthalmol Surg 21(8):544–549, 1990.
3. Elman MG, Bhatt AK, Quinlan PM, Enger C: The risk for systemic vascular diseases and mortality in patient with central retinal vein occlusion. Ophthalmology 97(11):1543–1548, 1990.
4. The Eye Disease Case-Control Study Group: Risk factors for central retinal vein occlusion. Arch Ophthalmol 114(5):545–554, 1996.
5. Trempe CL: Central retinal vein occlusion: prevention of rubeosis iridis by proper medical management. Symposium on Central Vein Occlusion, 10th Annual Macula Society Meeting, June 26, 1987, Cannes, France.
6. Hayreh SS, Zimmerman MB, Poldhajsky P: Incidence of various types of retinal vein occlusion and their recurrence and demographic characteristics. Am J Ophthalmol 117(4):429–441, 1994.
7. Giuffre G, Randazzo Papa G, Palumbo C: Central retinal vein occlusion in young people. Doc Ophthalmol 80(2):127–132, 1992.
8. Central retinal vein occlusion in young adults [published erratum appears in Surv Ophthalmol 38(1):88, 1993]. Surv Ophthalmol 37(6):393–417, 1993.
9. Walters RF, Spalton DJ: Central retinal vein occlusion in people aged 40 years or less: a review of 17 patients. Br J Ophthalmol 74(1):30–35, 1990.
10. Frucht J, Shapiro A, Merin S: Intraocular pressure in retinal vein occlusion. Br J Ophthalmol 68:26–28, 1984.
11. McGrath MA, Wechsler F, Hunyor ABL, Penny R: Systemic factors contributory to retinal vein occlusion. Arch Intern Med 138:216–220, 1978.
12. Gutman FA: Evaluation of a patient with central retinal vein occlusion. Ophthalmology 90:481, 1983.
13. Hitchings RA, Spaeth GL: Chronic retinal vein occlusion in glaucoma. Br J Ophthalmol 60:694, 1976.
14. Kohner EM, Cappin JM: Do medical conditions have an influence on central retinal vein occlusion? Proc R Soc Med 67:1052, 1974.
15. Ring CP, Pearson TC, Sanders MD, et al: Viscosity in retinal vein thrombosis. Br J Ophthalmol 60:397, 1976.
16. Slamovitis TI, Klingele TG, Burde RM, et al: Moyamoya disease with central retinal vein occlusion: case report. J Clin Neuroophthalmol 1:123, 1981.
17. Smith P, Green WR, Miller NR, et al: Central retinal vein occlusion in Reye's syndrome. Arch Ophthalmol 98:1256, 1980.
18. Stowe GC III, Zakov ZN, Albert DM: Central retinal vascular occlusion associated with oral contraceptives. Am J Ophthalmol 86:798, 1978.
19. Giuffre G, Vadala M, Manfre L: Retrobulbar anesthesia complicated by combined central retinal vein and artery occlusion and massive vitreoretinal fibrosis. Retina 15(5):439–441, 1995.
20. Allison RW, Linstrom SA, Sethi GK, Copeland JG: Central retinal vein occlusion after heart-lung transplantation. Ann Ophthalmol 25:58–63, 1993.
21. Winterkorn JM, Odel JG, Behrens MM, Hilal S: Large optic nerve with central retina artery and vein occlusion from optic neuritis/perineuritis rather than tumor. J Neuroophthalmol 14:157–159, 1994.
22. Chern S, Magargal LE, Brav SS: Bilateral central retinal vein occlusion as an initial manifestation of pseudotumor cerebri. Ann Ophthalmol 23(2):54–57, 1991.
23. Schaible ER, Golnik KC: Combined obstruction of the central retinal artery and vein associated with meningeal carcinomatosis. Arch Ophthalmol 111:1467–1468, 1993.
24. Giuffre G: Titled discs and central retinal vein occlusion. Graefes Arch Clin Exp Ophthalmol 231(1):41–42, 1993.
25. Austin JK: Optic disc drusen and associated venous stasis retinopathy. J Am Optom Assoc 66:91–95, 1995.
26. Gabsi S, Rekik R, Gritli N, et al: Occlusion of the central retinal vein in a 6 month pregnant woman. J Fr Ophthalmol 17:350–354, 1994.
27. Devin F, Roques G, Disdier P, et al: Occlusion of central retinal vein hepatitis B vaccination (Letter). Lancet 345:1625, 1996.

28. Ruby AJ, Jampol LM: Chrohn's disease and retinal vascular disease. Am J Ophthalmol 110:349–353, 1990.
29. Tashiro T, Takahashi H, Masuda H, et al: Complication of central retinal vein occlusion in iron deficiency anemia 19(3):437–42, 1990.
30. Hayasaka S, Ugomori S, Kodama T, et al: Central retinal vein occlusion in two patients with immunoglobulin G multiple myeloma associated with blood hyperviscosity. Ann Ophthalmol 25(5):191–194, 1993.
31. Wenzler EM, Rademakers AJ, Boers GH, et al: Hyperhomocysteinemia in retinal artery and retinal vein occlusion. Am J Ophthalmol 15:115(2):162–167, 1993.
32. Speicher L, Phillip W, Kunz FG: Factor XII deficiency and central retinal vein occlusion. Lancet 340:237, 1992.
33. Glacet-Bernard A, Bayani N, Chretein P: Antiphospholipid antibodies in retinal vascular occlusions. A prospective study of 75 patients. Arch Ophthalmol 112:790–795, 1994.
34. Bandello F, D'Angelo VS, Parlavecchia M, et al: Hypercoagulability and high lipoprotein (a) levels in patients with central retinal vein occlusion. Thromb Haemost 72(1):39–43, 1994.
35. Tavola A, D'Angelo SV, Bandello F, et al: Central retinal vein and branch artery occlusion associated with inherited plasminogen deficiency and high lipoprotein(a) levels: a case report. Thromb Res 80(4):327–331, 1995.
36. Prince HM, Thurlow PJ, Buchanan RC, et al: Acquired protein S deficiency in a patient with systemic lupus erythematosus causing central retinal vein thrombosis. J Clin Pathol 48(4):387–389, 1995.
37. Kruger K, Anger V: Ischemic occlusion of the central retinal vein and protein C deficiency. J Fr Ophthalmol 13(6–7):369–371, 1990.
38. Larson J, Olafsdottir E, Bauer B: Activated protein C resistance in young adults with central retinal vein occlusion. Br J Ophthalmol 80:200–202, 1996.
39. Yoshizumi MO, Townsend-Pico W: Essential thrombocythemia and central retinal vein occlusion with neovascular glaucoma. Am J Ophthalmol 121(6):728–730, 1996.
40. Primo S: Central retinal vein occlusion in a young patient with seropositive syphilis. J Am Optom Assoc 61(12):896–902, 1990.
41. Friedman SM, Margo CE: Bilateral central retinal vein occlusions in a patient with acquired immunodeficiency syndrome. Clinicopathologic correlation. Arch Ophthalmol 113(9):1184–1188, 1995.
42. Roberts SP, Haefs TM: Central retinal vein occlusion in a middle-aged man with HIV infection. Ophthalmol Vis Sci 69(7):567–569, 1992.
43. Battaglia Parodi M, Ramovecchi P, Ravalico G: Primary empty sella syndrome and central retinal vein occlusion. Ophthalmologica 209(2):106–108, 1995.
44. Shibuya Y, Hayasaka S: Central retinal vein occlusion in a patient with anorexia nervosa. Am J Ophthalmol 119(1):109–110, 1995.
45. Quinlan PM, Elman MJ, Bhatt, AK, et al: The natural course of central retinal vein occlusion. Am J Ophthalmol 110(2):118–123, 1990.
45a. The Central Retinal Vein Occlusion Study Group: Natural history and clinical management of central retinal vein occlusion. Arch Ophthalmol 115:486–491, 1997.
46. Hayreh SS, Klugman MR, Beri M, et al: Differentiation of ischemic from non-ischemic central retinal vein occlusion during the early acute phase. Graefes Arch Clin Exp Ophthalmol 228(3):201–217, 1990.
47. Coats G: A case of thrombosis of the central vein pathologically examined. Trans Ophthalmol Coc U K 24:161, 1903–1904.
48. Coats G: Der Verschluss der Zentralvene der Retina. Arch F Ophth 86:341, 1913.
49. Coats G: Discussion on retinal vascular disease: pathological aspect. Trans Ophthalmol Coc U K 33:30, 1913.
50. Leber T: Die Thrombose der Zentralvene und die Ha-

morrhagische Retinitis. In Graefe-Saemisch: Handbuch der Gesamten Augenheilkunde, Vol 7, Part 2. Leipzig, Wilhelm Engelmann, 1915, p 355.
51. Scheerer R: Ueber Veranderungen der Zentralvene bei Glaukomatosen Zustanden des Sehnervenkopfes und uber Kollateralbildung im Bereich des Vorderen des Zentralnervenstammes. Arch F Ophth 110:293, 1992.
52. Scheerer R: Die Entwickelung des verschlusses der Zentralvene. Arch F Ophthalmol 112:206, 1923.
53. Green WR, Chan CC, Hutchins GM, et al: Central retinal vein occlusion: a prospective histopathologic study of 29 eyes in 28 cases. Retina 1:27–55, 1981.
54. Masuyama Y, Kaodama Y, Matsuura Y, et al: Clinical studies on the occurrence and the pathogenesis of optociliary vein. J Clin Neuroophthalmol 10(1):1–8, 1990.
55. Anderson SF, Townsend JC, Selvin GJ, Jew RL: Congenital optociliary shunt vessels. J Am Optom Assoc 62(2):109–115, 1991.
56. Weinberg D, Jampol LM, Schatz H, Brady KD: Exudative retinal detachment following central and hemicentral retinal vein occlusions. Arch Ophthalmol 108(2):271–275, 1990.
57. Chan CC, Little HL: Infrequency of retinal neovascularization following central retinal vein occlusion. Ophthalmology 86:256, 1979.
58. Hayreh SS, Rojas P, Podhajsky P: Incidence of ocular neovascularization with retinal vein occlusion. Ophthalmology 90:488, 1983.
59. Laatikainen L, Kohner EM: Fluorescein angiography and its prognostic significance in central retinal vein occlusion. Br J Ophthalmol 60:411, 1976.
60. Hikichi T, Konno S, Trempe CL: Role of the vitreous in central retinal vein occlusion. Retina 15(5):29–33, 1995.
61. Hikichci T, Yoshide A, Konno S, Trempe CI: Role of the vitreous in central retinal vein occlusion. Nippon Ganka Gakkai Zasshi 100(1):63–68, 1996.
62. Akiba J, Kado M, Kakehashi A, Trempe CL: Role of the vitreous in posterior segment neovascularization in central retinal vein occlusion. Ophthal Surg 22(9):498–502, 1991.
63. Aiello LP, Avery RL, Arrigg PG, et al: Vascular endothelial growth factor in ocular fluid of patients with diabetic retinopathy and other retinal disorders. N Engl J Med 331(22):1480–1487, 1994.
64. Aiello LP, Northrup JM, Keyt BA, et al: Hypoxic regulation of vascular endothelial growth factor in retinal cells. Arch Ophthalmol 113(12):1538–1544, 1995.
65. Cao J, Wu L, Zhang H: Significance and detection of insulin-like growth factor I in vitreous with proliferative retinal disease by radioimmunoassay. Chung Hua Yen Ko Tsa Chih 31(2):122–125, 1995.
66. Magata T, Habuchi Y, Nakagami T: A case of central retinal vein occlusion accompanied by central retinal artery occlusion. Nippon Ganka Gakkai Zasshi 95(4):393–397, 1995.
67. Noble KG: Central retinal vein occlusion and cilioretinal artery infarction. Am J Ophthalmol 118(6):811–813, 1994.
68. Berler DR: Combined central retinal vein occlusion and cilioretinal artery occlusion associated with prolonged retinal arterial filling. Am J Ophthalmol 118(2):265, 1994.
69. Weber M, Kerrand E, Speeg-Schatz C, Flament J: X-shaped macular hemorrhage disclosing mixed occlusion of the cilioretinal artery and central retinal vein. J Fr Ophthalmol 17(2):133–137, 1994.
70. Keyser BJ, Duker JS, Brown GC, et al: Combined central retinal vein occlusion and cilioretinal artery occlusion associated with prolonged retinal arterial filling. Am J Ophthalmol 117(3):308–313, 1994.
71. Brazitikos PD, Pournaras CJ, Aumgratner A: Occlusion of a cilioretinal artery associated with occlusion of the central vein. Klin Monatsbl Augenheilkd 198(5):374–376, 1991.
72. Schatz H, Fong AC, McDonald HR, et al: Cilioretinal artery occlusion in young adults with central retinal vein occlusion. Ophthalmology 98(5):594–601, 1991.

73. Komiyama M, Yamanaka K, Nagata Y, Ishikawa H: Dural carotid-cavernous sinus fistula and central retinal vein occlusion; case report and review of the literature. Surg Neurol 34(4):255–259, 1990.

74. Schmidt D, Schumacher M: Central vein occlusion as a sequela of spontaneous arteriovenous fistula of the carotid artery to the cavernous sinus. Fortschr Ophthalmol 88(6):683–686, 1991.

75. Khairallah M, Allagui M, Chachia N: Congenital retinal arteriovenous fistula and central retinal vein occlusion. J Fr Ophthalmol 16(2):117–121, 1993.

76. Schatz H, Chang LF, Ober RR, et al: Central retinal vein occlusion associated with retinal arteriovenous malformation. Ophthalmology 100(1):24–30, 1993.

77. Bresnick GH, Korth K, Groo A, Palta M: Electroretinographic oscillatory potentials predict progression of diabetic retinopathy: preliminary report. Arch Ophthalmol 102:1307–1311, 1984.

78. Simonsen SE: The value of the oscillatory potential in selecting juvenile diabetics at risk of developing proliferative retinopathy. Metab Pediatr Ophthalmol 5:55–61, 1981.

79. Breton ME, Montzka DP, Brucker AJ, Quinn GE: Electroretinogram interpretation in central retinal vein occlusion. Ophthalmology 98(12):1837–1844, 1991.

80. Sabates R, Hirose T, McMeel JW: Electroretinography in the prognosis and classification of central retinal vein occlusion. Arch Ophthalmol 101:232, 1983.

81. Hayreh SS, Klugman RM, Podhajsky P, et al: Electroretinography in central retinal vein occlusion. Correlation of electroretinographic changes with pupillary abnormalities. Graefes Arch Clin Exp Ophthalmol 227:549, 1989.

82. Breton ME, Quinn GE, Keene SS, et al: Electroretinogram parameters at presentation as predictors of rubeosis in central retinal vein occlusion patients. Ophthalmology 96:1943, 1989.

83. Johnson MA, Marcus S, Elman MJ, et al: Neovascularization in central retinal vein occlusion: electroretinographic findings. Arch Ophthalmol 106:348, 1988.

84. Kay SB, Harding SP: Early electroretinography in unilateral central retinal vein occlusion as a predictor of rubeosis iridis. Arch Ophthalmol 106;353, 1988.

85. Elwyn H: Obstruction of central vein. In Elwyn H (ed): Diseases of the Retina. Philadelphia, The Blakinston Co, 1946.

86. The Central Vein Occlusion Study Group: Natural history and clinical management of central retinal vein occlusion. Arch Ophthalmol 115:480–491, 1997.

87. Sinclair SH, Gragoudas ES: Prognosis for rubeosis iridis following central retinal vein occlusion. Br J Ophthalmol 63:735, 1979.

88. Elman MJ, Bhatt AK, Quinlan PM, Enger C: The risk for systemic vascular diseases and mortality in patients with central retinal vein occlusion. Ophthalmology 97:1543–1548, 1990.

89. Graham EM: The investigation of patient with retinal vascular occlusion. Eye 4:464–468, 1990.

90. Johnston RL, Brucher AJ, Steinmann W, et al: Risk factors of branch retinal vein occlusion. Arch Ophthalmol 103:1831–1832, 1985.

91. Appiah AP, Trempe CL: Differences in contributory factors among hemicentral, central, and branch retinal vein occlusions. Ophthalmology 96:364–366, 1989.

92. Quinlan PM, Elman MJ, Kaur Bhatt A, et al: The natural course of central retinal vein occlusion. Am J Ophthalmol 110:118, 1990.

93. Weinberg DV, Seddon JM: Venous occlusive diseases of the retina. In Albert DM, Jakobiec FA (eds): Principles and Practice of Ophthalmology, Vol 2. Philadelphia, WB Saunders Co, 1994.

94. Brown GC: Central retinal vein obstruction with lipid exudate. Arch Ophthalmol 107:1001, 1989.

95. Central Vein Occlusion Study Group: Central vein occlusion study of photocoagulation therapy: manual of operations (Article). Online J Curr Clin Trials [serial online], 1993.

96. Central Vein Occlusion Study Group: Central vein occlusion study of photocoagulation therapy: design and baseline (Article). Online J Curr Clin Trials [serial online], 1993.

97. The Central Vein Occlusion Study Group: Baseline and early natural history report: the central vein occlusion study. Arch Ophthalmol 111:1087–1095, 1993.

98. The Central Vein Occlusion Study Group: A randomized clinical trial of early panretinal photocoagulation for ischemic central vein occlusion: The Central Vein Occlusion Study Group N report. Ophthalmology 102:1434–1444, 1995.

99. The Central Vein Occlusion Study Group: Evaluation of grid pattern photocoagulation for macular edema in central vein occlusion: the Central Vein Occlusion Group M report. Ophthalmology 102:1425–1433, 1995.

100. McAllister IL, Constable IJ: Laser-induced chorioretinal venous anastomosis for treatment of nonischemic central retinal vein occlusion. Arch Ophthalmol 113:456–462, 1995.

101. Kohner EM, Laatikainen L, Oughton J: The management of central retinal vein occlusion. Ophthalmology 90:484, 1983.

102. Laatikainen LT: Management of retinal vein occlusion. Curr Opin Ophthalmol 3:372, 1992.

103. Durand F, Delamaire M, Carre V, et al: Study of hemorheologic parameters in patients with retinal vein occlusion. Clin Haemorheol 11:533, 1991.

104. Hansen LL, Wiek J, Wiederholt M: A randomised prospective study of treatment of nonischaemic central retinal vein occlusion by isovolaemic haemodilution. Br J Ophthalmol 73:895, 1989.

105. Elman MJ, Quinlan P, Fine SL, et al: Thrombolitic therapy for central retinal vein occlusion. ARVO abstracts. Supplement to Invest Ophthalmol Vis Sci. Philadelphia, JB Lippincott, 1988, p 68.

106. Kreutzer A, Brunner R, Schaefer H, et al: Lysetherapie mit rt-PA bei patient mit Stamm-oder Zentralvenencclusion der retina. Fortschr Ophthalmol 85:511, 1988.

107. Gallasch G: Ergebnisse und Indikationsstellung Medikamentosertherapie bei Arteriellen und Venosen Gefabverschlussen der retina durch Erythroskerose. Fortschr Ophthalmol 82:102, 1985.

108. Sonkin PL, Sinclair SH, Hatchell DL: The effect of pentoxyfylline on retinal capillary blood flow velocity and whole blood viscosity. Am J Ophthalmol 115:775, 1993.

109. Lim JI, Flower RW: Pentoxifylline induced choroidal blood flow changes as determined by high speed digital ICG angiography. Invest Ophthalmol Vis Sci 34:1129, 1993.

110. Boisseau MR, Freyburger G, Busquet M, et al: Pharmacological aspects of erythrocyte aggregation. Effect of high doses of troxerutin. Clin Haemorheol 9:871, 1989.

111. Glacet-Bernard A, Coscas G, Chabanel A, et al: A randomized, double-masked study on the treatment of retinal vein occlusion with troxerutin. Am J Ophthalmol 118:421–429, 1994.

112. Glacet-Bernard A, Coscas G, Chabanel A, et al: Prognostic factors for retinal vein occlusion. A prospective study of 175 cases. Ophthalmology 103:551–560, 1996.

113. Suzuki Y, Matsumoto M, Katoh C, et al: Medical treatment for experimental retinal vein occlusion: thrombolytic effect of nasaruplase. Nippon Ganka Gakkai Zasshi 100:27–33, 1996.

114. Ota R, Okissaka S: Effects of anticoagulant therapy on retinal vein occlusion. Nippon Ganka Gakkai Zasshi 99:955–958, 1995.

115. Dodds EM, Lowder CY, Foster RE: Plasmapheresis treatment of central retinal vein occlusion in a young adult. Am J Ophthalmol 119:519–521, 1995.

116. Remky A, Wolf S, Hamid M, et al: Einfluss der Hamodilution auf die retinale Hamodynamik bei Venenastverschlussen. Ophthalmologe 91:288–292, 1994.

117. Wolf S, Arend O, Bertram B, et al: Hemodilution therapy in central retinal vein occlusion. One year result of a prospective randomized study. Graefes Arch Clin Exp Ophthalmol 232:33–39, 1994.
118. Schumman M, Hansen LL, Janknecht P, et al: Isovolamische Hamodilution bei Zentralvenenve rschlussen von patienten unter 50 jarhen. Klin Monatsbl Augenheilk 203:341–346, 1993.
119. Mach R: Izovolemicka hemodiluce: Jedna z moznosti lecby uzaveru ven sitnice. Cesk Oftalmol 49:308–312, 1993.
120. Haas A, Walzl M, Faulborn J, et al: Heparin-induzierte extracorporale LDL-Prazipitation (H.E.L.P.). Eine neue Therapiemoglichkeit bei Gefassverschlussen der Netzhatu: erste Ergebnisse. Ophthalmologe 91:283–287, 1994.
121. Yashima N, Takeshita M, Konomi I: Application of a disposable infusor to cervico-thoracic continuous epidural block for the treatment of retinal vein occlusion. Masui 43:753–757, 1994.
122. Masuda R, Yokoyama K, Kajivara K, et al: The effects of stellate ganglion block on conjunctival oxygen tension and intraocular pressure in patients with retinal vein occlusion. Masui 44:828–833, 1995.
123. Davydova NG, Mukha AI, Annamedow G: Results of the use of ticlid in the treatment of patients with post-thrombotic retinopathy. Vestn Oftalmol 108:22–24, 1992.
124. Myamoto H, Ogura Y, Honda Y: Hyperbaric oxygen treatment for macular edema after retinal vein occlusion: fluorescein angiographic findings and visual prognosis. Nippon Ganka Gakkai Zasshi 99:220–225, 1995.
125. Rodriguez A, Rodriguez FJ, Betancourt F: Presumed occlusion of posterior ciliary arteries following central retinal vein decompression surgery. Arch Ophthalmol 112:54–56, 1994.
126. Deng YP: The modality of Huoxue-Huayu in treatment of retinal vein occlusion. Chung Hua Yen Ko Tsa Chih 29:42–44, 1993.

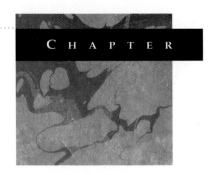

CHAPTER 25

Branch Retinal Vein Occlusion

Daniel Finkelstein, M.D.

Branch vein occlusion is a common retinal vascular disorder. Along with central vein occlusion, branch vein occlusion is second only to diabetic retinopathy as a cause of retinal vascular disturbance. Fortunately, the condition is usually unilateral, but for the 5 to 10% of patients with bilateral disease, the effect on visual function can be devastating. Prior to the Collaborative Branch Vein Occlusion Study, numerous investigators performed important pilot studies of the natural history and laser management of branch vein occlusion.[1-5] In this chapter, we will discuss the diagnosis of branch vein occlusion, as well as the laser management of perfused macular edema and the laser management for neovascularization, both of which have been proven beneficial in a multicenter randomized clinical trial. An investigative laser technique to bypass venous blockage by producing a chorioretinal anastomosis will also be mentioned. Lastly, we will summarize general recommendations for clinical management.

Branch vein occlusion always occurs at an arteriovenous crossing site when idiopathic. There are rare exceptions when a branch vein occlusion occurs associated with inflammatory disease, such as sarcoidosis, in which the vein occlusion may occur at a site other than an arteriovenous crossing site. Arteriovenous crossing sites are known to change anatomically in association with arteriosclerosis and hypertension; it has been suggested that hypertension and arteriosclerosis are risk factors,[6] but it is known that branch vein occlusion frequently occurs in those without hypertension as well.

DIAGNOSIS

Acute Phase

The diagnosis of branch vein occlusion in its acute phase, within the first 4 to 6 months of occurrence, is usually easy. Segmental intraretinal hemorrhage has its apex at approximately the location of the obstructed vein (Fig. 25–1). The hemorrhage generally follows the distribution of the obstructed venous system, but may extend somewhat beyond. Subretinal or vitreous hemorrhage during the acute phase is less common, but may occur infrequently to a mild or moderate degree. Depending upon the density of the intraretinal hemorrhage, secondary underlying retinal vascular changes may or may not be visible either with ophthalmoscopy or with fluorescein angiography. The intraretinal hemorrhage may also block view of the occlusion site itself. Cotton-wool spots may be scattered throughout the posterior aspect of the occluded segment, but are probably *not* a good indicator that widespread nonperfusion is present. Macular edema is frequently presumed when macular thickening with cystoid spaces appears. Macular thickening is frequent if the occluded vein subserves the macular circulation; macular thickening is infrequent if the vein does not subserve the macula, but rarely can occur as a distant effect[7] (Fig. 25–2). When macular thickening occurs in the acute phase of branch vein occlusion, it is essentially always with the appearance of cystoid spaces, often with layering of intraretinal hemorrhage within the cystoid spaces, with the largest cyst occurring in the center of the fovea.

Occasionally in the acute phase, in the presence of cystoid macular edema, a round yellow spot can appear in the center of the fovea that seems to have no prognostic significance with respect to visual acuity and that will fade after the first several months of the occlusion[8] (Fig. 25–3).

Chronic Phase

After the intraretinal hemorrhage has predominantly spontaneously absorbed (usually 9 to 12

HISTOPATHOLOGICAL FEATURES

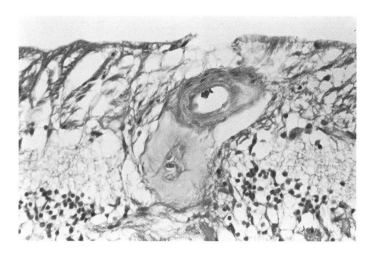

Branch vein occlusion. Area of occlusion with a single channel of recanalization of the branch of the superotemporal vein as it crosses under the arteriosclerotic artery. (From Vaghefi HA, Green WR, Kelly JS, et al: Correlation of clinicopathologic findings in a patient: congenital night blindness, branch retinal vein occlusion, cilioretinal artery drusen of the optic nerve head, and intraretinal pigmented lesion. Arch Ophthalmol 96:2097–2104, 1978. Copyright 1978, American Medical Association, with permission.)

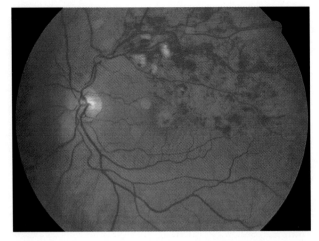

FIGURE 25–1 Photograph of an acute superotemporal branch vein occlusion.

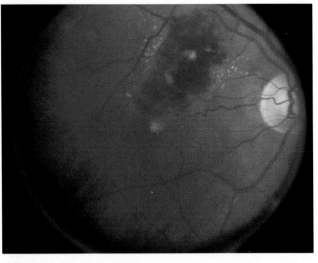

FIGURE 25–3 Photograph of an acute superotemporal branch vein occlusion with a yellow spot in the fovea.

months), as it always does, the pathognomonic picture of an acute branch vein occlusion is no longer apparent. However, underlying retinal vascular abnormalities essentially always remain and can be identified by ophthalmoscopy or fluorescein angiography. These abnormalities persist in a segmental pattern, presenting an appearance that is just as pathognomonic of a branch vein occlusion as the intraretinal hemorrhage in a segmental pattern offered for the acute phase (Fig. 25–4).

The retinal vascular abnormalities may include collateral vessels around the blockage site, collateral vessels across the temporal raphe, retinal capillary telangiectasia throughout the involved segment, and areas of capillary nonperfusion throughout the involved segment. In late phases of the fluorescein angiogram, one may identify perfused macular edema as fluorescein leakage from dilated capillaries with pooling of fluorescein dye in cystoid spaces involving the fovea and macula.

COMPLICATIONS OF BRANCH VEIN OCCLUSION

The complications of branch vein occlusion that are most common and potentially vision limiting include macular edema and retinal neovascularization. Less frequent complications, such as retinal detachment, will not be discussed here.

Perfused Macular Edema

Frequently, after there is sufficient intraretinal hemorrhage absorption such that high-quality fluorescein angiography can be obtained, it is seen that the macular capillaries are dilated if the occluded vein subserves that region. Often, the macular capillaries are dilated in a segmental pattern, but some-

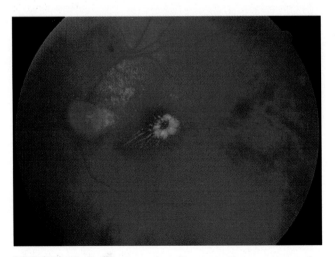

FIGURE 25–2 Photograph demonstrating a superior branch vein occlusion with a distant effect on the macula.

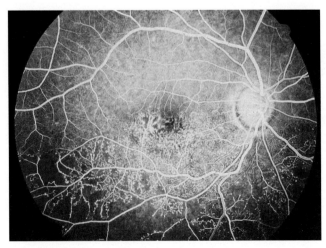

FIGURE 25–4 Fluorescein angiogram, transit phase, demonstrating inferior retinal vascular abnormalities in the chronic phase of a branch vein occlusion.

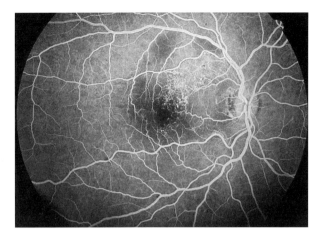

FIGURE 25-5   Fluorescein angiogram, transit phase, demonstrating segmental superior vascular dilatation involving the macula and extending beyond the drainage area to the inferior macula.

times the dilatation extends well beyond the drainage of the blocked vein, encircling the macula, for reasons that are unknown (Fig. 25–5). In the late phase of the angiogram, these dilated vessels are seen to leak fluorescein dye diffusely into cystoid spaces that may extend into the fovea (Fig. 25–6). Fluorescein accumulation in the fovea in a cystoid pattern is usually accompanied by decreased vision. It is not known why foveal edema causes decreased vision, but it is presumed that the fluid itself causes a structural change that reduces visual acuity, although other mechanisms are possible. Frequently when there is perfused macular edema and vision loss, the visual acuity will significantly improve with pinhole, but will not improve with refraction. In addition, visual acuity often is described as worse on arising in the morning and significantly improved later in the day.[9]

The Nationwide Collaborative Branch Vein Occlusion Study, a randomized clinical trial supported by the National Eye Institute, studied the natural history of vision loss from perfused macular edema. That study showed that about one third of patients with vision loss to 20/40 or worse and perfused macular edema showed improvement over the 3 years of follow-up.[10] Most other eyes with vision loss from macular edema will continue stable and a small percentage will worsen.

It is important to note that the cause of vision loss from perfused macular edema must be made carefully. One must first ascertain that there is no hemorrhage remaining in the fovea that can of itself reduce visual acuity. In addition, one must obtain high-quality fluorescein angiography that demonstrates perfused macular capillaries, without nonperfusion, and with leakage in the late phase of the angiogram extending into the center of the fovea.

Ischemic Macular Edema

Ischemic macular edema occurs when a segment of the macular circulation is nonperfused and there is no late leakage seen on the fluorescein angiogram (Fig. 25–7). Nevertheless, prominent cystoid macular edema may be *clinically* evident. It is presumed that retinal tissue ischemia results in a hypertonic environment that draws water into the tissue producing the cystoid edema. In a small pilot study that compared visual outcome in untreated perfused edema to untreated ischemic edema, the visual outcome was far better in those with ischemic edema.[11] As previously mentioned, about one third of patients with perfused edema will spontaneously improve somewhat, whereas 90% of those with ischemic edema improved somewhat.

If the macular ischemia is extensive, however, vision may be permanently reduced from the macular nonperfusion.

In some cases, there appears to be a mixture of perfused edema and ischemic edema. However,

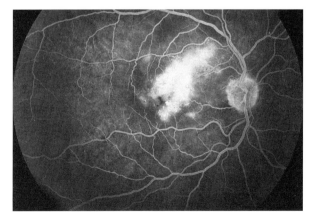

FIGURE 25-6   Fluorescein angiogram, late phase of Figure 25-5, demonstrating fluorescein dye leakage into cystoid spaces that extend into the center of the fovea.

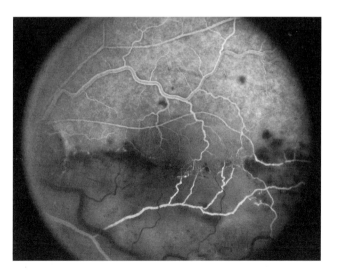

FIGURE 25-7   Fluorescein angiogram, transit phase, demonstrating inferior macular nonperfusion in an eye with *clinically* evident cystoid macular edema.

since ischemic edema usually seems to spontaneously resolve in 6 to 12 months, one may wait for the ischemic edema to resolve and then judge the potential outcome based on the remaining perfused edema.

Based upon the results of the Collaborative Branch Vein Occlusion Study, there is no evidence that cystoid macular edema in the first year produces structural damage that causes irreversible loss of vision; consequently, there is no evidence that there need be a rush in treating cystoid macular edema from branch vein occlusion in order to avoid irreparable damage.

Neovascularization as a Complication of Branch Vein Occlusion

As is the case in diabetic retinopathy and other retinal vascular disturbances associated with retinal capillary nonperfusion, retinal neovascularization from the disc and/or the peripheral retina is a common association with ischemic branch vein occlusion (Fig. 25–8). In branch vein occlusion, retinal neovascularization never occurs unless there is preceding ischemia. A segment of ischemia at least 5 disc diameters wide is required to produce retinal and/or disc neovascularization.

The diagnosis of neovascularization in branch vein occlusion can be difficult on occasion because the collaterals that form in branch vein occlusion can mimic neovascularization. When unclear, fluorescein angiography will show profuse leakage from neovascularization but no leakage or minimal staining only for collaterals.

From the Collaborative Branch Vein Occlusion Study, we know that 50% of eyes with a segment of capillary nonperfusion of 5 disc diameters or more will develop neovascularization.[12] It is interesting to note that 50% of eyes with this degree of ischemia will *not* develop neovascularization. (The

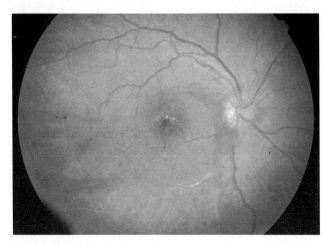

FIGURE 25–8 Photograph of neovascularization developing in association with an ischemic branch vein occlusion.

reason that some ischemic branch vein occlusions are at risk for neovascularization and that some are not at risk for neovascularization is not understood.) Of those eyes that develop neovascularization, 50% will develop vitreous hemorrhage. Other complications of neovascularization, such as traction retinal detachment, may occur as well. However, it appears unlikely that permanent and irrevocable retinal damage will occur from the consequences of branch vein occlusion neovascularization.[13]

When retinal neovascularization occurs, it is unlikely to occur in the first 4 months after a branch vein occlusion, but is most likely to begin to occur within the first year; however, neovascularization and subsequent vitreous hemorrhage can be identified as beginning even years after a branch vein occlusion.

Iris neovascularization is very unusual after a branch vein occlusion but appears to be more likely when large areas of ischemia occur or in patients with diabetes mellitus.

Neovascularization is more likely to occur in certain areas of the fundus. Such predilections occur at the optic nerve head and at the border zone between perfused and nonperfused retina. Neovascularization is unlikely to begin in normal segments of the fundus, but on those rare occasions when that circumstance occurs,[14] the neovascularization begins at arteriovenous crossing sites (Fig. 25–9).

LASER MANAGEMENT OF MACULAR EDEMA

Grid laser management of perfused macular edema has been demonstrated as useful in benefitting visual acuity when perfused macular edema has produced vision loss to 20/40 or worse that is not spontaneously improving.[10] For patients with a branch vein occlusion and visual loss to 20/40 or worse, when it is clear that vision is not spontaneously improving at successive visits and when foveal hemorrhage (i.e., a reversible cause of vision loss) has cleared, high-quality fluorescein angiography should be obtained to determine whether the cause of vision loss is from perfused macular edema. If perfused macular edema is identified on a high-quality fluorescein angiogram, one may consider the advisability of grid laser photocoagulation with the patient.

Using the fluorescein angiogram as a guide, grid laser photocoagulation is applied using a 50- or 100-μm spot at a duration of 0.1 second to produce a light to medium white burn at the level of the pigment epithelium (Fig. 25–10). The burns are placed one spot width apart. The grid treatment covers the area of the leaking capillaries and can extend as close to the fovea as the edge of the capillary-free zone and can extend as far as 2 disc diameters away from the center of the fovea. Gener-

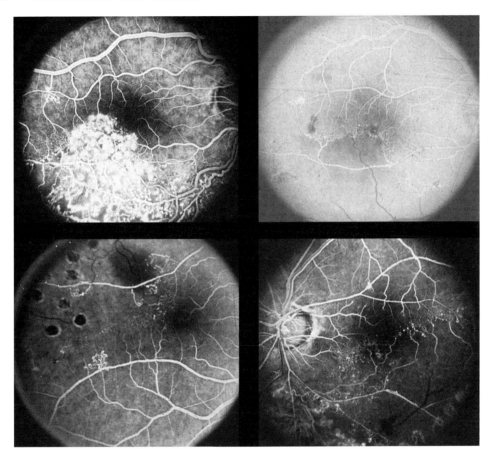

FIGURE 25-9 Composite fluorescein angiogram demonstrating development of neovascularization in a normal segment of the fundus, distant from the involved segment. Note that the neovascularization developed at arteriovenous crossing sites.

ally, the patient is re-evaluated at 2 to 4 months after the laser treatment. If the vision is improved, no action is taken. If the vision is not improved, a fluorescein angiogram is repeated; if there is continued fluorescein leakage into the fovea from vessels that are leaking and were not covered by the grid treatment on the first treatment, the grid treat-

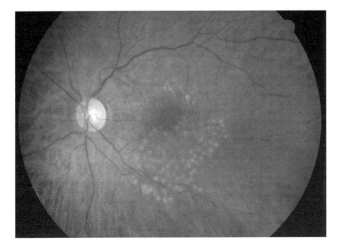

FIGURE 25-10 Photograph of grid laser photocoagulation for macular edema.

ment may be extended to the leaking area. At the first grid laser treatment, if the foveal landmarks are unclear at the laser, one may wish to remain a clearly safe distance away from the fovea and then judge treatment closer to the border of the avascular zone after a fluorescein angiogram is obtained at a future follow-up visit; in this way, a "graded" treatment can be performed with great safety, since the previous treatment spots will be visible as pigmented areas both on clinical examination and fluorescein angiography.

Although the mechanism for reducing edema and improving vision has not been established with certainty, experimental animal work has suggested that the grid laser photocoagulation may have its effect by thinning the retina, bringing retinal vessels closer to choroidal vessels, permitting the retinal vessels to constrict by autoregulation, thereby decreasing retinal blood flow and consequently decreasing edema, as one hypothesis.[15]

Before grid laser photocoagulation is performed, careful discussion with the patient is required regarding benefits and risks. It is important for the patient to understand that the average benefit to visual acuity is small, although on occasion very significant improvement can occur. The patient must understand that if the fellow eye is normal, the visual acuity improvement, if it occurs, will not be of functional significance, unless problems occur with the fellow eye, which is only likely to occur in 5 to 10% of cases. The likelihood of improvement in visual acuity is one third without laser photocoagulation and two thirds with grid photocoagulation. Even with grid photocoagulation, one third of cases will not improve at all. The risks of grid laser photocoagulation are small in experienced hands. However, scotoma formation from the laser grid photocoagulation almost always occurs, but the grid scotoma that appears immediately following the treatment in many cases often gradually fades and is visually nonsignificant after several months. However, on rare occasions, larger scotomas do occur that represent a visual handicap for the patient. Other complications, such as production of retinal fibrosis, can occur but are rare.

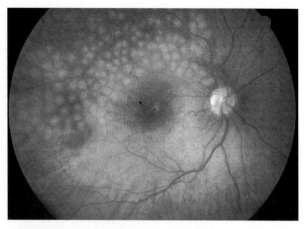

FIGURE 25–11   Photograph of scatter photocoagulation in the superotemporal quadrant as treatment for retinal neovascularization.

LASER MANAGEMENT OF RETINAL NEOVASCULARIZATION

It is recommended that laser photocoagulation in a scatter fashion be used to lessen the likelihood of vitreous hemorrhage if retinal neovascularization is developing. A prospective randomized clinical trial of laser photocoagulation for the management of neovascularization and branch vein occlusion has shown that, in the presence of 5 disc diameters in diameter of nonperfusion, scatter photocoagulation reduces the likelihood of development of neovascularization by 50% and reduces the likelihood of vitreous hemorrhage if neovascularization is already present by 50%.[12] (We know from natural history studies that the likelihood of neovascularization developing without laser treatment is 50% and the likelihood of development of vitreous hemorrhage if neovascularization is already present is 50%. Laser reduces each of these likelihoods by 50%.) It is *not* generally recommended that scatter photocoagulation be performed prior to the development of neovascularization, since one would be treating twice as many patients as need treatment; consequently, one may wait for the first sign of neovascularization and then introduce scatter photocoagulation.

Scatter photocoagulation is applied throughout the ischemic fundus area, beginning no closer to the fovea than 2 disc diameters distant and extending to the periphery, using 200- to 500-μm diameter spots at a duration of 0.1 to 0.2 second with a median white burn at the level of the pigment epithelium (Fig. 25–11). Although the mechanism of scatter photocoagulation is unknown, it is suspected that laser photocoagulation in some way changes ischemic retina to decrease the production of a diffusible angiogenesis material that causes the neovascularization.

Prior to performing scatter photocoagulation, a discussion with the patient should include careful discussion of the benefits and risks. A discussion of the risks should include the statement that scatter photocoagulation is safe in experienced hands, but could cause a decrease in the visual field being treated in some patients. Other complications can occur, but are quite rare.

Depending on the extent of the neovascularization when the scatter photocoagulation is performed, one normally re-evaluates patients in follow-up at 2 to 4 months to judge the adequacy of the photocoagulation. If the neovascularization is not lessened, further scatter photocoagulation could be considered in previously untreated ischemic zones.

HEMIRETINAL VEIN OCCLUSION

When an occlusion occurs at or near the optic nerve head, the entire superior half of the fundus or inferior half of the fundus may be involved, and that may be termed "hemiretinal vein occlusion." Such an occurrence may be a branch vein occlusion if the central retinal vein has already divided posterior to the blockage site. Under some circumstances, however, there may be two central retinal veins; the blockage of one of these at the location of the lamina cribrosa might be alternatively termed a "hemicentral retinal vein occlusion." It can be very difficult, or impossible, to determine in some cases whether a hemiretinal vein occlusion is a branch vein occlusion or a hemicentral retinal vein occlusion. No good studies have determined that there is a difference in outcome depending on whether the hemiretinal vein occlusion is a branch vein occlusion or a hemicentral retinal vein occlusion, so the clinical significance of the differentiation is not clear.

MEDICAL MANAGEMENT

Although it has been widely suggested that hypertension may play a role in precipitating branch retinal vein occlusion, it also seems clear that many, if not most, branch vein occlusions occur in persons who are systemically healthy. The average age for the appearance of a branch vein occlusion is 65, but there is a wide age distribution, with no strong evidence that differing precipitating factors are associated in younger patients.

Therapy with aspirin, Coumadin, heparin, or tissue plasminogen activator has never been shown to be beneficial in treating a branch vein occlusion or preventing a branch vein occlusion. Because of the potential complications of these therapies, they are often not recommended in the management of a branch vein occlusion.

LASER BYPASS

Recently, it was reported that a chorioretinal anastomosis can be produced by laser photocoagulation to bypass venous blockage and improve visual acuity outcome.[16] This procedure awaits further studies to confirm its benefit and demonstrate that complications can be minimized. However, the concept of bypassing the venous blockage by producing anastomosis with the choroid remains a most exciting and promising therapy for further investigation.[17,18]

SUMMARY RECOMMENDATIONS FOR MANAGEMENT OF BRANCH VEIN OCCLUSION

When a patient is first seen with an acute branch vein occlusion (seen within the first 6 months of symptoms) the patient is informed about the nature of a branch vein occlusion and that no acute management is recommended. At the second visit, 3 to 4 months later, if the vision is not improved and is 20/40 or worse, and if there is sufficient clearing of intraretinal hemorrhage to obtain high-quality fluorescein angiography, a fluorescein angiogram is obtained to judge the cause of the visual acuity loss. If the fluorescein angiogram shows perfused macular edema and the visual acuity is not spontaneously improving, grid laser photocoagulation could be considered with the patient, if there is sufficient clearing of intraretinal hemorrhage. If the fluorescein angiogram shows a large area (≥5 disc

diameters) of capillary nonperfusion, the patient should be followed every 4 months for the development of neovascularization. If neovascularization is seen, the advisability of scatter photocoagulation should be considered with the patient.

All management considerations deserve careful communication with the patient, particularly since benefits achieved are unlikely to be appreciated by the patient in this usually unilateral condition.

REFERENCES

1. Coscas G, Dhermy P: Occlusions veineuses retiniennes. Masson, 1978.
2. Orth DH, Patz A: Retinal branch vein occlusion. Surv Ophthalmol 22:357–376, 1978.
3. Gutman FA: Evaluation of vein occlusion. Ophthalmology 90:481–483, 1983.
4. Hayreh SS: Classification of central retinal vein occlusion. Ophthalmology 90:458–474, 1983.
5. Kohner EM, Laatikainen L, Oughton J: The management of central retinal vein occlusion. Ophthalmology 90:484–487, 1983.
6. Eye Disease Case Control Study Group: Risk factors for BRVO. Am J Ophthalmol 116:288–298, 1993.
7. Finkelstein D, Patz A: Distant effect of peripheral branch vein occlusion on the macula. Trans Am Ophthalmol Soc 86:380–388, 1988.
8. Finkelstein D, Patz A: Changes in the retinal pigment epithelium associated with cystoid macular edema. Trans Am Ophthalmol Soc 84:293–303, 1986.
9. Sternberg P, Fitzke F, Finkelstein D: Cyclic macular edema. Am J Ophthalmol 94:664–669, 1982.
10. Branch Vein Occlusion Study Group: Argon laser photocoagulation for macular edema and branch vein occlusion. Am J Ophthalmol 98:271–282, 1984.
11. Finkelstein D: Ischemic macular edema: recognition and favorable natural history in branch vein occlusion. Arch Ophthalmol 110:1427–1434, 1992.
12. Branch Vein Occlusion Study Group: Argon laser scatter photocoagulation for prevention of neovascularization and vitreous hemorrhage in branch vein occlusion: a randomized clinical trial. Arch Ophthalmol 104:34–41, 1986.
13. Patel A, Michels RG, Finkelstein D: BVO neovascularization: status following vitrectomy. Invest Ophthalmol Vis Sci 25(Suppl):252, 1984.
14. Finkelstein D, Clarkson J, Diddie K, et al, for the Branch Vein Occlusion Study Group: Branch vein occlusion: retinal neovascularization outside the involved segment. Ophthalmology 89:1357–1361, 1982.
15. Wilson D, Finkelstein D, Quigley H, Green W: Macular grid photocoagulation: an experimental study on the primate retina. Arch Ophthalmol 106:100–105, 1988.
16. McAllister I, Constable I: Laser-induced chorioretinal venous anastomosis for treatment of nonischemic central retinal vein occlusion. Arch Ophthalmol 113:456–462, 1995.
17. Finkelstein D, Clarkson J: Retinal vessel bypass: a promising new clinical investigative procedure. Arch Ophthalmol 113:421–422, 1995.
18. Fekrat S, Goldberg MF, Finkelstein D: Laser-induced chorioretinal venous anastomosis for nonischemic central or branch retinal vein occlusion. Arch Ophthalmol, in press.

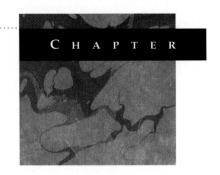

CHAPTER 26

Diabetic Retinopathy*

Lloyd M. Aiello, M.D.
Jerry D. Cavallerano, O.D., Ph.D.
Lloyd P. Aiello, M.D., Ph.D.
Sven-Erik Bursell, Ph.D.

Diabetic retinopathy and diabetic eye disease have surrendered many of their secrets since the landmark study of Waite and Beetham[1] in 1929. The advent of panretinal laser photocoagulation for the treatment of proliferative diabetic retinopathy[2] and the findings of the Diabetic Retinopathy Study (DRS),[3-16] the Early Treatment Diabetic Retinopathy Study (ETDRS),[17-30] the Diabetic Retinopathy Vitrectomy Study (DRVS),[31-35] and the Diabetes Control and Complications Trial (DCCT)[36-38] provide valuable insights into the understanding and management of diabetic retinopathy (a list or commonly used abbreviations is contained in Table 26–1). Proper treatment can reduce the 5-year risk of *severe visual loss* (SVL) (best corrected vision of 5/200 or worse) to less than 5% if a person with diabetic retinopathy approaching or just reaching high-risk proliferative retinopathy (defined below) has scatter (panretinal) laser photocoagulation surgery. Furthermore, individuals with *clinically significant diabetic macular edema* (CSME) can have the risk of *moderate visual loss* (MVL) (i.e., a doubling of the visual angle) reduced by 50% or more to approximately 12% or less if they have appropriate focal laser surgery. Since diabetic retinopathy is often asymptomatic when most amenable to treatment, early detection of diabetic retinopathy through regularly scheduled ocular examination is critical.

Despite recent advances, there is still much we do not know about diabetic retinopathy. We are unable to prevent its onset, and we have no cure for the condition. Half of the estimated 14 to 16 million Americans with diabetes mellitus (DM) are unaware that they have the disease, and about 50% of the 8 million Americans diagnosed with diabetes do not receive appropriate eye care.[39-44] Consequently, diabetic retinopathy (DR) remains a leading cause of new blindness in the United States today.[40,41] Blindness usually results from nonresolving vitreous hemorrhage, traction retinal detachment, or diabetic macular edema. Full implementation of the findings of the DRS, ETDRS, DRVS, and DCCT, in conjunction with annual eye exams, can result in significant saving of sight and reduction of societal costs. Also, current research continues to improve our understanding of DR, with hopes that DR can be prevented or cured in the future. Presently, however, clinical goals must concentrate on identifying eyes at risk of visual loss and ensuring that appropriate and timely laser surgery is offered to reduce the risk of visual loss.

This chapter reviews the natural history of DR, prognostic implications of the lesions of DR, and the risks of progression of retinopathy, with particular emphasis on identifying patients at risk of visual loss and in need of laser surgery. The laser

---

*Clinical information in this chapter is generally derived from the Diabetic Retinopathy Study, the Early Treatment Diabetic Retinopathy Study, and the Diabetic Retinopathy Vitrectomy Study. Portions of this chapter are from Aiello LP, Bursell SE: Diabetic eye disease. Endo Metab Clin North Am (in press). Portions of this chapter have been published previously in similar form in Aiello LM, Cavallerano JD: Ocular complications of diabetes mellitus. In Kahn CR, Weir GC (eds): Joslin's Diabetes Mellitus, 13th edition. Philadelphia, Lea & Febiger, 1994, pp 771–793, and in Aiello LM: Diabetes mellitus. In Albert DM, Jakobiec FA (eds): Clinical Practice: Principles and Practice of Ophthalmology. Philadelphia, WB Saunders Co, 1993.

HISTOPATHOLOGICAL FEATURES

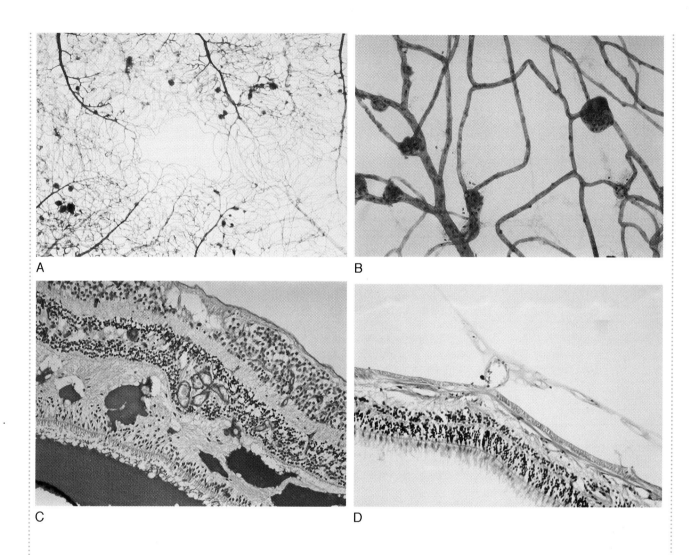

A, Trypsin digest preparation with numerous capillary microaneurysms in the juxtafoveal area in background diabetic retinopathy. *B*, Trypsin digest preparation discloses capillary microaneurysms adjacent to acellular capillaries in diabetic retinopathy. *C*, Marked diabetic macular edema with cluster of capillary microaneurysms. *D*, Proliferative diabetic retinopathy with retinal neovascularization extending into the partially detached vitreous. (From Green WR, Wilson DJ: Histopathology of diabetic retinopathy. In Franklin RM [ed]: Proceeding of the Symposium of Retina and Vitreous, New Orleans, 1993, New York, Kugler, 1993, with permission.)

TABLE 26-1 Abbreviations of Commonly Used Terms

Abbreviation	Term
PDR	Proliferative diabetic retinopathy
NPDR	Nonproliferative diabetic retinopathy
H/Ma	Hemorrhages and/or microaneurysms
HE	Hard exudates
SE or CWS	Soft exudates (cotton-wool spots)
VB	Venous beading
IRMAs	Intraretinal microvascular abnormalities
NVD	New vessels on or within 1 disc diameter (DD) of disc margin
NVE	New vessels elsewhere in the retina outside of disc and 1 DD from disc margin
FPD	Fibrous proliferation on or within 1 DD of disc margin
FPE	Fibrous proliferation elsewhere, not FPD
SVL	Severe visual loss: visual acuity ≤5/200 at two consecutive completed 4-month follow-up visits
MVL	Moderate visual loss: a doubling of the visual angle (e.g., 20/40 to 20/80 at two consecutive completed 4-month follow-up visits)
CSME	Clinically significant macular edema
DM	Diabetes mellitus
IDDM	Insulin-dependent diabetes mellitus
NIDDM	Non–insulin-dependent diabetes mellitus
DRS	Diabetic Retinopathy Study
ETDRS	Early Treatment Diabetic Retinopathy Study
DRVS	Diabetic Retinopathy Vitrectomy Study
DCCT	Diabetes Control and Complications Trial
NADH	Reduced Nicotinamide Adenine Dinucleotide
NAD	Nicotinamide Adenine Dinucleotide

treatment techniques are only generally described in this chapter, but are carefully detailed in ETDRS reports #3 and #4[19,20] and in Chapter 119 in this text.

EPIDEMIOLOGY OF DIABETIC RETINOPATHY

DM is a major medical problem in the United States and throughout the world. Fundamentally, diabetes is an abnormality of blood glucose metabolism due to altered insulin production or activity, clinically manifested by elevated levels of blood glucose. DM causes numerous long-term systemic complications that have considerable associated morbidity. Since the complications most commonly affect individuals in their economically productive years, the disease has enormous social and economic impact. It is estimated that societal costs associated with diabetes mellitus exceed $20 billion per year.[44]

Ten to 15% of the diabetic population have insulin-dependent diabetes mellitus (IDDM), also called type I diabetes, usually diagnosed before the age of 40. The majority of diabetic patients, however, have non–insulin-dependent diabetes mellitus (NIDDM), also called type II diabetes, usually diagnosed after the age of 40. These patients may or may not be treated with insulin. While those with type I diabetes experience a high incidence of severe ocular complications and are more likely to develop significant ocular problems during their lifetimes, those with type II diabetes make up the majority of clinical cases with diabetic eye disease because of their overall larger numbers. The ocular complications are similar in both groups and are discussed without distinction except where specifically indicated.[45,46]

Diabetic retinopathy is a highly specific vascular complication of both type I and type II DM. The duration of DM is a significant risk factor for the development of retinopathy. After 20 years of diabetes, nearly all patients with IDDM, and more than 60% with NIDDM, have some degree of retinopathy.[41,42,44] Diabetic retinopathy accounts for 12% of all new cases of blindness in the United States each year. At today's current levels of ophthalmic care for persons with diabetic retinopathy, it is estimated that over 220,000 person-years of sight are salvaged and over $471 million of savings to the federal government alone are realized each year. Savings of over 400,000 person-years of sight and $624 million in federal savings on an annual basis would result[47-50] if the currently available methods of ocular care were provided to *all* individuals with DM in the United States.

The prevalence of diabetic retinopathy in the general population has dramatically increased over the past 40 years. Improved care for DM allows patients to live longer and accounts for much of this increase. As a result, systemic complications that usually were manifest only after several decades of DM have become more prevalent. In the 1950s, the presence of proliferative diabetic retinopathy was closely associated with impending death, with the 5-year survival rate for patients with proliferative diabetic retinopathy being less than 30%. Today, survival rates are higher and advancements in retinopathy treatment have resulted in dramatically improved prognosis for the maintenance of visual potential in these patients.

Laser surgery and other surgical modalities help minimize the risk of MVL and SVL from DM, and, in some cases, restore useful vision for those who have suffered vision loss. These surgical modalities, particularly laser treatments, are most effective when initiated as a person *approaches* or just reaches *high risk proliferative diabetic retinopathy* (PDR), or before a person has lost visual acuity from diabetic macular edema.[25] Without laser treatment, the 5-year risk of SVL from high-risk PDR can be as high as 60%, and the risk of MVL from CSME may be as high as 25 to 30%.

Since proliferative retinopathy and macular edema may cause no ocular or visual symptoms when the retinal lesions are most amenable to treatment, it is imperative to identify eyes at risk of visual loss and ensure that patients receive laser surgery at the most appropriate time. Even minor errors in diagnosis of the level of retinopathy can result in a significant increase in the risk of visual loss. Furthermore, collateral health and medical

TABLE 26–2 Medical Complications

Condition	Comment
Risk Indicators of Diabetic Retinopathy	
Joint contractures	Association of retinopathy and contractures has been established. Eye examination is indicated. Care of joint contractures is important.
Neuropathy	Peripheral neuropathy may result in difficulty handling contact lenses. Neuropathy in lower extremities may alter mobility; therefore restoration and maintenance of as much vision as possible is important.
Conditions that May Affect the Course of Diabetic Retinopathy*	
Hypertension	Appropriate medical treatment is indicated for prevention of cardiovascular disease, stroke, and death. Hypertension itself may result in hypertensive retinopathy superimposed on diabetic retinopathy.
Elevated lipids	Appropriate management to normalize lipids is important. Proper diet and drug treatment may result in less retinal vessel leakage and hard exudate.
Proteinuria; elevated creatinine	Aggressive management of renal disease is indicated to avoid renal retinopathy which may increase risk of progression of diabetic retinopathy and of neovascular glaucoma.
Cardiovascular disease	Increased risk of peripheral vascular disease, particularly coronary vascular disease, is often associated with an increase in the attenuation and arteriosclerotic closure of the arterial system of the retina. A decreased risk of hemorrhage into the vitreous may result, but there also may be a decrease in retinal function with associated decrease in vision. Aggressive management of cardiovascular risk factors could theoretically relieve some of the ischemic process in the retina.

* There are no clinical trials that have specifically shown that control of systemic conditions (1–4 above) prevents the progression of diabetic retinopathy. However, clinical experience suggests that benefits result from appropriate treatment of these problems.

problems present a significant risk for the development and progression of diabetic retinopathy (Table 26–2). These factors include pregnancy,[51–54] chronic hyperglycemia,[55–58] hypertension,[59] renal disease,[57] and hyperlipidemia.[60,61] Patients with these conditions require careful medical evaluation and follow-up for the progression of diabetic retinopathy.

CLINICAL TRIALS OF DIABETIC RETINOPATHY

Three nationwide randomized clinical trials have largely determined the strategies for appropriate clinical management of patients with diabetic retinopathy.

The DRS (Table 26–3) conclusively demonstrated that scatter (panretinal) photocoagulation significantly reduces the risk of SVL from proliferative diabetic retinopathy, particularly when high-risk PDR is present. Although the DRS demonstrated the value of panretinal laser photocoagulation for eyes with high-risk PDR, guidelines for the timing of panretinal laser photocoagulation prior to the development of high-risk proliferative diabetic retinopathy were not clearly delineated.

The ETDRS provided valuable information concerning the timing of scatter (panretinal) laser surgery for advancing diabetic retinopathy and conclusively demonstrated that focal photocoagulation for CSME reduces the risk of MVL by 50% or more (Table 26–4). Furthermore, the ETDRS demonstrated that both early scatter (panretinal) laser sur-

gery (before high-risk PDR) and deferral of treatment "until and as soon as high-risk PDR developed" are effective in reducing the risk of SVL. Scatter laser surgery, therefore, should be considered as an eye approaches the high-risk stage and "usually should not be delayed if the eye has reached the high-risk proliferative stage."[25]

The DRVS provided guidelines for the most opportune time to consider vitrectomy surgery for type I and type II DM patients who suffered from vitreous hemorrhage or from severe PDR in eyes with useful vision (Table 26–5).[31–35] Early vitrectomy for eyes with recent severe vitreous hemorrhage and visual acuity less than 5/200 was beneficial, especially for patients with type I DM. Furthermore, the chance of achieving visual acuity 10/20 or better was increased by early vitrectomy in eyes with severe proliferating neovascular retinopathy, again especially for patients with type I DM.

The DCCT (Table 26–6) enrolled 1441 patients nationwide with insulin-dependent diabetes mellitus and minimal or no diabetic retinopathy. Two study questions were investigated:

1. *Primary prevention*: Does intensive insulin therapy prevent development of diabetic retinopathy and other diabetic complications compared with conventional therapy?
2. *Secondary intervention*: Does intensive therapy affect the progression of diabetic retinopathy and other diabetic complications compared with conventional therapy?

Patients assigned to intensive therapy used an insulin pump or took three or more injections of

---

TABLE 26–3 Diabetic Retinopathy Study (DRS)*

Major Eligibility Criteria
Visual acuity ≥20/100 in each eye.
PDR in at least one eye or severe NPDR in both eyes.
Both eyes suitable for photocoagulation.

Major Design Features
One eye of each patient was assigned randomly to photocoagulation (scatter [panretinal], local [direct confluent treatment of surface new vessels], and focal [for macular edema] as appropriate). The other eye was assigned to follow-up without photocoagulation.
The eye assigned to treatment was then randomly assigned to argon laser or xenon arc photocoagulation.

Major Conclusions
Photocoagulation reduced risk of severe visual loss by 50% or more (SVL = VA <5/200 at two consecutively completed 4-month follow-up visits).
Modest risks of decrease in visual acuity (usually only one line) and constriction of visual field (risks greater with xenon than argon).
Treatment benefit outweighs risks for eyes with high-risk PDR (50% 5-year rate of SVL in such eyes without treatment was reduced to 20% by treatment).

* Table prepared by Matthew D. Davis, M.D. and the ETDRS Research Group and for American Academy of Ophthalmology: Diabetes 2000 Program.

TABLE 26–4 Early Treatment Diabetic Retinopathy Study (ETDRS)*

Major Eligibility Criteria
  Visual acuity ≥20/40 (≥20/400, if reduction caused by macular edema).
  Mild NPDR to non–high-risk PDR, with or without macular edema.
  Both eyes suitable for photocoagulation.
Major Design Features
  One eye of each patient assigned randomly to early photocoagulation and the other to
    deferral (careful follow-up and photocoagulation if high-risk PDR develops).
  Patients assigned randomly to aspirin or placebo.
Major Conclusions
  Focal photocoagulation (direct laser for focal leaks and grid laser for diffuse leaks) re-
    duced risk of moderate visual loss (doubling of the visual angle) by 50% or more,
    and increased the chance of a small improvement in visual acuity.
  Both early scatter with or without focal photocoagulation and deferral were followed by
    low rates of severe visual loss (5-year rates in deferral subgroups were 2 to 10%, in
    early photocoagulation groups 2 to 6%).
  Focal photocoagulation should be considered for eyes with CSME.
  Scatter photocoagulation is not indicated for mild to moderate NPDR, but should be
    considered as retinopathy approaches the high-risk stage, and usually should not be
    delayed when the high-risk stage is present.

---

*Table prepared by Matthew D. Davis, M.D. and the ETDRS Research Group and for American Academy of Ophthalmology: Diabetes 2000 Program.

insulin each day. Frequent self-monitoring of blood glucose levels, hospitalization for the induction of therapy, strict adherence to meal plans, and frequent follow-up evaluations were provided.

The DCCT demonstrated[35–38] that intensive therapy reduced clinically meaningful DR by 35 to 74%; reduced the risk of severe nonproliferative diabetic retinopathy (NPDR), PDR, and laser treatment by 45%; and reduced the development of any DR by 27%. Additionally, intensive therapy reduced the development of microalbuminuria by 35%, clinical proteinuria by 56%, and clinical neuropathy by 60%. Adverse effects of intensive therapy included a threefold greater risk of hypoglycemia, catheter complications, weight gain, and ketoacidosis.

DIAGNOSIS, CLASSIFICATION, AND MANAGEMENT OF DIABETIC RETINOPATHY

Pathophysiology

The processes by which diabetes results in retinopathy and maculopathy are not fully understood. In studies with laboratory animals, insulin deficiency itself, even in animals that are not genetically diabetic, is sufficient to cause diabetic retinopathy.[61] The elevated blood glucose is accompanied by and probably causes structural, physiologic, and hormonal changes that affect the retinal capillaries, causing the capillaries to become functionally less competent.[63–65]

Six basic pathophysiologic processes are recognized in the development of the lesions of diabetic retinopathy:

1. Loss of pericyte function of retinal capillaries
2. Outpouching of capillary walls to form microaneurysms
3. Closure of retinal capillaries and arterioles
4. Breakdown of the blood/retinal barrier with increased vascular permeability of retinal capillaries
5. Proliferation of new vessels and fibrous tissue
6. Contraction of vitreous and fibrous proliferation with subsequent vitreous hemorrhage and retinal detachment due to traction.

Loss of function of intramural pericytes of retinal capillaries, either preceding or secondary to the development of nonperfusion of retinal capillaries, results in weakness of the capillary wall.[66–68] These changes, resulting in microaneurysm formation, are the earliest signs of diabetic retinopathy. At the cellular level, retinal pericytes, which are an endothelial-supporting cell, are classically lost in very early stages of the disease.[67,68] Although the precise chronology of change is unclear, the loss of the pericytes may result in abnormalities of their associated endothelial cells, possibly accounting for the eventual development of later complications. In addition, studies have determined that even in the earliest stages of DM, before the development of diabetic retinopathy, retinal blood flow is decreased,[69–73] although some have shown no significant changes in retinal blood flow in patients with no diabetic retinopathy.[74–76] In contrast, the au-

TABLE 26-5 Diabetic Retinopathy Vitrectomy Study (DRVS)*

Recent Severe Vitreous Hemorrhage (Group H)

Major Eligibility Criteria

Visual acuity (VA) ≤5/200.
Vitreous hemorrhage (VH) consistent with VA, duration 1–6 months
Macula attached by ultrasound.

Major Design Features

In most patients, only one eye is eligible. Eligible eye(s) assigned randomly to early vitrectomy or conventional management (vitrectomy if center of macula detaches or if
VH persists for 1 year, photocoagulation as needed and as possible).

Major Conclusions

Chance of recovery of VA ≥10/20 increased by early vitrectomy, at least in patients
with type 1 diabetes, who were younger and had more severe PDR (in most severe
PDR group, ≥10/20 at 4 years in 50% of early vitrectomy group vs. 12% in conventional management group).

Very severe PDR with Useful Vision (Group NR)

Major Eligibility Criteria

Visual acuity ≥10/200.
Center of macula attached.
Extensive, active, neovascular or fibrovascular proliferation.

Major Design Features

Same as group H (except conventional management included vitrectomy after a
6-month waiting period in eyes that developed severe VH).

Major Conclusions

Chance of VA ≥10/20 increased by early vitrectomy, at least for eyes with very severe
new vessels.

* Table prepared by Matthew D. Davis, M.D. and the ETDRS Research Group and for American
Academy of Ophthalmology: Diabetes 2000 Program.

toregulation of retinal blood flow is significantly impaired even in diabetic patients with no diabetic retinopathy.[77-79] This impairment in retinal auto-regulation may be linked to diabetes-associated loss in pericyte function.[67,80] Although the exact changes in retinal physiology during early stages of diabetes remain controversial, it is generally accepted that the measurements of retinal function, such as reti-nal blood flow or retinal autoregulation, can pro-vide a quantitative assessment of retinal status and subsequent risk for developing retinopathy.

Retinal Lesions

As the disease progresses, the clinically evident signs of early or nonproliferative diabetic retinop-athy appear. Eventually most diabetic persons will develop at least some degree of nonproliferative di-abetic retinopathy, with an incidence approaching 100% after 15 years of disease.[46,81] Various individ-ual retinal lesions identify the level of diabetic ret-inopathy and the risk of progression of retinopathy and visual loss[25,28] (Table 26–7). Consequently, the ability to determine the level of nonproliferative disease allows physicians to estimate prognosis and determine follow-up schedules.

The classic signs of NPDR are retinal microan-eurysms, small dot and blot retinal hemorrhages, cotton-wool spots (nerve fiber layer infarctions with associated stasis of axoplasmic flow), venous loops, venous caliber changes (venous tortuosity and beading) and retinal capillary dropout. The early clinical signs of diabetic retinopathy are *microaneu-rysms*, which are saccular outpouchings of retinal capillaries (Fig. 26–1). Ruptured microaneurysms,

TABLE 26–6 Diabetes Control and Complications Trial (DCCT)

Major Eligibility Criteria
  Age: 13–39 years.
  Primary Prevention:
    Duration insulin-dependent diabetes mellitus: 1–5 years.
    No diabetic retinopathy.
  Secondary intervention:
    Duration insulin-dependent diabetes mellitus: 1–15 years.
    Minimal nonproliferative diabetic retinopathy.
Major Design Features
  Patients were randomly assigned to conventional insulin therapy or intensive therapy.
  Study questions:
    Primary prevention: Does intensive therapy prevent the development of retinopathy
      and other complications compared with conventional therapy?
    Secondary intervention: Will intensive therapy affect the progression of retinopathy and
      other complications compared with conventional therapy?
Major Conclusions
  Intensive therapy reduced clinically meaningful DR by 35–74%; severe NPDR, PDR, and
    laser treatment by 45%; and the first appearance of any retinopathy by 27%.
  Intensive therapy reduced the development of microalbuminuria by 35%, clinical protein-
    uria by 56%, and clinical neuropathy by 60%.
  Risks of intensive therapy included hypoglycemia, catheter complications, weight gain,
    and ketoacidosis.

leaking capillaries, and intraretinal microvascular abnormalities result in *intraretinal hemorrhages* (Fig. 26–2). The clinical appearance of these hemorrhages reflects the architecture of the retinal level where the hemorrhage occurs. Hemorrhages in the nerve fiber layer assume a more flame-shaped appearance, reflecting the structure of the nerve fiber layer that runs parallel to the retinal surface. Hemorrhages deeper in the retina, where the arrangement of cells is more or less perpendicular to the surface of the retina, assume a pinpoint or dot shape and are more characteristic of diabetic retinopathy.

Intraretinal microvascular abnormalities (IRMA)

represent either new vessel growth within the retina or, more likely, pre-existing vessels with endothelial cell proliferation that become "shunts" through areas of nonperfusion. IRMAs may be seen adjacent to cotton-wool spots. Multiple IRMAs mark a severe stage of nonproliferative retinopathy, and frank neovascularization is likely to appear on the surface of the retina or optic disc within a short time.

Venous caliber abnormalities (Fig. 26–3) are indicators of severe retinal hypoxia. These abnormalities can be venous dilation, venous beading, or loop

TABLE 26–7 PDR at 1-Year Visit by Severity of Individual Lesion*

Lesion	Grade	PDR in 1 Year
H/Ma	Present 2–5 fields	9%
	Very severe	57%
IRMA	None	9%
	Moderate in 2–5 fields	57%
Venous beading	Absent	15%
	Present 2–5 fields	59%

* From the Early Treatment Diabetic Retinopathy Study Report Number 12: Fundus photographic risk factors for progression of diabetic retinopathy. Ophthalmology 98:823–833, 1991, with permission.

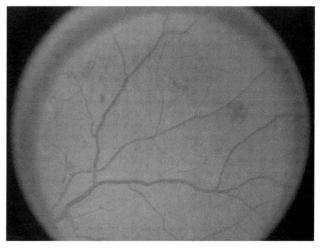

FIGURE 26–1 Standard photograph 2A of the Modified Airlee House Classification of Diabetic Retinopathy demonstrating a moderate degree of hemorrhage and/or microaneurysms (H/Ma).

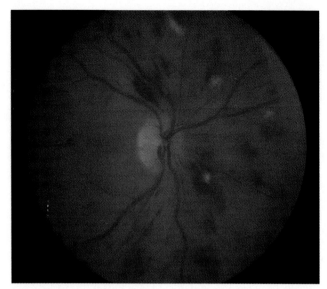

FIGURE 26–2 Flame-shaped hemorrhages occur in the nerve fiber layer of the retina, reflecting the architecture of the retina at this level; dot hemorrhages occur deeper in the retinal tissue, where the retinal structure is essentially perpendicular to the retinal surface. This photograph shows flame-shaped hemorrhages around the optic nerve head. There are also peripapillary soft exudates suggesting renal disease in this case. Flame-shaped hemorrhages may also be a part of early NPDR.

formation. There are areas of nonperfusion adjacent to the veins. Treatment with scatter (panretinal) photocoagulation may cause these abnormal veins to become less dilated and more regular.

With the development of nonproliferative diabetic retinopathy, the retinal blood flow begins to increase.[73,75,76] It is felt that this increase in retinal blood flow is associated with the development of capillary nonperfusion and increasing retinal ischemia. In addition, the impairment in retinal auto-

regulation increases as the level of diabetic retinopathy increases. Ultimately the increased retinal ischemia may provide the cellular triggers for the production of vasoproliferative factors and subsequent new vessel formation seen in proliferative diabetic retinopathy.

Proliferative retinopathy (Fig. 26–4) is marked by proliferating endothelial cell tubules. The rate of growth of these new vessels is variable. These vessels grow either at or near the optic disc (*neovascularization of the disc* [NVD]) or elsewhere in the retina (*neovascularization elsewhere* [NVE]). Translucent fibrous tissue often appears adjacent to the new vessels. This fibroglial tissue appears opaque and becomes adherent to the adjacent vitreous.

Active proliferation of new vessels on the retinal surface is apparently triggered by decreased oxygen levels as a result of capillary nonperfusion.[82–85] Neovascularization of the retina is most commonly observed at the borders of perfused and nonperfused retina and is more common and more severe in eyes that have more extensive nonperfusion. The neovascularization of the retina most commonly occurs along the temporal vascular arcades and at the optic nerve head. The new vessels propagate along the surface of the retina and along the vitreous "scaffold" afforded by the posterior vitreous hyaloid. These vessels themselves rarely cause visual loss, but they are fragile and prone to bleed (Fig. 26–5). As a result, vitreous hemorrhage is a major component of visual loss during this period. In severe cases, proliferation of new blood vessels may also occur in the anterior portion of the eye, especially on the iris and the anterior chamber angle. If the vessels obstruct the aqueous fluid outflow facilities of the eye, they can lead to neovascular glaucoma, a severe sight-threatening disorder. The stimulus for neovascularization is believed to be the

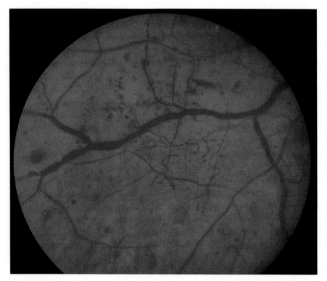

FIGURE 26–3 Standard photograph 6B of the Modified Airlee House Classification of Diabetic Retinopathy demonstrating venous caliber abnormalities. IRMA and venous shunts are also present.

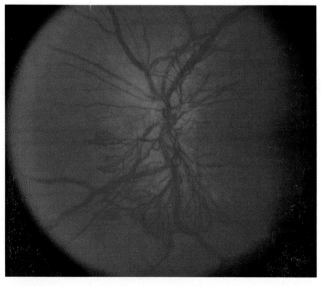

FIGURE 26–4 Proliferative diabetic retinopathy is marked by the growth of new vessels on the optic disc or elsewhere on the retina.

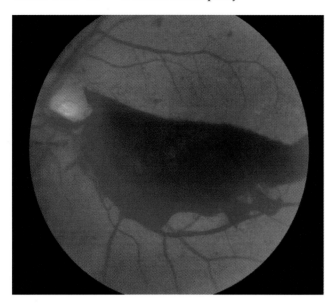

FIGURE 26–5   Preretinal hemorrhage from NVD.

release of growth factors from the retina in response to retinal ischemia. Significant progress has been made in characterizing some of these growth factors and such studies have implications for eventual novel treatment modalities as discussed later in this chapter.

The propensity for retinal neovascularization to become fibrotic and contract with time causes many complications of proliferative diabetic retinopathy (Fig. 26–6). Fibrovascular proliferation in diabetic retinopathy typically proceeds from the optic disc along the major temporal vascular arcades to encircle the macula with increasing traction. Such retinal traction can distort the normal retinal architecture causing macular traction and visual distortion. The traction itself can also induce edema of the central macula. In addition, fibrous tissue formation

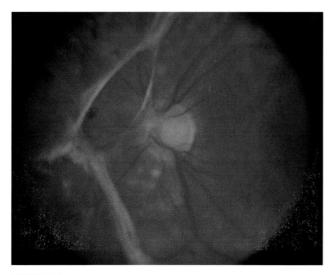

FIGURE 26–6   Fibrous tissue growth accompanies neovascularization and can cause traction on retinal tissue.

can cause traction retinal detachments. These traction retinal detachments may remain stable for many years and if present in nonvisually critical areas of the eye may be observed carefully without treatment. However, should the traction retinal detachment progress towards visually critical structures, or if the detachment involves these structures, pars plana vitrectomy surgery is indicated to relieve traction and allow anatomic reapproximation of the retina. The traction can also cause retinal tears or holes resulting in rhegmatogenous retinal detachments. If a retinal hole is discovered prior to significant retinal detachment, and there is relatively little tractional or subretinal fluid, then it is sometimes possible to seal such a hole with surrounding laser photocoagulation or cryotherapy. However, if the hole is large, significant traction still persists, or significant retinal detachment is present, then relief of traction, reapproximation of the retina, and sealing of the hole is required, often necessitating both pars plana vitrectomy surgery and scleral buckling procedures.

An additional, although unusual mode of visual loss may occur when fibrovascular proliferation forms across the visual axis. This proliferation may occur without distortion or traction on ocular structures. Since this fibrovascular sheet is opaque, significant visual loss can occur. However, because the ocular anatomy in these cases can be relatively undisturbed, removal of the fibrovascular membrane by pars plana vitrectomy may result in dramatic improvement of vision.

Levels of Diabetic Retinopathy

It is crucial to consider scatter (panretinal) laser photocoagulation as retinopathy approaches or reaches the high-risk stage of proliferative retinopathy. An eye is considered to be *approaching the high-risk stage* when there are retinal signs of severe or very severe NPDR, with or without early PDR (see below), or new vessels not quite fulfilling the definition of high-risk PDR (see below) associated with any level of NPDR. The baseline level of retinopathy indicates the risk of progression from NPDR stage to early proliferative diabetic retinopathy (early PDR) and to high-risk proliferative diabetic retinopathy (Tables 26–7 through 26–9).[28]

Nonproliferative Diabetic Retinopathy

Diabetic retinopathy is broadly classified as NPDR and PDR. Diabetic macular edema can occur with either NPDR or PDR and is discussed separately. Accurate diagnosis of a patient's "diabetic retinopathy level" is critical, since there is a varying risk of progression to PDR and high-risk PDR depending on specific NPDR level (Table 26–9 and Fig. 26–7). Regardless of the level of retinopathy, patients should be informed of the results of the

TABLE 26-8 Levels of Retinopathy*

Nonproliferative Diabetic Retinopathy (NPDR)

A. Mild NPDR
   At least one microaneurysm
   Definition not met for B, C, D, E, or F

B. Moderate NPDR
   Hemorrhages and/or MA > standard photo 2A (Fig. 26–1)
   Soft exudates, venous beading, and IRMA definitely present
      Definition not met for C, D, E, or F

C. Severe NPDR
   H/Ma > standard photo 2A (Fig. 26–1) in all 4 quadrants
   VB (venous beading) in two or more quadrants (Fig. 26–3)
      IRMA > standard photo 8A in at least one quadrant (Fig. 26–2)

D. Very Severe NPDR
   Any two or more of C above
   Definition not met for E or F

Proliferative Diabetic Retinopathy (PDR)

   Composed of:
   1. NVD or NVE
   2. Preretinal or vitreous hemorrhage
   3. Fibrous tissue proliferation

E. Early PDR
   New vessels
   Definition not met for F

F. High-Risk PDR
   1. NVD ≥1/3–1/2 DA (Fig. 26–4) *or*
   2. NVD and vitreous or preretinal hemorrhage *or*
   3. NVE ≥1/2 DA and preretinal or vitreous hemorrhage (Fig. 26–5)

Clinically Significant Diabetic Macular Edema

   1. Thickening of the retina located ≤500 μm from the center of the macula *or*
   2. Hard exudates with thickening of the adjacent retina located ≤500 μm from the center of the macula *or*
   3. A zone of retinal thickening, 1 DA or larger in size located ≤1 DA from the center of the macula

*From Early Treatment Diabetic Retinopathy Study Report Number 12: Fundus photographic risk factors for progression of diabetic retinopathy. Ophthalmology 98:823–833, 1991, with permission.

DCCT (Table 26–6) and the importance of control of blood glucose levels on the development and progression of DR.

Mild NPDR is marked by at least one retinal microaneurysm, but hemorrhages and microaneurysms are less than ETDRS standard photograph 2A (Fig. 26–1) in all four retinal quadrants (Table 26–8). No other significant retinal lesion or abnormality associated with diabetes is present. Those with mild NPDR have a 5% risk of progression to PDR within 1 year, and a 15% risk of progression to high-risk PDR within 5 years (Table 26–9).

Moderate NPDR (Table 26–8) is characterized by hemorrhages and/or microaneurysms greater than those pictured in ETDRS standard photograph 2A in at least one field but less than four retinal quadrants (Fig. 26–1). Cotton-wool spots (soft exudates), venous beading, and IRMAs are definitely present

to a mild degree (Fig. 26–8). The risk of progression to PDR within 1 year is 12 to 27%, and the risk of progression to high-risk PDR within 5 years is 33% (Table 26–9).

Patients with mild or moderate NPDR generally are not candidates for scatter (panretinal) laser surgery and can be followed safely at 6- to 12-month intervals as determined by the examiner. The presence of macular edema, even with mild or moderate degrees of NPDR, requires follow-up in a shorter period, and if CSME is present, focal laser treatment is advisable (Table 26–9). Coincident medical problems or pregnancy will influence the period of re-evaluation.

Severe NPDR, based on the severity of hemorrhages and/or microaneurysms (H/Ma), IRMA, and venous beading (VB), is characterized by any one of the following lesions (Table 26–8):

TABLE 26–9 General Management Recommendations

Level of Retinopathy	Natural Course/ Rate of Progression PDR 1 Yr	HRC 5 Yr	Evaluation Fundus Photo	FA	TX Strategies PRP	Focal	F/U (Mo)
1. Mild NPDR	5%	15%					
a. No macular edema			No	No	No	No	12
b. Macular edema			Yes	Occ	No	No	4–6
c. CSME			Yes	Yes	No	Yes	2–4
2. Moderate NPDR	12–27%	33%					
a. No macular edema			Yes	No	No	No	6–8
b. Macular edema (not CSME)			Yes	Occ	No	No	4–6
c. CSME			Yes	Yes	No	Yes	2–4
3. Severe NPDR	52%	60%					
a. No macular edema			Yes	No	Rarely	No	3–4
b. Macular edema (not CSME)			Yes	Occ	Focal	Occ	2–3
c. CSME			Yes	Yes	Occ after focal	Yes	2–3
4. Very Severe NPDR	75%	75%					
a. No macular edema			Yes	No	Occ	No	2–3
b. Macular edema (not CSME)			Yes	Occ	Occ after focal	Occ	2–3
c. CSME			Yes	Yes	Occ after focal	Yes	2–3
5. Non–high-risk PDR		75%					
a. No macular edema			Yes	No	Occ	No	2–3
b. Macular edema			Yes	Occ	Occ after focal	Occ	2–3
c. CSME			Yes	Yes	Occ after focal	Yes	2–3
6. High-risk PDR							
a. No macular edema			Yes	No	Yes	No	2–3
b. Macular edema			Yes	Yes	Yes	Usually	1–2
c. CSME			Yes	Yes	Yes	Yes	1–2

TX, treatment; HRC, high-risk characteristics; FA, fluorescein angiogram; PRP, scatter (panretinal) photocoagulation; F/U, follow-up; NPDR, nonproliferative diabetic retinopathy; CSME, clinically significant macular edema; occ, occasionally.

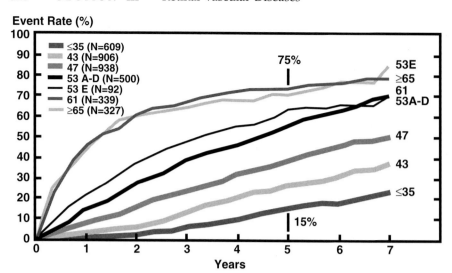

Event Rate (%)

≤35 (N=609)
43 (N=906)
47 (N=938)
53 A-D (N=500)
53 E (N=92)
61 (N=339)
≥65 (N=327)

75%

15%

Years

53E
≥65
61
53A-D

47

43

≤35

FIGURE 26–7 This graph from the ETDRS[24] shows the life-table cumulative event rates of high-risk PDR by level of retinopathy at baselines assigned to deferral of photocoagulation in the ETDRS: level ≤35, mild NPDR; level 43, moderate NPDR; level 47, moderate to severe NPDR; level 53 A–D, severe NPDR; level 53 E, very severe NPDR; level 61, early PDR; level 65, PDR less than high-risk PDR.

1. H/Ma greater than standard photo 2A (Fig. 26–1) in *four* quadrants *or*
2. Venous caliber abnormalities (VCAB) (Fig. 26–3) in *two* or more quadrants *or*
3. IRMAs greater than standard photo 8A in at least *one* quadrant.

This "4-2-1 rule" is a valuable clinical tool to diagnose the severe level of NPDR.

Eyes with severe NPDR have a 52% risk of developing PDR within 1 year, and a 60% risk of developing high-risk PDR within 5 years. These patients require follow-up evaluation in 2 to 4 months. Treatment of CSME is strongly indicated due to the risk of the development of PDR and high-risk PDR. Some eyes with macular edema, even if not clinically significant, may require focal treatment in preparation for impending scatter (panretinal) laser surgery, which may also be indicated as determined by the clinical judgment of the retinal specialist (Table 26–8).

Eyes with *very severe NPDR* (Table 26–8) have two or more lesions of severe NPDR, but no frank neovascularization (Fig. 26–9). There is a 75% risk of developing PDR within 1 year. Patients with very severe NPDR may be candidates for scatter (panretinal) laser surgery, and macular edema, if present, may require treatment. Very close follow-up evaluation at 2- to 3-month intervals is important (Table 26–9).

Proliferative Diabetic Retinopathy

Diabetic retinopathy marked by NVD (Fig. 26–10) or NVE (Fig. 26–11) on the retina, vitreous or preretinal hemorrhage, or fibrous tissue proliferation (Fig. 26–7) is designated PDR. *Early PDR* does not meet the definition of high-risk PDR (Table 26–8). Eyes with early PDR (less than high risk) have a

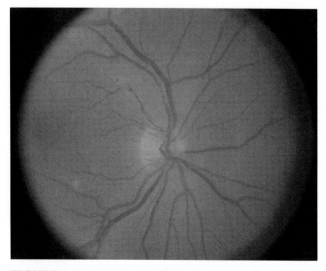

FIGURE 26–8   Moderate NPDR. This picture shows a mild to moderate degree of H/Ma and one soft exudate.

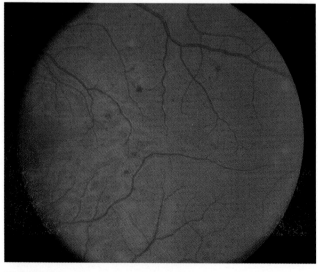

FIGURE 26–9   Very severe NPDR. Areas of IRMA and mild VCAB and moderate H/Ma are present in this picture.

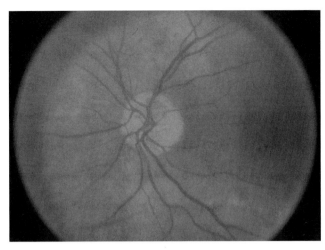

FIGURE 26–10 Standard photograph 10A of the Modified Airlee House Classification of Diabetic Retinopathy demonstrating neovascularization of the optic disc (NVD) covering approximately 1/4 to 1/3 of the disc area.

75% risk of developing high-risk PDR within a 5-year period. These eyes may require scatter (panretinal) laser surgery, and macular edema, even if not clinically significant, may benefit from focal treatment before scatter is initiated (Table 26–9).

In patients with early PDR (less than high-risk PDR) early scatter (panretinal) laser surgery should be considered if any of the associated findings are present:

- Any new vessels accompanied by severe or very severe NPDR
- Elevated new vessels
- NVD.

Patients with macular edema and severe NPDR or worse should be considered for focal treatment of macular edema regardless of whether the macular edema is clinically significant or not, since future need of scatter laser photocoagulation is imminent (Table 26–9). Subsequent scatter photocoagulation may exacerbate macular edema, and focal treatment prior to scatter photocoagulation may reduce this risk.

Patients with *high-risk PDR* generally require immediate scatter laser photocoagulation. High-risk PDR is characterized by any one or more of the following lesions:

1. NVD approximately 1/4 to 1/3 disc area or more in size (i.e., greater than or equal to NVD in standard photo 10A) (Fig. 26–10)
2. NVD less than 1/4 disc area in size if fresh vitreous or preretinal hemorrhage is present
3. NVE greater than or equal to 1/2 disc area in size if fresh vitreous or preretinal hemorrhage is present (Fig. 26–11).

Attention therefore must be paid to the presence or absence of new vessels, the location of new vessels, the severity of new vessels, and the presence or absence of preretinal or vitreous hemorrhages.[5]

Diabetic Macular Edema

Diabetic macular disease may be present at *any* level of retinopathy (Table 26–8) and alters the structure of the macula in any of the following manners, significantly affecting its function:

1. A collection of intraretinal fluid in the macula with or without lipid exudates and with or without cystoid changes (macular edema) (Fig. 26–12)
2. Nonperfusion of parafoveal capillaries with or without intraretinal fluid (Fig. 26–13)
3. Traction in the macula by fibrous tissue proliferation causing dragging of the retinal tissue, surface wrinkling, or detachment of the macula (Fig. 26–14)
4. Intraretinal or preretinal hemorrhage in the macula (Fig. 26–15)
5. Lamellar or full-thickness retinal hole formation (Fig. 26–16)
6. Combination of the above.

Clinically, *macular edema* is retinal thickening within 2 disc diameters of the center of the macula (*not* fluorescein leakage without thickening). Retinal thickening or hard exudates with adjacent retinal thickening that threaten or involve the center of the macula is considered to be clinically significant. CSME as defined by the ETDRS includes any *one* of the following lesions (Table 26–8):

1. Retinal thickening at or within 500 μm from the center of the macula (Fig. 26–17) *or*
2. Hard exudates at or within 500 μm from the center of the macula, if there is thickening of the adjacent retina (Fig. 26–18*A* and *B*) *or*

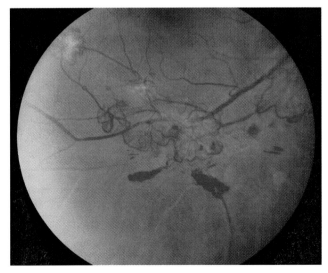

FIGURE 26–11 Standard photograph 7 of the Modified Airlie House Classification of Diabetic Retinopathy demonstrating neovascularization elsewhere (NVE) in the retina greater than 1/2 disc area with fresh hemorrhage present.

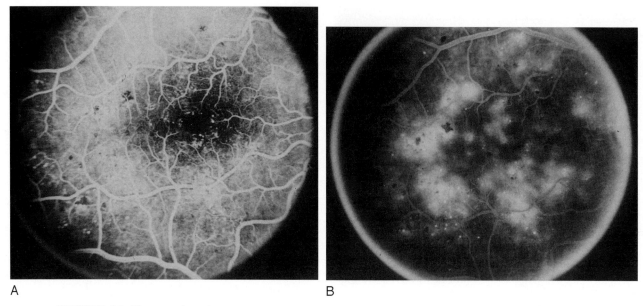

A   B

FIGURE 26–12   Macular edema. *A*, This early fluorescein angiogram shows areas of hyperfluorescence. There are microaneuryms around the fovea that are leaking into the macula. There are also areas of nonperfusion. *B*, The later angiogram shows accumulation of fluid in the macula area. Visual acuity is 20/25.

3. An area or areas of retinal thickening at least 1 disc area in size, at least part of which is within 1 disc diameter of the center of the macula (Fig. 26–19).

In managing CSME there are particular retinal lesions identified on fluorescein angiography that are amenable to treatment. These *treatable lesions* associated with macular edema include:

1. Focal leaks greater than 500 μm from the center of the macula thought to be causing retinal

thickening and/or hard exudates (Figs. 26–12 and 26–20)
2. Focal leaks 300 to 500 μm from the center of the macula thought to be causing retinal thickening or hard exudates if the treating ophthalmologist does not believe that treatment is likely to destroy the remaining perifoveal capillary network, and visual acuity is 20/40 or worse
3. Areas of diffuse leakage (Fig. 26–12) from extensive numbers of microaneurysms or from many IRMAs *or*
4. Avascular zones, other than the normal foveal avascular zone, not previously treated (Fig. 26–13).

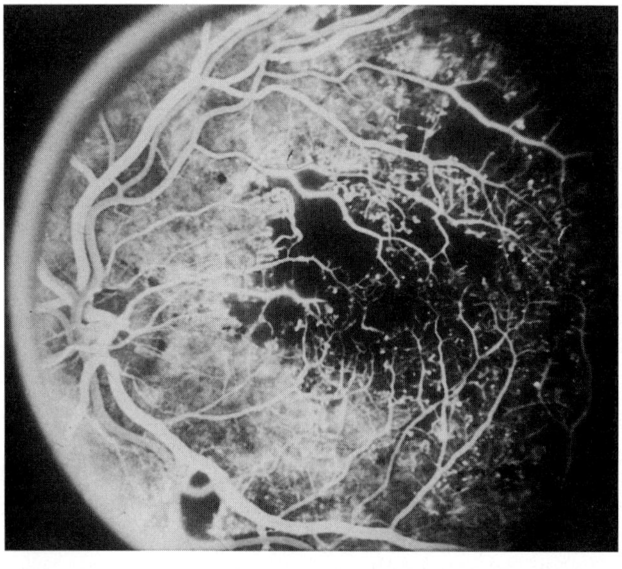

FIGURE 12–13   Nonperfusion of the macula. This fluorescein angiogram shows apparent gross enlargement of the foveal avascular zone, demonstrating nonperfusion in the macula area due to capillary dropout.

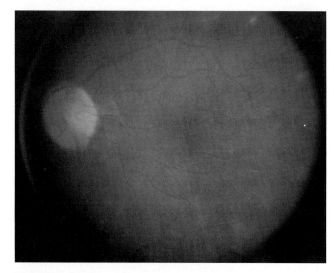

FIGURE 26–14   Fibrous tissue from the optic nerve head is causing traction in the macula area.

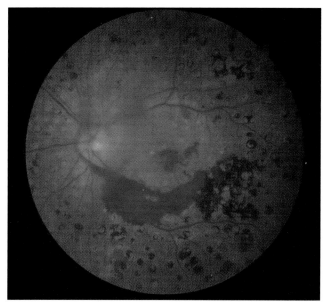

FIGURE 26–15   Hemorrhage has occurred in the macula area.

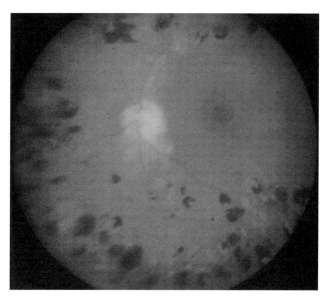

FIGURE 26–16   Formation of an epiretinal membrane over the macula has led to the formation of a retinal hole in the macula. Vision is 10/300.

Focal laser surgery for CSME consists of either "direct" laser treatment, "grid" laser treatment, or a "combination" of direct focal laser and grid laser treatment (Figs. 26–21 and 26–22). These treatment methods are described in detail elsewhere.[18,20] Table 26–9 summarizes the management recommendations for CSME at the various retinopathy levels.

Role of Clinical Fluorescein Angiography in the Management of Diabetic Retinopathy

Fluorescein angiography (FA) of the macula in the presence of CSME is fundamental for the detection of treatable lesions.[30] However, its use to identify lesions such as NVE or feeder vessels on NVD is not necessary, since scatter (panretinal) laser surgery is the method of choice for the treatment of DR as it approaches or reaches the high-risk proliferative stage.

Angiographic risk factors for progression of NPDR to PDR have been identified.[27,29,63–65] Analysis of data from the untreated (deferred) eyes in the ETDRS indicates that the following lesions are independently related to outcome: (1) fluorescein leakage; (2) capillary loss on FA; (3) capillary dilatation on FA; and (4) the color fundus photographic risk factors (a) IRMA, (b) VB, and (c) H/Ma. Hard and soft exudates (cotton-wool spots) have an inverse relationship to progression. It is widely accepted that capillary loss as documented on FA is a risk factor for progression of NPDR to PDR.[27,29,48,51,52] However, capillary dilatation on FA, fluorescein leakage, and capillary loss on FA, and the ETDRS color fundus photographic retinopathy severity levels are all closely correlated. Although

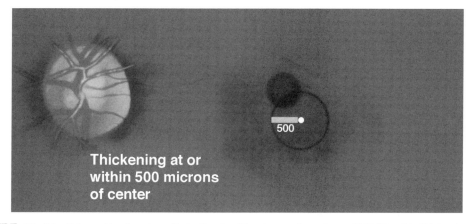

Thickening at or within 500 microns of center

500

FIGURE 26–17   Schematic showing clinically significant macular edema (CSME) with thickening of the macular less than 500 μm from the center of the macula. (Courtesy of Robert Murphy, M.D.)

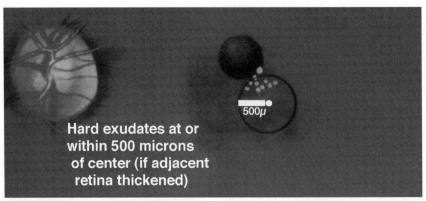

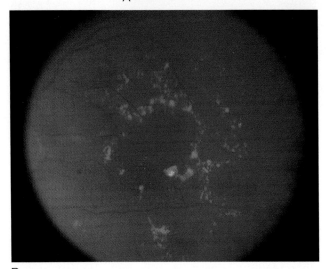

FIGURE 26–18 *A* and *B*, Clinically significant macular edema (CSME) with hard exudates at or within 500 µm from the center of the macula, with thickening of the retina adjacent to the exudates. (Courtesy of Robert Murphy, M.D.)

the FA abnormalities provide additional prognostic information, the color fundus photographic grading of retinopathy levels of both eyes give similar prognostic results.[28,29] Therefore, the increase in power to predict progression from NPDR to PDR by FA is "*not of significant clinical importance to warrant routine FA.*"[29]

Periodic follow-up retinal examinations, however, are necessary. The appropriate interval can be determined by skillful grading of 7 standard field

stereo color fundus photography and/or by retinal examination by an examiner experienced in the management of diabetic eye disease. Since the retinal level of DR derived from color fundus photography is predictive enough to establish frequency of follow-up, since FA classification cannot "identify all cases destined to progress," and since initiation of scatter (panretinal) laser photocoagulation should be considered as DR approaches or just as it reaches the high-risk stage, "periodic follow-up

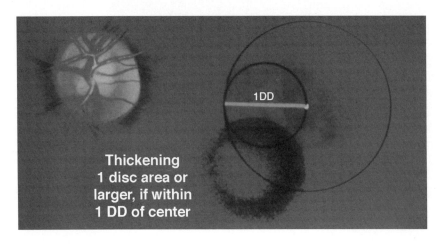

FIGURE 26–19 Schematic showing area of thickening 1 disc area in size, part of which is within 1 disc diameter of the center of the macula. (Courtesy of Robert Murphy, M.D.)

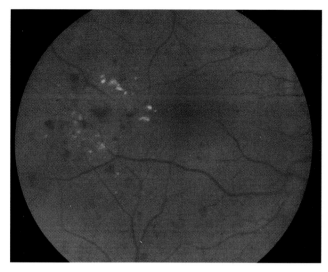

FIGURE 26–20 Clinical appearance of hard exudates less than 500 μm from the center of the macula. There is associated thickening of the adjacent retina, not appreciated without stereoscopic observation.

of all patients with diabetic retinopathy continues to be of fundamental clinical importance."[29] Table 26–9 summarizes the appropriate use of fundus photography and fluorescein angiography in monitoring and treating diabetic retinopathy and macular edema.

Follow-up Evaluations

Careful and lifelong follow-up evaluation of retinal status by an experienced examiner becomes crucial to reduce the risk of vision loss from diabetic retinopathy. Follow-up evaluations are determined by the baseline level of retinopathy (Table 26–8) and the presence of coincident medical conditions (Table 26–2) such as hypertension, renal disease, cholesterol level, and blood glucose control (Table 26–6). Patients should be informed of the need for careful follow-up and the importance of control of coincident medical conditions.

LASER PHOTOCOAGULATION

At all levels of retinopathy, it is important to be certain that the patient's overall diabetes status is under optimal control. The results from the DCCT[36–38] demonstrate that improved glycemic control delays the onset of any retinopathy and slows the progression of retinopathy when present. In addition, the DCCT demonstrated that improved glycemic control was associated with benefits in kidney, heart, and nerve function. Indeed, the only two currently proven methods by which the patient can positively affect the outcome of ocular disease is to achieve improved glucose control and rigor-

ously maintain regular lifelong ophthalmic follow-up with laser photocoagulation and/or vitrectomy as needed.

Timing of Photocoagulation

The 3-year risk of MVL from macular edema in the ETDRS without focal laser treatment was about 30%. Focal laser surgery for CSME reduced this risk to 15%,[17] reducing the risk of MVL by approximately 50%. Focal treatment also increased the chance of improvement in visual acuity of one line or more. On the other hand, scatter (panretinal) laser surgery was *not* effective in managing diabetic macular edema, and in some cases may have had a deleterious effect on the progression of macular edema.

Eyes with CSME and retinopathy that is approaching high-risk PDR are best treated first with focal photocoagulation of the macular edema 6 to 8 weeks before initiating scatter (panretinal) laser surgery. Eyes with mild or moderate NPDR and CSME respond best to prompt focal photocoagulation, with scatter treatment withheld unless very severe NPDR or high-risk PDR occurs. Delaying scatter photocoagulation while focal treatment is completed is unlikely to increase the risk of SVL, provided the retinopathy is not progressing rapidly and careful follow-up can be maintained. Delaying scatter photocoagulation while focal treatment is completed in eyes with high-risk PDR is usually not advisable.

Focal treatment was not attended by adverse effects on central visual field or color vision compared to eyes assigned to deferral of focal treatment in the ETDRS.[18] Any harmful effects of early photocoagulation reflected by constriction of the peripheral visual fields seem to be due mostly to scatter photocoagulation. Because the principal benefit of treatment is to prevent further decrease in visual acuity, focal laser surgery should be considered in all eyes with CSME, especially if the center of the macula is threatened or involved, even if normal visual acuity is present.

The DRS had demonstrated in 1976 that scatter (panretinal) photocoagulation was effective in reducing the risk of severe visual loss from high-risk PDR. However, the DRS did not provide a clear choice between prompt treatment or deferral of treatment unless there was progression to high-risk PDR. Thus, one question of concern for the ETDRS was whether earlier scatter photocoagulation, before the development of high-risk PDR, justified the side effects and risks of laser surgery (Table 26–10).

In the ETDRS, early treatment, compared with "deferral" of photocoagulation until high-risk PDR develops,[22] was associated with a small reduction in the incidence of SVL, but 5-year rates of SVL were low for both the early treatment group and the group assigned to "deferral" of treatment (2.6

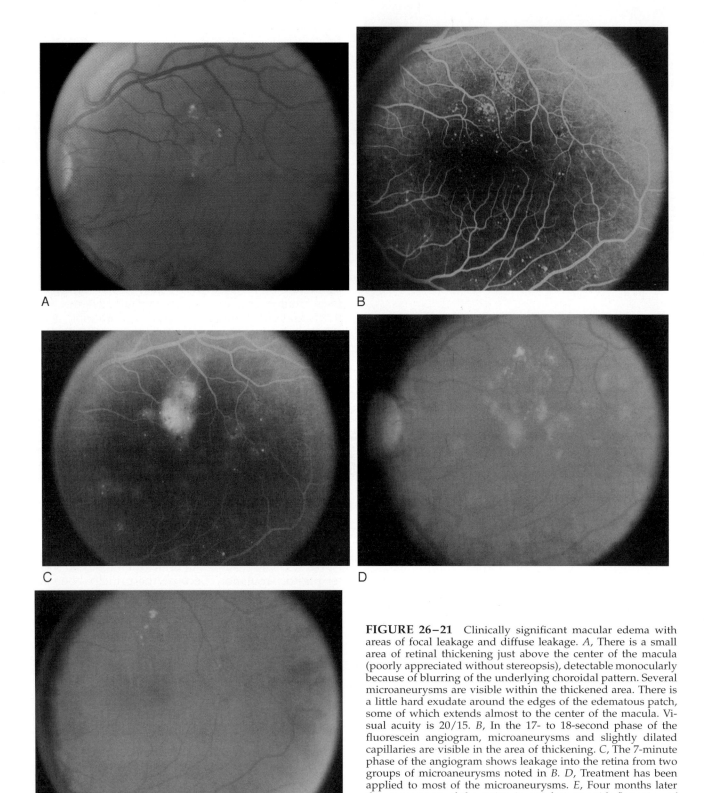

FIGURE 26–21 Clinically significant macular edema with areas of focal leakage and diffuse leakage. *A*, There is a small area of retinal thickening just above the center of the macula (poorly appreciated without stereopsis), detectable monocularly because of blurring of the underlying choroidal pattern. Several microaneurysms are visible within the thickened area. There is a little hard exudate around the edges of the edematous patch, some of which extends almost to the center of the macula. Visual acuity is 20/15. *B*, In the 17- to 18-second phase of the fluorescein angiogram, microaneurysms and slightly dilated capillaries are visible in the area of thickening. *C*, The 7-minute phase of the angiogram shows leakage into the retina from two groups of microaneurysms noted in *B*. *D*, Treatment has been applied to most of the microaneurysms. *E*, Four months later the appearance of the retina is satisfactory, with flattening of the center of the macula and disappearance of the thickening noted before treatment. Visual acuity remained at 20/15.

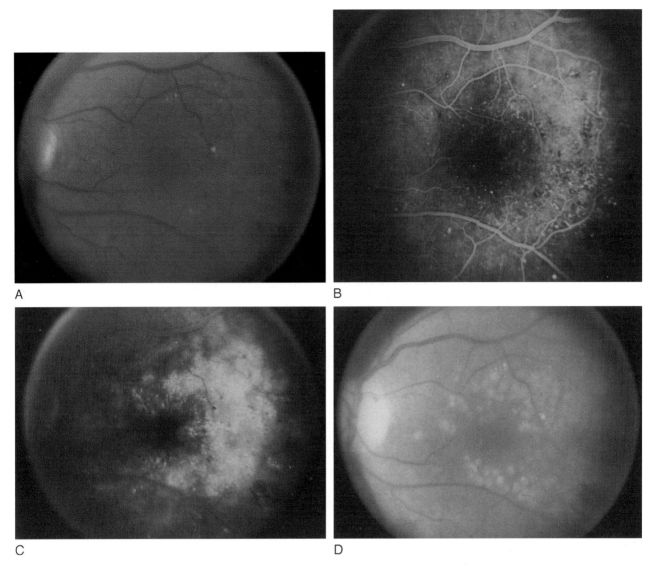

FIGURE 26–22   *A,* Clinical picture showing retinal thickening temporal to the center of the macula, extending just to the center. Visual acuity is 20/40. *B,* The early phase of the fluorescein angiogram shows capillary loss adjacent to the foveal avascular zone, capillary dilation, and scattered microaneurysms. *C,* The 7-minute phase of the angiogram shows extensive small cystoid spaces temporal to the center of the macula and above and below it. The center appears uninvolved. *D,* The microaneurysms have been treated focally and laser burns have been applied in a grid pattern in areas of diffuse leakage. *Illustration continued on following page*

and 3.7%, respectively). Provided careful follow-up can be maintained, scatter laser surgery is *not* recommended for eyes with mild or moderate NPDR.[25] When retinopathy is more severe (i.e., severe or very severe NPDR and early PDR), scatter photocoagulation should be "considered and usually should not be delayed if the eye has reached the high-risk proliferative stage."[25]

As retinopathy approaches the high-risk stage (very severe NPDR or early PDR), the benefits and risks of early photocoagulation may be roughly balanced; the benefit of a reduction of the risk of SVL from early photocoagulation may be more important in an eye that has almost a 50% risk of reaching high-risk stage within 1 year. Initiating scatter photocoagulation early in at least one eye seems par-

ticularly appropriate when both of a patient's eyes are approaching the high-risk stage, because optimal timing of photocoagulation may be difficult if both eyes simultaneously reach high-risk proliferative retinopathy and need photocoagulation. Also, prompt scatter photocoagulation should be considered for eyes with neovascularization in or threatening the anterior chamber angle, whether or not high-risk proliferative retinopathy is present.[25]

Treatment Protocol

The treatment program for diabetic retinopathy consists of (1) initial scatter laser photocoagulation

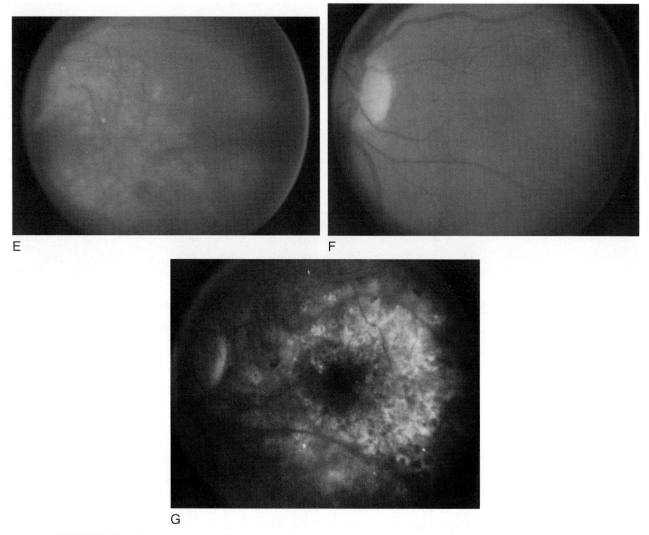

E

F

G

FIGURE 26–22 *Continued   E,* The temporal extent of the grid laser treatment. *F,* Four months later hemorrhages and hard exudates have decreased and the retinal thickening can no longer be detected. Visual acuity improved to 20/25. *G,* The 7-minute phase of the angiogram shows disappearance of most of the cystoid spaces visible in *C.*

surgery as the diabetic retinopathy approaches or reaches the high-risk stage, (2) careful follow-up at 4-month intervals following the treatment, (3) retreatment of persistent or recurrent treatable lesions, and (4) focal laser photocoagulation treatment for macular edema prior to scatter (panretinal) photocoagulation to reduce the risk of progression of macular edema secondary to scatter photocoagulation (see above). As high-risk PDR is reached, the major threat for SVL is traction retinal detachment, and a lesser threat is vitreous hemorrhage. The primary goal of the scatter laser surgery is the prevention of traction retinal detachment, particularly involving the macula, and the prevention of neovascular glaucoma.

Various strategies are involved in follow-up treatment. The ocular lesions to be considered for follow-up photocoagulation include new, flat neovascularization or elevated neovascularization; new, persistent, or recurrent CSME; and, rarely, feeder vessels to NVD. The treatment methods include additional scatter laser treatment; local laser to NVE; focal laser for CSME; pars plana vitrectomy, with or without endolaser, for recurrent hemorrhages with fibrovascular proliferation causing traction or, in some cases, for nonresponsive retinal or iris neovascularization; or perhaps merely continued observation. Further scatter treatment may be placed between previously placed laser scars as long as these scars do not become confluent and the extent of the scatter treatment is not such as to totally destroy retinal function.

While laser surgery is often considered painless, in younger patients some pain may be associated with the treatment. There also may be some discomfort or pain in all patients, especially when the peripheral retina is treated. Complications and side effects of laser photocoagulation are summarized in Table 26–10.

In summary, scatter treatment significantly reduces the risk of SVL from PDR. Both early scatter treatment prior to development of high-risk PDR and deferral of treatment until high-risk PDR develops reduce the risk of severe visual loss. The rates of SVL are low for each group. Consequently, it is recommended that scatter laser treatment *not* be used for mild to moderate NPDR. For severe NPDR and early PDR, scatter treatment is appropriate when close follow-up is unlikely or the disease process is progressing rapidly.

RESEARCH FRONTIERS IN DIABETIC RETINOPATHY

Present investigation of treatments for diabetic retinopathy address already established retinopathy in both early or late stages. Presumably, effective prevention of the early changes of diabetic retinopathy would also prevent the subsequent late sight-threatening pathology; however, the underlying mechanisms in the early processes are complex and clinical manifestations require several years to develop, thus making evaluation of treatment therapies slow.

The DCCT has shown conclusively that intensive diabetes control for persons with IDDM reduces the risk of onset and progression of early DR.[36–38] Another multicenter clinical trial, the Sorbinil Retinopathy Trial (SRT) (Table 26–11), tested whether a daily dose of sorbinil, an aldose reductase inhibitor (ARI), reduces the complications of diabetic retinopathy. Over a 3-year period the drug had no clinically beneficial effect on the course of diabetic retinopathy in adults with IDDM of moderate duration.[86] The group taking sorbinil, however, did show a slightly slower progression rate in microaneurysm count. There were complications of the use of the drug in the study population. Nearly 7% of the initial 202 participants had adverse reactions including toxic epidermal necrolysis, erythema multiforme, and Stevens-Johnson syndrome. It is unlikely that sorbinil will achieve prophylactic usage because of the hypersensitivity reactions and outcome similarities between the sorbinil-treated and control groups. Other ARIs, notably Tolrestat, which has a different chemical structure than sorbinil, are presently under investigation in the United States and Canada. Discouraging results of the Sorbinil Retinopathy Trial suggest that further research on the pharmacokinetics and side effects of ARIs is necessary before further human clinical trials are undertaken.[87–89]

Diabetes affects both large and small blood vessels. The most common pathologic changes occur in the microcirculation of the retina and the renal glomeruli, suggesting that systemic factors play a major role in the pathogenesis of diabetic vascular disease. Although diabetic vascular complications can affect almost every organ of the body, the observed histopathologies appear to be organ specific. Thus local factors might also be important in the development of vascular complications. Maintenance of euglycemia can prevent the onset of microvascular disease if it is initiated early in the course of the disease.[68,84] In fact, Engerman et al reported that maintenance of euglycemia in dogs by insulin at the initiation of diabetes will completely prevent the development of retinal vascular pathology. Retinopathy, however, will develop after 4 years of diabetes in dogs allowed to be hyperglycemic for the initial $2^1/_2$ years, followed by subsequent euglycemia, even though no vascular pathologies were detected at the halfway point. Further support for the necessity of early treatment has come from the study of retinopathy in diabetic patients who had achieved euglycemia with pancreatic transplants.[84] Their retinopathy progressed at a similar rate as traditional insulin therapy patients. In contrast, the results from the DCCT showed that patients with no diabetic retinopathy enrolled in the intensive insulin therapy group (primary intervention cohort) had a 76% reduction in the risk for developing retinopathy, while patients already exhibiting mild diabetic retinopathy (secondary intervention cohort) showed a 54% reduction in the risk for retinopathy progression.[36–38] These data strongly suggest that treatment to prevent vascular complications needs to be instituted early, before the onset of clinically overt vascular diseases, in order to realize maximal therapeutic benefit. Further, these studies suggest that some permanent biochemical or genetic alterations have already occurred in vascular tissues that are not detectable by current morphologic techniques.

Although genetic differences can modulate the severity of the vascular pathologies,[90] epidemiologic and animal studies suggest that one of the most important metabolic factors that may cause vascular dysfunction in diabetes is hyperglycemia.[36–38,91] The mechanisms eliciting the vascular abnormalities are not well characterized to date. It is generally accepted, however, that the adverse effects of hyperglycemia involve multiple mechanisms, as glucose and its metabolites are utilized by a number of different intracellular pathways. Several theories have been proposed to link observed effects with potential mechanisms. These include the aldose–reductase polyol pathway, nonenzymatic glycation, alteration of the redox potential, and the diacylglycerol–protein kinase C pathway.

Studies investigating the sorbitol–polyol pathway have shown in most cells exposed to high glucose levels that glucose can be converted to sorbitol by aldose reductase.[87] Sorbitol can be metabolized by sorbitol dehydrogenase into fructose with the production of NADH, but the rate of conversion of sorbitol is relatively slow, resulting in a cellular accumulation of sorbitol, as sorbitol does not diffuse across cell membranes.[87,88] Thus cellular damage can occur as a result of an increased osmotic stress. Such is the case in the lens of the eye where accumulation of sorbitol has been implicated in the development of cataracts in diabetes.[89] Sorbitol accumulation, however, can vary from tissue to tissue and may in some tissues never reach levels high enough to cause abnormalities. Studies in animal models of diabetes using aldose reductase inhibitors provided promising results in normalizing neurologic dysfunction and increased renal glomerular filtration rate in diabetic rats.[92,93] Subsequent clinical trials did not, however, demonstrate that aldose reductase inhibitors were effective in ameliorating human neuropathy or retinopathy and had significant side effects.[86] Further studies have focused on dogs and rats fed a high-galactose diet. Using this model it was felt that the accumulation of galactitol would mimic the effect of sorbitol and cause the development of vascular abnormalities independent of any other metabolic changes found in diabetes.[94-96] The results from these studies showed that formation of cataracts and early changes in the retinal microvessels similar to those seen in diabetes resulted from the accumulation of galactitol. Experiments involved with the use of aldose reductase inhibitors in the galactose model, however, were equivocal, as some studies showed an inhibition of the development of retinopathy while other studies were unable to demonstrate any significant effects.

Nonenzymatic glycation has also been proposed as a potential mechanism associated with the development of abnormal vascular cell function in diabetes. Nonenzymatic glycation refers to the ability of glucose to form covalent products by nucleophilic addition to protein amino groups and possibly DNA to form intermediate glycosylation products.[97,98] Further reactions of these intermediates lead to the formation of advanced glycosylation end products (AGE) in an irreversible chemical reaction. The half-life for the formation of AGE products can occur over many years, and the level of glucose and duration of exposure to glucose impact on the rate of AGE formation. Recent investigations have shown that infusion of AGE can mimic some of the vascular abnormalities noted in diabetes such as increased basement membrane thickening and alterations in vascular contractility, the latter mediated through a blunting of the effect of nitric oxide, which causes vasodilation or relaxation of contractile vessels. Studies are in progress investigating agents that can inhibit the formation of AGE such as aminoguanidine.[98-100] Early results have shown that chronic treatment with aminoguanidine may reduce basement membrane thickening and early changes in the retinal vasculature of diabetic rats.

Changes in the redox potential in association with high glucose levels have been shown to be the result of increased glucose metabolism via glycolysis or the polyol pathway resulting in an increase in the ratio of NADH to NAD.[101,102] Accordingly, the increased NADH/NAD ratio can lead to changes in other metabolic pathways such as the synthesis of diacylglycerol, DNA repair, and fatty acid oxidation. Studies investigating the normalization of the NADH/NAD ratio using pyruvate, for example, have shown a normalization of various vascular tissue functions in diabetic animals.[103,104]

The activation of protein kinase C (PKC) in diabetes has been the focus of a number of investigations. This interest is based in part by the fact that these regulatory enzymes and lipids affect a wide range of vascular functions such as permeability, contractility, coagulation, flow, hormone action, growth factor effects, and ultimately basement membrane synthesis and turnover.[105,106] All of these variables have been found to be abnormal in diabetes. In both chemically and genetically induced diabetes in rats it was found that PKC activities were elevated in many tissues such as the retina, aorta, heart, and renal glomeruli. Diacylglycerol (DAG) was found to increase in parallel with PKC activation in these tissues.[106,107] These results are consistent with the knowledge that DAG activates PKC, causing its translocation from the cytosol to the cell membrane. The membranous fraction of the PKC is the biologically active component. Studies have also shown that the *alpha* and *beta*-II isoforms predominate in vascular cells and that the *beta* isoform is preferentially elevated in retinal vascular cells in diabetes.[107,108] PKC and DAG changes are not modulated through osmotic changes or by changes in the sorbitol pathway, as PKC is unresponsive to aldose reductase. Studies in diabetic rats have shown a causal relationship between elevation of DAG, activation of PKC, and the development of abnormal retinal blood flow.[109] Preliminary clinical studies have also shown a relationship between retinal blood flow changes and elevations in DAG in diabetic patients with no diabetic retinopathy.[70,109] In addition, normalization of PKC activities in diabetes through the use of specific inhibitors has resulted in retinal blood flow normalization in diabetic rats.[110] Interestingly, the effects of elevated glucose in diabetes do not occur rapidly and are not easily reversed. Studies in diabetic rats showed, once PKC and DAG changes had been established over several weeks, that euglycemic control of the diabetic animals did not immediately reverse all the biochemical abnormalities.[107]

Ongoing investigations are addressing the modulation of retinal blood flow by vasoactive agents such as endothelin, angiotensin II, histamine, and oxygen. Inhibition of these processes with insulin therapy or islet cell transplants may normalize retinal blood flow in diabetes. The prevalence of antipericyte antibodies, a reflection of pericyte degeneration, may be related to early development of diabetic retinopathy.

Investigations focusing on different factors contributing to vascular abnormalities in diabetes have pointed the way to the development of various therapeutic agents aimed at inhibiting these abnormalities. For example, studies with vitamin E treatment have demonstrated a normalization of PKC levels and a normalization of retinal blood flow changes in diabetic rats.[66,111] With the increasing emphasis on investigating mechanisms associated with the development of diabetic retinopathy, a noninvasive method for quantitating changes in retinal physiology at the earliest stages of diabetes becomes essential for the rapid assessment of potential therapeutic agents used to ameliorate the risk for developing retinopathy. The investigation of the effects of locally or systematically generated vasoactive agents on the retinal vasculature and circulation is important, as these studies can provide insights into the in vivo biologic regulation of diabetic-related changes in the retina.

The noninvasive measurement of retinal blood flow provides a unique method for monitoring early physiologic function changes in diabetes. In addition, if the noninvasive measurement of retinal blood flow is correlated with the development of clinically observable pathologies, a means of characterization of the effects of early vascular changes on the physiologic function of the retina results. Generally, fluorescein angiography techniques and laser Doppler velocimetry (LDV) have been the methods of choice for noninvasive quantitation of retinal blood flow, as the measurements can be performed in both animal models and human subjects. If changes in retinal blood flow can provide a sensitive end point for assessing the effectiveness of therapeutic interventions, then the resulting advantage of providing an earlier end point than the clinically observed progression or development of diabetic retinopathy will permit shorter and less expensive clinical studies.

Researchers and clinicians have postulated for nearly 50 years that the proliferative component of diabetic retinopathy must be the result of growth factors released by the retina,[82,112] in response to retinal ischemia. Clinically, the development of retinal neovascularization at the borders of perfused and nonperfused zones, development of neovascularization at retinal sites remote from the nonperfused zones such as the optic nerve head, and development of neovascularization at distant sites in the eye such as the iris support this hypothesis. Numerous growth factors, some of which are capable of inducing capillary growth, have been isolated within the eye, including basic fibrovascular growth factor and insulin-like growth factor I.[112,113] Although sometimes elevated in eyes with proliferative diabetic retinopathy, these findings have not been consistent for these molecules. In addition, basic fibroblast growth factor does not possess a signal sequence capable of allowing it to be secreted from intact cells.[113,114] Since the finding of neovascularization at distant sites suggests that the responsible growth factor must be diffusable, it is difficult to envision how basic fibroblast growth factor could be the primary molecule involved.

Recent studies have focused on the angiogenic peptide called vascular endothelial growth factor (VEGF). This 45,000-dalton protein induces angiogenesis in numerous highly vascularized and rapidly proliferating tumors.[115,116] Its effect is endothelial cell-selective with receptors for the molecule primarily found on endothelial cells. Interestingly, its production is dramatically elevated under hypoxic conditions.[117] Recent studies have demonstrated that numerous retinal cells types including retinal pericytes, retinal endothelial cells, Müller cells, and retinal pigment epithelium can both produce VEGF and increase its production under hypoxic conditions.[83,118–120] In addition, retinal endothelial cells have been shown to possess more high-affinity VEGF receptors than any other cell type reported to date.[121] Clinical studies have demonstrated that VEGF levels are dramatically elevated in the aqueous and vitreous of patients with actively proliferating neovascularization from diabetic retinopathy, central retinal vein occlusion, rubeosis iridis, and other conditions.[85,125] Interestingly, VEGF is not elevated under these same conditions when neovascularization is quiescent. Specifically, in diabetic retinopathy, low levels of VEGF are noted during nonproliferative stages and during quiescent proliferative disease, while elevated concentrations are noted during the active proliferative periods. In addition, a posterior-to-anterior concentration gradient between the vitreous and aqueous fluids exists as would be expected for a retina-produced factor. Finally, following panretinal laser photocoagulation, which effectively reduces intraocular neovascularization, the VEGF levels were found to be reduced. These findings imply that vascular endothelial growth factor may play a major role in ischemia-induced neovascularization of the retina and anterior chamber as seen in diabetic retinopathy.

These findings suggest that inhibition of VEGF may result in suppression of neovascularization in vivo. Indeed, inhibition of VEGF in tumors in mice has suppressed tumor growth rates.[122] In vitro inhibition of VEGF can prevent VEGF-stimulated endothelial cell growth, hypoxic condition media–stimulated endothelial cell growth, and vitreous-stimulated cell growth when obtained from patients with actively proliferating diabetic retinopathy.[85,124] Recent studies have demonstrated that intravitreal injection of VEGF inhibitors in a mouse model of aggressive ischemia-induced neovascularization reduced the development of neovascularization by approximately 50%.[124,126] Similar results have been observed in primate models of iris neo-vascularization.[127] If similar growth factor inhibitors can be developed that permit noninvasive delivery, it may eventually be possible to provide novel treatment modalities for prevention of proliferative diabetic retinopathy that do not suffer from the intrinsic destructive nature of panretinal photocoagulation.

CLINICAL GUIDELINES

Until modalities are in place to prevent or cure diabetic retinopathy and other complications, the emphasis must be placed on identification, careful follow-up, and timely laser photocoagulation of patients with diabetic retinopathy and diabetic eye disease. Proper care will result in reduction of personal suffering for those involved as well as a substantial cost savings for the involved individuals, their families, and the country as a whole. Therefore, strict guidelines have been established for the ocular care of people with diabetes (Tables 26–9 through 26–12).

All diabetic patients should be informed of the possibility of developing retinopathy with or without symptoms and the associated threat of visual loss. The natural course and treatment of diabetic retinopathy should be discussed and the importance of routine examination should be stressed. Patients should be informed of the possible relationship between level of control of diabetes and the subsequent development of ocular and other medical complications. Their role as a partner in the health care team should be emphasized. Patients should be informed that diabetic nephropathy, as manifest by proteinuria, requires aggressive early treatment with proper diet and blood pressure control. The association of joint contractures, hypertension, cardiovascular disease, elevated lipid levels, and neuropathy with onset and progression of diabetic retinopathy should be discussed.

Diabetic women contemplating pregnancy should have a complete eye examination prior to conception. Pregnant women with diabetes should have their eyes examined early in each trimester of their pregnancy or more frequently as indicated by level of retinopathy. A postpartum examination 3 to 6 months following delivery is suggested. Since

TABLE 26–10   Complications and Side Effects of Scatter (Panretinal) Laser Photocoagulation

1. Field constriction and night blindness
   Depends upon extent of scatter
2. Foveal burn
   Landmarks may be difficult to identify
3. Macular edema
   About 10% risk of mild visual loss
4. Foveal traction
   Occurs with remission of PDR
   Occurs with burns applied over blood
5. Serous and/or choroidal detachment
   Acute angle closure glaucoma is possible
6. Anterior segment
   Posterior synechiae
   Cornea and lens burns
   Internal ophthalmoplegia
   Uncommon with multiple sessions, light to moderately intense burns, and use of laser instead of xenon
7. Pain
   Younger diabetic—more painful
   Peripheral retina—more painful
   Reassurance
   Retrobulbar anesthesia rarely needed
8. Retrobulbar hemorrhage due to retrobulbar anesthesia injection
   Laser surgery can continue
   More frequent without sedation
   Watch central retinal artery
9. Loss to follow-up:
   Importance of patient/doctor relationship

TABLE 26–11 Sorbinil Retinopathy Study (SRT)

SRT Evaluating
Effect on onset and progression of diabetic retinopathy
Effect on neuropathy and nephropathy
Safety and tolerance of sorbinil

SRT Design Features
Type I for 1–15 years
Random sorbinil/placebo
Follow-up for 3 years
250 mg daily

SRT Results (250 mg)
No effect on onset of diabetic retinopathy
No effect on progression of diabetic retinopathy
Hypersensitivity in 7%
Slightly less microaneurysm count
No effect on blood pressure, Hb A1C

Limitations of SRT
Diabetic retinopathy not early enough
Duration of SRT too short
Dosage (250 mg) too small
Unknown effect on retina
Pharmacokinetics still unclear

pregnancy may exacerbate existing retinopathy and be associated with hypertension, careful medical and ocular observation is crucial during pregnancy. In women with certain levels of proliferative retinopathy, cesarean section may be preferable to vaginal delivery to reduce the risk of Valsalva-induced vitreous hemorrhage. Close communication among the various members of the health care team is essential.

Patients with diabetic retinopathy, even in its mildest form, must be informed of the availability and benefits of early and timely laser photocoagulation therapy in reducing the risk of visual loss. The management program outlined in Table 26–9

is fundamental. Furthermore, patients with visual impairment of any degree, legal blindness, or total blindness, should be informed of the availability of visual, vocational, and psychosocial rehabilitation programs.

CONCLUSIONS

In its earliest stages, diabetic retinopathy usually causes no symptoms. Visual acuity may be excellent at the time of diagnosis and a patient may deny the presence of retinopathy. It is crucial at this stage for a patient's physician to initiate a careful program of education and medical and ocular follow-up.

If the retinal disease progresses, visual acuity may be compromised by macular edema or episodes of vitreous hemorrhage. These complications may cause difficulty in the work or home environment, resulting in continued denial, fear, or anger. Although ultimate visual acuity may improve, a patient may remain in a state of uncertainty and anxiety until retinopathy becomes quiescent, either secondary to laser treatment, vitreoretinal surgery, or the natural history of the disease process. Once the retinopathy is in remission and the vision stable, a patient is in a position to accept the situation and to make the appropriate psychological and social adjustments. At this time, visual and vocational rehabilitation is more likely to be successful.

Communication amongst all members of a patient's health care team is of paramount importance in dealing with the physical and psychological stresses of visual loss from diabetes. Faced with the current inability to prevent or cure diabetic retinopathy, the main concern of all doctors must now focus on early detection of diabetic retinopathy. Patient access, careful medical and ophthalmological follow-up, and timely laser photocoagulation are fundamental to the successful elimination of blindness in people with diabetes mellitus.

TABLE 26–12 Eye Examination Schedule

Type of Diabetes Mellitus	Recommendation Time of First Exam	Routine Minimum Follow-up*
Type I, IDDM	5 years after onset or during puberty	Yearly
Type II, NIDDM	At time of diagnosis	Yearly
During pregnancy	Prior to pregnancy for counseling	Each trimester
	Early in first trimester	More frequently as indicated
		3–6 months postpartum

* Abnormal findings dictate more frequent follow-up examinations (see Table 26–9).

REFERENCES

1. Waite JH, Beetham WP: The visual mechanism in diabetes mellitus: a comparative study of 2002 diabetics and 457 non-diabetics for control. N Engl J Med 212:367–379, 429–443, 1935.
2. Aiello LM, Beetham WP, Balodimos MC, et al: Ruby laser photocoagulation in treatment of diabetic proliferating retinopathy: preliminary report. In Goldberg MF, Fine S (eds): Symposium on the Treatment of Diabetic Retinopathy. Public Health Service Publication No. 1890. Washington, DC, US Government Printing Office, 1969, pp 437–463.
3. Diabetic Retinopathy Study Report Number 1: Preliminary report on effects of photocoagulation therapy. Am J Ophthalmol 81:1–14, 1976.
4. Diabetic Retinopathy Study Report Number 2: Photocoagulation of proliferative diabetic retinopathy. Ophthalmology 85:82, 1978.
5. Diabetic Retinopathy Study Report Number 3: Four risk factors for severe visual loss in diabetic retinopathy. Arch Ophthalmol 97:658, 1979.
6. Diabetic Retinopathy Study Report Number 4: A short report of long range results. Proceedings of the 10th Congress of International Diabetes Federation, Excerpta Medica, 1980.
7. Diabetic Retinopathy Study Report Number 5: Photocoagulation treatment of proliferative diabetic retinopathy. Relationship of adverse treatment effects to retinopathy severity. Dev Ophthalmol 2(39):1–15, 1981.
8. Diabetic Retinopathy Study Report Number 6: Design, methods, and baseline results. Invest Ophthalmol 21:149–209, 1981.
9. Diabetic Retinopathy Study Report Number 7: A modification of the Airlie House Classification of Diabetic Retinopathy. Invest Ophthalmol 21:210–226, 1981.
10. Diabetic Retinopathy Study Report Number 8: Photocoagulation treatment of proliferative diabetic retinopathy. Clinical application of Diabetic Retinopathy Study (DRS) findings. Ophthalmology 88:583–600, 1981.
11. Diabetic Retinopathy Study Report Number 9: Assessing possible late treatment effects in stopping clinical trials early: a case study by F. Ederer, MJ Podgor. Control Clin Trials 5:373–381, 1984.
12. Diabetic Retinopathy Study Report Number 10: Factors influencing the development of visual loss in advanced diabetic retinopathy. Invest Ophthalmol 26:983–991, 1985.
13. Diabetic Retinopathy Study Report Number 11: Intraocular pressure following panretinal photocoagulation for diabetic retinopathy. Arch Ophthalmol 105:807–809, 1987.
14. Diabetic Retinopathy Study Report Number 12: Macular edema in Diabetic Retinopathy Study patients. Ophthalmology 94:754–760, 1987.
15. Diabetic Retinopathy Study Report Number 13: Factors associated with visual outcome after photocoagulation for diabetic retinopathy. Invest Ophthalmol 30:23–28, 1989.
16. Diabetic Retinopathy Study Report Number 14: Indications for photocoagulation treatment of diabetic retinopathy. Int Ophthalmol Clin 27:239–253, 1987.
17. Early Treatment Diabetic Retinopathy Study Report Number 1: Photocoagulation for diabetic macular edema. Arch Ophthalmol 103:1796–1806, 1985.
18. Early Treatment Diabetic Retinopathy Study Report Number 2: Treatment techniques and clinical guidelines for photocoagulation of diabetic macular edema. Ophthalmology 94:761–774, 1987.
19. Early Treatment Diabetic Retinopathy Study Report Number 3: Techniques for scatter and local photocoagulation treatment of diabetic retinopathy. Int Ophthalmol Clin 27:254–264, 1987.
20. Early Treatment Diabetic Retinopathy Study Report Number 4: Photocoagulation for diabetic macular edema. Int Ophthalmol Clin 27:265–272, 1987.
21. Early Treatment Diabetic Retinopathy Study Case Reports Number 3 and 4: Case reports to accompany Early Treatment Diabetic Retinopathy Study Reports Numbers 3 and 4. Int Ophthalmol Clin J 27:273–333, 1987.
22. Early Treatment Diabetic Retinopathy Study Report Number 5: Detection of diabetic macular edema. Ophthalmoscopy versus photography. Ophthalmology 96:746–751, 1989.
23. Early Treatment Diabetic Retinopathy Study Report Number 7: Early Treatment Diabetic Retinopathy Study design and baseline patient characteristics. Ophthalmology 98:741–756, 1991.
24. Early Treatment Diabetic Retinopathy Study Report Number 8: Effects of aspirin treatment on diabetic retinopathy. Ophthalmology 98:757–765, 1991.
25. Early Treatment Diabetic Retinopathy Study Report Number 9: Early photocoagulation for diabetic retinopathy. Ophthalmology 98:766–785, 1991.
26. Early Treatment Diabetic Retinopathy Study Report Number 10: Grading diabetic retinopathy from stereoscopic color fundus photographs—an extension of the modified Airlie House Classification. Ophthalmology 98:786–806, 1991.
27. Early Treatment Diabetic Retinopathy Study Report Number 11: Classification of diabetic retinopathy from fluorescein angiograms. Ophthalmology 98:807–822, 1991.
28. Early Treatment Diabetic Retinopathy Study Report Number 12: Fundus photographic risk factors for progression of diabetic retinopathy. Ophthalmology 98:823–833, 1991.
29. Early Treatment Diabetic Retinopathy Study Report Number 13: Fluorescein angiographic risk factors for progression of diabetic retinopathy. Ophthalmology 98:834–840, 1991.
30. Early Treatment Diabetic Study Report Number 19: Focal photocoagulation treatment of diabetic macular edema: relationship of treatment effect to fluorescein angiographic and other retinal characteristics at baseline. Arch Ophthalmol 113:1144–1155, 1995.
31. Diabetic Retinopathy Vitrectomy Study Report Number 1: Two-year course of visual acuity in severe proliferative diabetic retinopathy with conventional management. Ophthalmology 92:492–502, 1985.
32. Diabetic Retinopathy Vitrectomy Study Report Number 2: Early vitrectomy for severe vitreous hemorrhage in diabetic retinopathy. Two-year results of a randomized trial. Arch Ophthalmol 103:1644–1652, 1985.
33. Diabetic Retinopathy Vitrectomy Study Report Number 3: Early vitrectomy for severe proliferative diabetic retinopathy in eyes with useful vision. Results of a randomized trial. Ophthalmology 95:1307–1320, 1988.
34. Diabetic Retinopathy Vitrectomy Study Report Number 4: Early vitrectomy for severe proliferative diabetic retinopathy in eyes with useful vision. Clinical application of results of a randomized trial. Ophthalmology 95:1331–1334, 1988.
35. Diabetic Retinopathy Vitrectomy Study Report Number 5: Early vitrectomy for severe vitreous hemorrhage in diabetic retinopathy. Four-year results of a randomized trial. Arch Ophthalmol 108:958–964, 1990.
36. DCCT Research Group: The effects of intensive treatment of diabetes on the development and progression of long-term complications in Insulin-Dependent Diabetes Mellitus. N Engl J Med 329:977–986, 1993.
37. DCCT Research Group: Are continuing studies on metabolic control and microvascular complications in insulin-dependent diabetes mellitus justified? N Engl J Med 318:246, 1988.
38. DCCT Research Group: Progression of retinopathy with intensive versus conventional treatment in the Diabetes Control and Complications Trial. Ophthalmology 102:647–661, 1995.
39. National Diabetes Data Group: National Institute of Diabetes and Digestive and Kidney Diseases, National Institutes of Health, 1994.

40. Klein HA, Moorehead HB: Statistics on Blindness in the Model Reporting Area, 1969–1970. [Bethesda, MD]: US Dept of Health, Education & Welfare, 1973 (DHEW Publ No [NIH] 73-427, 1970).

41. Klein R, Klein BEK: Vision disorders in diabetes. In National Diabetes Data Group. Diabetes in America: Diabetes Data Compiled 1984 [Bethesda, MD]: US Department of Health and Human Services, 1985, pp 1–2 (NIH Publ No 85-1468).

42. Klein R, Klein BEK, Moss SE, et al: The Wisconsin Epidemiologic Study of Diabetic Retinopathy. II. Prevalence and risk of diabetic retinopathy when age at diagnosis is less than 30 years. Arch Ophthalmol 102:520–526, 1984.

43. Klein R, Klein BEK, Moss SE, et al: The Wisconsin Epidemiologic Study of Diabetic Retinopathy. III. Prevalence and risk of diabetic retinopathy when age at diagnosis is 30 or more years. Arch Ophthalmol 102:527–532, 1984.

44. American Diabetes Association: 1994 Vital Statistics.

45. Aiello LM, Cavallerano JD: Ocular complications of diabetes mellitus. In Kahn CR, Weir GC (eds): Joslin's Diabetes Mellitus, 13th edition. Philadelphia, Lea & Febiger, 1994, pp 771–793.

46. Aiello LM, Rand LI, Briones JL, et al: Diabetes retinopathy in Joslin Clinic patients with adult-onset diabetes. Ophthalmology 88:619–623, 1981.

47. Javitt JC, Aiello LP, Bassi LJ, et al: Detecting and treating retinopathy in patients with type 1 diabetes mellitus. Ophthalmology 98:1565–1574, 1991.

48. Javitt JC, Aiello LP, Chiang YP, et al: Preventive eye care in people with diabetes is cost-saving to the federal government. Diabetes Care 17:909–917, 1994.

49. Javitt JC, Aiello LP, Bassi LJ, et al: Detecting and treating retinopathy in patients with type I diabetes mellitus. Savings associated with improved implementation of current guidelines. Ophthalmology 98:1565–1574, 1994.

50. Javitt JC, Aiello LP: Cost effectiveness of detecting and treating diabetic retinopathy. Ann Intern Med 124:164–168, 1996.

51. Moloney JBM, Drury MI: The effect of pregnancy on the natural course of diabetic retinopathy. Am J Ophthalmol 93:745–756, 1982.

52. Serup L: Influence of pregnancy on diabetic retinopathy. Acta Endocrinol 277:122–124, 1986.

53. Phelps RL, Sakol P, Metzger BE, et al: Changes in diabetic retinopathy during pregnancy; correlations with regulation of hyperglycemia. Arch Ophthalmol 104:1806–1810, 1986.

54. Klein BE, Moss SE, Klein R: Effect of pregnancy on progression of diabetic retinopathy. Diabetes Care 13:34–40, 1990.

55. The Kroc Collaborative Study Group: Blood glucose control and the evolution of diabetic retinopathy and albuminuria. N Engl J Med 311:365–372, 1984.

56. Grunwald JE, Riva CE, Martin DB, et al: Effect of insulin induced decrease in blood glucose on the human diabetic retinal circulation. Ophthalmology 94:1614–1620, 1987.

57. Chase HP, Jackson WE, Hoops SL, et al: Glucose control in the renal and retinal complications of insulin dependent diabetes. JAMA 261:1155–1160, 1989.

58. Brinchmann-Hansen O, Dahl-Jorgensen K, Hanssen KF, for the Oslo Study Group: Effects of intensified insulin treatment on various lesions of diabetic retinopathy. Am J Ophthalmol 100:644–653, 1985.

59. Krolewski AZ, Canessa M, Warram JH, et al: True disposition to hypertension and susceptibility to renal disease in insulin-dependent diabetes mellitus. N Engl J Med 318:140–145, 1988.

60. Stern MP, Patterson JK, Haffner SM, et al: Lack of awareness and treatment of hyperlipidemia in type II diabetes in a community survey. JAMA 262:360–364, 1989.

61. Chantry KH, Klein ML, Chew EY, for the Early Treatment Diabetic Retinopathy Study Group: Association of serum lipids and retinal hard exudates in patients enrolled in the Early Treatment Diabetic Retinopathy Study. Invest Ophthalmol Vis Sci 30(Suppl):434, 1989.

62. Engerman RL, Kern TS: Is Diabetic Retinopathy Preventable? Int Ophthalmol Clinic 28:225–229, 1988.

63. Bresnick GH: Background diabetic retinopathy. In Ryan SJ (ed): Retina, Vol 2. Medical Retina. St Louis, CV Mosby Co, 1989, pp 327–366.

64. Shimizu K, Kobayashi Y, Muraoka K: Midperipheral fundus involvement in diabetic retinopathy. Ophthalmology 88:601–612, 1981.

65. Takashi N, Muroka K, Shimizu K: Distribution of capillary nonperfusion in early-stage diabetic retinopathy. Ophthalmology 91:1431–1439, 1984.

66. Bursell S-E, Clermont AC, Oren B, et al: The in vivo effect of endothelins on retinal circulation in non-diabetic and diabetic rats. Invest Ophthalmol Vis Sci 36:596, 1995.

67. Kuwabara T, Cogan D: Studies of retinal vascular patterns. Part 1: normal architecture. Arch Ophthalmol 64:124, 1960.

68. Engerman RL, Kern TS: Progression of incipient diabetic retinopathy during good glycemic control. Diabetes 36:808, 1987.

69. Bertram B, Wolf S, Schulte K, et al: Retinal blood flow in diabetic children and adolescents. Graefes Arch Clin Exp Ophthalmol 98:996, 1991.

70. Bursell S-E, Clermont AC, Wald H, et al: Correlation between decreased retinal blood flow and increased diacylglycerol in patients with early diabetes. Invest Ophthalmol Vis Sci 35:2088, 1994.

71. Feke GT, Buzney SM, Ogasawara H, et al: Retinal circulatory abnormalities in type I diabetes. Invest Ophthalmol Vis Sci 35:2968, 1994.

72. Wolf S, Arend O, Toonen H, et al: Retinal capillary blood flow measurement with a scanning laser ophthalmoscope. Ophthalmology 98:996, 1991.

73. Yoshida A, Feke GT, Moralles-Stoppello J, et al: Retinal blood flow alteration during progression of diabetic retinopathy. Arch Ophthalmol 101:225, 1983.

74. Grunwald JE, Riva CE, Sinclair SH, et al: Laser Doppler velocimetry study of retinal circulation in diabetes mellitus. Arch Ophthalmol 104:991, 1986.

75. Grunwald JE, Riva CE, Baine J, et al: Total retinal volumetric flow rate in diabetic patients with poor glycemic control. Invest Ophthalmol Vis Sci 33:356, 1992.

76. Patel V, Rassam S, Kohner E, et al: Retinal blood flow in diabetic retinopathy. Br Med J 305:678, 1992.

77. Grunwald JE, Riva CE, Martin DB, et al: Effect of an insulin-induced decrease in blood glucose on the human diabetic retinal circulation. Ophthalmology 94:1614, 1987.

78. Grunwald JE, Riva CE, Petrig BL, et al: Effect of pure O_2-breathing on retinal blood flow in patients with background diabetic retinopathy. Curr Eye Res 3:239, 1984.

79. Riva CE, Grunwald JE, Sinclair SH: Laser Doppler velocimetry study of the effect of pure oxygen breathing on retinal blood flow. Invest Ophthalmol Vis Sci 24:47, 1983.

80. Winegrad AI: Banting Lecture: does a common mechanism induce the diverse complications of diabetes? Diabetes 36:396, 1987.

81. Rand LI, Krolewski AS, Aiello LM, et al: Multiple factors in the prediction of risk of diabetic retinopathy. N Engl J Med 313:1433, 1985.

82. Michaelson IC: The mode of development of the vascular system of the retina, with some observations on its significance for certain retinal diseases. Trans Ophthalmol Soc U K 68:137–180, 1948.

83. Aiello LP, Northrup JM, Keyt BA, et al: Hypoxic regulation of vascular endothelial growth factor in retinal cells. Arch Ophthalmol 113:1538–1544, 1995.

84. Ramsay RC, Goetz FC, Sutherland DER: Progression of diabetic retinopathy after pancreas transplantation for insulin-dependent diabetes mellitus. N Engl J Med 318:208, 1988.

85. Aiello LP, Avery RL, Arrigg PG, et al: Vascular endothelial growth factor in ocular fluid of patients with diabetic retinopathy and other retinal disorders. N Engl J Med 331:1480–1487, 1994.

86. Sorbinil Retinopathy Trial Research Group: A randomized

trial of sorbinil, an aldose reductase inhibitor in diabetic retinopathy. Arch Ophthalmol 108:1234–1244, 1990.

87. Greene DA, Lattimer SA, Sima AAF, et al: Sorbitol, phosphoinositides and sodium-potassium ATP-ase in the pathogenesis of diabetic complications. N Engl J Med 316:559, 1987.

88. Kador PF, Robison EG, Kinoshita JH: Pharmacology of aldose reductase inhibitors. Ann Rev Pharmacol Toxicol 25:691, 1985.

89. Kinoshita JH: Mechanisms initiating cataract formation. Invest Ophthalmol Vis Sci 13:713, 1974.

90. Seaquist ER, Goetz FC, Rich S, et al: Familial clustering of diabetic kidney disease. Evidence for genetic susceptibility to diabetic nephropathy. N Engl J Med 320:1161, 1989.

91. Pirart J: Diabetes mellitus and its degenerative complications: a prospective study of 4400 patients observed between 1947 and 1973. Diabetes Care 1:168, 1978.

92. Sutera SP, Chang K, Marvel J, et al: Concurrent increases in regional hematocrit and blood flow in diabetic rats: prevention by sorbinil. Am J Physiol 263:H945, 1992.

93. Williamson JR, Kawamura T, Kilo C, et al: Current concepts of the role of polyol metabolism and related metabolic abnormalities in diabetic complications. In Sakamoto N, Alberti KGMM, Hotta N (eds): Pathogenesis and Treatment of NIDDM and its Related Problems. Amsterdam, Elsevier Science BV, 1994, pp 75–81.

94. Robison WG, Tillis TN, Laver N, et al: Diabetes related histopathologies of the rat retina prevented with an aldose reductase inhibitor. Exp Eye Res 50:355, 1990.

95. Engerman RI, Kern TS: Experimental galactosemia produces diabetic-like retinopathy. Diabetes 33:97, 1984.

96. Engerman RI, Kern TS: Aldose reductase inhibition fails to prevent retinopathy in diabetic and galactosemic dogs. Diabetes 42:820, 1993.

97. Brownlee M, Cerami A, Vlassara H: Advanced glycosylation end products in tissue and the biochemical basis of diabetic complications. N Engl J Med 318:1315, 1988.

98. McCance DR, Dyer DG, Dunn JA, et al: Maillard reaction products and their relations to complications in insulin-dependent diabetes mellitus. J Clin Invest 91:2470, 1993.

99. Corbett JA, Tilton RG, Chang K, et al: Aminoguanidine, a novel inhibitor of nitric oxide formation, prevents diabetic vascular dysfunction. Diabetes 44:234, 1992.

100. Hammes H-P, Martin S, Federlin K, et al: Aminoguanidine treatment inhibits the development of experimental diabetic retinopathy. Proc Natl Acad Sci USA 88:1155, 1991.

101. Tilton RG, Baier LD, Harlow JE, et al: Diabetes-induced glomerular dysfunction: links to more reduced cytosolic ratio of NADH/NAD$^+$. Kidney Int 41:778, 1992.

102. Williamson JR, Chang K, Frangos M, et al: Hyperglycemia pseudohypoxia and diabetic complications. Diabetes 42:801, 1993.

103. Tilton WM, Seaman C, Carriero D, et al: Regulation of glycolysis in the erythrocyte: role of lactate/pyruvate and NAD/NADH ratios. J Lab Clin Med 118:146, 1991.

104. Van den Enden MK, Nyengaard JR, Ostrow E, et al: Elevated glucose levels increase retinal glycolysis and sorbitol pathway metabolism: implications for diabetic retinopathy. Invest Ophthalmol Vis Sci 36:1675, 1995.

105. Kikkawa U, Nishizuka Y: The role of protein kinase C in transmembrane signaling. Ann Rev Cell Biol 2:149, 1986.

106. King GL, Johnson S, Wu G: Possible growth modulators involved in the pathogenesis of diabetic proliferative retinopathy. In Westermark B, Betsholtz C, Hokfelt B (eds): Growth Factors in Health and Disease. New York, Excerpta Medica, 1990, p 303.

107. Inoguchi T, Battan R, Handler E, et al: Preferential elevation of protein kinase C isoform bII and diacylglycerol levels in the aorta and heart of diabetic rats: differential reversibility to glycemic control by islet transplantation. Proc Natl Acad Sci USA 89:11059, 1992.

108. Shiba T, Inoguchi T, Sportsman JR, et al: Correlation of diacylglycerol level and protein kinase C activity in rat retina to circulation. Am J Physiol 265(28):E783, 1993.

109. Clermont AC, Takagi C, Jirousek MR, et al: A PKC b isoform selective antagonist normalized retinal blood flow in STZ diabetic rats: first report of an oral agent selective for the PKC b isoenzyme. Invest Ophthalmol Vis Sci 35:S172, 1995.

110. Kunisaki M, Bursell S-E, Umeda F, et al: Normalization of diacyglycerol-protein kinase C activation by vitamin E in aorta of diabetic rats and cultured smooth muscle cells exposed to elevated glucose levels. Diabetes 43:1372, 1994.

111. Kunisaki M, Bursell S-E, Clermont AC, et al: Vitamin E treatment prevents diabetes-induced abnormality in retinal blood flow via the diacylglycerol-protein kinase C pathway. Am J Physiol 269:E239–E246, 1995.

112. Meyer-Schwickerath R, Pfeiffer A, Blum WF, et al: Vitreous levels of the insulin-like growth factors I and II, and the insulin-like growth factor binding proteins 2 and 3, increase in neovascular eye disease. J Clin Invest 92:2620–2625, 1993.

113. Muthukrishnan L, Warder E, McNeil PL: Basic fibroblast growth factor is efficiently released from cytosolic storage site through plasma membrane disruptions of endothelial cells. J Cell Physiol 148:1–16, 1991.

114. Vlodavsky I, Folkman J, Sullina R, et al: Endothelial cell-derived basic fibroblast growth factor: synthesis and deposition into subendothelial extracellular matrix. Proc Natl Acad Sci USA 84:2292–2296, 1997.

115. Plate KH, Breier G, Weich HA, Risau W: Vascular endothelial growth factor is a potential tumour angiogenesis factor in human gliomas in vivo. Nature 359:845–848, 1992.

116. Senger DR, Perruzzi CA, Feder J, Dvorak HF: A highly conserved vascular permeability factor secreted by a variety of human and rodent tumor cell lines. Cancer Res 46:5629–5632, 1986.

117. Shweiki D, Itin A, Soffer D, Keshet E: Vascular endothelial growth factor induced by hypoxia may mediate hypoxia-initiated angiogenesis. Nature 359:843–845, 1992.

118. Adamis AP, Shima DT, Yeo KT, et al: Synthesis and secretion of vascular permeability factor/vascular endothelial growth factor by human retinal pigment epithelial cells. Biochem Biophys Res Commun 193:631–638, 1993.

119. Pierce EA, Avery RL, Foley ED, et al: Vascular endothelial growth factor/vascular permeability factor expression in a mouse model of retinal neovascularization. Proc Natl Acad Sci USA 92:905–909, 1995.

120. Simorre-Pinatel V, Guerrin M, Chollet P, et al: Vasculotropin-VEGF stimulates retinal capillary endothelial cells through an autocrine pathway. Invest Ophthalmol Vis Sci 35:3393–3400, 1994.

121. Thieme H, Aiello LP, Takagi H, et al: Comparative analysis of vascular endothelial growth factor (VEGF) receptors on retinal and aortic microvascular endothelial cells. Diabetes 44:98–103, 1995.

122. Kim KJ, Li B, Winer J, et al: Inhibition of vascular endothelial growth factor-induced angiogenesis suppresses tumour growth in vivo. Nature 362:841–844, 1993.

123. West SK, Valmadrid CT: Epidemiology of risk factors for age-related cataract. Surv Ophthalmol 39:323–334, 1995.

124. Aiello LP, Pierce EA, Foley ED, et al: Suppression of retinal neovascularization in vivo by inhibition of vascular endothelial growth factor (VEGF) using VEGF-receptor chimeric proteins. Proc Natl Acad Sci USA 92:10457–10461, 1995.

125. Adamis AP, Miller JW, Bernal MT, et al: Increased vascular endothelial growth factor levels in the vitreous of eyes with proliferative diabetic retinopathy. Am J Ophthalmol 118:445–450, 1994.

126. Robinson GS, Pierce EA, Rook SL, et al: Oligodeoxynucleotides inhibit retinal neovascularization in a murine model of proliferative retinopathy. Proc Natl Acad Sci USA 93:4851–4856, 1996.

127. Adamis AP, Shima DT, Tolentino MJ, et al: Inhibition of vascular endothelial growth factor prevents retinal ischemia-associated iris neovascularization in nonhuman primate. Arch Ophthalmol 114:66–71, 1996.

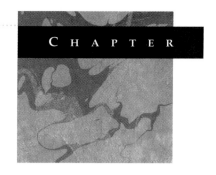

CHAPTER 27

Hypertensive Fundus Changes

Sohan Singh Hayreh, M.D., Ph.D.

In modern society, particularly in the industrialized world, the leading cause of death during the past half century has been cardiovascular disease. Arterial hypertension has been recognized as one of the most important risk factors. In the middle-aged and elderly population there is a trend towards a rise in blood pressure (BP) that often becomes steeper with age.[1] Systemic mortality and morbidity are markedly higher in hypertensives than in normotensives; for example, hypertensives are seven times as likely to develop stroke as normotensives, four times as likely to have congestive heart failure, three times as likely to have coronary artery disease, and twice as likely to have peripheral arterial disease; and the hypertensive's risk of total and cardiovascular mortality is twice that of the normotensive.[2] In malignant or accelerated arterial hypertension mortality and morbidity due to cardiovascular and other causes is even worse. Similarly, it is well established in the literature that hypertension plays an important role in the pathogenesis of a variety of ophthalmic conditions producing severe visual impairment[3-8]; also, ophthalmic manifestations may be the initial clinical presentation of hypertension, particularly of malignant hypertension. Recently emerging evidence indicates that in arterial hypertensives, particularly those treated aggressively with very potent hypotensive drugs, development of arterial hypotension (especially nocturnal hypotension) also plays an important role in the development of several systemic and visually crippling conditions.[9] In this chapter, I plan to discuss primarily fundus changes produced by malignant arterial hypertension because during the past two decades a good deal of new and important information has emerged on this very old subject.

Malignant arterial hypertension essentially produces its manifestations in the posterior segment of the eye, and hypertensive fundus changes constitute a very important part of the syndrome of malignant arterial hypertension.[10-24] Since 1859, when Liebreich[25] first described these fundus changes, a huge amount of literature has accumulated on the hypertensive fundus changes, drawn from both clinical and experimental studies. In spite of that, the subject still remains the center of many debates. While clinical observations and studies are extremely helpful in understanding a disease process, they have some serious limitations. Over recent years, (1) a better understanding of basic properties of the ocular and optic nerve head vascular beds (see below) and their response to malignant hypertension, (2) our ability to produce malignant arterial hypertension experimentally in primates,[12] (3) the advent of fluorescein fundus angiography and its application in hypertensive fundus changes,[13-15,18-21] and (4) other modern investigative techniques[10,11,26-29] have helped greatly to improve our understanding of the field, particularly about the pathology and pathogenesis of the various hypertensive fundus lesions.

First, in order to understand fully the mechanism of production of the various fundus lesions and their clinical pattern seen with malignant arterial hypertension, it is essential to comprehend some of the very basic anatomic and physiologic properties of the ocular vascular bed and their response to malignant arterial hypertension.

ANATOMIC AND PHYSIOLOGIC PROPERTIES OF THE RETINAL, CHOROIDAL, AND OPTIC NERVE HEAD VASCULAR BEDS

The relevant properties include the following:

345

Ocular Blood Flow

The blood flow in the retinal choroidal and optic nerve head (ONH) vascular beds is calculated by the following formula:

$$\text{Flow} = \frac{\text{perfusion pressure}}{\text{resistance to flow}}$$

where perfusion pressure is equal to mean blood pressure minus intraocular pressure. Perfusion pressure is also equal to mean arterial blood pressure minus venous pressure in a vascular bed. Normally, the central venous pressure is slightly higher than the intraocular pressure so that, for all practical purpose, intraocular pressure is a good index of the ocular venous pressure.

Mean blood pressure = diastolic blood pressure

+ 1/3 (systolic minus diastolic blood pressure)

From this formula, it is clear that the blood flow in the ONH depends upon the following three factors: (1) *mean blood pressure*, (2) *vascular resistance in the blood vessels*, and (3) *intraocular pressure*. The pathophysiology of factors controlling the blood flow is discussed in detail elsewhere.[30] Very briefly, the resistance to blood flow, according to Poiseuille's law, is directly proportional to blood viscosity and length of the vessel, and is inversely proportional to the fourth power of the radius of the vessel. Therefore, the resistance depends upon the state and caliber of the ocular arteries, which are in turn influenced by hypertensive arterial changes and efficiency of autoregulation of blood flow.

Autoregulation of Blood Flow

The object of blood flow autoregulation in a tissue is to keep the blood flow relatively constant during changes in its perfusion pressure. A number of studies have shown the presence of autoregulation in the retinal[31–38] and optic nerve head[39–42] blood vessels but not in the choroidal vascular bed.[34,35,38,43–46] The exact mechanism responsible for the autoregulation is still obscure except that it most probably operates by altering the vascular resistance. Generally, it is considered to be a feature of the terminal arterioles. With the rise or fall of blood pressure beyond the normal levels, the arterioles constrict or dilate, respectively, to regulate the blood flow. However, autoregulation becomes ineffective when the blood pressure rises or falls beyond critical range because of only a limited capacity in the arterioles to dilate or constrict. Recent studies suggest that vascular endothelium–derived vasoactive agents (e.g., endothelin-1, thromboxane A_2, and prostaglandin H_2 as *vasoconstrictors*; and nitric oxide as a *vasodilator*) profoundly modulate lo-

cal vascular tone[47] and, thereby, may play a role in autoregulation.[8]

Factors Causing Breakdown of Autoregulation

Autoregulation may be disrupted by alterations in blood pressure produced by a variety of local and systemic causes, including the following.

RISE OR FALL OF PERFUSION PRESSURE BEYOND THE CRITICAL AUTOREGULATORY RANGE. Autoregulation operates only over a critical range of perfusion pressure; with a rise or fall of perfusion pressure beyond the critical range, the autoregulation becomes ineffective and breaks down (Fig. 27–1). Thus, autoregulation does not protect the tissues all the time. If the perfusion pressure rapidly goes above the autoregulation range (as in malignant hypertension) it damages the tissue; and if it falls below the range (as in marked arterial hypotension) the tissue is subjected to a risk of ischemia.

ARTERIAL HYPERTENSION. With chronic malignant hypertension and essential arterial hypertension, the autoregulation adjusts itself to higher than normal levels as a compensatory mechanism.[48,49] In this, the range of autoregulation shifts to higher levels to adapt to high blood pressure[14] (Fig. 27–1). Although such an adjustment improves the patient's tolerance to high blood pressure, it makes that person correspondingly less tolerant to low blood pressure, so that a level of hypotension that would normally be quite safe becomes dangerous. Under such circumstances, a large, sudden fall of blood pressure in a hypertensive (spontaneously, as occurs during sleep, or because of overtreatment with hypotensive drugs) can cause the perfusion pressure to fall below the autoregulatory range and result in systemic and/or ocular vascular accidents[9,14]; these lesions may erroneously be attributed to hypertension because neither the physician nor the patient may be aware of episodes of marked hypotension (particularly nocturnal hypotension) in hypertensives.[9]

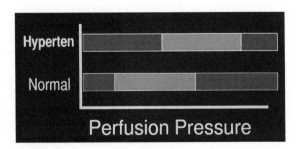

FIGURE 27–1   A diagrammatic representation of blood flow autoregulation range at different perfusion pressures in normal persons ("normal") and in hypertensives ("Hyperten"). The screened area represents the presence of autoregulation and solid area its absence. (From Hayreh SS: Systemic arterial blood pressure and the eye. Eye 10:5–28, 1996, with permission.)

CHANGES IN SIZE OF THE LUMEN OF THE PRECAP-ILLARY ARTERIOLES. The main factor normally regulating the blood flow is thought to be the size of the lumen of the precapillary arterioles. Arteriolar changes in hypertension are well known. These include vasospasm, vasodilation,[13] arteriolosclerosis,[18] drug-induced vasoconstriction or dilatation (by antihypertensive drugs—beta-blockers as vasoconstrictors and calcium-channel blockers as vasodilators), or vasoconstriction caused by angiotensin (leaked into ONH and choroid[14,15]; see below). All these arteriolar changes in hypertension can interfere with autoregulation.

CHANGES IN VASCULAR ENDOTHELIAL FUNCTION. These occur early in the course of vascular diseases. In hypertension, morphologic and functional alterations of endothelial cells occur and basal formation of nitric oxide (a vasodilator) is reduced.[50] Reduced formation of dilating agents by the endothelium may lead to unopposed action of endothelin (a powerful vasoconstrictor), causing vasoconstriction and interfering with autoregulation. Experimental data suggest that endothelial dysfunction develops as blood pressure increases and the dysfunction is related to the level of the blood pressure. Therefore, endothelial dysfunction may contribute to hypertensive vascular complications and accidents.[50] There is evidence to suggest that damage to vascular endothelium (associated with abnormalities in production of vascular endothelium–derived vasoactive agents) also occurs in arteriosclerosis, atherosclerosis, hypercholesterolemia, aging, diabetes mellitus, ischemia, and other so far unknown causes[8,47,50]; these conditions are often associated with arterial hypertension and would aggravate the situation.

Blood-Ocular Barrier

The presence of the blood-retinal barrier is well established. The choroid and optic nerve head, by contrast, do not possess blood-ocular barriers. The following account summarizes the bases for the presence or absence of the blood-ocular barrier in these tissues:

BLOOD-RETINAL BARRIER. This occurs at two levels.

In Retinal Blood Vessels. The blood-retinal barrier in these vessels is produced by the tight cell junctions between the endothelial cells of the vessels (due to the presence of extensive zonulae occludentes).[51,52] The tight interendothelial cell junctions block movement of macromolecules from the lumen toward the interstitial space. With a severe rise of blood pressure (i.e., above the level of autoregulation), the autoregulation breaks down, resulting in focal or generalized dilatation of arte-

rioles.[13] Morphologic studies have revealed discontinuity of the endothelial cell layer or interendothelial separation.[27] These changes result in the failure of the blood-retinal barrier and increased permeability.

At the Level of Retinal Pigment Epithelium. Tight cell junctions between the retinal pigment epithelium (RPE) cells also produce a blood-retinal barrier, preventing the leakage of fluid from the choroid into the retina. This barrier breaks down when the RPE cells are destroyed or subjected to ischemia, as in hypertensive choroidopathy.[15]

The retinal tissue itself has no barrier in its stroma, so fluid may be able to diffuse from one part to the adjacent areas.[15] Malignant hypertension may derange one or both the blood-retinal barriers.

Choroid. In contrast to the blood vessels in the retina, it is well established that choriocapillaris possesses no blood-ocular barrier because its endothelium shows the presence of numerous fenestrations. These make the choriocapillaris freely permeable,[45,53,54] with permeability to plasma proteins about five times that in the kidney, and choriocapillaris permeability to low-molecular-weight substances even higher than that to macromolecules.[55]

Optic Nerve Head. While the blood vessels in the optic nerve head, by virtue of tight cell junctions, have a blood-optic nerve barrier, it is important to remember that *the optic nerve head itself does not possess a blood-ocular barrier.* This is because the border tissue of Elschnig (separating the peripapillary choroid and optic nerve head) allows choroidal interstitial tissue fluid to leak into the optic nerve head from the peripapillary choroid.

Autonomic Nerve Supply

It is generally agreed that the vessels in the retina have no adrenergic vasomotor nerve supply.[56–58] In contrast to that, the choroidal vascular bed is richly supplied by the autonomic nerve supply—both sympathetic and parasympathetic nerves.[37,45,54,57,59–67]

Retinal Arterioles

In the retina the so-called retinal arteries are in fact arterioles, because they possess the following anatomic properties, typical of arterioles: (1) The widest part of the lumen of the retinal arterioles is near the optic disc and there its diameter is about 100 μm,[68] which is typically the diameter of an arteriole; and (2) unlike arteries, they possess neither an internal elastic lamina nor a continuous muscular coat.[68,69]

Blood Column of Retinal Vessels

As elsewhere in the blood vessels in the body, in the retinal blood vessels the blood flow is fastest in the axial part of the blood column, while it is almost stationary in the peripheral shell, which is in contact with the vessel wall. Also, the cells in the blood concentrate in the axial stream, the peripheral part of the blood column being mainly plasma. Ophthalmoscopy or color photographs of the retinal vessels show only the width of the central column of red blood cells. On the other hand, fluorescein fundus angiography reveals the entire width of the blood column, including the peripheral column of plasma. Moreover, periarteriolar retinal edema may partly mask the retinal arterioles, resulting in an ophthalmoscopic artifact of pseudonarrowing of retinal arterioles not seen on fluorescein fundus angiography (see below). *This shows the fallacy of making a judgment about the retinal arteriolar caliber on ophthalmoscopy.*

Thus, the retinal, choroidal, and optic nerve head blood vessels, because of their different anatomic and physiologic properties, respond differently to malignant arterial hypertension, thereby making hypertensive retinopathy, hypertensive choroidopathy, and hypertensive optic neuropathy three distinct and unrelated manifestations of malignant hypertension, a fact not fully appreciated in the past.

PATHOPHYSIOLOGY OF MALIGNANT ARTERIAL HYPERTENSION

To understand the pathogenesis of various fundus lesions in malignant arterial hypertension, it is also essential to have some idea of the latter's pathophysiology. This is still not fully understood. Arterial hypertension is considered a multifactorial disease secondary to the interaction of many abnormalities, including the following[70]:

1. *Abnormalities in cell membrane* resulting in defective membrane control over intracellular calcium concentration.
2. *Abnormalities of calcium metabolism* causing rise in cytoplasmic calcium which in turn causes increased tone of the arteriolar smooth muscle.
3. *Abnormalities of sodium metabolism* from inherited difficulty in the kidney's ability to eliminate sodium.
4. *Abnormalities of potassium metabolism* affect biosynthesis of aldosterone and renin release.
5. *Abnormalities of central nervous system* including abnormal release of humoral factors (e.g., natriuretic factor, vasopressin) increase sympathetic discharge and increase neurogenic vasomotor tone.
6. *Abnormalities of prostaglandins.*

7. *Abnormalities of vascular endothelium–derived vasoactive agents* (e.g., endothelin-1 [a powerful vasoconstrictor] and nitric oxide [a vasodilator]).
8. *Genetic effects* on blood pressure are polygenic in nature and play an important role in the development of arterial hypertension.
9. *Abnormalities of the renin-angiotensin-aldosterone system.* Available evidence strongly indicates that renin-angiotensin-aldosterone system abnormalities play an important role in the development and maintenance of renovascular malignant arterial hypertension.[12]

By some ill-understood mechanism(s), the levels of circulating endogenous vasoconstrictor agents (e.g., angiotensin II, epinephrine, vasopressin, and endothelin-1) increase. Kincaid-Smith[71] proposed the following schema for the various vascular changes seen in malignant arterial hypertension: Increase of endogenous vasoconstrictor agents → "sausage string" effect in arteries → turbulence and endothelial separation and damage → platelet deposition on endothelium → release of thromboxane, serotonin, histamine → microangiopathic hemolytic anemia and intravascular coagulation → further platelet and fibrin deposition → mitogenic and migration factors released by platelet aggregation → myointimal proliferation and organization of thrombi within vessels → renal ischemia → increase in vasoactive agents; thus a vicious circle is set up in malignant hypertension. Probably similar vascular changes in the ocular vessels may be developing and playing an important role in the development of hypertensive retinal, choroidal, and optic nerve head lesions.

Terminology Used for Hypertensive Fundus Changes

In 1859, Liebreich[25] first described fundus changes in malignant arterial hypertension under the title of "albuminuric retinitis." Since then a variety of terms have been suggested to describe these changes,[17] with "hypertensive retinopathy" being regarded as a universal term for all the fundus changes. However, from the above description of basic properties of the ocular and optic nerve head vascular beds and their response to malignant hypertension, it has become very evident that retinal, choroidal, and optic nerve head vascular beds respond very differently to malignant arterial hypertension. This was also confirmed by our recent studies on the subject.[10–21] All this newly emerged information has revealed that pathogenetically and clinically in fact fundus changes in malignant arterial hypertension fall into three very distinct categories: (1) *hypertensive retinopathy*, (2) *hypertensive choroidopathy*, and (3) *hypertensive optic neuropathy*. This is evident from the fact that lesions like Elschnig's spots, serous retinal detachment (RD), and the various RPE lesions represent hypertensive choroidopathy, while optic disc edema is a manifestation of hypertensive optic neuropathy—none of them are really due to hypertensive lesions of the retinal vascular bed, which means that the use of the term "hypertensive retinopathy" for all these lesions is misleading and not justified at all.

The following account of hypertensive fundus changes is essentially based on our recent experimental studies on the subject,[10-21] supplemented by my clinical experience in patients with malignant arterial hypertension.

HYPERTENSIVE RETINOPATHY

The primary factor responsible for the retinopathy is retinal vascular derangement caused by malignant hypertension.[17] The retinal lesions that make up hypertensive retinopathy can be divided for descriptive purposes into the following vascular and extravascular retinal lesions:

I. Retinal vascular lesions
  1. Retinal arteriolar changes[18]
  2. Focal intraretinal periarteriolar transudates (FIPTs)[13]
  3. Inner retinal ischemic spots (cotton-wool spots)[19]
  4. Retinal capillary changes[19]
  5. Retinal venous changes[16]
  6. Increased permeability of the retinal vascular bed[13,21]
II. Extravascular retinal lesions
  1. Retinal hemorrhages[16]
  2. Retinal and macular edema[18,21]
  3. Retinal lipid deposits (hard exudates)[20]
  4. Retinal nerve fiber loss[19]

The following is a brief account of these lesions.

Retinal Vascular Lesions

Retinal Arteriolar Hypertensive Changes

As discussed earlier, the so-called retinal arteries seen on ophthalmoscopy are in fact anatomically arterioles. Since the first description of "albuminuric retinitis" by Liebreich[25] in 1859, retinal arteriolar changes in malignant hypertension have been described as the main change in hypertensive retinopathy, with "spasm" of ophthalmoscopically seen retinal arterioles universally said to be the classic change. The other arteriolar changes described in the literature include generalized or focal narrowing, generalized or focal sclerosis, sheathing and occlusion of the arterioles, "arteriolar reflex change," "copper-wire arteries" and "silver-wire arteries."[18] In addition, almost all classifications of hypertensive retinopathy have been based essentially on retinal arteriolar changes.[22]

We recently investigated the subject by serial ophthalmoscopy and stereoscopic fundus photography and fluorescein angiography on long-term follow-up in our experimental studies. We have described our findings and the controversial issues on the subject in detail elsewhere.[18] It is best to discuss separately the changes involving (1) the ophthalmoscopically visible main arterioles and (2) the terminal arterioles, which are usually not readily seen on ophthalmoscopy. In our studies (described in detail elsewhere[13,18,19]) we particularly investigated the arteriolar changes in malignant hypertension.

CHANGES IN MAIN RETINAL ARTERIOLES. Narrowing and other changes in these arterioles on ophthalmoscopy have been described as classic manifestations of hypertensive retinopathy associated with malignant hypertension, with arteriolar "spasm" (localized or generalized) universally reported as typical. We were particularly interested in studying these changes, both during the early, acute phase of hypertensive retinopathy and later on during the chronic phase.[18]

During the Early, Acute Phase of Hypertension. In our studies, although some eyes on ophthalmoscopy showed an apparent narrowing of the retinal arterioles, no change in size from the baseline lumen width could be detected on fluorescein angiography in them (Figs. 27–2 through 27–4). Our fluorescein angiographic findings showed that the apparent ophthalmoscopically seen retinal arteriolar narrowing (generalized or focal) in these eyes was an ophthalmoscopic artifact, termed "pseudonarrowing." This pseudonarrowing was caused by the edematous retina masking a part of the retinal arterioles, giving an erroneous impression of spasm of the arterioles on routine ophthalmoscopy. Once the arteriolosclerotic changes developed, of course, the retinal arterioles showed a variable degree of arteriolar narrowing—but that is very different from the spasm during the acute phase stressed in the literature. Critics could argue that our observations in rhesus monkeys may not be valid for the human, but all the available evidence indicates that anatomically and physiologically the retinal vascular bed of rhesus monkeys behaves very much like that of man, so that our observations should apply to man as well. Cogan[72] stated that spasm seems unlikely because of the small amount of muscle in the retinal arterioles, the absence of any visible changes in the narrowing over a reasonable period of time, and the histologic evidence of hyalinization; he further added that "over-interpreting arterial narrowing in the fundus is a common failing. When one knows the patient has hypertension, one tends to attach undue significance to questionable changes." In fact, Pickering,[73] an authority on arterial hypertension, considered retinal arteriolar narrowing to be due to organic changes, and he stated that "so far as human observations are concerned, this problem (of

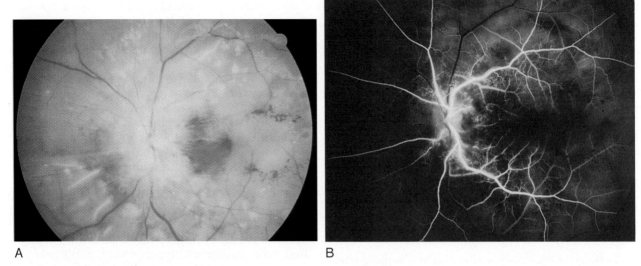

A   B

FIGURE 27–2 Fundus photograph (*A*) and fluorescein angiogram (*B*) of left eye of a hypertensive rhesus monkey with systolic BP 200 mm Hg. *A* shows marked attenuation of retinal arterioles, retinal and macular edema, many FIPTs, retinal hemorrhages and extensive serous RD. *B* shows normal caliber of the retinal arterioles (compare with marked narrowing of those seen on ophthalmoscopy in *A*). (*A* from Hayreh SS, Servais GE, Virdi PS: Fundus lesions in malignant hypertension IV. Focal intraretinal periarteriolar transudates. Ophthalmology 93:60–73, 1986; *B* from Hayreh SS, Servais GE, Virdi PS: Retinal arteriolar changes in malignant arterial hypertension. Ophthalmologica 198:178–196, 1989. Reproduced with permission of S. Karger AG, Basel.)

retinal arteriolar spasm) may now be said to be dead." Our studies fully support this view.

Thus, we could find no evidence of localized or generalized spasm in these retinal arterioles at any stage of development of hypertensive retinopathy. This contradicts the classic teaching on retinal arteriolar spasm or narrowing as the typical feature of malignant hypertension.

During the Chronic Phase of Hypertension. After prolonged hypertension, retinal arterioles show the following changes (Figs. 27–5 through 27–7):

1. Arteriolosclerosis (and associated localized or generalized narrowing and other changes) described as features of hypertensive retinopathy in the literature did develop *but were not*

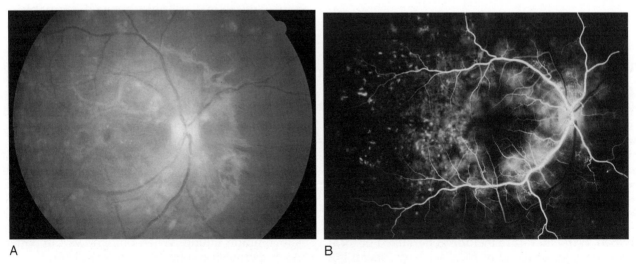

A   B

FIGURE 27–3 Fundus photograph (*A*) and fluorescein angiograms (*B*) of right eye of a hypertensive rhesus monkey with systolic BP 190 mm Hg. *A* shows extreme attenuation of retinal arterioles, microcystic macular edema, serous macular RD, multiple acute focal RPE lesions and hypertensive retinopathy lesions. *B* shows normal caliber of retinal arterioles, in spite of marked narrowing of the arterioles seen on ophthalmoscopy in *A*. (From Hayreh SS, Servais GE, Virdi PS: Retinal arteriolar changes in malignant arterial hypertension. Ophthalmologica 198:178–196, 1989. Reproduced with permission of S. Karger AG, Basel.)

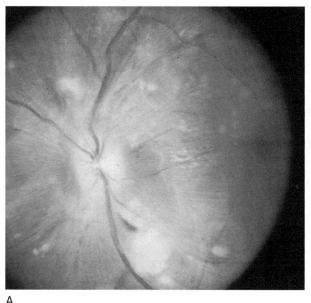

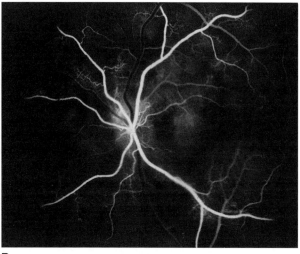

A   B

FIGURE 27–4   Fundus photograph (*A*) and fluorescein angiogram (*B*) of left eye of a hypertensive rhesus monkey with systolic BP 192 mm Hg. *A* shows segmental narrowing of retinal arterioles, FIPTs and IRISs. *B* shows markedly delayed filling of choroid and normal filling and caliber of retinal arterioles. (From Hayreh SS, Servais GE, Virdi PS: Fundus lesions in malignant hypertension IV. Focal intraretinal periarteriolar transudates. Ophthalmology 93:60–73, 1986; and Hayreh SS, Servais GE, Virdi PS: Fundus lesions in malignant hypertension V. Hypertensive optic neuropathy. Ophthalmology 93:74–87, 1986, with permission.)

early signs of hypertensive retinopathy (Figs. 27–5*A* through 27–7). Retinal arteriolosclerosis seen in chronic hypertension represents what has been described as copper-wire arteries in the literature because of increased ophthalmoscopic reflex from the wall of the sclerosed retinal arterioles (Fig. 27–5*B*).

2. Increased tortuosity of sclerotic arterioles may also be seen (Figs. 27–5 and 27–7).

3. Occlusion of a few of the fine arterioles in the distribution of the inner retinal ischemic spots (cotton-wool spots) may develop (Fig. 27–5). On ophthalmoscopy these look white and in the literature have been called silver-wire arteries.

The frequently mentioned "arteriolar reflex change," copper-wire arteries, and silver-wire arteries as signs of arterial hypertension are of little scientific validity, and Leishman[74] very appropriately remarked that "recording of clinical signs, such as copper-wire arteries, calibre variations, arteriovenous ratios, and the vagaries of the vascular light reflex, may become the self-imposed limit of legitimate clinical thought concerning the retinal vessels" in hypertension; he further added that these terms have been used by most ophthalmologists without "a clear conception of the meaning of these appearances." I feel that these terms, though picturesque, serve no useful purpose and should be discarded. In our study,[18] we found that the so-called silver-wire arteries in fact were completely occluded fine arterioles supplying the areas of multiple confluent inner retinal ischemic spots (cotton-

wool spots) (Fig. 27–5*B*) and the copper-wire arteries were the arterioles with marked degree of arteriolosclerosis and having a copper reflex (Fig. 27–5*B*).

CHANGES IN TERMINAL RETINAL ARTERIOLES. The retinal terminal arterioles are too small to be seen on ophthalmoscopy. During the early, acute phase of malignant hypertension, these arterioles may show two types of changes.

Dilatation of Terminal Arterioles. This is caused by failure of autoregulation secondary to accelerated hypertension to very high levels. Dilatation resulted in focal breakdown of the blood-retinal barrier and leakage (resulting in the development of FIPTs, described below)—the earliest lesion of hypertensive retinopathy seen in our study.[13]

Occlusion of Terminal Arterioles. This resulted in development of inner retinal ischemic spots (cotton-wool spots) and focal retinal capillary obliteration (see below).[19]

Focal Intraretinal Periarteriolar Transudate

This very specific retinal lesion, seen only in malignant arterial hypertension, was first discovered by us.[13] It is very common and one of the earliest retinal lesions in hypertensive retinopathy due to accelerated malignant arterial hypertension. FIPTs are round or oval in shape, varying in size from a pinpoint to about quarter of the optic disc diameter

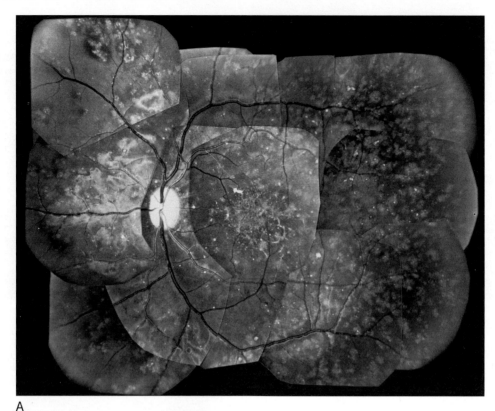

A

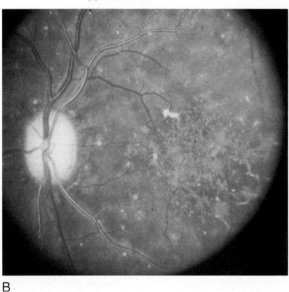

B

FIGURE 27–5 Fundus photographs: (*A*) a composite photograph and (*B*) a magnified view of the posterior pole of left eye of a hypertensive rhesus monkey with systolic BP 220 mm Hg. These show extensive RPE degeneration, drusen, retinal arteriolosclerosis, and optic atrophy. (*A* from Hayreh SS, Servais GE, Virdi PS: Fundus lesions in malignant hypertension VI. Hypertensive choroidopathy. Ophthalmology 93:1383–1400, 1986; *B* from Hayreh SS, Servais GE, Virdi PS: Retinal arteriolar changes in malignant arterial hypertension. Ophthalmologica 198:178–196, 1989. Reproduced with permission of S. Karger AG, Basel.)

(Figs. 27–8*A*, 27–9*A*, 27–11, and 27–12*A*). Sometimes they may fuse together to form a larger lesion. FIPTs are dull white when fresh and later fade away when resolving. They are typically located beside the major retinal arterioles and their main branches posteriorly, and in the deeper retinal layers. On fluorescein fundus angiography (Figs. 27–8 through 27–11), FIPTs show dilatation of the terminal retinal arterioles with focal leaking spots, appearing by the arteriovenous phase of angiography. During the late phase, these fluorescent spots are round in shape and spread out so that some of them may fuse together to form a large patch or a band of retinal staining along the retinal arterioles, with the original loci of lesions usually still evident as separate hyperfluorescent spots. No capillary obliteration is seen in the FIPTs. Fluorescein leaking spots on angiography appear before the ophthalmoscopically visible lesions. The lesions develop fully in about a week and last for 2 or 3 weeks. FIPTs usually appear in crops. On resolution, they leave no apparent microvascular, ophthalmoscopic, or fluorescein angiographic evidence of lesions.

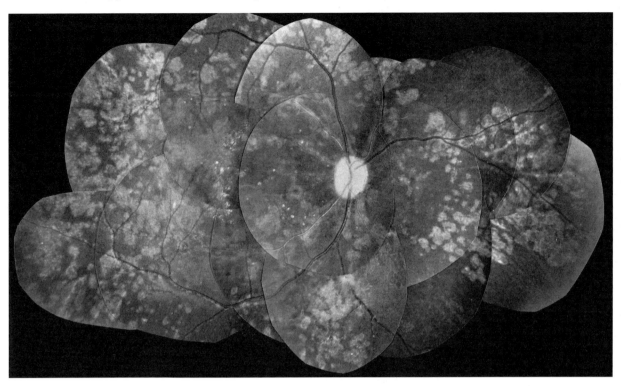

FIGURE 27–6 Composite fundus photograph of right eye of a hypertensive rhesus monkey with systolic BP 230 mm Hg. It shows extensive RPE degenerative lesions, optic atrophy, and retinal arteriolosclerosis. (From Hayreh SS, Servais GE, Virdi PS: Fundus lesions in malignant hypertension VI. Hypertensive choroidopathy. Ophthalmology 93:1383–1400, 1986, with permission.)

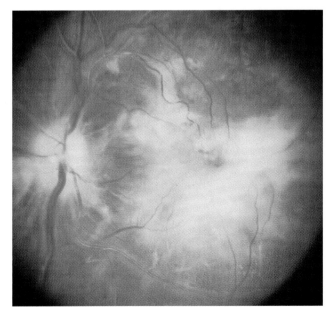

FIGURE 27–7 Fundus photograph of left eye of a hypertensive rhesus monkey with systolic BP 250 mm Hg. It shows whitish subretinal fibrosis in the macular region. (From Hayreh SS, Servais GE, Virdi PS: Fundus lesions in malignant hypertension VI. Hypertensive choroidopathy. Ophthalmology 93:1383–1400, 1986, with permission.)

The following sequence of events seems to be responsible for the development of FIPTs[13]: Severe rise of systemic arterial blood pressure → failure of retinal vascular autoregulation → focal dilatation of precapillary retinal arterioles (Fig. 27–10A) → separation of tight interendothelial cell junctions in the dilated arterioles → focal breakdown of the blood-retinal barrier → increased permeability of the dilated arterioles to plasmatic macromolecules → focal accumulation of plasmatic deposits in the retinal tissue (Figs. 27–10B and C and 27–13) → ophthalmoscopically seen white lesions and fluorescein leaking spots.

FIPTs in the past have been erroneously thought to be cotton-wool spots or precursors of cotton-wool spots.[27,75] The following account of cotton-wool spots will clearly demonstrate that FIPTs and cotton-wool spots are very different in nature.[13]

Inner Retinal Ischemic Spots (Cotton-Wool Spots)

Ever since the first clinical description of hypertensive retinopathy in 1859,[25] these lesions have been emphasized as an important classic feature of fundus lesions in malignant hypertension. It is well established now that these lesions are due to acute focal ischemia of the inner retina. In view of that,

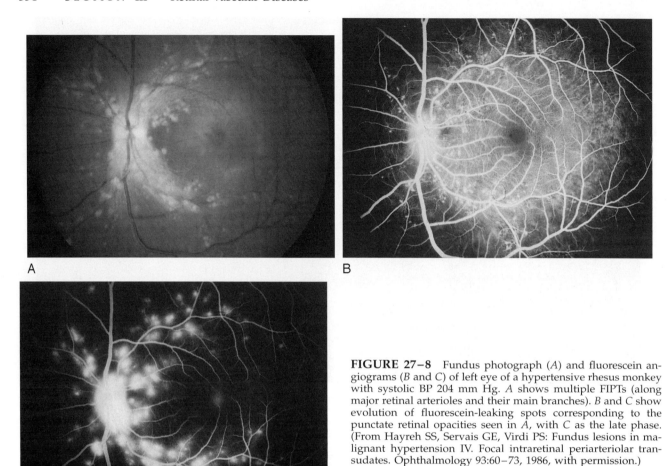

A

B

C

FIGURE 27–8 Fundus photograph (*A*) and fluorescein angiograms (*B* and *C*) of left eye of a hypertensive rhesus monkey with systolic BP 204 mm Hg. *A* shows multiple FIPTs (along major retinal arterioles and their main branches). *B* and *C* show evolution of fluorescein-leaking spots corresponding to the punctate retinal opacities seen in *A*, with *C* as the late phase. (From Hayreh SS, Servais GE, Virdi PS: Fundus lesions in malignant hypertension IV. Focal intraretinal periarteriolar transudates. Ophthalmology 93:60–73, 1986, with permission.)

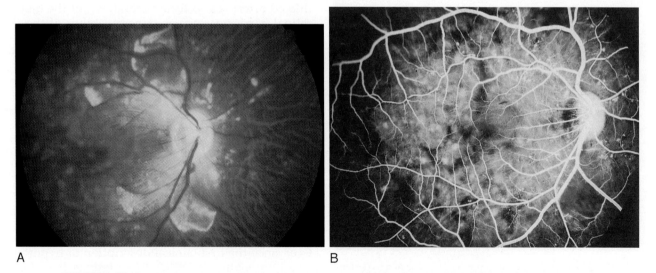

A

B

FIGURE 27–9 Fundus photograph (*A*) and fluorescein angiogram (*B*) of right eye of a hypertensive rhesus monkey with systolic BP 238 mm Hg. *A* shows multiple FIPTs, IRISs, and focal RPE lesions. *B* shows nonperfusion of retinal capillaries in the regions of IRISs, and late fluorescent spots correspond to either the FIPTs or focal RPE lesions. (From Hayreh SS, Servais GE, Virdi PS: Fundus lesions in malignant hypertension IV. Focal intraretinal periarteriolar transudates. Ophthalmology 93:60–73, 1986, with permission.)

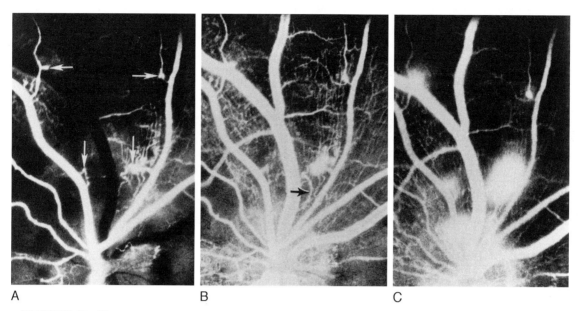

A   B   C

FIGURE 27–10   Fluorescein fundus angiograms of right eye of a hypertensive rhesus monkey after Gold-blatt's procedure with systolic BP 198 mm Hg. Magnified views from area just above optic disc during retinal arterial (*A*), late arteriovenous (*B*), and postvenous (*C*) phases; note dilated precapillary retinal arterioles at four sites (*white arrows*) in *A* and progressive fluorescein leakage at those sites, with normal filling of retinal capillaries in *B*, which also shows dilated venule draining one leaking spot (*black arrow*). (From Hayreh SS, Servais GE, Virdi PS: Fundus lesions in malignant hypertension IV. Focal intraretinal periarteriolar transu-dates. Ophthalmology 93:60–73, 1986, with permission.)

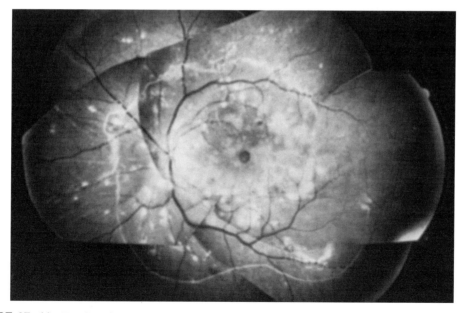

FIGURE 27–11   Fundus photograph of left eye of a hypertensive rhesus monkey with systolic BP 198 mm Hg. It shows serous RD (notice demarcation line outlining RD) with multiple acute focal RPE lesions, foveal cyst, and multiple FIPTs (along the retinal arterioles). (From Hayreh SS, Servais GE, Virdi PS: Fundus lesions in malignant hypertension VI. Hypertensive choroidopathy. Ophthalmology 93:1383–1400, 1986, with permission.)

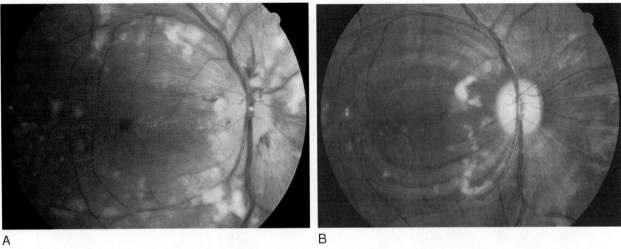

A   B

FIGURE 27–12   Fundus photographs of right eye, of a hypertensive rhesus monkey 57 (*A*) and 120 (*B*) days after Goldblatt's procedure with systolic BP 190 and 200 mm Hg, respectively. (*A*) shows multiple IRISs, FIPTs and acute focal RPE lesions, optic disc edema, macular retinal edema, and other lesions of hypertensive retinopathy. (*B*) shows resolution of old IRISs and appearance of new ones, with development of multiple areas of nerve fiber bundle loss (seen as dark semicircular bands in the macular region). Multiple focal RPE lesions are seen in temporal part of macular region in both photographs. (*A* from Hayreh SS, Servais GE, Virdi PS: Fundus lesions in malignant hypertension V. Hypertensive optic neuropathy. Ophthalmology 93: 74–87, 1986; and *B* from Hayreh SS: Systemic arterial blood pressure and the eye. Eye 10:5–28, 1996, with permission.)

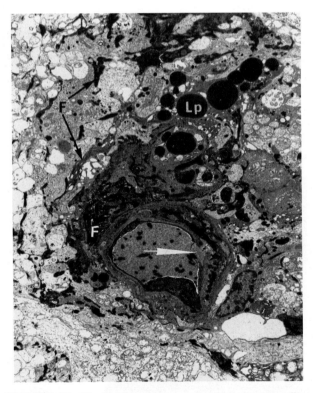

FIGURE 27–13   Electron micrograph of small precapillary retinal arteriole of a monkey with malignant arterial hypertension and hypertensive retinopathy, showing dilated lumen (L) and focal break (*arrow*) in endothelial lining. Arteriole is surrounded by fibrinous (F) and lipoidal (Lp) transudates in periarteriolar retina. (From Garner A, Ashton N, Tripathi R, et al: Pathogenesis of hypertensive retinopathy: an experimental study in the monkey. Br J Ophthalmol 59:3–44, 1975, with permission.)

a scientifically and pathogenetically valid term for this lesion is "inner retinal ischemic spot" (IRIS), instead of the commonly used term "cotton-wool spot" (which simply describes the ophthalmoscopic appearance during the acute phase, without giving any information about its true nature) or "soft exudates" (this term is absolutely wrong, since these are *not* exudative in nature but are ischemic in origin).[19]

Typically, on ophthalmoscopy, IRISs are fluffy white focal areas of retinal opacity, having irregular polymorphous shapes, frequently with somewhat feathery margins (Figs. 27–4*A*, 27–9*A*, 27–12, and 27–15*A*). They are located mostly in the nerve fiber layer of the retina, usually in the posterior pole (within a few disc diameters from the disc), essentially in the distribution of the radial peripapillary retinal capillaries[76,77] (Fig. 27–12*A*), and more closely related to the arterioles than to the venules. During the acute phase, they usually bulge slightly forward on the surface of the retina. The characteristic life cycle of an IRIS is that it starts as a gray film, expands as a white creamy fluffy cloud, and resolves into a dull fragmenting white patch before disappearing.[75] On fluorescein fundus angiography, IRISs show retinal capillary nonperfusion in their location, progressively becoming more marked, with usually no corresponding fluorescein leakage (Figs. 27–9, 27–14, and 27–15*B* and *C*). They usually last 3 to 6 weeks. Finally, on complete resolution, on ophthalmoscopy they leave a normal looking, transparent retina, with loss of retinal nerve fibers corresponding to the location of the spots (Fig. 27–12*B*), although fluorescein fundus angi-

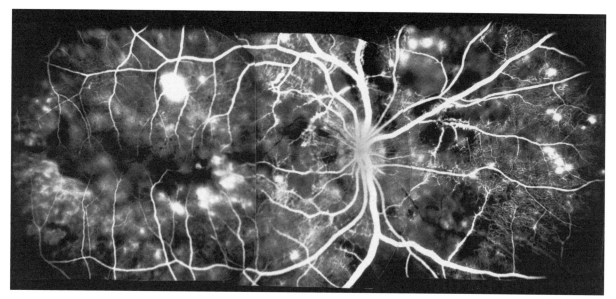

FIGURE 27–14   Fluorescein angiogram of right eye of a hypertensive rhesus monkey with systolic BP 214 mm Hg. It shows poor choroidal filling and patches of retinal capillary nonperfusion in the distribution of IRISs; fluorescein leaking spots in the nasal retina represent FIPTs. (From Hayreh SS: Classification of hypertensive fundus changes and their order of appearance. Ophthalmologica 198:247–260, 1989. Reproduced with permission of S. Karger AG, Basel.)

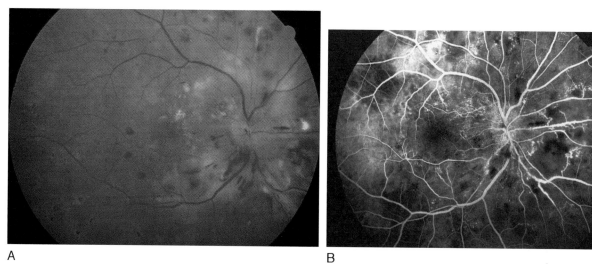

A

B

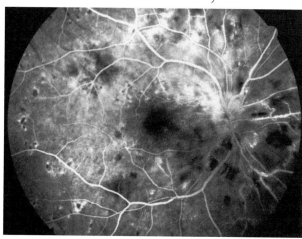

FIGURE 27–15   Fundus photograph (*A*) and fluorescein angiograms (*B* and *C*) of right eye of a 38-year-old male patient who, at initial visit to our clinic, complained of sudden onset of blurred vision in the left eye for 3 weeks and in the right eye for 1 week. On investigation he was discovered to have malignant hypertension (of which he was totally unaware and felt perfectly fit and healthy!) with BP 188/118 mm Hg. Fundus photograph (*A*), taken at the initial visit, shows optic disc edema, resolving IRISs, retinal hemorrhages, multiple focal RPE lesions (so-called Elschnig's spots), mild retinal and macular edema with a few fine lipid deposits, and serous RD in the lower periphery of the fundus (not seen in the photograph). *B* and *C* show markedly delayed filing of the choroid, patches of retinal capillary obliteration, retinal microaneurysms, and other intraretinal microvascular abnormalities; late-phase angiogram (*C*) shows multiple focal RPE lesions—with dark center and a fluorescent halo around that, and staining of the optic disc and endematous areas of the retina. (From Reinecke R (ed): Ophthalmology Annual. New York, Raven Press, 1989, pp 1–38, with permission.)

C

ography reveals permanent capillary nonperfusion on its location (Fig. 27–14).

The pathogenesis of IRISs is still not fully understood. In our studies,[19] we found occlusion of terminal retinal arterioles corresponding to the IRISs. Similarly, occlusion of precapillary retinal arterioles, produced either experimentally or by thromboembolic disorders in many systemic diseases, results in development of these spots. Thus, although all available clinical and experimental evidence shows that they represent foci of acute ischemia of the inner retina, the exact mechanism responsible for the occlusion of terminal retinal arterioles in the distribution of the radial peripapillary capillaries in malignant arterial hypertension is still not clear. We have discussed the subject at length elsewhere.[19]

Differential Diagnosis Between FIPTs and IRISs

In our studies, we investigated critically the relationship between FIPTs and IRISs, since in the earlier studies it had been stated or implied that FIPTs were precursors of IRISs, so that the two lesions represent a continuum.[27,75] Our studies, summarized above, clearly demonstrated that the two lesion are very different in nature, as is evident from the following:

Pathogenesis. FIPTs are due to focal leakage from dilated precapillary retinal arterioles lying in the deeper layers of the retina (Fig. 27–16). On the other hand, IRISs are due to acute focal ischemia of the surface nerve fiber layer produced by occlusion of the terminal arterioles in that layer (Fig. 27–16).

Location. FIPTs are located in the deeper retinal layers. The IRISs, by contrast, are located only in the surface nerve fiber layer.

Shape and Size. FIPTs are round or oval in shape, varying in size from pinhead to about a quarter of

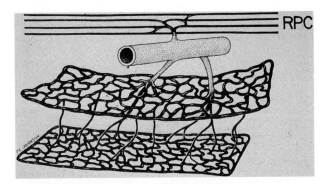

FIGURE 27–16 Schematic diagram of the blood supply to the retinal capillaries at the posterior pole of the eye. A retinal arteriole supplies both the radial peripapillary capillaries lying in the superficial nerve fiber layer (RPC) and the deeper capillary networks. (From Trans Am Acad Ophthalmol Otolaryngol 73:890–897, 1969, with permission.)

the optic disc diameter. The IRISs are of irregular polymorphous shapes, frequently with somewhat feathery margins, and are much larger than the FIPTs.

Color. FIPTs are dull white when fresh and later fade away when resolving. IRISs look white and fluffy when fresh, and during resolution phase they take on a white inspissated appearance.

Fluorescein Fundus Angiographic Pattern. FIPTs show dilatation of the terminal retinal arterioles with round, focal leakage in the deeper layers of the retina, appearing by the arteriovenous phase. No retinal capillary obliteration is seen in FIPTs. On the other hand, in the IRISs there is nonperfusion of the superficial retinal capillaries in the region of the lesion, with no fluorescein leakage, except very rarely, when some leakage may be seen along the peripheral margins of the IRISs.

Life Cycle. FIPTs last for about 2 to 3 weeks. In contrast, IRISs last much longer (about 4 to 6 weeks or even longer).

Resolution Pattern. FIPTs resolve rapidly, without leaving any permanent microvascular or retinal change. On the other hand, IRISs resolve much more slowly, leaving patches of retinal capillary obliteration and loss of retinal nerve fibers corresponding to the site of the IRISs.

Specificity of the Lesions. While IRISs are seen in a large variety of conditions and are not specific to malignant hypertension, FIPTs most probably are a very specific lesion of malignant hypertension.

Retinal Capillary Changes

Capillary obliteration is a hallmark of IRISs, and as such this is seen frequently in retinopathy with malignant hypertension, as discussed above. The retinal capillary obliteration may produce secondary intraretinal microvascular abnormalities, including microaneurysms, shunts around the areas of capillary obliteration, looped convoluted vessels, venous collaterals, and arteriovenous shunts[19] (Figs. 27–14 and 27–15B and C). Eyes with extensive retinal capillary nonperfusion may also develop optic disc and/or retinal neovascularization.

Retinal Venous Changes

These are an uncommon finding in hypertensive retinopathy due to malignant hypertension, and they do not represent an important part of the retinopathy. The various retinal venous changes may include venous nipping at the arteriovenous crossings of major vessels, dilatation and tortuosity of major retinal veins, or venous stasis retinopathy with marked retinal hemorrhages.[16]

Increased Permeability of the Retinal Vascular Bed

This is due to breakdown of the retina-blood barrier in malignant arterial hypertension. It plays an important role in the pathogenesis of FIPTs,[13] as discussed above. This is also responsible for the retinal and macular edema—a very common finding in hypertensive retinopathy, as discussed below.[21]

Extravascular Retinal Lesions

Retinal Hemorrhages

It is usually thought by ophthalmologists and is emphasized in the literature that retinal hemorrhages are an important, early manifestation of hypertensive retinopathy due to malignant hypertension. Wise et al[78] and Dollery[77] described small linear hemorrhages in the nerve fiber layer as one of the earliest features of accelerated hypertension. Ballantyne and Michaelson,[79] however, stated that "Haemorrhages are a familiar feature of the hypertensive fundus but they are not of pathognomic significance." They are described as usually striate, flame-shaped, occurring in the vicinity of the optic disc during the early stages, and later on they may be more widespread and seen even in deeper layers of the retina.

Our studies[16] revealed that retinal hemorrhages did not usually constitute either one of the earliest or one of the most conspicuous retinal lesions, but, on the contrary, were a minor feature of the retinopathy. We found that hemorrhages were usually situated in the nerve fiber layer, and could be located anywhere in the fundus but were usually found in the distribution of the radial peripapillary retinal capillaries (Figs. 27–2A and 27–15A). Their common occurrence at the latter site may be due to the distinctive features of the radial peripapillary capillaries[76] which, together with the much thicker nerve fiber layer in their distribution, could be factors in the production of retinal hemorrhages[16] as well as IRISs.[19] Optic disc edema and retinal edema in their distribution could interfere with the venous outflow from these long, straight, superficial capillaries, and result in development of hemorrhages. The possibility that pathologic changes in the capillaries (e.g., ischemic capillaropathy or other changes due to malignant hypertension) make them liable to hemorrhages cannot be ruled out. Dollery[77] also stated that the hemorrhages arise from the radial peripapillary capillaries, and he postulated that this is because these capillaries have a relatively high intravascular pressure.

Retinal and Macular Edema

Retinal edema is a well-known feature of hypertensive retinopathy due to malignant hypertension. It may be generalized or localized (usually in the macular region), and its severity may vary markedly from eye to eye. Our studies showed macular edema of variable degree as a common occurrence in malignant hypertension[21] (Figs. 27–2A, 27–3A, 27–8A, 27–11, 27–12A, 27–15A, 27–17A and B, 27–18A, and 27–20). Marked macular edema produces secondary macular changes, such as separation of nerve fibers by the serous fluid (usually in the retina between the fovea and optic disc), microcystic change, foveal cysts, and later on cystoid degeneration and rarely whitish subretinal fibrosis (Figs. 27–3A, 27–17A and B, 27–18A, 27–19, and 27–20). It has been postulated that generalized retinal edema can be due to autoregulatory failure, resulting in a rise in transmural pressure in the distal arterioles and proximal capillaries, which permits increased transudation of fluid into the retinal tissue.[26,27] Ultrastructural studies by Garner and coworkers[26,27] indicated that intracellular edema of ischemic origin is also of importance in the production of retinal edema in malignant hypertension. Our studies indicated that macular edema is usually *not* due to retinal vascular changes but represents to a great extent a manifestation of hypertensive choroidopathy[15] by the following sequence of events: hypertensive choroidopathy → breakdown of the blood retinal barrier in the RPE → serous RD → diffusion of subretinal fluid into the retinal tissue → macular edema.[15] Breakdown of the blood-retinal barrier may also contribute to macular edema. From this it would seem that macular and retinal edema may be due to one or more of the factors mentioned above, acting individually or collectively. The subject is discussed at length elsewhere.[21]

Retinal Lipid Deposits

"Macular star" has been described as a classic feature of hypertensive retinopathy; however, the deposits may not only assume a variety of shapes but also may be seen in other parts of the retina (Figs. 27–15A, 27–19, 27–20, and 27–21). In our studies,[20] we found that all eyes with lipid deposits had antecedent macular or retinal edema or serous retinal detachment. The deposits were ever changing, taking months or even more than a year to resolve. Our study suggested that in hypertensive retinopathy the lipid deposits are most probably the result of exudative and/or neural degenerative processes.[20] All the available evidence indicates that these deposits are composed of lipids. We also found that hyperlipidemia increased the extent of these deposits. In view of that it is more appropriate to call them lipid deposits than "hard exudates."

Retinal Nerve Fiber Loss

Ischemia in the distribution of IRISs (cotton-wool spots) damages the retinal nerve fibers in their location.[19] The loss of retinal nerve fibers starts to appear as the IRISs resolve. The location of the lost

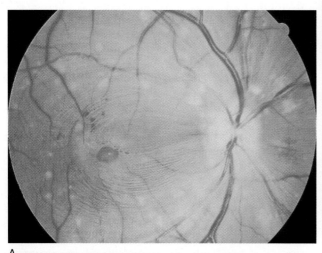

A

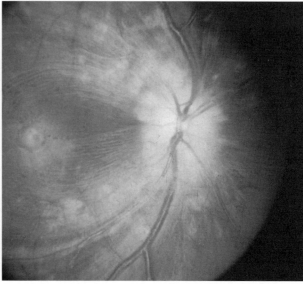

B

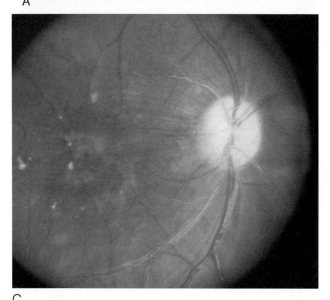

C

FIGURE 27–17 Fundus photographs of right eye of a hypertensive rhesus monkey 84 (*A*), 97 (*B*), and 320 (*C*) days after Goldblatt's procedure with systolic BP 190, 196, and 168 mm Hg, respectively. In *A* note optic disc edema, serous RD with separation of nerve fibers by edema, microcystic edema, foveal cyst, and focal RPE lesions (white spots in macular region). Notice marked optic disc edema in *B* and optic atrophy in *C*. (*A* from Hayreh SS, Servais GE, Virdi PS: Fundus lesions in malignant hypertension VI. Hypertensive choroidopathy. Ophthalmology 93:1383–1400, 1986, with permission.)

retinal nerve fibers corresponds to that of the IRISs (Fig. 27–12). Since these spots are usually situated in the area of radial peripapillary capillaries,[76] the loss of retinal nerve fibers is most marked in the superior and inferior temporal arcuate location. We found the nerve fiber loss usually progressive for some time initially.[19] It is possible that some of the nerve fiber loss could be due to ischemic damage to the optic nerve from hypertensive optic neuropathy.[14]

Early and Late Signs of Hypertensive Retinopathy

From this very brief account of hypertensive retinopathy in malignant arterial hypertension, it becomes apparent that the early signs are FIPTs, inner

retinal ischemic spots, a few punctate retinal hemorrhages, and macular edema. Cystoid macular changes, lipid deposits, retinal arteriolar changes, nerve fiber loss, and other retinal changes are late signs of retinopathy.[22] We found no evidence of retinal arteriolar spasm at any stage.[18]

HYPERTENSIVE CHOROIDOPATHY

While an enormous amount of literature has accumulated on "hypertensive retinopathy" since the first description of fundus changes in malignant hypertension in 1859,[25] there is practically no meaningful account of hypertensive choroidopathy in this disease. In fact, most of the lesions of hypertensive choroidopathy have erroneously been de-

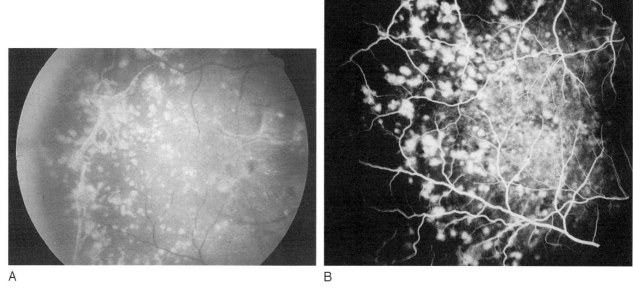

A   B

FIGURE 27–18   Fundus photograph (*A*) and fluorescein angiogram (*B*) of right eye of a hypertensive rhesus monkey with systolic BP 190 mm Hg. *A*, Fundus photograph of posterior fundus and temporal periphery, showing microcystic macular edema, serous macular RD, multiple acute focal RPE lesions, and hypertensive retinopathy lesions. *B* shows fluorescein staining of acute focal RPE lesions in late stages. (From Hayreh SS, Servais GE, Virdi PS: Fundus lesions in malignant hypertension VI. Hypertensive choroidopathy. Ophthalmology 93:1383–1400, 1986, with permission.)

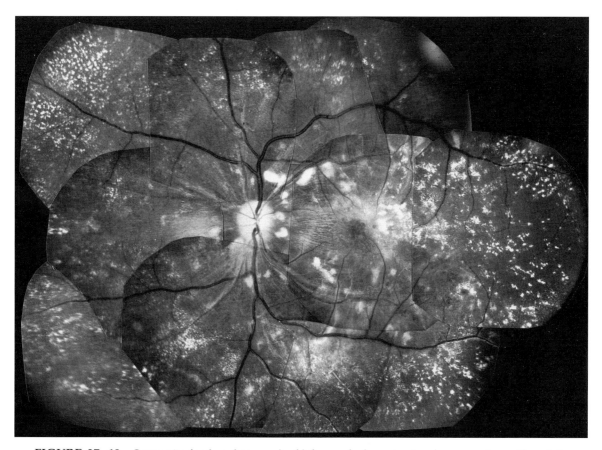

FIGURE 27–19   Composite fundus photograph of left eye of a hypertensive rhesus monkey with systolic BP 218 mm Hg. (From Hayreh SS, Servais GE, Virdi PS: Retinal lipid deposits in malignant arterial hypertension. Ophthalmologica 198:216–229, 1989. Reproduced with permission of S. Karger AG, Basel.)

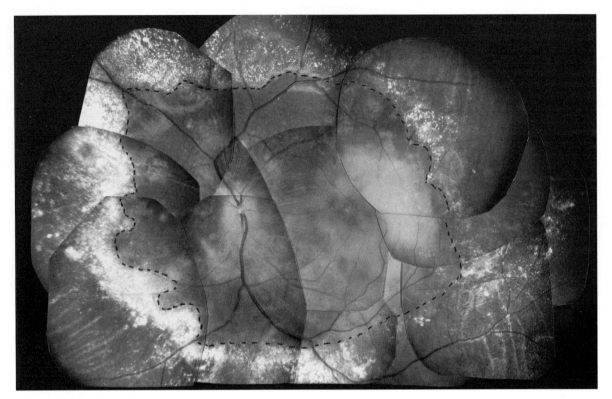

FIGURE 27–20   Fundus photograph of left eye of a hypertensive rhesus monkey with systolic BP 220 mm Hg showing serous RD of posterior pole (outlined by *dotted line*) associated with extensive lipid deposits peripheral to the RD and subretinal whitish proteinous deposit on the RPE in the macular region. (From Hayreh SS, Servais GE, Virdi PS: Fundus lesions in malignant hypertension VI. Hypertensive choroidopathy. Ophthalmology 93:1383–1400, 1986, with permission.)

scribed under retinopathy. Our studies have shown that, in malignant arterial hypertension, hypertensive choroidopathy is a distinct entity and is as important a clinical entity as hypertensive retinopathy, with a very different underlying pathogenetic mechanism. We have discussed hypertensive choroidopathy in detail elsewhere[10,15] and the following is a brief summary.

Pathogenesis of Hypertensive Choroidopathy

As discussed earlier, it is well established that choriocapillaris have numerous fenestrations in their endothelial cells so that there is no blood-ocular barrier, making them freely permeable to plasma proteins and other macromolecules. In malignant arterial hypertension, endogenous vasoconstrictor agents, including angiotensin II, epinephrine, and vasopressin, leak freely from the choriocapillaris into the choroidal interstitial fluid. Angiotensin II is one of the most powerful vasoconstrictor agents known, and it also potentiates the vasoconstrictor action of norepinephrine, which is released in excessive amounts due to angiotensin stimulating the sympathetic nervous system. The leaked vasoconstrictor agents act on the walls of the choroidal ves-

sels and result in choroidal vasoconstriction and ischemia. Sympathetic innervation of the choroidal arterioles may further make them susceptible to vasoconstriction. Our fluorescein angiographic[15] and pathologic[10] studies showed that choroidal ischemia initially is of an acute type and later becomes chronic; the effects of the two types of ischemia on the overlying RPE and retina vary. Thus the various lesions seen in hypertensive choroidopathy are due to choroidal ischemia.

Hypertensive Choroidopathy Lesions

These are described in detail elsewhere.[10,15] The following is a brief summary of that. Clinically, these consist of the following:

  I. Choroidal vascular bed abnormalities
 II. RPE lesions
    1. Acute focal RPE lesions
    2. RPE degenerative lesions
III. Serous retinal detachment

Choroidal Vascular Bed Abnormalities

Fluorescein angiography reveals these abnormalities best. Our studies revealed a marked interference with choroidal arterial circulation in all eyes

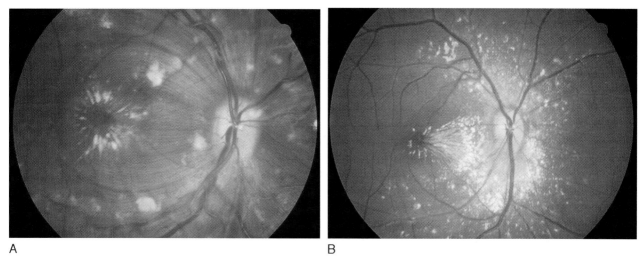

A   B

FIGURE 27–21 Fundus photographs of hypertensive rhesus monkeys and on atherogenic diet show extensive lipid deposits at the posterior pole, much more than seen in comparable hypertensive animals without atherogenic diet. (From Hayreh SS, Servais GE, Virdi PS: Retinal lipid deposits in malignant arterial hypertension. Ophthalmologica 198:216–229, 1989. Reproduced with permission of S. Karger AG, Basel.)

with choroidopathy that was particularly marked in the submacular choroid[10,15] (Figs. 27–3B, 27–4B, 27–9B, 27–14, 27–22, 27–23, and 27–24B). There is usually a generalized delayed filling of the choroidal vascular bed, mostly showing a patchy filling pattern, especially marked in the macular or foveal region.[15] We found choroidal circulatory insufficiency one of the earliest findings in malignant arterial hypertension, and also a significant ($p < .01$) correlation between the choroidal circulatory disturbances and the blood pressure level.[15] On ophthalmoscopy, there is evidence of choroidal vascular sclerosis in some eyes, particularly in those

associated with extensive RPE degeneration.[15] Our histopathologic studies revealed extensive choroidal vascular abnormalities and could be classified into three stages[10]:

ACUTE ISCHEMIC PHASE. The initial change in the choroidal vascular bed is constriction of arterioles, leading to acute ischemic changes in the regional choriocapillaris and overlying RPE.

CHRONIC OCCLUSIVE PHASE. During this stage, occlusive changes involve choroidal arteries and arterioles, and later on choriocapillaris (Fig. 27–25).

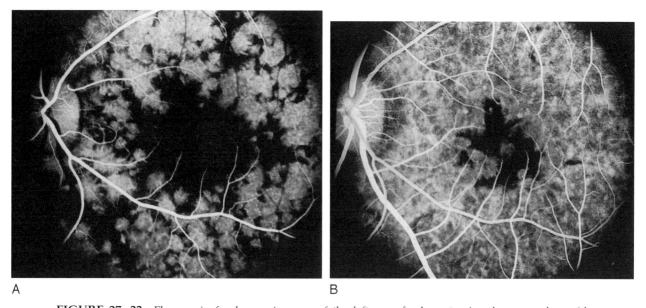

A   B

FIGURE 27–22 Fluorescein fundus angiograms of the left eye of a hypertensive rhesus monkey with systolic BP 205 mm Hg, during retinal (A) and late venous (B) phases, show marked delay in filling of the submacular choroid. (From Hayreh SS, Servais GE, Virdi PS: Fundus lesions in malignant hypertension VI. Hypertensive choroidopathy. Ophthalmology 93:1383–1400, 1986, with permission.)

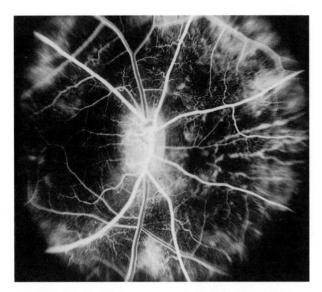

FIGURE 27–23 Fluorescein angiogram of right eye of a hypertensive rhesus monkey with systolic BP 170 mm Hg showing marked choroidal filling defect, particularly in the peripapillary choroid. (From Hayreh SS, Servais GE, Virdi PS: Fundus lesions in malignant hypertension V. Hypertensive optic neuropathy. Ophthalmology 93:74–87, 1986, with permission.)

CHRONIC REPARATIVE PHASE. In due course, recanalization of the choroidal vessels takes place. Arteriolization of the choriocapillaris, which seems to be a defensive mechanism to withstand the raised systemic blood pressure, also occurs.

Retinal Pigment Epithelial Lesions

These are ischemic in nature. They can be further classified into two types.

ACUTE FOCAL RPE LESIONS. Acute severe choroidal ischemia causes focal infarction of the overlying RPE and the outer retina. Clinically these lesions manifest almost routinely as pale or white punctate, round, focal, usually pinhead in size, and commonly distributed in groups, some of them associated with focal serous RD[15] (Figs. 27–2A, 27–3A, 27–9A, 27–11, 27–12A, 27–17A, and 27–24A). They are usually situated in the macular region and every so often elsewhere in the posterior fundus and in the periphery. With time these lesions increase in number.

On fluorescein angiography, at this stage, apart from the delayed and generally patchy filling of the choroidal vascular bed (especially marked in the macular or foveal region), there is staining of these lesions during the late phase[15] (Figs. 27–3B and 27–18B).

Pathologic studies showed that the initial choroidal arteriolar constriction caused acute focal necrosis of the choriocapillaris and the RPE, and focal subretinal exudate.[10]

On routine ophthalmoscopy, the acute focal RPE lesions[15] may be confused with FIPTs,[13] but on fluorescein angiography the RPE lesions stain less intensely and their staining persists for a much shorter duration than the FIPTs, in addition to the fact that RPE lesions are subretinal while FIPTs are intraretinal.

RPE DEGENERATIVE LESIONS. These can be further subdivided into two categories.[15]

Early RPE Degenerative Lesions. In 2 to 3 weeks the acute focal RPE lesions develop into focal RPE degenerative lesions—the two look very similar on ophthalmoscopy but fluorescein angiography shows unmasking of the underlying choroidal

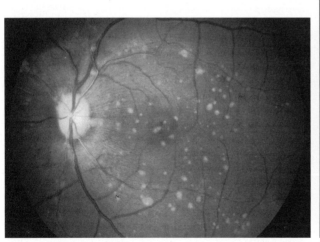

A

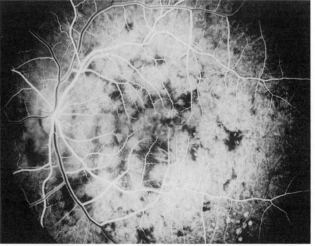

B

FIGURE 27–24 Fundus photograph (A) and fluorescein angiogram (B) of left eye of a hypertensive rhesus monkey with systolic BP 202 mm Hg. A shows multiple white acute focal RPE lesions, in addition to a few FIPTs (along the retinal arterioles). B shows delayed filling of the macular choroid. (A from Hayreh SS, Servais GE, Virdi PS: Fundus lesions in malignant hypertension VI. Hypertensive choroidopathy. Ophthalmology 93: 1383–1400, 1986, with permission.)

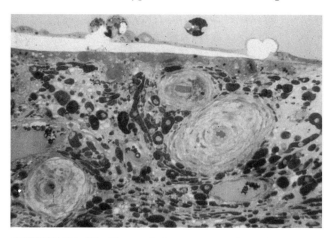

FIGURE 27–25 Histopathologic section of the choroid of a hypertensive monkey, showing choroidal arteries in chronic occlusive phase of hypertensive choroidopathy. Choroidal arteries and arterioles show marked hyperplastic arteriosclerosis. Lumens are extremely narrowed by thickened and laminated vessel wall. Choriocapillaris (top layer) is occluded by thrombus (toluidine blue stain). (From Kishi S, Tso MOM, Hayreh SS: Fundus lesions in malignant hypertension I. A pathologic study of experimental hypertensive choroidopathy. Arch Ophthalmol 103:1189–1197, 1985, Copyright 1985, American Medical Association, with permission.)

fluorescence with no late staining of the degenerative lesions. The acute lesions may become confluent and result in either ill-defined chorioretinal degenerative areas or fairly defined punched-out RPE degenerative lesions (the so-called Elschnig's spots) (Figs. 27–6, 27–12A, and 27–15). Since the acute lesions have only a short life span and change into degenerative lesions, the latter are far more numerous than the former.

Late RPE Degenerative Lesions. The degenerative lesions are almost invariably progressive in nature for a long time, so that they are far more extensive than the acute lesions. This would indicate that the progressive degenerative lesions are due to persistent chronic choroidal ischemia, not always preceded by acute lesions. These lesions are widely scattered throughout the fundus, being common in the macular and peripheral regions—the peripheral lesions are usually much more extensive than the those in the macular region—the temporal part of the macular region and the temporal part of the peripheral fundus are most extensively involved areas (Figs. 27–5 and 27–6). On ophthalmoscopy,[15] they are usually made up of polymorphic RPE atrophic areas as well as of diffuse pigmentary change, the latter giving a coarse granular or moth-eaten appearance to the RPE. The atrophic lesions may vary from being focal to confluent patches of varying sizes (e.g., geographic, triangular, irregular) (Figs. 27–5 and 27–6). Some eyes may show colloid or drusenoid degeneration of the RPE (Fig. 27–5). In the macular region, these changes may very much resemble those seen in age-related macular degeneration (Figs. 27–5 and 27–17C). In some

eyes with widespread RPE degeneration, the overall fundus appearance may very much resemble the late stages of the clinical entity called "birdshot retinopathy."

On fluorescein fundus angiography,[15] RPE degeneration is seen much more clearly and more extensively than on ophthalmoscopy because of unmasking of the underlying choroidal fluorescence in the degenerated areas (Figs. 27–15C). There is no late staining of these lesions. When the macular region is involved, the angiographic appearance may closely resemble age-related macular degeneration.

Pathologic studies[10] revealed that chronic occlusive changes involving the arteries, arterioles, and choriocapillaris result in diffuse patchy RPE degeneration and depigmentation, which follows the lobular arrangement of the choriocapillaris.

Serous Retinal Detachment

When hypertensive choroidopathy was seen in our studies,[15] macular and/or peripapillary serous RD of variable degree was almost always seen and was an important and prominent finding (Figs. 27–3A, 27–4A, 27–8A, 27–9A, 27–11, 27–12A, 27–17A and B, 27–18A, 27–19, 27–20, and 27–26). It involved the peripheral retina in about a third (Fig. 27–26). We could find no definite relationship between the development of serous RD and that of hypertensive retinopathy, indicating that etiologically the serous RD was not secondary to the retinopathy. However, the retina overlying the serous RD, particularly in the macular region, usually showed frank edematous changes, consisting of macular retinal edema, frequently with microcystic changes, and a prominent foveolar cyst developed in a quarter of them (Figs. 27–3A, 27–11, 27–12A, 27–17A and B, 27–18A, and 27–20). The subretinal fluid initially is usually clear but becomes progressively turbid, opaque, white and exudative in nature in marked cases with time, most marked in the foveal zone (Figs. 27–2A, 27–3A, 27–17B, 27–19, and 27–20), and later on once again it gradually clears up; some eyes develop subretinal fibrosis in the macular region (Fig. 27–7). The peripheral RD, when present, is usually bullous and may extend 360 degrees, and may lead to total RD, with subretinal fluid shifting with change of position of the head (Fig. 27–26). The serous RD resolves spontaneously in due course.

In our studies,[15] we found a good correlation between the early and late RPE changes and the onset, development, and severity of macular serous RD. We also found that all eyes with serous RD showed marked choroidal circulatory disturbance.[15] Thus, all the available clinical, angiographic, and morphologic evidence in our studies[10,15] showed that ischemia of the RPE causes breakdown of the normal retinal-blood barrier in RPE, resulting in leakage of fluid, proteins, and other materials from the choroid, through the RPE, into the subretinal space, and production of serous RD. Serous RD seen in eclampsia has the same mechanism.

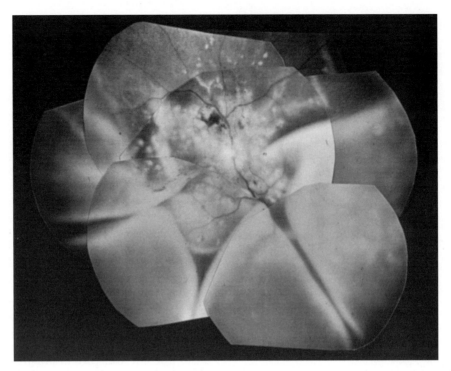

FIGURE 27–26   Composite fundus photograph of right eye of a hypertensive rhesus monkey with systolic BP 212 mm Hg. It shows marked attenuation of retinal arterioles, optic disc, retinal and macular edema, many FIPTs and IRISs, retinal hemorrhages, and massive bullous RD. (From Hayreh SS, Servais GE, Virdi PS: Fundus lesions in malignant hypertension VI. Hypertensive choroidopathy. Ophthalmology 93:1383–1400, 1986, with permission.)

Hypertensive Choroidopathy and Retinopathy: Two Independent and Unrelated Manifestations of Malignant Arterial Hypertension

The retinal and choroidal vascular beds have some fundamentally different anatomic and physiologic properties, as discussed above. For example, the choroidal vascular bed has (1) a profuse sympathetic nerve supply, (2) no autoregulation of blood flow, and (3) no blood-ocular barrier. By contrast, the retinal vascular bed has (1) no sympathetic nerve supply and (2) an efficient blood flow autoregulation as well as blood-retinal barrier. Hence, the two vascular systems respond very differently to malignant hypertension, making hypertensive retinopathy and choroidopathy two very different and entirely independent manifestations of malignant arterial hypertension.

HYPERTENSIVE OPTIC NEUROPATHY

The occurrence of optic disc edema in malignant arterial hypertension in the past has invariably been thought to point to a poor prognosis for the survival of the patient. For example, according to the Keith-Wagener-Barker[80] classification of hypertensive fundus changes, survival time for patients with optic disc edema (i.e., "grade IV hypertensive retinopathy") was only 4½ months, and Kincaid-Smith et al[71] found that 50% of the untreated patients in this group died within 2 months and 90% within a year. Therefore, presence of optic disc edema in malignant hypertension came to be regarded as an important, ominous, prognostic sign. However, McGregor et al,[81] in 96 consecutive patients with hypertensive retinopathy and optic disc edema, found on multivariate analysis that optic disc edema was not related to survival, and they concluded that optic disc edema is an unreliable physical sign and does not deleteriously influence the prognosis in hypertensive patients. They further held that optic disc edema should no longer be regarded as a necessary feature of malignant hypertension. Our studies support the views of McGregor et al.[81]

Apart from this clinical controversy on the importance of optic disc edema in malignant hypertension, its nature and pathogenesis have also remained contentious in the past. Our studies on the subject provide an important insight into the clinical course of optic disc edema, its evolution and other manifestations, and its pathogenesis.[14]

Hypertensive Optic Neuropathy Lesions

Our studies[14] showed that the initial optic disc change in malignant hypertension is edema which, on ophthalmoscopy, is indistinguishable from optic disc edema seen in many other conditions, such as intracranial hypertension (Figs. 27–2*A*, 27–4*A*, 27–7, 27–8*A*, 27–12*A*, 27–15*A*, 27–17*A* and *B*, and 27–21*A*). Fluorescein fundus angiography at this stage usually shows a variable amount of choroidal filling delay or choroidal circulatory disturbance in the posterior pole (Figs. 27–2*B*, 27–3*B*, 27–4*B*, 27–14, 27–22, 27–23, and 27–24*B*). On follow-up the disc edema usually resolves and is frequently followed by a variable degree of optic disc pallor (Figs. 27–5, 27–7, and 27–17*C*)—note gradual development of disc pallor in Figures 27–17*B* to 17*C*. Our pathologic studies[11] revealed vasoconstriction with subsequent axonal hydropic swelling, axolemma disruption, and glial swelling in the prelaminar region when the disc was edematous. In the retrolaminar region, the optic nerve showed more marked vasoconstriction, with endothelial swelling and pericytic degeneration, intramyelinic vacuoles, and glial swelling. These studies indicated that optic disc edema in these eyes was due to axonal hydropic swelling secondary to ischemia, followed by loss of axons and gliosis, so that ischemia seemed to play a major role in the pathogenesis of hypertensive optic neuropathy.

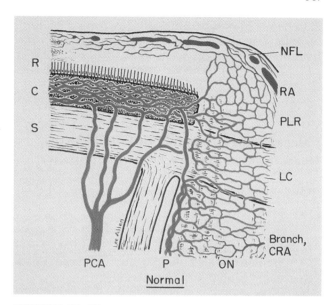

FIGURE 27–27   Schematic representations of blood supply of the optic nerve head and retrolaminar optic nerve. C, choroid; CRA, central retinal artery; LC, lamina cribrosa; NFL, surface nerve fiber layer of the disc; ON, optic nerve; P, pia; PCA, posterior ciliary artery; PLR, prelaminar region; R, retina; RA, retinal arteriole; S, sclera. (From Heilmann K, Richardson KT [eds]: Glaucoma: Conceptions of a Disease. Stuttgart, Thieme, 1978, pp 78–96, with permission.)

Pathogenesis of Hypertensive Optic Neuropathy

This has been a controversial subject in the past, and the various views put forward to explain it can be divided into the following four categories.

Optic Disc Edema Due to Raised Intracranial Pressure

During the early stages, optic disc edema in malignant hypertension is indistinguishable ophthalmoscopically from that seen in raised intracranial pressure. Many of these hypertensive patients may also have headache, vomiting, and other symptoms of raised intracranial pressure. Therefore, the major debate during the past 150 years has focused on whether optic disc edema in malignant hypertension is due to raised cerebrospinal fluid pressure. I have summarized the controversy elsewhere.[14,82] In our studies,[14] we found no evidence to support the theory that optic disc edema in malignant hypertension is due to raised cerebrospinal fluid pressure.

Optic Disc Edema Similar to Hypertensive Encephalopathy

In malignant arterial hypertension, hypertensive encephalopathy is seen in some cases. Since the optic nerve and brain circulations have many close similarities, it is but natural to consider the two organs as behaving identically in malignant hyper-

tension; however, there is an important difference between the two. The brain has an efficient autoregulation of the blood flow and blood-brain barrier. While the optic nerve head has been shown to have autoregulation of blood flow, it *does not have* a blood-optic nerve barrier because of leakage of fluid from the peripapillary choroid into the prelaminar region of the optic nerve through the border tissue of Elschnig, which separates the choroid from the optic nerve head[14] (Fig. 27–27). This absence of blood–optic nerve barrier plays an important role in the pathogenesis of hypertensive optic neuropathy (discussed below) and indicates that hypertensive optic neuropathy and encephalopathy are not identical in nature.

Optic Disc Edema a Part of Hypertensive Retinopathy

Since the main source of blood supply to the optic nerve head is the posterior ciliary artery circulation[30,83,84] and *not* retinal arterial circulation (Fig. 27–27), hypertensive optic neuropathy cannot be considered as a part of hypertensive retinopathy, apart from other considerations discussed below. Also, hypertensive retinopathy in our studies[12] appeared significantly ($p < .01$) earlier than hypertensive optic neuropathy or choroidopathy.

Optic Disc Edema is Ischemic in Nature

Pathologic findings in our studies[11] (discussed above) showed that hypertensive optic neuropathy is ischemic in nature. Similarly, the clinical patterns of optic disc edema and optic disc changes in malignant hypertension were found to be similar to those of anterior ischemic optic neuropathy.[14]

Mechanism of Ischemia of Optic Nerve Head in Hypertensive Optic Neuropathy

In the understanding of this, the following very important facts are to be borne in mind:

1. The primary source of blood supply to the optic nerve head is the posterior ciliary artery circulation, and peripapillary choroid is the major source[30,83,84] (Fig. 27–27).
2. There is no blood–optic nerve barrier because the choroidal interstitial fluid diffuses into the optic nerve head from the peripapillary choroid through the border tissue of Elschnig.[100]
3. As discussed above in pathogenesis of hypertensive choroidopathy, angiotensin II and other endogenous vasoconstrictor agents leak freely into the choroidal interstitial fluid.
4. In discussion of hypertensive choroidopathy, marked vasoconstriction of the choroidal arteries and arterioles, and consequent choroidal ischemia have been stressed. As a part of hypertensive choroidopathy, the peripapillary choroid also develops marked vasoconstriction and vaso-occlusive changes and consequent ischemia in its distribution.

From this brief discussion it is evident that optic nerve head ischemia in malignant hypertension is produced by a combination of the following two factors:

Involvement of the Peripapillary Choroid by Vasoconstriction and Vaso-occlusive Changes. Since peripapillary choroid is the main source of blood supply to the optic nerve head[30,83,84] (Fig. 27–27), these changes would secondarily cause ischemia of the optic nerve head.

Diffusion of Angiotensin II and Other Endogenous Vasoconstrictors into the Optic Nerve Head from the Peripapillary Choroid. These agents would produce vasoconstriction of the blood vessels in the optic nerve head by their direct action, resulting in ischemia.

Further evidence that these two mechanisms are responsible for hypertensive optic neuropathy is the fact that in our studies[12] there was no significant difference between the time of onset of hypertensive choroidopathy and optic neuropathy, whereas hypertensive retinopathy appeared significantly ($p < .01$) earlier than both of them.

Axoplasmic Flow Stasis in Hypertensive Optic Neuropathy

Our studies[11] revealed that optic disc edema in hypertensive optic neuropathy is essentially due to axoplasmic flow stasis in the optic nerve head. The axoplasmic flow stasis in turn is secondary to ischemia of the axons.

Thus, in conclusion, our studies[11,14] strongly suggest that optic disc edema in hypertensive optic neuropathy is due to ischemia, and that hypertensive optic neuropathy in fact represents anterior ischemic optic neuropathy. Our studies on a large population of patients with anterior ischemic optic neuropathy have shown that the severity of ischemia determines the severity of anterior ischemic optic neuropathy, which may vary from subclinical (with no clinically detectable visual disturbance other than optic disc edema and no or minimal residual optic disc pallor[85]) to severe (with marked visual loss and optic atrophy).[14]

Dangers of Precipitous Reduction of Blood Pressure in Patients with Hypertensive Optic Neuropathy

This is an extremely important consideration from the clinical management point of view. It has been shown that if blood pressure is lowered precipitously in patients with malignant arterial hypertension and optic disc edema, they may suffer immediate and permanent blindness or severe visual loss due to infarction of the optic nerve head[86–90] and may also develop acute ischemic neurologic lesions.[87,88,90,91] It has been postulated that this is due to ischemia of the optic nerve head, spinal cord, and/or brain due to marked hypotension in the presence of deranged autoregulation of blood flow in the respective organs. It is well established now that in patients with malignant hypertension of some duration, as an adaptive phenomenon, the range of blood flow autoregulation in the optic nerve head and brain shifts to a level higher than that of normal persons[48,49,55,92–97] (Fig. 27–1). Such an adjustment, although it improves the tolerance of such a person to very high blood pressures, makes them correspondingly less tolerant to low blood pressure also. As discussed above, the optic nerve head in hypertensive optic neuropathy is already ischemic; a precipitous reduction of blood pressure with a lack of autoregulation at lower levels of blood pressure (Fig. 27–1) would make such optic nerve heads extremely susceptible to severe acute ischemic damage. This could result in bilateral infarction of the optic nerve head. *Therefore, in such patients the blood pressure should be lowered gradually, over many hours or days, to give time for the autoregulation of blood flow to adapt to the falling blood pressure.*

CLASSIFICATION OF HYPERTENSIVE FUNDUS CHANGES

A large number of clinical classifications and methods of grading hypertensive fundus changes have been put forward since 1939.[29,72,74,80,98,99] All were based on ophthalmoscopic interpretation of the fundus changes, particularly retinal arteriolar changes. With a better understanding of the pathophysiology of the various hypertensive fundus lesions, the limitations of these various schemes have become apparent.

The first and most widely used classification has been that of Keith, Wagener, and Barker,[80] put forward in 1939. They graded the cases into four groups, based on histologic findings in the arterioles of pectoralis muscle biopsy and follow-up information. In the light of our current understanding of the subject and the multiple limitations in this and other classifications, which I recently discussed at length,[22] they have now become obsolete for clinical purposes.

From the previous discussion of the normal anatomic and physiologic properties of the retinal, choroidal, and optic nerve head vascular beds; the pathophysiologies of malignant arterial hypertension; and pathogenesis of hypertensive retinopathy, choroidopathy, and optic neuropathy, it becomes evident that various fundus lesions seen in malignant arterial hypertension defy any classification and grading of the type put forward in the past. Thus, I strongly discourage grading hypertensive fundus changes but recommend giving a descriptive account of the individual fundus lesions, revealed by ophthalmoscopy and fluorescein fundus angiography. That is far more informative and useful in follow-up and estimation of severity of hypertensive fundus changes than the various arbitrary grades advocated. Different hypertensive fundus lesions in a patient may have different severities, as indicated by our studies.[10-21] Moreover, because of differences in the pathogenesis of the various lesions in hypertensive fundus changes, different lesions have different degrees of significance.

Acknowledgments: I am grateful to my wife Shelagh for her help in the preparation of this manuscript, to Mrs. Georgiane Parkes-Perret for the secretarial help, and to our photography department for the illustrations. These studies were supported by NIH research grant EY-1576, and in part by an unrestricted grant from Research to Prevent Blindness, Inc.

REFERENCES

1. Page LB: Epidemiology of hypertension. In Genest J, Kuchel O, Hamet P, Cantin M (eds): Hypertension: Physiopathology and Treatment, 2nd edition. New York, McGraw-Hill, 683–699, 1983.
2. Kannel WB, Sorlie P: Hypertension in Framingham. In Paul O (ed): Epidemiology and Control of Hypertension. New York, Stratton, 553–592, 1975.
3. Hayreh SS: Anterior Ischemic Optic Neuropathy. New York, Springer-Verlag, 1975.
4. Hayreh SS: Pathogenesis of optic nerve damage and visual field defects. In Heilmann K, Richardson KT (eds): Glaucoma: Conceptions of a Disease. Stuttgart, Thieme, 1978, pp 104–137, 405–411.
5. Hayreh SS: Central retinal vein occlusion. In Mausolf FA (ed): The Eye and Systemic Disease. St Louis, CV Mosby Co, 1980, pp 223–275.
6. Hayreh SS: Die Bedeutung vasculaerer Faktoren in der Pathogenese des Glaukomschadens. In Pillunat LE, Stodtmeister R (eds): Das Glaukom. Heidelberg, Springer-Verlag, 1993, pp 34–58.
7. Hayreh SS, Joos KM, Podhajsky PA, Long CR: Systemic diseases associated with nonarteritic anterior ischemic optic neuropathy. Am J Ophthalmol 118:766–780, 1994.
8. Hayreh SS: Progress in the understanding of the vascular etiology of glaucoma. Curr Opin Ophthalmol 5:26–35, 1994.
9. Hayreh SS, Zimmerman BM, Podhajsky P, Alward WLM: Nocturnal arterial hypotension and its role in optic nerve head and ocular ischemic disorders. Am J Ophthalmol 117:603–624, 1994.
10. Kishi S, Tso MOM, Hayreh SS: Fundus lesions in malignant hypertension I. A pathologic study of experimental hypertensive choroidopathy. Arch Ophthalmol 103:1189–1197, 1985.
11. Kishi S, Tso MOM, Hayreh SS: Fundus lesions in malignant hypertension II. A pathologic study of experimental hypertensive optic neuropathy. Arch Ophthalmol 103:1198–1206, 1985.
12. Hayreh SS, Servais GE, Virdi PS, et al: Fundus lesions in malignant hypertension III. Arterial blood pressure, biochemical, and fundus changes. Ophthalmology 93:45–59, 1986.
13. Hayreh SS, Servais GE, Virdi PS: Fundus lesions in malignant hypertension IV. Focal intraretinal periarteriolar transudates. Ophthalmology 93:60–73, 1986.
14. Hayreh SS, Servais GE, Virdi PS: Fundus lesions in malignant hypertension V. Hypertensive optic neuropathy. Ophthalmology 93:74–87, 1986.
15. Hayreh SS, Servais GE, Virdi PS: Fundus lesions in malignant hypertension VI. Hypertensive choroidopathy. Ophthalmology 93:1383–1400, 1986.
16. Hayreh SS, Servais GE: Retinal hemorrhages in malignant arterial hypertension. Int Ophthalmol 12:137–145, 1988.
17. Hayreh SS: Hypertensive retinopathy: introduction. Ophthalmologica 198:173–177, 1989.
18. Hayreh SS, Servais GE, Virdi PS: Retinal arteriolar changes in malignant arterial hypertension. Ophthalmologica 198:178–196, 1989.
19. Hayreh SS, Servais GE, Virdi PS: Cotton-wool spots (inner retinal ischemic spots) in malignant arterial hypertension. Ophthalmologica 198:197–215, 1989.
20. Hayreh SS, Servais GE, Virdi PS: Retinal lipid deposits in malignant arterial hypertension. Ophthalmologica 198:216–229, 1989.
21. Hayreh SS, Servais GE, Virdi PS: Macular lesions in malignant arterial hypertension. Ophthalmologica 198:230–246, 1989.
22. Hayreh SS: Classification of hypertensive fundus changes and their order of appearance. Ophthalmologica 198:247–260, 1989.
23. Hayreh SS: Malignant arterial hypertension and the eye. Ophthalmol Clin North Am 5:445–473, 1992.
24. Hayreh SS: Systemic arterial blood pressure and the eye. Eye 10:5–28, 1996.
25. Liebreich R: Ophthalmoskopischer Befund bei Morbus Brightii. Albrecht von Graefes Arch Ophthalmol 5(2):265–268, 1859.

26. Ashton N: The eye in malignant hypertension. Trans Am Acad Ophthalmol Otolaryngol 76:17–40, 1972.

27. Garner A, Ashton N, Tripathi R, et al: Pathogenesis of hypertensive retinopathy: an experimental study in the monkey. Br J Ophthalmol 59:3–44, 1975.

28. de Venecia G, Wallow I, Houser D, et al: The eye in accelerated hypertension. I. Elschnig's spots in nonhuman primates. Arch Ophthalmol 98:913–918, 1980.

29. Tso MOM, Jampol LM: Pathophysiology of hypertensive retinopathy. Ophthalmology 89:1132–1145, 1982.

30. Hayreh SS: The optic nerve head circulation in health and disease. Exp Eye Res 61:257–272, 1995.

31. Porsaa K: Experimental studies on the vasomotor innervation of the retinal arteries. Acta Ophthalmol Suppl 18, 1941.

32. Dollery CT, Hill DW, Hodge JV: The response of normal retinal blood vessels to angiotensin and noradrenaline. J Physiol 165:500–507, 1963.

33. Russell RWR: Observations on intracerebral aneurysms. Brain 86:425–442, 1963.

34. Alm A, Bill A: The oxygen supply to the retina. II. Effects of high intraocular pressure and of increased arterial carbon dioxide tension on uveal and retinal blood flow in cats; a study with radioactively labelled microspheres including flow determinations in brain and some other tissues. Acta Physiol Scand 84:306–319, 1972.

35. Alm A, Bill A: Ocular and optic nerve blood flow at normal and increased intraocular pressures in monkeys (Macaca irus): a study with radioactively labelled microspheres including flow determinations in brain and some other tissues. Exp Eye Res 15:15–29, 1973.

36. Bill A: Effects of acetazolamide and carotid occlusion on the ocular blood flow in unanesthetized rabbits. Invest Ophthalmol 13:954–958, 1974.

37. Bill A, Sperber G: Aspects of oxygen and glucose consumption in the retina: effects of high intraocular pressure and light. Graefes Arch Clin Exp Ophthalmol 228:124–127, 1990.

38. Bill A, Sperber G: Control of retinal and choroidal blood flow. Eye 4:319–325, 1990.

39. Ernest JT: Autoregulation of optic-disk oxygen tension. Invest Ophthalmol 13:101–106, 1974.

40. Geijer C, Bill A: Effects of raised intraocular pressure on retinal, prelaminar, laminar, and retrolaminar optic nerve blood flow in monkeys. Invest Ophthalmol Vis Sci 18:1030–1042, 1979.

41. Sossi N, Anderson DR: Effect of elevated intraocular pressure on blood flow; occurrence in cat optic nerve head studied with iodoantipyrine I 125. Arch Ophthalmol 101:98–101, 1983.

42. Weinstein JM, Duckrow RB, Beard D, et al: Regional optic nerve blood flow and its autoregulation. Invest Ophthalmol Vis Sci 24:1559–1565, 1983.

43. Alm A, Bill A: Blood flow and oxygen extraction in the cat uvea at normal and high intraocular pressures. Acta Physiol Scand 80:19–28, 1970.

44. Alm A, Bill A: The oxygen supply to the retina. I. Effects of changes in intraocular and arterial blood pressures, and in arterial PO_2 and PCO_2 on the oxygen tension in the vitreous body of the cat. Acta Physiol Scand 84:262–274, 1972.

45. Bill A: Blood circulation and fluid dynamics in the eye. Physiol Rev 55:383–417, 1975.

46. Takats I, Leiszter F: Relationship between blood flow velocity in the choroid and intraocular pressure in rabbits. Acta Ophthalmol 57:48–54, 1979.

47. Haefliger IO, Meyer P, Flammer J, Luescher TF: The vascular endothelium as a regulator of the ocular circulation: a new concept in ophthalmology? Surv Ophthalmol 39:123–132, 1994.

48. Strandgaard S, Jones JV, MacKenzie ET, et al: Upper limit of cerebral blood flow autoregulation in experimental renovascular hypertension in the baboon. Circ Res 37:164–167, 1975.

49. Jones JV, Fitch W, MacKenzie ET, et al: Lower limit of

50. Luescher TF: The endothelium and cardiovascular disease—a complex relationship. N Engl J Med 330:1081–1083, 1994.

51. Cunha-Vaz JG: Studies on the permeability of the blood-retinal barrier. III. Breakdown of the blood-retinal barrier by circulatory disturbances. Br J Ophthalmol 50:505–516, 1966.

52. Shakib M, Cunha-Vaz JG: Studies on the permeability of the blood-retinal barrier. IV. Junctional complexes of the retinal vessels and their role in the permeability of the blood-retinal barrier. Exp Eye Res 5:229–234, 1966.

53. Bill A, Tornquist P, Alm A: Permeability of the intraocular blood vessels. Trans Ophthalmol Soc UK 100:332–336, 1980.

54. Bill A, Sperber G, Ujiie K: Physiology of the choroidal vascular bed. Int Ophthalmol 6:101–107, 1983.

55. Boisvert DJP, Jones JV, Harper AM: Cerebral blood flow autoregulation to acutely increasing blood pressure during sympathetic stimulation. Acta Neurol Scand 56(Suppl 64):46–47, 1977.

56. Malmfors T: The adrenergic innervation of the eye as demonstrated by fluorescence microscopy. Acta Physiol Scand 65:259–267, 1965.

57. Ehinger B: Adrenergic nerves to the eye and to related structures in man and in the cynomolgus monkey (Macaca irus). Invest Ophthalmol 5:42–52, 1966.

58. Laties AM: Central retinal artery innervation: absence of adrenergic innervation to the intraocular branches. Arch Ophthalmol 77:405–409, 1967.

59. Bill A: Autonomic nervous control of uveal blood flow. Acta Physiol Scand 56:70–81, 1962.

60. Ruskell GL: Facial parasympathetic innervation of the choroidal blood vessels in monkeys. Exp Eye Res 12:166–172, 1971.

61. Alm A, Bill A: The effect of stimulation of the cervical sympathetic chain on retinal oxygen tension and on uveal, retinal and cerebral blood flow in cats. Acta Physiol Scand 88:85–94, 1973.

62. Alm A: The effect of sympathetic stimulation on blood flow through the uvea, retina, and optic nerve in monkeys (Macaca irus). Exp Eye Res 25:19–24, 1977.

63. Matsusaka T: An evidence for adrenergic involvement in the choroidal circulation. Graefes Arch Clin Exp Ophthalmol 216:17–21, 1981.

64. Morgan TR, Green K, Bowman K: Effects of adrenergic agonists upon regional ocular blood flow in normal and ganglionectomized rabbits. Exp. Eye Res 32:691–697, 1981.

65. Bill A: Some aspects of the ocular circulation. Friedenwald Lecture. Invest Ophthalmol Vis Sci 26:410–424, 1985.

66. Alm A, Bill A: Ocular circulation. In Moses RA, Hart WM Jr (eds): Adler's Physiology of the Eye: Clinical Application, 8th edition. St Louis, CV Mosby Co, 1987, pp 183–203.

67. Grajewski AL, Ferrari-Dileo G, Feuer WJ, et al: Beta-adrenergic responsiveness of choroidal vasculature. Ophthalmology 98:989–995, 1991.

68. Hogan MJ, Alvarado JA, Weddell JE: Histology of the Human Eye: An Atlas and Textbook. Philadelphia, WB Saunders Co, 1971, pp 508–513.

69. Friedenwald JS, Wilder HC, Maumenee AE, et al: Ophthalmic Pathology: An Atlas and Textbook. Philadelphia, WB Saunders Co, 1952, p 310.

70. Genest J, Kuchel O, Hamet P, Cantin M: Physiopathology of experimental and human hypertension. In Hypertension: Physiopathology and Treatment, 2nd edition. New York, McGraw-Hill, 1983, pp 3–675.

71. Kincaid-Smith P: Malignant hypertension: mechanisms and management. Pharmacol Ther 9:245–269, 1980.

72. Cogan DG: Ophthalmic Manifestations of Systemic Vascular Disease. Philadelphia, WB Saunders Co, 1974, pp 74–78.

73. Pickering GW: High Blood Pressure, 2nd edition. London, Churchill, 1968, pp 342–343.

74. Leishman R: The eye in general vascular disease—hypertension and arteriosclerosis. Br J Ophthalmol 41:641–701, 1957.

75. Hodge JV, Dollery CT: Retinal soft exudates: a clinical study by colour and fluorescence photography. Q J Med 33:117–131, 1964.

76. Henkind P: New observations on the radial peripapillary capillaries. Invest Ophthalmol 6:103–108, 1967.

77. Dollery CT: Hypertensive retinopathy. In Genest J, Kuchel O, Hamet P, Cantin M (eds): Hypertension: Physiopathology and Treatment, 2nd edition. New York, McGraw-Hill, 1983, pp 723–832.

78. Wise GN, Dollery CT, Henkind P: The Retinal Circulation. New York, Harper & Row, 1971, p 331.

79. Ballantyne AJ, Michaelson IC: Textbook of the Fundus of the Eye. Edinburgh, Livingstone, 1970, p 179.

80. Keith NM, Wagener HP, Barker NW: Some different types of essential hypertension: their course and prognosis. Am J Med Sci 197:332–343, 1939.

81. McGregor E, Isles CG, Jay JL, et al: Retinal changes in malignant hypertension. Br Med J 292:233–234, 1986.

82. Hayreh SS: Optic disc edema in raised intracranial pressure. V. Pathogenesis. Arch Ophthalmol 95:1553–1565, 1977.

83. Hayreh SS: Blood supply of the optic nerve head and its role in optic atrophy, glaucoma and oedema of the optic disc. Br J Ophthalmol 53:721–748, 1969.

84. Hayreh SS: Blood supply of the optic nerve head in health and disease. In Lambrou GN, Greve EL (eds): Ocular Blood Flow in Glaucoma: Means, Methods and Measurements. Amsterdam, Kugler & Ghedini, 1989, pp 3–54.

85. Hayreh SS: Anterior ischemic optic neuropathy. V. Optic disc edema an early sign. Arch Ophthalmol 99:1030–1040, 1981.

86. Cove DH, Seddon M, Fletcher RF, et al: Blindness after treatment for malignant hypertension. Br Med J 2:245–246, 1979.

87. Hulse JA, Taylor DSI, Dillon MJ: Blindness and paraplegia in severe childhood hypertension. Lancet 2:553–556, 1979.

88. Pryor JS, Davies PD, Hamilton DV: Blindness and malignant hypertension. Lancet 2:803, 1979.

89. Wetherill JH: Blindness after treatment for malignant hypertension. Br Med J 2:550, 1979.

90. Taylor D, Ramsay J, Day S, et al: Infarction of the optic nerve head in children with accelerated hypertension. Br J Ophthalmol 65:153–160, 1981.

91. Ledingham JGG, Rajagopalan B: Cerebral complications in the treatment of accelerated hypertension. Q J Med 48:25–41, 1979.

92. Strandgaard S, Olesen J, Skinhoj E, et al: Autoregulation of brain circulation in severe arterial hypertension. Br Med J 1:507–510, 1973.

93. Fitch W, MacKenzie ET, Harper AM: Effects of decreasing arterial blood pressure on cerebral blood flow in the baboon; influence of the sympathetic nervous system. Circ Res 37:550–557, 1975.

94. Bill A, Linder J: Sympathetic control of cerebral blood flow in acute arterial hypertension. Acta Physiol Scand 96:114–121, 1976.

95. Edvinsson L, Owman C, Siesjo B: Physiological role of cerebrovascular sympathetic nerves in the autoregulation of cerebral blood flow. Brain Res 117:519–523, 1976.

96. Strandgaard S, MacKenzie ET, Jones JV, et al: Studies on the cerebral circulation of the baboon in acutely induced hypertension. Stroke 7:287–290, 1976.

97. MacKenzie ET, McGeorge AP, Graham DI, et al: Breakthrough of cerebral autoregulation and the sympathetic nervous system. Acta Neurol Scand 56(Suppl 64):48–49, 1977.

98. Wagener HP, Clay GE, Gipner JF: Classification of retinal lesions in the presence of vascular hypertension. Trans Am Ophthalmol Soc 45:57–73, 1947.

99. Scheie HG: Evaluation of ophthalmoscopic changes of hypertension and arteriolarsclerosis. Arch Ophthalmol 49:117–138, 1953.

100. Hayreh SS: Fluids in the anterior part of the optic nerve in health and disease. Surv Ophthalmol 23:1–25, 1978.

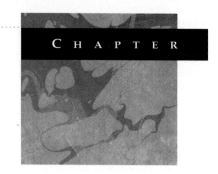

CHAPTER 28

Ocular Ischemic Syndrome

Gary C. Brown, M.D.

In 1963, Kearns and Hollenhorst[1] reported on the ocular symptoms and signs occurring secondary to severe carotid artery obstructive disease. They called the entity "venous stasis retinopathy" and noted that it occurred in approximately 5% of patients with severe carotid artery insufficiency or thrombosis. Some confusion has since arisen with this term because it has also been used to designate mild central retinal vein obstruction.[2] A number of additional alternative nomenclatures have been proposed, including ischemic ocular inflammation,[3] ischemic oculopathy,[4] and the ocular ischemic syndrome.[5,6] Histopathologic examination of eyes with the entity generally does not reveal inflammation,[7,8] and therefore the descriptive term that we prefer is the ocular ischemic syndrome.

BACKGROUND INFORMATION[1-8]

The mean age of patients with the ocular ischemic syndrome is about 65 years, with a range generally from the 50s to the 80s. No racial predilection has been identified, and males are affected more than females by a ratio of about 2:1. Either eye can be affected, and in approximately 20% of patients ocular involvement is bilateral. The prevalence of the disease has not been extensively studied, but from the work of Sturrock and Mueller[9] an annual estimate of 7.5 cases per million persons can be made. This number may be falsely low, since it is possible that a number of cases are misdiagnosed.

ETIOLOGY

In general, a 90% or greater stenosis of the ipsilateral carotid arterial system is present in eyes with the ocular ischemic syndrome.[6] It has been shown that a 90% carotid stenosis reduces the ipsilateral central retinal artery perfusion pressure by about 50%.[10,11] The obstruction can occur within the common carotid or internal carotid artery. In about 50% of cases the affected vessel is 100% occluded.[6]

Occasionally, obstruction of the ipsilateral ophthalmic artery can also be responsible.[6,12,13] Rarely, an isolated obstruction of the central retinal artery alone can mimic the dilated retinal veins and retinal hemorrhages seen in eyes with the ocular ischemic syndrome.[14]

Atherosclerosis within the carotid artery is the cause for the great majority of cases of the ocular ischemic syndrome.[6] Dissecting aneurysm of the carotid artery has been reported as a cause,[15] as has giant cell arteritis.[16] Hypothetically, entities such as fibromuscular dysplasia,[17] Behçet's disease,[18] trauma,[19] and inflammatory entities that cause carotid artery obstruction could lead to the ocular ischemic syndrome.

SYMPTOMS

Visual Loss

Greater than 90% of patients with the ocular ischemic syndrome relate a history of visual loss in the affected eye(s).[6] In two thirds of these it occurs over a period of weeks; it is abrupt in approximately 12%. In this latter group, with sudden visual loss there is often a cherry-red spot present on funduscopic examination.

Prolonged recovery following exposure to a bright light has been described in patients with severe carotid artery obstruction.[20] Concurrent attenuation of the visual evoked response has also been observed in these cases after light exposure. The phenomenon has been attributed to ischemia of the macular retina. In cases of bilateral, severe carotid artery obstruction, the visual loss after exposure to bright light occurs in both eyes, mimicking occipital lobe ischemia due to vertebrobasilar disease.[21]

Dissection of the internal carotid artery has been reported to cause scintillating scotomata that resemble a migraine aura.[22] While these could theoretically be associated with the classical ocular ischemic syndrome, they have not been observed by the author.

A history of amaurosis fugax is elicited in about 10% of ocular ischemic syndrome patients.[6] Amaurosis fugax, or fleeting loss of vision for seconds to minutes, is thought to be most commonly caused by emboli to the central retinal arterial system, although vasospasm may also play a role.[23] Although the majority of people with amaurosis fugax alone do not have the ocular ischemic syndrome, it can be an indicator of concomitant, ipsilateral carotid artery obstructive disease. About one third of patients with amaurosis fugax have an ipsilateral carotid artery obstruction of 75% or greater.[24] Rarely, it has been associated with a stenosis of the ophthalmic artery.[24]

Pain

Pain is present in the affected eye or orbital region in about 40% of cases,[6] and has been referred to as "ocular angina." Most often, it is described as a dull ache. It can occur secondary to neovascular glaucoma, but in those cases in which the intraocular pressure is normal the cause may be ischemia to the globe and/or ipsilateral dura.

SIGNS

Visual Acuity

Visual acuities at the time of presentation are variable in eyes with the ocular ischemic syndrome.[25] About 43% of affected eyes have vision ranging from 20/20 to 20/50, while in 37% vision is reduced to counting fingers or worse. Absence of light perception is generally not seen early, but can develop in the later stages of the disease, usually secondary to neovascular glaucoma. Among all eyes with the ocular ischemic syndrome at the end of 1 year of follow-up, including those with and without treatment, approximately 24% remain in the 20/20 to 20/50 group and 58% have counting fingers or worse vision.

Anterior Segment

Rubeosis iridis is encountered in approximately two thirds of eyes with the ocular ischemic syndrome at the time of presentation[6] (Fig. 28–1). Nevertheless, only slightly over half of these eyes have or develop an increase in intraocular pressure, even

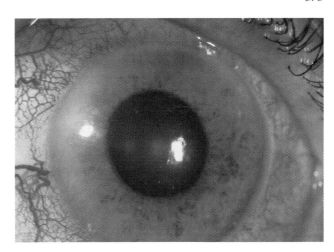

FIGURE 28–1 Rubeosis iridis and neovascular glaucoma. The eye is injected and new vessels can be seen on the peripheral iris nasally in this right eye.

if the anterior chamber angle is closed by fibrovascular tissue. Impaired ciliary body perfusion, with a subsequent decrease in aqueous production, probably accounts for this phenomenon.

Flare in the anterior chamber is usually present in most eyes with rubeosis iridis. An anterior chamber cellular response is seen in almost one fifth of eyes with the ocular ischemic syndrome,[6] but it rarely exceeds grade 2, as per the Schlaegel classification.[26] Keratic precipitates can be present, but are unusual.

In unilateral cases, there is generally little difference between the degree of lens opacification in each eye. As the disease advances, however, cataractous lens changes can develop. In advanced cases, the lens may become mature.

Although not an anterior segment sign, prominent collateral vessels are occasionally seen on the forehead. These vessels connect the external carotid system on one side of the head with the external carotid system on the other. They should not be mistaken for the enlarged tender vessels seen with giant cell arteritis and considered for temporal artery biopsy.

Posterior Segment

A list of the anterior and posterior segment signs found with the ocular ischemic syndrome is shown in Table 28–1.[1,3,4,6,9]

The retinal arteries are usually narrowed and the retinal veins are most often dilated, but not tortuous (Fig. 28–2). The venous dilation may be accompanied by beading, but usually not to the extent seen in eyes with marked preproliferative or proliferative diabetic retinopathy. Dilation of the veins is probably a nonspecific response to the ischemia from the inflow obstruction. Nevertheless, in some eyes both the retinal arteries and veins are narrowed. In contrast, eyes with central retinal vein

TABLE 28–1   Anterior and Posterior Segment Signs Seen in Eyes with the Ocular Ischemic Syndrome*

Signs	Frequency of Occurrence
Anterior segment	
Rubeosis iridis	67%
Neovascular glaucoma (rubeosis and intraocular pressure >22 mm Hg)	35%
Uveitis (cells and flare)	18%
Posterior segment	
Narrowed retinal arteries	Most
Dilated retinal veins	Most
Retinal hemorrhages	80%
Neovascularization	37%
Optic disc	−35%
Retina	−8%
Cherry-red spot	12%
Cotton-wool spot(s)	6%
Spontaneous retinal arterial pulsations	4%
Vitreous hemorrhage	4%
Cholesterol emboli	2%
Ischemic optic neuropathy	2%

* Adapted from Brown GC, Magaral LE: The ocular ischemic syndrome. Clinical, fluorescein angiographic and carotid angiographic features. Int Ophthalmol 11: 239–251, 1988. Reproduced with permission of Kluwer Academic Publishers.

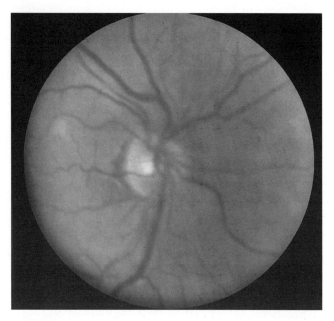

FIGURE 28–2   Right fundus of an eye with the ocular ischemic syndrome. The retinal arteries are narrowed and the retinal veins are dilated and beaded, but not tortuous.

obstruction usually also have dilated retinal veins, but they are often tortuous. The fact that the ocular ischemic syndrome occurs secondary to impaired inflow, while central retinal vein obstruction is usually associated with compromised outflow resulting from thrombus formation at or near the lamina cribrosa, may account for this difference.[27]

Retinal hemorrhages are seen in about 80% of affected eyes (Fig. 28–3).[6] They are most commonly present in the midperiphery, but can also extend into the posterior pole. While dot and blot hemorrhages are the most common variant, superficial retinal hemorrhages in the nerve fiber layer are occasionally seen. The hemorrhages probably arise secondary to leakage from the smaller retinal vessels that have sustained endothelial damage as a result of the ischemia. Similar to the case with diabetic retinopathy, they may also result from the rupture of microaneurysms. In general, the hemorrhages seen with the ocular ischemic syndrome are less numerous than those accompanying central retinal vein obstruction. They are almost never confluent.

Microaneurysms are frequently observed outside the posterior pole (Fig. 28–4), but can be seen in the macular region also. Hyperfluorescence with fluorescein angiography differentiates these abnormalities from hypofluorescent retinal hemorrhages. Retinal telangiectasia has also been described.[28]

Posterior segment neovascularization can occur at the optic disc or on the retina. Neovascularization of the disc (Fig. 28–5) is encountered in about 35% of eyes, while neovascularization of the retina is seen in about 8%.[6] Vitreous hemorrhage arising from traction upon the neovascularization by the vitreous gel has been reported to occur in 4% of eyes with the ocular ischemic syndrome in a retrospective study.[6] Rarely, the neovascularization

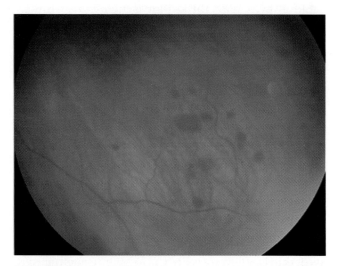

FIGURE 28–3   Ophthalmoscopic appearance of dot and blot hemorrhages in the left eye of a patient with the ocular ischemic syndrome secondary to a 100% common carotid artery obstruction.

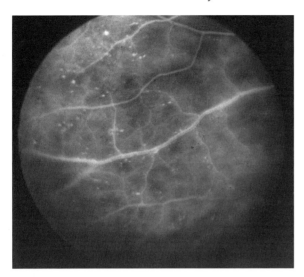

FIGURE 28–4   Fluorescein angiogram of the midperiphery of an eye with the ocular ischemic syndrome. Numerous hyperfluorescent microaneurysms are present. There is also staining of the retinal vessels.

can progress to severe preretinal fibrovascular proliferation.

A cherry-red spot is seen in approximately 12% of eyes with the ocular ischemic syndrome.[6] It can occur secondary to inner-layer retinal ischemia from embolic obstruction of the central retinal artery, but probably more often develops when the intraocular pressure exceeds the perfusion pressure within the central retinal artery, particularly in eyes with neovascular glaucoma.

Additional posterior segment signs[6] include cotton-wool spots in 6% of eyes, spontaneous retinal arterial pulsations in 4%, and cholesterol emboli within the retinal arteries in 2%. In contrast to spontaneous retinal venous pulsations, which are a normal variant and located at the base of the large veins on the optic disc, the arterial pulsations are usually more pronounced, and may extend 1 disc diameter or more out from the optic disc into the surrounding retina. Anterior ischemic optic neuropathy has also been reported in ocular ischemic syndrome eyes.[6,29,30] Acquired arteriovenous communications of the retina are rarely seen.[31]

ANCILLARY STUDIES

Fluorescein Angiography

The intravenous fluorescein angiographic signs associated with the ocular ischemic syndrome are listed in Table 28–2.[6]

Normally, the choroidal filling is completed within 5 seconds after the first appearance of dye. Sixty per cent of eyes with the ocular ischemic syndrome demonstrate patchy and/or delayed choroidal filling (Fig. 28–6). In some instances, the filling

is delayed for a minute or longer. Although not the most prevalent sign, an abnormality in choroidal filling is the most specific fluorescein angiographic sign in ocular ischemic eyes.

Prolongation of the retinal arteriovenous transit time is seen in 95% of eyes with the ocular ischemic syndrome, but can also be seen in eyes with central retinal artery obstruction and central retinal vein obstruction. Normally, the major retinal veins in the temporal vascular arcade are completely filled within 10 to 11 seconds after the first appearance of dye within the corresponding retinal arteries. In extreme cases of the ocular ischemic syndrome, the retinal veins fail to fill throughout the study.

Staining of the retinal vessels in the later phases of the study is seen in about 85% of eyes. both larger and smaller vessels can be involved (Figs. 28–5C and 28–7), the arteries generally more so than the veins. Chronic hypoxic damage to endothelial cells may account for the staining. In contrast, staining of the retinal vessels is uncommon with central retinal artery obstruction alone. With central retinal vein obstruction, the veins can demonstrate late staining, but the retinal arteries are generally not affected.

Macular edema with fluorescein angiography is seen in about one sixth of eyes with the ocular ischemic syndrome (Fig. 28–7).[32] Hypoxia, and subsequent endothelial damage, within the smaller retinal vessels, as well as leakage from microaneurysms, may account for this phenomenon. Dye accumulation may be mild or severe, and is usually associated with hyperfluorescence of the optic disc. The disc, however, is typically not swollen. Despite the prominent leakage with fluorescein angiography, the ophthalmoscopic cystic changes of macular edema are generally not as pronounced as those seen after ocular surgery or those associated with diabetic retinopathy.

Retinal capillary nonperfusion can be seen in some eyes (Fig. 28–8). Histopathologically, the absence of endothelial cells and pericytes within the retinal capillaries corresponds to the areas of nonperfusion seen with fluorescein angiography.[7,8,33]

Bilateral, simultaneous, intravenous fluorescein angiography is a technique that has been reported to be helpful diagnostically in patients with a unilateral ocular ischemic syndrome.[34] However, the technique requires specialized equipment and is not generally available.

Electroretinography

The electroretinogram often discloses a diminution of the amplitude, or absence, of both the a- and b-waves in eyes with the ocular ischemic syndrome (Fig. 28–9).[5,6] The b-wave corresponds to activity of the Müller and/or bipolar cells, and therefore to inner-layer retinal function, while the a-wave correlates with activity of the photoreceptors in the

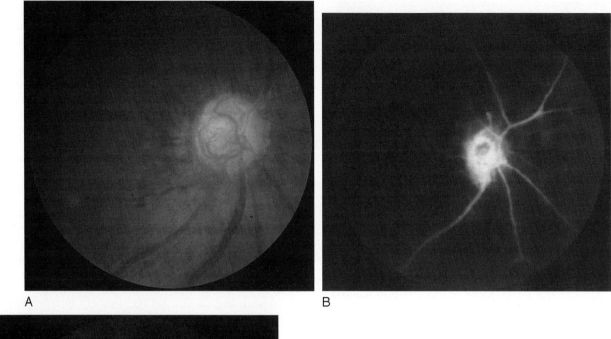

A

B

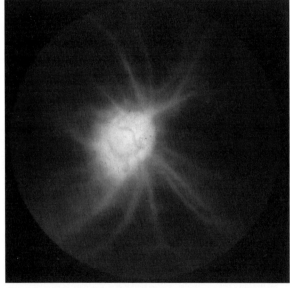

C

FIGURE 28–5 *A*, Neovascularization of the optic disc in a nondiabetic patient with a severe ipsilateral internal carotid artery stenosis. The retinal veins are dilated and beaded. *B*, Fluorescein angiogram corresponding to *A* at 32 seconds after injection. Hyperfluorescence on the optic disc is already present due to leakage of dye from the neovascularization. *C*, At 375 seconds after injection the disc hyperfluorescence has increased and there is prominent staining of the large retinal vessels, the arteries more so than the veins.

outer retina.[35,36] Therefore, with central retinal artery obstruction, in which there is essentially inner layer retinal ischemia, the b-wave amplitude is characteristically decreased. With the ocular ischemic syndrome there is both retinal vascular and choroidal compromise, leading to ischemia of the inner and outer retina, respectively. Thus, both the b-wave and the a-wave are affected.

Reduction in the amplitude of the oscillatory potential of the b-wave has been noted in eyes with retinal ischemia secondary to carotid artery stenosis.[37] This can be seen in patients with proven carotid artery disease, even in the presence of a normal fluorescein angiogram.

Carotid Artery Studies

Carotid angiography is generally undertaken when endarterectomy is being considered. Nevertheless, noninvasive tests, such as duplex ultrasonography and oculoplethysmography, have an accuracy of approximately 95% in detecting carotid stenosis of 75% or greater.[38,39]

Others

Visual evoked potentials have been used to study eyes with severe carotid artery stenosis. The re-

TABLE 28–2   Fluorescein Angiographic Signs
Seen in Eyes with the Ocular
Ischemic Syndrome

Signs	Frequency of Occurrence
Delayed and/or patchy choroidal filling	60%
Prolonged retinal arteriovenous transit time	95%
Retinal vascular staining	85%
Macular edema	17%
Other signs	
Retinal capillary nonperfusion	
Optic nerve head hyperfluorescence	
Microaneurysmal hyperfluorescence	

covery time of the amplitude of the major positive peak after photostress has been shown to improve in patients with severe stenosis after endarterectomy.[40]

Ophthalmodynamometry can be of benefit in detecting decreased ocular perfusion in cases of unilateral ocular ischemic syndrome.[10,41] In the absence of an ophthalmodynamometer, Kearns[40] has advocated light digital pressure on the upper lid of the affected eye during ophthalmoscopy. Retinal arterial pulsations can usually be readily induced in eyes with the ocular ischemic syndrome. This is generally not the case in eyes with central retinal vein obstruction, an entity that can be confused with the ocular ischemic syndrome.

SYSTEMIC ASSOCIATION

Diseases associated in one way or another with atherosclerosis are frequently seen in conjunction with the ocular ischemic syndrome. Systemic arterial hypertension has been reported in 73% of ocular ischemic syndrome patients and concomitant diabetes mellitus has been observed in 56%.[42] In an age-matched historical control population from the Framingham Study,[43] the corresponding prevalences for systemic arterial hypertension and diabetes mellitus were 26 and 6%, respectively.

At the time of presentation, almost one fifth of patients relate a history of having peripheral vascular disease for which previous bypass surgery was required.[42] The stroke rate for patients with the ocular ischemic syndrome is approximately 40% per year.[44]

Mortality data[42] have shown that the 5-year death rate for patients with the ocular ischemic syn-

drome is 40% (Fig. 28–9). The leading cause of death is cardiovascular disease, which accounts for about two thirds of cases. Stroke is the second leading cause of death. Thus, most patients with the ocular ischemic syndrome should probably be referred for cardiac evaluation, as well as a carotid work-up.

DIFFERENTIAL DIAGNOSIS

The entities that are most commonly confused with the ocular ischemic syndrome include mild central retinal vein obstruction and diabetic retinopathy. Features that differentiate these abnormalities are listed in Table 38–3.

In contrast to the ocular ischemic syndrome, the veins in eyes with mild, or nonischemic, central retinal vein obstruction are often dilated. Additionally, with light digital pressure on the lid it is difficult to induce retinal arterial pulsations in eyes with central retinal vein obstruction. While both entities usually have a prolonged retinal arteriovenous transit time, choroidal filling defects and prominent retinal arterial staining are usually absent on fluorescein angiography in eyes with central retinal vein obstruction.

Diabetic retinopathy can exist concomitantly with the ocular ischemic syndrome. The presence of hard exudate in the posterior pole usually suggests diabetic retinopathy, rather than the ocular ischemic syndrome. As is the case with central retinal vein obstruction, choroidal filling defects and retinal arterial staining are generally absent on fluorescein angiography in eyes with diabetic retinopathy.

In some cases of diabetic retinopathy, the ocular ischemic syndrome can exacerbate the proliferative changes. It has not been proven that carotid stenosis is protective against the development of proliferative diabetic retinopathy.[44]

TREATMENT

With regard to vision, the natural course of the ocular ischemic syndrome is uncertain. Nonetheless, most eyes with the fully developed entity probably have a poor long-term outcome. When rubeosis iridis is present, well over 90% of eyes become legally blind within a year of discovery.[25]

When a carotid artery is 100% obstructed, endarterectomy is usually ineffective, since a thrombus often propagates distally to the next major vessel. In these cases, extracranial-to-intracranial bypass surgery, usually from the superficial temporal artery to the middle cerebral artery, has been attempted to alleviate the obstruction. Although case reports suggest that this procedure can be of benefit initially in salvaging vision in eyes with the ocular

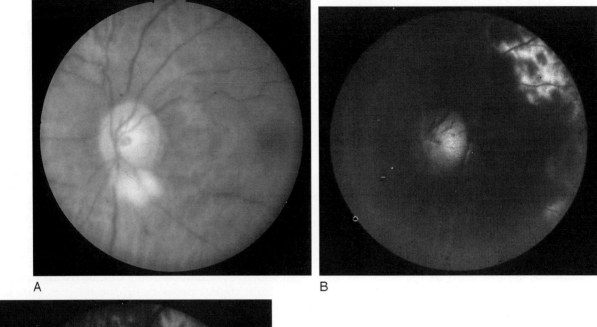

A

B

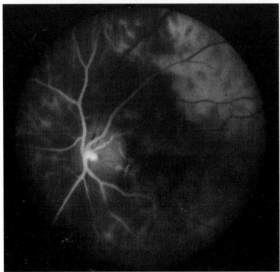

C

FIGURE 28–6   *A,* Fundus of an eye with the ocular ischemic syndrome secondary to a 100% internal carotid artery obstruction. Unrelated myelinated nerve fibers are present at the inferior border of the optic disc. The visual acuity was 20/20. *B,* Fluorescein angiogram corresponding to *A* at 37.7 seconds after injection. The retinal vessels are barely filled and minimal dye is present in the temporal choroid. *C,* At 56.6 seconds after injection the choroidal filling is still incomplete. A leading edge of dye is present in the retinal arteries. (Courtesy of Dr. Larry Magargal.)

ischemic syndrome,[45–50] as well as causing regression of neovascular glaucoma,[51] the visual prognosis at 1 year after the surgery is almost universally poor.[25] Additionally, the procedure has not been shown in a large randomized study to be of benefit in preventing the risk of ischemic stroke.[52]

Although there are no randomized studies that compare the natural history of the disease to the course after carotid endarterectomy, it appears that the best chance of stabilizing or improving the vision in ocular ischemic syndrome eyes occurs in patients who undergo successful endarterectomy prior to the development of rubeosis iridis.[25,53] Notwithstanding, the visual results are fair at best. In the series of Sivalingam et al,[42] at the end of 1 year, 7% of eyes with the ocular ischemic syndrome that underwent endarterectomy had visual improvement, 33% were unchanged, and 60% had worse vision. Among the 60 total ocular ischemic syn-

drome eyes in the group, an endarterectomy was performed for only three without rubeosis. At the end of 1 year follow-up, the vision was better in one, stable in one, and worse in the third. Endarterectomy appears to rarely cause regression or iris neovascularization in eyes with the ocular ischemic syndrome.[54]

It should be noted that eyes with the ocular ischemic syndrome will occasionally develop a severe increase in intraocular pressure after ipsilateral carotid endarterectomy.[55,56] This is most likely to occur in eyes with rubeosis iridis and anterior chamber angle compromise from fibrovascular tissue formation. Although aqueous outflow is impaired in such eyes, ciliary body perfusion and aqueous humor formation are also decreased secondary to the carotid stenosis. When the carotid obstruction is suddenly reversed, ciliary body perfusion and aqueous humor formation increase, but the outflow

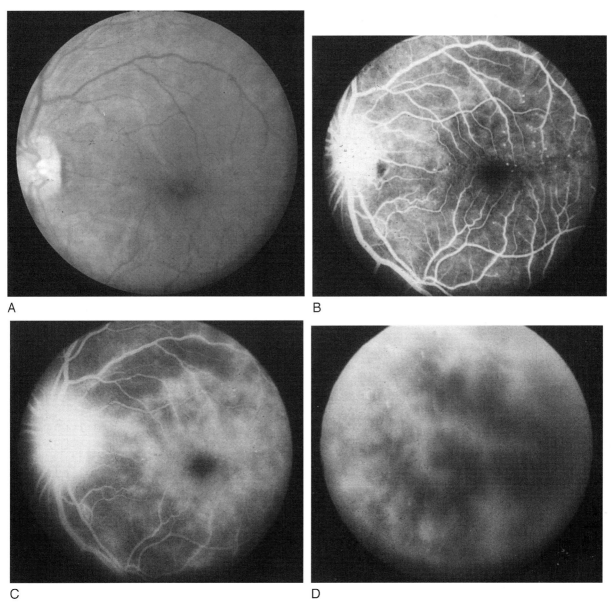

FIGURE 28–7   *A*, Foveolar cyst in the eye of a patient with a left 100% internal carotid artery obstruction and a visual acuity of 20/40. *B*, Fluorescein angiogram corresponding to *A* at approximately 70 seconds after injection demonstrates hyperfluorescent foci corresponding to microaneurysms. *C*, At over 7 minutes after injection there is prominent intraretinal leakage of dye. The optic disc is markedly hyperfluorescent. *D*, At approximately 7 minutes after injection there is marked staining of the midperipheral retinal vessels. (From Brown GC: Am J Ophthalmol 102:442–448, 1986. Copyright Ophthalmic Publishing Company, 1986, with permission.)

obstruction in the anterior chamber angle is still present. Thus, the intraocular pressure rises drastically. Ciliary body destructive procedures or glaucoma-filtering surgery may be required in these cases.

Several large randomized studies have recently been published concerning the indications for carotid endartertomy in general.[57–59] The group that has been proven to benefit from carotid endarterectomy includes patients with a 70 to 99% carotid stenosis who have had ischemic symptoms (nondisabling stroke, hemispheric transient ischemic attack, retinal transient ischemic attack). Among those studied by the North American Symptomatic Carotid Endarterectomy Trial Collaborators,[58] 9% of patients who underwent endarterectomy experienced a major stroke within 2 years after surgery; in the control group treated with antiplatelet therapy, the corresponding stroke rate was 26% within 2 years after randomization. The perioperative morbidity and mortality (within 30 days after surgery or randomization to medical therapy) was 2.1% for major stroke and death in the surgical group and 0.9% for major stroke and death in the control group. It should be noted that only surgeons who demonstrated expertise in the proce-

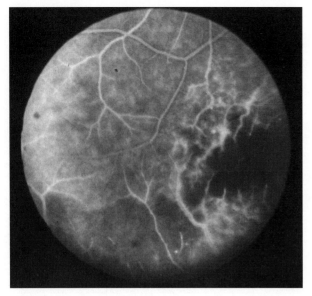

FIGURE 28–8   Fluorescein angiogram demonstrating inferior retinal capillary nonperfusion in an eye with the ocular ischemic syndrome.

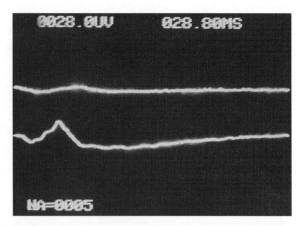

FIGURE 28–9   Electroretinographic findings in a normal left eye (*lower tracing*) and right eye with the ocular ischemic syndrome (*upper tracing*). The amplitudes of the a- and b-waves are reduced in the ocular ischemic syndrome eye.

dure were included in the study. The European Carotid Surgery Trial[57] demonstrated similar results for 70 to 99% stenosis, but also found that in the 0.29% stenosis group the early risks of surgery (2.3% died or had a disabling stroke within 30 days of surgery) outweighed the 3-year benefit when compared to medical therapy. Among 252 consecutive patients undergoing endarterectomy studied prospectively at the Mayo Clinic, the perioperative mortality was 0.7%.[60] The cumulative probability of ipsilateral stroke, transient ischemic attack, or reversible neurologic deficit in this latter series was

4% at 1 month and 8% at 5 years. Asymptomatic restenosis occurred in about 10% of cases.

Full-scatter panretinal laser photocoagulation has been advocated for ocular ischemic eyes with rubeosis iridis and/or posterior segment neovascularization.[53,61,62] This generally consists of 1500 to 2000 500-μm burns with the argon green laser. Unlike the situation when rubeosis iridis occurs secondary to diabetic retinopathy, in which there is regression in a majority of cases with full-scatter panretinal photocoagulation, approximately 36% of ocular ischemic syndrome eyes will demonstrate regression of the iris neovascularization after full-scatter treatment.[44] If the anterior chamber angle is completely closed by fibrovascular tissue and there is no posterior segment neovascularization, panretinal photocoagulation is probably not indicated

TABLE 28–3   Features that Differentiate the Ocular Ischemic Syndrome (OIS), Central Retinal Vein Obstruction (CRVO), and Diabetic Retinopathy (DR)

	OIS	CRVO	DR
Laterality	80% unilateral	Unilateral	Bilateral
Age	50s to 80s	50s to 80s	Variable
Fundus signs			
Veins	Dilated, beaded	Dilated, tortuous	Dilated, beaded
Optic disc	Normal	Swollen	Normal
Hard exudate	Absent unless DR also	Rare	Common
Retinal hemorrhages	Mild	Mild to severe	Mild to moderate
Microaneurysms	Midperiphery	Variable	Posterior pole
Retinal arterial perfusion pressure	Decreased	Normal	Normal
Fluorescein angiography			
Choroidal filling	Delayed, patchy	Normal	Normal
Arteriovenous transit time	Prolonged	Prolonged	Normal
Retinal vessel staining	Arterial	Venous	Usually absent

unless a glaucoma-filtering procedure is being considered.

REFERENCES

1. Kearns TP, Hollenhorst RW: Venous stasis retinopathy of occlusive disease of the carotid artery. Proc Mayo Clin 38: 304–312, 1963.
2. Hayreh SS: So-called central retinal vein occlusion. Venous-stasis retinopathy. Ophthalmologica 172:14–37, 1976.
3. Knox DL: Ischemic ocular inflammation. Am J Ophthalmol 60:995–1002, 1965.
4. Young LHY, Appen RE: Ischemic oculopathy, a manifestation of carotid artery disease. Arch Neurol 38:358–361, 1981.
5. Brown GC, Magargal LE, Simeone FA, et al: Arterial obstruction and ocular neovascularization. Ophthalmology 89:139–146, 1982.
6. Brown GC, Magargal LE: The ocular ischemic syndrome. Clinical, fluorescein angiographic and carotid angiographic features. Int Ophthalmol 11:239–251, 1988.
7. Michelson PE, Knox DL, Green WR: Ischemic ocular inflammation. A clinicopathologic case report. Arch Ophthalmol 86:274–280, 1971.
8. Kahn M, Green WR, Knox DL, Miller NR: Ocular features of carotid occlusive disease. Retina 6:239–252, 1986.
9. Sturrock GD, Mueller HR: Chronic ocular ischaemia. Br J Ophthalmol 68:716–723, 1984.
10. Kearns TP: Ophthalmology and the carotid artery. Am J Ophthalmol 88:714–722, 1979.
11. Kobayashi S, Hollenhorst RW, Sundt TM Jr: Retinal arterial pressure before and after surgery for carotid artery stenosis. Stroke 2:569–575, 1971.
12. Madsen PH: Venous-stasis insufficiency of the ophthalmic artery. Acta Ophthalmol 40:940–947, 1965.
13. Bullock J, Falter RT, Downing JE, Snyder H: Ischemic ophthalmia secondary to an ophthalmic artery occlusion. Am J Ophthalmol 74:486–493, 1972.
14. Magargal LE, Sanborn GE, Zimmerman A: Venous stasis retinopathy associated with embolic obstruction of the central retinal artery. J Clin Neuroophthalmol 2:113–118, 1982.
15. Duker JS, Belmont JB: Ocular ischemic syndrome secondary to carotid artery dissection. Am J Ophthalmol 106:750–752, 1988.
16. Hamed LM, Guy JR, Moster ML, Bosley T: Giant cell arteritis in the ocular ischemic syndrome. Am J Ophthalmol 113:702–705, 1992.
17. Effeney DJ, Krupski WC, Stoney RJ, Ehrenfeld WK: Fibromuscular dysplasia of the carotid artery. Aust N Z J Surg 53:527–531, 1983.
18. Dhobb M, Ammar F, Bensaid Y, et al: Arterial manifestations in Behçet's disease: four new cases. Ann Vasc Surg 1:249–252, 1986.
19. Sadun AA, Sebag J, Bienfang DC: Complete bilateral internal carotid artery occlusion in a young man. J Clin Neuroophthalmol 3:63–66, 1983.
20. Donnan GA, Sharbrough FW: Carotid occlusive disease. Effect of bright light on visual evoked response. Arch Neurol 39:687–689, 1982.
21. Wiebers DO, Swanson JW, Cascino TL, Whisnant JP: Bilateral loss of vision in bright light. Stroke 20:554–558, 1989.
22. Ramadan NM, Tietjen GE, Levine SR, Welch KM: Scintillating scotomata associated with internal carotid artery dissection: report of three cases. Neurology 41:1084–1087, 1991.
23. Winterkorn JM, Teman AJ: Recurrent attacks of amaurosis fugax treated with calcium channel blocker. Ann Neurol 30:423–425, 1991.
24. Aasen J, Kerty E, Russell D, et al: Amaurosis fugax: clinical, Doppler and angiographic findings. Acta Neurol Scand 77:450–455, 1988.
25. Sivalingam A, Brown GC, Magargal LE: The ocular ischemic syndrome. III. Visual Prognosis and the effect of treatment. Int Ophthalmol 15:15–20, 1991.
26. Schlaegel T: Symptoms and signs of uveitis. In Duane TD (ed): Clinical Ophthalmology, Vol 4. Hagerstown, MD, Harper & Row, 1983, pp 1–7.
27. Green WR, Chan CC, Hutchins GM, Terry JM: Central retinal vein occlusion. A prospective histopathologic study of 29 eyes in 28 cases. Retina 1:27–55, 1981.
28. Campo RV, Reeser FH: Retinal telangiectasia secondary to bilateral carotid artery occlusion. Arch Ophthalmol 101:1211–1213, 1983.
29. Waybright EA, Selhorts JB, Combs J: Anterior ischemic optic neuropathy with internal carotid artery occlusion. Am J Ophthalmol 93:42–47, 1982.
30. Brown GC: Anterior ischemic optic neuropathy occurring in association with carotid artery obstruction. J Clin Neuroophthalmol 6:39–42, 1986.
31. Bolling JP, Buettner H: Acquired retinal arteriovenous communications in occlusive disease of the carotid artery. Ophthalmology 97:1148–1152, 1990.
32. Brown GC: Macular edema in association with severe carotid artery obstruction. Am J Ophthalmol 102:442–448, 1986.
33. Dugan JD, Green WR: Ophthalmic manifestations of carotid occlusive disease. Eye 5:226–238, 1991.
34. Choromokos EA, Raymond LA, Sacks JG: Recognition of carotid stenosis with bilateral simultaneous retinal fluorescein angiography. Ophthalmology 89:1146–1148, 1982.
35. Henkes HE: Electroretinography in circulatory disturbances of the retina. II. The electroretinogram in cases of occlusion of the central retinal artery or one of its branches. Arch Ophthalmol 51:42–53, 1954.
36. Carr RE, Siegel JM: Electrophysiologic aspects of several retinal diseases. Am J Ophthalmol 58:95–107, 1964.
37. Coleman K, Fitzgerald D, Eustace P, Bouchier-Hayes D: Electroretinography, retinal ischaemia and carotid artery disease. Eur J Vasc Surg 4:569–573, 1990.
38. Bosley TM: The role of carotid noninvasive tests in stroke prevention. Semin Neurol 6:194–203, 1986.
39. Castaldo JE, Nicholas GG, Gee W, Reed JF: Duplex ultrasound and ocular pneumoplethysmography concordance in detecting severe cartoid stenosis. Arch Neurol 46:518–522, 1989.
40. Banchini E, Franchi A, Magni R, et al: Carotid occlusive disease. An electrophysiological investigation. J Cardiovasc Surg 28:524–527, 1987.
41. Kearns TP: Differential diagnosis of central retinal vein obstruction. Ophthalmology 90:475–480, 1983.
42. Sivalingham A, Brown GC, Magargal LE, Menduke H: The ocular ischemic syndrome II. Mortality and systemic morbidity. Int Ophthalmol 13:187–191, 1989.
43. Kannel WB, Gordon T (eds): The Framingham Study. Public Health Service Publication No. NIH 77-1247, Section 6, Tables 6–9, Section 29, Tables A-22 and A-23, Section 32, pp 84–85.
44. Duker J, Brown GC, Bosley TM, et al: Asymmetric proliferative diabetic retinopathy and carotid artery disease. Ophthalmology 97:869–874, 1990.
45. Kearns TP, Younge BR, Peipgras PG: Resolution of venous stasis retinopathy after carotid artery bypass surgery. Proc Mayo Clin 55:342–346, 1980.
46. Kiser WD, Gonder J, Magargal LE, et al: Recovery of vision following treatment of the ocular ischemic syndrome. Ann Ophthalmol 15:305–310, 1983.
47. Higgins RA: Neovascular glaucoma associated with ocular hypoperfusion secondary to carotid artery disease. Aust J Ophthalmol 12:155–162, 1984.
48. Katz B, Weinstein PR: Improvement of photostress recovery testing after extracranial-intracranial bypass surgery. Br J Ophthalmol 70:277–280, 1986.
49. Shibuya M, Suzuki Y, Takayasu M, Sugita K: Effects of STA-MCA anastamosis for ischaemic oculopathy due to occlusion of the internal carotid artery. Acta Neurochir 103:71–75, 1990.

50. Edwards MS, Chater NL, Stanley JA: Reversal of chronic ischaemia by extracranial-intracranial arterial by-pass. Neurosurgery 7:480–483, 1980.
51. Kearns TP, Siebert RG: The ocular aspects of carotid artery surgery. Trans Am Ophthalmol Soc 76:247–265, 1978.
52. The EC/IC Bypass Study Group: Failure of extracranial-intracranial arterial bypass to reduce the risk of ischemic stroke. Results of an international randomized trial. N Engl J Med 313:1191–1200, 1985.
53. Johnston ME, Gonder JR, Canny CL: Successful treatment of the ocular ischemic syndrome with panretinal photocoagulation and cerebrovascular surgery. Can J Ophthalmol 23:114–119, 1988.
54. Hauch TL, Busuttil RW, Yoshizumi MO: A report of iris neovascularization. An indication for carotid endarterectomy. Surgery 95:358–362, 1984.
55. Coppeto JR, Wand M, Bear L, Sciarra R: Neovascular glaucoma and carotid artery obstructive disease. Am J Ophthalmol 99:567–570, 1985.
56. Melamed S, Irvine J, Lee DA: Increased intraocular pressure following endarterectomy. Ann Ophthalmol 19:304–306, 1987.
57. European Carotid Surgery Trialists' Collaborative Group: MRC European carotid surgery trial: interim results for symptomatic patients with severe (70–99%) or with mild carotid stenosis. Lancet 337:1235–1243, 1991.
58. North American Symptomatic Carotid Endarterectomy Trial Collaborators: Beneficial effect of carotid endarterectomy in symptomatic patients with high-grade carotid stenosis. N Engl J Med 325:445–453, 1991.
59. Mayberg MR, Wilson SE, Yatsu F, et al., for the Veterans Affairs Cooperative Studies Program 309 Trialist Group: Carotid endarterectomy and prevention of cerebral ischemia in symptomatic carotid stenosis. JAMA 266:3289–3294, 1991.
60. Sundt TM, Whisnant JP, Houser OW, Fode NC: Prospective study of the effectiveness and durability of carotid endarterectomy. Mayo Clin Proc 65:625–635, 1990.
61. Eggleston TF, Bohling CA, Eggleston HC, Hershey FB: Photocoagulation for ocular ischemia associated with carotid artery occlusion. Ann Ophthalmol 12:84–87, 1980.
62. Carter JE: Panretinal photocoagulation for progressive ocular neovascularization secondary to occlusion of the common carotid artery. Ann Ophthalmol 16:572–576, 1984.

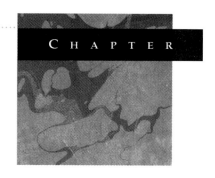

CHAPTER 29

Retinal Arterial Macroaneurysms

M. Madison Slusher, M.D.

Retinal arterial macroaneurysms are acquired fusiform or round arteriolar dilations occurring in the posterior pole within the first three orders of retinal arterial bifurcation (Fig. 29–1). Historically, Loring[1] is attributed with publishing the first report of an isolated retinal arterial macroaneurysm or "peculiar bulging" of the inferotemporal artery, in 1880. And although several isolated reports also appeared in the ophthalmic literature between 1917 and 1920,[2-4] Robertson's description of 13 patients in 1973 authoritatively defined this entity and established the term retinal macroaneurysm.[5] Macroaneurysms have also been described in other retinal affectations such as angiomatosis retinae, Eales' disease, Leber's miliary aneurysms, and Coats' disease. They have also been recognized as secondary vascular alterations in longstanding retinal branch venous occlusion and occasionally, diabetic retinopathy.

Acquired macroaneurysms are most frequently observed in the sixth and seventh decades of life and, beginning with Robertson's observations, published series over the past 20 years have shown that there are often associated vascular problems and diseases in patients with retinal macroaneurysms in terms of hypertension and generalized arteriosclerotic vascular disease (Table 29–1). Elevation of serum lipids and abnormalities in lipoproteins have also been reported.[6] A large collaborative study by Schatz and co-workers,[7] as well as other sizeable series listed in Table 29–1, noted that there is a marked female preponderance in the incidence of retinal arterial macroaneurysms.[6,8-10] Macroaneurysms are infrequently bilateral (10%).[11]

Although retinal arterial macroaneurysms may often be detected on routine funduscopic exam, since the patients may be visually asymptomatic, the most common presenting symptom is that of an acute loss of vision. The mechanisms of visual loss in patients with macroaneurysms are several, but the most frequent presentation is that of a shallow serous macular detachment with leakage of proteinaceous and lipid exudates that deposit in the macula in a typical circinate retinopathy (Figs. 29–1 and 29–2). However, bleeding into the retina or beneath the internal limiting membrane may be the predominant clinical features; vitreous hemorrhage is also observed (Figs. 29–3 through 29–6). Some investigators have attempted to classify these clinical features into two basic groups: group I denotes an acute aneurysmal decompensation in which hemorrhage is the predominant clinical feature, while group II is characterized by perianeurysmal and macular exudation.[12]

Recent morphometric analyses of acquired retinal arterial macroaneurysms tend to support such observations, since they show hemorrhagic macroaneurysms tend to be greater in diameter, located on larger arterioles, and located closer to the optic disc, whereas exudative macroaneurysms are smaller in diameter and, if located within 3 mm of the fovea, leakage tends to exceed the clearing capacity of the venous net and gravitates into the foveal avascular zone leading to severe visual loss[13,14] (Fig. 29–2). Recognized as likely to occur at the bifurcation of retinal arterioles, macroaneurysms have also have been noted to occur with some frequency proximal to retinal emboli which, in such cases, are probably correctly considered causative[8,15-17] (Figs. 29–6).

Histopathologically, these aneurysms demonstrate linear breaks in the vascular wall surrounded by a laminar-fibrin platelet clot associated with varying amounts of hemorrhage, lipid-laden macrophages, hemosiderin, and fibroglial reaction[11,18] (Fig. 29–7). When the hemorrhagic subretinal and

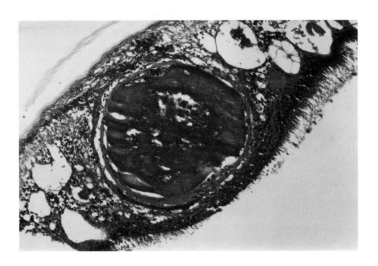

Thrombosed arterial macroaneurysm in an 81-year-old man with hypertension.

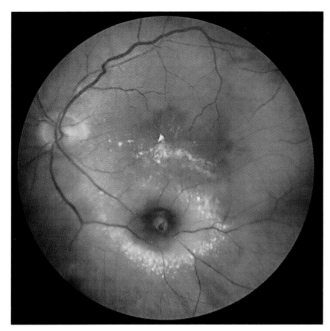

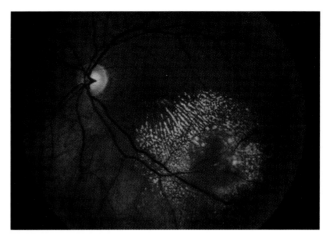

FIGURE 29–2 A red-free fundus photograph accentuates a distinctly sclerotic or hyalinized macroaneurysm that may be seen centered in the circinate configuration of lipid and protein deposits. Note the migratory pattern of the lipid-rich exudative material into the foveal avascular zone along the distribution of retinal nerve fibers.

FIGURE 29–1 A retinal arterial macroaneurysm is located along the inferior temporal retinal artery in a hypertensive 74-year-old female. Visual acuity is reduced to 20/300 secondary to sensory macular detachment and lipoprotein deposits in the foveal avascular zone as part of a circinate figure surrounding the macroaneurysm.

subhyaloid component of this entity is dominant, the clinical presentation of such patients can become confusing and misdiagnosis, specifically age-related macular degeneration, is a distinct possibility and probably a frequent occurrence.[19] And if extravasated blood is sufficiently extensive, hemorrhagic macroaneurysms have been documented as having been confused with malignant melanoma.[20]

The typical arterial macroaneurysm fluoroangiographically completely fills in the early phase of the dye transit but hyperfluorescence may be totally or partially blocked by both exudate and surrounding hemorrhage (Fig. 29–8). If there is an associated se-

rous detachment of the macula, massive lipid deposition in the macula and foveal avascular zone may also block fluorescein. Fluorescein angiography is specifically useful in demonstrating associated changes in the arterial vasculature, such as attenuation in the caliber of the proximal and distal arteriole; a Z-shaped kink at the site of the aneurysm after closure has also been documented by fluorescein studies[12] (Figs. 29–9 and 29–10). Other salient features which are best demonstrated by fluorescein angiography are affectations in the perfusion of the periarterial capillary beds such as microvascular abnormalities, capillary dilatations, microaneurysms, and capillary bed nonperfusion. Leakage is usually from the macroaneurysm itself rather than the microvascular abnormalities in the immediately surrounding capillary beds.[11] In cases of extensive retinal hemorrhage and in which fluorescein may be clinically perceived as unlikely to identify a possible macroaneurysm as the etiology,

TABLE 29–1 Retinal Arterial Macroaneurysms: Demographics*

Author	(Year)	Cases	Mean Age	Sex M	F	Percentage of Patients with Hypertension
Robertson[5]	(1973)	13	65	6	7	33%
Cleary et al[6]	(1974)	20	68	8	12	65%
Lewis et al[8]	(1976)	16	66	6	10	81%
*Schatz et al[7]	(1980)	132	71	33	99	67%
Lavin et al[9]	(1987)	40	66	12	28	47%
Rabb et al[10]	(1988)	60	71	12	48	78%

* Presented at the American Academy of Ophthalmology, November 1980.

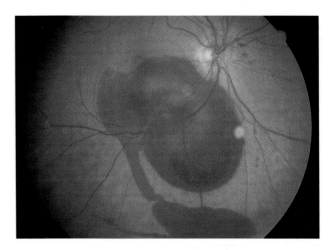

FIGURE 29–3 The retinal arterial macroaneurysm is obscured in this 78-year-old male due to hemorrhage that is more profuse in the deeper retinal layers. A portion of the hemorrhage has broken through into the preretinal space inferiorly and obscures the retinal vessels. Visual acuity is 20/70.

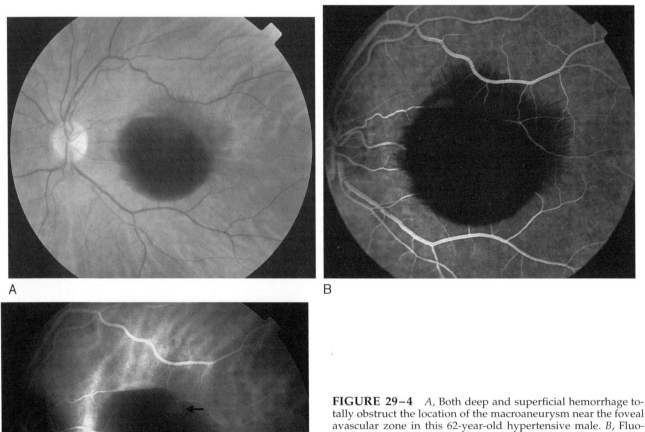

A

B

C

FIGURE 29–4 *A,* Both deep and superficial hemorrhage totally obstruct the location of the macroaneurysm near the foveal avascular zone in this 62-year-old hypertensive male. *B,* Fluorescein angiography fails to demonstrate the location of the associated macroaneurysm due to extensive preretinal hemorrhage blocking details of the dye transit. *C,* Indocyanine green (ICG) dye transit clearly demonstrates hyperfluorescense from the macroaneurysm, clarifying the etiology of the hemorrhage as well as the anatomic location of the arterial macroaneurysm.

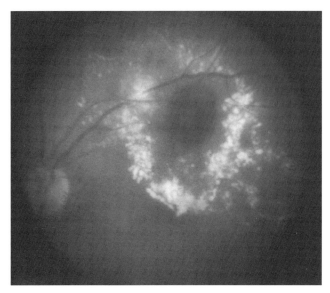

FIGURE 29-5   Both hemorrhagic and exudative features of retinal arterial macroaneurysms are present in the left eye of this 71-year-old male. Vision is reduced to 20/400; this dramatic presentation has been termed a "blow-out" by some authors.

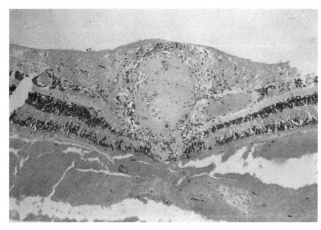

FIGURE 29-7   Rupture of a large arterial macroaneurysm into the subretinal space, creating an extensive hemorrhagic macular detachment. Whorls of fibrinous exudate surround the macroaneurysm and cause swelling of the surrounding retina. (Hematoxylin-eosin stain.) (Courtesy of Dr. W. Richard Green.)

recent reports suggest that indocyanine green (ICG) may be successful in locating the characteristic hyperfluorescence through the associated hemorrhage[21] (Fig. 29-4).

Since macroaneurysms can lead to significant loss of vision, multiple investigators have attempted to determine the natural history of this disease and particularly how it may relate to treatment modalities and rationale.[12,22] Robertson and succeeding investigators have emphasized that the majority of macroaneurysms resolve spontaneously, allowing retention of good visual function.[5,6,11,23] However, a substantial number of pa-

tients may experience reduced central vision due to retinal damage from macular involvement secondary to hemorrhage or lipoprotein exudation prior to spontaneous resolution. This recognition has stimulated attempts to classify macroaneurysms according to location,[15] as well as predominant clinical features (i.e., hemorrhage vs. macular edema and exudation), in an effort to identify individuals who might benefit from photocoagulation treatment.[10,12] The treatment techniques that have been advocated have been both direct photocoagulation to the macroaneurysm and indirectly to the perianeurysmal capillary beds and have traditionally included xenon arc and argon laser photocoagulation.[8,9,12,23] More recently, theoretical advantages of the improved absorption of krypton yellow wave-

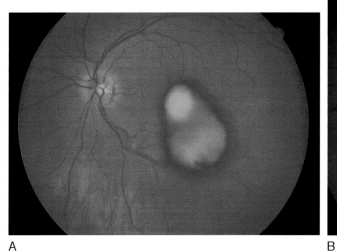

A

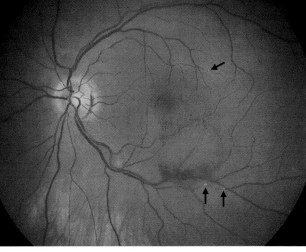

B

FIGURE 29-6   A, A chronic subhyaloid and superficial retinal hemorrhage in the macula associated with a macroaneurysm reduced this 72-year-old male's vision to 20/300 for more than 4 months. B, The precise location of the arterial macroaneurysm is still somewhat obscured by hemorrhagic residues, but multiple emboli are visible in the arterioles (arrows). The hemorrhage has cleared spontaneously; vision is 20/20.

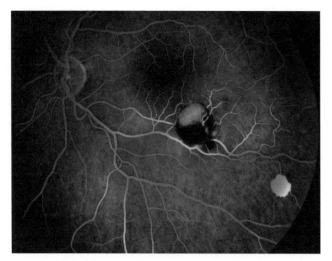

FIGURE 29–8   Active fluorescein leakage is evident at the site of the macroaneurysm, which is partially obscured by hemorrhage. Figure 29–11A is a fundus photograph of this same eye: note that the hemorrhage is essentially subhyaloid and that while the exudative reaction extends into the fovea, hyperfluorescence is blocked and is absent on the dye transit photograph. A second, distal hyalinized macroaneurysm fills but does not display leakage.

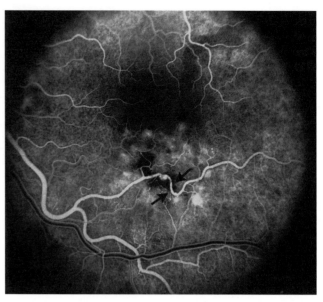

FIGURE 29–10   Arrows denote a Z-shape configuration in the arteriole associated with a small macroaneurysm. The macroaneurysm has been "closed" with direct laser photocoagulation; gentle laser treatment has also been applied to the perianeurysmal capillary beds in an effort to reduce associated exudation. Visual acuity is 20/60.

length by hemoglobin and oxyhemoglobin have led to advocacy of direct treatment with this modality[24–26] (Fig. 29–11). Despite the seeming logic of photocoagulation treatment, however, in terms of preventing hemorrhage and exudation into the macula, or shortening of the duration of such events, significant confusion and controversy remain regarding the advocacy of such therapy as

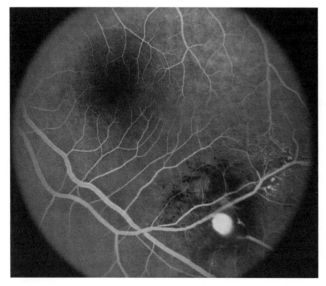

FIGURE 29–9   Complete filling of an unobscured retinal arterial macroaneurysm in arteriovenous phase shows a typical location at the arterial bifurcation and also demonstrates characteristic changes in the periarterial capillary beds consisting of microaneurysms, perfusion defects, and capillary dilatations.

favorably and predictably affecting the ultimate visual outcome.[27] Moreover, direct treatment to retinal arterial macroaneurysms has the potential of leading to additional hemorrhage by rupturing the aneurysm itself, and secondary occlusion of the distal arteriole has also been reported.[26] This latter complication is extremely important to consider when treating a macroaneurysm associated with an arteriole that supplies the foveal avascular zone.

Other therapeutic considerations should be listed for those rare macroaneurysms associated with extensively dense, premacular, submacular, and vitreous hemorrhage. As a rare but recognized cause of spontaneous vitreous hemorrhage, retinal arterial macroaneurysms may be associated with chronic, nonclearing hemorrhage of initially unrecognized etiology; posterior vitrectomy may be necessitated to establish the diagnosis as well as improve vision.[28] Similarly, in instances of persisting dense premacular hemorrhage of uncertain etiology, neodymium:yttrium-aluminum-garnet (Nd: YAG) laser treatment has been proposed as a method of shortening the duration of such hemorrhage and preventing tractional macular detachment by perforating the internal limiting membrane or an associated fibrotic epiretinal membrane and releasing the trapped blood into the vitreous, thus allowing rapid clearing of the hemorrhage.[29] Submacular surgery and removal of thick submacular hemorrhage probably has a legitimate role in improving an otherwise dismal visual prognosis in rare cases of such hemorrhage in patients with retinal arterial macroaneurysms.[30]

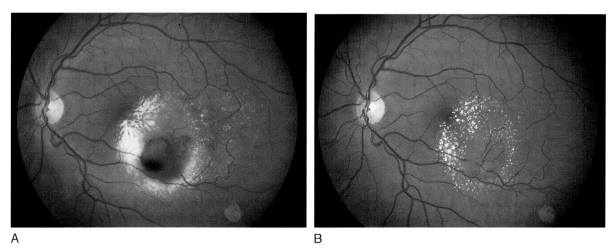

A   B

FIGURE 29–11 *A*, Visual acuity is 20/200 in the left eye of a 59-year-old hypertensive male secondary to lipoprotein exudate gravitating into the foveal avascular zone from the associated macroaneurysm. *B*, The macroaneurysm has been closed by treatment with direct laser photocoagulation, obviously reducing the exudative deposits. Vision eventually improved to 20/40.

REFERENCES

1. Loring FB: Peculiar anatomical development of one of the central arteries of the retina. Trans Am Ophthalmol Soc 16:40–42, 1880.
2. Pringle JA: A case of multiple aneurysms of the retinal arteries. Br J Ophthalmol 1:87–89, 1917.
3. Fernadez FM: Multiple aneurysm of retinal arteries. Am J Ophthalmol 3:641–643, 1920.
4. Jennings JE: Aneurysms of the retinal arteries. Am J Ophthalmol 1:12–13, 1918.
5. Robertson DM: Macroaneurysms of the retinal arteries. Trans Am Acad Ophthalmol Otolaryngol 77: 55–67, 1973.
6. Cleary PE, Kohner EM, Hamilton AM, and Bird AC: Retinal macroaneurysms. Br J Ophthalmol 59:355–361, 1975.
7. Schatz H, Gitter K, Yannuzzi L, Irvine A: Retinal arterial macroaneurysms: a large collaborative study. Presented at the American Academy of Ophthalmology Annual Meeting, Chicago, November, 1980.
8. Lewis RA, Norton EWD, Gass JDM: Acquired arterial macroaneurysms of the retina. Br J Ophthalmol 60:21–30, 1976.
9. Lavin MJ, Marsh RJ, Pert S, Raehman A: Retinal arterial macroaneurysms: a retrorespective review of 40 patients. Br J Ophthalmol 71:817–825, 1987.
10. Rabb MF, Gagliano DA, Teske MP: Retinal arterial macroaneurysms. Surv Ophthalmol 33:73–96, 1988.
11. Gass JDM: Stereoscopic Atlas of Macular Diseases: Diagnosis and Treatment. 3rd edition, Vol 1. St Louis, CV Mosby Co, pp 362–367.
12. Abdel-Khalek MN, Richardson J: Retinal macroaneurysm: natural history and guidelines for treatment. Br J Ophthalmol 70:2–11, 1986.
13. Tezel TH, Gunalp I, Tezel G: Morphometrical analysis of retinal arterial macroaneurysms. Doc Ophthalmol 88:113–125, 1994.
14. Tezel TH, Gunalp I, Tezel G: Morphometric analysis of exudative retinal arterial macroaneurysms: a geometrical approach to exudate curves. Ophthalmic Res 26:332–339, 1994.
15. Palestine AG, Robertson DM, Goldstein MG: Macroaneurysms of the retinal arteries. Am J Ophthalmol 93:164–171, 1982.
16. Kahil M, Lorenzetti DWC: Acquired retinal macroaneurysms. Can J Ophthalmol 14:163–168, 1979.
17. Wiznia RA: Development of a retinal artery macroaneurysm at the site of a previously detected retinal artery embolus. Am J Ophthalmol 14:642–643, 1992.
18. Fichte C, Streeten BW, Friedman AL: A histopathologic study of retinal arterial macroaneurysms. Am J Ophthalmol 85:509–518, 1978.
19. Irvine AR: The diagnoses most commonly missed by ophthalmologists referring patients for fluorescein angiography. Ophthalmology 93:1216–1221, 1986.
20. Perry HD, Zimmerman LE, Benson WE: Hemorrhage from isolated aneurysm of a retinal artery: a report of two cases simulating malignant melanoma. Arch Ophthalmol 95: 281–283, 1977.
21. Parodi MB, Ravalico G: Detection of retinal arterial macroaneurysms with indocyanine-green video-angiography. Graefes Arch Clin Exp Ophthalmol 233:119–121, 1995.
22. Panton RW, Goldberg MF, Farber MD: Retinal arterial macroaneurysms: risk factors and natural history. Br J Ophthalmol 74:595–600, 1990.
23. Nadel AJ, Gupta KK: Macroaneurysms of the retinal arteries. Arch Ophthalmol 94:1092–1096, 1976.
24. Joondeph BC, Joondeph HC, Blair MP: Retinal macroaneurysms treated with the yellow-dye laser. Retina 9:187–192, 1989.
25. Mainster MA, Whitacre MM: Dye-yellow photocoagulation of retinal arterial macroaneurysms. Am J Ophthalmol 105:97–98, 1988.
26. Russell SR, Folk JC: Branch artery occlusion after dye-yellow photocoagulation of an arterial macroaneurysm. Am J Ophthalmol 104:186–187, 1987.
27. Brown DM, Sobol WM, Folk JC, Weingeist TA: Retinal arteriolar macroaneurysms: long-term visual outcome. Br J Ophthalmol 78:534–538, 1994.
28. Lindgren G, Sjodell L, Lindblom B: A prospective study of dense spontaneous vitreous hemorrhage. Am J Ophthalmol 119:458–465, 1995.
29. Raymond LA: Neodymium:YAG laser treatment for hemorrhages under the internal limiting membrane and posterior hyaloid of the macula. Ophthalmology 102:406–411, 1995.
30. Ibanez HE, Williams DF, Thomas MA, et al: Surgical management of submacular hemorrhage. A series of 47 consecutive cases. Arch Ophthalmol 113:62–69, 1995.

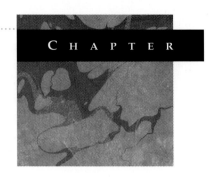

Coats' Disease

Naresh Mandava, M.D.
Lawrence A. Yannuzzi, M.D.

HISTORY

Coats' disease is an idiopathic condition that was first characterized by George Coats in 1908.[1] Coats described this entity as abnormal telangiectatic or aneurysmal retinal vessels associated with intraretinal and subretinal exudates. He classified the disease into three groups. Group I had massive subretinal exudates, no vascular abnormalities, and a choroidal mononuclear infiltrate. Group II eyes also had massive subretinal exudates, but in addition, retinal vascular abnormalities with intraretinal hemorrhages and no choroidal mononuclear infiltrate. Group III also had massive exudates with arteriovenous malformations. Von Hippel later characterized this group III as a distinct entity, angiomatosis retinae, which led Coats to remove it from his classification.[2] Later, Leber described a disease, Leber's multiple miliary aneurysms, that had the same vascular abnormalities as Coats' disease but lacked the massive subretinal exudates.[3] The idea that this was a nonprogressive or early form of Coats' disease was confirmed when Reese documented a case of presumptive multiple miliary aneurysms that eventually developed massive subretinal exudation typical of Coats'.[4] He was also the first to use the term "retinal telangiectasis," which many authors feel better describes the disease and its wide spectrum of presentation and severity.

DEMOGRAPHICS

Coats' is predominantly a disease of childhood, although it less commonly can affect adults. The majority of cases are diagnosed by age 20, with a peak incidence at the end of the first decade.[5,6] The earliest reported case is at 4 months of age.[7] Males are affected up to four times as frequently as females.[5] There is no racial or ethnic predisposition. Over 80% of cases are unilateral. Bilateral cases have been reported.[5,6,8–10]

ETIOLOGY

Historically, infectious and inflammatory processes were implicated in Coats' disease. Coats thought exudates were caused by resorption of hemorrhages while others thought the mononuclear infiltrate was associated with an infectious process.[2] A vascular etiology has also been described. The presence of PAS positive material and thickening of endothelial basement membrane supports this.[11] Preparation of vascular specimens after trypsin digestion reveals dilated capillaries and microaneurysmal formation. Also, histopathologic specimens reveal a dilated, thin walled microvasculature. Importantly, these histopathologic and morphologic changes may only be a common endpoint to another etiology. For example, an endocrine disturbance for Coats' disease has been suggested based upon the similarity in basement membrane disease to diabetes and pregnancy related vascular diseases. Other systemic abnormalities have been investigated. A defect in cholesterol transport has been proposed.[12] The known association between hypercholesterolemia and the adult form of Coats' may be further evidence of a serum lipid abnormality.[13]

CLINICAL PRESENTATION

Congenital retinal telangiectasis is a disease of the retinal vasculature that principally affects one eye

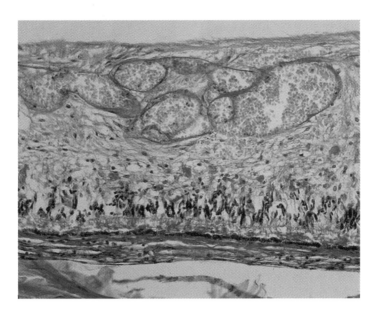

Telangiectatic vessels of Coats' disease. (From Green WR: Bilateral Coats' disease. Arch Ophthalmol 77:378–385, 1967, Copyright 1967, American Medical Association, with permission.)

of male patients.[1,2,5,6,8,14–17] From the files of the Manhattan Eye, Ear, and Throat Hospital and the private practice of Lawrence A. Yannuzzi, M.D., we have not seen one convincing case of bilateral Coats' disease appearing in the classic congenital form. Traditionally, Coats' disease describes the aggressive form of a spectrum of disease involving a yellowish, green subretinal exudation and retinal detachment.[18] Children and infants can present with leukokoria secondary to subretinal lipid deposition in the posterior pole or exudative retinal detachment. Strabismus often ensues secondary to poor visual acuity. Because of the common presentation of leukokoria and strabismus in other childhood diseases, other diagnoses must be entertained (Table 30–1).[18–20]

Detailed ophthalmoscopy is crucial in making the diagnosis. Primarily, retinal capillaries are involved with telangiectasis, increased tortuosity, and exudation from incompetence of small-caliber vessels; however, larger vessels including large arteries and veins can be affected with sheathing, aneurysmal dilations, anomalous channels, and exudation (Fig. 30–1). Preretinal neovascularization in the periphery or at the disc is rare despite the presence of capillary nonperfusion and adjacent relatively normal blood vessels. It is speculated that these eyes may lack the chemical stimulus for neovascularization typical of other disease processes. Vitreous hemorrhage and frank neovascularization can be seen when larger zones of capillary nonperfusion are present or in the setting of a concomitant retinal detachment. An understanding of the spectrum of disease severity and the remitting and exacerbating nature of the disease is crucial. Although rare, complete remissions have been reported.[21,22] The rare patient with bilateral disease typically presents with only mild involvement of the second eye, often, to a clinically insignificant level.[8]

Adult-onset disease is typically less severe, with telangiectasis and intraretinal exudation often simulating other diseases (Fig. 30–2). Visual loss is secondary to leakage of perifoveal telangiectasias

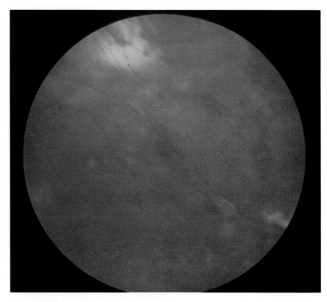

FIGURE 30–1   Retinal vascular aneurysmal and telangiectatic changes associated with lipid exudation and hemorrhage.

causing cystoid macular edema and often a circinate pattern of lipid deposition around the macula. The ophthalmoscopic and angiographic picture in the adult form of disease is often difficult to differentiate from other perifoveal microvascular abnormalities (Table 30–2). Exudative retinal detachments are rare in adult-onset Coats'.

The aggressive form of the disease is seen in children and infants. Severe retinal vascular leakage eventually causes subretinal deposition of protein and lipid-rich exudate (Fig. 30–3). In turn, massive subretinal exudation creates gravitation of yellow-

TABLE 30–1   Differential Diagnosis of Childhood Disease (Leukokoria or Exudative Retinal Detachment)

Retinoblastoma
Persistent hyperplastic primary vitreous
Retinopathy of prematurity
Familial exudative vitreoretinopathy
Norrie's disease
Toxocariasis
Von Hippel-Lindau (angiomatosis retinae)
Acquired peripheral capillary angioma
Incontinentia pigmenti
Pars planitis
Retinitis pigmentosa with Coats'-like response

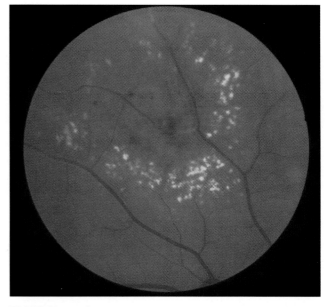

FIGURE 30–2   A localized area of microaneurysmal and telangiectatic change at the center of a circinate area of lipid. This is a mild presentation of a disease most commonly seen in adults.

TABLE 30-2 Parafoveal Telangiectasis with or without Lipid Exudation

Diabetic vasculopathy
Branch retinal vein occlusion
Idiopathic perifoveal telangiectasis
Epiretinal membrane with secondary vascular
 leakage
Sickle cell retinopathy
Radiation retinopathy
Acquired inflammatory diseases

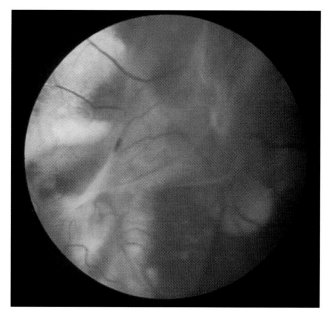

FIGURE 30-4 Massive lipid exudation into the macula (a Coats' response in the macula). There is also an area of secondary choroidal neovascularization in the inferotemporal macula with disciform scar formation. Note the preretinal membrane formation extending into the macula.

ish material inferiorly, causing the bullous retinal detachment characteristic of Coats' disease. In time, nonresolving subretinal lipid deposition can lead to fibrovascular tissue formation and even choroidal neovascularization (Fig. 30-4). Often, a disciform scar is the end result. Disciform scars are most common in the macular region, as even peripheral exudative lesions tend to track lipid towards the macula. In fact, disciform scars are most common in children and infants with broader zones of peripheral involvement.[14]

Complications from longstanding retinal detachments are numerous. Rarely, organization of subretinal fluid in longstanding detachments can lead to a clinical picture simulating other diseases. Coalescence of intraretinal cystic spaces in unresolved detachments have reportedly led to hemorrhagic retinal macrocysts.[23] There is also a report of an orbital cellulitis developing from the transscleral leakage of subretinal toxins in a child with advanced Coats' disease.[24] Most importantly longstanding retinal detachments in general can lead to cataract formation, iridocyclitis, and even neovascular glaucoma, often leading to phthisis bulbi.

Although no conclusive evidence of a genetic transmission of Coats' disease has been proven, multiple associations with systemic and ocular diseases have been reported. Alport's disease,[25] tuberous sclerosis,[26] Turner's syndrome,[27] Senior-Loken syndrome,[28] and the ichthyosis hystrix variant of epidermal nevus syndrome[29] have all anecdotally been reported to be associated with a Coats'-like response. Multiple reports of an association with muscular dystrophy, and more recently with fascioscapulohumeral dystrophy exist.[30-33] In 1956, Zamorani was the first to report an association of retinitis pigmentosa to Coats' disease.[34] Morgan and others have since described multiple cases of a Coats'-like response in retinitis pigmentosa patients.[35] Khan et al report 46 cases of retinitis pigmentosa associated with a Coats'-like response in the literature.[36] It remains the most common disease entity to present with a Coats'-like response. The adult form of Coats' disease has been associated with hypercholesterolemia as discussed earlier.

FLUORESCEIN ANGIOGRAPHY

Fluorescein angiography demonstrates the vascular origin of Coats' disease. Both children and adults present with the same angiographic findings. Large-vessel involvement is seen as saccular aneurysmal dilations, anomalous vascular communications, and telangiectasias. Occasionally, beading of vessel walls is seen.[14] Capillary involvement is demonstrated by telangiectasias as well as capillary nonperfusion. Large areas of capillary nonperfusion are typically associated with neighboring abnormal large vessels with aneurysmal dilations[14]

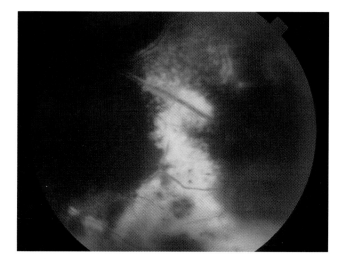

FIGURE 30-3 Intraretinal and subretinal lipid exudation in Coats'. Note the aneurysmal dilation of small vessels inferiorly. The predominance of lipid over hemorrhage is a hallmark of Coats'.

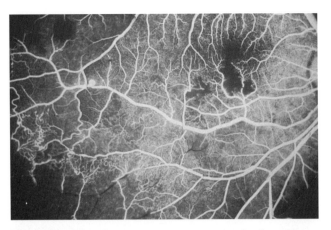

FIGURE 30–5   Fluorescein angiogram. Peak phase shows scattered microvascular abnormalities mostly in the mid-periphery but also some abnormalities in the macula. Note the microaneurysms, telangiectasis, and collateral formation. Characteristically, there is a large zone of peripheral nonperfusion with no evidence of retinal neovascularization.

(Fig. 30–5). These areas of vascular pathology have a tendency to occur in the temporal and superotemporal portions of the retina.[8] Fluorescein dye does leak into the subretinal space but only stains minimally. Large zones of exudative retinal detachment distal to the telangiectasias do not stain. However, fluorescein dye does fill intraretinal cystic spaces, often showing a pattern characteristic of cystoid macular edema.[14] Interestingly, many cases with exudation originally reported as not having a frankly visible vascular origin have since been shown to have associated vascular anomalies by fluorescein angiography. There may be some benefit to fluorescein angiography in differentiating Coats' disease from retinoblastoma.[14] Endophytic retinoblastomas may have a feeder vessel leading to the subretinal mass. The treatment of Coats' disease has been enhanced by fluorescein angiography. Unsuspected areas of vascular leakage can readily be identified, and photocoagulation or cryotherapy applied.[8]

DIFFERENTIAL DIAGNOSIS AND DIAGNOSTIC TESTING

The differential diagnosis in the childhood form of Coats' presenting with leukokoria or exudative retinal detachment is quite extensive (Table 30–1).[18] Most importantly, retinoblastoma must be ruled out, as it is life threatening. In Howard and Ellsworth's report, 3.9% of 254 children initially thought to have retinoblastoma were found to have Coats' disease.[37] A thorough history and clinical exam are most important for an accurate diagnosis. As discussed elsewhere, Coats' disease is primarily a disease of males and has no genetic predisposition, unlike retinoblastoma and angiomatosis retinae (von Hippel's lesion).[18] Typically, Coats' disease presents with more lipid exudation than retinoblas-

toma. Angiomatosis retinae and the acquired capillary peripheral angioma can present with significant lipid exudation. Angiomatosis retinae also has a high rate of bilaterality and often has a dilated feeder and draining vessels, unlike the Coats' lesion.[18] The acquired capillary peripheral angioma is, perhaps, the most troublesome to differentiate between Coats' disease, as it also does not have a dilated feeder vessel and can present with heavy lipid exudation, serous detachment, epiretinal membrane disease, and telangiectatic vascular change.

Ancillary tests may be pivotal in the differentiation of Coats' from retinoblastoma. Radiologic testing is a useful adjunct to the clinical exam in the diagnosis of Coats' disease. Haik reports ultrasound and computed tomography (CT) imaging are crucial in the detection of subretinal calcification, which is typical of retinoblastoma.[38] The radiologic diagnosis is more difficult in poorly calcified retinoblastoma.[38–40] Also, thin sections with contrast CT imaging can detect vascularization of the subretinal space sometimes found in retinoblastoma lesions. Fluorescein angiography may also be useful in evaluating the vasculature of an endophytic mass.[14] Retinoblastomas can present with a feeder vascular stalk seen by angiography. Aqueous lactate dehydrogenase (LDH) and isoenzyme levels have not assisted in the diagnosis. However, the presence of cholesterol-laden macrophages in the subretinal fluid is unique to Coats' disease but is of little help in the clinical noninvasive setting.[38]

Localized telangiectasis and leakage is seen in the adult form of Coats' disease. Gass classified these patients into group 1A: unilateral congenital parafoveolar telangiectasis.[14] The differential diagnosis includes all parafoveal retinal microvascular abnormalities that can present with or without leakage (Table 30–2). Certainly, diabetic vasculopathy and venous occlusive disease present more commonly in this manner than Coats'. Idiopathic perifoveal telangiectasis (group II by Gass' classification) can have minimal intraretinal serous exudation but does not have lipid exudation by definition.[41] It is typically a bilateral disease and has no sex predilection. Other important manifestations of idiopathic perifoveal telangiectasis are an absence of nonperfusion and microaneurysms, and the presence of vascular anastomoses from the retina to the choroidal circulation and crystalline deposits in the inner retina. The presence of foveal atrophy

TABLE 30–3   Localized Telangiectasis with Arterial or Venous Aneurysms

Cavernous hemangioma of retina
Idiopathic retinal vasculitis aneurysm and neuroretinitis (IRVAN)
Acquired arterial macroaneurysm

greater than edema is unique to idiopathic peri-foveal telangiectasis. Capillary nonperfusion and parafoveal microvascular disease seen in the adult form of Coats' are also seen in radiation retinopathy and sickle cell retinopathy. Cavernous hemangiomas appear as grape-like clusters that have no vascular leakage by fluorescein angiography. Acquired arterial macroaneurysms have a zone of leakage surrounding the lesion by angiography. Idiopathic retinal vasculitis aneurysms and neuroretinitis (IRVAN) presents with a constellation of findings not typical of Coats' (Table 30–3).

HISTOPATHOLOGY

Because of improvements in diagnostic testing, enucleations of eyes afflicted with Coats' are far fewer. Most histopathologic reports of Coats' disease are from earlier studies. By light microscopy, all reports describe abnormal telangiectatic vessels that leak plasma and exudate into retinal tissues as well as subretinally[11,42–44] (Fig. 30–6). Lipid-engorged macrophages are found in the subretinal space. Green reports that it is uncertain whether these macrophages originate from retinal vessels and migrate subretinally or travel from the choroidal circulation to phagocytize lipid in the subretinal space.[43]

Electron microscopy confirms abnormalities at the level of the retinal vascular endothelium in Coats' eyes.[45] In addition, Egbert demonstrated retinal vascular aneurysms and deposition of periodic acid–Schiff (PAS)–positive material in retinal vascular walls after trypsin digestion in 10 eyes[11] (Fig. 30–7). Trypsin digestion in 62 eyes at the AFIP demonstrated diffuse involvement of capillaries even in peripheral retina.[42]

Chronic lipid deposition leads to the growth of fibrovascular tissue and eventually a disciform scar clinically. Histopathologically, retinal pigment epi-

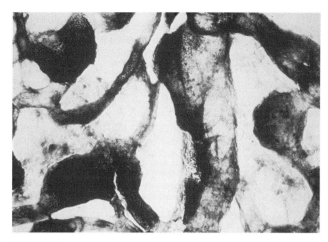

FIGURE 30–7 Trypsin digest preparation of the retina demonstrates dilated capillaries and microaneurysm formation. The variety of microvascular abnormalities seen in Coats' are demonstrated well with trypsin digestion.

thelial hyperplasia is often seen overlying this organized subretinal fibrovascular tissue.[43] Fibrous metaplasia of the retinal pigment epithelium (RPE) has been reported with the occasional presence of calcium and even bone in these organized fibrous nodules.[42,46]

MANAGEMENT

Multiple treatment strategies have been proposed for the management of Coats' disease. Early treatments for the disease with adrenocorticotropic hormone (ACTH), steroids, and antibiotics were unsuccessful. Although some authors reported an occasional benefit to transscleral diathermy and x-ray irradiation, it was not until Meyer-Schwickerath applied his new laser techniques to Coats' disease that significant cure rates were established.[47]

In the 1970s, treatments of vascular lesions in Coats' disease by xenon arc, argon laser photocoagulation, or cryotherapy were minimally successful. The major prognostic factor despite the most aggressive treatment was the area of involvement of disease.[8,15,48] Egerer and Tasman reported success in visual improvement only in eyes with two or less quadrants of pathology.[8] Harris' previous report echoed this finding.[15] Harris also concluded that lipid deposition in the macula was irreversible. Later, Spitznas reported several cases of Coats' with resolution of lipid deposition in the macula after treatment.[49] However, he surmised that early treatment was preferred, as more severe lipid deposition did not resolve and often led to permanent visual loss. Most investigators deduced that early treatment of vascular lesions before lipid accumulation in the macula was beneficial.[8,15,48,49]

In 1982, in a retrospective review of 41 patients,

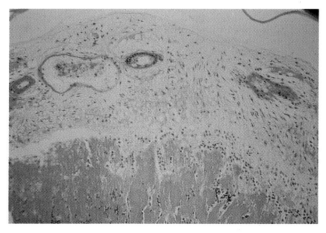

FIGURE 30–6 Histopathology demonstrates abnormal dilated, thin-walled microvasculature.

Ridley et al reported more severe disease in Coats' patients less than 4 years of age.[16] Their report suggested that aggressive treatment with photocoagulation, cryotherapy, and repair of retinal detachments was beneficial. In fact, in children over 4 years of age, only 25% of those untreated maintained at least their previous visual acuity, while over 70% of those children who underwent aggressive treatment maintained their previous acuity. The visual outcomes were worse for children less than 4 years of age; however, aggressive treatment still carried a better prognosis. A combination of successful retinal detachment repair with adequate external or internal drainage of subretinal fluid is necessary to achieve successful application of laser photocoagulation or cryotherapy to leaking vessels.[8,16,49] Machemer and Williams reported two patients with traction retinal detachments secondary to Coats' disease who developed spontaneous retinal reattachment and resolution of exudates after vitrectomy surgery using modern vitreoretinal surgical techniques. Adequate treatment of leaking vessels prevented further exudation and membrane formation.[50]

Complications of laser photocoagulation of these angiomatous lesions include vitreous hemorrhage secondary to destruction of vascular walls and macular pucker secondary to vitreous contraction.[8,15,16] Rarely, progressive fibrosis and traction retinal detachments can develop.[27] As such, laser energy should be used sparingly to avoid these complications. We use laser photocoagulation whenever possible, as it minimizes epiretinal membrane formation when compared to cryotherapy. Treatment of the aneurysms directly or scatter treatment in the distribution of the telangiectasias works.

Our preference is to treat the aneurysms in the course of scatter treatment. Multiple sessions of laser photocoagulation are often necessary to treat residual leaking vessels, which may become visible when exudates clear. In addition, recurrences have been reported up to 5 years after complete resolution of the Coats' process.[8] This necessitates close observation of all Coats' patients even after stabilization of the disease process.

REFERENCES

1. Coats G: Forms of retinal disease with massive subretinal exudation. R Lond Ophthalmic Hosp Rep 17:440–525, 1908.
2. Coats G: Ueber retinitis exudativa (retinitis hemorrhagiga externa). Graefes Arch Ophthalmol 81:275–327, 1912.
3. Leber TH: Verber ein durch Yorkommen miltipler Miliaraneurisimen characterisierte Form von Retinal-degeneration. Graefes Arch Clin Exp Ophthalmol 81:1–14, 1912.
4. Reese AB: Telangiectasis of the retina and Coats' disease. Am J Ophthalmol 42:1–8, 1956.
5. Gomez MA: Coats' disease. Natural history and results of treatment. Am J Ophthalmol 60:855, 1965.
6. Spitznas M, Joussen F, Wessing A, Meyer-Schwickerath G: Coats' disease: an epidemiologic and fluorescein angiographic study. Graefes Arch Clin Exp Ophthalmol 195(4):241–50, 1975.
7. Dow DS: Coats' disease: occurrence in a 4-month old infant. South Med J 66:836–838, 1973.
8. Egerer I, Tasman W, Tomer TL: Coats' disease. Arch Ophthalmol 92:109-112, 1974
9. Green WR: Bilateral Coats' disease. Massive gliosis of the retina. Arch Ophthalmol 77:378, 1967.
10. Mcgettrick PM, Loeffler KU: Bilateral Coats' disease in an infant. Eye 1:136–145, 1987.
11. Egbert PR, Chan CC, Winter FC: Flat preparations of the retinal vessels in Coats' disease. J Pediatr Ophthalmol 13(6):336–339, 1976.
12. Yeung J, Harris GS: Coats' disease: a study of cholesterol transport in the eye. Can J Ophthalmol 11(1):61–68, 1976.
13. Woods AC, Duke J: Coats' disease. Review of the literature, diagnostic criteria, clinical findings, and plasma lipid studies. Br J Ophthalmol 47:385–412, 1963.
14. Gass JDM: Stereoscopic Atlas of Macular Diseases: Diagnosis and Treatment, 3rd edition. St Louis, CV Mosby Co, 1987, pp 384–397.
15. Harris GS: Coats' disease, diagnosis and treatment. Can J Ophthalmol 5:311, 1970.
16. Ridley ME, Shields JA, Brown GL: Coats' disease: evaluation and management. Ophthalmology 89:1381–1387, 1982.
17. Pauleikhoff D, Kruger K, Heinrich T, Wessing A: Epidemiologic features and therapeutic results in Coats' disease. Invest Ophthalmol 29:335, 1988.
18. Tasman WS: Clinical Decisions in Medical Retinal Disease. St Louis, CV Mosby Co, 1994.
19. Shields JA: Diagnosis and Management of Intraocular Tumors. St Louis, CV Mosby Co, 1983.
20. Harley RD: Pediatric Ophthalmology, 2nd edition. Philadelphia, WB Saunders Co, 1983.
21. Campbell FP: Coats' disease and congenital vascular retinopathy. Trans Am Ophthalmol Soc 24:365–372, 1976.
22. Deutsch TA, Rabb MF, Jampol LM: Spontaneous regression of retinal lesions in Coats' disease. Can J Ophthalmol 17:169, 1982.
23. Goel SD, Augsburger JJ: Hemorrhagic retinal macrocysts in advanced Coats' disease. Retina 11:437–440, 1991.
24. Judisch GF, Apple DJ: Orbital cellulitis in an infant secondary to Coats' disease. Arch Ophthalmol 98:2004, 1980.
25. Kondra L, Cangemi FE, Pitta CG: Alport's syndrome and retinal telangiectasia. Ann Ophthalmol 15:550, 1983.
26. Blum M, Alexandridis E, Rating D: Cerebral tuberous sclerosis and Coats' disease (German). Ophthalmologe 91(3):377–379, 1994.
27. Asdourian G: Vascular anomalies of the retina. In Peyman GA, Sanders DR, Goldberg MF (eds): Principles and Practices of Ophthalmology, Vol 2. Philadelphia, WB Saunders Co, 1980, pp 1299–1324.
28. Schuman JS, Lieverman KV, Friedman A, et al: Senior-Loken syndrome (familial retinal dystrophy) and Coats' disease. Am J Ophthalmol 100:822, 1985.
29. Burch JV, Leveille AS, Morse PH: Ichthyosis hystrix (epidermal nevus syndrome) and Coats' disease. Am J Ophthalmol 89:25, 1980.
30. Chijiiwa T, Nishimura M, Inomata H: Ocular manifestations of congenital muscular dystrophy (Fukuyama type). Ann Ophthalmol 15:921, 1983.
31. Gurwin EB, Fitzsimons RB, Sehmi KS, Bird AC: Retinal telangiectasia in fascioscapulohumeral muscular dystrophy with deafness. Arch Ophthalmol 103:1695, 1985.
32. Small RG: Coats' disease and muscular dystrophy. Trans Am Acad Ophthalmol Otolaryngol 72:225, 1968.
33. Taylor DA, Carroll J, Smith ME: Fascioscapulohumeral dystrophy associated with hearing loss and Coats' syndrome. Ann Neurol 12:395–398, 1982.
34. Zamorani G: A rare association of Coats' and retinitis pigmentosa (Italian). G Ital Oftal 9:429–443, 1956.
35. Morgan WE III, Crawford JB: Retinitis pigmentosa and Coats' disease. Arch Ophthalmol 79:146, 1968.

36. Khan JA, Ide CH, Strickland MP: Coats'-type retinitis pigmentosa. Surv Ophthalmol 32:317–332, 1988.

37. Howard GM, Ellseworth RM: Differential diagnosis of retinoblastoma: a statistical survey of 500 children. I. Relative frequency of the lesions which simulate retinoblastoma. Am J Ophthalmol 60:610–617, 1965.

38. Haik BG: Advanced Coats' disease. Trans Am Ophthalmol Soc 89:371–476, 1991.

39. Katz NN, Margo CE, Dorwart RH: Computed tomography with histopathologic correlation in children with leukocoria. J Pediatr Ophthalmol 21(2):50–56, 1984.

40. Jaffe MS, Shields JA, Canny CL: Retinoblastoma simulating Coats' disease: a clinicopathologic report. Ann Ophthalmol 9(7): 863–868, 1977.

41. Gass JDM, Oyakawa RT: Idiopathic juxtafoveolar retinal telangiectasis. Arch Ophthalmol 100:769, 1982.

42. Chang MM, McLean IW, Merritt JC: Coats' disease: a study of 62 histologically confirmed cases. J Pediatr Ophthalmol 21(5):163–168, 1984.

43. Green WR: Congenital variations and abnormalities. In Spencer WH (ed): Ophthalmic Pathology, 3rd edition. Philadelphia, WB Saunders, 1985, pp 624-630.

44. Farkas TG, Potts AM, Boone C: Some pathologic and biochemical aspects of Coats' disease. Am J Ophthalmol 75: 289, 1973.

45. Tripathi R, Ashton N: Electron microscopical study of Coats' disease. Br J Ophthalmol 55:289, 1971.

46. Senft SH, Hidayat AA, Cavender JC: Atypical presentation of Coats' disease. Retina 14(1):36–38, 1994.

47. Meyer-Schwickerath G: Light Coagulation. St Louis, CV Mosby Co, 1960, p 103.

48. McGrand JC: Photocoagulation in Coats' disease. Trans Am Ophthalmol Soc 90:47, 1970.

49. Spitznas M: Coats' disease: an epidemiologic and fluorescein angiographic study. Graefes Arch Clin Exp Ophthalmol 199:31, 1976.

50. Machemer R, Williams JM: Pathogenesis and therapy of traction detachment in various retinal vascular diseases. Am J Ophthalmol 105:170–181, 1988.

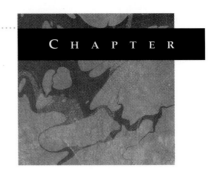

Parafoveal Telangiectasis

Gaetano R. Barile, M.D.
Lawrence A. Yannuzzi, M.D.

Reese originally applied the term telangiectasis to the developmental vascular abnormalities seen in Coats' disease and Leber's military aneurysms.[1] Gass observed that retinal telangiectasis could be confined to the capillaries of the parafoveal region and noted the importance of fluorescein angiography in diagnosing these cases.[2] Bilateral, acquired forms of parafoveal retinal telangiectasis of unclear etiology were later described.[3-6] These cases had a common pattern of focal microaneurysmal or saccular dilatation of some portion of the perifoveal capillary network. Gass and Oyakawa expanded the spectrum of this disorder, terming the condition idiopathic juxtafoveolar retinal telangiectasis and classifying the cases on the basis of clinical findings.[7] Additional experience with this condition led Gass and Blodi to revise previous classifications in 1993.[8]

Telangiectasis of the parafoveal capillary network may occur secondarily in a number of retinal vascular diseases and other systemic diseases,[9-13] but the condition here refers to primary, idiopathic forms of parafoveal telangiectasis. At the most basic level, one may distinguish between two forms of parafoveal telangiectasis: a developmental vascular anomaly that tends to occur unilaterally in male patients (along the spectrum of Coats' disease); and an acquired vascular disease that tends to present bilaterally without any sex predilection. The disorder may then be further subdivided, modifying the scheme of Gass and Blodi.

GROUP 1 (VISIBLE TELANGIECTASIS WITH EXUDATION)

These patients have parafoveal telangiectatic blood vessels that are readily visible on biomicroscopic and fluorescein angiographic examination. These patients are typically male, and they have unilateral disease in the vast majority of cases. A hallmark of their clinical disease is the presence of yellow exudates along the outer margin of the telangiectatic vessels, sometimes taking the shape of a ring in more dramatic cases.[8] Less severe exudation may result in the typical biomicroscopic appearance of cystoid macular edema (CME). There is normally minimal or no capillary occlusion seen during fluorescein angiography in these cases.

Patients with this form of telangiectasis present around 40 years of age with mild visual loss due to CME or lipid exudate. Despite the relatively late onset of symptoms, most authorities consider patients in group 1 to have a mild variant of congenital retinal telangiectasis or Coats' disease. Consistent with this notion is the observation that extramacular telangiectasis is present in numerous cases.[8,14] For unknown reasons, these developmentally abnormal capillaries may be patent for many years before decompensating with exudative manifestations.

Gass and Blodi further categorize group 1 disease on the basis of extent of telangiectasis. Patients in group 1A typically have retinal capillary telangiectasis in the temporal half of the macula involving the superior and inferior portions of the horizontal raphe. Group 1A patients have at least 1 disc diameter (DD) of telangiectasis and usually have more than 2 DDs of disease. Group 1B patients have the telangiectatic process localized 2 clock hours or less of the perifoveal capillary network. The demographics, unilateral predilection, and clinical and angiographic findings in these two sets of group 1 patients are otherwise quite similar.

The natural history of patients with this form of telangiectasis is variable. Some patients are asymptomatic for many years, while others develop fluc-

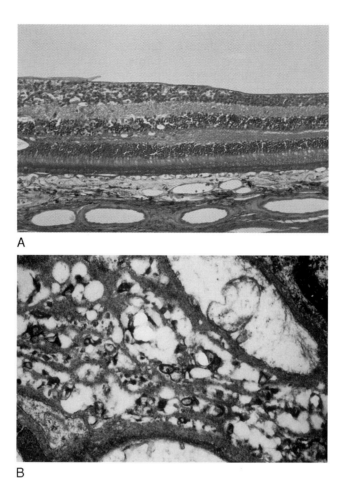

A, Parafoveal telangiectasia. Temporal parafoveal area with edema involving full thickness of the retina. *B*, Parafoveal telangiectasia. The retinal capillaries are not telangiectatic but the walls were thickened, had replication of basement membrane, and had deposits of lipid material like that seen in diabetes. (From Green WR, Quigley HT, de la Cruz Z, Cohen B: Parafoveal retinal telangiectasia: light and electron microscopy studies. Trans Ophthalmol Soc U K 100:162–170, 1980, with permission.)

tuating visual loss in the 20/25- to 20/40-range coincident with variations in exudative findings. A few patients will develop more severe and progressive visual deterioration. Particularly for these patients, the judicious application of laser photocoagulation to the telangiectatic capillaries appears to be beneficial, with most uncontrolled case series reporting stabilized or improved visual function.[2,7,8,14]

The differential diagnosis of this form of parafoveal telangiectasis includes other retinal capillary diseases associated with vascular incompetence and exudation. Diabetic maculopathy with accordant CME or lipid exudation may resemble group 1 telangiectasis, but more extensive retinal disease with microaneurysms, hemorrhages, and cotton-wool spots is usually evident. Similar findings may occur with radiation retinopathy, but a history of ocular or head irradiation should facilitate this diagnosis. Any cause of vitreous cellular infiltration, including Irvine-Gass syndrome, tapetoretinal dystrophies, and pars planitis, may result in dilation of the perifoveal capillary network and macular edema.[10] In contrast, intraocular inflammation is not a feature of parafoveal telangiectasis.

Probably the most common disorder that may be confused with group 1 disease is capillary telangiectasis secondary to branch retinal vein occlusion (BRVO). The capillary bed drained by the obstructed vein may develop dilation, telangiectasis, and chronic edema. Two adjacent venules may occasionally be involved in the macular region. Telangiectasis due to a BRVO can be distinguished from group 1 parafoveal telangiectasis by careful examination of the involved vasculature. In a BRVO, the obstruction site occurs at an arteriovenous crossing point and, therefore, the entire capillary bed distal to this point demonstrates vascular changes. Such precise localization does not occur in parafoveal telangiectasis, particularly in group 1A disease where the affected vasculature crosses the horizontal raphe. In addition to BRVO, retinal arterial macroaneurysms with chronic exudation may also be associated with secondary capillary telangiectasis. Particularly in older hypertensive patients, a macroaneurysm should be considered in the differential diagnosis of primary parafoveal telangiectasis.[15]

GROUP 2 (OCCULT TELANGIECTASIS WITH MINIMAL EXUDATION)

Gass and Blodi subdivide this group into an adult form (group 2A) and a juvenile, familial form of disease (group 2B). As the most common form of parafoveal telangiectasis, group 2A disease is sometimes simply referred to as idiopathic perifoveal telangiectasis (IPT).[15] IPT is a bilateral, acquired disease that presents in the fifth or sixth decade of life without any sex predilection.[8,14] The pattern of telangiectasis in IPT is typically symmetric in each eye, and there is involvement of the temporal parafoveal region in all cases (Fig. 31–1). The region of telangiectasis is usually less than 1 DD in area, but the entire perifoveal capillary network may be affected in some cases. The median visual acuity at presentation is 20/40, and funduscopic examination at this stage may only reveal a grayish sheen to the involved retina.[8] The "occult" telangiectatic capillaries are best detected during the early frames of the fluorescein angiogram, with later frames re-

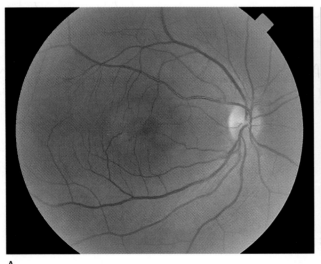
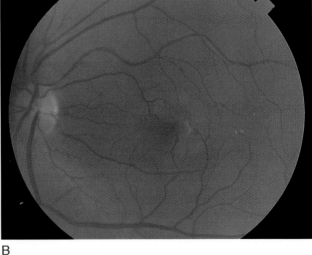

A   B

FIGURE 31–1   A 49-year-old woman with idiopathic perifoveal telangiectasis (group 2A disease). Visual acuity is 20/70 OD and 20/30 OS. Telangiectasis is most apparent superotemporally (OD > OS). The right fundus reveals moderate retinal thickening of the parafoveal region with a grayish loss of transparency; a small intraretinal hemorrhage is visible inferotemporal to the fovea. The left fundus has mild parafoveal thickening with a macular pseudohole. A few superficial crystalline deposits are also visible.

vealing retinal staining within the zone of telangiectasis (Fig. 31–2). IPT is associated with minimal macular edema in biomicroscopy, contrasting these patients to those with group 1 telangiectasis. The development of a cystoid pattern of macular edema or lipid exudation in IPT usually reflects the presence of subretinal neovascularization.

Further progression of this disease may lead to other characteristic findings in IPT. Many patients will develop mildly dilated retinal venules that bend posteriorly at right angles to drain a network of telangiectatic capillaries within the outer retina (Fig. 31–3B). Focal atrophy of the foveal retina is a common finding in IPT and may resemble a lamellar macular hole in some cases (Fig. 31–1B).[8,16] A hyperplastic retinal pigment epithelial response may occur within the neurosensory retina, some-

times producing stellate plaques of pigment alongside the draining retinal venules (Fig. 39–4). Fibrous metaplasia may also be seen in advanced disease (Fig. 31–3A). Late stages of IPT may be complicated by the development of subretinal neovascularization (SRN) with accordant exudation, hemorrhage, and disciform scarring (Fig. 31–5). The exact origin of these new blood vessels is unclear, with some investigators suggesting an intraretinal vascular origin and others a choroidal neovascular process. In contrast to age-related macular degeneration, patients with IPT who develop SRN rarely manifest retinal pigment epithelial detachment as part of their disease process. A common end point of SRN in IPT is the formation of a retinochoroidal anastomosis.

In almost half of the patients with IPT, numerous

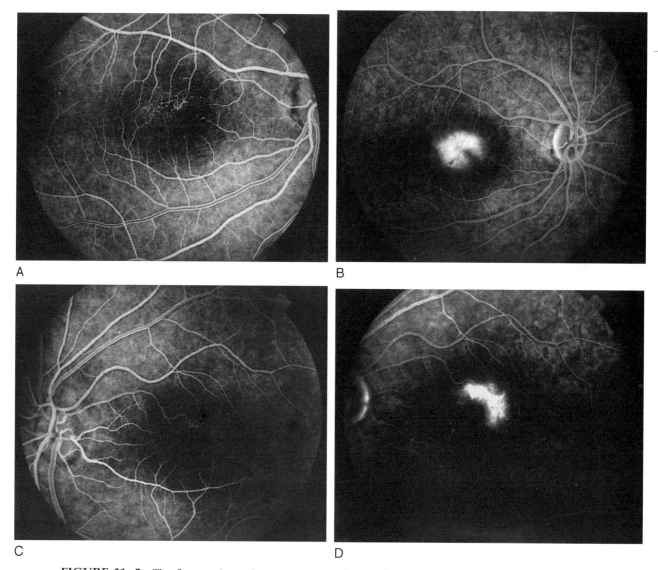

A

B

C

D

FIGURE 31–2 The fluorescein angiogram corresponding to the patient in Figure 31–1. Capillary telangiectasis of the parafoveal region is apparent in the early stages of the angiogram (OD > OS). There is late staining within the retina (OD > OS). The intraretinal hemorrhage visible in Figure 31–1A blocks fluorescence in Figure 31–2B. Despite the presence of hemorrhage in this patient, there was no evidence of neovascularization.

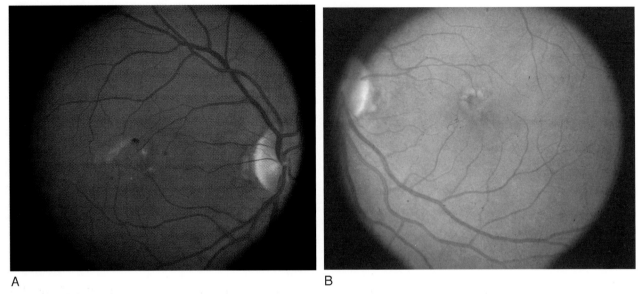

A   B

FIGURE 31–3   This patient exhibits later fundus changes characteristic of IPT. There is foveal atrophy (OD > OS). Plaques of pigment epithelial hyperplasia and fibrous metaplasia are visible OD. A characteristic right-angle venule is present in the left fundus, along with a plaque of fibrous metaplasia.

golden refractile opacities appear along the inner retinal surface in the region of telangiectasis (Fig. 31–6).[8,17] The etiology of the crystalline deposits is unclear, but their presence may aid in the diagnosis of subtle forms of IPT. On rare occasions, some patients with IPT develop an oval or round 0.25- to 0.33-DD central yellow lesion within the outer retinal layers. This lesion resembles the vitelliform lesion associated with perifoveal leakage described as pseudovitelliform macular degeneration by Fishman et al.[18] Parafoveal capillary telangiectasis, however, was not reported in these patients.

The natural course of IPT is quite variable, with prognosis varying with extent of parafoveal capillary involvement, degree of vascular incompetence, and the presence of atrophy or neovascularization. Despite persistent fluorescein staining and/or loss of retinal transparency in the parafoveal region, many patients preserve useful vision in at least one eye for several years.[8,14] Progressive central visual loss occurs in some eyes due to gradual atrophy of the involved retina. Patients with IPT may acutely lose vision due to exudative disease associated with subretinal neovascularization. The occurrence of SRN in one eye appears to increase the risk for the development of disciform disease in the fellow eye.[14]

In the series of Gass and Blodi, foveal atrophy was the most common etiology of severe visual loss (20/200 or less visual acuity) in group 2A telangi-

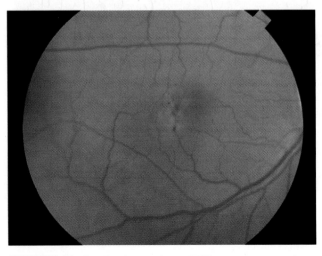

FIGURE 31–4   The hyperplastic RPE response sometimes produces stellate lesions along the venule in IPT.

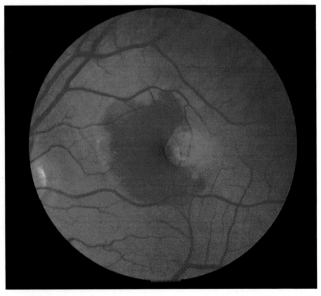

FIGURE 31–5   This patient with IPT developed subretinal hemorrhage and fluid due to a temporal neovascular complex.

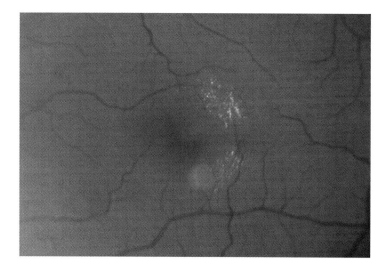

FIGURE 31–6 Glistening crystalline deposits are sometimes present in IPT.

ectasis or IPT.[8] In their experience, CME or lipid exudation was not a cause of visual loss except in association with SRN. For these reasons, focal laser photocoagulation of the juxtafoveal telangiectatic capillaries is unlikely to be beneficial in the treatment of these patients. While laser photocoagulation may be considered in those patients who develop SRN, the frequent subfoveal location of the neovascular process limits the potential benefit of laser treatment.

The pathogenesis and etiology of IPT is unknown. Gass and Blodi propose that the initial disease process occurs within the capillary walls of the deep perifoveal capillary network.[8] In this model, chronic metabolic damage rather than exudation leads to atrophy of the sensory retinal layers and late pigmentary disease. Casswell et al noted fluorescein staining at the level of the retinal pigment epithelium (RPE) in the early stages of IPT, prior to the development of leakage from the telangiectatic capillaries.[14] This finding led these investigators to suggest that IPT could be a primary disease of the RPE with secondary outer retinal vascular changes.

The histopathologic features of one case of IPT were reported by Green and colleagues.[19] No telangiectatic capillaries or abnormalities of the RPE were demonstrated in this study. Instead, there was narrowing of the capillary lumens associated with endothelial cell basement membrane proliferation (Fig. 31–7). Many capillaries demonstrated a multilayered basement membrane, the lamina of which were separated by cellular debris from degenerated endothelial cells and pericytes and by membranous lipid material (Fig. 31–8). These findings were most prominent in the clinically affected temporal parafoveal region, but they were also present diffusely throughout the retina. There were occasional areas of focal endothelial cell disruption, which the investigators proposed were sites of fluorescein diffusion into capillary walls with subsequent leakage into surrounding retina. The histopathologic changes observed were consistent with primary en-

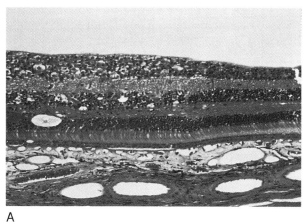

A

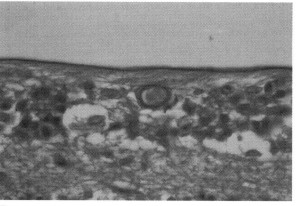

B

FIGURE 31–7 Light microscopic specimens of a retina from a patient with IPT. The temporal foveal retina reveals thickening and edema of the inner retinal layers. The RPE is normal. The capillaries in this specimen exhibited capillary wall thickening. (From Green WR, Quigley HA, de la Cruz Z, Cohen B: Parafoveal retinal telangiectasis: light and electron microscopy studies. Trans Ophthalmol Soc U K 100:162–170, 1980, with permission.)

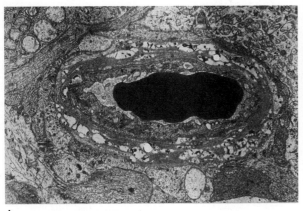
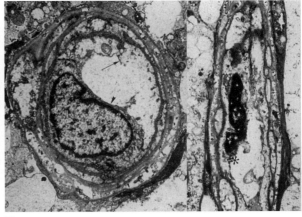

A   B

FIGURE 31–8   Electron microscopy of this specimen revealed a multilayered basement membrane, with the layers separated by cellular debris and membranous lipid material. (From Green WR, Quigley HA, de la Cruz Z, Cohen B: Parafoveal retinal telangiectasis: light and electron microscopy studies. Trans Ophthalmol Soc U K 100:162–170, 1980, with permission.)

dothelial cell degeneration and regeneration and secondary loss of pericytes. In particular, the histopathologic findings in the capillaries of this patient closely resemble those found in diabetic patients. While the patient studied had no clinical evidence of diabetes mellitus, she had refused diagnostic studies, such as a glucose tolerance test, for the presence of diabetes.

These histopathologic changes first suggested a relationship of IPT with diabetes mellitus. Other associations of IPT with abnormal glucose metabolism and diabetic retinopathy have since been reported. Chew and associates described five patients with diabetes mellitus, nonproliferative retinopathy, and visual loss due to leakage of parafoveal telangiectatic capillaries.[20] All five patients had bilateral telangiectasis, and each patient demonstrated plaques of pigment epithelial hyperplasia typical of IPT. Abnormal glucose tolerance tests have also been observed in association with parafoveal telangiectasis, leading some investigators to recommend that such testing be considered in these patients.[21,22] At this time, however, the possibility that some patients with IPT are in a prediabetic state or have an abnormal glucose metabolism remains a point of speculation. Further studies are required to elucidate the possible role of diabetes mellitus in IPT.

In addition to diabetic retinopathy, the differential diagnosis of IPT or group 2A telangiectasis includes the other retinal diseases discussed with group 1 disease. Due to the subtle nature of the vascular changes, early stages of IPT may be misdiagnosed as central serous chorioretinopathy. As noted above, other clinical features of IPT may be confused with such diverse retinal disorders as lamellar macular hole, crystalline retinopathies, and vitelliform dystrophies. The hyperplastic RPE response seen in IPT may suggest an underlying in-

flammatory choroidopathy. The development of SRN and disciform scarring in IPT may mimic age-related macular degeneration and other diseases associated with choroidal neovascularization. In short, IPT may present with a variety of funduscopic findings. The accurate diagnosis of this condition ultimately requires recognition of its characteristic features along with a high level of clinical suspicion for its underlying presence.

GROUP 3 (VISIBLE TELANGIECTASIS WITH CAPILLARY OCCLUSION AND MINIMAL EXUDATION)

This group of patients with parafoveal telangiectasis have the least frequently encountered findings. Biomicroscopically visible telangiectasis is present in the parafoveal region, and some cases reveal subtle telangiectatic changes outside the macular region. Fluorescein angiography reveals an enlargement of the capillary-free zone and with minimal late dye leakage in these patients. Patients with this occlusive form of parafoveal telangiectasis usually have an associated systemic disease that may be related to their retinal findings.

Group 3A comprised three women in Gass and Blodi's series.[8] Despite the presence of prominent parafoveal capillary ischemia, there was relatively minimal visual loss (visual acuity 20/20 to 20/50) in these patients. Concordant medical illnesses present in these women included gout, polycythemia, and/or hypoglycemia, and one patient had a sibling with similar retinal findings. A similar familial pattern of occlusive parafoveal telangiectasis without exudation was described by Ehlers and

Jensen, though some of these patients also had re-fractile deposits suggestive of IPT.[23]

The group 3B classification refers to the association of similar occlusive and telangiectatic disease with evidence of a central nervous system vasculopathy.[8] These patients have various neurologic findings, including an exaggeration of tendon reflexes and disturbances in gait. Neuroimaging may reveal multiple cerebral infarcts, and affected patients may have family members with similar disease. The patients with a familial pattern of group 3B disease probably have cerebroretinal vasculopathy, a recently recognized hereditary syndrome.[24] This autosomal dominant condition presents with bilateral occlusion of the perifoveal capillary bed and parafoveal vascular changes resembling telangiectasis. Scattered areas of peripheral capillary occlusion are occasionally present, and some cases may be complicated by the development of retinal neovascularization. While a variety of neurologic symptoms may occur, affected individuals typically develop mass lesions in the frontoparietal lobe. Biopsy specimens and neuropathologic studies of these lesions reveal fibrinoid necrosis of involved vessels, a variable perivascular inflammatory infiltrate, and chronic infarctions predominantly affecting the white matter.

The differential diagnosis of group 3 occlusive parafoveal telangiectasis includes several ocular and systemic diseases. Capillary obliteration is frequently associated with diabetic retinopathy, and diabetes mellitus should be considered in all forms of parafoveal telangiectasis. Severe hypertensive retinopathy may similarly result in an ischemic maculopathy. Branch retinal vein occlusions may also be complicated by capillary nonperfusion, but the localization to the involved vein distinguishes this condition from the diffuse perifoveal occlusion seen in group 3 telangiectasis. The late effects of ocular irradiation may result in similar parafoveal disease; however, more diffuse involvement of the retina is usually present along with the history of radiation treatment.[10] Sickling hemoglobinopathies may also alter the vasculature of the posterior pole to produce telangiectasis and an enlargement of the foveal avascular zone.[11] These patients generally have peripheral signs of sickle retinopathy and/or well-documented hematologic disease. An important disease to consider in patients with occlusive telangiectasis in the parafoveal region is carotid artery obstruction, which in some cases presents with bilateral disease.[10,12] A delay in the perfusion of dye in the retinal arterial circulation is apparent during fluorescein angiography in cases of carotid artery occlusion. Collagen vascular diseases may also produce vascular occlusions in the posterior pole, though there is usually more extensive retinal involvement. Systemic lupus erythematosis, in particular, may present with retinal and central nervous system vaso-occlusive disease and should be considered in patients with group 3B telangiectasis.[24]

SUMMARY

The term "parafoveal telangiectasis" refers to several well-recognized clinical syndromes of unclear etiology characterized by the presence of dilated and ectatic capillaries of the parafoveal region. One disorder occurs predominantly as a unilateral condition in men and is probably a variant of Coats' disease. The most common form of parafoveal telangiectasis is IPT, a bilateral disease of middle-aged adults that has characteristic clinical features. An occlusive variant of telangiectasis has also been observed, usually in association with an underlying medical or neurologic disease.

REFERENCES

1. Reese AB: Telangiectasis of the retina and Coats' disease. Am J Ophthalmol 42:1–8, 1956.
2. Gass JDM: A fluorescein angiographic study of macular dysfunction secondary to retinal vascular disease. V. Retinal telangiectasis. Arch Ophthalmol 80:592–605, 1968.
3. Gass JDM: Stereoscopic Atlas of Macular Diseases, 2nd edition. St Louis, CV Mosby Co, 1977.
4. Hutton WL, Snyder WB, Fuller D, Vaiser A: Focal parafoveal retinal telangiectasis. Arch Ophthalmol 96:1362–1367, 1978.
5. Chopdar A: Retinal telangiectasis in adults: angiographic findings and treatment by argon laser. Br J Ophthalmol 62:243–250, 1978.
6. Schatz H, Burton TC, Yannuzzi LA, Rabb MF: Interpretation of fundus fluorescein angiography. St Louis, CV Mosby Co, 1978.
7. Gass JDM, Oyakawa RT: Idiopathic juxtafoveolar retinal telangiectasis. Arch Ophthalmol 100:769–780, 1982.
8. Gass JDM, Blodi BA: Idiopathic juxtafoveolar retinal telangiectasis: update of classification and follow-up study. Ophthalmology 100:1536–1546, 1993.
9. Frenkel M, Russe HP: Retinal telangiectasia associated with hypogammaglobulinemia. Am J Ophthalmol 63:215–220, 1967.
10. Gass JDM: A fluorescein angiographic study of macular dysfunction secondary to retinal vascular disease. VI. X-ray irradiation, carotid artery occlusion, collagen vascular disease, and vitritis. Arch Ophthalmol 80:606–617, 1968.
11. Stevens TS, Busse B, Lee CB, et al: Sickling hemoglobinopathies: macular and perimacular vascular abnormalities. Arch Ophthalmol 92:455–463, 1974.
12. Campo RV, Reeser FH: Retinal telangiectasia secondary to bilateral carotid artery occlusion. Arch Ophthalmol 101:1211–1213, 1983.
13. Gurwin EB, Fitzsimmons RB, Sehmi KS, Bird AC: Retinal telangiectasis in fascioscapulohumeral muscular dystrophy with deafness. Arch Ophthalmol 103:1695–1700, 1985.
14. Casswell AG, Chaine G, Rush P, Bird AC: Paramacular telangiectasis. Trans Ophthalmol Soc U K 105:683–692, 1986.
15. Yannuzzi LA (ed): Laser Photocoagulation of the Macula. Philadelphia, JB Lippincott Co, 1989.
16. Patel B, Duval J, Tullo AB: Lamellar macular hole associated with idiopathic juxtafoveolar telangiectasia. Br J Ophthalmol 72:550–551, 1988.
17. Moisseiev J, Lewis H, Bartov E, et al: Superficial retinal refractile deposits in juxtafoveal telangiectasis. Am J Ophthalmol 109:604–605, 1990.
18. Fishman GA, Trimble S, Rabb MF, Fishman M: Pseudovitelliform macular degeneration. Arch Ophthalmol 95:73–76, 1977.

19. Green WR, Quigley HA, de la Cruz Z, Cohen B: Parafoveal retinal telangiectasis: light and electron microscopy studies. Trans Ophthalmol Soc U K 100:162–170, 1980.
20. Chew EY, Murphy RP, Newsome DA, Fine SL: Parafoveal telangiectasis and diabetic retinopathy. Arch Ophthalmol 104:71–75, 1986.
21. Millay RH, Klein ML, Handelman IL, Watzke RC: Abnormal glucose metabolism and parafoveal telangiectasia. Am J Ophthalmol 102:363–370, 1986.
22. Brown GC: Discussion of idiopathic juxtafoveolar retinal telangiectasis. Ophthalmology 100:1546, 1993.
23. Ehlers N, Jensen VA: Hereditary central retinal angiopathy. Acta Ophthalmol 51:171–178, 1973.
24. Grand MG, Kaine J, Fulling K, et al: Cerebroretinal vasculopathy: a new hereditary syndrome. Ophthalmology 95:649–659, 1988.

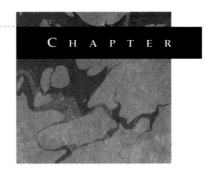

Retinopathy of Prematurity: Stages 1 Through 3

Philip J. Ferrone, M.D.

Michael T. Trese, M.D.

In the Cryotherapy for Retinopathy of Prematurity (Cryo-ROP) trial, in which infants with a birth weight of less than 1251 g were evaluated with ophthalmologic exams starting 4 to 6 weeks after birth, it was found that 66% of the 4099 infants examined eventually developed retinopathy of prematurity (ROP). This percentage was as high as 82% if the birth weight of the infant was less than 1000 g. The incidence of retinography of prematurity increased as birth weight decreased or gestational age decreased. It was found that black infants were less susceptible than nonblack infants. The timing of the retinal changes consistent with retinopathy of prematurity correlated more with the postconceptional age than with the patient's postnatal age. This was interpreted to reflect that the disease is influenced more by the patient's level of maturity than by postnatal environmental influences.[1] The incidence of threshold retinopathy of prematurity in this study was 6% of infants.

Retinopathy of prematurity was first described as retrolental fibroplasia in 1941 by Terry. At that time it was noted to be more prevalent in the more "modern" nurseries. This led to the suspicion that this may be partially an organic disease. Subsequently, there was a study by Kinsey in 1956 which showed that premature infants that did not have lung disease and were given oxygen at a concentration higher than 50% for 4 weeks showed a threefold increase in the development of retinopathy of prematurity.[2] After this study was published, the concentration of inspired oxygen in newborn nurseries was limited to a maximum of 40%. This in turn led to a dramatic decrease in the incidence of retinopathy of prematurity until the late 1960s. This approach also led to a dramatic increase in

mortality for premature infants with lung disease, since the maximum inspired oxygen concentration was 40%. Then in the 1970s, as neonatal intensive care units were formed, the survival rates for premature infants increased. Consequently, as the number of premature infants increased, so did the incidence of retinopathy of prematurity. It is estimated that retinopathy of prematurity causes complete visual loss in as many as 2 to 4% of infants with a birth weight of less than 2 lb.[3]

FACTORS ASSOCIATED WITH RETINOPATHY OF PREMATURITY

The greatest risk factor for retinopathy of prematurity is prematurity itself. Infants at risk are those who have a birth weight of less than 1500 g or a gestational age of less than 32 weeks. Developing retinopathy of prematurity at a higher birth weight or a longer gestational age is uncommon. One instance in which the birth weight can be misleading is if the patient has hydrops and prematurity.[4] Of course, these patients have a higher birth weight, but still may show the same retinal prematurity of a lower birth weight infant for a particular gestational age.

Other factors that are reportedly associated with retinopathy of prematurity, but for which there is no definitive evidence of association, include corticosteroid usage in the infants, light exposure, and surfactant use.[5-13] In one study, indomethacin was found to have an influence on patients developing retinopathy of prematurity. It was found that in-

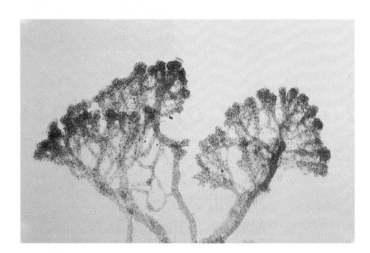

Trypsin digest preparation discloses intraretinal neovascularization sea-fan-like configurations in retinopathy of prematurity. (From Chui HC, Green WR: Acute retrolental fibroplasia: a clinicopathologic correlation. Md Med J 26:71–74, 1977, with permission.)

TABLE 32–1   Stages of Retinopathy of Prematurity

Stage No.	Characteristic
1	Demarcation line
2	Ridge
3	Ridge with extraretinal fibrovascular proliferation
4	Subtotal retinal detachment
	A. Extrafoveal
	B. Retinal detachment including fovea
5	Total retinal detachment

	Funnel:	Anterior	Posterior
		open	open
		narrow	narrow
		open	narrow
		narrow	open

fants who were given indomethacin were 1.5 times more likely to develop ROP in this study, which involved 338 infants.[14] There is also no definitive evidence for vitamin E therapy or elevated bilirubin acting in an antioxidant role to help prevent the development of retinopathy of prematurity.[15,16]

A well-controlled, but not randomized, study that examined the role of oxygen administration and its influence in the development of retinopathy of prematurity was performed by Flynn and colleagues.[17] In this study it was found that a significant association existed between the amount of time an infant's arterial oxygen tension was equal to or exceeded 80 mm Hg and the incidence and severity of retinopathy of prematurity. The association was stronger when the elevated arterial oxygen levels occurred during the second through the fourth week of an infant's life. Nevertheless, it appears from this and other studies that retinopathy of pre-

maturity is not simply a preventable disease caused by inappropriate oxygen administration.[17–20]

CLASSIFICATION OF RETINOPATHY OF PREMATURITY

In the mid 1980s retinopathy of prematurity was classified by an international committee.[21,22] The classification contains five stages (Table 32–1), three zones (Fig. 32–1), and the absence or presence of plus disease.

Stage 1 consists of a demarcation line (Fig. 32–2). This line lies in the plane in the retina. It is white in color and is relatively flat. It separates avascular from vascularized retina. Stage 2 consists of a ridge (Fig. 32–3). It is a progression of stage 1 with a line that now has height and volume. It extends up from the plane of the retina. It may have a white or pinkish color. Stage 3 consists of a ridge with extraretinal fibrovascular proliferation (Fig. 32–4). From this ridge that extends out of the plane of the retina emanates extraretinal blood vessels; these may have a ragged brush border appearance or frankly extend out into the vitreous as pronounced neovascular fronds. Stage 4 consists of a retinal detachment. This retinal detachment may be effusive or tractional, or both. Sometimes these retinal detachments may be difficult to detect due to their shallowness. They can often be detected even when shallow by seeing a loss of choroidal pattern on fundus examination. Stage 4A does not involve the fovea, while stage 4B does involve the fovea. Stage 5 is a total retinal detachment that may be narrow or open in configuration. The narrowness or openness of the retinal detachment is judged in the anterior retina and posterior retina.

The retinal area is divided into three zones. Each zone is centered on the optic disc rather than on

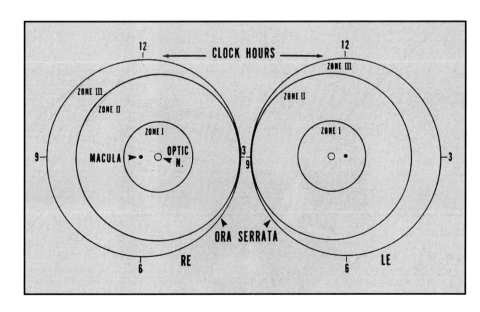

FIGURE 32–1   The three zones of retinopathy of prematurity with clock hours. (From The International Committee for the Classification of Retinopathy of Prematurity: An international classification of retinopathy of prematurity. Arch Ophthalmol 102:1130–1134, 1984. Copyright 1984, American Medical Association, with permission.)

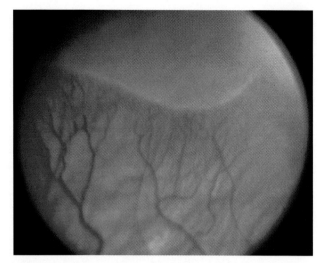

FIGURE 32–2 Stage 1 retinopathy of prematurity with demarcation line. (From Oregon Health Sciences University, Department of Ophthalmology, Portland, OR and from Focal Points: Clinical Modules for Ophthalmologists, Vol XI: No. 3, March, 1993, Module 12. San Francisco, Am Acad Ophthalmol, Chicago, IL, 1988, with permission.)

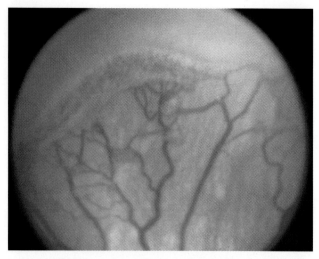

FIGURE 32–4 Stage 3 retinopathy consisting of a ridge with extraretinal fibrovascular proliferation. (From Oregon Health Sciences University, Department of Ophthalmology, Portland, OR and from Focal Points: Clinical Modules for Ophthalmologists, Vol XI: No. 3, March, 1993, Module 12. San Francisco, Am Acad Ophthalmol, Chicago, IL, 1988, with permission.)

the macula. Zone I consists of a circle with a radius of 30 degrees, and extends from the disc to twice the disc-fovea distance for 360 degrees around the optic nerve head. Zone II extends from the edge of zone I peripherally to the ora serrata nasally. Temporally it extends to approximately the equator of the globe. Zone III consists of the residual area temporally between zone II and the ora serrata. This is typically the last area vascularized in the premature infant's eye.

The extent of disease is specified as the disease involved retina by clock hours with there being 12 total clock hours in an eye. Plus disease is charac-

terized by posterior venous and arterial tortuosity and dilation (Fig. 32–5).[21–23]

SCREENING

Screening is recommended for infants with a birth weight of less than 1500 g, or a gestational age of less than 32 weeks. The first dilated fundus examination is performed between 4 and 6 weeks after birth. Examinations are then performed at least every 2 weeks until the retina is fully vascularized.

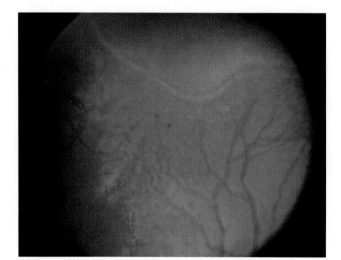

FIGURE 32–3 Stage 2 retinopathy of prematurity consisting of a ridge. (From Oregon Health Sciences University, Department of Ophthalmology, Portland, OR and from Focal Points: Clinical Modules for Ophthalmologists, Vol XI: No. 3, March, 1993, Module 12. San Francisco, Am Acad Ophthalmol, Chicago, IL, 1988, with permission. Courtesy of Dr. E.A. Palmer.)

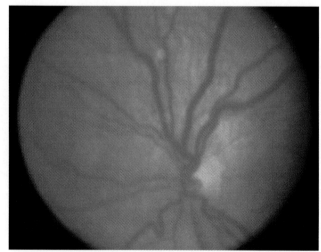

FIGURE 32–5 Plus disease in retinopathy of prematurity characterized by posterior venous and arterial tortuosity and dilation. (From Cryotherapy for Retinopathy of Prematurity Cooperative Group: Multicenter trial of cryotherapy for retinopathy of prematurity; preliminary results. Arch Ophthalmol 106[4]:471–479, 1988. Copyright 1988, American Medical Association, with permission.)

Infants who develop prethreshold retinopathy of prematurity (defined as zone I retinopathy of prematurity at any stage less than threshold; zone II retinopathy of prematurity at stage 2+; or zone II retinopathy of prematurity stage 3 without plus disease; or zone II retinopathy of prematurity stage 3+ with fewer than the threshold number of clock hours) are recommended to have examinations on at least a weekly basis.

Dilated fundus examinations are performed using a lid speculum and Flynn scleral depressor when it is not possible to see the vascularized retinal and nonvascularized retinal junction.[1] After the infant's retina has fully vascularized, it is recommended that they follow-up with a pediatric ophthalmologist approximately 5 to 6 months after their last retinal exam for evaluation of the possible development of myopia and/or strabismus.

In infants with retinopathy of prematurity that does not reach threshold, it is common for these eyes not to show complete vascularization of the retina at term.[24] In posterior retinopathy of prematurity with stage 3, vascularized retina does not often reach zone III until after a postconceptional age of 42 weeks. In some of these patients permanent vascular sequelae are seen, with the most common change being failure to vascularize the temporal peripheral retina completely.[25]

Appropriately timed screening of retinopathy of prematurity has been predicted to result in a gain of 3899 to 4648 quality-adjusted life-years, and a net government savings of $38.3 to $64.9 million for each annual U.S. birth cohort of 28,321 premature infants (500 to 1249 g). Proper screening most importantly is estimated to save at least 320 infants per year from a lifetime of blindness.[26]

THRESHOLD DISEASE

Threshold retinopathy of prematurity is defined as five or more contiguous or eight cumulative clock hours of stage 3+ retinopathy of prematurity in either zone I or zone II. As soon as threshold retinopathy of prematurity is diagnosed, it is recommended that peripheral retinal ablation be performed within 72 hours. This may be accomplished by using either cryotherapy or laser treatment. More recently, laser has become a preferred method of treatment. In the Cryo-ROP study in which 4099 infants were studied with a birth weight of less than 1251 g, 6% of these children were diagnosed with threshold retinopathy of prematurity.[1] The median time for developing threshold disease was 36.9 weeks postconceptional age, with threshold being diagnosed as early as 31 weeks postconceptional age, and 95% of infants who reached threshold did so by 42 weeks postconceptional age.[1] The 3-month outcome of the Cryo-ROP study showed that cryotherapy to the avascular retinal periphery for threshold retinopathy of prematurity in zone I

or zone II cut the risk of an unfavorable outcome approximately in half. Initially, unfavorable outcomes were reported in 43% of the untreated patients and in 22% of the cryotherapy-treated patients.[27] An unfavorable outcome was defined as a posterior retinal detachment, a retinal fold in the macula, or retrolental tissue. These were the preliminary results from the 3-month study. The final results from the 3-month Cryo-ROP study reported an unfavorable structural outcome with 51% of untreated eyes and only 31% of cryotherapy-treated eyes.[28] A subsequent report of the 1-year structural outcome from the Cryo-ROP study showed an unfavorable outcome with 47% of untreated and 26% of cryotherapy-treated eyes.[29] The $3\frac{1}{2}$-year structural outcome report reported an unfavorable posterior pole status in 45% of the untreated group and only 26% of the cryotherapy treated group.[30] The $5\frac{1}{2}$-year structural outcome Cryo-ROP report reported that untreated eyes had a 45% unfavorable outcome, while cryotherapy-treated eyes had a 27% unfavorable outcome.[31]

The percentages of unfavorable function outcome at 1 year from the Cryo-ROP study showed untreated eyes had a 56% unfavorable functional outcome, while cryotherapy-treated eyes had a 35% unfavorable functional outcome.[29] The $3\frac{1}{2}$-year Cryo-ROP report, which evaluated HOTV letter acuity and Teller grading acuity, showed an unfavorable functional outcome for the untreated group in 58% of patients, while the cryotherapy-treated group had an unfavorable functional outcome in 47% of patients as measured by HOTV letter acuity. In the same study, the untreated group had an unfavorable functional outcome in 66% of patients, and the cryotherapy-treated group had an unfavorable functional outcome in 52% of patients as measured by Teller grading acuity.[30] The $5\frac{1}{2}$-year Cryo-ROP functional outcome data showed that untreated eyes had a 62% unfavorable outcome, while cryotherapy-treated eyes had a 47% unfavorable outcome. In the $5\frac{1}{2}$-year Cryo-ROP data analysis, favorable visual acuity was defined as a Snellen visual acuity of better than 20/200. In this follow-up study of 234 eyes, blind eyes were reported in 48% of untreated eyes and 31.5% of cryotherapy-treated eyes. Blindness was defined as vision too poor to quantify.[31]

Factors that influenced the risk of developing threshold of retinopathy of prematurity in the Cryo-ROP study were as follows: (1) lower birth weight, (2) younger gestational age, (3) white race, (4) multiple birth, and (5) being born outside of a Cryo-ROP study nursery. Factors that influenced the risk of having an unfavorable macular outcome include (1) zone I retinopathy of prematurity, (2) plus disease, (3) severity of stage of retinopathy of prematurity, (4) amount of circumferential involvement of retinopathy of prematurity, and (5) a rapid rate of progression to prethreshold disease. The postconceptional age at which retinopathy of prematurity was first noted did not influence the risk of an unfavorable macular outcome.[32] In a natural history study of retinopathy of prematurity from the Cryo-ROP trial, an unfavorable outcome was found in 59% of zone I stage 3 eyes, 44% of zone II stage 3+ eyes which had involvement of 9 to 12 clock hours, and less than 1% of zone II eyes without plus disease or zone III retinopathy of prematurity. From these data it was concluded that the more posterior the zone of the retinopathy of prematurity and the greater the extent of stage 3+ involvement, the greater the chance of an unfavorable outcome.[33]

The Cryo-ROP study used exocryotherapy to treat the avascular peripheral retina. More recently, the diode and argon indirect lasers have been used to ablate this avascular retinal tissue. There are numerous studies that show the diode laser to be as effective as exocryotherapy; it is also better tolerated by the patient and is technically easier to administer.[34-40]

One problem reported more frequently with the argon laser, as opposed to the diode indirect laser, is the complication of cataract formation from absorption of laser energy in the residual tunica vasculosa lentis or pigment on the crystalline lens.[41-43] Transient lens changes have been reported after diode indirect laser, for retinopathy of prematurity, but these are very infrequent.[39,44] Rare potential complications of the indirect laser photocoagulation include corneal burns, iris burns, lens burns, choroidal hemorrhages with subsequent subretinal neovascularization, inadvertent photocoagulation of the fovea, and late-onset rhegmatogenous retinal detachments.[45] Cryotherapy itself has been associated with significant complications, which include respiratory arrest and cardiorespiratory arrest.[46] Rhegmatogenous retinal detachments can also occur after cryotherapy secondary to tears occurring at the junction of treated and untreated retina.[47]

OBSERVATIONS AFTER RETINOPATHY OF PREMATURITY

Numerous structural changes can be seen in the periphery and posterior retina after retinopathy of prematurity has regressed. Peripheral changes include failure to vascularize the peripheral retina, abnormal nondichotomous branching of retinal vessels, telangiectatic vessels, and vascular arcades with circumferential anastomoses. Peripheral changes can also include pigmentary changes, vitreoretinal interface abnormalities, abnormally thin retina, peripheral retinal folds, vitreous membranes with and without attachment to the retina, lattice-like degeneration, retinal breaks, and traction/rhegmatogenous retinal detachments.[21] Posterior changes after retinopathy of prematurity can include vascular tortuosity, straightening of retinal vessels with temporal or (less commonly) nasal

dragging, pigmentary changes, ectopia of the macula, and dragging of the retina over the optic nerve head.[21]

Myopia, strabismus, and amblyopia have been reported following retinopathy of prematurity.[48-55] The Cryo-ROP study evaluated patients with a birth weight of less than 1251 g in which no cryotherapy was performed. A 20% incidence of myopia was found at 3 months, 12 months, and 24 months. The percentage of high myopia (defined as ≥5 diopters) doubled between the 3- and 12-month examinations (2 to 4.6%). Low birth weight and increased severity of retinopathy of prematurity were strong predictors of myopia and high myopia in this population.[54] In another study, it was found that myopia from regressed retinopathy of prematurity is most commonly due to increased corneal curvature, as opposed to an increased axial length, which is seen more commonly in full-term myopia patients.[48] Strabismus has been reported in 14 to 40% of retinopathy of prematurity affected eyes, while myopia has been reported in 16 to 50% of these eyes, and amblyopia in 6 to 33% of these eyes.[49-51,56,57] It is for these reasons among others that close follow-up with a pediatric ophthalmologist is recommended.

Late traction retinal detachments and rhegmatogenous retinal detachments have also been seen in these eyes. Prolonged retinal traction may lead to the development of retinal holes located in the fragile, anterior, nonvascularized retina.[47,58-60] This is another reason why these patients need to be followed closely life long.

Visual fields can also be affected by retinopathy of prematurity with and without peripheral retinal ablation being performed.[61-63] Stage 3 retinopathy of prematurity itself can cause constriction of the visual field or delay visual field development without peripheral retinal ablation being performed.[62] In a study which used Goldmann visual field testing (II-4-e target and V-4-e target) to compare eight eyes treated with exocryotherapy for severe retinopathy of prematurity and six control eyes with untreated severe retinopathy of prematurity, the cryotherapy-treated eyes had slightly smaller visual fields compared to the untreated regressed ROP eyes. The visual field in the cryotherapy-treated eyes decreased by approximately 10 degrees for the two targets mentioned above.[63]

REFERENCES

1. Palmer EA, Flynn JT, Hardy RJ, et al: Incidence and early course of retinopathy of prematurity. The Cryotherapy for Retinopathy of Prematurity Group. Ophthalmology 98(11): 1628–1640, 1991.
2. Kinsey VE: Retrolental fibroplasia: cooperative study of retrolental fibroplasia and the use of oxygen. Arch Ophthalmol 56:481–543, 1956.
3. Phelps DL: Retinopathy of prematurity. Pediatr Rev 16(2): 50–56, 1995.
4. Trese MT, Batton DG: Ocular examination schedule for in-

fants with fetal hydrops (Letter). Am J Ophthalmol 108(4): 459, 1989.

5. Ramanathan R, Siassi B, de Lemos RA: Severe retinopathy of prematurity in extremely low birth weight infants after short-term dexamethasone therapy. J Perinatol 15(3):178–182, 1995.

6. McGinnity FG, Girschek PK, Morin JD, et al: Bovine surfactant therapy and retinopathy of prematurity. J Pediatr Ophthalmol Strabismus 31(4):238–241, 1994.

7. Seiberth V, Linderkamp O, Knorz MC, Liesenhoff H: A controlled clinical trial of light and retinopathy of prematurity. Am J Ophthalmol 118(4):492–495, 1994.

8. Holmes JM, Cronin CM, Squires P, Myers TF: Randomized clinical trial of surfactant prophylaxis in retinopathy of prematurity. J Pedatr Ophthalmol Strabismus 31(3):189–191, 1994.

9. Wright K, Wright SP: Lack of association of glucocorticoid therapy and retinopathy of prematurity. Arch Pediatr Adolesc Med 148(8):848–851, 1994.

10. Baerts W, Wildervanck de Blecourt-Devilee M, Sauer PJ: Ambient light, ophthalmic artery blood flow velocities and retinopathy of prematurity. Acta Paediatr 82(9):719–722, 1993.

11. Repka MX, Hardy RJ, Phelps DL, Summers CG: Surfactant prophylaxis and retinopathy of prematurity. Arch Ophthalmol 111(5):618–620, 1993.

12. Tubman TR, Rankin SJ, Halliday HL, Johnson SS: Surfactant replacement therapy and the prevalence of acute retinopathy of prematurity. Biol Neonate 1(Suppl 61):54–58, 1992.

13. Rankin SJ, Tubman TR, Halliday HL, Johnson SS: Retinopathy of prematurity in surfactant treated infants. Br J Ophthalmol 76(4):202–204, 1992.

14. Darlow BA, Horwood LJ, Clemett RS: Retinopathy: risk factors in a prospective population-based study. Paediatr Perinatal Epidemiol 6(1):62–80, 1992.

15. Fauchere JC, Meier-Gibbons FE, Koerner F, Bossi E: Retinopathy of prematurity and bilirubin—no clinical evidence for a beneficial role of bilirubin as a physiological anti-oxidant. Eur J Pediatr 153(5):358–362, 1994.

16. Romeo MG, Tina LG, Scuderi A, et al: Variations of blood bilirubin levels in the newborn with and without retinopathy of prematurity (ROP). Pediatr Med Chir 16(1):59–62, 1994.

17. Flynn JT, Banclari E, Snyder ES, et al: A cohort study of transcutaneous oxygen tension and the incidence and severity of retinopathy of prematurity. N Engl J Med 326:1050–1054, 1992.

18. Bancalari E, Flynn J, Goldberg RN, et al: Influence of transcutaneous oxygen monitoring on the incidence of retinopathy of prematurity. Pediatrics 79:663–669, 1987.

19. Flynn JT, Bancalari E, Bawol R, et al: Retinopathy of prematurity: a randomized, prospective trial of transcutaneous oxygen monitoring. Ophthalmology 94:630–683, 1987.

20. Flynn JT, Bancalari E, Bachynski BN, et al: Retinopathy of prematurity: diagnosis, severity, and natural history. Ophthalmology 94:620–629, 1987.

21. The International Committee for the Classification of the Late Stages of Retinopathy of Prematurity: An international classification of retinopathy of prematurity. Arch Ophthalmol 105(7):906–912, 1987.

22. The International Committee for the Classification of Retinopathy of Prematurity: An international classification of retinopathy of prematurity. Arch Ophthalmol 102:1130–1134, 1984.

23. Flynn JT: An international classification of retinopathy of prematurity; clinical experience. Ophthalmology 92(8):987–994, 1985.

24. Jandeck C, Kellner U, Helbig H, et al: Natural course of retinal detachment in preterm infants without threshold retinopathy. Ger J Ophthalmol 4(3):131–136, 1995.

25. Preslan MW, Butler J: Regression pattern in retinopathy of prematurity. J Pediatr Ophthalmol Strabismus 31(3):172–176, 1994.

26. Javitt J, Dei Cas R, Chiang YP: Cost-effectiveness of screening and cryotherapy for threshold retinopathy of prematurity. Pediatrics 91(5):859–866, 1993.

27. Cryotherapy for Retinopathy of Prematurity Cooperative Group: Multicenter trial of cryotherapy for retinopathy of prematurity; preliminary results. Arch Ophthalmol 106(4):471–479, 1988.

28. Cryotherapy for Retinopathy of Prematurity Cooperative Group: Multicenter trial of cryotherapy for retinopathy of prematurity; three month outcome. Arch Ophthalmol 108(2):195–204, 1990.

29. Cryotherapy for Retinopathy of Prematurity Cooperative Group: Multicenter trial of cryotherapy for retinopathy of prematurity; one year outcome—a structure and function. Arch Ophthalmol 108(10):1408–1416, 1990.

30. Cryotherapy for Retinopathy of Prematurity Cooperative Group: Multicenter trial of cryotherapy for retinopathy of prematurity; three-and-one-half year outcome—structure and function. Arch Ophthalmol 111(3):339–344, 1993.

31. Cryotherapy for Retinopathy of Prematurity Cooperative Group: Snellen visual acuity and structural outcome at $5^1/_2$ years after randomization. Arch Ophthalmol 114:417–424, 1996.

32. Schaffer DB, Palmer EA, Plotsky DF, et al: Prognostic factors in the natural course of retinopathy of prematurity; the Cryotherapy for Retinopathy Cooperative Group. Ophthalmology 100(2):230–237, 1993.

33. Cryotherapy for Retinopathy of Prematurity Cooperative Group: The natural ocular outcome of premature birth and retinopathy; status at one year. Arch Ophthalmol 112(7):903–912, 1994.

34. Hunter DG, Repka MX: Diode laser photocoagulation for threshold retinopathy; a randomized study. Ophthalmology 100(2):238–244, 1993.

35. McNamara JA, Tasman W, Vander JF, Brown GC: Diode laser photocoagulation for retinopathy of prematurity; preliminary results. Arch Ophthalmol 110(12):1714–1716, 1992.

36. Ling CS, Fleck BW, Wright E, et al: Diode laser treatment for retinopathy of prematurity; structural and functional outcome. Br J Ophthalmol 79(7):637–641, 1995.

37. Goggin M, O'Keefe M: Diode laser for retinopathy of prematurity; early outcome. Br J Ophthalmol 77(9):559–562, 1993.

38. Seiberth V, Linderkamp O, Vardarli I, et al: Diode laser photocoagulation for threshold retinopathy of prematurity in eyes with tunica vasculosa lentis. Am J Ophthalmol 119(6):748–751, 1995.

39. Benner JD, Morse LS, Hay A, Landers MB III: A comparison of argon and diode photocoagulation combined with supplemental oxygen for the treatment of retinopathy of prematurity. Retina 13(3):222–229, 1993.

40. McNamara JA, Tasman W, Brown GC, Federman JL: Laser photocoagulation for stage 3+ retinopathy of prematurity. Ophthalmology 98(5):576–580, 1991.

41. Campolattaro BN, Lueder GT: Cataract in infants treated with argon laser photocoagulation for threshold retinopathy of prematurity (Letter). Am J Ophthalmol 120(2):264–266, 1995.

42. Christiansen SP, Bradford JD: Cataract in infants treated with argon laser photocoagulation for threshold retinopathy of prematurity. Am J Ophthalmol 119(2):175–180, 1995.

43. Pogrebniak AE, Bolling JP, Stewart MW: Argon laser-induced cataract in an infant with retinopathy of prematurity (Letter). Am J Ophthalmol 117(2):261–222, 1994.

44. Capone A Jr, Drack AV: Transient lens changes after diode laser retinal photocoagulation for retinopathy of prematurity (Letter). Am J Ophthalmol 118(4):533–535, 1994.

45. Hunt L: Complications of indirect laser photocoagulation. Insight 19(4):24–25, 1994.

46. Brown GC, Tasman WS, Naidoff M, et al: Systemic complications associated with retinal cryoablation for retinopathy of prematurity. Ophthalmology 97(7):855–858, 1990.

47. Greven CM, Tasman W: Rhegmatogenous retinal detachment following cryotherapy in retinopathy of prematurity. Arch Ophthalmol 107(7):1017–1018, 1989.

48. Gallo JE, Fagerholm P: Low-grade myopia in children with regressed retinopathy of prematurity. Acta Ophthalmol 71(4):519–523, 1993.
49. Page JM, Schneeweiss S, Whyte HE, Harvey P: Ocular sequelae in premature infants (Review). Pediatrics 92(6): 787–790, 1993.
50. Maly E: Frequency and natural history of retinopathy of prematurity; a prospective study in a Swedish city, 1986–1990. Acta Ophthalmol 210(Suppl):52–55, 1993.
51. Nissenkorn I, Yasur Y, Mashkowski D, et al: Myopia in premature babies with and without retinopathy of prematurity. Br J Ophthalmol 67(3):170–173, 1983.
52. Ben-Sira I, Nissenkorn I, Weinberger D, et al: Long-term results of cryotherapy for active states of retinopathy of prematurity. Ophthalmology 93(11):1423–1428, 1986.
53. Robinson R, O'Keefe M: Follow-up study on premature infants with and without retinopathy of prematurity. Br J Ophthalmol 77(2):91–94, 1993.
54. Quinn GE, Dobson V, Repka MX, et al: Development of myopia in infants with birth weights less than 1251 grams; the Cryotherapy for Retinopathy of Prematurity Cooperative Group. Ophthalmology 99(3):329–340, 1992.
55. Cats BP, Tan KE: Prematures with or without regressed retinopathy of prematurity; comparison of long-term (6–10 years) ophthalmological morbidity. J Pediatr Ophthalmol Strabismus 26(6):271–275, 1989.
56. Summers G, Phelps DL, Tung B, Palmer EA: Ocular cosmesis in retinopathy of prematurity; the Cryotherapy for Retinopathy of Prematurity Cooperative Group. Arch Ophthalmol 110(8):1092–1097, 1992.
57. Snir M, Nissenkorn I, Sherf I, et al: Visual acuity, strabismus, and amblyopia in premature babies with and without retinopathy of prematurity. Ann Ophthalmol 20:256–258, 1988.
58. Mintz-Hittner HA, Kretzer FL: Postnatal retinal vascularization in former preterm infants with retinopathy of prematurity. Ophthalmology 101(3):548–558, 1994.
59. Machemer R: Late traction detachment in retinopathy of prematurity or ROP-like cases. Graefes Arch Clin Exp Ophthalmol 231:389–394, 1993.
60. Sneed SR, Pulido JS, Blodi CF, et al: Surgical management of late-onset retinal detachments associated with regressed retinopathy of prematurity. Ophthalmology 97(2):179–183, 1990.
61. Takayama S, Tachibana H, Yamamoto M: Changes in the visual field after photocoagulation or cryotherapy in children with retinopathy of prematurity. J Pediatr Ophthalmol Strabismus 28(2):96–100, 1991.
62. Luna B, Dobson V, Carpenter NA, Biglan AW: Visual field development in infants with stage 3 retinopathy of prematurity. Invest Ophthalmol Vis Sci 30(3):580–582, 1989.
63. Quinn GE, Miller DL, Avins JA, et al: Measurement of Goldmann visual fields in older children who received cryotherapy as infants for threshold retinopathy of prematurity. Arch Ophthalmol 114:425–428, 1996.

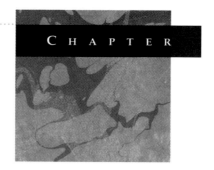

CHAPTER 33

Eales' Disease

Hermann D. Schubert, M.D.

Eales' disease is an idiopathic occlusive vasculopathy that affects the peripheral retinal vasculature, leading to retinal nonperfusion, extraretinal neovascularization, and vitreous hemorrhage.

The disease is quite rare in America, more common in India and parts of the Middle East, and definite regional variations in prevalence seem to exist. Since the etiology of this condition is unknown, the reasons for the variation remain speculative, even though it has been often linked to the prevalence of tuberculous infection.

Another reason for its rarity in some locations may be the increasing identification of secondary causes of peripheral retinal neovascularization making the primary disease less frequent after extensive medical surveys. One might therefore assume that the eponym has long outlived its usefulness, yet it has remained in widespread use and may reveal to be an attractive diagnosis in the age of managed care. Since for the above reasons the eponym may be here to stay, we should re-examine what Eales actually described in his two publications.[1,2]

THE DISEASE ACCORDING TO EALES

"Cases of retinal hemorrhage, associated with epistaxis and constipation" (1880) contains a description of the original five patients (Table 33–1), subsequently summarized and reinterpreted.[2] The cases shared the symptoms of constipation, epistaxis, and tortuous distended retinal vessels; however, "in no case was there any evidence of primary retinitis, or any constitutional disease, such as syphilis, leucocythaemia, anaemia, to account for the hemorrhage."[1] The constipation was considered as the starting point of all other phenomena, females were saved by their menstruation.[1]

"Primary retinal hemorrhage in young men" (1882) contains a summary of four of the above patients and three less completely recorded ones. Eales emphasized the recurrent nature of the hemorrhages, the glistening patches of retinal degeneration, the vascular fullness and corkscrew pattern, as well as elevated veins. He felt that the hemorrhages originated from the venous radicles or capillaries. There were no associated systemic findings, except for dyspepsia, low spirits, want of energy, feelings of lassitude, and frequent frontal headaches, "a neurosis inherited in the male line." Most importantly, however, "in no case has any condition like retinitis been seen to precede or accompany these hemorrhages."[2]

THE PROBLEMATIC DEFINITIONS OF VASCULITIS, SHEATHING, AND VITRITIS

It is the more surprising that the angiopathy without features of inflammation that Eales actually described and the vasculitis that he did not describe have become synonymous.

The main two areas of inconsistency in subsequent publications concern the concepts of sheathing of vessels and of vitritis.

Sheathing is derived from sheath: a tubular structure enclosing or surrounding some organ or part[3] and refers to a whitish appearing perivascular accumulation of cells. These cells can be either mainly inflammatory or mainly glial depending on the number of cells, intensity, and stage of the disease process. Any repair following vaso-obliteration must share some features of inflammation in the acute and subacute stage and the end result should be glial sheathing of obliterated vessels, vascular remodeling, and reactive gliosis of the avascular ischemic retina.

415

TABLE 33-1 Clinical Findings in Eales' Original Five Patients (1880)

A	B	C	D	E	F
Case	1	2	3	4	5
Age	16	19	20	14	29
Epistaxis	+	+	+	+	+
Constipation	+	+	+	+	−
Syphilis	−	−	−	?	−
Symptoms	−	Bilious attack	Headache	Headache	Alcoholism
Ocular findings	Cloud OS, Full, threadlike vessels, glaucoma	Blind OS, Veins full, recurrent hemorrhages	Vitreous opacities	Opacities OS, Full, tortuous vessels, hemorrhages	Blind OD, Full, tortuous vessels OS opacities
Vasculitis	None	None	None	None	None

OS, left eye; OD, right eye.

It is of note that Eales did not describe perivasculitis, arteriolitis, or phlebitis.[1,2] Neither did he describe vitritis per se, even though any hemorrhage into the vitreous represents a breakdown of the blood ocular barrier and, depending on duration and infiltration by macrophages, may be interpreted as mild vitritis.

Keeping the above in mind, when using the eponym, one is somewhat bound by the original description in judging idiopathic recurrent vitreous hemorrhages that are related to peripheral retinal nonperfusion after an extensive negative medical work-up.

Eales' disease therefore should be reserved for the *idiopathic* peripheral occlusive vasculopathy. Phenotypically it should be a *noninflammatory* disorder of retinal vascular walls, leading to atrophy, remodeling, and glial sheathing of the peripheral vasculature (Fig. 33-1).

EALES' DISEASE (TRUE EALES')

Spitznas identified a subgroup of peripheral vasculopathy that closely resembled Eales' original description and called it "true Eales."[4] The angiography of these patients revealed microaneurysms, capillary dilation, and remodeling in a rope-ladder pattern as well as vascular tortuosity. The avascular areas were associated with formation of new vessels in 84% and vitreous hemorrhage in 54%. The patients were mostly males (3:1) of an average age at presentation of 41 years and the disease was mostly bilateral. There was no evidence of inflammation.

IDIOPATHIC PERIPHERAL RETINAL VASCULITIS (SO-CALLED EALES')

Spitznas juxtaposed a second group of patients. Just as in true Eales', the peripheral vasculitis remained idiopathic after an extensive medical work-up and it led to recurrent vitreous hemorrhages. The main difference was seen in the extent of sheathing and the infiltration of the vitreous by inflammatory cells. The sheathing of predominantly veins was massive, broad, and fluffy; there was perivascular exudate, which spilled into the vitreous. The inflammatory process led to secondary obliteration of vessels, retinal nonperfusion, neovascularization, and vitreous hemorrhage. Unilateral involvement was more frequent, and unlike true Eales', the sex distribution was equal.[4]

THE CLINICAL MANIFESTATION OF MANY DISEASED CONDITIONS (EALES'-LIKE)

Duke Elder and the majority of authors considered the clinical entity of Eales' disease[6] more like a clinical spectrum[5] at the core of which was idiopathic peripheral retinovascular occlusion (inflammatory or not) followed by extraretinal neovascularization and vitreous hemorrhage.

This approach lumped all peripheral occlusive vasculopathies and separated them from phenotypically similar conditions that were often not limited to the eye and for which an etiology or at least association could be found (see "Differential Diagnosis" below).

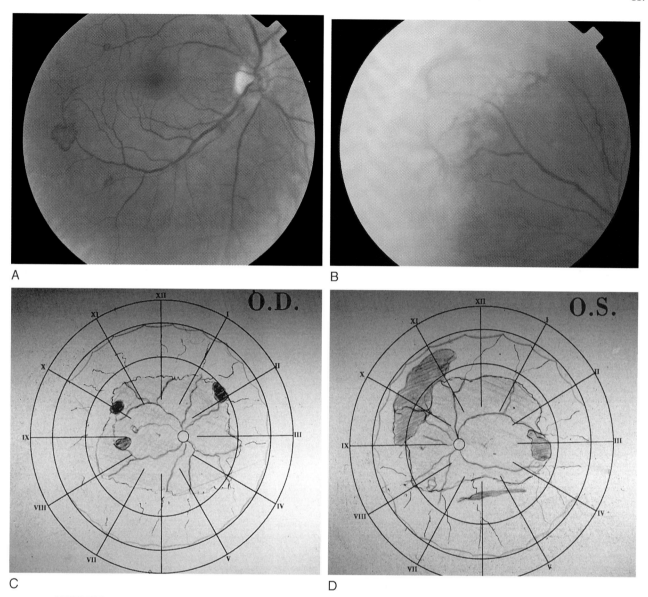

FIGURE 33–1   A 31-year-old woman who presented with a vitreous hemorrhage in her left eye. *A* and *B*, Funduscopic photos show the flat and elevated extraretinal neovascularization. *C* and *D*, Fundus drawings show the extent of peripheral nonperfusion. *Illustration continued on following page*

Since this approach (albeit somewhat removed from Henry Eales) is not only widespread but is also of practical use, it will provide the frame of the discussion of the clinical manifestations of Eales'-like peripheral occlusive vasculopathies.

PRESENTATION

Typically, an otherwise healthy young man notices blurring or a vitreous floater in one eye. Most frequently the symptom occurs upon awakening or after periods of relative quietness, but has also been noted after exertion (this is where hemorrhages in constipated individuals, prone to Valsalva mechanisms, may fit in). The age of onset ranges from 17 to 44 years[6–8] with a mean at age 30[4] or 40.[9]

The presentation is usually unilateral but will involve the second eye in half to two thirds of cases[6] or as frequently as in 29 of 32 cases.[9] Bilateral involvement suggests Eales' disease as opposed to a primary vasculitic process.[4] The interval between the involvement of the first and second eye was found to be 2.9 years by Elliot.[6] Eventually, the typical case of Eales therefore is bilateral.

COURSE

Since the retinal abnormality is peripheral and does not involve the macula, central visual acuity is determined by the extent and density of the vitreous opacity. This makes visual acuity a poor indicator

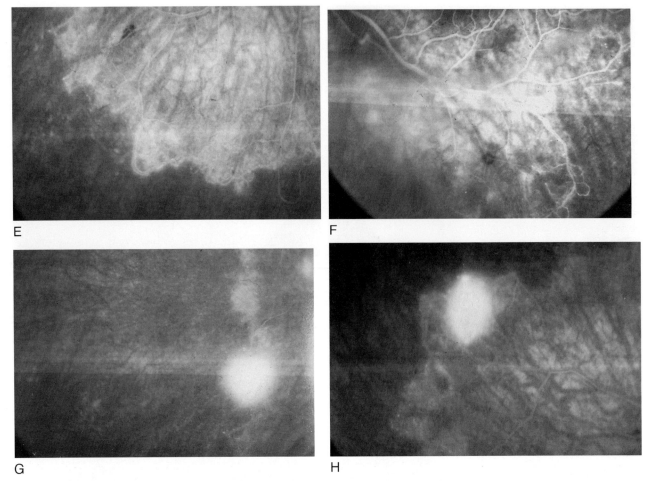

E   F

G   H

FIGURE 33–1 *Continued   E* through *H*, The angiogram demonstrates the vascular remodeling, sharp border of perfused to nonperfused retina, as well as neovascularization. Note the absence of vitritis and sheathing in quiet eyes that see 20/25. Whereas the presentation is one of true Eales', it must be considered Eales'-like after the discovery of anticardiolipin antibody. Even better, it should be called an occlusive peripheral vasculopathy associated with anticardiolipin syndrome.

of the overall extent of retinal disease.[6] With increasing duration, however, recurrent hemorrhages that never completely clear are the rule.

PROGNOSIS

Prior to vitrectomy the prognosis was considered serious.[5] In a long-term study of 46 eyes, Elliot found 54% of patients to have good vision (20/20 to 20/50), 20% with fair vision (20/60 to 20/200), and 26% with poor (<20/200) vision.[6] In a more recent report, 16% of patients were legally blind.[9] The visual outcome after modern vitrectomy and endolaser should be substantially better but has not been reported.

BIOMICROSCOPIC FINDINGS

Typically, there should be no signs of anterior uveitis and the vitreous should contain red not white cells. The pertinent findings should be found in the peripheral (temporal) retina and include venous tortuosity, vascular remodeling, vascular occlusions, and sheathing of arteries and veins. There is no firm rule as to what represents sheathing (see above) or whether or not arteries should be involved. Both phenomena may be modified by the time course, the stage at presentation, and the intensity of the disease process. It is possible that initially there is only vascular occlusion/incompetence, followed by sheathing to ultimately result in a glial scar. Mild inflammation might prefer veins, more severe inflammation might also involve arteries.

The presentation may include hemorrhages in the retina and vitreous as well as exudates.[6–9] Hemorrhage may occur from dilated tortuous vessels. New extraretinal vessels may form in the periphery; however, they are not necessary to induce a hemorrhage.

STAGES

The course of the disease is somewhat predictable and has been arbitrarily divided into four stages.[10]

Eales' 1 is characterized by ladder-like capillaries and mild periphlebitis in the retinal periphery. Larger vessels are involved in stage 2. Eales' 3 features new vessels and hemorrhages into retina and vitreous. Stage 4 involves the formation of scar tissue possibly leading to retinal detachment.

ANGIOGRAPHY

The angiogram shows most elements of a branch vein occlusion,[11] including vascular dilation, tortuosity, staining, occlusion, areas of nonperfusion, microaneurysms, and vascular remodeling. The dilations of capillaries have been termed rope-ladder-like.[4] New vessels are frequently found (84%), often associated with hemorrhage (58%), which will make angiography impossible in many cases.[4]

PATHOLOGY

Since Eales' is a disease of otherwise healthy young people, little pathologic material has become available, particularly of the early stages, which might give reliable pathogenetic clues. Elliot[6] found little if any inflammatory reaction in the retinal vessels in the early stages. The only abnormality was hyaline thickening of the walls of small vessels. Most studies show the late stages in which perivascular mononuclear infiltrates and vascular occlusions in addition to the secondary changes of hemorrhages, exudation, and cicatrization are predominant.[6] Traction rhegmatogenous retinal detachment and hemorrhagic or neovascular glaucoma are rare final events.

DIFFERENTIAL DIAGNOSIS

The differential diagnosis of peripheral occlusive vasculopathy is extensive and even more so after inclusion of peripheral vasculitides. A practical short list would include the more frequent and/or treatable entities like peripheral vein occlusions, sarcoidosis, lupus erythematosus, temporal arteritis, multiple sclerosis, pars planitis, and familial exudative vitreoretinopathy.

A basic work-up should include fasting blood glucose, chest radiograph, erythrocyte sedimentation rate, antinuclear antibody, rheumatoid factor, LE cell preparation, and tuberculoprotein sensitivity testing.[9] Another approach emphasizes a careful history and physical examination. If the patient has no signs or symptoms of an associated disease, then the evaluation should be limited to a fluorescein angiogram, complete blood count, erythrocyte sedimentation rate, urinalysis, fluorescent treponemal antibody absorption test (FTA-ABS), rapid plasma reagent, and a chest roentgenogram.[12] More guided

tests were not only found to be more cost effective but fewer tests also reduced the risk of false positives, potentially complicating the "shotgun" approach.

More comprehensive are the following pathogenetic subgroups:

> *Embolism*: Cardiac valvular disease,[13] mitral valve prolapse,[14] atrial myxoma, cardiac dysrhythmia, atheromatous disease[15]
> *Blood dyscrasias*: Clotting disorders,[16] protein C deficiency (Fig. 33–1), sickle cell disease, leukemia
> *Vasculitis*: Sarcoidosis, tuberculosis, syphilis, systemic viral infections, pars planitis, temporal arteritis, polyarteritis nodosa, Takayasu's disease, lupus erythematosus, Wegener's disease, multiple sclerosis, Behçets'disease, toxoplasmosis, cytomegalic inclusion disease,[17] polymyositis, dermatomyositis, Whipple's disease, Crohn's disease, multiple sclerosis[12]
> *Developmental*: Retinopathy of prematurity, familial exudative vitreoretinopathy

ASSOCIATION

A link to multiple sclerosis has not been confirmed.[9] An association with vestibulocochlear disease has been described[9,18] thought to be due to microangiopathy[19] that affects both eye and ear. In "true" Eales', however, there should be no associated systemic finding.[2]

ETIOLOGY

The etiology is obscure. An allergy to tuberculoprotein has been implicated most frequently and remains the most commonly held "aetiological belief of the observer." A detailed historical review of these suppositions has been provided by Donders.[5]

TREATMENT

Since the etiology is not known, there is no specific therapy. After the appearance of favorable reports using diathermy even without visualization of the fundus (coagulation à ciel couvert),[20] Meyer-Schwickerath pioneered light coagulation in eyes where a view of the fundus could be obtained.[21] With a follow-up of 2.9 years, 124 of 143 eyes had no recurrence of vitreous hemorrhage. At 5 years 91% had anatomic and 87% had visual stabilization. The incidence of macular pucker was 3%. Hemorrhage and retinal detachment were infrequent complications of the coagulation.[22]

Most of the literature on Eales' disease predates modern vitreoretinal treatment methods. The introduction of vitrectomy and argon endolaser has brought further improvements in a disease that formerly often led to long-term hospitalization in a sanatorium for chronic eye diseases.[5] Donders reviewed 44 sometimes drastic treatment methods, including bloodletting, cobra venom, splenectomy, radiation, intravitreal hemolysin, and ligation of the common carotid artery.[5] The anecdotal reports of hemolysin and radiation treatment are of note in view of the renewed interest in the use of plasmin and radiation for ocular neovascular conditions.

THE CONTINUING STRUGGLE WITH THE DEFINITION OF EALES' DISEASE

It was Elliot's opinion that "the original descriptions by Eales' in his classic report have not been improved on,"[8] which implies that the original description was clear to everybody and unambiguous. In subsequent publications the disease has been termed not only classic,[14] true,[4] and documented[9] but also atypical,[14] so-called,[21] sometimes referred to as Eales.[17] Others felt that it was a long-recognized but poorly understood disease.[9]

Therefore the student of Eales' disease will find formulations such as "when we say Eales' disease," "we include,"[5] "is now considered to be,"[15] "our current understanding of,"[12] all suggesting that our concept is indeed evolving. A working definition that is close to Eales' description might be helpful as a home base in a time of change.

CONCLUSION

Eales' disease is an idiopathic occlusive vasculopathy that affects the peripheral retinal vessels. As such, it should remain a diagnosis of exclusion.

To deserve the eponym (instead of the more descriptive "occlusive peripheral vasculopathy of unknown origin") it should occur in the "young" (around 40), should have no signs of anterior uveitis, and suffer recurrent vitreous hemorrhages. The overall funduscopic finding should be consistent with a primary noninflammatory disorder of retinal vascular walls (i.e., a vasculopathy characterized by only mild sheathing and without vitritis). Bilateral involvement would also support a diagnosis of Eales' disease.

Eales'-like conditions including peripheral vasculitis with vitreous hemorrhage should be differentiated from (true) Eales' disease. Eales'-like conditions would tend to be unilateral and would

either be idiopathic ("primary") or associated with a known cause.

Only the first idiopathic and "noninflammatory" group, however, should carry the eponym until more is known about retinal vasculopathies and a more definitive diagnosis can be made.

REFERENCES

1. Eales, H: Cases of retinal haemorrhage, associated with epistaxis and constipation. Birmingham Med Rev 9:262–273, 1880.
2. Eales, H: Primary retinal hemorrhage in young men. Ophthalmol Rev 1:41–46, 1882.
3. Dorlands Illustrated Medical Dictionary, 25th edition. Philadelphia, WB Saunders Co, 1974.
4. Spitznas M, Meyer-Schwickerath G, Stephan B: The clinical picture of Eales disease. Graefe's Arch Klin Exp Ophthalmol 194:73–85, 1975.
5. Donders PC: Eales' disease. Doc Ophthalmol 12:1–74, 1958.
6. Elliot AJ: Recurrent intraocular hemorrhage in young adults (Eales's disease). A report of thirty-one cases. Trans Am Ophthalmol Soc 52:811–875, 1954.
7. Elliot AJ, Harris GS: The present status of the diagnosis and treatment of periphlebitis retinae (Eales' disease). Can J Ophthalmol 4:117–122, 1969.
8. Elliot AJ: 30-year observation of patients with Eales's disease. Am J Ophthalmol 80:404–408, 1975.
9. Renie W, Murphy R, Anderson K, et al: The evaluation of patients with Eales' disease. Retina 3:243–248, 1983.
10. Charamis J: On the classification and management of the evolutionary course of Eales' disease. Trans Ophthalmol Soc UK 85:157–160, 1965.
11. Wise G, Dollery C, Henkind P: The Retinal Circulation. New York, Harper & Row, 1971, pp 377–381.
12. George R, Walton C, Whitcup S, Nussenblatt R: Primary retinal vasculitis. Systemic associations and diagnostic evaluation. Ophthalmology 103:384–389, 1996.
13. Kelley J, Randall H: Peripheral retinal neovascularization in rheumatic fever. Arch Ophthalmol 97:81–83, 1979.
14. Caltrider N, Irvine A, Kline H, Rosenblatt A: Retinal emboli in patients with mitral valve prolapse. Am J Opthalmol 90:534–539, 1980.
15. Patrinely J, Green W, Randolph M: Retinal phlebitis with chorioretinal emboli. Am J Ophthalmol 94:49–57, 1982.
16. Savir H, Wender T, Creter, Djaldetti M: Bilateral retinal vasculitis associated with clotting disorders. Am J Ophthalmol 84:542–547, 1977.
17. Jampol L, Isenberg S, Goldberg M: Occlusive retinal arteriolitis with neovascularization. Am J Ophthalmol 81:583–589, 1976.
18. Delaney W, Torrisi P: Occlusive retinal vascular disease and deafness. Am J Ophthalmol 82:232–236, 1976.
19. Pfaffenbach D, Hollenhorst R: Microangiopathy of the retinal arterioles. JAMA 225:480–483, 1973.
20. Franceschetti A: Coagulation diathermique transclerale dans la maladie d'Eales. Probl Actuels Ophthalmol 4:2–9, 1966.
21. Meyer-Schwickerath G: Eales' disease treatment with light coagulation. Mod Probl Ophthalmol 4:10–18, 1966.
22. Spitznas M, Meyer-Schwickerath G, Stephan B: Treatment of Eales' disease with photocoagulation. Graefes Arch Klin Exp Ophthalmol 194:193–198, 1975.

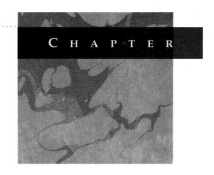

Familial Exudative Vitreoretinopathy

Carl D. Regillo, M.D.

Familial exudative vitreoretinopathy (FEVR) is a hereditary disorder first described by Criswick and Schepens[1] in 1969. They reported six cases from two families with bilateral vitreoretinal abnormalities that resembled various stages of retinopathy of prematurity (ROP), but lacked a history of premature birth or perinatal problems. The major ocular manifestations included peripheral neovascularization, peripheral retinal traction with temporal dragging, falciform folds or detachments, and lipid exudation. The familial nature of the condition and presence of active, progressive neovascularization at an older age in some patients served to help distinguish this previously unrecognized entity from ROP.

Two years later, in 1971, Gow and Oliver[2] published a report on a large pedigree with multiple members affected by FEVR. They identified an autosomal dominant hereditary pattern and expanded upon the spectrum of ocular findings. They emphasized the importance of the peripheral vascular abnormalities and were concerned about the potential for progression, regardless of the patient's age. A three-stage clinical classification was proposed.

In 1976, Canny and Oliver[3] demonstrated peripheral retinal nonperfusion in four cases of FEVR. This supported the concept that the condition was primarily vascular in nature, with the various vitreal changes and traction on the retina probably representing a secondary phenomenon, analogous to ROP. The zone of avascular peripheral retina was later verified by several other investigators and the important role of fluorescein angiography to help identify mildly affected eyes became apparent.[4–7]

Since 1980, many other articles have appeared in the literature on FEVR. Over 200 cases from more than 30 families have been reported. Much has been learned about the genetics, the various phenotypic expressions, and the natural history of the condition. However, despite these advances, pathogenesis and management remain uncertain.

CLINICAL FEATURES

From the first descriptions, it was recognized that the fundus manifestations of FEVR vary greatly among affected patients. Gow and Oliver[2] divided their findings into three clinical stages. Originally, however, this classification scheme did not incorporate what is now known to be the hallmark of the disease, an avascular peripheral retina. It has, therefore, since been modified to include this sometimes subtle peripheral finding which is consistently present, even in the earliest stages.[3,5] The three stages describe the mild, moderate, and severe forms of FEVR, respectively, and can be seen in patients of any age.[7–9] Although most eyes exhibit progression if followed long enough, the rate varies considerably and not all eyes progress through all stages.[6,7,10] The disease is a bilateral process, but because there can be intrapatient progression rate variability, asymmetry is not unusual.[10]

Stage 1

In this mildest form of FEVR, patients typically have good visual acuity and are asymptomatic. Nonproliferative, peripheral retinal vascular abnormalities are essentially all that manifest at this stage. A variably sized zone of avascular retina is consistently present and is most prominent in the temporal periphery, but may extend for 360 de-

421

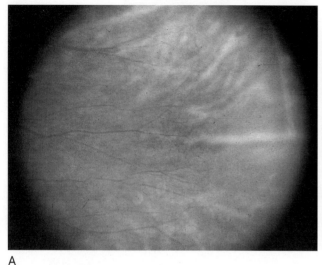
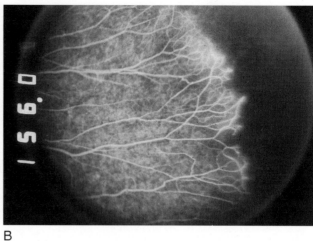

A   B

FIGURE 34–1   The temporal periphery of an asymptomatic patient of FEVR. *A,* The avascular zone is seen as a gray area on the right side of the fundus photograph. *B,* Lack of retinal perfusion is confirmed with fluorescein angiography. Note the straightening and increased branching of the peripheral vessels and the arteriovenous shunts at the border that exhibit mild leakage of fluorescein dye. (Courtesy of Jerry Shields, M.D.)

grees.[4,7,11] In many cases, the temporal zone, especially when broad, assumes a V shape with the apex of the V located in the horizontal meridian and pointed posteriorly.[12]

Near the border of the avascular zone, a variety of associated nonproliferative vascular changes can be seen. There is usually excessive branching of retinal blood vessels, with the increased number of vessels assuming a near parallel or straightened appearance as they approach the border (Fig. 34–1).[1,6,12,13] Vascular sheathing or dilation is sometimes present (Fig. 34–2). At the border itself, vessels either end in a brush-like configuration or form variable caliber arteriovenous shunts.[4–7,12,13] Angiographically, there is typically leakage of fluorescein

dye from the capillaries or shunts at the margin of vascularized and nonvascularized retina (Fig. 34–1).[3–5,7,12,13] Angiographic studies have also shown the presence of mildly dilated capillaries in the posterior pole which can exhibit late leakage in the macular and peripapillary regions.[4,6]

Ophthalmoscopically, the peripheral vascular changes may be difficult to appreciate. Detection of the avascular zone itself may be facilitated with the use of a green filter over the light source of the indirect ophthalmoscope as the resultant red-free light accentuates the color difference between vascularized and nonvascularized retina.[7] Although fluorescein angiography will help establish the lack of peripheral retinal vascularization along with some of the associated retinal vascular changes, adequate peripheral views can be technically difficult and will not be feasible in very young patients unless under anesthesia.

In a recent series by Benson[10] with 39 patients in 22 families, stage 1 changes alone were identified in 34 of 78 (44%) eyes (Table 34–1). Early reports, especially before the value of angiography was realized, may have underestimated the prevalence of this stage, as these mildly affected family members can be easily overlooked. An important difference between this stage of FEVR and a similar appearing stage of ROP is that the peripheral retina in FEVR never vascularizes over time, unlike the majority of ROP cases.

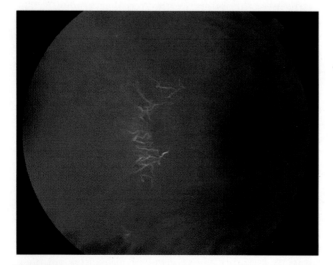

FIGURE 34–2   Sclerosed retinal vessels marking the border of perfused and nonperfused retina in the temporal periphery of an eye with stage 1 FEVR.

Stage 2

In this stage, both proliferative and exudative changes are encountered. Limited traction or exu-

TABLE 34–1 Presenting Ocular Features of Familial Exudative Vitreoretinopathy*

Ocular Findings	Percentage of Eyes Involved
Avascular zone only	44%
Active peripheral neovascularization	18%
Subretinal or intraretinal lipid exudation	22%
Localized peripheral retinal detachment	15%
Falciform fold	26%
Total retinal detachment	13%

* Adapted from Benson WE: Familial exudative vitreoretinopathy. Trans Am Ophthalmol Soc 93:473–521, 1995, with permission.

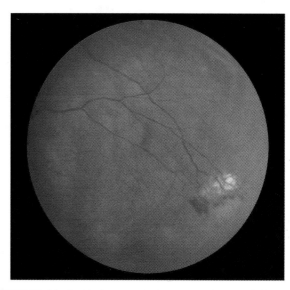

FIGURE 34–3 Early stage 2 disease with a small focus of fibrovascular tissue evident in the peripheral retina.

dative retinal detachments can also be seen. In addition to the avascular zone and associated retinal vascular abnormalities present in stage 1, retinal neovascularization at the border of perfused and nonperfused retina is the feature common to most of the manifestations in this stage (Figs. 34–3 and 34–4).[3,5] Frank extraretinal fibrovascular proliferation has been reported to be present in 17 to 20% of eyes in various large FEVR series.[10,11,13] In younger patients, the vascular component typically predominates, appearing reddish in color. In older patients, it takes on a more fibrotic character, but is not necessarily completely regressed or inactive.[10,11] The neovascularization sometimes assumes a large, fibrovascular mass configuration. Pigmentary alter-

ations are sometimes seen around these larger, neovascular foci, probably related to either traction or leakage with secondary retinal pigment epithelial disruption.[5]

The presence of neovascularization is often associated with changes that can affect visual acuity such as traction with retinal dragging or detachment, intra- or subretinal exudation, and hemorrhage (Figs. 34–5 and 34–6). The neovascularization itself in some cases may not be evident, as these secondary manifestations may predominate and obscure its presence.[10,11] Although neovascularization is likely to lead to such vision-threatening complications, especially when extensive or mass-like, it does not always portend a poor prognosis.[10] There have been several reports of patients, espe-

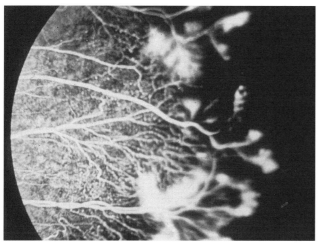

A

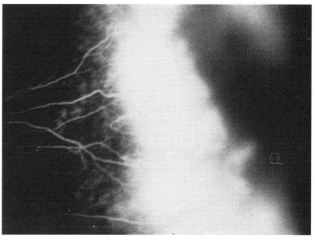

B

FIGURE 34–4 The left eye of an asymptomatic patient with FEVR. Early- (A) and late- (B) phase fluorescein angiogram photographs showing extensive leakage of dye from multiple fronds of retinal neovascularization along the border of perfused and nonperfused retina. (Courtesy of Jerry Shields, M.D.)

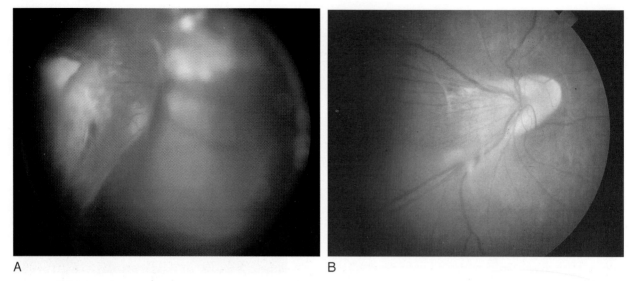

A   B

FIGURE 34–5   The right eye of a 19-year-old female with FEVR and 20/60 visual acuity. Advanced fibro-vascular proliferation is evident in the temporal periphery associated with (A) localized traction retinal detachment, lipid exudation, preretinal hemorrhage, and (B) temporal dragging of the macula and peripapillary retina. (Courtesy of James Augsburger, M.D.)

cially of older age, with isolated peripheral neovascularization and no significant ocular sequelae on limited follow-up.[6,8,14]

Strong vitreoretinal adhesion with evidence for traction is commonly found in this stage. Some degree of temporal dragging of the retina is seen in 18 to 49% of affected eyes.[11,13] Peripheral nonrhegmatogenous retinal detachment is another common manifestation of this stage, reported to be present in 15 to 17% of eyes.[10,13] Although both traction and exudative retinal detachments have been described, some element of both typically coexist, and, therefore, published reports tend to group them together. Such a mixed pattern of detachments is not unique to FEVR, as it has also been seen in ROP and juvenile retinoschisis.[15,16] Intraretinal or sub-

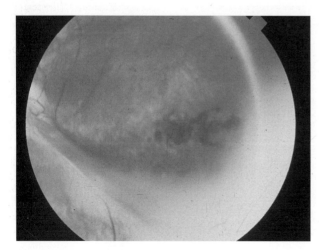

FIGURE 34–6   A prominent falciform fold in a child with FEVR. The inferotemporally directed fold is associated with marked retinal pigment epithelial disruption in the posterior pole. (Courtesy of William Tasman, M.D.)

retinal lipid exudate is present in FEVR without frank retinal detachment in 9% of eyes.[11] The presence of any lipid exudate in all affected eyes, however, is as high as 22% (Table 34–1).[10]

Stage 3

This stage represents the most severely affected eyes. It consists mainly of various types of retinal detachments or dragging that involves the macula and results in poor visual outcomes. In some cases, the temporally located peripheral vitreoretinal traction progresses primarily in an anteroposterior direction and causes increasing retinal elevation that spreads into the macula or involves the whole retina. In others, the traction has a more prominent tangential component and culminates in massive temporal retinal dragging or falciform fold formation (Fig. 34–6).[17-19] The traction phenomenon can also lead to retinal holes and rhegmatogenous detachments (Fig. 34–7). The subretinal exudation, which also typically starts in the temporal periphery, may become so extensive as to dominate the presentation and cause total retinal detachments that resemble Coats' disease. Visually significant vitreous hemorrhage from retinal neovascularization is a surprisingly rare manifestation.[11] Anterior segment changes such as cataract, neovascular glaucoma, and band keratopathy are secondary in nature and may be seen in FEVR as with other conditions that lead to longstanding, total retinal detachments.

Retinal detachment, in general, is relatively common in FEVR. The prevalence of all types of retinal detachments in published series ranges from 20 to 32%, with total detachment found in about 13% of

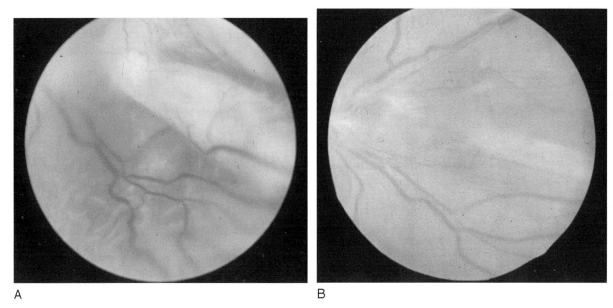

A   B

FIGURE 34–7   *A*, An acute rhegmatogenous retinal detachment in the left eye of an 18-year-old patient with known FEVR and pre-existing temporal dragging. *B*, After scleral buckling surgery, the retina is completely flat, but significant temporal dragging of the macula persists. (From Benson WE: Familial exudative vitreoretinopathy. Trans Am Ophthalmol Soc 93:473–521, 1995, with permission.)

cases.[10,13,20,21] Nonrhegmatogenous retinal detachments are more common in younger patients, often presenting by the end of the first decade of life, whereas rhegmatogenous detachments are more often found in older individuals.[21] Some series suggest that rhegmatogenous detachments may be more common than nonrhegmatogenous ones.[13,21] The causative breaks are typically small atrophic holes in avascular retina, but flap tears of various sizes, even giant retinal tears, may also be found.[5,11,20] Advanced proliferative vitreoretinopathy has been reported in the spectrum of rhegmatogenous retinal detachments.[20] Overall, retinal detachments, regardless of the type, are rarely seen presenting beyond the third decade of life.[12,20]

Presentation and Prognosis

When FEVR was first recognized as a distinct clinical entity, investigators were concerned that the disease would prove to be progressive in most affected eyes and that visual prognosis would be universally poor.[1,2,9] As more data accumulated, great variability in both presenting manifestations and long-term outcome became evident.[6–8,10,11,13] Initial clinical findings based on the recently published series of patients with FEVR by Benson[10] are summarized in Table 34–1.

In general, about one half of all patients with FEVR are asymptomatic and the condition is recognized in these individuals after a family screening or, less often, routine examination.[6–8,10,11] They are found to have stage 1 or mild stage 2 disease. Infants usually present for evaluation of poor fixa-

tion, true or pseudostrabismus, or nystagmus. A more advanced stage of disease is present and this usually takes the form of a large nonrhegmatogenous retinal detachment or prominent falciform fold. Rarely, leukocoria from a total retinal detachment is the presenting sign (Fig. 34–8). Decreasing vision will bring the older patient to attention and this is typically from progressive retinal detachment (traction or rhegmatogenous), temporal retinal dragging, or lipid exudate extending into the macula. Of note is that some patients with macular ectopia do not experience reduced visual acuity

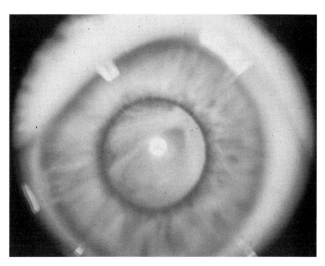

FIGURE 34–8   Leukocoria in an infant with FEVR. Note the clear lens and dense retrolental fibrovascular tissue. A total retinal detachment was evident ultrasonographically. (Courtesy of William Tasman, M.D.)

and only manifest pseudoexotropia with a positive angle kappa.[14]

Ultimate visual outcome is strongly influenced by age at onset of signs or symptoms. The extent and rate of deterioration is typically greatest in the youngest age group. Benson[10] found only 2 of 28 patients whose onset of symptoms were prior to their third birthday with a final visual acuity of 20/200 or better. Although progressive disease is well documented in older individuals, it tends to be relatively slow or limited in most, and major loss of vision is less common in those first presenting after the third decade of life.[6,7,10,11,20] Furthermore, in adults that do exhibit significant deterioration, the overall prognosis for retention of good visual acuity in at least one eye is fair, as the process tends to be more asymmetric than in the younger patients, and, therefore, one eye is often spared from an advanced stage of disease.[10]

HISTOPATHOLOGY

Histopathologic findings from both enucleated globes and vitrectomy specimens of patients with FEVR have been reported.[10,22–26] The globes analyzed to date were enucleated for indications of end-stage neovascular glaucoma, nonneovascular angle-closure glaucoma (from massive subretinal hemorrhage and secondary forward displacement of the lens-iris diaphragm), phthisis, and suspected retinoblastoma. All of these eyes, along with those in which tissue was obtained from vitrectomy surgery alone, had extensive retinal detachment and other stage 3 findings evident clinically.

In addition to changes in common to chronic detachments of any etiology, all of the enucleated globes examined histopathologically thus far have shown the presence of peripherally located, preretinal fibrovascular membranes. Intraretinal and subretinal exudates have been demonstrated in two cases.[24] Multiple adhesions of prominent preretinal or vitreous membranes to the peripheral retina with significant retinal folding was seen in one case.[22] Two cases also had evidence for necrosis and acute inflammation within the peripheral retina, the significance of which is unclear.[23,24] Other findings, mostly of the anterior segment, appeared secondary in nature and were not felt to be unique or directly related to the underlying disease.

Specimens obtained from vitrectomy surgery were epiretinal membranes in cases of traction retinal detachments.[10,26] As seen in the enucleated globes, the membranes were fibrovascular in nature. Electron microscopic analysis in two cases revealed the presence of myofibrocytes, fibrous astrocytes, and, surprisingly, blood vessels lined by endothelium with tight junctions.[26] The finding of nonfenestrated blood vessels in such tissue is difficult to explain given the ophthalmoscopic and angiographic evidence for at least some degree of vascular incompetence in affected eyes.

Unfortunately, no clinicopathologic correlations are available from eyes with earlier stages of disease. Without microscopic data on the full spectrum of presentations in FEVR, our understanding of the disease process is likely to remain limited.

PATHOGENESIS

Abnormal peripheral retinal vascularization appears to represent the primary pathobiologic feature of FEVR. This is based on the clinical observation that all affected eyes have a peripheral zone of avascularized retina and that the various stages of disease most resemble ROP. The difference in terms of time course and natural history of these two conditions probably resides in what triggers the cessation of retinal vascularization, which is permanent with FEVR and, in most cases, temporary with ROP.

The persistent avascular zone in FEVR translates into a continued risk for neovascularization throughout the life of the patient, and the larger the area of nonvascularized retina, the higher the likelihood of developing a significant degree of progressive neovascularization with secondary traction and late-stage manifestations.[10]

While searching for other factors that may contribute to disease progression, Chaudhuri and coworkers[27] found reduced platelet aggregation to arachidonic acid in patients with FEVR. They suggested that this defect could lead to reduced production of thromboxane A_2, a prostaglandin that may have a protective effect on immature retinal blood vessels. Abnormal platelet function, however, has not been corroborated by other investigators.[11,28,29]

GENETICS

The classic and still most commonly identified mode of inheritance in FEVR is that of an autosomal dominant transmission pattern.[2,4–8,10,14,25,30] Studies indicate nearly 100% penetrance with marked variation in expressivity.[6,25] Linkage analysis strongly suggests that the gene for the dominant form of the disease resides on the long arm of chromosome 11.[31,32] A genetic defect in this region that results in abnormal peripheral retinal vascularization is further supported by a recently reported isolated case of an infant with an 11q− syndrome that had bilateral retinal vascular abnormalities resembling FEVR.[33]

X-linked recessive inheritance and sporadic cases of FEVR have also been reported.[11,13,34–38] Plager and colleagues[34] were the first to recognize an X-linked recessive form of FEVR in a report published in 1992 and suggested that some earlier publications,

TABLE 34-2 Differential Diagnosis of Familial Exudative Vitreoretinopathy

Primary Ocular Manifestation	Diseases
Avascular peripheral retina (infancy)	ROP, IP
Total retinal detachment (infancy)	ROP, PHPV, Norrie's, IP, XLJR, idiopathic retinal dysplasia
Retinal dragging or folds	ROP, PHPV, Norrie's, IP, XLJR, toxocara, congenital falciform fold
Peripheral neovascularization (adults)	Sickle, Eales', pars planitis, miscellaneous retinovascular occlusive diseases
Intra- or subretinal lipid exudation	Coats', angiomatosis retinae, pars planitis

ROP, retinopathy of prematurity; IP, incontinentia pigmenti; XLJR, X-linked juvenile retinoschisis; PHPV, persistent hyperplastic primary vitreous.

including the original Criswick and Schepens series, had evidence for this mode of inheritance. Linkage analysis by Fullwood and associates[35] confirmed involvement of the X chromosome in a report published in 1993. They identified two possible loci on the X chromosome, one of which is the same as that of the Norrie's disease gene, and proposed that the phenotypes of both X-linked FEVR and Norrie's disease can come about from defects in the same gene. This concept was further supported by the findings of Chen and associates,[38] who later identified a specific mutation of the Norrie's disease gene in a FEVR pedigree. A recent review of all the reported FEVR cases suggested that the prognosis may be worse with the X-linked form of disease than with the autosomal dominant form.[39]

DIFFERENTIAL DIAGNOSIS

Familial exudative vitreoretinopathy can resemble many ocular conditions depending on the present-ing stage of disease and age of the patient. The differential diagnosis by the primary ocular manifestation is summarized in Table 34-2. The conditions that can most closely resemble or sometimes pose the greatest challenge to differentiate from FEVR are discussed in detail below and highlighted in Table 34-3.

Overall, the spectrum of findings in FEVR, especially when presenting in infancy, is most similar to ROP. Unlike ROP, patients with FEVR are expected to have a normal gestational length, birth weight, and neonatal history. Furthermore, in FEVR, there is frequently a history of visual loss or known disease in the family or various relatives found to be affected by formal screening examinations. Marked asymmetry and active neovascularization after infancy is unusual in ROP. Regression with vascularization of the peripheral retina is common in ROP but never observed in FEVR.[40,41] Lipid exudation is much more typical of FEVR than ROP.[10] Although high myopia is probably more common in ROP, reports show wide variation in refractive error in both conditions, and, therefore,

TABLE 34-3 Features of the Major Disorders that Most Closely Resemble Familial Exudative Vitreoretinopathy (FEVR)

Feature	FEVR	Retinopathy of Prematurity	Incontinentia Pigmenti	Norrie's Disease	Persistent Hyperplastic Primary Vitreous
Sex	Males = females	Males = females	Females only	Males only	Males = females
Inheritance	Dominant or X-linked recessive	None	X-linked dominant	X-linked recessive	None
Prematurity	No	Yes	No	No	No
Laterality	Bilateral	Bilateral	Bilateral	Bilateral	Unilateral
Microphthalmia	No	No	No	±	Yes
Avascular periphery	Yes	Yes	Yes	±	No
Retinal detachment	Yes	Yes	Yes	Yes	±
Systemic associations	No	±	Yes	Yes	No

contrary to what some investigators have suggested in the past, refractive error would not be expected to be a useful differentiating feature.[42]

Incontinentia pigmenti (IP) is a hereditary condition that can present with an avascular peripheral retina, with or without neovascularization, in both infancy and later in life. Both conditions can have rapidly progressive disease that results in retinal dragging or detachment and ocular findings that can be very asymmetric.[10,43-45] Although both diseases may be inherited in an X-linked fashion, IP is lethal in males and, therefore, only seen in females. The key to differentiating the two conditions, however, is the recognition of the systemic manifestations of IP, the most notable of which is the characteristic blistering skin changes that occur in the neonatal period.[44] It is important to note that the blisters are transient and the depigmentation that ensues often fades with time and may be inapparent in older children. Other systemic features of IP, which sometimes may also be subtle, include central nervous system abnormalities, dental hypoplasia, and alopecia.[44,45]

Juvenile retinoschisis and FEVR have in common peripheral vitreoretinal traction phenomenon that can result in dragged or detached retinas and vitreous hemorrhage.[46,47] Although both conditions are hereditary and lack systemic findings, juvenile retinoschisis is strictly X-linked. Ocular features of juvenile retinoschisis that serve to differentiate it from FEVR include the hallmark "spoke-wheel" foveal changes, the consistently decreased electroretinogram b wave, and the commonly seen inferior retinal schisis cavities.[46,47] Furthermore, peripheral neovascularization and lipid exudation, common in FEVR, are unusual findings in X-linked juvenile retinoschisis.[10,15,16,48]

When lipid exudation and exudative retinal detachment dominate the clinical picture, differentiating FEVR from Coats' disease can be sometimes difficult. Although peripheral retinal vascular abnormalities such as dilatation and nonperfusion are present in both conditions, "light-bulb"–shaped vascular outpouchings are characteristic of Coats' disease, whereas frank fibrovascular proliferation and secondary vitreoretinal traction are typical of FEVR.[49-51] Demographically, they also differ with Coats' disease, being nonfamilial, more common in males, and usually unilateral.

Both FEVR and persistent hyperplastic primary vitreous (PHPV) can present with total retinal detachment and retrolental fibrovascular tissue. The leukocoria that results, however, is typically present at birth with PHPV, and there are no other family members affected. Furthermore, PHPV is nearly always unilateral and usually associated with microphthalmia and ciliary processes that appear dragged toward the pupillary center.[52,53]

Norrie's disease is an uncommon, X-linked condition that can also closely resemble the advanced stages of FEVR. Bilateral falciform folds or retinal detachments in infancy are presentations common to both conditions.[54] Although microphthalmia and corneal opacification may sometimes be seen in Norrie's disease, the diagnosis may not be possible on the basis of the ocular exam alone if they are not evident. The clinician may have to rely on the associated findings of mental retardation and deafness with Norrie's disease to distinguish the two conditions.[55,56] Histopathologically, the diagnosis of Norrie's disease can be confirmed by demonstrating retinal dysplasia, a feature that has not been seen with FEVR. In the future, genetic analysis may be of further diagnostic utility in differentiating FEVR from Norrie's disease and other inherited diseases.

MANAGEMENT

All affected members of a given family with FEVR must be identified. The inheritance pattern can then be determined from the pedigree and appropriate genetic counseling then rendered.

Patients with stage 1 or early stage 2 disease in both eyes typically will be asymptomatic and will require close observation to monitor for progression. Patients must be followed for life and never considered free of risk for potentially serious late complications. Although older individuals are more likely to have a relatively stable course, good visual acuity into the teens or later is no guarantee that deterioration will not occur later in life. In the series of 39 patients with FEVR by Benson,[10] 5 patients developed retinal detachments 6 to 17 years after apparent stabilization.

Treatment to the avascular zone with cryotherapy or laser photocoagulation, analogous to ROP, should be considered in eyes with active fibrovascular proliferation, especially when there is progressive enlargement of the neovascular tissue or associated vision-threatening features such as lipid exudation or vitreous hemorrhage. Unfortunately, unlike ROP, there are no controlled clinical trials definitively demonstrating the efficacy of such treatments at any stage of FEVR. Successful stabilization or regression of the neovascularization or exudative sequelae has been reported by a number of investigators with the therapy directed to the avascular zone, the neovascular tissue, or both.[2,3,7,10,14,17,25] However, cases have been reported in which there has been no apparent effect despite aggressive ablation with both cryotherapy and laser therapy, and the treatment itself may occasionally lead to retinal breaks and detachments.[1,10,17] Because of the potential for complications with this treatment and because spontaneous regression can occur, small fronds of neovascularization should be observed.

Also like ROP, both scleral buckling and vitrectomy surgery have been utilized in FEVR cases to repair various types of retinal detachments that involve or threaten the macula. Together, several reports indicate that rhegmatogenous retinal detachments in FEVR have a reasonably good prognosis for reattachment and visual recovery with scleral buckling alone, despite the sometimes prominent vitreous traction component.[1,5,10,17,25] If, however, buckling fails to adequately support the breaks, vitrectomy with membrane peeling or dissection will be needed in combination with the scleral buckle. The success of either vitrectomy or scleral buckling for nonrhegmatogenous detachments has been variable.[10,11,14,25,34,57-60] A recently published series that utilized newer, lens-sparing techniques in children with FEVR showed encouraging anatomic and visual results in six eyes with macula involving traction retinal detachments.[26] Regardless of the type of detachment and the surgical technique utilized to repair it, eyes must be followed closely in the postoperative period for reproliferation of fibrovascular tissue or proliferative vitreoretinopathy, both of which can lead to redetachment.

REFERENCES

1. Criswick VG, Schepens CL: Familial exudative vitreoretinopathy. Am J Ophthalmol 68:578–594, 1969.
2. Gow J, Oliver GL: Familial exudative vitreoretinopathy: an expanded view. Arch Ophthalmol 86:150–155, 1971.
3. Canny CL, Oliver GL: Fluorescein angiographic findings in familial exudative vitreoretinopathy. Arch Ophthalmol 94:1114–1120, 1976.
4. Nijhuis FA, Deutman AF, Aan de Kerk AL: Fluorescein angiography in mild stages of dominant exudative vitreoretinopathy. Mod Probl Ophthalmol 20:107–114, 1979.
5. Laqua H: Familial exudative vitreoretinopathy. Graefes Arch Clin Exp Ophthalmol 213:121–133, 1980.
6. Ober RR, Bird AC, Hamilton AM, Sehmi K: Autosomal dominant exudative vitreoretinopathy. Br J Ophthalmol 64:112–120, 1980.
7. Tasman W, Augsburger JJ, Shields JA, et al: Familial exudative vitreoretinopathy. Trans Am Ophthalmol Soc 79:211–226, 1981.
8. Gitter KA, Rothschild H, Waltman DD, et al: Dominantly inherited peripheral retinal neovascularization. Arch Ophthalmol 96:1601–1605, 1978.
9. Slusher MM, Hutton WE: Familial exudative vitreoretinopathy. Am J Ophthalmol 87:152–156, 1979.
10. Benson WE: Familial exudative vitreoretinopathy. Trans Am Ophthalmol Soc 93:473–521, 1995.
11. van Nouhuys CE: Signs, complications, and platelet aggregation in familial exudative vitreoretinopathy. Am J Ophthalmol 111:34–41, 1991.
12. Miyakubo H, Inohara N, Hashimoto K: Retinal involvement in familial exudative vitreoretinopathy. Ophthalmologica 185:125–135, 1982.
13. Miyakubo H, Hashimoto K, Miyakubo S: Retinal vascular pattern in familial exudative vitreoretinopathy. Ophthalmology 91:1524–1530, 1984.
14. Feldman EL, Norris JL, Cleasby GW: Autosomal dominant exudative vitreoretinopathy. Arch Ophthalmol 101:1532–1535, 1983.
15. Greven CM, Moreno RJ, Tasman W: Unusual manifestations of X-linked retinoschisis. Trans Am Ophthalmol Soc 88:211–228, 1990.
16. Regillo CD, Tasman WS, Brown GC: Surgical management of complications associated with X-linked retinoschisis. Arch Ophthalmol 111:1080–1086, 1993.
17. Dudgeon J: Familial exudative vitreo-retinopathy. Trans Ophthalmol Soc U K 99:45–49, 1979.
18. Nishimura M, Yamana T, Sugino M, et al: Falciform retinal fold as sign of familial exudative vitreoretinopathy. Jpn J Ophthalmol 27:40–53, 1983.
19. van Nouhuys CE: Congenital retinal fold as a sign of dominant exudative vitreoretinopathy. Graefes Arch Clin Exp Ophthalmol 217:55–67, 1981.
20. van Nouhuys CE: Juvenile retinal detachment as a complication of familial exudative vitreoretinopathy. Fortschr Ophthalmol 86:221–223, 1989.
21. Hashimoto K, Miyakubo H, Inohara N, Tada H: Juvenile retinal detachment and familial exudative vitreoretinopathy. Jpn J Clin Ophthalmol 37:797–803, 1983.
22. Brockhurst RJ, Albert DM, Zakov N: Pathologic findings in familial exudative vitreoretinopathy. Arch Ophthalmol 99:2143–2146, 1981.
23. Nicholson DH, Galvis V: Crsiwick-Schepens syndrome (familial exudative vitreoretinopathy): study of a Colombian kindred. Arch Ophthalmol 102:1519–1522, 1984.
24. Boldrey EE, Egbert P, Gass DM, Friberg T: The histopathology of familial exudative vitreoretinopathy: a report of two cases. Arch Ophthalmol 103:238–241, 1985.
25. van Nouhuys CE: Dominant exudative vitreoretinopathy and other vascular developmental disorders of the peripheral retina. Doc Ophthalmol 54:1–414, 1982.
26. Glazer LC, Maguire A, Blumenkranz MS, et al: Improved surgical treatment of familial exudative vitreoretinopathy in children. Am J Ophthalmol 120:471–479, 1995.
27. Chaudhuri PR, Rosenthal AR, Goulstine DB, et al: Familial exudative vitreoretinopathy associated with familial thrombocytopathy. Br J Ophthalmol 67:755–758, 1983.
28. Friedrich CA, Francis KA, Kim HC: Familial exudative vitreoretinopathy (FEVR) and platelet dysfunction (Letter). Br J Ophthalmol 73:477–478, 1989.
29. Gole GA, Goodall K, James MJ: Familial exudative vitreoretinopathy (Letter). Br J Ophthalmol 69:76, 1985.
30. Saraux H, Laroche L, Koenig F: Exudative retinopathy with dominant transmission. Report of a new pedigree. J Fr Ophtalmol 8:155–158, 1985.
31. Li Y, Muller B, Fuhrmann C, et al: The autosomal dominant familial exudative vitreoretinopathy locus maps on 11q and is closely linked to D11S533. Am J Hum Genet 51:749–754, 1992.
32. Li Y, Fuhrmann C, Schwinger E, et al: The gene for autosomal dominant familial exudative vitreoretinopathy (Criswick-Schepens) on the long arm of chromosome 11 (Letter). Am J Ophthalmol 113:712–713, 1992.
33. Uto H, Shigeto M, Tanaka H, et al: A case of 11q− syndrome associated with abnormalities of retinal vessels. Ophthalmologica 208:233–236, 1994.
34. Plager DA, Orgel IK, Ellis FD, et al: X-linked recessive exudative vitreoretinopathy. Am J Ophthalmol 114:145–148, 1992.
35. Fullwood P, Jones J, Bundey S, et al: X-linked exudative vitreoretinopathy: clinical features and genetic linkage analysis. Br J Ophthalmol 77:168–170, 1993.
36. Shasty BS, Trese MT: X-linked familial exudative vitreoretinopathy (FEVR): results of DNA analysis with candidate genes (Letter). Am J Med Genet 45:111–113, 1993.
37. Shasty BS, Hartzer MK, Trese MT: Familial exudative vitreoretinopathy: multiple modes of inheritance (Letter). Clin Genet 44:275–276, 1993.
38. Chen ZY, Battinelli EM, Fielder A, et al: A mutation in the Norrie disease gene (NDP) associated with X-linked familial exudative vitreoretinopathy. Nat Genet 5:180–183, 1993.
39. Clement F, Beckford CA, Corral A, Jimenez R: X-linked familial exudative vitreoretinopathy. Report of one family. Retina 15:141–145, 1995.
40. Cryotherapy for Retinopathy of Prematurity Cooperative Group. Multicenter trial of cryotherapy for retinopathy of prematurity: one-year outcome-structure and function. Arch Ophthalmol 108:1408–1416, 1990.
41. Cryotherapy for Retinopathy of Prematurity Cooperative Group: Multicenter trial of cryotherapy for retinopathy of prematurity: 3 1/2-year outcome-structure and function. Arch Ophthalmol 111:339–344, 1993.

42. Campo RV: Similarities of familial exudative vitreoreti-nopathy and retinopathy of prematurity (Letter). Arch Ophthalmol 101:821, 1983.
43. Watzke RC, Stevens TS, Carney RG Jr: Retinal vascular changes of incontinentia pigmenti. Arch Ophthalmol 94:743–746, 1976.
44. Carney RG: Incontinentia pigmenti. A world statistical analysis. Arch Dermatol 112:535–542, 1976.
45. Goldberg MF, Custis PH: Retinal and other manifestations of incontinentia pigmenti (Bloch-Sulzberger syndrome). Ophthalmology 100:1645–1654, 1993.
46. Deutman AF: The Hereditary Dystrophies in the Posterior Pole of the Eye. Assen, the Netherlands, Van Gorcum, 1971, pp 48–99.
47. George NDL, Yates JRW, Moore AT: Clinical features in affected males with X-linked retinoschisis. Arch Ophthalmol 114:274–280, 1996.
48. Keunen JE, Hoppenbrouwers RW: A case of sex-linked juvenile retinoschisis with peripheral vascular anomalies. Ophthalmologica 191:146–149, 1985.
49. Egerer I, Tasman W, Tomer TL: Coats' disease. Arch Ophthalmol 92:109–112, 1974.
50. Tarkkanen A, Laatikainen L: Coats' disease: clinical, angiographic, histopathological findings and clinical management. Br J Ophthalmol 67:766–776, 1983.
51. Woods AC, Duke J: Coats' disease. I. Review of the liter-ature, diagnostic criteria, clinical findings, and plasma lipid studies. Br J Ophthalmol 47:385–412, 1963.
52. Reese AB: Persistent hyperplastic primary vitreous. Am J Ophthalmol 40:317–331, 1955.
53. Haddad R, Font RL, Reeser F: Persistent hyperplastic primary vitreous. A clinicopathologic study of 62 cases and review of the literature. Surv Ophthalmol 23:123–134, 1978.
54. Jacklin HN: Falciform fold, retinal detachment, and Norrie's disease. Am J Ophthalmol 90:76–80, 1980.
55. Hausen AC: Norrie's disease. Am J Ophthalmol 66:328–332, 1968.
56. Townes PL, Roca PD: Norrie's disease (hereditary oculo-acoustic-cerebral degeneration). Am J Ophthalmol 76:797–803, 1973.
57. Treister G, Machemer R: Results of vitrectomy for rare proliferative and hemorrhagic diseases. Am J Ophthalmol 84:394–412, 1977.
58. Machemer R, Williams JM Sr: Pathogenesis and therapy of traction detachment in various retinal vascular diseases. Am J Ophthalmol 105:107–181, 1988.
59. Bergen RL, Glassman R: Familial exudative vitreoreti-nopathy. Ann Ophthalmol 15:275–276, 1983.
60. Maguire AM, Trese MT: Visual results of lens-sparing vitreoretinal surgery in infants. J Pediatr Ophthalmol Strabismus 30:28–32, 1993.

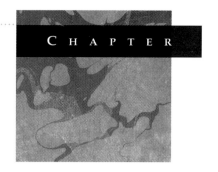

CHAPTER 35

Frosted Branch Angiitis

Richard F. Spaide, M.D.

In the diagnosis of a systemic vasculitis, a physician starts with the history and the examination of the patient. Later, appropriate laboratory tests are ordered. After these are reviewed, it is common to perform a biopsy and use histopathologic examination to help diagnose and classify the vasculitis. The diagnosis of a retinal vasculitis also starts with a history and examination. With the retinal vasculitides we have the advantage of actually being able to see the inflamed vessels. The vasculitis may involve any or all elements of the vascular circuit, including the arterioles, capillaries, and venules. The proper diagnosis of retinal vasculitis frequently depends on pattern recognition, as many conditions do not have supportive laboratory testing available. In addition, biopsy of the intraocular contents usually is impractical or overly invasive.

The retinal vasculitides are usually split into two large groups: those with primarily localized ocular problem and those with a systemic disease that may also have a retinal vasculitis as a component (Table 35–1). On occasion a patient with a systemic disease, such as sarcoidosis or leukemia, may present with a retinal vasculitis as their first sign of disease. Many patients with a retinal vasculitis as part of a systemic disease have a known systemic diagnosis on presentation to the ophthalmologist. The remaining patients with a retinal vasculitis presenting to an ophthalmologist have a localized ocular problem.

Some patients present with an incredible sheathing of the retinal vessels, to the extent that the blood column is obscured by a coat of perivasculitis. In 1976 Ito and associates[1] examined a 6-year-old boy who had bilateral uveitis with profound sheathing of the retinal vessels. Based on the ophthalmoscopic appearance, and not on the pathophysiology or histopathology, the retinal vasculitis was called frosted branch angiitis (Fig. 35–1). Since then a number of additional cases have been reported with additional features. The focus of this chapter is retinal vasculitis with severe perivascular accumulation giving the ophthalmoscopic appearance of frosted branch angiitis. A classification system of frosted branch angiitis based on clinical course, proposed etiology, and treatment will be presented.

IDIOPATHIC FROSTED BRANCH RETINAL ANGIITIS

The first cases of frosted branch angiitis were described in Japanese children who had a rapid decrease in their visual acuity associated with the frosted branch angiitis.[1-3] These children had involvement of both the retinal arteries and veins. Medical evaluation of these patients did not reveal an etiologic agent. Treatment with corticosteroids was thought to be beneficial.[3] The cases reported from Japan primarily involved children.

Kleiner and associates[4] described three patients from the United States who had pronounced sheathing of retinal vessels and decreased visual acuity. These patients differed from the Japanese patients in that their age ranged from 23 to 29 years old and they had a periphlebitis without retinal arteriolar involvement. One patient had an elevated antistreptolysin O titer that was normal on repeat testing 6 days later; otherwise no systemic abnormality was found in any patient. Of special interest, all viral studies in their patients were negative: the first patient had negative urine and blood cultures for virus, and had a negative human immunodeficiency virus (HIV) titer. The second patient was found to have negative acute and convalescent viral antibody titers, while the third had negative cytomegalovirus (CMV) titers.[4] All patients showed rapid improvement of their signs and symptoms when treated with oral corticosteroid therapy.[4]

TABLE 35–1 Classification of the Retinal Vasculitides

		Presentation	Associated Ocular Findings	Systemic Abnormalities	Treatment
Primary (idiopathic) frosted branch angiitis	Children	Acute onset Sheathing of arteries and veins	Cells in vitreous Swelling of disc Exudative detachment (rare)	No systemic abnormalities	Corticosteroids, in most cases
	Adults	Acute onset Sheathing of veins	Cells in vitreous Swelling of disc	No systemic abnormalities	Corticosteroids, in most cases
Secondary frosted branch angiitis					
CMV Retinitis	Adults	Subacute onset Sheathing of veins	Retinitis Swelling of disc	Immuno-compromised Usually AIDS	Anti-CMV treatment (ganciclovir, foscarnet)
Leukemia	Usually adults	Subacute onset Sheathing of arteries and veins	Cells in vitreous Swelling of disc White-centered hemorrhages	Leukemia	Treatment of underlying malignancy

Sugin and associates described two patients,[5] one 32 and the other 26 years old, who had unilateral frosted branch angiitis associated with ipsilateral decreased visual acuity. The first patient was hospitalized 5 weeks prior to his loss of vision for what was thought to be a viral syndrome. However, his white blood cell count at the time of admission was 20,000 cells/mm[3] with 80% polymorphonuclear leukocytes, which is a degree of granulocytosis not commonly seen in viral infections. The second patient had no systemic abnormality and was seronegative for antibodies against HIV. Both patients seemed to have an improvement in their signs and symptoms after treatment with oral corticosteroids.[5] Vander and Masciulli[6] reported one case of bilateral frosted branch angiitis in a 33-year-old patient who had decreased visual acuity. The patient had an unrevealing systemic work-up including negative studies for CMV and HIV. The visual acuity in this patient improved to 20/30 with topical corticosteroid treatment. Browning[7] reported one patient with mild frosted branch angiitis who responded to a single subconjunctival injection of triamcinolone. Hamed and associates[8] reported a 5-year-old child with a severe periphlebitis, who had a negative systemic work-up including negative CMV cultures, and who had a good clinical response to only topical corticosteroids. Even after improvement of the visual acuity, the photopic and scotopic electroretinograms showed decreased voltage and increased latency.

For the most part, patients described in reports from the United States were young adults who primarily had involvement of the retinal veins. Like the Japanese patients, treatment with corticosteroids appeared to cause a resolution of the retinal vasculitis.

CYTOMEGALOVIRUS RETINITIS

Several reports,[9–11] in quick succession, described frosted branch angiitis in patients with the acquired immune deficiency syndrome (AIDS) with low CD4+ T-lymphocyte counts and early CMV retinitis (Figs. 35–2 and 35–3). These patients primarily had sheathing of the retinal veins throughout the retina, even in sites remote from the CMV retinitis. In one report the patient responded to oral corticosteroids.[9] In other reports the patients showed a rapid response to intravenous treatment for the CMV retinitis without the need for corticosteroids.[10,12] A later report described a heart transplant patient with frosted branch angiitis associated with CMV retinitis.[13] This patient was initially treated with intravenous ganciclovir and a reduction in immunosuppressive medications. The patient developed signs of cardiac rejection and was given increased corticosteroids. With the combination of increased corticosteroids and ganicilovir the patient had a resolution of the retinal vascular sheathing.[13]

In patients with AIDS and CMV retinitis the sheathing of the vessels generally resolves after less than 2 weeks of induction treatment for the CMV, which was sooner than the retinal opacification cleared.[10] Frosted branch angiitis has only been seen on presentation of the CMV retinitis and does not occur with reactivation of CMV retinitis infec-

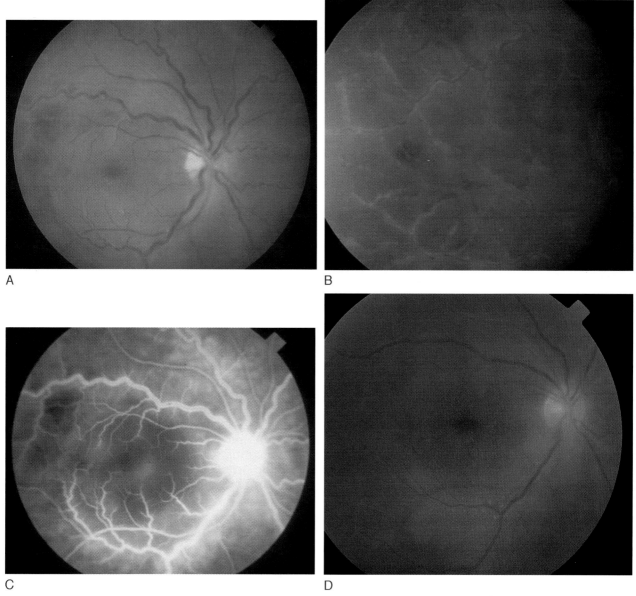

FIGURE 35–1   Acute frosted branch angiitis of a 9-year-old boy affecting both eyes. *A*, The sheathing of the vessels in the posterior pole was not prominent. There also was swelling of the disc, a subtle neurosensory detachment, and dilation of the retinal veins. His visual acuity was 20/200. *B*, In the periphery he had sheathing of both the arteries and veins, much like the cases of children with frosted branch angiitis reported from Japan. *C*, Fluorescein angiography shows leakage and staining of the nerve head as well as retinal vascular leakage. *D*, His medical work-up was negative. He was treated with oral corticosteroids, which caused a marked decrease in the amount of perivascular sheathing, a decrease in the amount of subretinal fluid, and a macular star. His right eye continued to show some retinal vascular sheathing until he was given a subtenon injection of 20 mg of triamcinolone. His visual acuity improved to 20/20 in each eye.

tions. Although the frosted appearance of the vessels may occur remote from the site of infection, the frosting occurs only in the eye with active retinitis.[10]

LEUKEMIA

A fundus picture suggesting an atypical frosted branch angiitis has been seen in patients with leukemia. Kim and associates[14] treated one patient with acute lymphoblastic leukemia who had cells in the vitreous, disc swelling, diffuse retinal whitening, and perivascular sheathing of the retinal vessels. The patient had a positive lumbar puncture for lymphoblastic cells. The patient received radiation and chemotherapy and had a prompt resolution of the ocular findings. The patient later developed similar ocular findings that were retreated successfully with radiation and chemotherapy. Kohno and associates[15] described a patient with adult T-cell leukemia/lymphoma associated with human T-

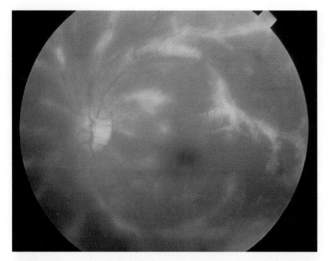

FIGURE 35–2 Frosted branch angiitis associated with a newly diagnosed case of cytomegalovirus retinitis in a patient with AIDS.

lymphotropic virus type I, a retrovirus endemic in certain portions of Japan. This man had intense intraocular inflammation with areas of retinitis that were heralded by severe retinal vasculitis.

Patients with leukemia and sheathing of the retinal vessels usually have a number of concurrent ocular findings not seen in patients with frosted branch angiitis. These include infiltration of the vitreous, retina, and choroid; scattered retinal hemorrhages (that frequently are white-centered); and clumping of the retinal pigment epithelium (RPE) cells. Patients with typical cases of frosted branch

angiitis show pronounced sheathing of the retinal vessels, have no systemic abnormalities, and respond quickly to corticosteroids and do not have recurrences.

OTHER ENTITIES

Retinal vasculitis may be part of the clinical picture for a number of ocular and systemic diseases. It is rare, however, for the vasculitis to be as prominently evident as in frosted branch angiitis. Prominent arteritis and phlebitis have been seen in a biopsy-proven case of Crohn's disease.[16] Retinal phlebitis has been reported in patients with syphilis.[17,18] Patients with syphilis and phlebitis may also have other fundus findings such as yellow placoid outer retinal opacification or disc edema.

Retinal phlebitis, particularly of the peripheral retinal veins, is not uncommon in patients with multiple sclerosis.[19] The phlebitis seen in multiple sclerosis usually is not particularly severe, but on occasion, the phlebitis may not only be prominent but may also be associated with signs of vascular occlusion.[20] The phlebitis may be chronic and can reflect changes in the activity of the systemic disease.[19] In one study patients with multiple sclerosis demonstrated tissue-bound IgG on retinal ganglion cells.[21] A study of ten patients with idiopathic retinal vasculitis who had a positive family history of multiple sclerosis found that three had magnetic resonance imaging (MRI) abnormalities of the brain

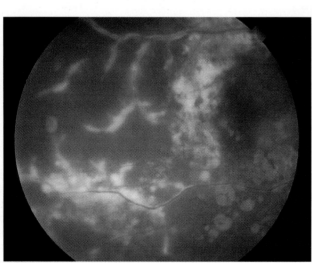

A

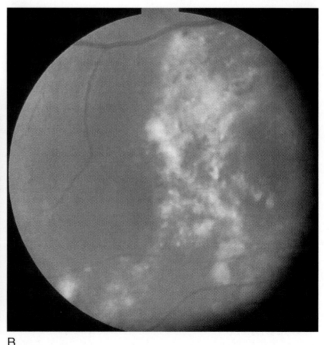

B

FIGURE 35–3 Frosted branch angiitis secondary to CMV retinitis in a patient with AIDS. *A*, On initial presentation the patient had marked sheathing of the retinal vessels. Note the area of active retinitis. *B*, After 10 days of intravenous ganciclovir the frosted appearance diminished, but the retinitis continued to be present.

and two had optic nerve lesions characteristic for multiple sclerosis.[22]

POSSIBLE PATHOPHYSIOLOGIC MECHANISMS

The histopathology of systemic vasculitides has been characterized, and varies with the disease. For example, Wegener's granulomatosis produces a necrotizing granulomatous vasculitis that primarily affects small arteries and veins of the respiratory tracts associated with glomerulonephritis. Polyarteritis nodosa causes necrotizing inflammation of small- and medium-sized muscular arteries with neutrophil and monocyte infiltration. Hypersensitivity vasculitis, which represents a group of allied entities, generally causes inflammation of small vessels, particularly postcapillary venules with infiltration by neutrophils, monocytes, and eosinophils. Temporal arteritis causes inflammation of predominantly medium- and large-sized arteries with monocyte and multinucleated giant cell infiltration, destruction of the internal elastic lamina, and proliferation of the intima.

By comparison, the histopathology of retinal vasculitis is largely unknown. A case of retinal phlebitis examined histopathologically has shown perivascular lymphocytic infiltration with some extension of cells into the vitreous.[23] No cases of the histopathology of frosted branch retinal angiitis have been published. This lack of histopathology makes any theory about pathogenesis particularly speculative.

The sheathing around the vessels in frosted branch angiitis probably represents infiltration of leukocytes, possibly lymphocytes. The rapid response to corticosteroids in idiopathic frosted branch angiitis and to anticytomegalovirus therapy in frosted branch angiitis secondary to CMV retinitis argues against a more permanent structural alteration such as glial proliferation.

The control of lymphocyte trafficking from the blood into tissue occurs by a sequential multiple-step process.[24,25] Cellular adhesion molecules are proteins expressed on cell membranes that mediate critical interactions in the extravascularization of lymphocytes. These molecules are generally classified into three major groups according to their molecular structure: selectins, integrins, and the immunoglobulin supergene family. In the multistep model, lymphocytes first form a loose attachment, called a rolling attachment, to the endothelial cell wall through interactions with selectins. The next step occurs when the rolling lymphocytes are further activated to form a strong adhesion, mediated by integrins, by factors in their microenvironment such as the cytokines tumor necrosis factor-α (TNF-α), interleukin-1 (IL-1), and interferon-gamma (IFN-γ). Depending on the nature of the stimulatory signals present, the lymphocytes may then migrate across the vessel wall. This transmigration is mediated by molecules in the integrin and immunoglobulin supergene family.

Lymphocyte migration occurs through a tightly controlled, orchestrated process that is regulated at multiple points.[24,25] At each step of the process there is opportunity for either inhibition or ensuing sequential activation of the lymphocyte transmigration process compelling the lymphocyte to move out of the vessel. For lymphocytes to accumulate around the retinal vessel wall, specific stimuli are necessary and must be sufficient to direct the movement of the lymphocyte in a directed process through the multiple checkpoints.

The stimulus for the accumulation of the cellular infiltration in frosted branch angiitis associated with CMV retinitis appears to be related to the CMV itself. The perivascular infiltrate seen in these patients may have been the result of direct CMV infection of the retinal vessels or the retina immediately surrounding the vessels. Indeed, CMV has a certain tropism for vascular endothelial cells.[26,27] The rapid resolution of the perivascular infiltrate with intravenous antiviral treatment may result from higher tissue levels of antiviral in the vascular and perivascular regions. There are several reasons that argue against direct infection of the perivascular space, however. The vessels of the retina seemed to be globally involved, not just in areas contiguous with CMV retinitis. Resolution of the areas of sheathing is not accompanied by any discernible retinal atrophy or retinal pigment epithelial scarring one might expect if the perivascular areas were directly infected with CMV.[10] When these patients have a reactivation of their retinitis, the infection spreads from past areas of clinically evident retinitis, but not from the perivascular areas.

CMV retinitis is probably anteceded by a systemic CMV infection. The frosted branch angiitis in patients with CMV retinitis, though, does not appear to be secondary to an ocular manifestation of a systemic hypersensitivity process. The vascular sheathing only occurrs in the eye infected with CMV. In addition, the patients involved do not have any other signs of a hypersensitivity vasculitis such as purpura, urticaria, bullae, myalgias, polyarthralgias, or the like.

It is possible that viral antigens released as part of CMV retinitis may be the inciting stimulus in the production of frosted branch angiitis in patients with AIDS. The eye has a unique anatomy—the posterior segment is in many ways a hollow structure. Viral antigens diffusing from a retinal source have the potential to come into contact with vessels over a large expanse of retina. These antigens initially may incite a vigorous outpouring of leukocytes causing the vascular sheathing through stimulation by the antigen itself or by antigen-antibody reactions. The rapid resolution of the perivascular infiltrate with intravenous ganciclovir may be the result of lowering the intraocular antigen load through antiviral treatment. Corticosteroids have profound effects on the immune response, altering both the cellular and humoral arms. It is possible that corticosteroids reduce the cellular response to antigen or antigen-antibody complexes. It is also possible that corticosteroids may lessen regional antibody concentrations in the eye reducing the amount of immune-complex formation and thereby lessening the amount of perivascular infiltrate.

Patients with idiopathic frosted branch angiitis have prominent perivascular sheathing, but these patients have no observable retinal pathology as an inciting event. It has been suggested that the inflammatory exudate around the retinal vessels in idiopathic frosted branch angiitis may be related to antigen-antibody complex deposition.[5] The source of the antigen is not known. The cases of frosted branch angiitis reported in the literature did not seem to have signs of a systemic vasculitis or a systemic hypersensitivity reaction, but rather had signs and symptoms limited to the eye; indeed, some cases were unilateral.[5] This suggests that the production of the inciting antigen in conventional frosted branch angiitis might occur within the eye. It is possible that the inciting antigen is normally found within the retina, but it is difficult to explain unilateral cases of frosted branch angiitis. Although not every case reported in the literature was tested, immunocompetent patients with frosted branch angiitis do not have abnormal CMV titers, positive CMV cultures, or findings suggestive of CMV retinitis. This suggests that frosted branch angiitis in patients without AIDS may be caused by agents or factors other than CMV.

Patients with idiopathic frosted branch angiitis respond to corticosteroids, sometimes with amazing swiftness. The rapid resolution of frosted branch angiitis in patients without AIDS using corticosteroid treatment might be the result of dampening a specific antibody response decreasing any antigen-antibody complexes formed or by reducing the inflammatory response to any inflammatory stimulus such as immune-complex deposition. In any case the sheathing resolves, often without sequela, and does not return.

Frosted branch angiitis is an uncommon syndrome that has been previously reported to occur as a primary disorder in immunocompetent patients. Frosted branch angiitis appears to have occurred as a secondary phenomenon in patients with AIDS and CMV retinitis. Other forms of secondary frosted branch angiitis may occur in other disease states. Some conditions, such as leukemia, can produce prominent sheathing of the retinal vessels, but often there are concomitant changes in the eye that are not consistent with idiopathic frosted branch angiitis. The most efficient treatment strategy for patients with frosted branch angiitis hinges on establishing the proper diagnosis. Patients with typical idiopathic frosted branch angiitis, who are otherwise in good health, probably need little in the way of any medical work-up. This is similar to pa-

tients with idiopathic retinal vasculitis.[28] Treatment of this primary form with corticosteroids appears to be an effective means of therapy. Differentiating the primary form from secondary types, such as those associated with CMV retinitis or pseudo-forms such as those associated with leukemia, can be done using both the ophthalmoscopic and systemic examinations. Corticosteroids would seem to be unnecessary in the secondary form of frosted branch angiitis associated with CMV retinitis in patients with AIDS. Such patients already have profound immune suppression and they respond quickly to anti-CMV therapy. Patients with leukemia require therapy specifically tailored to their needs.

REFERENCES

1. Ito Y, Nakano M, Kyu N, Takeuchi M: Frosted-branch angiitis in a child. Jpn J Ophthalmol 30:797, 1976.
2. Yamane S, Nishiuchi T, Nakagawa Y, et al: A case of frosted-branch angiitis of the retina. Folia Ophthalmol Jpn 6:1822, 1985.
3. Watanabe Y, Takeda N, Adachi-Usami E: A case of frosted-branch angiitis. Br J Ophthalmol 71:553, 1987.
4. Kleiner R, Kaplan HJ, Shakin JL, et al: Acute frosted retinal periphlebitis. Am J Ophthalmol 106:27, 1988.
5. Sugin SL, Henderly DE, Friedman SM, et al: Unilateral frosted branch angiitis. Am J Ophthalmol 111:682, 1991.
6. Vander JF, Masciulli L: Unilateral frosted branch angiitis. Am J Ophthalmol 112:477, 1991.
7. Browning DJ: Mild frosted branch angiitis. Am J Ophthalmol 114:505–506, 1992.
8. Hamed LM, Fang EN, Fanous MM, et al: Frosted branch angiitis: the role of systemic corticosteroids. J Pediatr Ophthalmol Strabismus 29(5):312–313, 1992.
9. Geier SA, Nasemann J, Klauss V, et al: Frosted branch angiitis associated with cytomegalovirus retinitis. Am J Ophthalmol 114(4):514–516, 1992.
10. Spaide RF, Vitale AT, Toth IR, Oliver JM: Frosted branch angiitis associated with cytomegalovirus retinitis. Am J Ophthalmol 113:522–528, 1992.
11. Rabb MF, Jampol LM, Fish RH, et al: Retinal periphlebitis in patients with acquired immunodeficiency syndrome with cytomegalovirus retinitis mimics acute frosted retinal periphlebitis. Arch Ophthalmol 110:1257–1260, 1992.
12. Mansour AM, Li HK: Frosted retinal periphlebitis in the acquired immunodeficiency syndrome. Ophthalmologica 207:182–186, 1993.
13. Cortina P, Diaz M, Espana E, et al: Acute frosted retinal periphlebitis associated with cytomegalovirus retinitis in a heart transplant patient (Letter). Retina 14(5):463–464, 1994.
14. Kim TS, Duker JS, Hedges TR III: Retinal angiopathy resembling unilateral frosted branch angiitis in a patient with relapsing acute lymphoblastic leukemia. Am J Ophthalmol 117:806–808, 1994.
15. Kohno T, Uchida H, Inomata H, et al: Ocular manifestations of adult T-cell leukemia/lymphoma. A clinicopathologic study. Ophthalmology 100:1794–1799, 1993.
16. Garcia-Diaz M, Mira M, Nevado L, et al: Retinal vasculitis associated with Crohn's disease. Postgrad Med J 71:170–172, 1995.
17. Halperin LS, Berger AS, Grand MG: Syphilitic disc edema and periphlebitis. Retina 10:223–225, 1990.
18. Lobes LA Jr, Folk JC: Syphilitic phlebitis simulating branch vein occlusion. Ann Ophthalmol 13:825, 1981.
19. Tola MR, Granieri E, Casetta I, et al: Retinal periphlebitis in multiple sclerosis: a marker of disease activity? Eur Neurol 33:93–96, 1993.

20. Vine AK: Severe periphlebitis, peripheral retinal ischemia, and preretinal neovascularization in patients with multiple sclerosis. Am J Ophthalmol 113:28–32, 1992.
21. Lucarelli MJ, Pepose JS, Arnold AC, Foos RY: Immunopathologic features of retinal lesions in multiple sclerosis. Ophthalmology 98:1652–1656, 1991.
22. Gass A, Graham E, Moseley IF, et al: Cranial MRI in idiopathic retinal vasculitis. J Neurol 242:174–177, 1995.
23. Patrinely JR, Green WR, Randolph ME: Retinal phlebitis with chorioretinal emboli. Am J Ophthalmol 94:49–57, 1982.
24. Springer TA: Adhesion receptors of the immune system. Am J Infect Dis 346:425–436, 1990.
25. Springer TA: Traffic signals for lymphocyte recirculation and leukocyte emigration: the multistep paradigm. Cell 76:301–314, 1994.
26. Ho DD, Rota TR, Andrews CA, Hirsh MS: Replication of human cytomegalovirus in endothelial cells. J Infect Dis 150:956, 1984.
27. van Dorp WT, Jonges E, Bruggeman CA, et al: Direct induction of MHC class I but not class II expression on endothelial cells by cytomegalovirus infection. Transplantation 48:467, 1989.
28. George RK, Walton RC, Whitcup SM, Nussenblatt RB: Primary retinal vasculitis. Systemic associations and diagnostic evaluation. Ophthalmology 103:384–389, 1996.

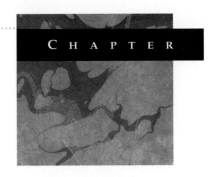

Hemoglobinopathies

Sharon Fekrat, M.D.

Gerard Lutty, Ph.D.

Morton F. Goldberg, M.D.

In each erythrocyte, normal hemoglobin A consists of four polypeptide chains, two α and two β chains, each with a central ferroprotoporphyrin heme ring. A patient with a hemoglobinopathy has by definition abnormal hemoglobin in his red blood cells. In sickle cell and related hemoglobinopathies, one or more of the β polypeptide chains is a product of a point mutation, where the glutamic acid residue, in position six on the β chain, is replaced by either lysine to form hemoglobin C or valine to form hemoglobin S. This abnormal hemoglobin can occur in combination with normal hemoglobin A or abnormal hemoglobin S or C, producing various hemoglobinopathies, including hemoglobin AS (sickle cell trait), hemoglobin SS (sickle cell disease or anemia), hemoglobin SC (sickle cell hemoglobin C disease), and hemoglobin AC (hemoglobin C trait). An inadequate rate of synthesis of either the α or β polypeptide chain (globin) may produce a thalassemia that, when combined with sickle hemoglobin, results in a hemoglobinopathy termed "sickle cell thalassemia" or "SThal disease."

As observed in 1910, erythrocytes containing the abnormal hemoglobin may assume a sickle shape upon deoxygenation.[1] When exposed to hypoxia, acidosis, or hyperosmolarity, hemoglobin S polymerizes within the erythrocyte and transforms it into a sickle shape.[2,3] This results in decreased cell pliability, increased hemolysis and blood viscosity, and vaso-occlusion. Vaso-occlusion in the peripheral retinal vasculature begins the cascade of events in proliferative sickle cell retinopathy that may culminate in traction and/or rhegmatogenous retinal detachment.

EPIDEMIOLOGY

Sickle cell hemoglobinopathies originated in and are most prevalent in both central and west Africa; however, they are also found in patients from countries in the Mediterranean such as Greece, Italy, Israel, and Saudi Arabia. In North America, about 10% of African descendents have abnormal hemoglobin. 8.5% of these have sickle cell trait (AS), 2.5% have hemoglobin C trait (AC), 0.4% have sickle cell disease (SS), 0.2% have sickle cell hemoglobin C disease (SC), and 0.03% have sickle cell thalassemia (SThal)[4,5] (Table 36–1). One study reported as many as 0.5 to 1.0% with SThal disease.[6]

The onset of clinically detectable proliferative sickle cell retinopathy may begin in the first decade of life, but more commonly occurs between 15 and 30 years of age.[7] Proliferative retinopathy occurs in about 33% of patients with SC disease, 14% of patients with SThal hemoglobinopathies, and 3% of patients with SS disease[8–10] (Table 36–1). With aging, retinopathy occurs more commonly in SS subjects.[8] A causative relationship between AS and AC hemoglobinopathies and proliferative retinopathy has been suggested but is unclear.[11–14]

SYSTEMIC MANIFESTATIONS

Patients with more abnormal hemoglobin within their erythrocytes and an increased propensity for the abnormal hemoglobin to sickle under adverse conditions may be more likely to exhibit the systemic manifestations of the disease.[15,16] The sys-

HISTOPATHOLOGICAL FEATURES

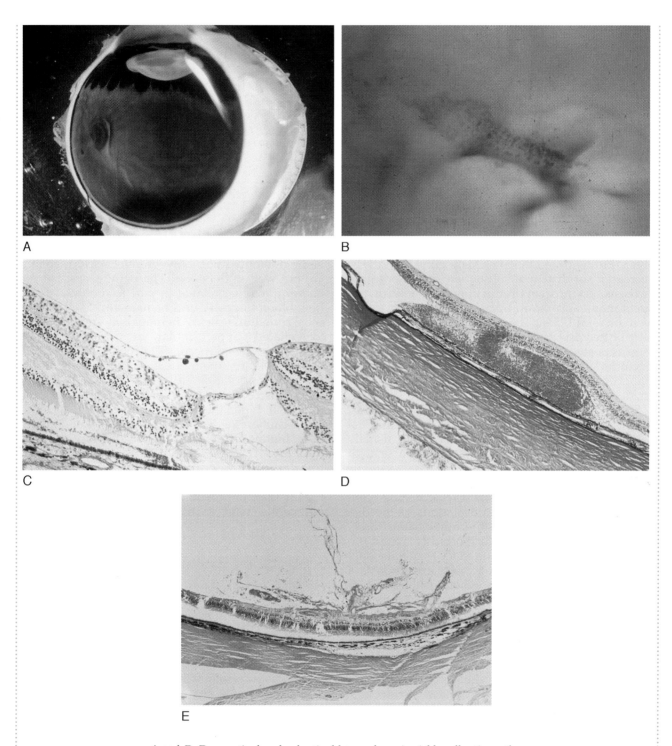

A and D, Deep retinal and subretinal hemorrhage in sickle cell retinopathy (Salmon patch). B, Iridescent spot in the macula has a brown rust appearance. C, Iridescent spots are found in an acquired area of schisis from a resolved sub–internal limiting hemorrhage with residual hemosiderin. D, Retinal hemorrhage with extension into the subretinal space. E, Localized retinal neovascularization (sea fan) in an eye of a patient with SC disease. (From Romayananda N, Goldberg MF, Green WR: Histopathology of sickle cell retinopathy. Trans Am Acad Ophthalmol Otolaryngol 77:652–676, 1973, with permission.)

TABLE 36–1 Sickle Cell Hemoglobinopathies in North America

Type	Incidence	Proliferative Sickle Retinopathy (Approximate %)
Any abnormal hemoglobin	10%	—
Sickle cell trait (AS)	8.5%	Unclear, but very low
Hemoglobin C trait (AC)	2.5%	Unclear, but very low
Sickle cell disease (SS)	0.4 %	3%
Sickle cell hemoglobin C (SC)	0.2%	33%
Sickle cell thalassemia (SThal)	0.03%	14%

temic effects are the most severe in patients with SS disease, and may be due, in part, to the presence of more than 90% hemoglobin S within their erythrocytes. In patients with SS disease, intravascular sickling may occur in the microvascular circulations, leading to red blood cell sludging, hemolysis, decreased survival, and subsequent anemia despite increased erythrocyte production. Bone marrow infarcts may cause bony trabeculation and sclerosis seen on skull, long bone, and vertebrae x-rays. Aseptic necrosis of the femoral head may also occur from repeated bony infarcts. Sickling in precapillary arterioles may result in painful joints, abdominal pain, pulmonary infarcts, and cerebrovascular accidents.[15]

Systemic manifestations are less likely in SC, SThal, and especially in AS subjects. SC and SThal heterozygotes are only mildly anemic and usually have an uneventful or mild systemic course with very few crises per year. Despite minimal systemic findings, however, SC and SThal patients are the most likely of all patients with sickle hemoglobinopathies to have ocular manifestations of the disease. AS heterozygotes, on the other hand, rarely experience systemic or ocular morbidity, except under severe hypoxic conditions, since they have only 50% abnormal hemoglobin S.[17] An exception is a hyphema in an AS patient in whom ocular morbidity may be just as severe as in more serious systemic hemoglobinopathies.[18] The discrepancy between the severity of systemic and ocular findings in the various hemoglobinopathies has not yet been clearly explained.

CLINICAL FEATURES AND PATHOPHYSIOLOGY

Erythrocyte sickling can occur in any microvascular network of the eye. Depending on the anatomical location of the vaso-occlusion(s), visual function may or may not be affected. One site of vaso-occlusion that may be used for a diagnostic clue is the conjunctival vasculature, where vaso-occlusions result in characteristic comma signs[19] (Fig. 36–1).

The comma sign is seen most commonly in SS subjects (about 70%) and in only 34% of SC and 17% of SThal patients.

SC and SThal patients are more likely to exhibit retinal manifestations than are patients with other hemoglobinopathies; however, the reasons for this are not well understood. The pathogenesis of retinopathy may be related in part to the rate of sickling, blood viscosity, and hematocrit.[5,16,20] When red cells containing sickle hemoglobin traverse a deoxygenated, hyperosmolar, or acidotic capillary bed, sickling may occur. The increased rigidity of sickled cells hampers effective circulation through the microvasculature and increases blood viscosity. Blood viscosity is determined by the most abundant cell type, the erythrocyte, especially in the small-caliber vessels.[21] Sickling in those patients with higher hematocrits leads to an even higher viscosity.[20] The marked increase in viscosity contributes to vaso-occlusive events. For example, the hematocrit in SC and SThal patients is significantly higher than in SS subjects. Thus, SC or SThal heterozygotes tend to have greater blood viscosity

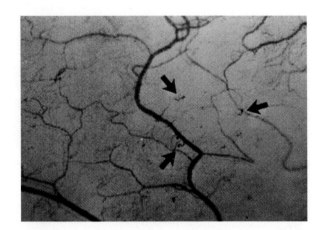

FIGURE 36–1 Vaso-occlusions within the conjunctival vasculature may produce the comma sign (*arrows*) and may be used as a diagnostic tool. (From Nagpal KC, Asdourian GK, Goldbaum MH, et al: The conjunctival sickling sign, hemoglobin S, and irreversibly sickled erythrocytes. Arch Ophthalmol 95:808–811, 1977. Copyright 1977, American Medical Association, with permission.)

during a sickling episode than SS homozygotes and, therefore, may experience more vaso-occlusive events in the retinal microvasculature where red blood cell characteristics play a crucial role. Despite the large number of sickled red cells in SS subjects, their lower hematocrit, and thus lower viscosity, may provide relative protection against vaso-occlusion in retinal vessels. The relationship of sickling, vessel wall adhesion, and the presence of various serum factors in predisposing and/or promoting vaso-occlusion in various hemoglobinopathies is currently being investigated.

RETINAL MANIFESTATIONS

The retinal manifestations may be categorized into nonproliferative and proliferative changes.

Nonproliferative Changes

Retinal findings referred to as nonproliferative or background sickle cell retinopathy include the salmon patch hemorrhage, iridescent spots, and black sunburst lesion. These three changes may be pathogenetically related. Other nonproliferative changes, described below, include abnormalities in the retinal vasculature, macula, choroid, vitreoretinal interface, and optic disc, among others.

Salmon Patch Hemorrhage

A salmon patch hemorrhage[22] is an oval or round collection of preretinal or superficial intraretinal blood that is up to 1 disc diameter in size with a flattened or dome-shaped appearance and well-defined borders. Such hemorrhages occur commonly in the midperiphery adjacent to an intermediate-sized retinal arteriole. They may form due to sudden arteriolar occlusion by sickled erythrocytes with subsequent vessel rupture. The blood is initially red (Fig. 36–2A), but may evolve into a red-orange or salmon color over time (Fig. 36–2B). The patch may be localized beneath the internal limiting membrane or may hydraulically dissect into the vitreous or subretinal space.

Iridescent Spots

As the salmon patch hemorrhage resorbs, the retina may revert to normal, may have a faint indentation outlined by the internal limiting membrane light reflex, or, following resorption of the intraretinal portion of the hemorrhage, may develop a small retinoschisis cavity containing yellowish granules (Fig. 36–3) that represent multiple hemosiderin-laden macrophages.[23] The glistening spots within the cavity are termed "iridescent spots." In selected patients, the cavity was observed in 33% of SC, 18% of SThal, and 13% of SS patients,[24–26] although its incidence varies among reports.[5,10,27]

Histopathologic examination demonstrates a small retinoschisis space following resorption of the intraretinal blood,[23] and both intra- and extracellular iron can be identified. The cavity is lined by the internal limiting membrane anteriorly and by the sensory retina posteriorly.

Black Sunburst

The black sunburst[5] is a round or oval patch of hyperplastic retinal pigment epithelium (RPE) that

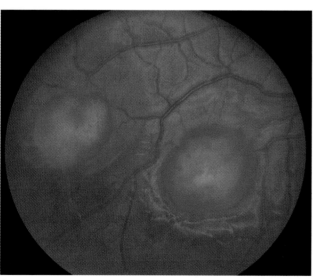

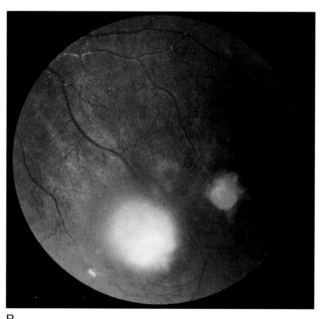

A   B

FIGURE 36–2 *A,* A salmon patch hemorrhage may initially be red in color. *B,* Over time, it may adopt a whitish or salmon color.

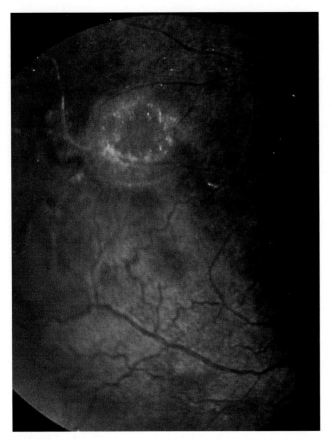

FIGURE 36–3 Iridescent spots are found in a retinoschisis cavity following resorption of an intraretinal salmon patch hemorrhage.

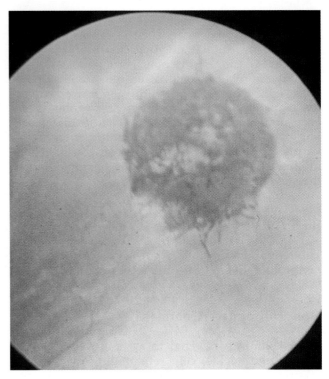

FIGURE 36–4 A black sunburst lesion may be round as shown or oval. (From Welch RB, Goldberg MF: Sickle-cell hemoglobin and its relation to fundus abnormality. Arch Opthalmol 75:353–362, 1966. Copyright 1966, American Medical Association, with permission.)

has migrated into the sensory retina. Romayananda and co-workers hypothesized that RPE migration into the retina may be stimulated by blood that had dissected into the subretinal space.[23] The lesion is about 1/2 to 2 disc diameters in size, and its borders are stellate or spiculate due to perivascular pigment accumulation (Fig. 36–4). Refractile granules similar to those of iridescent spots may be present. Histologically the black sunburst lesion represents areas of focal RPE hypertrophy, hyperplasia, and migration (Fig. 36–5A and B). The overlying sensory retina is usually thinned and degenerated. Pigment and hemosiderin-laden macrophages and diffuse deposits of iron may be found.[23] The reported incidence may be up to 41% in SC subjects,[25] 35% in SS patients,[24] and 20% in SThal patients.[26]

The pathogenesis of the black sunburst may be multifactorial. The black sunburst may evolve directly from a salmon patch hemorrhage, depending on the plane of dissection of the resulting hemorrhage,[28,29] as has been clearly demonstrated in a 17-year-old man with SC disease during a 6-year follow-up period.[29] However, others have demonstrated choroidal neovascularization (CNV) that has occurred within the black sunburst lesion,[30,31] and it may be related to the formation of the black

sunburst. The black sunburst may also develop following a localized vascular occlusion in the choroid.[32,33]

Retinal Vasculature

In the posterior pole, the major retinal vessels usually appear normal. Increased vascular tortuosity may be present in up to 47% of SS and 32% of SC subjects[5] (Fig. 36–6). It is not common in AS and SThal heterozygotes. The pathogenesis has not been elucidated, but it has been attributed to arteriovenous shunting in the retinal periphery.

In the periphery, the major retinal vessels may end abruptly, often in hairpin loops[34] (Fig. 36–7). Peripheral microvascular occlusions have been observed in SS subjects as young as 2 years of age.[34] The nonperfused areas observed in middle-aged subjects may represent an aggregation of multiple vaso-occlusive events.

Despite the generally normal appearance of the retinal vasculature in the posterior pole of these eyes, vascular occlusions may occur and range from perifoveal capillary dropout to central retinal artery occlusion (Fig. 36–8). Central, branch, and macular retinal artery occlusions have been reported.[24,28,35–47] An increased risk of central or branch retinal vein occlusion in sickle cell patients has not been demonstrated.

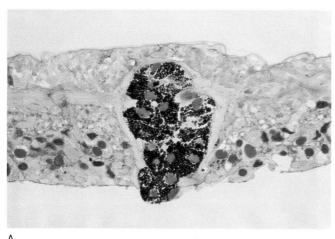
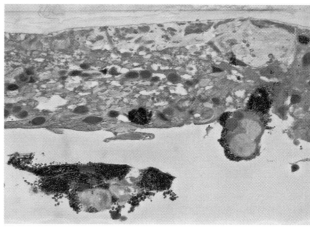

A   B

FIGURE 36–5 Cross sections of a black sunburst lesion at the border of perfused and nonperfused retina in a 54-year-old SC subject (A) demonstrate a cluster of retinal pigment epithelium-like (RPE-like) cells in this atrophic area of retina. (B), In some areas of this lesion, the RPE-like cells appeared to ensheath cores of basement membrane material that appear to have been blood vessels.

Macula

Vascular changes may occur in the macula. Macular arteriolar occlusion and subsequent nonperfusion are common in SS homozygotes (Fig. 36–9) and may precede the development of retinal thinning and atrophy. The thinning and atrophic changes may produce a concave area that appears as a dark circle or oval with a bright central reflex[48] and may be associated with a mild decrease in visual acuity. This is known as the macular depression sign.

Abnormalities in the macula and/or temporal vascular raphe have been described in 32% of SS subjects, 36% of SC subjects, and 20% of SThal sub-

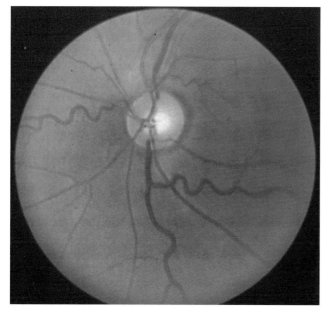

FIGURE 36–6 Increased vascular tortuosity. Its pathogenesis in sickle hemoglobinopathies has not been elucidated but has been speculatively attributed to arteriovenous shunting in the retinal periphery.

jects in 100 consecutive cases.[49–51] The abnormalities may consist of microaneurysmal dots, enlarged precapillary arterioles and capillary segments, cotton-wool spots, hairpin venous loops with adjacent capillary dropout, and foveal avascular zone irregularities. Paramacular vessel abnormalities may represent the early vaso-occlusive phase that may progress to enlargement of the foveal avascular zone (Fig. 36–9).[51] These chronic remodeling changes in the parafoveal vasculature, however, do not necessarily result in significant functional visual loss.[9] Symptomatic ischemic maculopathy would be expected in patients with sickle cell hemoglobinopathies if these changes were progressive; however, no cases have been reported. The lack of reported cases may be attributed to the shortened lifespan in patients with sickle cell hemoglobinopathies.[52]

The temporal horizontal vascular raphe extends from the fovea temporally to the periphery. The terminal arteriolar branches that meet in this anatomic area may also become occluded with sickled erythrocytes. There is no strong correlation between the amount of nonperfusion along the raphe and that in the periphery, despite the vascular similarities in the two areas.[50]

Choroidal Occlusions

Choroidal occlusions have been described in patients with sickle cell hemoglobinopathies[34,53–55] and may have some pathogenetic relationship to the formation of choroidal neovascularization[30,31] and/or the black sunburst lesion.[32,33] Lutty and associates have histopathologically observed apparent choroidal vaso-occlusion associated with impacted erythrocytes, increased fibrin, and platelet-fibrin thrombi.[34,57] Choroidal nonperfusion may result in outer retinal atrophy and RPE hypertrophy.

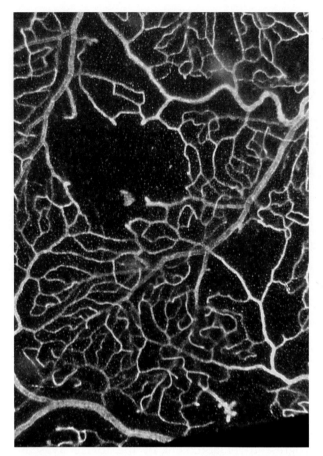

FIGURE 36–7 Hairpin loops in a small nonperfused area of a 54-year-old SC subject. In this piece of adenosine diphosphatase (ADPase) flat-embedded retina, the ADPase (lead) reaction product in blood vessels is white against a black background. The periphery is at the top.

Vitreoretinal Interface

Areas of whitening of the peripheral retina similar to white-without-pressure in these eyes[24–26,58,59] may represent areas of stronger or abnormal vitreoretinal adhesion. The peripheral whitening may be seen in up to 93% of SS, 83% of SC, and 82% of SThal subjects[24] and has been suggested to correlate inversely with the severity of the peripheral vascular changes.[59] The described vitreoretinal interface change may not be a separate entity occurring in sickle cell patients and may just be similar to white-without-pressure seen in the general population.[60]

Brown patches within the retina have been reported in patients with SS and SC hemoglobinopathies.[61] These transient areas have been described in the posterior pole and midperiphery and leave no trace of their presence after their disappearance. They are homogeneous, geographical, flat, and brown in color and have been termed "dark-without-pressure."[61] The underlying choroid is normal ophthalmoscopically and angiographically in the affected area, and thus these lesions are not thought to be associated with hemorrhage[61] as had been

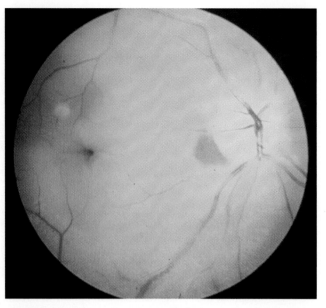

FIGURE 36–8 Central retinal artery occlusion in a 15-year-old SS female. The cloudy swelling clearly outlines the cherry red spot. (From Acacio I, Goldberg MF: Peripapillary and macular vessel occlusions in sickle cell anemia. Am J Ophthalmol 75:861–866, 1973. Ophthalmic Publishing Company, with permission.)

previously suggested.[24] The pathogenesis of these lesions is unknown.

Optic Nerve Head

Transient small red spots on the optic disc have been reported in 9 of 80 sickle cell patients, 7 of whom were SS subjects, in one study,[48] and in 17 of 74 SS patients in another study.[24] These spots are referred to as the sickle disc sign and represent

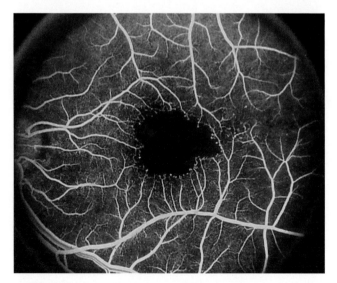

FIGURE 36–9 Macular arteriolar occlusion and subsequent nonperfusion are common in SS homozygotes. Note the 'pruned' vessels along the border of the enlarged foveal avascular zone.

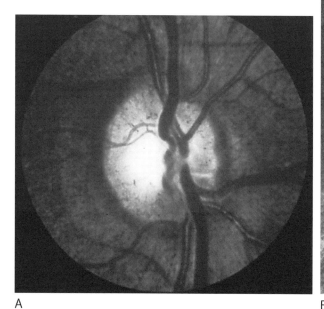
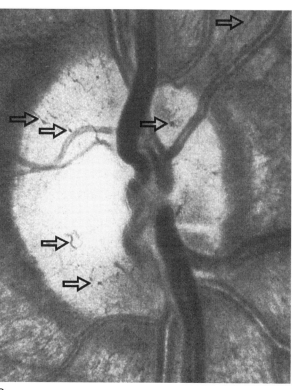

A   B

FIGURE 36–10   *A* and *B*, Sickle disc sign. The *arrows* demonstrate the plugs of sickled erythrocytes within precapillary arterioles and capillaries on the disc surface as seen on the red-free photographs. (From Goldbaum MH, Jampol LM, Goldberg MF: The disc sign in sickling hemoglobinopathies. Arch Ophthalmol 96: 1597–1600, 1978. Copyright 1978, American Medical Association, with permission.)

plugs of sickled erythrocytes within precapillary arterioles and capillaries on the disc surface. They may be linear or may adopt a Y-shaped configuration and usually do not alter visual function (Figs. 36–10*A* and *B*).

Neovascularization of the disc has been reported in four SC patients[7,62–64] and one SS patient.[24]

Angioid Streaks

The incidence of angioid streaks (Fig. 36–11), grayish lines that are deep to the retinal vessels and extend radially from the optic disc, has been reported to be about 1 to 2% in various sickle hemoglobinopathies.[60,65–67] Angioid streaks may be more common in SS homozygotes and have been described in up to 22% of Hb SS Jamaican patients over 40 years old, compared to only 2% in patients younger than 40 years old.[65] The clinical course is usually unremarkable.[60,65–67]

Proliferative Changes

Proliferative sickle retinopathy (Fig. 36–12) is a peripheral retinal vascular disease and should be included in the differential diagnosis of peripheral neovascularization of the fundus. The initiating pathogenetic event is peripheral retinal arteriolar

occlusion resulting, eventually, in sea fan neovascularization. Elevated sea fans are more likely than flat fans to predispose to vitreous hemorrhage and subsequent tractional vitreous membrane forma-

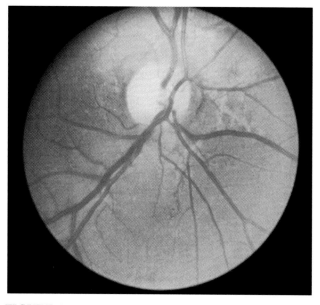

FIGURE 36–11   Angioid streaks often have an unremarkable course in patients with sickle cell hemoglobinopathies.

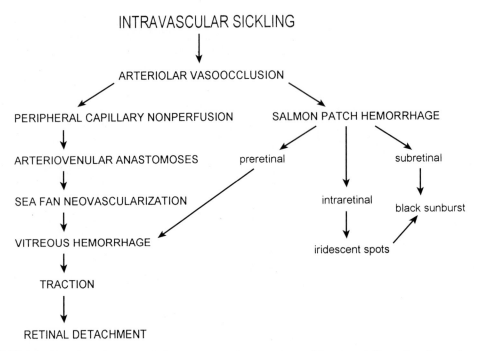

INTRAVASCULAR SICKLING

↓

ARTERIOLAR VASOOCCLUSION

PERIPHERAL CAPILLARY NONPERFUSION　　　SALMON PATCH HEMORRHAGE

ARTERIOVENULAR ANASTOMOSES　　preretinal　　　　　subretinal

SEA FAN NEOVASCULARIZATION　　　　　intraretinal　　black sunburst

VITREOUS HEMORRHAGE

TRACTION　　　　　iridescent spots

RETINAL DETACHMENT

FIGURE 36–12　Flow diagram of the sequence of events in proliferative sickle cell retinopathy. (From Romayanada N, Goldberg MF, Green WR: Histopathology of sickle cell retinopathy. Trans Am Acad Ophthalmol Otolaryngol 77:652–657, 1973, with permission.)

tion, which may lead to tractional and/or rhegmatogenous retinal detachment.[68]

Originally described by Goldberg,[69] the following classification of proliferative sickle cell retinopathy has been widely adopted.

Goldberg Stage I

The ophthalmoscopic and angiographic alteration that sets the stage for subsequent proliferative sickle retinopathy is peripheral arteriolar occlusion (Fig. 36–13). Such occlusions characterize stage I. The peripheral retinal vasculature may be predisposed to sickling and vaso-occlusion because of the longer arteriovenous transit times and decreased blood flow. These vaso-occlusions occur mostly in the precapillary arterioles, as demonstrated in fluorescein angiographic studies[9] and in more recent dual-perspective histologic analyses.[34] The sickled erythrocytes act as microemboli and impede local blood flow or cause intravascular thromboses. Arteriolar flow is terminated, and the capillary bed and venules that drain the affected retina become nonperfused. Thus, areas of peripheral capillary nonperfusion develop.

Goldberg Stage II

Stage II is characterized by vascular remodeling at the border of the perfused and nonperfused retina, with the formation of peripheral arteriovenous anastomoses (Fig. 36–14). These abnormal vessels shunt blood from the occluded arterioles to nearby medium-sized venules anterior to the equator.

These anastomoses retain intraluminal fluorescein during angiography, unlike true neovascular tissue that invariably leaks dye. Thus, these vessels appear to represent the creation of preferential vascular channels from pre-existing retinal vasculature by enlargement of pre-existing capillaries[62] instead of true neovascularization. The blood flow through these connections is slow, and the deoxygenation during one passage may be sufficient to induce

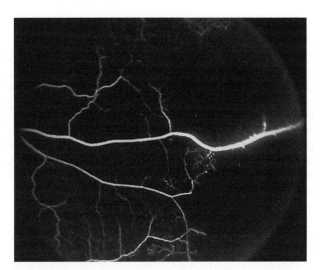

FIGURE 36–13　Peripheral arteriolar occlusions characterize stage I proliferative sickle cell retinopathy (PSR). Arteriolar flow is sharply terminated in affected areas, and peripheral areas of capillary nonperfusion develop as seen on this fluorescein angiogram. Compare with Figure 36–15B.

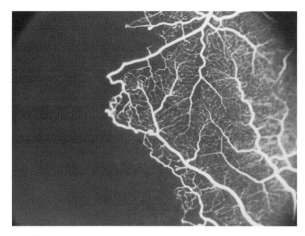

FIGURE 36–14 Peripheral arteriovenous anastomosis formation characterizes stage II PSR and is well demonstrated on this fluorescein angiogram.

more sickling and further vaso-occlusion. The formation of these abnormal arteriolar–venular connections may be a hydrostatic response to the occlusion of the distal vessels and precedes the development of sea fan formation.[62]

Goldberg Stage III

The hallmark of stage III is peripheral neovascularization or sea fan formation. Individual sea fans appear an average of 18 months after the formation of arteriovenous anastomoses.[62] A sea fan is a tuft of preretinal neovascular tissue that resembles the marine invertebrate *Gorgonia flabellum* and arises from the venous side of arteriovenous anastomoses, growing from perfused retina toward peripheral nonperfused retina[8] (Figs. 36–15*A*, *B*, and *C*). The ischemic peripheral retina may elaborate factors that initiate and promote the growth of the neovascular tissue.[8] Lutty and co-workers observed elevated basic fibroblast growth factor (bFGF) in peripheral nonperfused areas[57] and increased vascular endothelial growth factor (VEGF) in a patient with sickle cell retinopathy.[70]

Once occlusions occur in the precapillary arterioles, altered blood flow patterns may then stimulate the formation of more vaso-occlusive events anywhere within the vascular tree, such as in the venous system.[34] Occlusion within a portion of a vein may exert substantial back-pressure within the proximal vessel and result in focal vascular extrusion.[34] This vessel may further enlarge as the elevated intraluminal pressure persists. Stretching of the vascular structures may contribute to endothelial cell proliferation[71] and neovascularization.[72]

The new capillaries initially grow into a fan-shape, forming fine red channels that may be overlooked on indirect ophthalmoscopy because of their small size and coloration that is similar to that of the fundus. The peripheral superotemporal quadrant is most frequently involved, followed by the inferotemporal, superonasal, and inferonasal quadrants. Sea fans are usually equatorial and rarely encroach on the ora serrata or posterior pole. Initially, the sea fan is flat and grows on the internal surface of the retina between the posterior hyaloid and internal limiting membrane and may be sustained by one feeding arteriole and draining venule. The feeder vessels may have large luminal diameters (Fig. 36–16). Further growth with the addition of more feeding and draining vessels may result in a larger, arborizing neovascular lesion (Fig. 36–17) that may form a peripheral traction band in the vitreous by its circumferential growth. Due to an inadequate blood-retinal barrier, chronic transudation into the vitreous from the sea fans may result in early vitreous degeneration, collapse, and traction, and prompt the onset of stages IV and V.

Goldberg Stage IV

Vitreous hemorrhage characterizes stage IV. Vitreous hemorrhage occurs most commonly in those patients with hemoglobin SC (21 to 23%) and less often in patients with hemoglobin SS (2 to 3%).[5,24,67] Vitreous hemorrhage in patients with other sickle hemoglobinopathies may be even less frequent.[5,67,73] Evaluation of untreated eyes with sickle retinopathy suggested three risk factors for subsequent vitreous hemorrhage: the presence of hemoglobin SC, any vitreous hemorrhage in the eye on initial examination, and more than 60 total degrees of active neovascular lesions[74] (Table 36–2). If there are greater than 60 degrees of circumferential neovascularization, the risk of a vitreous hemorrhage is increased.[74]

Sea fans may grow or may be pulled into the vitreous cavity. Traction on the delicate neovascular tissue from the adherent vitreous may result in hemorrhage. Sea fans may bleed at irregular intervals for several years as a result of minor ocular trauma, vitreous movement, vitreous syneresis, or contraction of vitreous bands induced by or exacerbated by previous hemorrhages. The hemorrhage may be asymptomatic and remain localized to the area surrounding the sea fan or may break into the vitreous gel and interfere with visual function. Plasma and blood may also chronically leak from the neovascular fronds and stimulate vitreous strand and fibroglial membrane formation, sometimes culminating in retinal detachment or stage V.

Goldberg Stage V

Stage V is characterized by traction and/or rhegmatogenous retinal detachment. Retinal detachment occurs most commonly in SC double heterozygotes,[5] since proliferative disease is most common in these patients. Retinal detachment has been rarely described in patients with AS[75] and SS[24,76] hemoglobinopathies.

Traction on the retina caused by vitreous bands

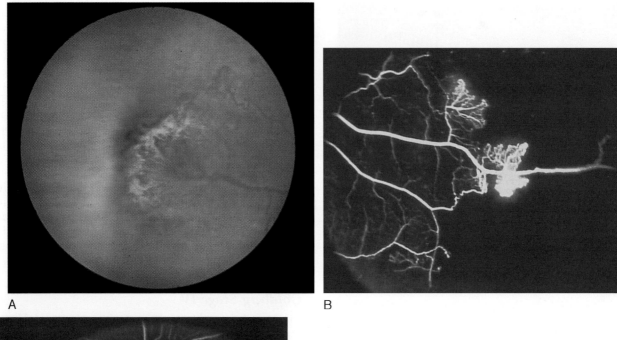

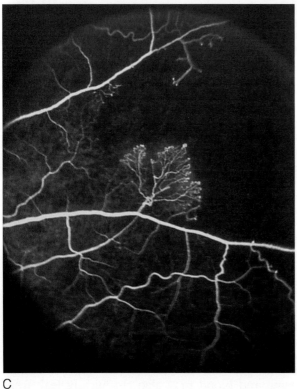

FIGURE 36-15 Peripheral neovascularization or sea fan formation characterizes stage III PSR. *A*, This tuft of neovascular tissue resembles the marine invertebrate *Gorgonia flabellum* and grows toward peripheral nonperfused retina. *B*, Fluorescein angiography clearly defines sea fan neovascularization. Compare this to the earlier angiogram in Figure 36–13. *C*, Sea fan formation usually develops in areas of peripheral arteriolar occlusion.

and/or fibroglial membranes may result in retinal breaks and detachment[77] (Fig. 36–18). These bands and membranes represent the effects of chronic transudation into the vitreous and repeated vitreous hemorrhages from the peripheral sea fans. Retinal breaks are usually located adjacent to fibrovascular lesions and may even be hidden by these lesions or by blood, making the break difficult to find in some detachments. In the absence of vitreoretinal traction, retinal breaks may also occur from

retinal atrophy due to retinal ischemia and may also result in a retinal detachment.

DIFFERENTIAL DIAGNOSIS

Peripheral neovascularization has been reported in various disorders[78] (Table 36–3). A thorough patient and family history and clinical examination are

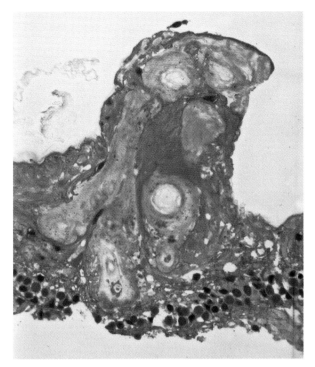

FIGURE 36–16 Cross section of an autoinfarcted sea fan in peripheral, atrophic retina from a 54-year-old SC subject. The feeder vessel had a large luminal diameter.

usually sufficient to make the correct diagnosis. Adjunctive blood tests such as a sickle cell screening test or hemoglobin electrophoresis will usually confirm the suspicion.

Management

Autoinfarction

The natural course of proliferative retinopathy may include autoinfarction of the sea fan lesion at a rate of up to 60%[7,79–81]; however, vitreous traction and retinal detachment may still occur. The pathophysiology of autoinfarction has not been well delineated; however, repeated sickling and thromboses within the neovascular lesion, decreased production of angiogenic substances, vitreous traction with kinking of the sea fan and decreased blood supply, and/or avulsion by vitreous traction may contribute to the spontaneous regression of the neovascular tissue.[81,82] Moreover, the slow blood flow in the neovascular formations may make them more susceptible than normal retinal vessels to vaso-occlusion. Sea fans may autoinfarct in one area of the retina (Fig. 36–19), while in another area of the same eye, a sea fan may continue to enlarge, and stage III may escalate into stage V. Thus, even though some sea fans may autoinfarct spontaneously, many neovascular fronds are potentially dangerous and most should probably be treated.

Indications

Because autoinfarction may occur and because some retinas do not demonstrate progressive sea fan growth, the precise indications for treatment are not always clear. However, patients with bilateral proliferative retinopathy, large elevated sea fan(s), rapid growth of a sea fan, evidence of vitreous hemorrhage, or those who have already lost one eye to proliferative disease are candidates for therapeutic intervention. If only one eye has a small sea fan, the patient and physician may opt to follow it closely and initiate treatment when growth of, or hemorrhage from, the lesion has been documented.

Since vitrectomy and scleral buckling surgery carry a high risk of complications in patients with sickle cell hemoglobinopathies as discussed below,[68,82–84] our goal of management has emphasized early treatment of proliferative manifestations seen in stage III by causing involution of the neovascular lesion(s) before the secondary complications of stages IV and V become manifest. Various treatment techniques have been explored, such as diathermy, cryotherapy, and laser photocoagulation. Among these, photocoagulation is widely available and has the fewest side effects. Application techniques include feeder vessel photocoagulation, local scatter photocoagulation with or without focal treatment of the sea fan, and 360-degree scatter application.[64,79,80,85,86]

Laser Photocoagulation

FEEDER VESSEL PHOTOCOAGULATION. Feeder vessel laser photocoagulation has been demonstrated to induce sea fan closure in 88% of patients with direct, heavy treatment to the feeding arteriole(s) and draining venule(s) of each sea fan in a controlled clinical trial[79] (Fig. 36–20). Both argon and xenon arc lasers have been effective in decreasing the incidence of vitreous hemorrhage and secondary visual loss. Further feeder vessel photocoagulation, or other supplemental methods of treatment such as scatter photocoagulation[85] or cryotherapy,[87,88] may be necessary if the posttreatment examination or fluorescein angiogram suggests that one or more neovascular fronds remain perfused.

Preferred treatment parameters to the arteriole and venule include use of the argon laser with a slitlamp delivery system and a spot size of 500 μm, 0.2 to 0.5-second duration, and a power adequate to facilitate closure of the feeding arteriole (usually starting at about 500 mW)[86] (Table 36–4). If the laser burn to the arteriole does not produce complete interruption of the blood column, the power level may be increased by 50 to 100 mW to achieve arteriolar segmentation. If the blood column still does not segment, the arteriole may be retreated within the prior laser burn with a smaller 50-μm spot size at higher power settings, or at a lower power set-

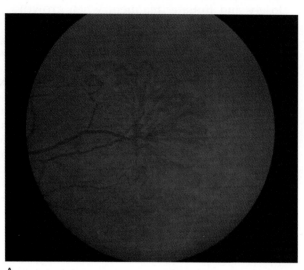

A

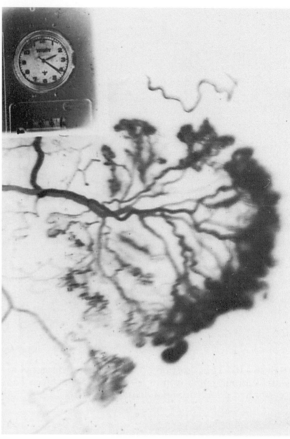

B

FIGURE 36–17   *A*, A large arborizing sea fan may result from continued growth with the addition of more feeding and draining vessels. *B*, Fluorescein angiography outlines an arborizing sea fan. (From Goldberg MF: Sickle cell retinopathy. In Duane TD, Jaeger EA (eds): Clinical Ophthalmology, Vol 3. Philadelphia, Harper & Row Publishers, Inc, 1979, with permission.)

ting 2 weeks later, when the prior laser burn has developed pigmentation and overlying retinal thinning.[82] Complications of feeder vessel treatment (Table 36–5) have been observed in 32% of treated patients within 6 months after treatment in one study.[79] Moreover, argon laser photocoagulation, applied in this manner, may be associated with an increased risk of retinal detachment in treated eyes.[74]

SCATTER PHOTOCOAGULATION. Scatter laser photocoagulation around the sea fan(s) has a lower complication rate than feeder vessel treatment and effectively reduces the incidence of vitreous hemorrhage and visual loss in patients with proliferative disease.[80] In a randomized, clinical trial of scatter photocoagulation, complete or partial sea fan closure occurred in 81% of the sea fans treated once, with complete closure in 30% of treated eyes, and with minimal treatment complications. Spontaneous regression occurred in only 46% of the untreated eyes and complete autoinfarction occurred in only 22%.[80] The rate of vitreous hemorrhage with scatter treatment is similar to that with feeder vessel treatment.[79,80] Local scatter treatment may not be

as successful in promoting sea fan shrinkage if the sea fan is elevated.[85]

The laser spots are applied locally in a scatter pattern (Fig. 36–21) to surround the sea fan using suggested parameters (Table 36–4). The spots are placed about one burn width apart. Treatment is applied for approximate distances of 1 disc diameter anterior to and posterior to the sea fan and 1 clock hour to either side of the treated lesions. The theory supporting the use of this approach is that the localized ischemia that develops from periph-

TABLE 36–2   Risk Factors for Vitreous Hemorrhage in Eyes with Proliferative Sickle Cell Retinopathy*

The presence of hemoglobin SC genotype
Any vitreous hemorrhage in the eye on initial examination
More than 60 total degrees of active sea fans

*Data derived from Condon et al.[74]

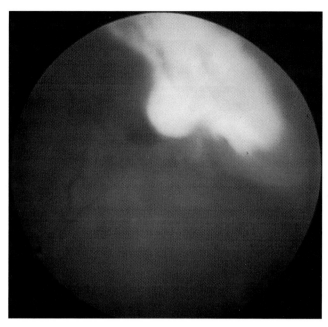

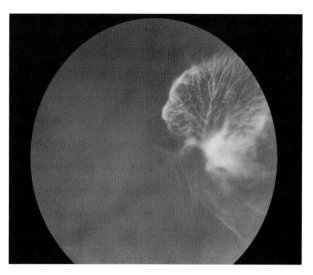

FIGURE 36–19   An autoinfarcted sea fan. Note the fibrotic changes in the elevated frond.

FIGURE 36–18   Traction-rhegmatogenous retinal detachment characterizes stage V PSR. Traction on the retina caused by vitreous bands and/or fibroglial membranes may result in a retinal break and detachment.

eral arteriolar nonperfusion may create a concentration gradient of vasoproliferative factors that promote sea fan growth. Local scatter treatment may reduce vasoproliferative factor production and secondarily lead to sea fan involution. The laser

TABLE 36–3   Differential Diagnosis of Peripheral Retinal Neovascularization*

Central and branch retinal vein occlusion
Chronic myelogenous leukemia
Chronic retinal detachment
Diabetic retinopathy
Eales' disease
Familial exudative vitreoretinopathy
Hyperviscosity syndromes
Idiopathic occlusive arteriolitis
Incontinentia pigmenti
Pars planitis
Posterior uveitides
Radiation retinopathy
Retinopathy of prematurity
Rheumatic fever
Sarcoidosis
Sickle cell retinopathy
Talc embolization

*Data derived from Jampol and Goldbaum.[78]

scar also induces chorioretinal adhesions that may prevent or minimize subsequent retinal detachment. Direct laser treatment of the sea fan itself may be attempted alone or in addition to local scatter treatment if the sea fan is not elevated (Fig. 36–22). If scatter or even direct treatment does not induce adequate regression of the neovascularization and if vitreous hemorrhage begins or continues, feeder vessel treatment may be used to supplement the initial treatment.

Whether or not to initiate scatter photocoagulation when there is only one or two sea fans in an eye is not clear, because the development of a vitreous hemorrhage and/or visual loss in eyes with 60 degress or less of circumferential proliferative disease is low.[74] However, since the risks of scatter treatment are also low, it should probably be initiated in most patients when any proliferative changes are noted.[80] One exception may be for SS homozygotes over the age of 40. Treatment may not always be necessary in this subset of patients, because 86% with neovascular sea fans may remain stable or demonstrate regression.[95]

If the patient is reliable and can return for scheduled follow-up examinations, then a local scatter treatment may be performed with or without direct treatment of any flat sea fans. If new lesions subsequently develop, then further scatter treatment may be added. If the patient is unreliable for regular follow-up, however, then a 360-degree technique of scatter treatment may be considered,[96] since new sea fans may develop in up to 34% of eyes in other areas despite previous local scatter treatment.[80] The available evidence, however, does not convincingly suggest that circumferential treatment is better than either the clinical course of the disease when left untreated or sector peripheral scatter treatment to definite neovascular fronds alone.[82,85]

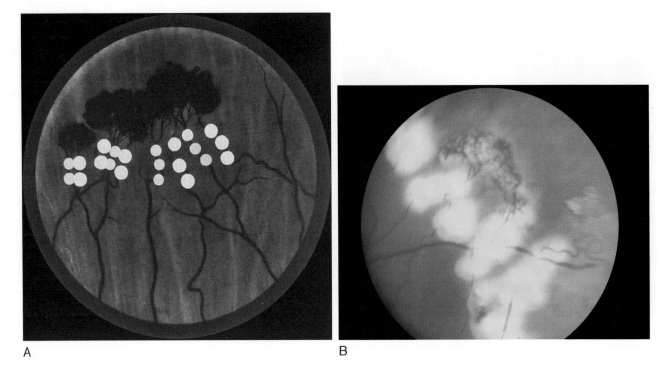

FIGURE 36–20   *A*, Feeder vessel laser photocoagulation to active sea fan neovascularization is depicted schematically. *B*, A clinical photograph following feeder vessel treatment is shown. (From Goldberg MF, Jampol LM: Treatment of neovascularization, vitreous hemorrhage, and retinal detachment in sickle cell retinopathy. In Symposium on Medical and Surgical Diseases of the Retina and Vitreous; Transactions of the New Orleans Academy of Ophthalmology. St Louis, CV Mosby Co, 1983, pp 53–81, with permission.)

Cryotherapy

Lenticular and/or vitreous opacities may make visualization and laser photocoagulation of some sea fans difficult or even preclude it altogether. In these cases, transconjunctival cryotherapy may be necessary. The sea fan to be treated can usually be visualized using indirect ophthalmoscopy; however, concurrent fluorescein angioscopy may be needed for better visualization in eyes with a dense vitreous hemorrhage.[82] With one application, about 70% of sea fans may be effectively treated.[87] The treatment end point is to surround the sea fan with cryotherapy application(s) (Fig. 36–23). There should be no overlap of adjacent applications. Excessive cryotherapy (defined as retreatment in the same area) may cause retinal breaks and detachment.

Pars Plana Vitrectomy

The source of a vitreous hemorrhage should be identified and treated with laser photocoagulation whenever possible; however, the vitreous hemorrhage itself may initially be treated conservatively.[82] Fluorescein angiography may elucidate the source of the hemorrhage; however, adequate angiography may be hampered by the hemorrhage. Angioscopy may better locate a perfused sea fan, because fluorescein leaks into the vitreous and is more readily seen. The sea fan may then be treated with laser photocoagulation if visualization is adequate or with cryotherapy if the media are too hazy for photocoagulation. Close follow-up during resolution of the hemorrhage is important. If the vitreous hemorrhage does not clear within 6 months, and if laser

TABLE 36–4   Suggested Sea Fan Laser Photocoagulation Parameters*

	Feeder vessel	Local scatter
Spot size	500 μm	500 μm
Duration	0.2 second–0.5 second	0.2 second
Power	500 mW—titrate for vessel closure	Modest intensity burn

*Data derived from Jampol et al.[86]

TABLE 36–5 Complications of Sea Fan Feeder Vessel Photocoagulation*

Choroidal ischemia
Choroidal hemorrhage
Choroidal neovascularization
Choriovitreal neovascularization
Epiretinal membrane
Macular hole
Retinal break
Rhegmatogenous retinal detachment
Subretinal fibrosis
Tractional retinal detachment
Vitreous hemorrhage

*Data derived from Condon et al,[74] Jacobson et al,[79] Dizon-Moore et al,[89] Goldbaum et al,[90] Condon et al,[91] Carney et al,[92] Fox et al,[93] and Galinos et al.[94]

Scleral Buckling

Retinal detachment surgery in patients with sickle cell hemoglobinopathies is performed only if absolutely necessary. It cannot be delayed if the detachment is rhegmatogenous. However, surgery may be postponed in eyes with tractional retinal detachments unless progression is documented. If a vitreous hemorrhage and severe vitreous traction coexist, a pars plana vitrectomy may also be necessary.

Surgery in these patients poses an increased risk of intraoperative and postoperative complications compared to nonsicklers undergoing similar surgery[82]; however, improved vitrectomy techniques may decrease potential surgical complications. Complications include, but are not limited to, anterior segment ischemia,[97] optic nerve and macular infarctions when intraocular pressures are only 25 mm Hg or greater, and intraoperative sickle cell crises during general anesthesia (Table 36–6). Precautions should be taken to reduce the risk of developing surgical complications. An exchange transfusion may be considered preoperatively[98] to obtain hemoglobin A levels of 50 to 60% (by electrophoresis) and a hematocrit of 35 to 40%. However, if elevated intraocular pressure develops postoperatively, the safety margin provided by the preoperative exchange transfusion is reduced. A preoperative exchange transfusion is no longer considered routine,[99] however, due to the potential risk of acquiring hepatitis or the human immunodeficiency virus (HIV). Its use should be individualized

or cryotherapy is not possible, a vitrectomy with endolaser photocoagulation may be necessary.[82,84] If the fundus cannot be visualized at any time following the development of the hemorrhage, B-scan ultrasonography may be necessary to exclude a concurrent retinal detachment. If a retinal detachment is identified initially or during serial ultrasonography, surgical intervention is needed.

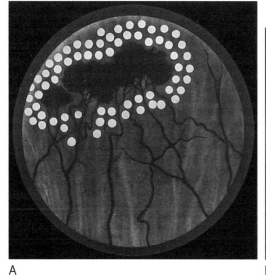

A

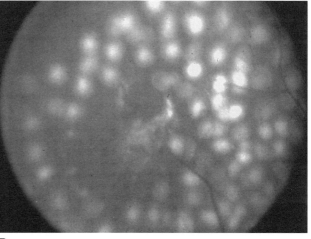

B

FIGURE 36–21 *A,* Local scatter laser photocoagulation to active sea fan neovascularization is depicted schematically. (From Goldberg MF, Jampol LM: Treatment of Neovascularization, Vitreous Hemorrhage, and Retinal Detachment in Sickle Cell Retinopathy. In Symposium on Medical and Surgical Diseases of the Retina and Vitreous; Transactions of the New Orleans Academy of Ophthalmology. St Louis, CV Mosby Co, 1983, pp 53–81, with permission.) *B,* A clinical photograph following local scatter laser treatment is shown.

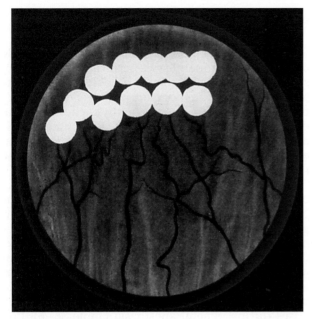

FIGURE 36–22 Focal laser photocoagulation to flat sea fans, depicted schematically here, may complement local scatter treatment. For small flat sea fans, this technique can occasionally be used alone. (From Goldberg MF, Jampol LM: Treatment of neovascularization, vitreous hemorrhage, and retinal detachment in sickle cell retinopathy. In Symposium on Medical and Surgical Diseases of the Retina and Vitreous; Transactions of the New Orleans Academy of Ophthalmology. St Louis, CV Mosby Co, 1983, pp 53–81, with permission.)

for each patient while considering coexistent ocular disorders, the condition of the contralateral eye, the operative procedure, and the anesthetic regimen. An alternative to an exchange transfusion may be the use of hyperbaric oxygen during the scleral buckling procedure[100]; however, widespread availability of this equipment is lacking. In most circum-

TABLE 36–6 Intraoperative Complications with Retinal Detachment Surgery in Patients with Sickle Cell Hemoglobinopathies*

Anterior segment ischemia/necrosis
Optic nerve and macular infarctions with intraocular pressures $\geq$25 mm Hg
Sickle cell crises during general anesthesia

---

*Data derived from Goldberg and Jampol[82] and Ryan and Goldberg.[97]

stances, an exchange transfusion can be avoided with modern surgical techniques.

Additional precautions include the preoperative closure (by photocoagulation) of large sea fans that might bleed intraoperatively; avoidance of any recurrently applied sympathomimetic agents; the administration of intra- or postoperative oxygen; avoidance of unnecessary traction on, or removal of, rectus muscles and of transscleral coagulation in the horizontal meridian; maintenance of a low intraocular pressure intraoperatively to facilitate vascular perfusion; the use of transscleral cryotherapy instead of diathermy; the drainage of subretinal fluid when placing the scleral buckle (to prevent marked elevation of the intraocular pressure)[83]; hyperoxygenation both intra- and postoperatively; and preoperative hematologic consultation (Table 36–7).

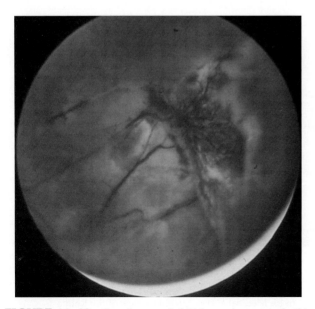

FIGURE 36–23 Cryotherapy (whitish area) surrounds this active sea fan.

TABLE 36–7 Recommended Preoperative and Intraoperative Precautions for Patients with Sickle Cell Hemoglobinopathies*

Preoperative closure of sea fans if possible
Avoid recurrently applied sympathomimetic agents
Intraoperative and postoperative oxygen
Avoid unnecessary traction on or removal of rectus muscles
Avoid transscleral coagulation in the horizontal meridian
Maintain low intraoperative intraocular pressures
Use cryotherapy instead of diathermy
Drain subretinal fluid when placing the scleral buckle
Preoperative hematologic consultation

---

*Data derived from Cohen et al.[83]

FUTURE INVESTIGATIONS

Progress in the treatment of sickle cell disease and the associated retinopathy has been hindered in the past by a lack of animal models for sickle cell disease. Recently, transgenic animal technology has permitted the creation of animal models of sickle cell disease. Constructs of the different variants in human β^s globin and the human α-globin gene have been inserted into fertilized mouse eggs.[101] Some of the animals expressed the human genes but at low levels. By subsequently breeding the transgenic mice into a background of mouse β^{major} deletion, the equivalent of β-thalassemia, the resultant mice expressed high levels of the human genes but were not thalassemic. The erythrocytes of these mice sickle, however, and Lutty and co-workers have observed a severe form of sickle cell retinopathy in one of these transgenic mouse lines.[31]

Retinal pathologic changes were observed in the $\alpha^H\beta^s[\beta^{MDD}]$ transgenic mouse line of Fabry and colleagues that was established by simultaneously injecting $\mu LCR\text{-}\beta^s$ and $\mu LCR\text{-}\alpha^H$ (LCR = locus control region) constructs into C57BL/6J mice and breeding the transgenics with mice that were homozygous for the mouse β^{major} deletion.[102] The mice in this line have 80% human β^s-globin genes, have spleen and lung pathology, and many hematologic characteristics in common with human sickle cell disease.[103] The retinas of these transgenic mice demonstrate vaso-occlusive processes that result in loss of precapillary arterioles, capillaries, and venules. Intra- and extraretinal neovascularization was observed and was associated mostly with veins, venules, and arteriovenous anastomoses. Pigmented lesions resembling human black sunburst lesions were observed and consisted mostly of blood vessels that often appeared to be of choroidal origin (Fig. 36–24) and were ensheathed by RPE-like cells (Fig. 36–25). Chorioretinopathy was bilateral and occurred in 30% of the animals examined. The in-

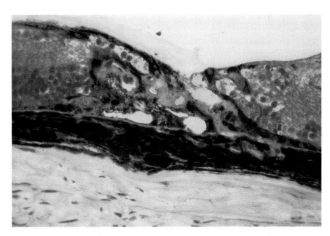

FIGURE 36–25   Pigmented lesions resembling human black sunburst lesions were also observed in the $\alpha^H\beta^s[\beta^{MDD}]$ transgenic mouse line. As in the human lesions, RPE-like cells have migrated into retina and may be associated with schisis cavities. RPE-like cells ensheathed blood vessels, some of which may be of choroidal origin. The apparent photoreceptor loss was often observed in animals with severe chorioretinopathy.

cidence increased with age. This model is probably the only available genetically derived animal model for retinal and choroidal neovascularization.[31]

The retinopathy that occurs in this mouse line is similar to human retinopathy, because occlusions, intra- and extraretinal neovascularization, choroidal neovascularization, and pigmented lesions occur. The retinopathy in the transgenic mice differs from human retinopathy, however, in that occlusions are not predominantly in peripheral retina, and hemorrhages are observed infrequently. Also, unlike the human, choroidal neovascularization was more common than retinal neovascularization. In the human, photoreceptor degeneration occurs in areas of retinal and choroidal nonperfusion only, whereas in advanced retinopathy in the mice all photoreceptors degenerate. In a second study from Lutty's laboratory, photoreceptor atrophy and choroidal neovascularization were associated with choroidal nonperfusion, as determined with a vascular tracer.[104]

Animal models to study the mechanism of vaso-occlusion in sickle cell disease have also recently been developed. Initially, vasculatures like mesocecum and mesoappendix were used, so that vital examination of sickled erythrocyte adhesion and vascular obstruction could be performed.[105] Recently, Wajer and colleagues have introduced a model to evaluate the retention of sickle red cells in the retinal vasculature.[106] Rats were administered fluorescently labeled human sickled erythrocytes intravenously, and retention of the cells within the vasculature was evaluated in retinal flat mounts. This model is currently being used by Lutty and associates to determine which cell population adheres within retinal vessels and under what physiologic conditions.[107]

With the advent of animal models, the mechanisms of vaso-occlusion in the sickle cell retina can

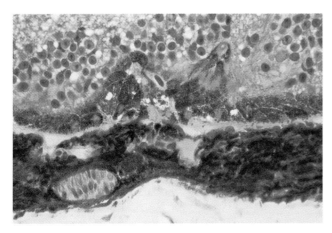

FIGURE 36–24   Choroidal neovascularization was frequently observed in the $\alpha^H\beta^s[\beta^{MDD}]$ transgenic mouse line. New vessels are ensheathed with RPE-like cells as they enter this area with outer retinal atrophy.

be determined. Therapeutic interventions addressing these mechanisms could then be evaluated in the transgenic mouse lines to determine if the treatments can prevent or allay vaso-occlusive processes in sickle cell retinopathy. Like diabetic retinopathy,[108] if the vaso-occlusive processes can be prevented, subsequent proliferative vasculopathy may be avoided.

Acknowledgements: This work was supported in part by an unrestricted research grant from Research to Prevent Blindness, Inc, New York, the Guerrieri Fund, and by Core Grant No 2-P30-EY01765–19 from the National Eye Institute, and by the Heed and Heed/Knapp Fellowship Foundation.

REFERENCES

1. Herrick JB: Peculiar elongated and sickle-shaped red blood corpuscules in a case of severe anemia. Arch Intern Med 6:517–621, 1910.
2. Eaton WA, Hofrichter J: Hemoglobin S gelation and sickle cell disease. Blood 70:1245–1266, 1987.
3. Noguchi CT, Schechter AN: The intracellular polymerisation of hemoglobin and its relevance to sickle cell disease. Blood 58:1057–1068, 1981.
4. Necheles TF, Allen DN, Finkel HE: Clinical Disorders of Hemoglobin Structure and Function. New York, Appleton-Century-Crofts, 1969.
5. Welch RB, Goldberg MF: Sickle-cell hemoglobin and its relation to fundus abnormality. Arch Ophthalmol 75:353–362, 1966.
6. Pearson HA: Hemoglobin S-thalassemia syndrome in Negro children. Ann NY Acad Sci 165:83–92, 1969.
7. Condon PI, Serjeant GR: Behaviour of untreated sickle retinopathy. Br J Ophthalmol 64:404–411, 1980.
8. Goldberg MF: Retinal neovascularization in sickle cell retinopathy. Trans Am Acad Ophthalmol Otolaryngol 83:409–431, 1977.
9. Goldberg MF: Retinal vaso-occlusion in sickling hemoglobinopathies. Birth Defects 12:475–515, 1976.
10. Goldberg MF: Natural history of untreated proliferative sickle retinopathy. Arch Ophthalmol 85:428–437, 1971.
11. Abrams LS, Goldberg MF: Retinopathy associated with hemoglobin AC. Arch Ophthalmol 112:1410–1411, 1994.
12. Rummeld R: Hamoglobinanomalien in der ophthalmologischen praxis. Klin Monatsbl Augenheilkd 166:644–650, 1975.
13. Nagpal KC, Asdourian GK, Rabb M, et al: Proliferative retinopathy in sickle cell trait. Report of seven cases. Arch Intern Med 137:325–328, 1977.
14. Moschandreou M, Galinos SO, Valenzuela R, et al: Retinopathy in hemoglobin C trait (AC hemoglobinopathy). Am J Ophthalmol 77:465–471, 1974.
15. Bloch RS: Hematologic disorders. In Duane TD, Jaeger EA (eds): Clinical Ophthalmology, Vol 5. Philadelphia, Harper & Row Publishers Inc, 1984.
16. Goldberg MF: Sickle cell retinopathy. In Duane TD, Jaeger EA, (eds): Clinical Ophthalmology, Vol 3. Philadelphia, Harper & Row Publishers Inc, 1979.
17. Serjeant GR: Sickle Cell Disease. Oxford, Oxford University Press, 1985.
18. Goldberg MF: Sickled erythrocytes, hyphema, and secondary glaucoma: I. The diagnosis and treatment of sickled erythrocytes in human hyphemas. Ophthalmic Surg 10:17–31, 1979.
19. Paton D: The conjunctival sign in sickle cell disease. Arch Ophthalmol 68:627–632, 1962.
20. Charache S, Conley CL: Rate of sickling of red cells during deoxygenation of blood from persons with various sickling disorders. Blood 24:25–34, 1964.
21. Horne MK III: Sickle cell anemia as a rheologic disease. Am J Med 70:288–98, 1981.
22. Gagliano DA, Goldberg MF: The evolution of salmon patch hemorrhages in sickle cell retinopathy. Arch Ophthalmol 107:1814–1815, 1989.
23. Romayananda N, Goldberg MF, Green WR: Histopathology of sickle cell retinopathy. Trans Am Acad Ophthalmol Otolaryngol 77:652–657, 1973.
24. Condon PI. Serjeant GR: Ocular findings in homozygous sickle cell anemia in Jamaica. Am J Ophthalmol 73:533–543, 1972.
25. Condon PI, Serjeant GR: Ocular findings in hemoglobin SC disease in Jamaica. Am J Ophthalmol 74:921–931, 1972.
26. Condon PI, Serjeant GR: Ocular findings in sickle cell thalassemia in Jamaica. Am J Ophthalmol 74:1105–1109, 1972.
27. Levine RA, Kaplan AM: The ophthalmoscopic findings in C + S disease. Am J Ophthalmol 59:37–42, 1965.
28. Asdourian GK, Nagpal KC, Goldbaum M, et al: Evolution of the retinal black sunburst in sickling haemoglobinopathies. Br J Ophthalmol 59:710–716, 1975.
29. van Meurs JC: Evolution of a retinal hemorrhage in a patient with sickle cell-hemoglobin C disease. Arch Ophthalmol 113:1074–1075, 1995.
30. Liang JC, Jampol LM: Spontaneous peripheral chorioretinal neovascularization in association with sickle cell anaemia. Br J Ophthalmol 67:107–110, 1983.
31. Lutty GA, McLeod DS, Pachnis A, et al: Retinal and choroidal neovascularization in a transgenic mouse model of sickle cell disease. Am J Pathol 145:490–497, 1994.
32. Cogan DG: Ophthalmic Manifestations of Systemic Vascular Disease. Philadelphia, WB Saunders, 1974.
33. Wise GN, Dollery CT, Henkind P: The retinal circulation. New York, Harper & Row Publishers Inc, 1971.
34. McLeod DS, Goldberg MF, Lutty GA: Dual-perspective analysis of vascular formations in sickle cell retinopathy. Arch Ophthalmol 111:1234–1245, 1993.
35. Kabakow B, Van Weimokly SS, Lyons HA: Bilateral central retinal artery occlusion. Arch Ophthalmol 54:670–677, 1955.
36. Goodman G, von Sallmann L, Holland MG: Ocular manifestations of sickle cell disease. Arch Ophthalmol 58:657–682, 1957.
37. Lieb WA, Geeraets WJ, Guerry D: Ocular and systemic manifestations of sickle cell disease. Acta Ophthalmol 58(Suppl):25–45, 1951.
38. Conrad WC, Penner R: Sickle cell trait and central retinal artery occlusion. Am J Ophthalmol 63:465–468, 1967.
39. Condon PI, Whitelocke RAF, Bird AC, et al: Recurrent visual loss in homozygous sickle cell disease. Br J Ophthalmol 69:700–706, 1985.
40. Asdourian GK: Central retinal artery occlusion. Am J Ophthalmol 79:374–380, 1975.
41. Klein ML, Jampol LM, Condon PI, et al: Central retinal artery occlusion without retrobulbar hemorrhage after retrobulbar injection. Am J Ophthalmol 93:573–577, 1982.
42. Weissman H, Nadel AJ, Dunn M: Simultaneous bilateral retinal arterial occlusions treated by exchange transfusions. Arch Ophthalmol 75:353–362, 1979.
43. Appen RE, Wray SH, Cogan DG: Central retinal artery occlusion. Am J Ophthalmol 79:381–384, 1975.
44. Chopdar A: Multiple major retinal vascular occlusions in sickle-cell hemoglobin C disease. Br J Ophthalmol 59:493–499, 1975.
45. Ryan SJ: Occlusion of macular capillaries in sickle cell hemoglobin C disease. Am J Ophthalmol 77:459–461, 1974.
46. Knapp JW: Isolated macular infarction in sickle cell (SS) disease. Am J Ophthalmol 73:857–859, 1972.
47. Acacio I, Goldberg MF: Peripapillary and macular vessel occlusions in sickle cell anemia. Am J Ophthalmol 75:861–866, 1973.

48. Goldbaum MH: Retinal depression sign indicating a retinal infarct. Am J Ophthalmol 86:45–55, 1978.

49. Asdourian GK, Nagpal KC, Busse B, et al: Macular and perimacular vascular remodeling in sickling hemoglobinopathies. Br J Ophthalmol 60:431–453, 1976.

50. Stevens TS, Busse B, Lee C, et al: Sickling hemoglobinopathies. Macular and perimacular abnormalities. Arch Ophthalmol 92:455–463, 1974.

51. Marsh RJ, Ford SM, Rabb MF, et al: Macular vasculature, visual acuity and irreversibly sickled cells in homozygous sickle cell disease. Br J Ophthalmol 66:155–160, 1982.

52. Platt OS, Brambilla DJ, Rosse WF, et al: Mortality in sickle cell disease: life expectancy and risk factors for early death. N Engl J Med 330:1639–1644, 1994.

53. Stein MR, Gay AJ: Acute chorioretinal infarction in sickle cell trait. Arch Ophthalmol 84:485–490, 1970.

54. Condon PI, Serjeant GR, Ikeda H: Unusual chorioretinal degeneration in sickle cell disease. Br J Ophthalmol 57:81–88, 1973.

55. Dizon RV, Jampol LM, Goldberg MF, Juarez C: Choroidal occlusive disease in sickle cell hemoglobinopathies. Surv Ophthalmol 23:297–306, 1973.

56. Lutty GA, Goldberg MF: Ophthalmologic complications. In Embury SH, Hebbel RP, Mohandas N, Steinberg MH (eds): Sickle Cell Disease: Basic Principles and Clinical Practice. New York, Raven Press Ltd, 1994.

57. Lutty GA, Merges C, Crone S, McLeod S: Immunohistochemical insights into sickle cell retinopathy. Curr Eye Res 13:125–138, 1994.

58. Nagpal KC, Huamonte F, Constantaras A, et al: Migratory white-without-pressure retinal lesions. Arch Ophthalmol 94:576–579, 1976.

59. Condon PI, Serjeant GR: The progression of sickle cell eye disease in Jamaica. Doc Ophthalmol 39:203–210, 1975.

60. Nagpal KC, Asdourian G, Goldbaum M, et al: Angioid streaks and sickle hemoglobinopathies. Br J Ophthalmol 37:325–328, 1977.

61. Nagpal KC, Goldberg MF, Asdourian GK, et al: Dark-without-pressure fundus lesions. Br J Ophthalmol 59:476–479, 1975.

62. Raichand M, Goldberg MF, Nagpal KC, et al: Evolution of neovascularization in sickle cell retinopathy. Arch Ophthalmol 95:1543–1552, 1977.

63. Ober RR, Michels RG: Optic disc neovascularization in hemoglobin SC disease. Am J Ophthalmol 85:711–714, 1978.

64. Kimmel AS, Magargal LE, Tasman WS: Proliferative sickle retinopathy and neovascularization of the disc: regression following treatment with peripheral retinal scatter laser. Ophthalmic Surg 17:20–22, 1986.

65. Condon PI, Serjeant GR: Ocular findings in elderly cases of homozygous sickle-cell disease in Jamaica. Br J Ophthalmol 60:361–364, 1976.

66. Clarkson JG, Altman RD: Angioid streaks. Surv Ophthalmol 26:235–246, 1982.

67. Clarkson JG: The ocular manifestations of sickle-cell disease: a prevalence and natural history study. Trans Am Ophthalmol Soc 90:481–504, 1992.

68. Jampol LM, Green JR, Goldberg MF, Peyman GA: An update on vitrectomy surgery and retinal detachment repair in sickle cell disease. Arch Ophthalmol 100:591–593, 1982.

69. Goldberg MF: Classification and pathogenesis of proliferative sickle retinopathy. Am J Ophthalmol 71:649–665, 1971.

70. Lutty GA, McLeod DS, Merges C, et al: Localization of VEGF in human retina and choroid. Arch Ophthalmol 114:971–977, 1996.

71. Curtis ASG, Seehar GM: The control of cell division by tension or diffusion. Nature 274:52–53, 1978.

72. van Meurs JC: Ocular findings in sickle cell disease on Curacao. Nijmegen, the Netherlands: Catholic University of Nijmegen; 1990, Thesis.

73. Goldberg MF, Charache S, Acacio I.: Ophthalmologic manifestations of sickle cell thalassemia. Arch Intern Med 128:33–39, 1971.

74. Condon PI, Jampol LN, Farber MD, et al: A randomised clinical trial of feeder vessel photocoagulation of proliferative sickle cell retinopathy: II. Update and analysis of risk factors. Ophthalmology 91:1496–1498, 1984.

75. Isbey HK, Clifford GO, Tanaka KR: Vitreous hemorrhage associated with sickle-cell trait and sickle-cell hemoglobin C disease. Am J Ophthalmol 45:870–879, 1958.

76. Kearney WF: Sickle-cell ophthalmopathy. NY State J Med 65:2677–2681, 1965.

77. Carney MD, Jampol LM: Epiretinal membranes in sickle cell retinopathy. Arch Ophthalmol 105:214–217, 1987.

78. Jampol LM, Goldbaum MH: Peripheral proliferative retinopathies. Surv Ophthalmol 25:1–14, 1980.

79. Jacobson MS, Gagliano DA, Cohen SB, et al: A randomized clinical trial of feeder vessel photocoagulation of sickle cell retinopathy. A long-term follow-up. Ophthalmology 98:581–585, 1991.

80. Farber MD, Jampol LM, Fox P, et al: A randomized clinical trial of scatter photocoagulation of proliferative sickle cell retinopathy. Arch Ophthalmol 109:363–367, 1991.

81. Nagpal KC, Patrianakos D, Asdourian GK, et al: Spontaneous regression (autoinfarction) of proliferative sickle retinopathy. Am J Ophthalmol 80:885–892, 1975.

82. Goldberg MF, Jampol LM: Treatment of neovascularization, vitreous hemorrhage, and retinal detachment in sickle cell retinopathy. In Symposium on Medical and Surgical Diseases of the Retina and Vitreous; Transactions of the New Orleans Academy of Ophthalmology. St Louis, CV Mosby Co, 1983, pp 53–81.

83. Cohen SB, Fletcher ME, Goldberg MF, Jednock NJ: Diagnosis and management of ocular complications of sickle hemoglobinopathies: Part V. Ophthalmic Surg 17:369–374, 1986.

84. Goldbaum MH, Peyman GA, Nagpal KC, et al: Vitrectomy in sickling retinopathy: report of five cases. Ophthalmic Surg 7:92–102, 1976.

85. Rednam KRV, Jampol LM, Goldberg MF: Scatter retinal photocoagulation for proliferative sickle cell retinopathy. Am J Ophthalmol 93:594–599, 1982.

86. Jampol LM, Farber M, Rabb MF, Serjeant GR: An update on techniques of photocoagulation treatment of proliferative sickle cell retinopathy. Eye 5:260–263, 1991.

87. Lee CB, Woolf MB, Galinos SO, et al: Cryotherapy of proliferative sickle cell retinopathy. I. Single freeze-thaw cycle. Ann Ophthalmol 7:1299–1308, 1975.

88. Hanscom TA: Indirect treatment of peripheral retinal neovascularization. Am J Ophthalmol 93:88–91, 1982.

89. Dizon-Moore RV, Jampol LM, Goldberg MF: Chorioretinal and choriovitreal neovascularization. Their presence after photocoagulation of proliferative sickle cell retinopathy. Arch Ophthalmol 99:842–849, 1981.

90. Goldbaum MH, Galinos SO, Apple D, et al: Acute choroidal ischemia as a complication of photocoagulation. Arch Ophthalmol 94:1025–1035, 1976.

91. Condon PI, Jampol LM, Ford SM, Serjeant GR: Choroidal neovascularization induced by photocoagulation in sickle cell disease. Br J Ophthalmol 65:192–197, 1981.

92. Carney MD, Paylor RR, Cunha-Vaz JG, et al: Iatrogenic choroidal neovascularization in sickle cell retinopathy. Ophthalmology 93:1163–1168, 1986.

93. Fox PD, Acheson RW, Serjeant GR: Outcome of iatrogenic choroidal neovascularization in sickle cell disease. Br J Ophthalmol 74:417–420, 1990.

94. Galinos SO, Asdourian GK, Woolf MB, et al: Choroidovitreal neovascularisation after argon laser photocoagulation. Arch Ophthalmol 93:524–530, 1975.

95. Fox PD, Vessey SJR, Forshaw ML, Serjeant GR: Influence of genotype on the natural history of untreated proliferative sickle retinopathy—an angiographic study. Br J Ophthalmol 75:229–231, 1991.

96. Kimmel AS, Magargal LE, Stephens RF, Cruess AF: Peripheral circumferential retinal scatter photocoagulation for the treatment of proliferative sickle retinopathy. An update. Ophthalmology 93:1429–1434, 1986.

97. Ryan SJ, Goldberg MF: Anterior segment ischemia follow-

ing scleral buckling in sickle cell hemoglobinopathy. Am J Ophthalmol 72:35–50, 1971.

98. Brazier DH, Gregor ZJ, Blach RK, et al: Retinal detachment in patients with proliferative sickle cell retinopathy. Trans Ophthalmol Soc U K 105:100–105, 1986.

99. Pulido JS, Flynn HW, Clarkson JG, Blankenship GW: Pars plana vitrectomy in the management of proliferative sickle retinopathy. Arch Ophthalmol 106:1553–1557, 1988.

100. Freilich DB, Seelenfreund MH: Long-term follow-up of scleral buckling procedure with sickle cell disease and retinal detachment treated with the use of hyperbaric oxygen. Mod Probl Ophthalmol 18:368–372, 1977.

101. Fabry ME: Transgenic animal models of sickle cell disease. Experentia 49:28–36, 1993.

102. Fabry ME, Nagel RL, Pachnis A, et al: High expression of human β^s and α-globins in transgenic mice: hemoglobin composition and hematological consequences. Proc Natl Acad Sci USA 89:12150–12154, 1992.

103. Fabry ME, Constantini F, Pachnis A, et al: High expression of human β^s- and α-genes in transgenic mice: eryth-rocyte abnormalities, organ damage, and the effect of hypoxia. Proc Natl Acad Sci USA 89:12155–12159, 1992.

104. Merges C, McLeod DS, Crone S, et al: Retinal and choroidal nonperfusion precedes neovascularization and outer retinal atrophy in a transgenic mouse model of sickle cell disease. Curr Eye Res (in press), 1997.

105. Kaul D, Fabry M, Nagel R: Microvascular sites and characteristics of sickle cell adhesion to vascular endothelium in shear flow conditions: pathological implications. Proc Natl Acad Sci USA 86:3356–3360, 1989.

106. Wajer SD, McLeod DS, Fabry M, et al: Confocal microscopic imaging of fluorescently-labeled human sickle erythrocytes in ADPase flat-mounted rat retinas. Invest Ophthalmol Vis Sci 33(Suppl):1949, 1992.

107. Lutty GA, Phelan A, McLeod DS, et al: A rat model for sickle cell-mediated vaso-occlusion in retina. Microvascular Res. 52:270–280, 1996.

108. Kohner E, Porta M: Vascular abnormalities in diabetes and their treatment. Trans Ophthalmol Soc UK 100:440–444, 1980.

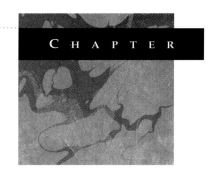

CHAPTER 37

Plasma Protein Risk Factors for Retinal Vascular Occlusive Disease

Antonio P. Ciardella, M.D.

David R. Guyer, M.D.

Lawrence A. Yannuzzi, M.D.

Retinal vascular occlusive disease is typically a disease of older patients associated with hypertension, diabetes, hyperlipidemia, and open angle glaucoma. In recent years, an increasing attention has developed towards newly recognized risk factors for retinal vascular thrombotic episodes in young patients.

PROTEIN C DEFICIENCY AND RESISTANCE TO ACTIVATED PROTEIN C

Protein C is a vitamin K–dependent plasma protein that acts as a physiologic anticoagulant. It consists of heavy and light chain polypeptides linked by sulfydryl groups.[1] Protein C circulates as an inactive zymogen, and is activated by enzymatic cleavage on the surface of endothelial cells by a complex of thrombin and thrombomodulin. Activated protein C (APC) is a potent anticoagulant that inhibits the coagulation cascade by selectively degrading factors V and VIII activated (Va and VIIIa) in the presence of phospholipid, calcium, and protein S, a vitamin K–dependent cofactor.[2,3]

Protein C deficiency can be caused by both reduction of the total amount of circulating protein C or by reduced activity in the presence of normal blood concentration. Both congenital and acquired forms of protein C deficiency are found.

Congenital protein C deficiency may be inherited as an autosomal recessive or dominant trait.

Homozygous protein C deficiency is inherited in an autosomal recessive fashion and is a severe condition. Affected individuals have almost no detectable protein C activity, less than 1% (normal, 70 to 140%),[5] causing massive venous thrombosis in the newborn, or neonatal purpura fulminans[6] in the first few days of life. Severe protein C deficiency causes disseminated systemic thromboses and hemorrhages and is a life-threatening condition that requires prompt diagnosis and immediate therapy with protein C substitutes.

Heterozygous protein C deficiency is inherited as an autosomal dominant disorder and is associated with concentration around 50% of normal and a tendency to thrombosis. Since the first description in 1981[7] of a case of venous thrombosis associated with protein C deficiency, several family pedigrees have been reported, where heterozygous individuals had a history of recurrent thrombotic episodes associated with reduced serum levels of protein C.[8] The most common clinical manifestations of heterozygous protein C deficiency are recurrent deep vein thrombosis at an early age and recurrent superficial thrombophlebitis. Cerebral vein thrombosis, pulmonary embolism, and arterial thrombosis have been reported as well.[9] About one third of individuals with heterozygous deficiency are asymptomatic during life.[10]

The acquired form of protein C deficiency is associated with liver disease[11]; anticoagulant ther-

459

apy[12]; disseminated intravascular coagulopathy[13]; severe infection and septic shock[14]; the postoperative state[15]; breast cancer patients receiving cyclophosphamide, methotrexate, and 5-fluorouracil[16]; in association with L-asparaginase therapy[17]; and adult respiratory distress syndrome,[18] and it is found also in preterm neonates.[5]

Recently, a new condition of familial thrombosis characterized by normal plasma level of protein C and inherited defect in the anticoagulant response to APC has been described.[19-23] This condition has been termed "resistance to activated protein C"

(APC resistance). The phenotype of APC resistance has been shown, by polymerase chain reaction (PCR) analysis of genomic DNA, to be due to heterozygosity or homozygosity for a point mutation in the factor V gene (FV Q506) inherited as an autosomal dominant trait. A defect in factor V involving the mutation of Arg506 to Gln506 (Arg506Gln) is, in fact, most often the cause of activated protein C resistance.[20,21] This is the site at which activated protein C cleaves factor Va, and this sequence alteration makes the mutant factor Va molecule biochemically resistant to inactivation by activated

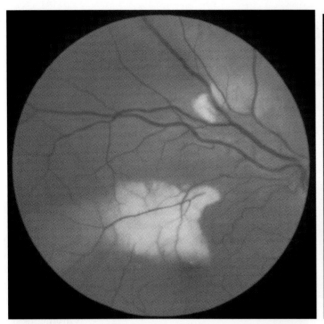

A

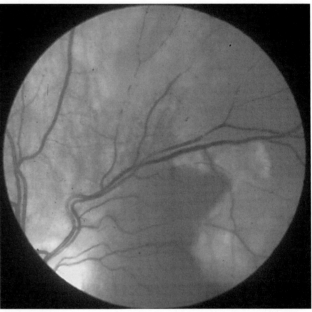

B

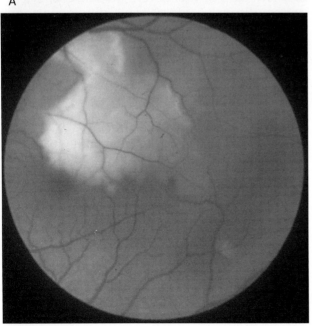

C

FIGURE 37-1 Protein C (PC) deficiency–branch retinal arteriole occlusion. Recurrent branch retinal artery occlusion in a 34-year-old woman with PC deficiency. The patient had a family history of thrombotic disease. *A*, The patient presented complaining of a defect in the visual field of her right eye in September 1986. She was 3 months postpartum. A clinical photograph shows a superotemporal branch arteriole occlusion with retinal pallor above the macula. A microinfarct is shown in relation to the superotemporal retinal vein. *B* and *C*, In April 1987 she became pregnant and began warfarin to prevent further thrombosis. Postnatally, anticoagulation was continued for 10 weeks with warfarin, maintaining the international normalized ratio (INR) between 2 and 3. One week after discontinuing warfarin, in March 1988, she developed a visual field defect in the left eye. Clinical photographs show a superotemporal retinal arteriole occlusion. Segmentation of the blood column in the occluded arteriole is visible. (From Nelson ME, Talbot JF, Preston FE: Recurrent multiple-branch retinal arteriolar occlusion in a patient with protein C deficiency. Graefes Arch Clin Exp Ophthalmol 227:443–447, 1989, with permission. Courtesy of Drs. Michael E. Nelson, John F. Talbot, and F. Eric Preston.)

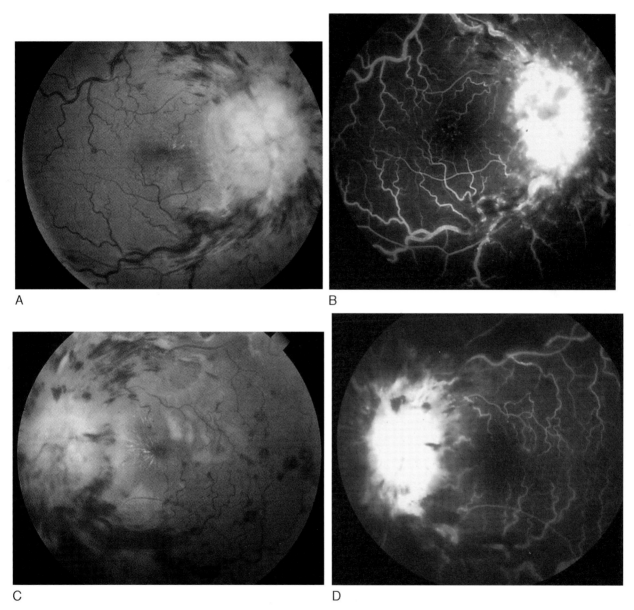

FIGURE 37–2   Protein C (PC) deficiency–central retinal vein occlusion. A 38-year-old black female presented complaining of blurring vision, headaches, and intermittent double vision. Past history was significant for multiple deep venous thrombosis and family history of strokes in a young sister and a paternal niece. She was found to have PC deficiency. *A*, Clinical photograph of the right eye shows marked disc edema, intraretinal hemorrhages and exudates, and tortuosity of the retinal veins. *B*, Fluorescein study reveals staining and leakage of the optic nerve, blockage of the retinal hemorrhages, telangiectatic capillaries in the superior macula, and marked vessel tortuosity. *C*, Clinical photograph of the posterior pole of the left eye shows a similar picture. Roth's spots are visible temporally. A partial nasal macular star of exudates is also evident. Patchy areas of retinal microinfarction are present in the superotemporal macula. *D*, Fluorescein angiogram of the left eye. Staining and leakage of the disc, and vessel tortuosity are evident. *Illustration continued on following page*

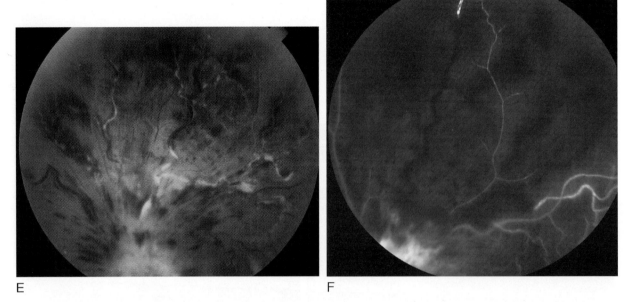

E   F

FIGURE 37–2 *Continued E,* Clinical photograph of the superotemporal quadrant of the left eye shows the presence of white yellowish material in the retinal veins. This is probably dehemoglobinized blood trapped in the nonperfused vessels. *F,* Fluorescein study of the same area confirms the presence of marked nonperfusion of the retinal veins. (Courtesy of Dr. Wendall C. Bauman, Chief Retina Service, Brooke Army Medical Center, San Antonio, TX.)

protein C. Svensson and Dahlaback[22] in 1994 reported on three families with various forms of venous thrombosis, in which an inherited APC resistance was present. APC resistance has been found in 21%[23] of patients with an idiopathic predisposition to thromboembolic disease and in 5%[23] of normal controls.

OCULAR MANIFESTATIONS

Ophthalmic manifestations of homozygous protein C deficiency have been reported[24,25] in newborns in the first days of life and are usually associated with the typical systemic manifestations of purpura fulminans (necrotic skin lesions). They consist of vitreous hemorrhage, retinal hemorrhages, and retinal vein and artery occlusion. Anterior segment examination may disclose subconjunctival hemorrhages, nonreactive pupils, and signs of inflammation as cells and flare in the anterior chamber, ectropion uveae, and posterior synechiae. The same clinical picture is common to the acquired form of protein C deficiency found in preterm newborns.

Heterozygous protein C deficiency has been associated with ocular vascular occlusion in young patients (<40 years of age). Smith and Ens[26] reported a case of amaurosis fugax in 1987. Philipp and Mayer[27] described a case of a 34-year-old woman who presented bilateral recurrent multiple-branch retinal arteriolar occlusions (Fig. 37–1). Bauman (personal communication) presented a case of

bilateral central retinal vein occlusion in a 38-year-old black female (Fig. 37–2). She had a past medical history positive for multiple deep venous thrombosis and a family history of strokes. Amaro (personal communication) saw a 29-year-old male with unilateral central retinal vein occlusion (Fig. 37–3). Past medical history and family history were negative for thrombotic disease. An extensive medical work-up was completely nonrevealing except for a serum level of protein C of 40%. Both these two cases of central retinal vein occlusion were characterized by a fundus picture of frosted angiitis, with extensive perivenous retinal exudates and marked optic disc swelling (Figs. 37–2 and 37–3).

APC resistance may also be complicated by ocular thrombotic disease (Fig. 37–4). Dhote et al reported a case of central retinal vein occlusion (CRVO) in a 49-year-old female who was found to be heterozygous for the factor V gene mutation.[28] Muller et al[29] found a prevalence of 10.6% heterozygous carriers of the FV Q506 mutation in a population of 95 patients with retinal vascular occlusive disease. Among these patients, 26% had central retinal artery occlusion, 10% had branch retinal artery occlusion, 30% had CRVO, 11% had branch retinal vein occlusion, and 23% had anterior ischemic optic neuropathy. In the same study, the prevalence of FV Q506 among 196 normal controls was significantly less frequent (4.3%).

These data suggest that APC resistance may be a causative factor in retinal vascular occlusive diseases, but since the same FV Q506 mutation is found also in healthy individuals without any his-

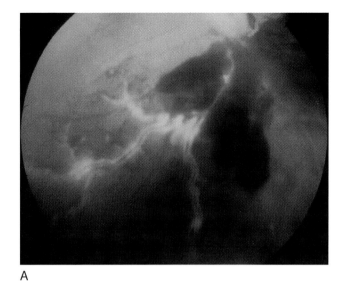

FIGURE 37–3 Protein C (PC) deficiency–central retinal vein occlusion. A 28-year-old male presented with central retinal vein occlusion in the left eye. Past history and family history were negative for thrombotic disease. A complete medical work-up was not revealing except for reduced blood level of protein C (47%). *A*, Clinical photograph of the inferonasal quadrant of the left eye shows retinal hemorrhages and marked sheathing of the retinal veins. Note the diffuse retinal whitening along the course of the vessels. This is usually believed to be due to intraretinal inflammatory cell infiltrates, and it is more typically seen in inflammatory retinal diseases such as sarcoidosis and frosted angiitis. *B*, Wide-field composite photograph of the same eye demonstrates the presence of large peripapillary retinal hemorrhages, optic nerve edema, and a macular star of exudates. (Courtesy of Dr. Miguel Hage Amaro.)

A

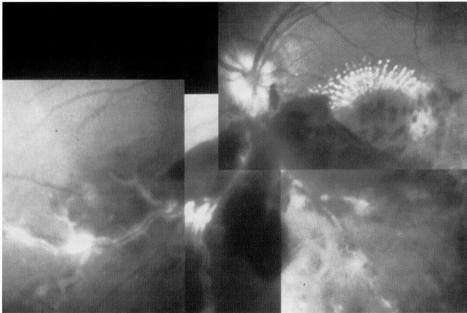

B

tory of thrombotic episodes, further studies are necessary to establish the real relationship between retinal vascular occlusive disease and APC resistance.

DIAGNOSIS

Protein C deficiency should be suspected in any case of retinal vascular occlusive disease in young patients. A past medical history of deep vein thrombosis, recurrent superficial thrombophlebitis, and a positive family history for thrombosis should always be investigated. A fundus picture of CRVO with frosted angiitis and recurrent bilateral branch retinal arteriolar occlusive episodes are also suggestive of this condition. A variety of immunologic

and functional techniques are available to measure protein C levels in plasma samples. Protein C normally circulates in human plasma at an average concentration of 4 μg/ml.[30] The levels of protein C antigen in healthy adults are log normally distributed with, 95% of the values ranging from 70 to 140%. Patients with a protein C value of less than 55% are very likely to have the genetic abnormality, while levels from 55 to 65% are consistent with either a deficiency state or the lower end of the normal distribution.[30] To document the presence of protein C deficiency, it is useful to obtain repeated laboratory determinations as well as to perform family studies to identify an autosomal dominant inheritance pattern.[31] Patients with homozygous protein C deficiency and autosomal recessive in-

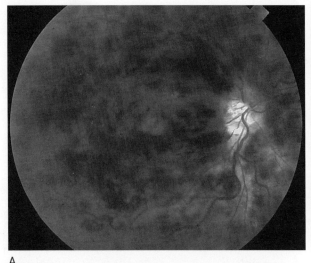

A

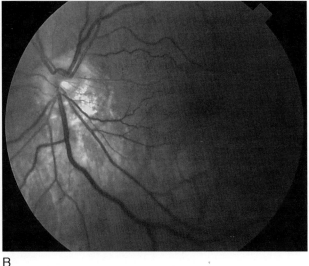

B

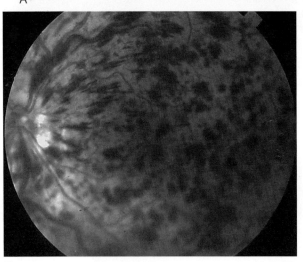

C

FIGURE 37–4 Activated protein C (APC) resistance–central retinal vein occlusion. A 46-year-old man in excellent health developed a central retinal vein thrombosis in the right eye. He was subsequently started on aspirin, 81 mg/day and was well until 2 years later, when he developed a central retinal vein occlusion in the fellow eye. The family history was significant for coronary artery disease in his father and in his male uncles. The patient's own history was negative for previous thrombotic diseases. An extensive work-up included protein C and S evaluations, antithrombin III levels, anticardiolipin antibodies, plasminogen levels, APC resistance assay, and factor V analysis. The studies were significant only for increased APC resistance; however, molecular analysis did not reveal any mutation in factor V. *A,* Clinical photograph of the right eye shows the presence of central retinal vein occlusion. *B,* Clinical photograph of the left eye on the same day does not reveal any abnormality. *C,* Clinical photograph of the left eye 2 years later shows the presence of a central retinal vein occlusion, which occurred despite the anticoagulant therapy with aspirin.

heritance pattern have very low serum levels of protein C of about 1%.[5]

When resistance to activated protein C is suspected, in the presence of normal levels of protein C antigen, several laboratory tests are also available. An APC resistance test (a modified activated partial thromboplastin time test) measures the anticoagulant response to the addition of a standard amount of APC.[22] DNA analysis with PCR may reveal a point mutation in factor V (FV Q506).[20,21]

THERAPY

Homozygous protein C deficiency in newborns, as well as severe acquired deficiency in preterm neonates, requires substitutive therapy with frozen plasma or a highly purified protein C concentrate, which facilitates the rapid and complete normalization of plasma protein C levels.[24]

Management of patients with heterozygous protein C deficiency is achieved with anticoagulants.

However, anticoagulant therapy should be used only in symptomatic patients, or in situations such as pregnancy and surgery. Short-term control for acute thrombotic episodes is with heparin. Long-term therapy is with oral anticoagulant vitamin K antagonists.[32] Attention must be paid when therapy with a vitamin K antagonist such as warfarin is started, because protein C is a vitamin K–dependent factor too. Warfarin-induced skin necrosis, in fact, is caused by a rapid decrease in the levels of protein C, in the first day of anticoagulant therapy. For this reason, it is advisable to start with heparin and then switch to warfarin.[33] No therapy is recommended for APC resistance.

ANTIPHOSPHOLIPID–PROTEIN ANTIBODIES

Antiphospholipid–protein antibodies (APA) are a family of autoimmune immunoglobulins (IgG, IgM, IgA, or mixtures) that recognize protein phospho-

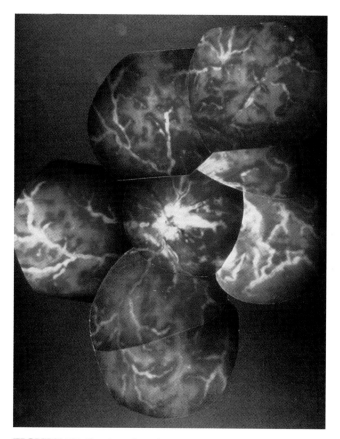

FIGURE 37–5 Antiphospholipid antibodies. A 15-year-old boy with systemic lupus erythematosus (SLE) and positive anticardiolipin antibodies noted a sudden decrease in vision in his left eye. Fundus examination revealed edematous optic disc, tortuous veins, and nearly invisible arteries because of severe constriction. There were also extensive perivenous exudates and intraretinal hemorrhages. (From Snyders B, Lambert M, Hardy JP: Retinal and choroidal vaso-occlusive disease in systemic lupus erythematous associated with antiphospholipid antibodies. Retina 10:255–260, 1990, with permission.)

malignancy, acquired immunodeficiency syndrome, infectious diseases, and drug ingestion (including chlorpromazine, hydralazine, procainamide, quinidine, phenytoin, interferon, and cocaine).[38] However, in the majority of cases LA and ACA are not associated with any systemic disease, and are found in otherwise healthy patients. These persons are classified as having primary, rather than secondary, APA syndrome.

The exact mechanism of action of APA is not known. It is probably due to action on phospholipid components of platelet membranes and vascular endothelium as well as on natural anticoagulant proteins such as antithrombin III, protein C, and protein S.[39]

Both primary and secondary APA syndromes have been associated with branch and central retinal artery and vein occlusions in young adults (Figs. 37–5 through 37–8). While ACA are associated with both arterial and venous thrombosis, LA are more often associated only with venous thrombosis. ACA are also five times more frequent than LA.[38]

APA syndrome has been associated with retinal and choroidal vascular occlusive events in earlier reports.[40,41]

In a recent study of a series of patients with vascular occlusive disease, APA has been found only in 5% of the patients without a significant difference with the control group.[42] It seems that they may be especially implicated in retinal vascular occlusive disorders in young patients with SLE or clinical features associated with the APA syndrome. Anticoagulant therapy is advisable for symptomatic patients with APA in order to prevent new occlusive episodes.

lipid complexes in in vitro laboratory test systems. They actually consist of two different antibodies the lupus anticoagulant (LA) and the anticardiolipin antibody (ACA).

LA was first found in patients with systemic lupus erythematosus (SLE),[34,35] and since the patient's plasma did not coagulate appropriately using in vitro phospholipid coagulation assays, it was termed lupus anticoagulant. Ironically, the patients had no evidence of clinical bleeding, but instead had a predisposition to thrombotic events.[36] Subsequently, it was discovered that the majority of patients with LA did not have SLE.

ACA was first described in 1983 with a radioimmunoassay test that utilized cardiolipin as antigen.[37]

Both antibodies, LA and ACA, may be associated with arterial and venous thrombosis, spontaneous abortion due to placental vessel occlusion, and thrombocytopenia. Both these antiphospholipid syndromes can be seen in association with SLE, other connective tissue and autoimmune disorders,

OTHER RISK FACTORS

Other risk factors of retinal occlusive disease in young patients includes a hypercoagulability state caused by a deficiency of natural anticoagulants such as protein S[43] (Fig. 37–9), antithrombin III, and heparin cofactor II. Increased blood viscosity should also be investigated; it may be caused by an elevation of hematocrit (Fig. 37–10), plasma viscosity, and fibrinogen. Increased red blood cell aggregation has been found as a possible cause of increased blood viscosity in patients with CRVO.[44,45] Systemic cause of increased blood viscosity such as malignancy, paraproteinemia, nephrotic syndrome, leukemia, polycythemia, and thrombocythemia should also be investigated. Other diseases that have been associated with retinal vascular occlusive disease are hyperhomocysteinemia,[46] homocystinuria,[47–50] migraine, trauma, sickle cell hemoglobinopathy, cardiac disorders such as mitral valve prolapse, oral contraceptives, pregnancy, sarcoidosis, and intravenous drug abuse.[50–53]

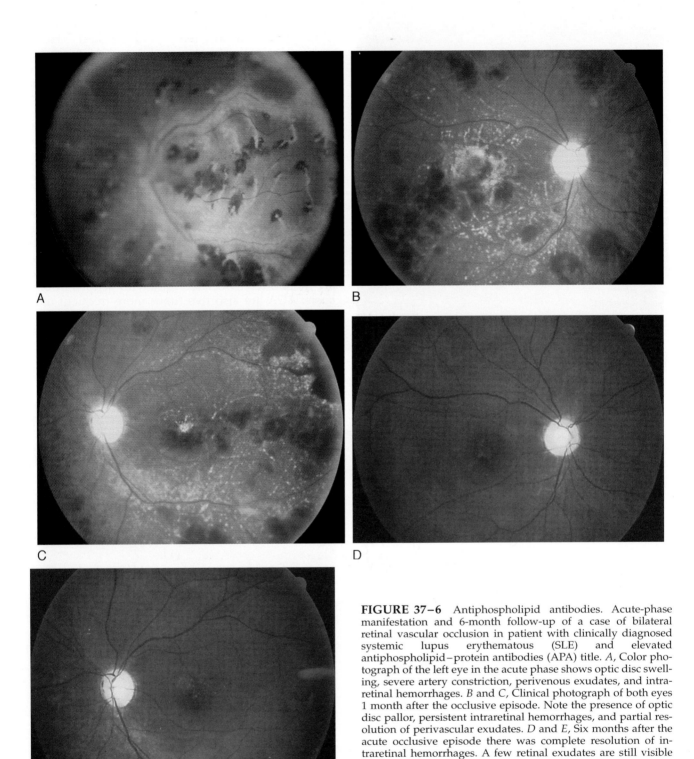

FIGURE 37–6 Antiphospholipid antibodies. Acute-phase manifestation and 6-month follow-up of a case of bilateral retinal vascular occlusion in patient with clinically diagnosed systemic lupus erythematous (SLE) and elevated antiphospholipid–protein antibodies (APA) title. *A,* Color photograph of the left eye in the acute phase shows optic disc swelling, severe artery constriction, perivenous exudates, and intraretinal hemorrhages. *B* and *C,* Clinical photograph of both eyes 1 month after the occlusive episode. Note the presence of optic disc pallor, persistent intraretinal hemorrhages, and partial resolution of perivascular exudates. *D* and *E,* Six months after the acute occlusive episode there was complete resolution of intraretinal hemorrhages. A few retinal exudates are still visible in the macula of both eyes. Note the marked narrowing of retinal arteries and optic disc atrophy.

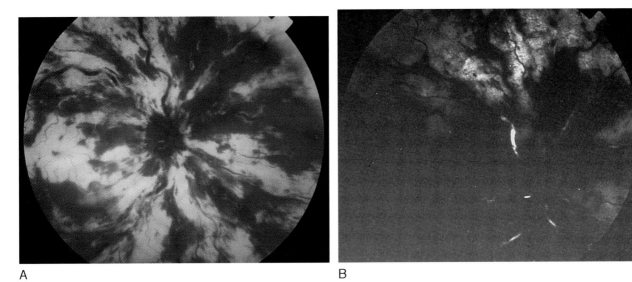

A   B

FIGURE 37–7   Antiphospholipid antibodies (APA). *A* and *B*, A 9-year-old black female experienced acute central artery and vein occlusion. A medical work-up revealed elevated title of APA in a patient with SLE. *A*, Clinical photograph of the right fundus shows massive retinal infarction and intraretinal hemorrhages. Note the tortuosity of the retinal vasculature. *B*, Fluorescein study of the same patient reveals marked nonperfusion of both retinal veins and arteries. (Courtesy of Dr. Lee M. Jampol.)

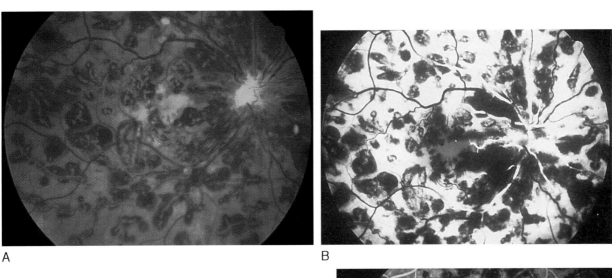

A   B

FIGURE 37–8   Antiphospholipid antibodies. A 29-year-old female complained of sudden decrease of vision in her right eye. Findings on examination included vision of hand motion in her right eye and 20/20 in her left eye. Anterior segment examination was unrevealing. The patient had a laboratory evaluation including an erythrocyte sedimentation rate of 80. The CBC, PY, PTT, ANA, protein C and protein S, ECG, chest x-ray, and MRI of the brain were normal. Infectious disease and rheumatology consultations found no other organ system involvement. APA title was elevated. *A*, Clinical photograph of the right fundus demonstrates marked perivenous whitening, outlined by intraretinal hemorrhage. Blood flow in the retinal vessels was so slow that intravascular cellular movement could be easily observed with fundus biomicroscopy. *B*, Fluorescein study of the same eye better demonstrates the presence of a very slow blood flow in the retinal vasculature. *C*, Fluorescein study of the peripheral retina reveals diffuse capillary nonperfusion. (Courtesy of Dr. Travis A. Meredith.)

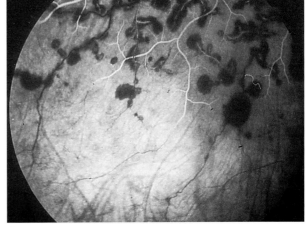

C

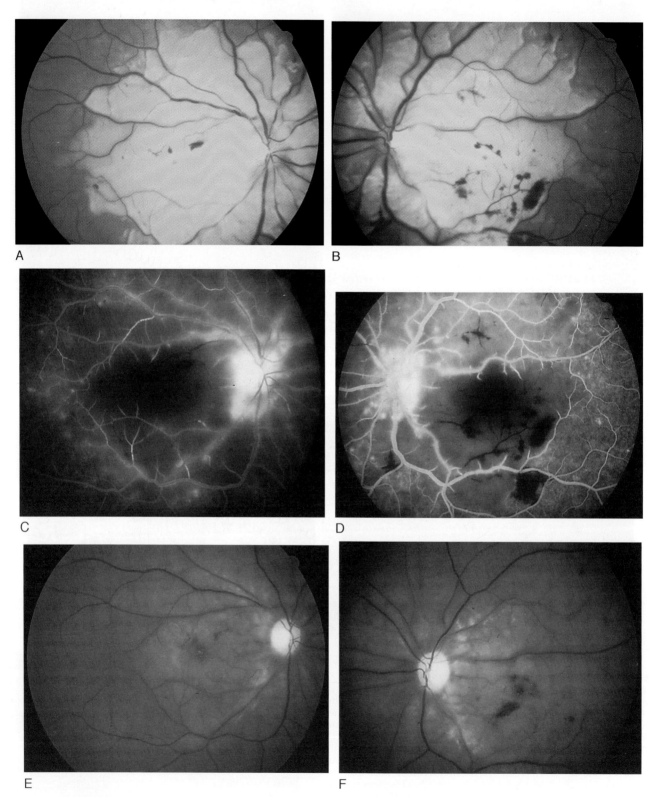

FIGURE 37–9   Protein S deficiency–retinal arteriole occlusion. Purtcher's-like retinopathy after pregnancy in a patient with protein S deficiency. *A* and *B*, Clinical photographs of both eyes in the acute phase reveal massive whitening of the posterior pole, swollen disc, and intraretinal hemorrhages. *C* and *D*, Fluorescein angiography in the acute phase shows marked arteriolar and capillary nonperfusion in the corresponding areas and optic nerve staining. *E* and *F*, Clinical photographs 2 weeks later show partial resolution of the cotton-wool patches and optic disc pallor in both eyes. *Illustration continued on opposite page*

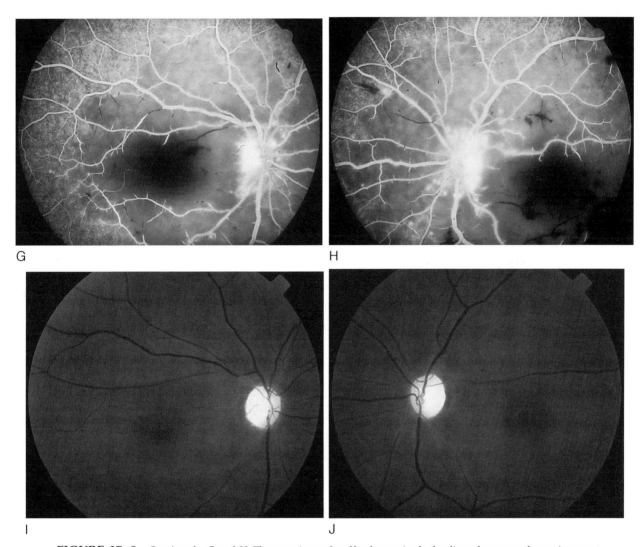

FIGURE 37–9 *Continued* *G* and *H*, Fluorescein study of both eyes in the healing phase reveals persistence of extensive arteriolar and capillary occlusion. *I* and *J*, Clinical photographs several years later showing long-term sequelae: arteriolar narrowing and optic disc atrophy in both eyes. (Courtesy of Leonard Joffe, M.D., F.R.C.S.)

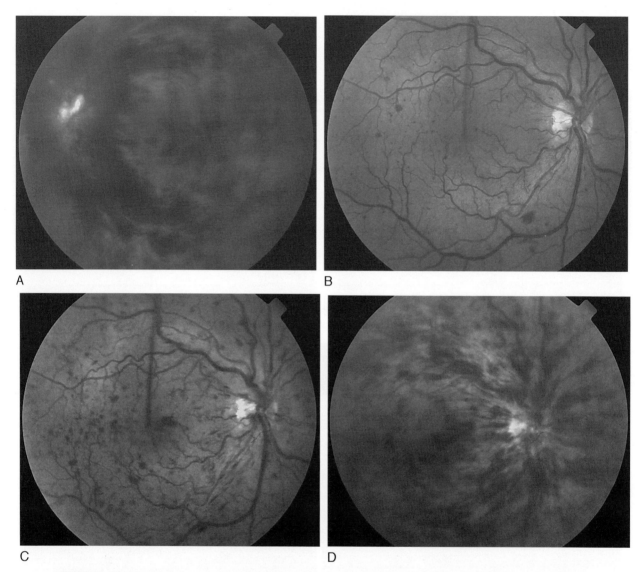

FIGURE 37–10 High hematocrit level–central retinal vein occlusion. A 65-year-old woman developed bilateral ischemic central retinal vein occlusion over a period of 8 months. She had a complete medical work-up, including laboratory testing, rheumatologic testing, internal medicine testing, cardiology consult, and hematologic consult. A fatty liver was noted on liver biopsy. No other systemic diseases were noted at that time. Subsequently, repeated laboratory testing revealed elevation of the hematocrit. *A,* The patient presented on June 8, 1995 for decreased vision in the left eye. At this time visual acuity was 20/30 in the right eye and 20/400 in the left eye. She had an ischemic central retinal vein occlusion in the left eye that was treated with panretinal photocoagulation (PRP). *B,* Her right eye also had a few intraretinal hemorrhages. *C,* Throughout the next few months, the intraretinal hemorrhages in the right eye increased. *D,* On February 28, 1996 she developed a full-blown central retinal vein occlusion in her right eye; there was cystoid macular edema present as well. Her vision deteriorated to 20/200. *Illustration continued on opposite page*

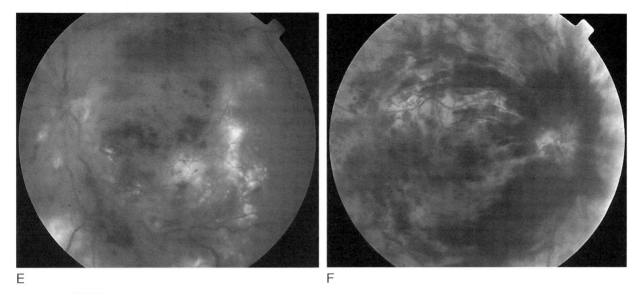

E   F

FIGURE 37–10   *Continued   E*, On last examination (May 22, 1996) visual acuity was 5/100 in the left eye. Ophthalmoscopic examination revealed remnants of ischemic vein occlusion status post-PRP. *F*, At the same date, visual acuity in the right eye was decreased to 20/400 and she had developed vitreous hemorrhage and increased macular edema. PRP in the right eye was advised.

CONCLUSION

In conclusion the ophthalmologist must be aware of the possibility that a retinal occlusive episode, especially in a young patient, may be associated with one of the above discussed risk factors. It is, in fact, important to recognize these conditions, because sometimes new thrombotic episodes may be avoided with anticoagulant therapy.

A newborn with clinical signs of purpura fulminans and ocular vascular thromboses and hemorrhages must be investigated for protein C deficiency, since a prompt diagnosis and an immediate initiation of therapy with protein C substitutes may be life-saving.

REFERENCES

1. Firie B, Furie BC: The molecular basis of blood coagulation. Cell 53:505–518, 1988.
2. Davie EW, Fujikawa K, Kisiel W: The coagulation cascade: initiation, maintenance, and regulation. Biochemistry 30:10363–10370, 1991.
3. Esmon CT: The roles of protein C and thrombomodulin in the regulation of blood coagulation. J Biol Chem 264:4743–4746, 1989.
4. Dahlback B, Stenflo J: The protein C anticoagulant system. In Stamatoyanopoulus G, Nienhuis AW, Majerus PW, Varmus H (eds): The Molecular Basis of Blood Diseases. 2nd edition. Philadelphia, WB Saunders Co, 1994, pp 599–627.
5. Marlar RA, Montgomery RR, Broekmans AW: Diagnosis and treatment of homozygous protein C deficiency. J Pediatr 114:528–534, 1989.
6. Manco-Johnson MJ, Marlar RA, Jacobson LJ, et al: Severe protein C deficiency in newborn infants. J Pediatr 113:359–363, 1988.
7. Griffin JH, Evatt B, Zimmerman TS, et al: Deficiency of protein C in congenital thrombotic disease. J Clin Invest 68:1370–1373, 1981.
8. Horellou MH, Conard J, Bertina RM, Samama M: Congenital protein C deficiency and thrombotic disease in nine French families. Br Med J 289:1285–1287, 1984.
9. Mannucci PM, Owen WG: Basic clinical aspects of protein C and S. In Bloom AL, Thomas DP (eds): Haemostasis and thrombosis, 2nd edition. Edinburgh Harlow, New York, Churchill Livingstone, 1987, pp 452–464.
10. Clouse LH, Clomp PC: The regulation of haemostasis: the protein C System. N Engl J Med 314:1298–1304, 1986.
11. Broekmans AW, Veltkamp JJ, Bertina RM: Congenital protein C deficiency and venous thromboembolism. A study of three Dutch families. N Engl J Med 309:340, 1983.
12. D'Angelo SV, Comp PC, Esmon CT, D'Angelo A: Relationship between protein C antigen and anticoagulant activity during oral anticoagulation and in selected disease states. J Clin Invest 77:416, 1986.
13. Malar RA, Enders-Brooks J, Miller C: Serial studies of protein C and its plasma inhibitor in patients with disseminated intravascular coagulation. Blood 66:59, 1985.
14. Mannucci PM, Vigano S: Deficiences of protein C, an inhibitor of blood coagulation. Lancet 2:463, 1982.
15. Blamey SL, Lowe GDO, Bertina RM, et al: Protein C levels in major abdominal surgery: relationship to deep vein thrombosis, malignancy and treatment with stanazolol. Thromb Haemost 54:622, 1985.
16. Marlar RA: Protein C in thromboembolic disease. Semin Thromb Hemost 11:387, 1985.
17. Rodeghiero F, Mannucci PM, Vigano S, et al: Liver dysfunction rather than intravascular coagulation as the main cause of low protein C and antithrombin III in acute leukemia. Blood 63:965, 1984.
18. Broekmans AW, Bertina RM, Loeliger EA, et al: Protein C and the development of skin necrosis during anticoagulant therapy. Thromb Haemost 49:251, 1983.
19. Dahlback B, Carlsson M, Svensson PJ: Familial thrombophilia due to a previously unrecognized mechanism characterized by poor anticoagulant response to activated protein C: prediction of a coofactor to activated protein C. Prot Natl Acad Sci USA 90:1004–1008, 1993.
20. Griifin JH, Evatt B, Widerman C, Fernandez JA: Anticoagulant protein C pathway in majority of thrombophilic patients. Blood 82:1989–1993, 1993.
21. Zoller B, Dahlback B: Linkage between inherited resistance to activated protein C and factor V gene mutation in venous thrombosis. Lancet 343:1536–1538, 1994.

22. Svensson PJ, Dahlback B: Resistance to activated protein C as a basis for venous thrombosis. N Engl J Med 330:517–522, 1994.
23. Koster T, Roosendal FR, de Ronde H, et al: Venous thrombosis due to poor anticoagulant response to activated protein C: Leiden Thrombophilia Study. Lancet 342:1503–1506, 1993.
24. Cassels-Brown A, Minford AMB, Chatfield SL, Bradbury JA: Ophthalmic manifestations of neonatal protein C deficiency. Br J Ophthalmol 78:486–487, 1994.
25. Pulido JS, Lingua RM, Cristol S, Byrne SF: Protein C deficiency associated with vitreous hemorrhage in a neonate. Am J Ophthalmol 104:546–547, 1987.
26. Smith DB, Ens GE: Protein C deficiency: a cause of amaurosis fugax. J Neurol Neurosurg Psychiatry 50:361–362, 1987.
27. Nelson ME, Talbot JF, Preston FE: Recurrent multiple-branch retinal arteriolar occlusion in a patient with protein C deficiency. Graefes Arch Clin Exp Ophthalmol 227:443–447, 1989.
28. Dhote R, Bachmayer C, Horellou MH, et al: Central retinal vein thrombosis associated with resistance to activated protein C. Am J Ophthalmol 120:388–389, 1995.
29. Muller HM, Hoffmann M, Nauck M, et al: Increased frequency of a factor V gene mutation associated with resistance to activated protein C in patients with retinal vascular occlusion. Poster presentation, ARVO 1996, Fort Lauderdale.
30. Bertina RM, Broeckmans AW, Krommenhoek C, et al: The use of a functional and immunological assay for plasma protein C in the study of the heterogeneity of congenital protein C deficiency. Thromb Haemost 51:1–5, 1984.
31. Bertina RM, Broekmans AW, Linden IK, Mertens K: Protein C deficiency in a Dutch family with thrombotic disease. Thromb Haemost 48:1–5, 1982.
32. Samama M, Horellou MH, Soria J, et al: Successful progressive anticoagulation in a severe protein C deficiency and previous skin necrosis at the initiation of oral anticoagulant therapy. Thromb Haemost 51:132–133, 1984.
33. Francis RB, McGehee WG: Defibrination during warfarin therapy in a man with protein C deficiency. Thromb Haemost 53:249–251, 1985.
34. Mueller JF, Ratnoff O, Heinle RW: Observations on the characteristic of an unusual circulating anticoagulant. J Lab Clin Med 38:254–261, 1951.
35. Conley CL, Hartmann RC: A haemorrhagic disorder caused by circulating anticoagulants in patients with disseminated lupus erythematosus. J Lab Clin Invest 31:621–622, 1952.
36. Bowie EJW, Thompson JH, Pascuzzi CA, et al: Thrombosis in systemic lupus erythematosus despite circulating anticoagulants. J Lab Clin Med 62:416–430, 1963.
37. Feinstein DI, Rapaport SI: Acquired inhibitors of blood coagulation. Prog Hemost Thromb 1:79–95, 1972.
38. Bick RL: The antiphospholipid thrombosis syndromes. Am J Clin Pathol 100:477–479, 1993.
39. Triplett DA: Antiphospholipid protein antibodies: laboratory detection and clinical relevance. Thrombosis Res 78:1–31, 1995.
40. Snyers B, Lambert M, Hardy JP: Retinal and choroidal vaso-occlusive disease in systemic lupus erythematosus associated with antiphospholipid antibodies. Retina 10:255–260, 1990.
41. Asherson RA, Merry P, Acheson JF, et al: Antiphospholipid antibodies: a risk factor for ocular vascular disease in systemic lupus erythematosus and the primary antiphospholipid syndrome. Ann Rheum Dis 48:358–361, 1989.
42. Glacet-Bernard A, Bayani N, Chretien P: Antiphospholipid antibodies in retinal vascular occlusions. Arch Ophthalmol 112:790–795, 1994.
43. Greven CM, Weaver RG, Owen J, Slusher MM: Protein S deficiency and bilateral branch retinal artery occlusion. Ophthalmology 98:33–34, 1991.
44. Chabanel A, Glact-Bernard A, Lelong F, et al: Increased red blood cell aggregation in retinal vein occlusion. Br J Haematol 75:127–131, 1990.
45. Glacet-Bernard A, Chabanel A, Lelong F, et al: Elevated erythrocyte aggregation in patients with CRVO and without conventional risk factors. Ophthalmology 101:1483–1487, 1994.
46. Wenzler EM, Rademakers AJJM, Boers GHJ, et al: Hyperhomocystinemia in retinal artery and retinal vein occlusion. Am J Ophthalmol 115:162–167, 1993.
47. Mukuno K, Matsui K, Haraguchi H: Ocular manifestation of homocystinuria, report of two cases. Acta Soc Ophthalmol Jpn 71:66, 1967.
48. Grobe H: Homocystinuria (cystathionine synthase deficency). Results of treatment in late diagnosed patients. Eur J Pediatr 135:199, 1980.
49. Wilson RS, Ruiz RS: Bilateral central retinal artery occlusion in homocystinuria. Arch Ophthalmol 82:267–268, 1969.
50. Van den Berg W, Verbraak FD, Bos PJM: Homocystinuria presenting as central retinal artery occlusion and long-standing thromboembolic disease. Br J Ophthalmol 74:696–697, 1990.
51. Brown GC, Magaral LE, Shields J, et al: Retinal arterial obstruction in children and young adults. Ophthalmology 88:18–25, 1981.
52. Gitting JW: Branch retinal artery occlusion in a young woman. Surv Ophthalmol 30:52–58, 1985.
53. Greven CM, Slusher MM, Weaver RG: Retinal arterial occlusion in young adults. Am J Ophthalmol 120:776–783, 1995.

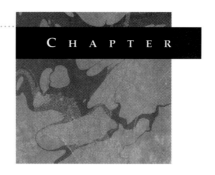

CHAPTER 38

Disseminated Intravascular Coagulopathy

Gaetano R. Barile, M.D.

David R. Guyer, M.D.

Disseminated intravascular coagulopathy (DIC) is a disorder of hemostasis that may serve as an intermediary mechanism of disease in association with numerous well-defined clinical disorders. DIC is a systemic disorder of hemorrhage and thrombosis that may affect every organ system. While DIC and associated multisystem end-organ damage may lead to irreversible morbidity and mortality, some patients with less fulminant disease states may develop a more chronic or subacute form of compensated DIC. Ophthalmologists should, therefore, be familiar with the ocular manifestations and characteristic funduscopic findings of DIC.

ETIOLOGY

DIC is usually associated with a well-defined underlying clinical disorder, perhaps the most familiar being septicemia. Systemic sepsis with meningococcus was one of the first infections to be linked with DIC (Waterhouse-Friderichsen syndrome). Other gram-negative bacteria were later recognized in association with DIC, the common mechanism being initiation of coagulation with bacterial coat lipopolysaccharide (endotoxin). Gram-positive organisms may also induce DIC with their bacterial coat mucopolysaccharides. In addition to systemic bacteremia, DIC is associated with many viremias, the responsible mechanism apparently involving activation of factor XII with circulating antigen–antibody complexes. The exanthemous viral illnesses (varicella, rubella, rubeola, variola), herpetic family of viruses (herpes simplex, herpes zoster, cytomegalovirus), viral hemorrhagic fevers (dengue, hantaan), hepatitis, and human immunodeficiency virus (HIV) infection may all produce clinical syndromes typical of DIC.[1,2]

The syndrome of DIC was first recognized in complications of pregnancy. Obstetric complications such as placenta previa, placenta abruptio, amniotic fluid embolism, fetal death, toxemia of pregnancy, and abortion with retention of gestational products may all lead to DIC. While many of these complications are fulminant, some women may initially develop a low-grade, compensated form of DIC in which ophthalmologic symptoms and findings occur.[1]

DIC is common in malignancy, particularly in prostatic carcinoma, pancreatic carcinoma, leukemia, and metastatic disease of any solid tumor. Cardiovascular disease, including myocardial infarction, prosthetic heart valves, and aortic aneurysm, may also be associated with DIC, usually as a chronic or subacute form of the syndrome. An important peripheral vascular disorder that may precipitate DIC is the Kasabach-Merritt syndrome with large cavernous hemangioma. In this syndrome, platelets and fibrinogen concentrate within the tumefaction where they contribute to an intralesional thrombosis that may subsequently activate the clotting process systemically.[2]

Intravascular hemolysis of any etiology is a common precipitating cause of DIC. The acute hemolytic transfusion reaction or multiple transfusions may stimulate the release of red blood cell membrane phospholipoprotein and activate the coagulation cascade. Patients with trauma, crush injuries with tissue necrosis, extensive burns, acidosis, and severe hepatic disease are all predisposed to the development of DIC. The syndrome, usually in a compensated form, is also seen in the collagen vascular diseases or other vasculitides, particularly in the presence of small vessel involvement. DIC may occur in sarcoidosis, amyloidosis, and the acquired immunodeficiency syndrome (AIDS). In short, rarely does a patient develop DIC in which a well-recognized underlying clinical disease entity is not apparent.[1-3]

PATHOPHYSIOLOGY

The diverse circumstances that are associated with the syndrome of DIC have in common the systemic activation of circulating thrombin and circulating plasmin. While numerous unrelated pathophysiologic insults may generate these enzymes through many potential mechanisms, the simultaneous activation of thrombin and plasmin is necessary for the development of DIC. Stimulation of both the procoagulant arm (thrombin) and the fibrinolytic arm (plasmin) of the coagulation system leads to the concomitant development of thrombosis and hemorrhage in patients with DIC.[2,3] Recalling the central roles these two enzymes play in the coagulation system allows a more thorough understanding of the apparently paradoxic events that occur in DIC.

The extrinsic and intrinsic pathways of coagulation have in common the generation of circulating thrombin from its precursor prothrombin. Circulating thrombin cleaves fibrinopeptides A and B from fibrinogen, leaving fibrin monomer, which may polymerize into fibrin clot. In DIC the systemic activation of thrombin leads to extensive deposition of fibrin clot in the vasculature. This systemic clot formation sequesters platelets and causes a consumptive thrombocytopenia. Thrombotic events occur in the microcirculation and sometimes larger vessels, resulting in substantial end-organ ischemia and dysfunction.[2,3]

Plasmin is a proteolytic enzyme with a broad spectrum of activity. The generation of plasmin from its inert proenzyme plasminogen leads to degradation of circulating fibrinogen and fibrin clot, creating fibrin(ogen) degradation products (FDPs). A large number of circulating FDPs accumulate in DIC, and these products may combine with circulating fibrin monomer to impair their polymerization and clot formation. In addition, FDPs interfere with platelet function, leaving circulating platelets not consumed in clot formation dysfunctional. Plasmin may also degrade clotting factors that normally participate in the extrinsic and intrinsic pathways of coagulation. Any of these plasmin-mediated events may impair hemostasis and lead to clinically significant hemorrhage.[2,3]

OCULAR MANIFESTATIONS

Like other organs in the body, the eye may be affected by the thrombotic and hemorrhagic events seen in DIC. While any portion of the globe's vasculature may be compromised by these events, the preferential involvement of the choroidal vessels in the posterior pole accounts for the typical funduscopic findings of DIC (Fig. 38-1). Thrombotic occlusion of these vessels may result in an exudative detachment of the neurosensory retina and/or hemorrhage within the choroid.[4] While retinal and vitreous hemorrhages occasionally occur in adult patients with DIC, these findings seem to occur predominantly in infants with DIC.[5-7]

The classic ocular histopathologic findings of DIC were reported by Cogan in his series of seven adult patients.[4] Platelet-fibrin clots were observed in the choriocapillaris and adjacent arterioles and venules in these patients (Figs. 38-2 and 38-3). These findings were primarily localized in the submacular and peripapillary regions of the choroid. Thrombotic occlusion of larger choroidal vessels as they entered the choroid was seen in one patient, but the peripheral choroid, posterior ciliary vessels, retinal vasculature, and optic nerves were generally spared of occlusive disease. Overlying the foci of choriocapillary occlusion were variably disrupted retinal pigment epithelium (RPE) cells (Figs. 38-2 and 38-3). In some cases, transudates of serum visibly dissected through the RPE and resulted in a serous detachment of the retina. Choroidal hemorrhage, seen in three of the seven cases, often surrounded the thrombotic processes in such cases.

Additional clinical reports amplify Cogan's classic findings. Samples and Buettner described the presence of yellowish gray plaque-like lesions (Fig. 38-2), some with adjacent hemorrhage, in the posterior choroid of a patient who ultimately died from complications of DIC.[8] On histopathologic examination, these plaques corresponded to fibrin thrombi within the vasculature of the posterior choroid (Figs. 38-2 and 38-3). The thrombosed vessels were sometimes surrounded by hemorrhage and

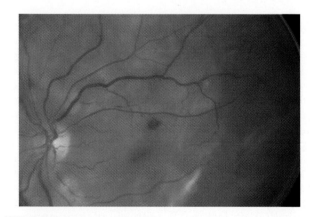

FIGURE 38-1 Fundus photograph of a patient who ultimately died from complications of disseminated intravascular coagulopathy. An exudative detachment of the neurosensory retina is present, along with a few intraretinal hemorrhages. Some subtle plaque-like lesions at the level of the retinal pigment epithelium may be appreciated along the superotemporal arcade. (Courtesy of Alan Friedman, M.D.)

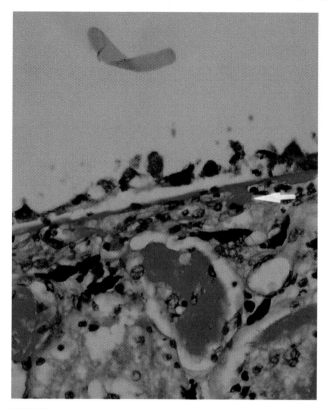

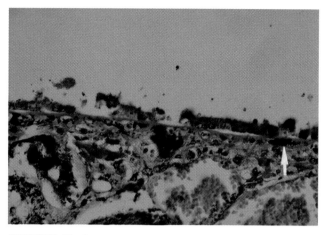

FIGURE 38–3 Histopathologic photomicrograph of the posterior choroid and RPE from the eye seen in Fig. 38–1 (phosphotungstic acid hematoxylin). Fibrin clots (blue) are demonstrated within larger choroidal vessels and a choriocapillaris vessel (arrow). The RPE is disrupted. (Courtesy of Alan Friedman, M.D.)

FIGURE 38–2 Histopathologic photomicrograph of the posterior choroid and retinal pigment epithelium from the eye seen in Fig. 38–1 (hematoxylin-eosin). Larger choroidal vessels and a choriocapillaris vessel (arrow) are occluded with fibrin thrombi, and the overlying RPE is attenuated and disrupted. (Courtesy of Alan Friedman, M.D.)

hemosiderin-laden macrophages. Hoines and Buettner later described fluorescein angiographic findings in a patient who developed DIC as a complication of abruptio placentae.[9] Serous retinal detachments were present in both eyes of this patient. Fluorescein angiography revealed markedly delayed filling in the posterior choroid with late patchy leakage in some regions. These angiographic findings and exudative detachments resolved 4 weeks after cesarean section.

The thrombotic occlusion of the choriocapillaris and adjacent vessels in DIC is responsible for the delay in choroidal filling seen on fluorescein angiography. The sudden deceleration of blood flow of the ciliary arteries as they enter the large vascular bed of the choriocapillary sinusoids may favor the deposition of clots in the submacular region.[4] The resultant occlusion may result in acute necrosis of the overlying RPE, compromising the outer blood-retinal barrier and allowing a serous exudate to accumulate in the subretinal space. Progression of this process may result in a more extensive exudative detachment of the neurosensory retina. These events may also occur in other diseases that cause choroidal infarction, such as malignant hypertension, chronic renal disease, collagen vascular disease, and toxemia of pregnancy.[10,11] Resolution of

these infarctions may result in typical Elschnig's spots or a general mottling of the RPE.[12]

In addition to serous retinal detachments, patients with DIC may develop choroidal hemorrhage. A diffuse and relatively flat hemorrhage in the choroid may occur, resulting in a dark funduscopic reflex. In some cases, white streaks may appear against this background hemorrhage, the streaks presumably representing occlusion of larger choroidal vessels.[4] This funduscopic appearance is relatively unique to DIC and thrombotic thrombocytopenic purpura, a closely related condition that some hematologists consider to be a milder form of DIC. More extensive choroidal hemorrhages have also been described as a complication of DIC.[13]

Infants with DIC may develop more extensive ocular findings. In addition to the choriocapillaris involvement, fibrin clot formation has been observed in the ciliary body, iris, and retinal vessels in cases of neonatal DIC.[7] The more diffuse involvement of the globe's vasculature in infants with DIC may account for the more widespread hemorrhagic events seen in these eyes compared to their adult counterparts. Hemorrhages in the periorbita, conjunctiva, anterior chamber, vitreous body, subhyaloid space, retinal layers, subretinal space, and subdural space surrounding the optic nerve (resulting in optic nerve swelling) have been noted in neonatal cases of DIC.[5-7] The reasons for the more extensive involvement of the neonatal vasculature in the eye in DIC are not clear.

The incidence of ocular findings and possible relation to prognosis in cases of DIC is not known. The more severe systemic disease due to DIC typically overshadows ocular symptoms and signs of disease, but on occassion the ocular findings may constitute initial symptoms of this hematologic process. Chronic, compensated forms of this disorder occur in certain diseases, and in these cases ophthalmologists may especially aid in the diagnosis of DIC.

REFERENCES

1. Baker WF: Clinical aspects of disseminated intravascular coagulation: a clinician's point of view. Semin Thromb Hemost 15:1–57, 1989.
2. Bick RL, Kunkel LA: Disseminated intravascular coagulation syndromes. Int J Hematol 55:1–26, 1992.
3. Bick RL: Disseminated intravascular coagulation. Med Clin North Am 78:511–543, 1994.
4. Cogan DG: Ocular involvement in disseminated intravascular coagulopathy. Arch Ophthalmol 93:1–8, 1975.
5. Azar P, Smith RS, Greenberg MH: Ocular findings in disseminated intravascular coagulation. Am J Ophthalmol 78:493–496, 1974.
6. Wiznia RA, Price, J: Vitreous hemorrhages and dissemi-nated intravascular coagulation in the newborn. Am J Ophthalmol 82:222–226, 1976.
7. Ortiz JM, Yanoff M, Camerson JD, Schaeffer D: Disseminated intravascular coagulation in infancy and the neonate: ocular findings. Arch Ophthalmol 100:1413–1415, 1982.
8. Samples JR, Buettner H: Ocular involvement in disseminated intravascular coagulation. Ophthalmology 90:914–916, 1983.
9. Hoines J, Buettner H: Ocular complications of disseminated intravascular coagulation in abruptio placentae. Retina 9:105–109, 1989.
10. Gaudric A, Coscas G, Bird AC: Choroidal ischemia. Am J Ophthalmol 94:489–498, 1982.
11. Klein BA: Ischemic infarcts of the choroid (Elschnig spots): a cause of retinal separation in hypertensive disease with renal insufficiency. Am J Ophthalmol 66:1069–1074, 1968.
12. Morse PH: Elschnig's spots and hypertensive choroidopathy. Am J Ophthalmol 66:844–852, 1968.
13. Allinson RW, Fante RG, List AF: Recurrent hemorrhagic choroidal detachment associated with disseminated intravascular coagulation. Ann Ophthalmol 24:72–74, 1992.

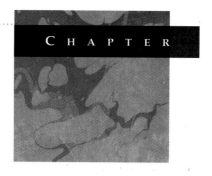

CHAPTER 39

Radiation Retinopathy

Peter K. Kaiser, M.D.

Evangelos S. Gragoudas, M.D.

Injury to the eye may result from direct radiation of intraocular tumors or when the ocular structures are within the treatment beam for extraocular tumors. Radiation damage has been reported following external beam radiotherapy for the treatment of orbital disorders including tumors[1,2] and Graves' disease[3-7]. It is also seen after treating uveal melanomas with episcleral plaque therapy[8-10] and proton beam irradiation.[11-14] In addition, it is a known complication of radiation treatment of retinoblastoma,[15-17] intracranial lesions,[18-20] nasal and paranasal tumors,[21] and following total body irradiation in bone marrow transplant patients.[22]

The anterior ocular structures are very sensitive to radiation damage. Externally, eyelid telangiectasia, erythema, and permanent loss of lashes can occur.[23,24] Over time trichiasis, ectropion, entropion, and even epiphora may develop.[24,25] Corneal edema, keratitis, corneal ulcers, chronic conjunctivitis, keratoconjunctivitis sicca, and a permanent loss of secretions from lacrimal gland damage are frequent complications.[23,26,27] Cataracts, classically of the posterior subcapsular type, are the most common anterior segment finding owing to the inherent radiosensitivity of the lens, especially in the germinative zone of the equatorial region.[12,28]

Radiation retinopathy is a slowly progressive retinal vascular disorder with characteristic fundus abnormalities. The structure and permeability of the retinal and optic nerve vessels are affected by radiation exposure. The damage to the vasculature appears ophthalmoscopically as microaneurysms, retinal telangiectases, dot and blot intraretinal hemorrhages, cotton-wool spots, macular exudates, macular edema, intraretinal microvascular abnormalities, neovascularization, vitreous hemorrhage, pigmentary changes, and retinal vasculature occlusions. Visual loss results from anterior or posterior segment changes, although the main culprits are cataracts, macular edema, macular ischemia, disc edema, and optic atrophy. In the late stages, neovascular glaucoma, retinal neovascularization, traction retinal detachments, and vitreous hemorrhage may further affect visual acuity.

Since the clinical findings found in radiation retinopathy are similar to those found in several other common diseases, it is important to carefully query the patient about previous radiation exposure. A complete past history with emphasis on any prior radiotherapy must be undertaken to identify radiation exposure.

HISTORY

Radiation therapy has been used to treat tumors for many years. The first reported ocular complications from radiation treatment were in the late 19th century.[29,30] It was not until 1933 that radiation retinopathy was first recognized, when Stallard described retinal exudates in a circinate pattern in patients treated with radon seeds for retinoblastoma and retinal capillary hemangioma.[31] Many other case reports quickly followed.[32-35] Optic neuropathy was not a known complication of radiation treatment until the 1950's.[36,37] In 1956, Forrest and associates described four patients who developed optic neuropathy after implantation of radon seeds, and in 1957, two patients developed optic neuropathy after external beam irradiation.[36,37] Optic neuropathy and radiation retinopathy are now well-described complications of radiation therapy.

EPIDEMIOLOGY AND ETIOLOGY

It has been difficult to effectively estimate the incidence of radiation retinopathy and the morbidity from ocular radiation, since several confounding variables made it difficult to analyze older studies. Without the aid of modern imaging techniques, the exact location of central nervous system (CNS) tumors or tumors close to the CNS could not be appreciated, and thus, accurate dosimetry was difficult to determine. Consequently, the radiation dose delivered to ocular structures was hard to calculate. Earlier papers often failed to differentiate patients treated with adjunctive chemotherapy from those who received radiation alone or only reported patients with visually significant retinopathy without regard for the total number of patients treated.[23] Thus, accurate dosimetry and epidemiologic studies have only recently been completed.

There is a latent period between radiation exposure and the development of radiation retinopathy. In general, it is uncommon for the retinopathy to occur within 6 months after the ocular irradiation or more than 3 years after treatment.[19,38,39] In one study, the average time before onset was 14.6 months in cobalt plaque–treated patients (brachytherapy) with a range of 4 to 32 months.[39] In patients who received external beam irradiation (teletherapy), the mean time before onset of retinopathy was 18.7 months with a range of 7 to 36 months.[39] Other studies have found retinopathy occurring in as little as 1 month after treatment and as late as 15 years after treatment.[9,31] The mean time before radiation optic neuropathy after cobalt plaque treatment was 12.6 months with a range of 3 to 22 months.[40] Like the retinopathy, it took longer for the optic neuropathy to develop after external beam irradiation, averaging 19.3 months with a range of 5 to 36 months.[40] This effect is due to the delivery method and does not represent a differing risk between the methods of irradiation.

The probability of developing radiation retinopathy rises as the total dose of radiation to the retina increases (Table 39–1). There is no threshold therapeutic radiation dose where radiation retinopathy will always occur. In general, radiation retinopathy is rare for total doses less than 4500 cGy at 180 to 200 cGy per fraction. One study found all patients developed retinopathy after receiving 4000 to 5000 cGy external beam irradiation for sinus cancer, but none of the patients exhibited visual loss.[41] Brown and associates found a total mean dose of 4900 cGy was required before patients developed radiation retinopathy.[39] There have been a few scattered reports of patients developing retinopathy with doses lower than 4000 cGy; however, these were most likely due to dosimetry errors such that a larger intended dose was administered,[4] larger dose fractions were received than anticipated,[4,6] or the total dose delivered was difficult to estimate owing to the treatment plan.[42] In one study, retinopathy was reported with a dose of 2000 cGy in ten fractions; however, the treatment plan indicated that the retina may not have been within the irradiation field; therefore, other factors may have been involved than reported.[5]

Most current studies indicate that dosages in the 4500- to 5500-cGy range delivered to half or more of the retina would be likely to produce radiation retinopathy. Although the exact rate cannot be estimated due to differences in dose specifications, the rate has been estimated to be anywhere from 9 to 53%, averaging around 22%.[33,43–45] As the total dose gets larger, the likelihood of developing retinopathy increases exponentially.[43] As many as 88% of patients developed retinopathy with doses of 5750 to 6300 cGy, and 100% of patients receiving 6500 to 7400 cGy in one study[43]; 50% of patients receiving 6000 cGy developed retinopathy in another report, and 85 to 95% developed retinopathy after doses of 7000 to 8000 cGy.[46] Finally, another study mirrored these results with 89% of patients suffering from retinopathy after receiving 7000 cGy in five fractions of proton beam irradiation.[14]

The threshold for radiation retinopathy also depends on the fractionation scheme. Unfortunately, only a few reports on fraction size in the development of radiation retinopathy are available. Larger fractions are generally more damaging when delivering the same dose.[23] This is confirmed in studies of radiation optic neuropathy where increased risk of developing papillopathy occurred with increasing doses per fraction.[47,48] One recent study found radiation retinopathy developed in patients receiving just 3000 cGy in 300-cGy fractions.[6] The current recommended individual dose fraction to the retina should not exceed 180 to 200 cGy.[43] Fraction sizes greater than 250 cGy will predispose the retina to greater damage.[47,48]

The radiation delivery system also plays a role in the probability of developing radiation retinopathy. Much higher doses of local therapy must be delivered to produce retinal vascular damage than with external beam treatment. In one study, the total dose required to produce the retinopathy was three times greater in the cobalt plaque–treated group as compared to the external beam–irradiated patients.[39] Others have found similar results.[28] Furthermore, the larger the area of retina irradiated, the lower the threshold for radiation retinopathy. External beam radiotherapy usually produces a more diffuse retinopathy that is more evident in the posterior pole than local therapy.[39]

Patients with diabetes mellitus have a substantially increased risk of developing radiation retinopathy compared to patients without diabetes.[49,50]

TABLE 39–1 Risk Factors for Developing Radiation Retinopathy

Total radiation doses >4500 cGy
Fractionated radiation doses >250 cGy
Diabetes mellitus
Concurrent adjunctive chemotherapy and/or bone
  marrow transplantation

In addition, patients who have pre-existing diabetic retinopathy are at particularly high risk of developing proliferative radiation retinopathy.[39] Viebahn and associates reported a case of a diabetic patient with minimal background diabetic retinopathy developing radiation retinopathy with loss of vision to the hand motion range after a dose of just 3000 cGy in 15 fractions over 3 weeks.[49] Other studies have shown higher dosages (4500 cGy) are still required to produce radiation retinopathy in diabetic patients.[39,43,50] Other systemic diseases that may predispose to radiation retinopathy include collagen vascular disease and hypertension. It is believed that patients with these risk factors are more likely to suffer from visually significant radiation retinopathy with lower doses of irradiation, although other studies have not found similar results.[5,44]

The administration of adjunctive chemotherapy and bone marrow transplantation in close temporal proximity to irradiation can increase the risk of developing radiation retinopathy.[22,33,39,44] In one study, patients developed radiation retinopathy after an average total dose of only 2736 cGy.[22] The patients were all taking high-dose cytarabine HCl in preparation for bone marrow transplantation. Similar results were found in patients with metastatic breast cancer who were receiving concurrent chemotherapy after total radiation doses of 2500 to 3000 cGy.[51] Another study showed a fourfold increase in the risk of retinopathy after receiving intra-arterial 5-fluorouracil and radiation therapy.[33] Unfortunately, it has proven difficult to differentiate the changes due to radiation treatment and those due to the chemotherapeutic agents. Thus, the etiology behind this effect is not yet known. Finally, simultaneous treatment with external beam radio-therapy and hyperbaric oxygen has also been shown to raise the probability of developing radiation retinopathy.[52,53]

CLINICAL FEATURES

Patients can present with all spectrums of symptoms ranging from metamorphopsia to abrupt, complete loss of vision. Visual loss depends on the area affected by the retinopathy. Peripheral changes often go unnoticed, while blurred central vision, with some patients noting a faint central scotoma, can occur with posterior pole pathology.[23,38,54] Patients may also describe floaters and visual distortions.

The ophthalmoscopic features of radiation retinopathy are very characteristic and follow a defined pattern. Early microvascular changes include microaneurysms, retinal telangiectasia, dot and blot intraretinal hemorrhages, cotton-wool spots, macular exudates, macular edema, perivascular sheathing, and intraretinal microvascular abnormalities (Figs. 39–1A and 39–2A). The retinal hemorrhages are thought to be due to vascular occlusions with telangiectasia arising in areas of nonperfusion to serve as collateral channels.[55] As the retinopathy progresses and extensive retinal vascular occlusion occurs, proliferative neovascularization of the disc, retina, and iris, as well as retinal vascular occlusions, can occur. This may lead to vitreous hemorrhage, neovascular glaucoma, and traction retinal detachments.[28] In addition, subretinal neovascular membranes originating from the telangiectatic retinal vessels have been described.[56] Over time, pig-

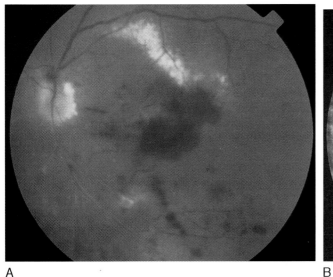
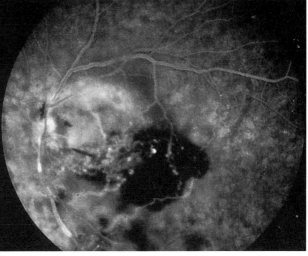

A   B

FIGURE 39–1   *A*, Fundus photograph of an eye treated with proton beam irradiation for choroidal melanoma. Microaneurysms, macular exudates, retinal hemorrhages, vascular occlusion, and retinal edema are present. Vascular sheathing is present along the inferotemporal arcade. *B*, Fluorescein angiogram of the same eye illustrating the microvascular changes including capillary nonperfusion, microaneurysms, and telangiectasia.

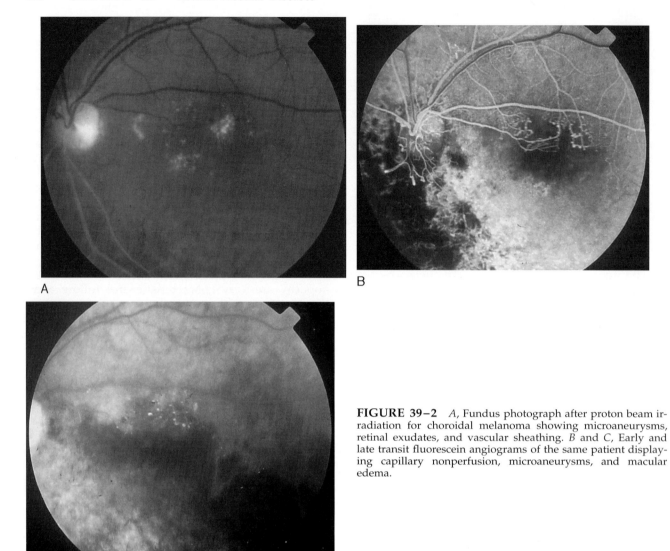

FIGURE 39–2 *A,* Fundus photograph after proton beam irradiation for choroidal melanoma showing microaneurysms, retinal exudates, and vascular sheathing. *B* and *C,* Early and late transit fluorescein angiograms of the same patient displaying capillary nonperfusion, microaneurysms, and macular edema.

mentary changes appear, including retinal pigment epithelial atrophy and generalized abnormalities in a salt-and-pepper pattern.[57]

According to a study by Guyer and associates, the earliest and most common macular finding in radiation retinopathy is macular edema.[14] Telangiectasia and microaneurysms were the next to appear and intraretinal hemorrhages, hard exudates, nerve fiber layer infarcts, and capillary nonperfusion followed slowly thereafter.[14] The least common finding was vascular sheathing.[14] Other studies have shown similar findings with hard exudates and intraretinal hemorrhages being the first abnormalities seen after cobalt plaque treatment, and intraretinal hemorrhages and hard exudates being the most common findings after external beam irradiation.[39] Other microvascular events including telangiectasia, cotton-wool spots, and vascular sheathing appeared next. The interesting difference between the groups was the early appearance of hard exudates in the brachytherapy patients that

was not seen till later in the teletherapy group. Although the doses were higher in the plaque group, Brown and associates postulate that this is due to some intrinsic factor released from tumors that enhances vascular leakage in the brachytherapy group.[39] Finally, neovascularization was more common in the teletherapy group.[39] The higher frequency of neovascularization was thought to be secondary to the larger surface area of the retina affected by the radiation.[39]

Several authors have proposed categorizing radiation retinopathy into three forms: background, preproliferative, and proliferative (Table 39–2). Each category has distinctive features and would theoretically have different treatment and prognostic implications. Background radiation retinopathy is similar to nonproliferative diabetic retinopathy. It is defined as one or more retinal capillary microaneurysms associated with biomicroscopically identifiable retinal edema and/or retinal exudates.[38] Patients may also exhibit a few cotton-wool spots

TABLE 39–2 Ophthalmic Complications of Radiation Exposure

Anterior Segment Changes
Eyelid erythema and telangiectasia
Loss of lashes
Trichiasis
Ectropion or entropion
Corneal edema
Corneal ulcers
Chronic conjunctivitis
Keratoconjunctivitis sicca
Cataracts
Background Radiation Retinopathy
Microaneurysms
Retinal telangiectasia
Dot and blot intraretinal hemorrhages
Few cotton-wool spots
Macular exudates and/or edema
Preproliferative Radiation Retinopathy
Intraretinal microvascular abnormalities
Venous beading
Multiple cotton-wool spots
Proliferative Radiation Retinopathy
Neovascularization of the disc or elsewhere in the retina
Vitreous hemorrhage
Neovascular glaucoma
Traction retinal detachment
Radiation Optic Neuropathy
Optic disc edema
Circumpapillary subretinal fluid and/or exudates
Optic atrophy

and dot and blot intraretinal hemorrhages. Preproliferative radiation retinopathy is defined as having the fundus abnormalities of background radiation retinopathy with the addition of retinal venous beading, multiple cotton-wool spots, and prominent intraretinal microvascular abnormalities (IRMA).[38] Finally, proliferative radiation retinopathy is present when patients exhibit neovascularization of the disc or elsewhere in the retina.

Radiation retinopathy is commonly associated with radiation optic neuropathy.[40,59] However, radiation papillopathy may occur as a separate disorder without the concurrent retinal changes.[40,59] During the acute stages of radiation optic neuropathy, patients usually complain of acute, painless, monocular decrease in visual acuity.[40,59,60] Visual field abnormalities are common.[59] One may see nerve fiber bundle defects, central scotomas, altitudinal defects, generalized constriction, or even temporal field cuts that mimic a chiasmal syndrome.[61] Two types of optic neuropathy can occur after radiation—anterior ischemic optic neuropathy and retrobulbar ischemic optic neuropathy. Both types are thought to be due to vascular occlu-

sion preventing blood from nourishing the optic nerve.[62] The appearance of the optic disc is dependant on what portion of the nerve received the highest radiation dose.[23] The disc can be normal or slightly pale after radiation to posterior orbital structures or retrobulbar optic neuropathy. Radiation directly to the eye often produces hyperemic optic disc swelling, circumpapillary exudative subretinal fluid and exudates, cotton-wool spots, enlarged tortuous vessels, and intraretinal hemorrhages (Figs. 39–3A and 39–4).

The optic nerve is more radiosensitive than the other cranial nerves.[23,63] One study found a total threshold dose of 5500 cGy was required before radiation optic neuropathy developed.[40] However, it appears that daily fraction size is the important determinant in developing optic neuropathy, not the total dose.[47] One study found that 18% of patients treated with more than 250 cGy in daily fractionated doses developed visually significant damage.[47] None of the patients who received less than 250 cGy developed optic neuropathy despite receiving 4500 to 5000 cGy total doses. Another study warned that lower fractionated dosages of 150 to 180 cGy may increase the risk of optic neuropathy.[48] Similar to radiation retinopathy, the optic neuropathy is more likely to occur in patients receiving concurrent chemotherapy.[62,64] In addition, increasing age may also create a greater chance of injury.[62] Older patients were more likely to suffer from disc hemorrhages and nerve fiber layer infarcts, but were less likely to have nerve pallor.[13] This effect is thought to be due to the presumed vascular basis of the optic neuropathy.

FLUORESCEIN ANGIOGRAPHY

The most consistent finding on fluorescein angiography is capillary nonperfusion (Figs. 39–1B and 39–2B and C).[39,55,65–67] The capillary dropout was greatest overlying the tumor and surrounding the tumor base in patients with intraocular tumors treated with plaque therapy.[39,55] In addition, capillary leakage, tortuous macular vessels with aneurysmal and saccular dilation, capillary closure, and neovascularization may be seen.[43,66,67] A less specific finding was transmission hyperfluorescence corresponding to the areas of retinal pigment epithelial atrophy.[54] When radiation optic neuropathy is present, ischemia of the optic nerve head with superficial areas of nonperfusion and/or leakage can be seen (Fig. 39–3B).[40] There is also a loss of vessels in both the superficial and deep vascular networks.[62]

PATHOLOGIC FEATURES

Radiation retinopathy is due to vascular damage to the retinal and optic nerve vessels.[39,46,68] With low dosages, the endothelial cells' intracellular tight

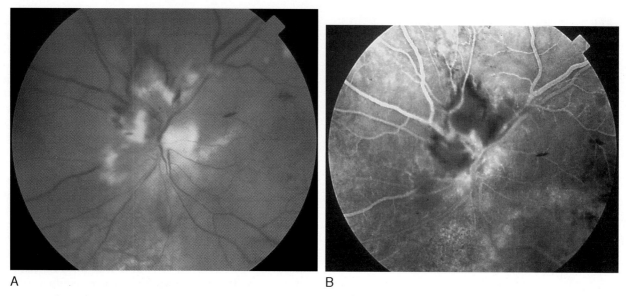

A   B

FIGURE 39–3   *A*, Radiation papillopathy with disc edema, cotton-wool spots, hemorrhages, and hard exudates after proton beam irradiation for choroidal melanoma. *B*, Fluorescein angiogram of the same eye exhibiting leakage from the optic disc.

junctions lose their integrity, causing an increase in vascular permeability; retinal edema and exudation results. If the radiation dose is larger, the endothelial cells die, causing the vascular channels to become occluded; cotton-wool spots and capillary nonperfusion then develops.[38] Histopathologic examination of vascular damage has shown thickening of arteriolar capillary walls; accumulation of fine fibrillar material within the walls of the vessels; myointimal proliferation; swelling of the endothelium; an enlarged elastic lamina; narrowing and occlusion of the vessel lumen; degeneration of the media and adventitia; and swelling and loss of muscular, elastic, and collagenous compo-

nents.[12,16,69,70] In addition, trypsin digestion studies show loss of pericytes and endothelial cells.[56] The retinal hemorrhages are likely due to the vascular occlusion, and telangiectasia arise as collateral channels in areas of nonperfusion.[55] Subretinal neovascularization has been reported to originate from telangiectatic retinal vessels.[56]

Animal studies have outlined the progression of vascular damage seen in radiation retinopathy.[58,71] Capuchin monkeys were irradiated with a single dose of 3000 cGy to the posterior segment.[58] The earliest changes were focal loss of capillary endothelial cells leading to microinfarcts. These areas appeared as cotton-wool spots on fundus examination that faded over time, leaving areas of capillary nonperfusion on fluorescein angiography. Capillary loss was multifocal and irregular. The damage started with deeper, smaller vessels, but progressively spread to larger vessels. As the vascular damage continued, recanalization, microaneurysms, and eventually neovascularization developed. Thirty to 42 months after irradiation, the monkeys developed rubeosis iridis and neovascular glaucoma. Other animal studies have shown similar findings in New Zealand white rabbits.[71]

One recent report has examined the acute effects of radiation on retinal cells.[72] A single dose of 200 to 2000 cGy was delivered to Lister rat retinas that were examined 1 hour to 1 month after irradiation.[72] The most sensitive retinal cells were the rod photoreceptors, which developed membrane abnormalities within 1 hour of receiving 200 cGy. The amount of membrane damage was dose dependant. Doses greater than 1000 cGy caused photoreceptor cell death. Furthermore, studies using New Zealand white rabbits and guinea pigs receiving 200 cGy found cessation of function in a large part of

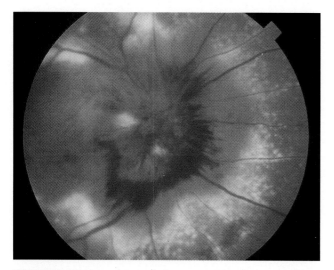

FIGURE 39–4   Severe radiation papillopathy with disc edema, hemorrhages, and exudation after proton beam irradiation for choroidal melanoma. There is extensive lipid exudation surrounding the optic disc.

the rod cell population as evidenced by electroretinogram (ERG) recordings.[71] The rod cell nuclei were pyknotic and the cells were disorganized.[71] The cone photoreceptors appeared to be more resilient to radiation damage. The retinal pigment epithelium manifested damage with doses greater than 500 cGy, although cell death did not occur till levels reached 2000 cGy.[72] In addition, glial cell proliferation was seen. Clinical studies have exhibited areas of retinal ganglion cell loss and nerve fiber layer thinning.[39,56] Similarly, histopathologic studies have found cystic changes in the inner nuclear layers and retinal ganglion cell loss.[16,69,70,73,74] In general, there is preferential damage to the inner retinal layers owing to their dependance on the retinal circulation.

The histopathologic damage seen in radiation optic neuropathy is similar to the retinopathy. Early changes include perivascular lymphocytic cuffing and hyalinization with subsequent fibrosis, thrombosis, and infarction of the neural tissue.[40,60] This leads to loss of axonal bundles, demyelinization, and gliosis.

Radiation damage appears to affect the DNA of the retinal vascular endothelium and pericytes.[75,76] Radiation has been shown to cause radiolysis of water into oxygen free radicals and hydroxyl ions that can interact with the sugar phosphate backbone of DNA resulting in strand scission.[75,77] This leads to fragmentation of the DNA and prevents cell replication. Since radiation damage is cumulative, as the dosage increases, the body's compensatory mechanisms are overwhelmed and can no longer correct the mistakes formed in the DNA, leading to cell death.

CLINICAL COURSE AND PROGNOSIS

The clinical course of radiation retinopathy is slow and variable, with one end of the spectrum being stabilization of the retinal vascular abnormalities and an improvement of retinal function. In one report, spontaneous improvement in clinical symptoms and fundus abnormalities over a few months has been demonstrated.[78] On the other hand, progression usually occurs with increased edema; capillary nonperfusion; and occasionally formation of neovascularization, traction retinal detachments, and neovascular glaucoma. Disease progression is usually seen within 3 to 6 months after the initial diagnosis of radiation retinopathy.[39] Nerve fiber infarcts showed the highest rate of resolution in one study with two thirds of the lesions resolved by the last follow-up examination.[14] Unfortunately, macular edema rarely cleared. Guyer and associates found that 95% of patients still had some macular edema by the last follow-up exam.[14] Furthermore, capillary nonperfusion, microaneurysms, and telangiectasia rarely resolved spontaneously.[14]

Radiation optic neuropathy often stabilizes within 2 to 12 months.[13,40,62] As the papillopathy stabilizes, the disc swelling subsides and the hemorrhages and exudate resolve, leaving a pale and sometimes, atrophic disc[13] (Fig. 39–5). A corresponding decline in visual acuity mirrors the optic atrophy with patients having count fingers to no light perception vision.[40] Occasionally, if the optic neuropathy is not severe, visual acuity may improve slightly as the disc edema resolves; however, final acuities rarely recover to their original levels[40] (see Fig. 39–6). The visual loss is usually monocular, although there have been a few reported cases of the irradiated contralateral nerve being affected months to years later.[59,61]

DIFFERENTIAL DIAGNOSIS

The retinopathy seen after radiation treatment is similar to other retinal vascular diseases including diabetic retinopathy, previous retinal arterial or venous occlusions, idiopathic or acquired parafoveal telangiectasia, Eales' disease, and hypertensive retinopathy (Table 39–3). The fundus changes seen in diabetic retinopathy most closely resemble radiation retinopathy. History holds the clue to differentiate the two disorders, since patients with diabetic retinopathy have longstanding diabetes mellitus and no history of prior ocular irradiation. In addition, diabetic retinopathy is usually a bilateral disease and fibrovascular proliferation is more common. Other diagnosis may appear similar to radiation retinopathy; however, the history of radiation exposure is usually enough to differentiate between the entities. Although this seems self-evident, patients often do not volunteer previous radiation treatment for nonocular tumors unless a careful history is taken.

TREATMENT

There have been no large, randomized clinical trials to evaluate treatment strategies for radiation retinopathy. Owing to the similarity between diabetic and radiation retinopathy, the rationale and treatment criteria for diabetes has been adopted to treat radiation retinopathy (Table 39–4). Much like diabetic retinopathy, photocoagulation should not be undertaken if there is extensive ischemic maculopathy.

Background retinopathy without any signs of macular edema or exudates can be followed. When the retinopathy progresses and focal macular edema or exudates appear, the patients can be treated with focal laser photocoagulation.[18,54,79] Argon green, krypton red, and tunable dye lasers can be used for photocoagulation. Laser settings of 0.05 to 0.1 second to produce burn diameters of 50 to 100 μm are generally used to treat leakage sites

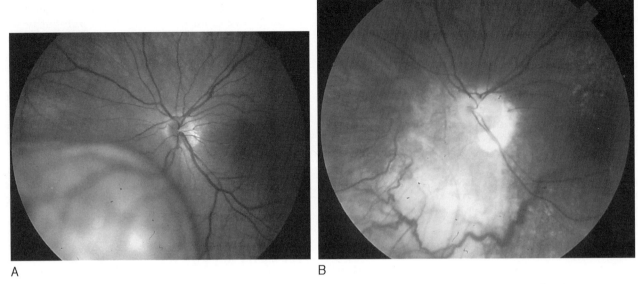

FIGURE 39–5 *A*, Patient with choroidal melanoma before treatment with proton beam irradiation. *B*, Fundus photograph of the same patient after treatment showing optic atrophy, vascular attenuation, and retinal exudates.

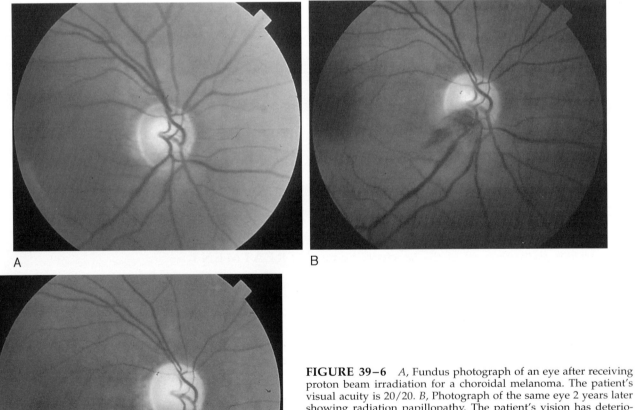

FIGURE 39–6 *A*, Fundus photograph of an eye after receiving proton beam irradiation for a choroidal melanoma. The patient's visual acuity is 20/20. *B*, Photograph of the same eye 2 years later showing radiation papillopathy. The patient's vision has deteriorated to 20/200. *C*, Six months later, photographs of the same eye show resolution of the disc edema and sectoral optic disc pallor. The patient's visual acuity has recovered to 20/50.

TABLE 39–3 Differential Diagnosis

Diabetic retinopathy
Hypertensive retinopathy
Branch or central retinal artery occlusion
Branch or central retinal vein occlusion
Eales' disease
Idiopathic or acquired parafoveal telangiectasia

TABLE 39–4 Treatment of Radiation Retinopathy

Background and Preproliferative Radiation Retinopathy
  Background retinopathy without macular edema or exudates—follow
  Focal macular edema or exudates—focal laser photocoagulation
  Diffuse macular edema or exudates—grid laser photocoagulation
Proliferative Radiation Retinopathy
  Neovascularization of the disc or retina—Panretinal photocoagulation
  Nonclearing vitreous hemorrhage and traction retinal detachments—pars plana vitrectomy
Radiation optic neuropathy
  No effective treatment

identified on fluorescein angiograms.[54] Amoaku and Archer noted that telangiectatic vessels adjacent to retinal burns collapsed and failed to perfuse fluorescein after macular photocoagulation.[18] In addition, microaneurysms decreased in size and often disappeared after treatment. Unfortunately, no reperfusion of ischemic retinal areas was demonstrated.

If the retinopathy is more severe and the patients have diffuse macular edema, grid treatment can be performed in addition to focal photocoagulation. Grid treatment should be spaced one burn width apart starting 2 disk diameters from the center of the macula. Kinyoun and associates found a 2 line increase in vision in 60% of patients after grid photocoagulation over a 3- to 22-month follow-up period.[54] None of the patients experienced a decrease in vision. After receiving focal or grid treatment, patients should be followed monthly. If the macular edema persists, retreatment may be necessary after a few months.

When preproliferative and proliferative radiation retinopathy changes become apparent, scatter or panretinal retinal photocoagulation should be used.[54,65] Laser settings of 0.1 second exposures with 500- to 1000-μm burn diameters spaced one to two burn widths apart may be used. An end point of mild to moderate retinal whitening is appropriate. The intensity of the burns and the number of spots depends on the degree of proliferation. In the experience of the authors, radiation proliferative retinopathy generally responds better to photocoagulation than diabetic proliferative retinopathy. Discrete areas of neovascularization can be treated directly. Forty-three per cent of patients in one study had regression of neovascularization after scatter photocoagulation during the follow-up period of 19 to 66 months.[54] The photocoagulation may also prevent the development or progression of neovascular glaucoma.[65]

Traction retinal detachment, fibrovascular proliferation, and nonclearing vitreous hemorrhages may require surgery. Standard pars plana vitrectomy techniques may be utilized to treat these problems. In one series of three patients with nonclearing vitreous hemorrhages, pars plana vitrectomies were performed.[54] After the vitreous hemorrhage was removed, fibrovascular proliferation and localized traction retinal detachments were found and treated. During the follow-up examinations, none

of the patients had recurrent growth of new vessels or vitreous hemorrhages.[54] Unfortunately, the postoperative vision was still impaired by macular edema and ischemia, as well as optic neuropathy.

At this time there is no effective treatment for radiation papillopathy. One report on the use of hyperbaric oxygen therapy was encouraging.[60] In two of four patients treated with hyperbaric oxygen within 3 days of the diagnosis of radiation optic neuropathy, a return of vision to baseline levels was noted.[60] Unfortunately, larger studies have not produced similar results.[40,61] Roden and associates treated 13 patients immediately to 1 month after diagnosis of radiation papillopathy with corticosteroids and repeated hyperbaric oxygen treatment using 100% oxygen at 2 atmospheres for 2-hour periods. During the follow-up period, none of the patients had any improvement in visual function.[61] In fact, 25% of patients continued to deteriorate more than 2 lines from pretreatment levels despite the hyperbaric oxygen therapy.[61] Furthermore, one study found exacerbation of the radiation retinopathy with the use of hyperbaric oxygen.[53] Thus, until a proven therapy for radiation optic neuropathy is developed, prevention is the most important treatment. This can be accomplished only by reducing as much as possible the radiation dose to the optic nerve through accurate planning and selecting the appropriate radiotherapeutic modalities.

PREVENTION

As our knowledge about radiation retinopathy and papillopathy improves, the design of radiation treatment protocols are being updated to minimize the side effects of the therapy. Ophthalmologists need to work with the oncologists and radiation therapists to ensure that ocular structures receive only limited amounts of radiation. Improved imaging techniques, computerized planning programs, highly localized dose distribution achieved with the use of heavy particles like protons and helium ions, and better and more accurate delivery systems will hopefully decrease the incidence of radiation retinopathy in the future.

REFERENCES

1. Bessell EM, Henk JM, Whitlocke RAF, Wright JE: Ocular morbidity after radiotherapy of orbital and conjunctival lymphoma. Eye 1:90–96, 1987.
2. Heyn R, Ragab A, Raney B, et al: Late effects of therapy in orbital rhabdomyosarcoma in children. Cancer 57: 1738–1743, 1986.
3. Kinyoun JL, Orcutt JC: Radiation retinopathy (Letter). JAMA 258:610, 1987.
4. Kinyoun JL, Kalina RE, Brower SA, et al: Radiation retinopathy after orbital irradiation for Graves' ophthalmopathy. Arch Ophthalmol 102:1473–1476, 1984.
5. Miller ML, Goldberg SH, Bullock JD: Radiation retinopathy after standard radiotherapy for thyroid-related ophthalmopathy. Am J Ophthalmol 112:600–601, 1991.
6. Nikoskelainen E, Joensuu H: Retinopathy after irradiation for Graves' ophthalmopathy. Lancet 2:690–691, 1989.
7. Brennan MW, Leone CR, Janaki L: Radiation therapy for Graves' disease. Am J Ophthalmol 96:195–199, 1983.
8. Bedford MA, Bedotto C, MacFaul PA: Radiation retinopathy after the application of cobalt plaque. Br J Ophthalmol 54:505–509, 1970.
9. Char DH, Lonn LI, Margolis LW: Complications of cobalt plaque therapy of choroidal melanomas. Am J Ophthalmol 84:536–541, 1977.
10. Moura RA, McPherson AR, Easley J: Malignant melanoma of the choroid: treatment with episcleral 198 Au plaque and xenon-arc photocoagulation. Ann Ophthalmol 17: 114–125, 1985.
11. Gragoudas ES, Seddon JM, Goitein M, et al: Current results of proton beam irradiation of uveal melanomas. Ophthalmology 92:284–291, 1985.
12. Gragoudas ES, Zakov NZ, Albert DM, Constable IJ: Long-term observations of proton-irradiated monkey eyes. Arch Ophthalmol 97:2184–2191, 1979.
13. Mukai S, Guyer DR, Eagan KM, et al: Radiation papillopathy after proton beam irradiation of choroidal melanoma. Ophthalmmology 98(Suppl):116, 1991.
14. Guyer DR, Mukai S, Eagan K, et al: Radiation maculopathy following proton beam irradiation for choroidal melanoma. Ophthalmology 99:1278–1285, 1992.
15. Egbert PR, Donaldson SS, Moazed K, Rosenthal AR: Visual results and ocular complications following radiotherapy for retinoblastoma. Arch Ophthalmol 96:1826–1830, 1978.
16. Egbert PR, Fajardo LF, Donaldson SS, Moazed K: Posterior ocular abnormalities after irradiation for retinoblastoma: a histopathologic study. Br J Ophthalmol 64:660–665, 1980.
17. Martin H, Reese AB: Treatment of bilateral retinoblastoma (retinal glioma) surgically and by irradiation. Am J Ophthalmol 33:429–439, 1945.
18. Amoaku WMK, Archer DB: Cephalic radiation and retinal vasculopathy. Eye 4:195–203, 1990.
19. Bagan SM, Hollenhurst RW: Radiation retinopathy after irradiation of intracranial lesions. Am J Ophthalmol 88: 694–697, 1979.
20. Tomsak RL, Smith JL: Radiation retinopathy in a patient with lung carcinoma metastatic to brain. Ann Ophthalmol 12:619–622, 1980.
21. Midena E, Segato T, Piermarocchi S, et al: Retinopathy following radiation therapy of paranasal sinus and nasopharyngeal carcinoma. Retina 7:142–147, 1987.
22. Lopez PF, Sternberg P, Dabbs CK, et al: Bone marrow transplant retinopathy. Am J Ophthalmol 112:635–646, 1991.
23. Gordon KB, Char DH, Sagerman RH: Late effects of radiation on the eye and ocular adnexa. Int J Radiat Oncol Biol Phys 31:1123–1139, 1995.
24. Fitzpatrick PJ, Thompson GA, Easterbrook WM, et al: Basal and squamous cell carcinoma of the eyelids and their treatment by radiotherapy. Int J Radiat Oncol Biol Phys 10: 449–454, 1984.
25. Sagerman RH, Fariss AR, Chung CT, et al: Radiotherapy for nasolacrimal tract epithelial cancer. Int J Radiat Oncol Biol Phys 29:177–181, 1994.
26. Bahrassa F, Datta R: Postoperative beta radiation treatment of pterygium. Int J Radiat Oncol Biol Phys 9:679–684, 1983.
27. Parsons JT, Bova FJ, Fitzgerald CR, et al: Severe dry eye syndrome following beam irradiation. Int J Radiat Oncol Biol Phys 30:775–780, 1994.
28. MacFaul PA, Bedford MA: Ocular complications after therapeutic irradiation. Br J Ophthalmol 54:237–247, 1970.
29. Chalupecky H: Ueber die wirkung der rontgenstrahlen auf das Auge und die haut. Zentralbl Augenheilkd 21:234, 1897.
30. Birch-Hirschfeld A: Die wirkung der rontgen-und radium-strahlen auf das auge. Graefes Arch Ophthalmol 59:229–310, 1904.
31. Stallard H: Radiant energy as (a) pathogenic (b) a therapeutic agent in ophthalmic disorders. Br J Ophthalmol 6(Suppl):1–126, 1933.
32. Moore RF: Presidential address. Trans Ophthalmol Soc U K 55:3–26, 1935.
33. Chan RC, Shukovsky LJ: Effects of irradiation on the eye. Radiology 120:673–675, 1976.
34. Cogan DG: Lesions of the eye from radiant energy. JAMA 142:145–151, 1950.
35. Flick JJ: Ocular lesions following the atomic bombing of Hiroshima and Nagasaki. Am J Ophthalmol 31:137–154, 1948.
36. Forrest APM, Brown DAP, Morris SR, Illingworth CFW: Pituitary radon implant for advanced cancer. Lancet 270: 399–401, 1956.
37. Buys NS, Kerns TC: Irradiation damage to the chiasm. Am J Ophthalmol 44:483–486, 1957.
38. Augsberger JJ: Radiation retinopathy. In Tasman WS (ed): Clinical Decision in Medical Retinal Diseases. Philadelphia, Mosby, 1994, pp 216–275.
39. Brown GC, Shields JA, Sanborn G, et al: Radiation retinopathy. Ophthalmology 89:1494–1501, 1982.
40. Brown GC, Shields JA, Sanborn G, et al: Radiation optic neuropathy. Ophthalmology 89:1489–1493, 1982.
41. Nakissa N, Rubin P, Strohl R, Keys H: Ocular and orbital complications following paranasal sinus malignancies and review of literature. Cancer 51:980–986, 1983.
42. Elsås T, Thorud E, Jetne V, Conradi IS: Retinopathy after low dose irradiation for an intracranial tumor of the frontal lobe. Acta Ophthalmol (Copenh) 66:65–68, 1988.
43. Parsons JT, Bova FJ, Fitzgerald CR, et al: Radiation retinopathy after external-beam irradiation: analysis of time-dose factors. Int J Radiat Oncol Biol Phys 30:765–773, 1994.
44. Wara WM, Irvine AR, Neger RE, et al: Radiation retinopathy. Int J Radiat Oncol Biol Phys 5:81–83, 1979.
45. Shukovsky LJ, Fletcher GH: Retinal and optic nerve complications in a high dose irradiation technique of ethmoid sinus and nasal cavity. Radiology 104:629–634, 1972.
46. Merriam GR, Szechter A, Focht EF: The effects of ionizing radiations on the eye. Front Radiat Ther Oncol 6:346–385, 1972.
47. Harris JR, Levene MB: Visual complications following irradiation for pituitary adenomas and craniopharyngiomas. Radiat Med 120:167–171, 1976.
48. Aristizabal S, Caldwell WL, Avila J: The relationship of time-dose fractionation factors to complications in the treatment of pituitary tumors by irradiation. Int J Radiat Oncol Biol Phys 2:667–673, 1977.
49. Viebahn M, Barricks ME, Osterloh MD: Synergism between diabetic and radiation retinopathy: case report and review. Br J Ophthalmol 75:629–632, 1991.

50. Dhir SP, Joshi AV, Banerjee AK: Radiation retinopathy in diabetes mellitus. Acta Radiol (Oncol) 21:111–113, 1982.
51. Mewis L, Tang RA, Salmonsen PC: Radiation retinopathy after "safe" levels of irradiation. Invest Ophthalmol Vis Sci 22:222, 1982.
52. Weaver RG, Chauvenet AR, Smith TJ, Schwartz AC: Ophthalmic evaluation of long-term survivors of childhood acute lymphoblastic leukemia. Cancer 58:963–968, 1986.
53. Stanford MR: Retinopathy after irradiation and hyperbaric oxygen. J R Soc Med 77:1041–1043, 1984.
54. Kinyoun JL, Chittum ME, Wells CG: Photocoagulation treatment of radiation retinopathy. Am J Ophthalmol 105:470–478, 1988.
55. Hayreh SS: Postradiation retinopathy: a fluorescence fundus angiographic study. Br J Ophthalmol 54:705–714, 1970.
56. Boozalis GT, Schachat AP, Green WR: Subretinal neovascularization from the retina in radiation retinopathy. Retina 7:156–161, 1987.
57. Mukai S, Guyer DR, Gragoudas ES: Radiation retinopathy. In Albert DA, Jakobiec FA (eds): Principles and Practice of Ophthalmology: Clinical Practice, 1st edition. Philadelphia, WB Saunders Co, 1994, pp 1038–1041.
58. Irvine AR, Wood IS: Radiation retinopathy as an experimental model for ischemic proliferative retinopathy and rubeosis iridis. Am J Ophthalmol 103:790–797, 1987.
59. Kline LB, Kim JY, Ceballos R: Radiation optic neuropathy. Ophthalmology 92:1118–1126, 1985.
60. Guy J, Schatz N: Hyperbaric oxygen in the treatment of radiation-induced optic neuropathy. Ophthalmology 93:1083–1088, 1986.
61. Roden D, Bosley TM, Fowble B, et al: Delayed radiation injury to the retrobulbar optic nerves and chiasm. Clinical syndrome and treatment with hyperbaric oxygen and corticosteroids. Ophthalmology 97:346–351, 1990.
62. Parsons JT, Bova FJ, Fitzerald CR, et al: Radiation optic neuropathy after megavoltage external-beam irradiation: analysis of time-dose factors. Int J Radiat Oncol Biol Phys 30:755–763, 1994.
63. Tishler RB, Loeffler JS, Lunsford LD, et al: Tolerance of cranial nerves of the cavernous sinus to radiosurgery. Int J Radiat Oncol Biol Phys 27:215–221, 1993.
64. Fishman ML, Bean SC, Cogan DG: Optic atrophy following prophylactic chemotherapy and cranial radiation for acute lymphocytic leukemia. Am J Ophthalmol 82:571–576, 1976.
65. Chaudhuri PR, Austin DJ, Rosenthal AR: Treatment of radiation retinopathy. Br J Ophthalmol 65:623–625, 1981.
66. Chee PHY: Radiation retinopathy. Am J Ophthalmol 66:860–865, 1968.
67. Gass JDM: A fluorescein angiographic study of macular dysfunction secondary to retinal vascular disease: x-ray irradiation, carotid artery occlusion, collagen vascular disease, and vitritis. Arch Ophthalmol 80:606–617, 1968.
68. Archer DB, Amoaku WMK, Gardiner TA: Radiation retinopathy: clinical, histopathological, ultrastructural, and experimental correlations. Eye 5:589–593, 1991.
69. Seddon JM, Gragoudas ES, Albert DM: Ciliary body and choroidal melanomas treated by proton beam irradiation. Arch Ophthalmol 101:1402–1408, 1983.
70. Kincaid MC, Folberg R, Torczynski E, et al: Complications after proton beam therapy for uveal malignant melanoma. A clinical and histopathologic study of 5 cases. Ophthalmology 95:982–991, 1988.
71. Cibis PA, Noell WK, Eichel V: Ocular effects produced by high-intensity x-radiation. Arch Ophthalmol 53:651–663, 1955.
72. Amoaku WMK, Frew L, Mahon GJ, Gardiner TA: Early ultrastructural changes after low dose x-irradiation in the retina of the rat. Eye 3:638–646, 1989.
73. Ferry AP, Blair CJ, Gragoudas ES, Volk SC: Pathologic examination of ciliary body melanoma treated with protein beam irradiation. Arch Ophthalmol 103:1849–1853, 1985.
74. Saornil MA, Egan KM, Gragoudas ES, et al: Histopathology of uveal melanomas treated by proton beam irradiation: a comparison study. Arch Ophthalmol 110:1112–1118, 1992.
75. Ahnstrom G, Erixon K: Radiation induced strand breakage in DNA form mammalian cells. Strand separation in alkaline solution. Int J Radiat Biol 23:285, 1973.
76. Hiss EA, Preston RJ: The effect of cytosine arabinoside on the frequency of single strand breaks in DNA of mammalian cells following irradiation or chemical treatment. Biochem Biophys Acta 478:1, 1977.
77. Phillips RA, Tolmach LJ: Repair of potentially lethal damage in x-irradiated HeLa cells. Radiat Res 29:413, 1966.
78. Noble KG, Kupersmith MJ: Retinal vascular remodeling in radiation retinopathy. Br J Ophthalmol 68:475–478, 1984.
79. Axer-Siegel R, Kremer L, Ben-Sira I, Weiss J: Radiation retinopathy treated with krypton red laser. Ann Ophthalmol 21:272–276, 1989.

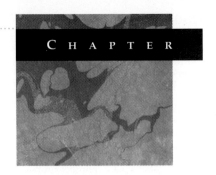

Bone Marrow Transplant Retinopathy

Peter K. Kaiser, M.D.

Evangelos S. Gragoudas, M.D.

Bone marrow transplantation (BMT) is the treatment of choice for both malignant and nonmalignant disorders of the bone marrow including aplastic anemia, acute/chronic myelogenous leukemia, acute/chronic lymphocytic leukemia, and lymphoma.[1,2] BMT is also used in combination with high-dose chemotherapy for patients with metastatic or high-risk primary breast cancer.[3] In preparation for the transplantation, patients usually undergo cytoreductive chemotherapy and total body irradiation (TBI) to eradicate all host malignant cells and suppress the host immune response and thus minimize rejection of the donor marrow. They then receive either an allogenic (HLA compatible donor, such as a sibling), syngeneic (donor is a monozygotic twin), or autologous (patient's own stored marrow) bone marrow transplant to reconstitute the patients hematologic function. BMT results in significant morbidity and mortality owing to the underlying disease process, conditioning regimen, graft-versus-host (GVH) disease, infections, immunodeficiency, and hematologic complications.

There are numerous anterior segment complications from bone marrow transplantation (Table 40–1). Most are related to GVH disease, where immunocompetent donor lymphocytes from the transplanted marrow react immunologically to the genetically determined differences in the host tissue and mount an immunologic attack against the host. Acute GVH disease occurs in more than 50% of successful graft recipients, while chronic GVH disease is seen in 25 to 45% of long-term survivors.[4–6] Keratoconjunctivitis sicca,[7–13] pseudomembranous conjunctivitis,[8,13,14] conjunctival GVH disease,[15] superficial punctate keratitis, massive denudement of corneal epithelium, and sterile and/or infectious

corneal ulceration[13,16] have been reported secondary to GVH disease and bone marrow transplantation. Cataracts, mainly posterior subcapsular opacification, also develop as late complications.[12,13,16,17] During the early posttransplant period, patients are usually immunocompromised secondary to the severe marrow aplasia and are at increased risk of developing ocular infections including both viral and bacterial keratitis and conjunctivitis.[16]

Posterior segment complications of BMT can be divided into three groups: infectious, hematologic, and an occlusive microvascular retinopathy. Similar to the anterior segment complications, retinal infections are seen during the immediate posttransplant period. One study found that 2% of 397 patients developed either fungal retinitis, viral retinitis, or endophthalmitis after BMT.[18] Fungal infections with *Candida* or *Aspergillus* were observed within 120 days of transplantation, while viral infections with varicella zoster or cytomegalovirus and parasitic infections with *Toxoplasma gondii* occurred later. Another study reported 1% of 785 patients developed CMV retinitis after BMT.[19]

During the early posttransplant period, hematologic abnormalities including anemia, hyperviscosity, and thrombocytopenia are common.[20] This transplantation-induced bone marrow aplasia has been blamed for vitreous hemorrhages, intraretinal hemorrhages, and other hemorrhagic complications.[9,12,18] Coskuncan and associates found that 3.5% of their patients developed hemorrhagic complications, on average, 51 days after BMT.[18] These patients had mean platelet counts of 27×10^9/liter, mean hematocrit levels of 0.27, and their hemorrhages cleared as the pancytopenia resolved without any long-term sequelae. Hemorrhages in other

TABLE 40–1 Ophthalmic Complications of Bone Marrow Transplantation

Anterior Segment Changes
Dry eyes
Keratoconjunctivitis sicca
Pseudomembranous conjunctivitis
Conjunctival graft-versus-host disease
Bacterial and viral conjunctivitis
Superficial punctate keratitis
Sterile and infectious corneal ulceration
Keratitis
Cataracts
Posterior Segment Changes
Fungal and viral retinitis
Endophthalmitis
Vitreous hemorrhages
Bone marrow transplantation retinopathy
Multiple, bilateral cotton-wool spots
Retinal telangiectases
Microaneurysms
Small intraretinal hemorrhages
Macular edema
Hard exudates
Vascular attenuation
Retinal neovascularization
Optic disc edema

ocular structures including the conjunctiva have also been reported during the pancytopenic phase after BMT.[9]

Bone marrow transplantation retinopathy was first reported in 1983.[8,9,21] Multiple, bilateral cotton-wool spots and retinal hemorrhages were described in patients who had received bone marrow transplants. The BMT retinopathy occurs after a characteristic latent period and usually resolves after a few weeks. This occlusive microvascular retinopathy is now a recognized complication of BMT.

EPIDEMIOLOGY AND ETIOLOGY

The reported incidence of BMT retinopathy after transplantation has varied from 1% to 62%; however, most large series indicate the true incidence is probably closer to the lower rate.[3,14,18,22,23] Bernauer and associates published a prospective study in which 10.3% of 127 patients developed BMT retinopathy.[14] Two other large studies reported lower incidence rates of 3.5% of 397 patients and 5.5% of 72.[18,23] The varying incidence rates may reflect the use of different preparative regimens, since the patients in the three studies did not receive similar pretreatments. For instance, Bernauer and associates used TBI and cyclosporine in their patients before BMT, while Coskuncan and associates did not use irradiation (see discussion below). Another possible reason for the varying incidence rates is the

fact that most patients after BMT are significantly ill and subtle visual changes may go unnoticed during this time period.

BMT retinopathy occurs, on average, within 6 months of bone marrow transplantation.[8,14,16,18,21,22,24–26] The earliest reported case of BMT retinopathy was 3 months and the longest latent period was 25 months. The development of BMT retinopathy was not influenced by age, sex, or race of the transplant recipients.[14]

The etiology of BMT retinopathy is unclear, and is believed to be multifactorial (Table 40–2).[22,26] Cyclosporine toxicity, TBI, and pre- or posttransplant chemotherapeutic drugs have all been implicated in BMT retinopathy.[14,22,24] Additional potential etiologic factors include reactivation of the primary disease, hematologic abnormalities, infections, immunodeficiency, hypertension, and chronic GVH disease.

All patients who developed BMT retinopathy had malignant disorders as the underlying disease process.[3,14] Nonmalignant conditions such as severe aplastic anemia never resulted in BMT retinopathy. The type of malignancy and stage of the underlying disease were not significant risk factors.[14] However, even though patients with malignant diseases developed BMT retinopathy, the fundus lesions are not manifestations of the underlying malignancy. Histopathologic studies did not reveal any malignant cells in the posterior segment of patients with BMT retinopathy.[26] Thus, although malignant hematologic disorders play a role in the pathogenesis of BMT retinopathy, the malignancies alone do not cause the disorder.

Leukemia can cause hematologic abnormalities including anemia, hyperviscosity, and thrombocytopenia which can cause ocular abnormalities even without BMT therapy.[20,26] In addition, during the immediate posttransplant period, patients often exhibit hematologic abnormalities, which can produce posterior segment lesions. Thus, it has been proposed that the cotton-wool spots seen in BMT retinopathy may represent a hypercoagulable state due to the underlying disease.[24] However, this is

TABLE 40–2 Possible Risk Factors for Developing Bone Marrow Transplantation Retinopathy

Underlying malignant disorders
Infections
Hematologic abnormalities
Posttransplantation immunodeficiency
Cyclosporine
Hypertension
Total body irradiation
Conditioning chemotherapeutic drugs
Graft-versus-host disease

unlikely because hematologic testing did not reveal any coagulation disorders, thrombocytopenia, or severe anemia when the characteristic cotton-wool spots appeared.[24] Furthermore, the lesions appear after the marrow aplasia resolves and the transplanted marrow is capable of producing functional hematopoietic cells.

The immunodeficient state in the early posttransplant period predisposes the entire body to infections, leading some authors to suggest an infectious etiology for BMT retinopathy. Serologic testing in BMT retinopathy patients has universally been negative, including tests for cytomegalovirus, herpesvirus, Epstein-Barr virus, hepatitis virus, and human immunodeficiency virus (HIV).[14,24] Further evidence against an infectious cause is the observed improvement after steroid treatment in patients with BMT retinopathy, whereas an infectious source would likely worsen with this treatment. Finally, the complete absence of both anterior and posterior segment cells virtually excludes an infectious etiology for BMT retinopathy.

In HIV retinopathy, cotton-wool spots have been observed[27] and some investigators have suggested that there is a link between the immunodeficient state in the early post-BMT period and HIV.[24] This seems rather doubtful given the lack of the distinctive lesions in renal and cardiac transplant patients who suffer from similar immune deficiency after transplantation.[28-30] In addition, HIV-positive patients do not develop BMT retinopathy after bone marrow transplantation, and patients with BMT retinopathy are HIV-negative on serologic testing.[14] Thus, it is rather unlikely that BMT retinopathy is related to an immunodeficient state.

Cyclosporine, also known as cyclosporin A, is a potent immunosuppressive drug that prolongs survival of allogenic transplant patients by preventing and treating GVH disease. The drug attacks the endothelium of the vascular system and is known to cause a characteristic, dose-limiting nephrotoxicity.[14,29,31-33] Cyclosporine has also been implicated as a cause of a variety of neurologic abnormalities including seizures, encephalopathy, cerebellar and spinal syndromes, dysarthria, tremor, coma, cortical blindness, increased intracranial pressure, and increased cerebral spinal fluid (CSF) protein.[34,35] These neurologic side effects are usually reversible with reduction or discontinuation of cyclosporine.[28,36] Given its neurotoxic side effects, cyclosporine has been proposed as a possible etiologic factor in BMT retinopathy.[12,14,24,35] Bernauer and associates found that all their patients with BMT retinopathy received cyclosporine during their conditioning regimen and that the use of cyclosporine and TBI was a significant risk factor for the development of BMT retinopathy.[14] Toxic levels of cyclosporine or elevated levels of creatinine were not discovered in any of their patients. Another study reported that all 13 patients who developed BMT retinopathy, out of 127 total patients, were pretreated with cyclosporine and TBI.[12] Conversely, two recent reports

demonstrated BMT retinopathy in patients who did not receive cyclosporine.[3,26] In one study, the patients received campath 1G, a monoclonal antibody of the IgG 2b subclass used to deplete donor lymphocytes and prevent GVH disease, as well as reduce the probability of graft failure.[26] In the other, the patients received autologous BMT and, therefore, did not require prophylaxis against GVH disease.[3] Other studies have also described BMT retinopathy in patients who did not receive cyclosporine.[18,22,37] Moreover, cyclosporine has never been shown to produce BMT retinopathy in autologous or syngeneic bone marrow recipients, or in renal transplant recipients.[3,14,24,30,38] Thus, cyclosporine alone cannot produce BMT retinopathy. Since both cyclosporine and campath 1G inhibit the function of T cells, it has been suggested that normal T-cell function may be necessary to protect the retinal endothelium.[26] The loss of this protection may render the retinal vessels more susceptible to other insults including radiation damage and retinal ischemia.

Malignant hypertension can produce hypertensive retinopathy, which is associated with cotton-wool spot formation.[39-41] Furthermore, a known side effect of cyclosporine is hypertension, although the elevation in blood pressure is usually mild.[29,32] Thus, some authors have postulated that BMT retinopathy is a manifestation of systemic hypertension. Other studies have disputed this argument noting that any elevation in blood pressure seen in BMT retinopathy patients was usually mild and easily controlled with antihypertensive medications.[24,32,33] Moreover, higher threshold blood pressures and longer periods of elevated pressure are usually required before the development of hypertensive retinopathy.[39-41] Thus, it is doubtful that hypertension plays a role in BMT retinopathy.

Many patients who develop BMT retinopathy also received TBI and/or supplemental cranial radiation, leading some authors to suggest that BMT retinopathy is simply a form of radiation retinopathy.[22] In one report, only patients who received TBI developed BMT retinopathy.[14] Similarly, the likelihood of developing BMT retinopathy increased with increasing radiation dose in another study, and patients who received both prophylactic cranial radiation and TBI were more likely to develop BMT retinopathy than those receiving TBI alone.[22] The authors believe that radiation damages the retinal microvasculature, producing the characteristic findings of ischemic microangiopathy. However, it is unlikely that radiation is the only factor, since BMT retinopathy has been described in patients who did not receive TBI or local head irradiation.[3,18] Additional evidence against radiation being the only etiologic factor for BMT retinopathy is provided by the fact that BMT retinopathy has not been described in cardiac or renal allograft recipients who received similar radiation dosages.[28-30] Furthermore, the total radiation dose in TBI is considerably lower than the 4000 cGy usually required to produce radiation retinopathy. The average total radiation dose in one study was 27 cGy and two patients developed the retinopathy after just 12 cGy total irradiation.[22] Finally, the classic picture of radiation retinopathy does not resemble BMT retinopathy. Unlike BMT retinopathy, radiation retinopathy does not respond well to treatment and is usually progressive. Thus, BMT retinopathy may share some common findings with radiation retinopathy, but other factors must be involved to create the ischemic retinopathy of BMT.

Conditioning chemotherapeutic drugs have also been implicated as possible etiologic factors in BMT retinopathy. Ocular toxicity from cisplatin has been described previously. Toxic side effects include papilledema, retrobulbar optic neuritis, transient cortical blindness, temporary homonymous hemianopsia, and central retinal artery occlusions.[42-48] Similarly, optic neuroretinitis, intraretinal hemorrhages, arterial narrowing, and nerve fiber layer infarcts have been described with carumstine toxicity.[48-50] Thus, one report postulated that the BMT retinopathy seen in their patients was secondary to cisplatin and carumstine toxicity.[3] However, BMT retinopathy has been described in patients who did not receive either chemotherapeutic. Vogler and associates noted BMT retinopathy in patients receiving both cytosine arabinoside and TBI.[38] Other reports describe BMT retinopathy in patients receiving TBI and high-dose cyclophosphamide.[18,24] This prompted Gloor and associates to hypothesize that the chemotherapeutics shift the radiation dose response curve to the left, producing more retinal damage at any given radiation dose.[24] These authors believe that chemotherapeutic drugs prevent retinal cells from repairing radiation damage and lower dosage of radiation may generate retinal toxicity. Evidence against this theory comes from studies that describe BMT retinopathy in patients who did not receive TBI. Thus, in all the studies, various combinations of chemotherapeutics were used and no single chemotherapeutic drug can be singled out as the cause of BMT retinopathy.

Another theory involves the possibility that GVH disease may play a role in BMT retinopathy. To date, ischemic retinopathy is not a recognized feature of GVH disease[8,14,25]; however, a recent study cited chronic GVH disease as a possible risk factor for the development of cotton-wool spots.[18] In the report the authors used multivariate analysis to determine the relative odds ratios for various risk factors in the development of BMT retinopathy. Cyclosporine, Bisulfan, and TBI were not significant risk factors in their study patients. Interestingly, chronic GVH disease was a significant risk factor ($p<.05$), although it did not fully account for the development of the ischemic retinopathy.[18] Conversely, other studies have shown very low or no GVH disease activity in patients with BMT retinopathy.[14] Thus, while chronic GVH disease may play a role in the development of BMT retinopathy, further studies are needed to verify this fact.

The pathogenesis of BMT retinopathy is most likely multifactorial. Patients receiving bone marrow transplants often have multiple organ abnormalities and complex medical problems requiring multiple medical therapies. Implicating one of these therapies as the primary etiologic factor is difficult. Cyclosporine, TBI, preparative chemotherapeutics, and GVH disease alone cannot produce BMT retinopathy. Therefore, a combination of pathologic mechanisms is presumably the culprit.

CLINICAL FEATURES

Patients with BMT retinopathy may appear without any symptoms; however, they usually present complaining of decreased visual acuity or describing visual field losses. In one study, 77% of the BMT retinopathy patients presented with decreased visual acuity.[14] In another study, visual acuity ranged from 20/20, when there was no macular edema present, to 20/200 when macular edema was severe.[22] Patients may note the acute appearance of paracentral scotomas that can be quantified on an Amsler grid,[24] and multiple, localized, shallow scotomas on visual field testing.[14] When optic disc edema is present without the retinopathy, patients were usually asymptomatic; however, further scrutiny often revealed decreased color vision.[35] Defects on visual field testing may range from an enlarged blind spot to moderate field loss in a diffuse or arcuate pattern.[35] None of the patients develop an afferent pupillary defect (APD).

The funduscopic findings in bone marrow transplant retinopathy are generally bilateral and symmetric (Table 40–1). The first signs are multiple, bilateral cotton-wool spots (Fig. 40–1C and D).[3,12,14] Cotton-wool spots are small, whitish opacities with feathery edges that represent microinfarctions of the small retinal arterioles.[51] The cotton-wool patches develop, on average, 150 days after bone marrow transplantation.[18] Retinal telangiectasia, microaneurysms, and small hemorrhages are also seen usually at the edge of the foveal avascular zone or scattered throughout the midperiphery (Fig. 40–1A and B). Macular edema in a diffuse, rather than circinate, pattern occasionally develop near the areas of telangiectases. Later, hard exudates and vascular attenuation are seen.[12] No vitreous cells or vascular sheathing is observed. One study noted the late development of retinal neovascularization and a subhyaloid hemorrhage in one patient.[22] It is unclear if these proliferative changes are part of BMT retinopathy because no other studies have reported similar changes.[12,14] Until other studies find similar proliferative changes, it seems likely that BMT retinopathy does not progress beyond the ischemic microvascular stage.

In general there are no optic disc changes in the microvascular retinopathy seen after BMT, but some patients may present with bilateral disc

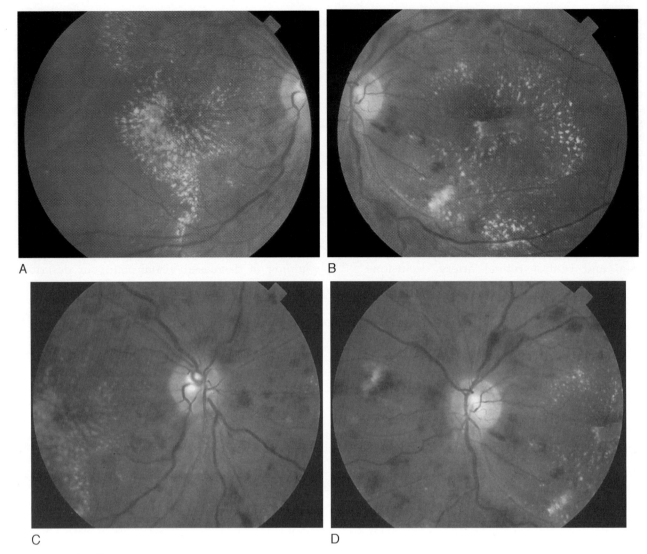

FIGURE 40–1 *A* and *B,* Fundus photographs of a patient 8 months after receiving a bone marrow transplant (BMT) for chronic myelogenous leukemia. The patient received total body irradiation (200-cGy fractions over 7 days for a total dose of 1400 cGy) and Cytoxan (60 mg/kg) before the BMT. The photographs show extensive hard exudates and retinal hemorrhages. There is subretinal fibrosis present in the left macula. *C* and *D,* Disc photographs of the same patient showing cotton-wool spots and retinal hemorrhages. No disc edema or neovascularization is present. The patient's visual acuity is 20/320 OD and 20/500 OS. (Courtesy of Donald J. D'Amico, M.D.)

edema. Coskuncan and associates noted that 2% of their patients had bilateral optic disc edema.[18] The authors attributed the disc edema to cyclosporine, and noted that when the cyclosporine dose was decreased or discontinued the disc edema resolved.[18] Another study found 2.5% of 323 patients developed bilateral disc edema.[35] In 87.5% of these patients, discontinuing cyclosporine produced an improvement in the disc edema. Extensive neurologic work-up including computed tomography, magnetic resonance imaging, CSF analysis, and lumbar punctures failed to reveal central nervous system infections, malignancies, or elevated intracranial pressure in any of these patients.[14,18,35] It is interesting to note that the disc edema occurs on average 148 days after BMT, which is similar to the latent period for development of the retinopathy.[18] At this time, it is unclear if the optic disc edema is part of BMT retinopathy or simply a side effect of cyclosporine treatment.

FLUORESCEIN ANGIOGRAPHY

Fluorescein angiographic examination of BMT retinopathy patients demonstrated capillary nonperfusion in the areas of the cotton-wool spots and adjacent retinal capillary beds (Fig. 40–2).[3,14,26] The cotton-wool spots themselves appear hypofluorescent due to both blocked fluorescence from cellular debris and arteriolar nonperfusion. Near the edges

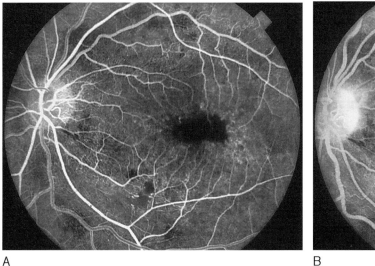

A

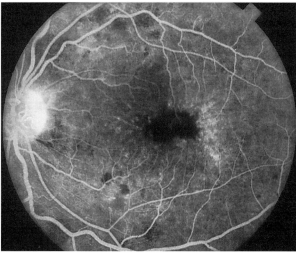

B

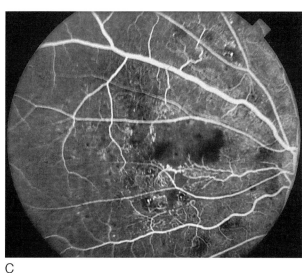

C

FIGURE 40–2 *A* and *B*, Early and midtransit fluorescein angiograms OS of the same patient described in Figure 40–1, illustrating microaneurysms, blocked fluorescence from intraretinal hemorrhages, telangiectatic vessels and enlargement of the foveal avascular zone. *C*, Peripheral view during the arteriovenous phase of the fluorescein angiogram showing capillary dropout, microaneurysms, and telangiectasia. (Courtesy of Donald J. D'Amico, M.D.)

of the nonperfused areas, intraretinal microvascular abnormalities and microaneurysms were noted. In a minority of patients, there was fluorescein leakage around the fovea corresponding to areas of macular edema. When optic disc edema was present, leakage of the fluorescein about the optic disc was appreciated in the late phases of the angiograms.

PATHOLOGIC FEATURES

Light microscopy of histopathologic specimens taken from patients with BMT retinopathy revealed edematous nerve fiber layers with focal swelling of the retinal fibers forming cytoid bodies.[14,26] Ischemic retinal ganglion cells and shrunken, eosinophilic neurons in the inner plexiform layers were also noted.[14,26] In the areas surrounding the cotton-wool spots, small hemorrhages, saccular microaneurysms, and focal, ectatic retinal capillaries were

present.[14] The outer retinal layers were normal. Step-serial sections did not show any abnormalities of the blood vessels supplying the areas with cotton-wool spots.[24] Electron microscopy indicated abnormal transport of cellular debris from degenerating mitochondria and other intracellular organelles. The disruption of axoplasmic flow produced axonal swelling and the characteristic whitish appearance of the cotton-wool spots.[26] The surrounding capillaries were filled with clumped erythrocytes, and showed loss of endothelial cells with relative preservation of pericytes.[26] There was no evidence of malignant cells, infectious organisms, or any inflammatory cell infiltration in any specimen.[24,26]

DIFFERENTIAL DIAGNOSIS

The appearance of cotton-wool spots in the retina is nonspecific and usually indicates a systemic vascular disease (Table 40–3). Cotton-wool spots are common in diabetic retinopathy, hypertensive retinopathy, and retinal vascular occlusions. The progressive nature of diabetic retinopathy and the presence of elevated glucose levels differentiates it from BMT retinopathy. Blood pressures were slightly elevated in some patients with BMT retinopathy, leading some authors to postulate that BMT retinopathy is a manifestation of hypertensive changes. This is unlikely because higher threshold blood pressures and longer periods of elevated pressure are usually required before the development of hypertensive retinopathy.[39–41] Finally, patients with retinal vascular occlusions can exhibit cotton-wool spots and retinal hemorrhages; however, the presence of retinal edema and characteristic fluorescein angiograms aid in making the diagnosis.

The microvascular abnormalities in radiation retinopathy may mimic BMT retinopathy and has also been suggested to play a role in the pathogenesis. Nonetheless, the history of bone marrow transplantation serves to distinguish the two disorders. Likewise, recurrence of leukemia is a feared complication after transplantation and it can appear similar to BMT retinopathy. Sometimes a vitrectomy is required to confirm the diagnosis. Malignant cells were never identified in any patient with BMT retinopathy, making the likelihood of a recurrence of the underlying disease improbable. Although hemorrhagic complications following BMT are common, none of the patients with BMT retinopathy had any hematologic abnormalities that would classify them as a retinopathy associated with blood anomalies. This list includes retinopathy of anemia, polycythemia, and dysproteinemias that can produce hemorrhages, cotton-wool spots, and optic disc hyperemia. Retinal manifestations of collagen vascular diseases may simulate BMT retinopathy; however, the lack of inflammation, absence of collagen vascular disease, and the short recovery period separates the diseases. HIV retinopathy presents with multiple cotton-wool spots and scattered hemorrhages, microaneurysms, and other microvascular changes. The picture is very similar to BMT retinopathy, leading some authors to postulate a similar pathogenesis; however, none of the patients with BMT retinopathy were HIV-positive, making the diagnosis unlikely. Leber's idiopathic stellate neuroretinitis resembles BMT retinopathy with disc edema and macular exudates; however, the lack of APD, inflammation, and bilaterality observed in BMT retinopathy differentiates the two entities. Finally, rare causes of cotton-wool spots include Purtscher's retinopathy, retinopathy from acute pancreatitis, and retinopathy of toxemia of pregnancy. Each of these disorders has characteristic systemic findings that help make the diagnosis. Obviously, the history of a malignant hematologic disorder and bone marrow transplantation should point clinicians toward the diagnosis of BMT retinopathy, effectively minimizing the need to explore the other entities in the differential diagnosis.

TREATMENT AND PROGNOSIS

In most studies, patients with BMT retinopathy generally respond to treatment over a period of weeks to months. Patients receiving cyclosporine either discontinued or decreased the dosage of the drug.[14,18,26] In addition, most authors started oral prednisone with initial dosages up to 100 mg/day for 14 days followed by a slow tapering of the medication. The cotton-wool spots and retinal hemorrhages usually regress and disappear clinically over the next few months (Fig. 40–3). In one report, 69% of patients had complete resolution of the fundus lesions.[14] The visual acuity recovered completely in 46% of patients, and visual field defects were completely reversible in 50% of patients and partially reversible in the other 50%. Other studies have reported complete visual recovery in 100% of patients with only rare hard exudates and scattered retinal hemorrhages remaining on fundus examination.[3,24] Similarly, patients with bilateral optic disc edema have been treated with oral prednisone and decreasing or discontinuing cyclosporine doses.[14,24] In almost all the patients, the optic disc edema resolved over a few weeks without sequelae. Of note, two patients with breast cancer eventually developed optic atrophy with progressive visual field loss despite steroid treatment.[3] The authors postulate that the permanent optic nerve damage seen in these patients was due either to a direct toxic effect of the chemotherapeutic drugs or an indirect effect resulting from ischemia. Some patients have had spontaneous recovery of visual function and resolution of the fundus lesions without any treat-

TABLE 40–3   Differential Diagnosis

Diabetic retinopathy
Hypertensive retinopathy
Retinal artery occlusion
Radiation retinopathy
Leukemic retinopathy
Retinopathy of anemia
Retinopathy of polycythemia vera
Retinopathy of dysproteinemias
Retinopathy of collagen vascular diseases
Human immunodeficiency virus retinopathy
Leber's idiopathic stellate neuroretinitis
Purtscher's retinopathy
Retinopathy of acute pancreatitis
Retinopathy of toxemia of pregnancy

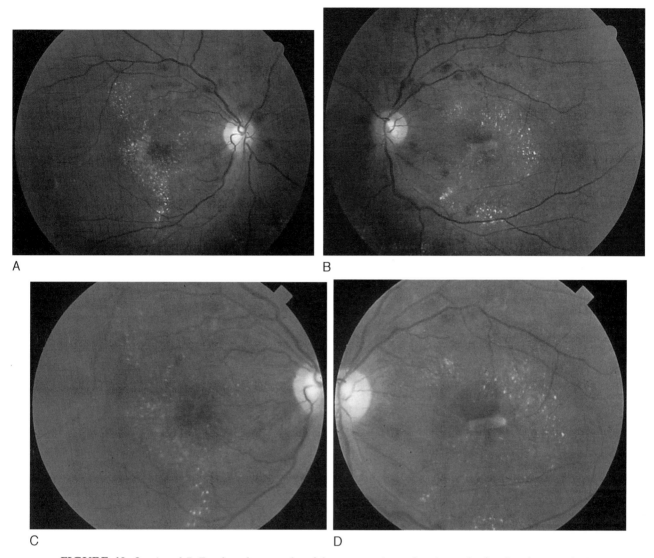

FIGURE 40-3 *A and B,* Fundus photographs of the same patient taken 1 month after the photographs in Figure 40–1. The patient has not received any treatment for the fundus lesions. There is resolution of the cotton-wool spots and decrease of the macular exudates and retinal hemorrhages. *C and D,* Three months after the original photographs. Subretinal fibrosis is present in both macula and there is almost complete resolution of the retinal hemorrhages. The retinal exudates have been reduced in both eyes. (Courtesy of Donald J. D'Amico, M.D.)

ment.[26] This is an important consideration, since withdrawal of cyclosporine may be fatal when GVH disease is present; therefore, extreme care must be undertaken to balance the need for cyclosporine with the risk of BMT retinopathy.

One study outlined the use of laser photocoagulation for the treatment of complications of BMT retinopathy.[22] Panretinal photocoagulation was used to treat retinal neovascularization seen in one patient with subsequent involution of the new vessels.[22] Patients with diffuse macular edema were treated using grid photocoagulation.[22] Since recovery of visual function has been observed in patients with BMT retinopathy without any treatment, pho-

tocoagulation should only be considered in patients with longstanding macular edema.

PREVENTION

Given the potential for developing bone marrow transplant retinopathy after BMT and the ability to successfully treat the disorder by decreasing and/or discontinuing medications, regular funduscopic examination is indicated for these patients. Ophthalmic examination should be undertaken in all patients even when cyclosporine, TBI, and other etiologic factors were not used, given the multifactorial nature of BMT retinopathy. In addition, close ophthalmic observation and care may help identify the underlying etiology of the disorder.

REFERENCES

1. Goldman JM, Apperley JF, Jones L, et al: Bone marrow transplantation for patients with chronic myeloid leukemia. N Engl J Med 314:202–207, 1986.
2. Elfenebin GJ, Mellits ED, Santos GW: Patients with aplastic anemia: engraftment and survival after allogenic bone marrow transplantation for severe aplastic anemia. Transplant Proc 15:1412–1416, 1983.
3. Khawly JA, Rubin P, Petros W, et al: Retinopathy and optic neuropathy in bone marrow transplantation for breast cancer. Ophthalmology 103:87–95, 1996.
4. Slavin RE, Santos GW: The graft-versus-host reaction in man after bone marrow transplantation: pathology, pathogenesis, clinical features, and implications. Clin Immunol Immunopathol 1:472–498, 1973.
5. Tutschka PJ, Bortin MM: Graft versus host disease. Transplant Proc 13:1267–1269, 1981.
6. Wingard JR, Piantadosi S, Vogelsang GB: Predictors of death from chronic graft-versus-host disease after bone marrow transplantation. Blood 74:1428–1435, 1989.
7. Hanada R, Ueoka Y: Obstruction of nasolacrimal ducts closely related to graft-versus-host disease after bone marrow transplantation. Bone Marrow Transplant 4:125, 1989.
8. Hirst LW, Jabs DA, Tutschka PJ, et al: The eye in bone marrow transplantation. I. Clinical study. Arch Ophthalmol 101:580–584, 1983.
9. Jabs DA, Hirst LW, Green WR, et al: The eye in bone marrow transplantation. II. Histopathology. Arch Ophthalmol 101:585–590, 1983.
10. Jack MK, Jack GM, Sale GE, et al: Ocular complications of graft vs host disease. Arch Ophthalmol 101:1080–1084, 1983.
11. Franklin RM, Kenyon KR, Tutschka PJ, et al: Ocular manifestations of graft versus host disease. Ophthalmology 90:4, 1983.
12. Tichelli A: Late ocular complications after bone marrow transplantation. Nouv Rev Fr Hematol 36(Suppl):79–82, 1994.
13. Bray LC, Carey PJ, Proctor SJ, et al: Ocular complications of bone marrow transplantation. Br J Ophthalmol 75:611–614, 1991.
14. Bernauer W, Gratwohl A, Keller A, Daicker B.: Microvasculopathy in the ocular fundus after bone marrow transplantation. Ann Intern Med 115:925–930, 1991.
15. Jabs DA, Wingard J, Green WR, et al: The eye in bone marrow transplantation. III. Conjunctival graft vs host disease. Arch Ophthalmol 107:1343–1348, 1989.
16. Jack MK, Hicks JD: Ocular complications in high dose chemoradiotherapy and marrow transplantation. Ann Ophthalmol 6:709–711, 1981.
17. Dunn JP, Jabs DA, Wingard J, et al: The eye in bone marrow transplantation V. Cataracts after bone marrow transplantation. Arch Ophthalmol 111:1367–1373, 1993.
18. Coskuncan NM, Jabs DA, Dunn JP, et al: The eye in bone marrow transplantation. VI. Retinal complications. Arch Ophthalmol 112:372–379, 1994.
19. Wingard JR, Piantadosi S, Burns WH, et al: Cytomegalovirus infections in bone marrow transplant recipients given intensive cytoreductive therapy. Rev Infect Dis 12(Suppl):793–804, 1990.
20. Rosenthal AR: Ocular manifestations of leukemia: a review. Ophthalmology 90:899–905, 1983.
21. Gratwhol A, Gloor B, Hahn H, Speck B: Retinal cotton wool patches in bone marrow transplant recipients. N Engl J Med 308:1101, 1983.
22. Lopez PF, Sternberg P, Dabbs CK, et al: Bone marrow transplant retinopathy. Am J Ophthalmol 112:635–646, 1991.
23. Stuckenschneider BJ, Meiler WF: Ocular findings following bone marrow transplantation (Abstract). Ophthalmology 92(Suppl):152, 1992.
24. Gloor B, Gratwohl A, Hahn H, et al: Multiple cotton wool spots following bone marrow transplantation for treatment of acute lymphatic leukemia. Br J Ophthalmol 69:320–325, 1985.
25. Livesey SJ, Holmes JA, Whittaker JA: Ocular complications of bone marrow transplantation. Eye 3:271–276, 1989.
26. Webster AR, Anderson JR, Richards EM, Moore AT: Ischaemic retinopathy occurring in patients receiving bone marrow allografts and campath-1G: a clinicopathological study. Br J Ophthalmol 79:687–691, 1995.
27. Pepose JS, Holland GN, Nestor MS, et al: Acquired immune deficiency syndrome. Pathologic mechanisms of ocular disease. Ophthalmology 92:472–484, 1985.
28. Wilczek H, Ringden O, Tyden G: Cyclosporine-associated central nervous system toxicity after renal transplantation. Transplantation 39:110, 1985.
29. Walfe JA, McCann RL, Sanfilippo F: Cyclosporine-associated microangiopathy in renal transplantation: a severe but potentially reversible form of early graft injury. Transplantation 41:541–544, 1986.
30. Oechslin M, Thiel G, Landmann J, Gloor B: Cotton-wool exudates not observed in recipients of renal transplants treated with cyclosporine. Transplantation 41:60–62, 1986.
31. Dieterle A, Gratwohl A, Nizze H, et al: Chronic cyclosporine-associated nephrotoxicity in bone marrow transplant patients. Transplantation 49:1093–1100, 1990.
32. Hamilton DV, Carmichael DJ, Evans DB, Calne RY: Hypertension in renal transplant recipients on cyclosporine A and corticosteroids and azathioprine. Transplant Proc 14:597–600, 1982.
33. Joss DV, Barrett AJ, Kendra JR, et al: Hypertension and convulsions in children receiving cyclosporine A. Lancet 1:906, 1982.
34. Reece DE, Frei-Lahr DA, Shepard JD, et al: Neurologic complications in allogenic bone marrow transplant patients receiving cyclosporine. Bone Marrow Transplant 8:393–401, 1991.
35. Avery R, Jabs DA, Wingard JR, et al: Optic disc edema after bone marrow transplantation: possible role of cyclosporine toxicity. Ophthalmology 98:1294–1301, 1991.
36. Atkinson K, Biggs J, Darveniza P, et al: Cyclosporine-associated central nervous system toxicity after allogenic bone marrow transplantation. Transplantation 38:34–37, 1984.
37. Coccia P, Strandjord SE, Warkentin PI, et al: High-dose cytosine arabinoside and fractionated total body irradiation: an improved preparative regimen for bone marrow transplantation of children with acute lymphoblastic leukemia in remission. Blood 71:888–893, 1988.
38. Vogler WR, Winton EF, Heffner LT, et al: Ophthalmological and other toxicities related to cytosine arabinoside and total body irradiation as preparative regimen for bone marrow transplantation. Bone Marrow Transplant 6:405–409, 1990.
39. Hayreh SS, Servais GE, Virdi PS: Macular lesions in malignant arterial hypertension. Ophthalmologica 198:230–246, 1989.
40. Hayreh SS, Servais GE, Virdi PS: Retinal arteriolar changes in malignant arterial hypertension. Ophthalmologica 198:178–196, 1989.
41. Hayreh SS, Servais GE, Virdi PS: Cotton-wool spots in malignant arterial hypertension. Ophthalmologica 198:197–215, 1989.
42. Wilding G, Caruso R, Lawrence TS, et al: Retinal toxicity after high-dose cisplatin therapy. J Clin Oncol 3:1683–1689, 1985.
43. Urba S, Forastiere AA: Retrobulbar neuritis in a patient treated with intraarterial cisplatin for head and neck cancer. Cancer 62:2094–2097, 1988.
44. Pippitt CH, Muss HB, Homesley HD, Jobson VW: Cis-

platin associated cortical blindness. Gynecol Oncol 12:253–255, 1981.
45. Berman IJ, Mann MP: Seizures and transient cortical blindness with cis-platinum (II) diamminedichloride (PDD) therapy in a thirty year old man. Cancer 45:764–766, 1980.
46. Becher R, Schutt P, Osieka R, Schmidt CG: Peripheral neuropathy and ophthalmologic toxicity after treatment with cis-dichlorodiammineplatinum (II). J Cancer Res Clin Oncol 96:219–222, 1980.
47. Ostrow S, Hahn D, Wiernik PH, Richards RD: Ophthalmologic toxicity after cis-dichlorodiammineplatinum (II) therapy. Cancer Treat Rep 62:1591–1594, 1978.
48. Kupersmith MJ, Seiple WH, Holopigian K, et al: Maculopathy caused by intra-arterially administered cisplatin and intravenously administered carmustine. Am J Ophthalmol 113:435–438, 1992.
49. McLennan R, Taylor HR: Optic neuroretinitis in association with BCNU and procarbazine therapy. Med Pediatr Oncol 4:43–38, 1978.
50. Shingleton BJ, Bienfang DC, Albert DM, et al: Ocular toxicity associated with high-dose carmustine. Arch Ophthalmol 100:1766–1772, 1982.
51. Destro M, Gragoudas ES: Arterial occlusions. In Albert DA, Jakobiec FA (eds): Principles and Practice of Ophthalmology: Clinical Practice, 1st edition. Philadelphia, WB Saunders Co, 1994.

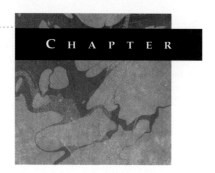

CHAPTER 41

Retinal Diseases in Pregnancy

Janet S. Sunness, M.D.
Arturo Santos, M.D.

In the early part of this century, the appearance of the retina in patients with such diseases as preeclampsia[3-5] and diabetes[6,7] was used as a measure of the systemic status and fetal viability. Now that modern medical and obstetric means of monitoring and managing pregnant women are available, the retina is only rarely used as a measure of risk for the fetus.[8] Current interest has focused instead on the effects of pregnancy on the retina of the mother, both in health and in illness. Pregnancy is associated with the development of retinal disease in patients with no pre-existing ocular disorder, and may modify the course of pre-existing disorders such as diabetic retinopathy. Most of the changes associated with pregnancy tend to resolve, in part or completely, by several months postpartum. However, some changes, such as retinal arteriolar occlusions associated with pregnancy-induced hypertension, may have permanent sequelae of reduced vision.

This chapter will review what is known about the impact of pregnancy on diseases of the retina. Though there is overlap between groups, for the sake of organizing the discussion of the various conditions, they have been divided into those conditions developing de novo in the context of a normal pregnancy, changes in pre-existing retinal conditions during pregnancy, and changes arising out of pregnancy-related systemic disease or associated with labor and delivery. Considerations in using diagnostic pharmacologic agents for retinal evaluation during pregnancy will also be discussed.

RETINAL CHANGES IN THE CONTEXT OF A NORMAL PREGNANCY, WITHOUT PRE-EXISTING EYE DISEASE

An early study reported that the retinal arterioles, venules, and capillary bed appear normal in normal pregnancies.[9] There are some pathologic retinal conditions that develop during normal pregnancy, perhaps with greater frequency than in the nonpregnant state. These include central serous chorioretinopathy, uveal melanoma, and other less common conditions.

Central Serous Chorioretinopathy

Central serous chorioretinopathy (CSC) is a relatively common macular disorder characterized by a localized serous detachment of the neurosensory retina. This condition usually occurs between the ages of 20 and 45 years, with an 80 to 90% male predominance.[10,11] Pathophysiologically, there is a functional discontinuity in the retinal pigment epithelium (RPE), allowing choroidal fluid to enter the subretinal space. Central serous chorioretinopathy may be asymptomatic when the fovea is not involved or if the episode occurs in the nondominant eye. When the fovea is involved, the patient usually has a mild to moderate decrease in visual acuity, along with symptoms of metamorphopsia, micropsia, color changes, and/or darkness of the central visual field. In most cases, CSC resolves spontaneously within a few months and visual acuity returns to 20/25 or better, although patients may continue to experience the other visual symptoms to some degree. Twenty to 30% of patients have one or more recurrences in the same eye, and one third of patients have focal RPE changes in the fellow eye, suggesting previous involvement of the fellow eye. A small number of patients, estimated at 5%, may develop the severe form of CSC, with prolonged and/or recurrent episodes of sensory retinal detachment, large areas of detachment, and occasional severe visual loss.[10] Laser photocoagulation of the leak may be indicated in specific cases to hasten resolution of the detachment.[10]

Specific attention has been given to patients who develop CSC during pregnancy (Fig. 41–1). Twenty-three cases of CSC in pregancy were reported from 1974 to 1996.[12–19] With the exception of one patient who was 22 years old, all patients were between ages 27 and 36 years, with an overall mean age of 31.1 years. All patients were in good systemic health. Seven patients developed CSC during their first pregnancy, and 11 were multiparas who had not had CSC in prior pregnancies (one patient's history was unknown). Sixty-one per cent of the patients developed CSC in their third trimester of pregnancy, and the remainder were divided between the first (13%) and second trimesters (26%). There is a report of one patient developing CSC 1 month postpartum in two successive pregnancies.[12] All patients for whom final acuity is reported (19 patients) had resolution of CSC, with return of visual acuity to 20/20 or better toward the end of the pregnancy or within several months after delivery. CSC was bilateral in one patient.[19]

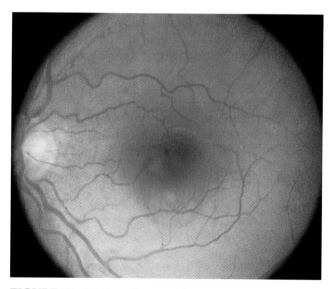

FIGURE 41–1 Central serous chorioretinopathy presenting in the seventh month of pregnancy. There is a circular white subretinal exudate within the inferior aspect of the detachment. There was resolution shortly before delivery. (From Sunness JS, Haller JA, Fine SL: Central serous chorioretinopathy and pregnancy. Arch Ophthalmol 111:360–364, 1993. Copyright 1993, American Medical Association, with permission.)

There has been discussion in the literature as to whether there is a racial risk factor for this disorder.[16–18] Of the 23 patients described in the literature to date, nine were white (Caucasian), three were Hispanic, three were Oriental, two were black (African-American), and one was Native American; the race of five is unknown. The number of cases reported overall is still quite small, and it is difficult to draw any definite conclusion as to a racial association in this disorder.

Subretinal exudates have been seen in a high proportion of both white and nonwhite patients with CSC in pregnancy[16,18,19] (Fig. 41–1). The reason for increased subretinal exudation is not clear, but an awareness of its occurrence may aid in correct diagnosis.

There have been two reports of patients who developed CSC in subsequent pregnancies; one woman developed CSC in four consecutive pregnancies,[13] and the other woman developed CSC in two consecutive pregnancies.[14] More recently, Sunness[18] reported a patient with a subsequent pregnancy not complicated by maternal CSC; a second patient in this study had two subsequent pregnancies uncomplicated by CSC (J. Sunness, unpublished data). Thus, the development of CSC during pregnancy does not imply that it will definitely recur in subsequent pregnancies. There is also a case in which CSC that developed during pregnancy recurred or persisted in a nonpregnant state.[18]

Although there is no evidence that fluorescein angiography during pregnancy adversely affects the fetus (see discussion below), there is in general no indication to perform fluorescein angiography during pregnancy in cases of uncomplicated CSC in view of the spontaneous resolution and good visual acuity outcome of the cases reported in the literature.

The number of cases thus far reported is too small to answer the question of whether CSC in pregnancy is a separate disorder or merely typical CSC that coincidentally occurs during pregnancy. Some characteristics of CSC in pregnancy suggest that pregnancy may influence the manifestations of this disorder. There is a higher rate of subretinal white exudates in CSC during pregnancy.[16,18] In addition, no severe case of CSC has been associated with this subset of patients with CSC, and two of the three patients who experienced recurrences had these develop only in the context of subsequent pregnancy. Some authors have suggested that the very special conditions of pregnancy, including hemodynamic[15] and hormonal[13] alterations, hypercoagulability,[15] and changes in prostaglandins[16] may be implicated in the development of CSC in pregnancy. Quillen and associates[19] hypothesized that cortisol directly or indirectly may play a role in the development of CSC. Cortisol concentrations may increase in late pregnancy, returning to normal after delivery.[20] The possible mechanism by which cortisol may influence this condition is unclear. Typical CSC not associated with pregnancy has been associated with stress and type A personality[21]; it may be that the very special stresses of pregnancy may cause susceptible women to develop CSC in this framework alone.

Uveal Melanoma

There are a number of reports in the literature of uveal melanomas presenting or growing rapidly during pregnancy.[22-29] Shields[30] reported their experience with 16 cases of uveal melanoma that were diagnosed and managed during pregnancy; this represented 0.4% of 3706 consecutive patients with uveal melanoma seen over a 17-year period, and 7.5% of all women with uveal melanomas between the ages of 15 and 44. All patients were white. In this series, seven pre-existing stable choroidal tumors were found to grow during pregnancy. Whether this apparent change in the tumor was merely coincidental with the pregnancy or represented true growth, vascular engorgement, or some other factor associated with the pregnant state is unknown. However, histopathologic findings appear to suggest that tumor enlargement is real and caused by cellular growth. All 16 patients had a moderate amount of subretinal fluid seen ophthalmoscopically; the presence of subretinal fluid associated with uveal melanoma generally suggests that the tumor is actively growing, although fluid retention related to pregnancy may be a factor as well.[30] Pregnancy may theoretically influence melanoma-associated survival by one of several mechanisms. Pregnancy is associated with a diminution of both cell-mediated and humoral immunity, which may allow proliferation of cancerous cells. Pregnancy also is accompanied by a general increase in circulating hormone levels, including estrogens, progesterone, and melanocyte-stimulating hormone.[31]

One study suggested that there is a trend toward a larger than expected number of uveal melanomas recognized during pregnancy.[25] Hartge et al[32] reported a case-control study that compared 238 women with uveal malignant melanoma with 223 matched control women with detached retinas to evaluate the effects of hormones on the risk of uveal melanoma. Women who had a past history of pregnancy or estrogen replacement therapy had an increased risk of uveal melanoma (relative risk, 1.4), whereas those who had oophorectomy had a decreased risk (relative risk, 0.6).

There is no evidence that termination of pregnancy is of any benefit in this disorder. In the series reported by Shields,[30] all of the patients who elected to carry the pregnancy to term (14 of 16) delivered healthy babies with no placental or infant metastases.

Shields[30] suggests that the early survival for pregnant women with posterior uveal melanoma is no worse than their nonpregnant counterparts. In their series, the 5-year survival rate using the life table method in pregnant women with posterior uveal melanoma was 71% and was similar to the survival of nonpregnant women with posterior uveal melanoma reported in other series. Egan and co-workers[33] evaluated survival in relation to pregnancy and oral contraceptive use after diagnosis in a series of female patients with choroidal melanoma who were of reproductive age and still menstruating at the time of diagnosis. In addition, they considered whether there are any male/female differences in survival among younger persons with uveal melanoma. A total of 24 full-term pregnancies were reported among the 139 women still menstruating at diagnosis. Metastases developed in 15 of the 139 women. Compared with other women in the series, rates of metastases were not higher among the women who reported pregnancies or oral contraceptive use after diagnosis. The overall rate of metastasis among women was similar to that of men followed during the same interval. Although this study was based on relatively few exposed women and occurrences of metastases, and limited follow-up after pregnancy, results suggest that the hormonal environment has no appreciable influence on risk of metastases in younger women with uveal melanoma. Estrogen and progesterone receptors have not been found in 27 ocular melanomas that have been studied using immunohistochemistry; this included one melanoma from a pregnant woman.[26,34] The lack of estrogen or progesterone receptors in melanomas thus is consistent with the epidemiologic evidence that has failed to demonstrate a large or consistent effect of either giving exogenous or having increased levels of endogenous estrogens and progesterones.

Other Retinal Conditions Arising During a Normal Pregnancy

An association between pregnancy and *unilateral acute idiopathic maculopathy* has been reported.[35] In this condition, there is a profound loss of central vision with spontaneous improvement and nearly complete visual recovery. It may be confused with idiopathic choroidal neovascularization or central serous chorioretinopathy. There is a case report of a *choroidal osteoma* with associated *choroidal neovascularization* developing toward the end of pregnancy, with resolution of fluid by 6 months postpartum.[10]

RETINAL CHANGES IN THE CONTEXT OF PRE-EXISTING RETINAL DISEASE

The most important disease in this category, both because of its prevalence and because of pregnancy's impact on it, is diabetic retinopathy.

Diabetic Retinopathy

Diabetes 2000, the program for educating internists and primary care physicians about diabetic retinopathy and associated preventable visual loss, has targeted pregnancy as one of the factors requiring more careful follow-up for progression of retinopathy. Until the development of modern medical and obstetric management of the pregnant diabetic patient, along with laser photocoagulation for proliferative diabetic retinopathy, the prognosis both for the mother's vision and for fetal viability were limited. These new methods have had a significant positive impact on the outcome of pregnancy for the fetus as well as for the mother and the preservation of her vision. For this reason, studies in the literature must be interpreted based on the nature of the medical management, with special emphasis on the degree of blood-glucose control before and during pregnancy.

Blood-glucose control (as reflected by glycosylated hemoglobin A1c and blood-glucose) instituted before conception and maintained throughout the pregnancy may reduce the risk of spontaneous abortion,[36] congenital anomalies, and fetal morbidity.[37] A recent study suggest that the severity of diabetic retinopathy may be a significant factor in predicting an adverse fetal outcome, even after correction for blood glucose control,[8] but another study suggests that good glucose control may counteract the adverse fetal effects of proliferative retinopathy or nephropathy.[38] The importance of blood-glucose control overrides concerns regarding transient worsening of retinopathy that has occurred with sudden imposition of tight control.[39,40] The Diabetes Control and Complications Study has shown in nonpregnant insulin-dependent diabetics that there is a marked benefit of intensive treatment in terms of a decreased rate of progression.[40]

A diabetic woman's ophthalmologic status should also be evaluated and stabilized before pregnancy. This is particularly important for patients with proliferative retinopathy, since treatment of proliferative disease with laser photocoagulation before pregnancy leads to less likelihood of progression during pregnancy itself.[1] It may also be important to stabilize diabetic macular edema prior to pregnancy, but there is inadequate information in the literature about this. The frequency of ophthalmologic evaluation for a diabetic patient during pregnancy is determined by her baseline status, ideally assessed prepartum or if necessary in the first trimester.[1,41]

Progression of Retinopathy During Pregnancy

The duration of diabetes and the patient's level of retinopathy at the start of the pregnancy are the major determinants of the progression of retinopathy.[1,42-45] It has been recommended for this rea-

son that diabetic women try to have their families early in their married life.[6] Other factors such as the induction of intensive insulin therapy[45,46] in patients not previously well controlled and the presence of a coexistent hypertensive disorder[45] have also been described.

A meta-analysis of a large number of studies of diabetic retinopathy in pregnancy that were published from 1978 to 1988 was included in Sunness' earlier review of pregnancy and its impact on the mother's eye.[1] A review by Rodman[47] of studies published from 1948 to 1978 documented in general a lower rate of progression of retinopathy, since the early studies used more coarse measures of progression, while the studies from 1978 and since have used photographic documentation to count microaneurysms, assess the amount of neovascularization present, and in general subdivide retinopathy into smaller units. The discussion in this chapter bases itself on Sunness' summary and recent studies; interested readers are referred to the original reviews[1,47] for details and references regarding the individual studies included in the meta-analysis.

The discussion of the progression of retinopathy during pregnancy will be subdivided by the baseline level of retinopathy present. The classification for most studies did not use the recent nonproliferative, severe nonproliferative, etc, terminology recommended by the Early Treatment Diabetic Retinopathy Study[48]; where possible the results have been converted to the new classification.

NO INITIAL RETINOPATHY. Sunness[1] summarized nine studies that included 484 pregnant diabetic women with no initial retinopathy. Twelve per cent of these patients developed some background change during pregnancy and one patient (0.2%) developed proliferative retinopathy. In the 23 cases with progression in which postpartum follow-up was available, there was some regression of the background change in 57%.

One recent study[49] found that 7% of 94 patients with no initial retinopathy developed retinopathy during pregnancy. Another recent study found that 23% of eyes with no retinopathy at baseline progressed to some retinopathy.[45]

Vingolo[50] performed adaptoelectroretinography, that is the b2/b1 ratio (the ratio of the rod-mediated–to–cone-mediated b-wave 7 minutes after a retinal bleach) on patients with no diabetic retinopathy at baseline. Their subject groups included 1A, patients with insulin-dependent diabetes who had had good metabolic control for the 6 months prior to pregnancy; 1B, patients with non–insulin-dependent diabetes and gestational diabetes; and 2, control patients. They found that the b2/b1 ratio for group 1B was markedly abnormal, while that for group 1A was not significantly different from the control group. They also found a tight correlation with glycemic control, progression of retinopathy, and fetal outcome. These findings suggest that the glycemic control is a major factor in retinal and fetal outcome. It is not clear whether gestational diabetics progressed in this study.

A 12-year prospective survey on diabetic retinopathy in pregnancy[51] concluded that patients with gestational diabetes do not appear to be at risk for diabetic retinopathy. However, more recent work has found increased retinal vascular tortuosity in gestational diabetics, that has persisted at 5 months' postpartum.[52] There is also a recent case report[53] of a 24-year-old nulliparous woman with an unremarkable medical history who was first diagnosed as having diabetes at 8 weeks' gestation. Rapid glucose control was achieved by insulin therapy, with a decrease of the initially high hemoglobin A1c level of 16.2% to normal values within 12 weeks. At 31 weeks, severe bilateral proliferative diabetic retinopathy developed. The markedly elevated hemoglobin A1c suggests that the patient may have had diabetes prior to the pregnancy, rather than being a gestational diabetic.

MINIMAL INITIAL RETINOPATHY. In two studies including 24 women with fewer than ten microaneurysms and dot hemorrhages and no exudate in either eye, there was an 8% rate of developing more microaneurysms and a 0% incidence of proliferative disease.[1]

INITIAL NONPROLIFERATIVE RETINOPATHY. Ten studies tabulated by Sunness[1] included 258 pregnant women with background diabetic retinopathy. Forty-seven per cent of patients developed an increase in the amount of background change during the course of the pregnancy. This is a significantly higher rate than was found in earlier studies[47]; the difference is probably attributable to a more detailed quantification of change (increase in microaneurysms, etc), along with changes associated with imposition of tight glucose control. The course of background change often waxes and wanes during the pregnancy, with improvement late in the third trimester and in the postpartum period. Five per cent of the women developed proliferative change during pregnancy.

Two additional studies including 124 patients reported a 12% rate of progression in nonproliferative retinopathy.[49,54] Only 2 of 12 patients had improved by 6 weeks postpartum.[49] One study reported 3 of 39 eyes with nonproliferative retinopathy (in 28 patients) developing proliferative retinopathy during pregnancy.[54] A recent study found a progression rate of 41% in eyes with nonproliferative diabetic retinopathy at baseline, and a regression rate of 25% by 6 to 12 weeks postpartum.[45]

DIABETIC MACULAR EDEMA. Diabetic macular edema is probably the greatest diagnostic dilemma in terms of retinal disease during pregnancy. For nonpregnant patients with clinically significant diabetic macular edema, focal laser photocoagulation is recommended to preserve the patient's visual acuity; in only about 20% of cases is there an improvement in visual acuity following focal photocoagulation.[55] In patients who develop diabetic macular edema during pregnancy, one may see return of visual acuity to normal or near-normal levels following delivery and resolution of the edema. Thus, the same considerations that may be operant for eyes with diabetic macular edema outside the context of pregnancy may not be applicable to pregnant women. More detailed and systematic study of diabetic macular edema in pregnancy is required to give clear, scientifically based recommendations for management.

Macular edema may be prominent during pregnancy,[56] with spontaneous resolution thereafter. In a recent study, 16 (29%) of 56 eyes of pregnant diabetic women with initial nonproliferative or proliferative retinopathy developed cystoid macular edema during pregnancy. Fourteen (88%) of the 16 eyes had return of visual acuity and resolution of the macular edema postpartum without laser treatment.[54] One study showed that eight of nine patients who developed cystoid macular edema had proteinuria of more than 1 g/day.[57]

In general, pregnant women with diabetic macular edema should not be treated during pregnancy, given the high rate of spontaneous recovery postpartum. Possible exceptions might include cases in which lipid is threatening the fovea, and cases in which macular edema begins early in pregnancy and persists with decreasing visual acuity during pregnancy. Anecdotally, even in these latter cases there may be spontaneous resolution of the edema postpartum with visual recovery.

PREPROLIFERATIVE RETINOPATHY. In three studies of 90 pregnant women with initial background retinopathy (and no initial cotton-wool spots), new cotton-wool spots developed in 43% of patients who had not previously had them.[1] Three (8%) of these patients with new cotton-wool spots went on to develop proliferative retinopathy.

The appearance of cotton-wool spots in some patients may be related to the imposition of tight glucose control,[46] and two studies[42,58] suggest that cotton-wool spots and blot hemorrhages may be transient changes that resolve postpartum. One study[59] described the retinopathy status of 13 patients placed on insulin pump treatment during pregnancy. Seven of the patients had at most minimal retinopathy at baseline; on the insulin pump five were unchanged and two developed mild background retinopathy. Of the six patients with background retinopathy at baseline, four remained unchanged and two patients, with rapid decreases in the hemoglobin A1c level, developed acute ischemic changes and ultimately proliferative retinopathy.

INITIAL PROLIFERATIVE RETINOPATHY. Sunness tabulated 12 studies including 122 women with proliferative retinopathy at baseline; 46% of them developed progression in their proliferative disease during pregnancy, when measured using fundus findings (rather than visual acuity change) as a criterion.[1] Optimal treatment of proliferative disease prior to pregnancy may play an important role in the likelihood of progression during pregnancy. In Sunness' study,[1] those patients who had no laser treatment prior to pregnancy had a 58% progression rate, whereas those who had any laser photocoagulation before pregnancy had a 26% progression rate. In this series, those patients with total regression of proliferative disease prior to pregnancy, either spontaneously or related to scatter laser photocoagulation, did not progress during pregnancy.[1]

In a recent study, there was a 63% rate of progression in eyes with proliferative retinopathy at baseline.[45] In another recent study,[60] half the patients identified as having proliferative retinopathy at baseline who underwent laser treatment prior to pregnancy required laser treatment during pregnancy, and 65% of patients who had proliferative disease during pregnancy required photocoagulation postpartum. In this study, the four patients with proliferative disease who did not undergo photocoagulation prior to pregnancy did not require photocoagulation during pregnancy; this is presumably a group with only early proliferative disease not indicating a need for photocoagulation. No patient had proliferative disease that was unresponsive to laser photocoagulation.[60]

Proliferative disease may regress, in part or completely, near the end of pregnancy or in the postpartum period. One study found that four of five women who developed proliferative retinopathy during pregnancy had spontaneous regression to nonproliferative retinopathy within 2 months postpartum.[61] However, another study of 8 women with proliferative disease reported no spontaneous regression of proliferative change by 12 weeks postpartum.[45]

Scatter laser photocoagulation is effective during pregnancy in inducing regression of proliferative retinopathy[62]; nor do prior pregnancies appear to modify the effectiveness of scatter photocoagulation.[63] Thirty of 35 patients (86%) who were treated with scatter photocoagulation and for whom posttreatment results were available had some regression of their proliferative disease.[1] Since proliferative disease may also regress spontaneously late in pregnancy or postpartum, there are a number of different opinions regarding treatment of proliferative disease during pregnancy. Almost all retinal specialists would aggressively treat patients with high-risk proliferative retinopathy as defined by the Diabetic Retinopathy Study.[64] In patients with proliferative diabetic retinopathy that does not meet the high-risk criteria, some would treat one or both eyes, given the fact that some patients have progressed rapidly during pregnancy.[44] One study suggests waiting 8 to 12 months postpartum before treating.[61]

Five women with proliferative diabetic retinopathy have been reported to develop vitreous hemorrhage during labor and delivery.[65] However, in this era of availability of vitrectomy for nonclearing vitreous hemorrhage, there is not enough evidence to justify a cesarean section on the basis of proliferative retinopathy alone.[1]

PROGRESSION IN PREGNANT WOMEN COMPARED WITH NONPREGNANT WOMEN. In determining whether pregnancy is associated with progression of diabetic retinopathy, one must separately consider short-term changes from long-term changes in that there is a high rate of regression postpartum.

To evaluate the relative rate of short-term progression, a nonpregnant control group against which to compare rates of progression is necessary. This has been achieved in several ways. One study of 16 women with no or background retinopathy compared progression during pregnancy with progression between 6 and 15 months in the same women postpartum.[66] Little change in the number of microaneurysms was seen until the 28th week of pregnancy. Between the 28th and 35th weeks, there was a rapid increase in the number of microaneurysms. Six months postpartum the number of microaneurysms had decreased from the maximum but was in most cases still higher than the baseline level. The number remained stable over the 9-month subsequent nonpregnant interval.

Three other studies used separated control groups of nonpregnant women to compare with the progression in women during pregnancy. One study[67] compared the course of diabetic retinopathy in 93 pregnant women and 98 diabetic nonpregnant women. Worsening of initial retinal lesions was observed in 16% of the pregnant group, statistically higher than the 6% rate of nonpregnant women showing similar worsening. More of the nonpregnant group (32%) had retinopathy at baseline than did the pregnant group (22%), making these findings more significant. A second study compared 39 nonpregnant women, 46% of whom had retinopathy at baseline, with 53 pregnant diabetic women, 57% of whom had retinopathy at baseline.[42] In the nonpregnant group, over a 15-month follow-up period, microaneurysms remained stable, streak or blob hemorrhages appeared in three patients (8%), and no cotton-wool spots developed. In the pregnant group, one patient with background retinopathy developed proliferative retinopathy, and in general microaneurysms increased moderately, and streak and blob hemorrhages and cotton-wool spots increased markedly. In the third study,[68] there were 133 pregnant and 241 nonpregnant women. Initially, no difference existed between the two groups in terms of severity of retinopathy. Within each quartile of glycosylated hemoglobin, pregnant women had a greater tendency to have worsening of retinopathy and the nonpregnant women had a greater tendency to have improvement in their level of diabetic retinopathy during the follow-up interval. One author[69] proposed that the worsening retinopathy seen during pregnancy is partly due to increased retinal blood flow without autoregulation of blood vessel diameter. The diabetic retinal microcirculation is unable to cope with the added stress, and there are deleterious consequences for the diabetic damage that may already exist. Those patients who progressed in their retinopathy were those who had increased retinal blood flow during pregnancy.[69]

Thus, diabetic retinopathy does progress more rapidly during pregnancy than it does in the nonpregnant state. However, considering the high rate of regression of retinopathy in the postpartum period, the long-term effects of pregnancy on diabetic retinopathy must be separately determined. There are only limited data available on this. When duration of diabetes is taken into account, the number of prior pregnancies does not appear to be a factor in the severity of retinopathy present.[70,71]

In one study of 40 women followed for a full year postpartum,[61] 19 had no retinopathy at baseline. Somewhat less than one third of these women developed mild background retinopathy during the second and third trimesters. None had retinopathy 1 year postpartum. Of the remaining 21 women with retinopathy at baseline, 11 worsened during pregnancy, with 2 developing neovascularization of the disc. None of these women regressed to her initial eye status at 1 year postpartum, but one of the patients with new proliferative retinopathy had spontaneous full regression of her proliferative retinopathy.

Maternal Retinopathy and Fetal Well-Being

The outcome of a diabetic pregnancy is much improved relative to the past due to improved medical and obstetric management. Also, since diabetes is a risk factor for pre-eclampsia, better management of this condition has also improved the outcome in diabetic pregnancies. The presence of diabetic retinopathy, which may reflect the systemic status, has been looked at as a risk factor for adverse fetal outcome. Background retinopathy in the mother may not place the pregnancy at higher risk.[47] However, a recent study found an adverse fetal outcome in 43% of 28 women with proliferative retinopathy as compared with 13% of 131 women with at most nonproliferative retinopathy.[8] In one study of 22 pregnancies complicated by retinopathy and/or nephropathy in which good glycemic control was present prepartum and throughout pregnancy, there were no infant deaths and only one infant with perinatal disease (mild respiratory distress in a 33-week infant delivered due to severe pre-eclampsia).[38] A recent study[60] looked at the retinal and pregnancy outcomes of 20 pregnancies (in 17 women) complicated by proliferative di-

abetic retinopathy. Among these 20 pregnancies, spontaneous abortion occurred in 2 (10%) and stillbirth in 1 (5%); the remaining 17 (85%) pregnancies culminated in live births at a mean gestational age of 36 weeks, with a mean birth weight of 2620 g. Three infants had major congenital anomalies, two with tetralogy of Fallot and ventricular septal defect, and one with meconium peritonitis, later requiring temporary ileostomy. The authors concluded that retinal status should not preclude pregnancy, since contemporary methods of management can result in satisfactory retinal and pregnancy outcomes even in the presence of advanced diabetic microvascular disease.[60]

Other Changes Seen in Association with Diabetes

Optic disc edema has been reported in pregnant women[72] and appears no different from its appearance in a nonpregnant patient. Diabetes is a risk factor for pregnancy-induced hypertension (pre-eclampsia/eclampsia), and its attendant complications (see "Pregnancy-Induced Hypertension," below).

Oral contraceptives do not appear to be a risk factor for the development of early diabetic retinopathy or nephropathy.[73]

Toxoplasmosis

Active ocular toxoplasmosis in pregnant women was reported to have been treated by 22 of 57 members of the American Uveitis Society who were surveyed.[74] Patients are treated with the goal of preserving vision, with 82% of respondents using the same indications for beginning treatment in a pregnant woman as for a nonpregnant woman. Three quarters of the respondents change their therapy during pregnancy; few use pyrimethamine during pregnancy due to possible teratogenic effects. Most respondents used sulfadiazine either alone or in combination with corticosteroids, or clindamycin.[74]

One concern of pregnant patients with toxoplasmosis retinochoroiditis is whether toxoplasmosis can be transmitted to the fetus. In general, the answer to this is no. Congenital toxoplasmosis in the fetus generally results only from active infection of the mother that develops during that pregnancy. The presence of focal toxoplasmic retinochoroiditis or scars in the mother is evidence that *she* was infected congenitally. Therefore, the fetus should not be at risk for contracting congenital toxoplasmosis and forms its related birth defects. Eighteen pregnant women with active toxoplasmic retinochoroiditis or scars, some of whom had high stable toxoplasmosis titers, did not transmit toxoplasmosis to their fetuses.[75] (No patient in this group had increasing titers during pregnancy however.)

There are, however, endemic areas in which people often eat uncooked meat and have repeated re-infections with toxoplasmosis, where evidence of prior infection with toxoplasmosis will not guarantee lack of exposure of the fetus.[76]

Other Pre-existing Retinal Diseases

There is limited information relating to the impact of pregnancy on other pre-existing retinal diseases. One study of 50 *high myopes* before and after delivery found that none developed a retinal detachment associated with labor and delivery.[77] A report of 16 pregnancies in 13 women with prior *retinal detachment surgery* found no retinal complications.[78] The authors felt there was no evidence that a spontaneous vaginal delivery is a contraindication for patients with previous retinal detachment surgery,[78] although a survey of British obstetricians in 1990 found that three quarters of the respondents felt retinal detachment to be an indication for obstetric intervention (cesarean section, forceps) during labor. Pregnant women with *pseudoxanthoma elasticum* have not been found to experience worsening of their retinal status, though cardiac and gastrointestinal complications have been associated with pregnancy.[79,80] *Choroidal hemangiomas* have been reported to undergo rapid growth during pregnancy,[81] and may regress postpartum.[82]

Conditions with an immunologic component may undergo temporary remission during pregnancy due to the relative immunosuppressive effect of pregnancy and the high corticosteroid levels present in the mother. There may be a flare-up in the postpartum period. This pattern has been seen in *sarcoidosis*,[83,84] although one study reported three patients with sarcoid uveitis who showed no change during pregnancy.[83] The same pattern has been seen in *Vogt-Koyanagi-Harada* (VKH) syndrome,[85,86] although one study reported two previously undiagnosed cases of VKH first presenting in the second half of a normal pregnancy and remitting postpartum.[87] A study of 27 *uveitis* patients with a variety of conditions treated during pregnancy reported that in 92%, visual acuity was maintained or improved. Postpartum exacerbations within 8 weeks of delivery were common.[88]

Retinitis pigmentosa (RP) does not always progress uniformly; periods of more rapid worsening and periods of relatively little change may occur. It therefore becomes difficult to interpret whether changes reported during pregnancy are merely coincidental, or whether they are related to pregnancy. Five to 10% of women with RP reported worsening during pregnancy,[1,89] without improvement postpartum[1]; there is one other report in the literature of visual field worsening during pregnancy that regressed postpartum.[90] One case of worsening of *pericentral retinal degeneration* during pregnancy has also been reported.[91]

RETINAL CHANGES ASSOCIATED WITH PREGNANCY-RELATED DISEASE AND WITH LABOR AND DELIVERY

Pregnancy-Induced Hypertension (Pre-eclampsia/Eclampsia, Toxemia)*

Pregnancy-induced hypertension includes pre-eclampsia and eclampsia, conditions formerly called toxemia. Pre-eclampsia develops in the second half of pregnancy, and is defined by the presence of hypertension, edema, and proteinuria. Eclampsia is pre-eclampsia plus convulsions. In otherwise healthy women, pre-eclampsia is seen in about 5% of first pregnancies. Risk factors for pre-eclampsia include multifetal pregnancy, very young and very old maternal age, hemolytic disease of the newborn, and such systemic conditions as diabetes mellitus, chronic hypertension, and renal disease.[31] Visual disturbances, including scotoma, diplopia, dimness, and photopsia, were reported in 1952 to be present in 25% of patients with severe pre-eclampsia and in as many as 50% of patients with eclampsia.[3] Visual changes may be a sign of impending seizure.[92] Stimulation with bright lights may predispose susceptible patients to seizures, but the benefit of an ophthalmoscopic exam outweighs this risk when such an examination is indicated.[93]

Three major visual manifestations have been described, in addition to less common associations (Table 41–1).

Retinopathy

A retinopathy similar to hypertensive retinopathy is the most common change seen. This is characterized by focal arteriolar narrowing and later by generalized narrowing of the retinal arterioles.[94] In early studies, the focal findings were seen in 40 to 100% of patients with pre-eclampsia,[5,95,96] but more recent studies found these changes in about 5% of pre-eclamptic patients[97] and in 30% of pregnant women with pre-existing chronic hypertension.[97,98] The lower frequency of these changes is presumably accounted for by improved medical management of the hypertension in pre-eclampsia. The changes are more common in severe pre-eclamptics than in mild pre-eclamptics, and the changes cannot distinguish mild pre-eclampsia from a normal pregnancy.[99] The vessel caliber changes are reversible in most patients.[5,94] In the past, changes in retinal vessels were used as a risk factor for placental

---

*The interested reader is referred to a more comprehensive discussion by Sunness.[1]

TABLE 41–1 Ocular Findings in Pre-eclampsia/
Eclampsia

Retinopathy
  Focal arteriolar narrowing
  Generalized arteriolar narrowing
  Cotton-wool spots, hemorrhages, edema, papil-
    ledema (mainly in patients with pre-existing
    systemic disease)
  Retinal arteriolar occlusions
**Serous Retinal Detachment (Thought to be on
  Choroidal Basis)**
  Bilateral bullous or cyst-like detachments
Late Findings Following Serous Detachment
  Elschnig's spots
  Pigmentary changes mimicking retinitis pigmen-
    tosa or macular dystrophy
  Optic atropy (rare)
Cortical Blindness (Transient)
Other Findings
  Conjunctival ischemia
  Pupillary alterations
  Ptosis
  Papillophlebitis
  Peripheral neovascularization
  Vitreous hemorrhage

insufficiency and fetal mortality, and an indication for delivery.[3–5,100]

Other changes associated with hypertensive retinopathy including hemorrhages, cotton-wool spots, retinal edema, and papilledema are seen primarily in patients with an underlying chronic systemic disease. An old and a recent study of patients with pre-eclampsia and eclampsia found that the group with retinal hemorrhages and cotton-wool spots had a higher rate of fetal mortality.[101,102]

Serous Retinal Detachment

Serous detachments of the retina are seen in about 1% of severe pre-eclamptics and 10% of eclamptics.[94,103] These exudative detachments are usually bilateral and bullous, although localized cyst-like detachments have been reported.[104,105] Though there was early controversy about the cause of the detachments, current thought is that these are related to changes in the choroidal vasculature. Fluorescein angiography has shown leakage deep to the retina (Fig. 41–2), and limited histopathology and the presence of Elschnig's spots on resolution point to choroidal vascular changes.[93,104,106–110] Yellow opaque foci at the level of the retinal pigment epithelium have been reported; these may progress to chorioretinal atrophy or may resolve.[111] Retinal detachments can occur independent of the retinopathy described above.[110] Retinal detachment does not appear to be a risk factor for adverse fetal outcome,[5] unlike severe retinopathy. The detachment typically

occurs late in pregnancy, and may develop in the early postpartum period. In one study, those patients developing serous retinal detachment had significant decreases of platelet count and fibrinogen, suggesting a mild form of disseminated intravascular coagulopathy.[102] There are rare reports of exudative detachments in pregnant women without pre-eclampsia.[112,113]

The detachments can cause a marked loss of vision, but most patients recover spontaneously to normal vision within a few weeks. In some patients, however, there is residual pigmentary change of the retinal pigment epithelium[114–116] that can mimic a macular dystrophy or retinitis pigmentosa (Fig. 41–3).[116] Rarely, a patient develops optic atrophy.[103]

Cortical Blindness

Cortical blindness may appear late in pregnancy or in the early postpartum period.[117–122] It is thought to be related to cerebral edema of the occipital lobes.[118] It is transient, with recovery of vision.

Other Changes Associated with Pre-eclampsia/Eclampsia

Conjunctival ischemia,[9] pupillary changes,[123] ptosis,[123] ischemic papillophlebitis,[124] and peripheral neovascularization[125] have been reported in association with pre-eclampsia/eclampsia. White-centered retinal hemorrhages were seen in one patient as an early sign of pre-eclampsia, thought perhaps to be the result of spasm leading to a cotton-wool spot surrounded by a hemorrhage.[126]

In addition, patients with pre-eclampsia are at risk of developing vascular occlusions. These are discussed below.

The HELLP syndrome[127] is associated with severe pre-eclampsia or eclampsia, and consists of *he*molysis, *e*levated *l*iver enzymes, and *l*ow *p*latelets, along with upper abdominal pain. Serous retinal detachments, with yellow-white subretinal opacities,[128] vitreous hemorrhage,[129] and reversible cortical blindness have been reported in association with this condition, but they may be associated with the severe pre-eclampsia/eclampsia, rather than a special change related to the HELLP syndrome.[130]

Occlusive Vascular Disease

Pregnancy is a hypercoagulable state, in that clotting factors and clotting activity are increased.[31] Thrombosis and embolization may also occur. In one review, ischemic cerebrovascular disease was found to be 13 times more common in pregnant women than in nonpregnant patients.[131] These disorders affect the retina and choroid as well, although many patients who develop occlusive vas-

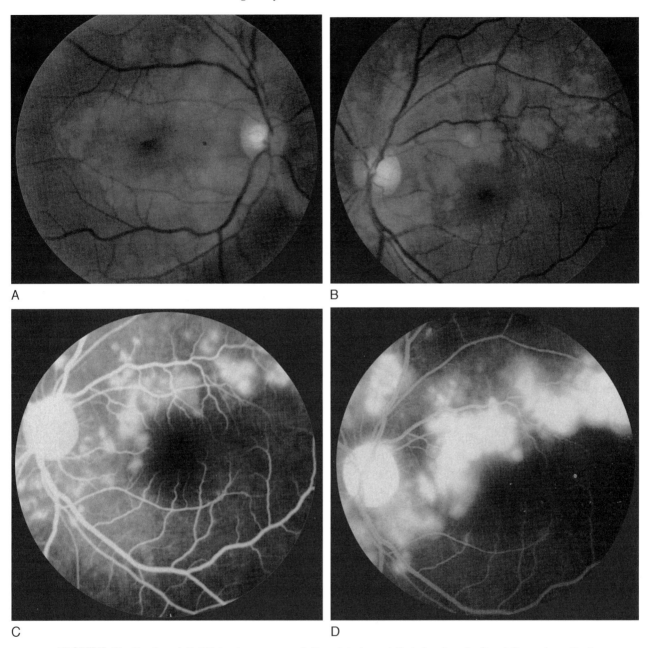

A   B   C   D

FIGURE 41–2   *A* and *B,* Bilateral serous exudative detachment that developed after delivery in patient with pre-eclampsia/eclampsia. Yellow-white deposits are present at the level of the retinal pigment epithelium. *C* and *D,* Fluorescein angiography after delivery shows multiple leaks at the level of the retinal pigment epithelium. (Courtesy of Dr. Guy Barile and Mr. Jose Martinez.)

cular disease during pregnancy appear to have an underlying systemic cause, such as a change in clotting factor level, the presence of pre-eclampsia, or an obstetric complication.

Retinal Artery Occlusion

Retinal artery occlusion has been reported during pregnancy, and also during or after labor and delivery.

Of the patients reported with retinal artery occlusion during pregnancy, one had a history of migraine,[132] one had a history of migraine and an in-creased plasma factor VIII level,[132] one had a history of migraine and hypertension,[133] one had a decreased level of protein S and diabetes,[133] two had anticardiolipin antibody,[133,134] and two patients with papillophlebitis and a branch retinal artery occlusion had no identifiable risk factos.[133,135] Four women on oral contraceptives developed a retinal artery occlusion, and two of these had a history of migraine.[133]

Retinal artery occlusions during or after labor and delivery have been reported. The presentation has been described as a Purtscher's-like retinopathy, with nerve fiber layer infarctions and multiple

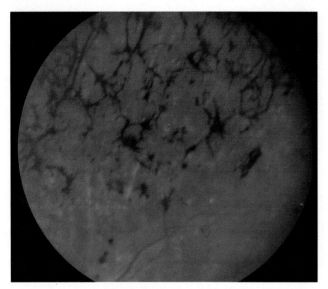

FIGURE 41–3 Late pigmentary alterations following bilateral serous detachments from pre-eclampsia/eclampsia. The appearance mimics retinitis pigmentosa. (From Gass JDM, Pautler SE: Toxemia of pregnancy pigment epitheliopathy masquerading as a heredomacular dystrophy. Trans Am Ophthalmol 83:114, 1985, with permission.)

acuity improved to near-normal levels, though patients may still have a scotoma in their field. However, at times the occusion can cause irreversible visual loss and severe vision loss. One patient in Blodi's study had a loss of perfusion to both maculas, and was left with permanent legal blindness in both eyes (Fig. 41–4).[136]

Retinal Vein Occlusion

One patient with a central retinal vein occlusion during pregnancy was found to have wide diurnal swings of intraocular pressure.[139] Cases of retinal papillophlebitis, suggestive of early central retinal vein occlusions, have been reported[135,140]; one of these also had a branch retinal artery occlusion.[135] In the early literature, there are reports of central retinal vein and artery occlusions during or immediately after delivery, but some of these were related to general anesthesia.[141]

One patient with a bilateral branch retinal vein occlusion during pregnancy had no known risk factors. The occlusions resolved. The patient had a subsequent uneventful pregnancy (J. Wroblewski, personal communication, 1996).

Disseminated Intravascular Coagulopathy

Disseminated intravascular coagulopathy (DIC) may develop in association with obstetric complications such as severe pre-eclampsia, abruptio placentae, intrauterine fetal death, and complicated abortion.[142–144] The major impact of DIC is on the choroid, where there is thrombotic occlusion of the choroidal vessels and choriocapillaris. This may cause serous retinal detachments, which resolve with restoration of vision and residual pigmentary change. DIC may be the underlying cause

retinal arteriolar occlusion.[10,136] Three patients reported with this condition were pre-eclamptic (and one of these also had cerebral infarcts),[136] one had protein C deficiency (with occlusion 2 months postpartum),[137] and one had protein S deficiency.[136] Three patients were reported to develop this without a predisposing condition during pregnancy,[136,138] though one of these patients was 16 years old, had labor induced, and suffered a generalized seizure 2 hours postpartum.[136]

The initial decrease of vision is dependent upon the site(s) of occlusion. In many patients, visual

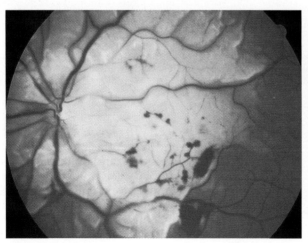

A

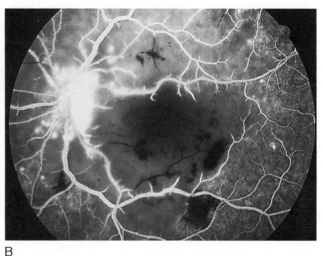

B

FIGURE 41–4 Bilateral retinal arteriolar occlusion shortly after delivery leading to infarction of the macula in both eyes. A, Fundus appearance. B, Fluorescein angiographic appearance. (From Blodi BA, Johnson MW, Gass JDM, et al: Purtscher's-like retinopathy after childbirth. Ophthalmology 97:1654–1659, 1990, with permission.)

of serous detachments in cases of pre-eclampsia/eclampsia.[102]

Thrombotic Thrombocytopenic Purpura

Thrombotic thrombocytopenic purpura (TTP) may develop in association with pregnancy. Visual symptoms occur in about 10% of patients, generally related to serous retinal detachment, arteriolar constriction, and disc edema. Other ocular findings may be seen, such as subconjunctival hemorrhage, anisocoria, motility disturbances, ischemic optic neuropathy, homonymous hemianopia, and scintillating scotoma.[145]

Amniotic Fluid Embolism

This is a catastrophic event that presents in a strong labor, and is associated with DIC and with a high mortality.[146] One patient developed bilateral retinal arteriolar occlusions, thought to be related to particles from the amniotic fluid.[147] One patient had extensive blood loss, and developed ischemia of both the retina and the choiroid, leading to a blind eye.[148]

Other Vascular Changes

Intracranial venous thrombosis[141,149,150] and ischemic optic neuropathy[95,151,152] have been reported in association with pregnancy.

Other Changes Associated with Pregnancy-Related Disease

Retinal hemorrhages may be seen in association with severe vomiting during pregnancy (hyperemesis gravidarum).[9]

Other Changes Related to Labor and Delivery

Endogenous candidal endophthalmitis has been reported postpartum[153,154] and also following spontaneous abortion[155]; this has been thought to be related to intravascular dissemination around the time of delivery. *Valsalva maculopathy, acute macular neuroretinopathy*, and *cystoid macular edema associated with vitritis* have been reported in the immediate postpartum period.[10]

THE USE OF DIAGNOSTIC PHARMACOLOGIC AGENTS DURING PREGNANCY

Fluorescein Angiography

Sodium fluorescein crosses the placenta and enters the fetus; this has been observed in humans[156] as well as in animals.[157] However, no teratogenic or embryocidal effects have been seen in rats, mice, or rabbits, and no reports of teratogenic effects in humans have been reported to the National Registry of Drug-Induced Ocular Side Effects (M. Meyer, personal communication). There are widely differing views on the use of fluorescein angiography during pregnancy in the United States as compared to Europe. European investigators have performed research studies administering fluorescein (without specific clinical indication) to 22 pregnant diabetic women to quantify the change in the number of microaneurysms during pregnancy[66]; no adverse effects on the fetus were seen. A survey of retinal specialists, primarily from the United States, found that nearly 80% had never knowingly performed a fluorescein angiogram on a pregnant woman.[158] Some retinal specialists have treated well-defined extrafoveal choroidal neovascular membranes during pregnancy without obtaining a fluorescein angiogram.[28] In a study of neonatal outcomes in 105 pregnant women who underwent fluorescein angiography during pregnancy,[158] it was felt that there was not an increased rate of adverse fetal outcome over what might be expected in the absence of fluorescein angiography. In this group, there were four fetal or neonatal deaths, two of which were related to the presence of eclampsia. One infant had syndactyly and one had an undescended testicle. Eight infants of mothers with hypertension had low birth weights. However, a criticism of this study has been raised in that only 41 patients underwent fluorescein angiography in the first trimester, which is the time of organogenesis, and the time at which congenital malformations would be more likely.[159]

Thus, there is no evidence in the literature to date that fluorescein adversely affects the fetus, though it clearly crosses the placenta. The conditions for which one might perform a fluorescein angiogram, such as diabetes and pre-eclampsia, are associated with an increased rate of adverse fetal outcome and a fluorescein angiogram might be only an incidental occurrence in a patient at otherwise increased risk. For vision-threatening conditions, such as choroidal neovascularization that one would consider treating, the benefit of a fluorescein angiogram would seem clearly to be greater than the undemonstrated risk of fluorescein administration. For conditions such as diabetic macular edema, it would seem that the physician should define whether the results of a fluorescein angiogram would change the management of the condition in terms of whether to perform laser treatment or how to treat, and make the decision about performing the angiogram accordingly.

The situation in nursing mothers is somewhat different. After the neonate is born, it must rely on its own decreased neonatal clearance capacity for fluorescein ingested in breast milk. Fluorescein has been detected in breast milk for at least 76 hours following maternal fluorescein angiography,[160,161] and it has even been detected in breast milk following a single topical application.[160] Fluorescein (in large doses) has been reported to induce a phototoxic reaction in a premature infant undergoing phototherapy for hyperbilirubinemia.[162] Therefore, fluorescein angiography should be performed in a nursing mother only when a clear benefit to her care is anticipated, and consideration should be given to having the mother temporarily discontinue breastfeeding for the first hours to a few days following angiography.

Topical Anesthetics and Dilating Drops

No cases of teratogenic effects related to the use of topical anesthetics or dilating drops have been reported. However, a recent review of ophthalmic medications during pregnancy categorized dilating drops as being relatively contraindicated,[163] because minor fetal malformations have been reported in association with systemic administration of phenylephrine, atropine, and homatropine early in pregnancy. Fetal hypoxia has been reported late in pregnancy or during labor in women receiving parenteral phenylephrine. The conditions for which these drugs were used systemically may have been etiologic factors in the adverse events, rather than the drugs themselves.

These medications then should be used when there is clear indication; when indicated, precautions should be taken to minimize systemic absorption (such as pressure on the puncta).

SUMMARY

Pregnancy may have an impact on the course of a pre-existing retinal disease, or may be associated with the development of a retinal disorder. Pregnancy is associated with a variety of systemic changes that can have an impact on the mother's retinal and choroidal status. Though most disorders reverse at least in part by several months postpartum, some may have a permanent effect on vision. It is helpful to understand the effect of pregnancy in order to treat the patient appropriately. Much remains to be learned regarding the effect of pregnancy; for example, it is difficult to give recommendations currently regarding the use of laser photocoagulation for severe diabetic macular edema during pregnancy, and the long-term impact of pregnancy on diabetes is not known. As more is understood about the causes of specific changes during pregnancy, it is likely that insights into the disease processes themselves will follow.

Acknowledgment: This work is supported in part by the Gillingham Pan-American Fellowship and the Retina Research Foundation (Arturo Santos, M.D.).

REFERENCES

1. Sunness JS: The Pregnant Woman's Eye. Surv Ophthalmol 32:219–238, 1988.
2. Sunness JS: Pregnancy and the eye. Ophthalmol Clin North Am 5:623–640, 1992.
3. Dieckmann WJ: The Toxemias of Pregnancy, 2nd edition. St Louis, CV Mosby Co, 1952.
4. Sadowsky A, Serr DM, Landau J: Retinal changes and fetal prognosis in the toxemias of pregnancy. Obstet Gynecol 8:426–431, 1956.
5. Wagener HP: Arterioles of the retina in toxemia in pregnancy. JAMA 101:1380–1384, 1933.
6. Beetham WP: Diabetic retinopathy in pregnancy. Trans Am Ophthalmol Soc 48:205–219, 1950.
7. White P, Gillespie L, Sexton L: Use of female sex hormones therapy in pregnant diabetic patients. Am J Obstet Gynecol 71:57–69, 1956.
8. Klein BEK, Klein RK, Meuer SM, et al: Does the severity of diabetic retinopathy predict pregnancy outcome? Diabet Complicat 2:179–184, 1988.
9. Landesman R: Retinal and conjunctival vascular changes in normal and toxemic pregnancy. Bull NY Acad Med 31:376–390, 1955.
10. Gass JDM: Stereoscopic Atlas of Macular Diseases: Diagnosis and Treatment, St Louis, Mosby-Year Book, 1987, pp 46–59, 178–179, 346–347, 380–383, 512–513, 564–565.
11. Gilbert CM, Owens SL, Smith PD, Fine SL: Long-term follow-up of central serous chorioretinopathy. Br J Ophthalmol 68:815–820, 1984.
12. Bedrossian RH: Central serous retinopathy and pregnancy. Am J Ophthalmol 78:152, 1974.
13. Chumbley LC, Frank RN: Central serous retinopathy and pregnancy. Am J Ophthalmol 77:158–160, 1974.
14. Cruysberg JR, Deutman AF: Visual disturbances during pregnancy caused by central serous choroidopathy. Br J Ophthalmol 66:240–241, 1982.
15. Fastenberg DM, Ober RR: Central serous choroidopathy in pregnancy. Arch Ophthalmol 101:1055–1058, 1983.
16. Gass JDM: Central serous chorioretinopathy and white subretinal exudation during pregnancy. Arch Ophthalmol 109:677–681, 1991.
17. Ko W: Central serous chorioretinopathy associated with pregnancy. J Ophthalmic Nurs Technol 11:203–205, 1992.
18. Sunness JS, Haller JA, Fine SL: Central serous chorioretinopathy and pregnancy. Arch Ophthalmol 111:360–364, 1993.
19. Quillen DA, Gass JDM, Brod RD, et al: Central serous retinochoroidopathy in women. Ophthalmology 103:72–79, 1996.
20. Allolio B, Hoffman J, Linton EA, et al: Diurnal salivary cortisol patterns during pregnancy and after delivery: relationship to plasma corticotrophin-releasing-hormone. Clin Endocrinol 33:279–289, 1990.
21. Yannuzzi LA: Type A behavior and central serous chorioretinopathy. Trans Am Ophthalmol Soc 84:799–845, 1986.
22. Borner R, Goder G: Melanoblastom der Uvea and Schwangerschaft. Klin Monatsbl Augenheilkd 149:684–693, 1966.
23. Frenkel M, Klein HZ: Malignant melanoma of the choroid in pregnancy. Am J Ophthalmol 62:910–913, 1966.
24. Pack GT, Scharnagel IM: The prognosis for malignant melanoma in the pregnant woman. Cancer 4:324–334, 1951.
25. Reese AB: Tumors of the Eye. Hagerstown, MD, Harper & Row, 1976, pp 235–236.
26. Seddon JM, MacLaughlin DT, Albert DM, et al: Uveal melanomas presenting during pregnancy and the investigation of oestrogen receptors in melanomas. Br J Ophthalmol 66:695–704, 1982.
27. Siegel R, Amslie WH: Malignant ocular melanoma during pregnancy. JAMA 185:542–543, 1963.

28. Sunness JS, Gass JDM, Singerman LJ, et al: Retinal and choroidal changes in pregnancy. In Singerman LJ, Jampol LM (eds): Retinal and Choroidal Manifestations of Systemic Disease. Baltimore, Williams & Wilkins, 1991, pp 251–286.

29. Jay M, McCartney ACE: Familial malignant melanoma of the uvea and p53: a Victorian detective story. Surv Ophthalmol 37:457–462, 1993.

30. Shields CL, Shields JA, Eagle RCJ, et al: Uveal melanoma and pregnancy. Ophthalmology 98:1667–1673, 1991.

31. Pritchard JA, MacDonald PC, Grant NF: Williams Obstetrics. Norwalk, CT, Appleton-Century-Crofts, 1985, pp 188–191, 191–194, 609.

32. Hartge P, Tucker MA, Shields JA, et al: Case-control study of female hormones and eye melanoma. Cancer Res 49: 4622–4625, 1989.

33. Egan KM, Walsh SM, Seddon JM, Gragoudas ES: An evaluation of the influence of reproductive factors on the risk of metastases from uveal melanoma. Ophthalmology 100: 1160–1166, 1993.

34. Foss AJE, Alexander RA, Guille MJ, et al: Estrogen and progesterone receptor analysis in ocular melanomas. Ophthalmology 102:431–436, 1995.

35. Yannuzzi LA, Freund KB: The expanding clinical spectrum of unilateral acute idiopathic maculopathy. The Macula Society Scientific Program, 1995, p 154.

36. Mills J, Simpson JL, Driscoll SG, and the National Institute of Child Health and Human Development-Diabetes in Early Pregnancy Study: Incidence of spontaneous abortion among normal women and insulin-dependent diabetic women whose pregnancies were identified within 21 days of conception. N Engl J Med 319:1617–1623, 1988.

37. Miller E, Clogerty JP, et al: Elevated maternal hemoglobin A1C in early pregnancy and major congenital anomalies in infants of diabetic mothers. N Engl J Med 304:1331–1334, 1981.

38. Jovanovic R, Jovanovic L: Obstetric management when normoglycemia is maintained in diabetic pregnant women with vascular compromise. Am J Obstet Gynecol 149:617–623, 1984.

39. Kroc Collaborative Study Group: Blood glucose control and the evolution of diabetic retinopathy and albuminuria. N Engl J Med 311:365–372, 1984.

40. Diabetes Contol and Complications Trial Research Group: The effect of intensive diabetes treatment on the progression of diabetic retinopathy in insulin-dependent diabetes mellitus. Arch Ophthalmol 113:36–51, 1995.

41. Kentucky Diabetic Retinopathy Group: Guidelines for eye care in patients with diabetes mellitus. Arch Intern Med 149:769–770, 1989.

42. Moloney JBM, Drury MI: The effect of pregnancy on the natural course of diabetic retinopathy. Am J Ophthalmol 93:745–756, 1982.

43. Aiello LM, Rand LI, Briones JC, et al: Nonocular clinical risk factors in the progression of diabetic retinopathy. In Little HL, et al (eds): Diabetic Retinopathy. New York, Thieme-Stratton, 1983, pp 21–32.

44. Dibble CM, Kochenour NK, Worley RJ, et al: Effect of pregnancy on diabetic retinopathy. Obstet Gynecol 59: 699–704, 1982.

45. Rosenn B, Miodovnik M, Kranias G, et al: Progression of diabetic retinopathy in pregnancy: association with hypertension. Am J Obstet Gynecol 166:1214–1218, 1992.

46. Phelps RL, Sakol P, Metzger BE, et al: Changes in diabetic retinopathy during pregnancy. Arch Ophthalmol 104: 1806–1810, 1986.

47. Rodman HM, Singerman LJ, Aiello LM, Merkatz IR: Diabetic retinopathy and its relationship to pregnancy. In Merkatz IR, Adam PAJ (eds): The Diabetic Pregnancy: A Perinatal Perspective. New York, Grune & Stratton, 1979, pp 73–91.

48. Early Treatment Diabetic Retinopathy Study Research Group: Fundus photographic risk factors for progression of diabetic retinopathy. Ophthalmology 98:823–833, 1991.

49. Berk MA, Miodovnik M, Mimouni F: Impact of pregnancy on complications of insulin-dependent diabetes mellitus. Am J Perinatol 5:359–367, 1988.

50. Vingolo E, Rispoli E, Zicari D, et al: Electrophysiologic monitoring of diabetic retinopathy in pregnancy. Retina 13:99–106, 1993.

51. Horvat M, MacLean H, Goldberg L, Crock GW: Diabetic retinopathy in pregnancy: a 12-year prospective study. Br J Ophthalmol 64:398–403, 1980.

52. Boone MI, Farber ME, Jovanovic-Peterson L, Peterson CM: Increased retinal vascular tortuosity in gestational diabetes mellitus. Ophthalmology 96:251–254, 1989.

53. Hagay Z, Schachter M, Pollack A, Levy R: Development of proliferative retinopathy in a gestational diabetes patient following rapid metabolic control. Eur J Obstet Gynecol Reprod Biol 57:211–213, 1994.

54. Stoessel KM, Liao PM, Thompson JT, Reece AE: Diabetic retinopathy and macular edema in pregnancy. Ophthalmology 98(Suppl):146, 1991.

55. Early Treatment Diabetic Retinopathy Study Research Group: Photocoagulation for diabetic macular edema. Arch Ophthalmol 103:1796–1806, 1985.

56. Sinclair SH, Nesler C, Foxman B, et al: Macular edema and pregnancy in insulin-dependent diabetes. Am J Ophthalmol 97:154–167, 1984.

57. Chang S, Fuhrmann M, Diabetes in Early Pregnancy Study Group: Pregnancy, retinopathy, normoglycemia: a preliminary analysis. Diabetes 34(Suppl):39a, 1985.

58. Ohrt V: The influence of pregnancy on diabetic retinopathy with special regard to the reversible changes shown in 100 pregnancies. Acta Ophthalmol 62:603–616, 1984.

59. Laatikainen L, Teramo K, Hieta-Heikurainen H, et al: A controlled study of the influence of continuous subcutaneous insulin infusion treatment on diabetic retinopathy during pregnancy. Acta Med Scand 221:367–376, 1987.

60. Reece E, Lockwood C, Tuck S, et al: Retinal and pregnancy outcomes in the presence of diabetic proliferative retinopathy. J Reprod Med 39:799–804, 1994.

61. Serup L: Influence of pregnancy on diabetic retinopathy. Acta Endocrinol Suppl (Copenh) 277:122–124, 1986.

62. Hercules BL, Wozencroft M, Gayed I: Peripheral retinal ablation in the treatment of proliferative diabetic retinopathy during pregnancy. Br J Ophthalmol 64:87–93, 1980.

63. Singerman LJ: Diabetic retinopathy in juvenile-onset diabetes 1. Laser therapy in high-risk proliferatives 2. Effects of pregnancy. In Fine SL, Owens SL (eds): Management of Retinal Vascular & Macular Disorders. Baltimore, Williams & Wilkins, 1983, pp 43–46.

64. Diabetic Retinopathy Study Research Group: Four risk factors for severe visual loss in diabetic retinopathy. Arch Ophthalmol 97:654–655, 1979.

65. Kitzmiller JL, Aiello LM, Kaldany LM, Younger MD: Diabetic vascular disease complicating pregnancy. Clin Obstet Gynecol 24:107–123, 1981.

66. Soubrane G, Canivet J, Coscas G: Influence of pregnancy on the evolution of background retinopathy: preliminary results of a prospective fluorescein angiography study. In Ryan JJ, Dawson AK, Little HL (eds): Retinal Diseases. New York, Grune & Stratton, 1985, pp 15–20.

67. Ayed S, Jeddi A, Dagfous F, et al: Aspects evolutifs de la retinopathie diabetique pendant la grossesse. J Fr Ophthalmol 15:474–477, 1992.

68. Klein BEK, Moss SE, Klein R: Effect of pregnancy on progression of diabetic retinopathy. Diabetes Care 13:34–40, 1990.

69. Chen H, Newsom R, Patel V, et al: Retinal blood flow changes during pregnancy in woman with diabetes. Invest Ophthalmol Vis Sci 35:3199–3208, 1994.

70. Klein BEK, Klein R: Gravidity and diabetic retinopathy. Am J Epidemiol 119:564–569, 1984.

71. Lipman MJ, Kranias G, Bene CH, Khoury J: The effect of multiple pregnancies on diabetic retinopathy. Ophthalmology 100(Suppl):141, 1993.

72. Ward SC, Woods DR, Gilstrap LC, Hauth J: Pregnancy and acute optic disc edema of juvenile-onset diabetes. Obstet Gynecol 64:816–818, 1984.

73. Garg SK, Chase HP, Marshall G, et al: Oral contraceptives and renal and retinal complications in young women with insulin-dependent diabetes mellitus. JAMA 271:1099–1102, 1994.

74. Engstrom REJ, Holland GN, Nussenblatt RB, Jabs DA: Current practices in the management of ocular toxoplasmosis. Am J Ophthalmol 111:601–610, 1991.

75. Oniki S: Prognosis of pregnancy in patients with toxoplasmic retinochoroiditis. Jpn J Ophthalmol 27:166–174, 1983.

76. Silveira C, Belfort R, Burnier M, Nussenblatt R: Acquired toxoplasmic infection as the cause of toxoplasmic retinochoroiditis in families. Am J Ophthalmol 106:362–364, 1988.

77. Neri A, Grausbord R, Kremer I, et al: The management of labor in high myopic patients. Eur J Obstet Gynecol Reprod Biol 19:277–279, 1985.

78. Inglesby DV, Little BC, Chignell AH: Surgery for detachment of the retina should not affect a normal delivery. Br Med J 300:980, 1990.

79. Berde C, Willis DC, Sandberg EC: Pregnancy in women with pseudoxanthoma elasticum. Obstet Gynecol Surv 38:339–344, 1983.

80. Lao TT, Walters BNJ, DeSwiet M: Pseudoxanthoma elasticum and pregnancy. Two case reports. Br J Obstet Gynaecol 91:1049–1050, 1984.

81. Reese AB: Tumors of the Eye. New York, Harper & Row, 1963, pp 366–370, 411–412.

82. Pitta C, Bergen R, Littwin S: Spontaneous regression of a choroidal hemangioma following pregnancy. Ann Ophthalmol 11:772–774, 1979.

83. Mayock RL, Sullivan RD, Greening RR, et al: Sarcoidosis and pregnancy. JAMA 164:158–163, 1957.

84. Chumbley LC, Kearns TP: Retinopathy of sarcoidosis. Am J Ophthalmol 73:123–131, 1972.

85. Snyder DA, Tessler HH: Vogt-Koyanagi-Harada syndrome. Am J Ophthalmol 90:69–75, 1980.

86. Steahly LP: Vogt-Koyanagi-Harada syndrome and pregnancy. Ann Ophthalmol 22:59–62, 1990.

87. Friedman Z, Granat M, Neumann E: The syndrome of Vogt-Koyanagi-Harada and pregnancy. Metab Pediatr Ophthalmol 4:147–149, 1980.

88. Chavis PS, Tabbara KF, Al-Rajhi AA, Wafai MZ: Uveitis during pregnancy and postpartum. Ophthalmology 99(Suppl):139, 1992.

89. Yoser SL, Heckenlively JR, Friedman L, Oversier J: Evaluation of clinical findings and common symptoms in retinitis pigmentosa. Invest Ophthalmol Vis Sci 28(Suppl):112, 1987.

90. Wagener H: Lesions of the optic nerve and retina in pregnancy. JAMA 103:1910–1913, 1934.

91. Hayasaka S, Ugomori S, Kanamori M, Setogawa T: Pericentral retinal degeneration deteriorates during pregnancies. Ophthalmologica 200:72–76, 1990.

92. Watson DL, Sibai BM, Shaver DC, et al: Late postpartum eclampsia. South Med J 76:1487–1489, 1983.

93. Folk JC, Weingeist TA: Fundus changes in toxemia. Ophthalmology 88:1173–1174, 1981.

94. Hallum AV: Eye changes in hypertensive toxemia of pregnancy. JAMA 106:1649–1651, 1936.

95. Beck RW, Gamel JW, Wilcourt RJ, Berman G: Acute ischemic optic neuropathy in severe preeclampsia. Am J Ophthalmol 90:342–346, 1980.

96. Mussey RD, Mundell BJ: Retinal examinations: a guide in the management of the toxic hypertensive syndrome of pregnancy. Am J Obstet Gynecol 37:30–36, 1939.

97. Schreyer P, Tzadok J, Sherman DJ, et al: Fluorescein angiography in hypertensive pregnancies. Int J Gynaecol Obstet 34:127–132, 1990.

98. Saito Y, Omoto T, Kidoguchi K, et al: The relationship between ophthalmoscopic changes and classification of toxemia in toxemia of pregnancy. Acta Soc Ophthalmol Jpn 94:870–874, 1990.

99. Jaffe G, Schatz H: Ocular manifestations of preeclampsia. Am J Ophthalmol 103:309–315, 1987.

100. Riss B, Riss P, Metka M: Die prognostische Wertigkeit von Veranderungen am Augenhintergrund bei Eph-Gestose. Z Geburtshilfe Perinatol 187:276–279, 1983.

101. Landesman R, Douglas RG, Snyder SS: Retinal changes in the toxemias of pregnancy. Am J Obstet Gynecol 63:16–27, 1952.

102. Uto M, Uemura A: Retinochoroidopathy and systemic state in toxemia of pregnancy. Acta Soc Ophthalmol Jpn 95:1016–1019, 1991.

103. Fry WE: Extensive bilateral retinal detachment in eclampsia with complete reattachment. Arch Ophthalmol 1:609–614, 1929.

104. Gitter KA, Houser BP, Sarin LK, Justice J: Toxemia of pregnancy. An angiographic interpretation of fundus changes. Arch Ophthalmol 80:448–454, 1968.

105. Saito T, Shimizu S: Fluorescence fundus angiography of cyst-like elevations associated with toxemias of pregnancies. Folia Ophthalmol Jpn 31:152–156, 1980.

106. Fastenberg DM, Fetkenhour CL, Choromokos E: Choroidal vascular changes in toxemia of pregnancy. Am J Ophthalmol 89:362–368, 1980.

107. Kenny GS, Cerasol JR: Color fluorescein angiography in toxemia of pregnancy. Arch Ophthalmol 87:383–388, 1972.

108. Klien BA: Ischemic infarcts of the choroid (Elschnig spots). Am J Ophthalmol 66:1069–1074, 1968.

109. Mabie WC, Ober RR: Fluorescein angiography in toxemia of pregnancy. Br J Ophthalmol 64:666–671, 1980.

110. Oliver M, Uchenik D: Bilateral exudative retinal detachment in eclampsia without hypertensive retinopathy. Am J Ophthalmol 90:792–796, 1980.

111. Saito Y, Omoto T, Fukuda M: Lobular pattern of choriocapillaris in pre-eclampsia with aldosteronism. Br J Ophthalmol 74:702–703, 1990.

112. Bosco JAS: Spontaneous nontraumatic retinal detachments in pregnancy. Am J Obstet Gynecol 82:208–212, 1961.

113. Brismar G, Schimmelpfennig W: Bilateral exudative retinal detachments in pregnancy. Acta Ophthalmol 67:699–702, 1989.

114. Ballantyne AJ, Michaelson IC: Textbook of the Fundus of the Eye, 2nd edition. Baltimore, Williams & Wilkins, 1970.

115. Crowther WL, Hamilton JB: Eclampsia with amaurosis due to detachment of the retina. Med J Aust 2:177–178, 1932.

116. Gass JDM, Pautler SE: Toxemia of pregnancy pigment epitheliopathy masquerading as a heredomacular dystrophy. Trans Am Ophthalmol Soc 83:114–130, 1985.

117. Arulkumaran S, Gibb DMF, Rauff M, et al: Transient blindness associated with pregnancy-induced hypertension. Br J Obstet Gynaecol 93:847–849, 1985.

118. Beeson JH, Duda EE: Computed axial tomography scan demonstration of cerebral edema in eclampsia preceded by blindness. Obstet Gynecol 60:529–532, 1982.

119. Goodlin RC, Strieb E, Sun SF, et al: Cortical blindness as the initial symptom in severe preeclampsia. Am J Obstet Gynecol 147:841–842, 1983.

120. Grimes DA, Ekbrah LE, McCartney WH: Cortical blindness in preeclampsia. Int J Gynaecol Obstet 17:601–603, 1980.

121. Gyr T, Ramzin MS, Zimmerli W: Postpartuale Amaurose bei Patientinnen mit Praeklampsie. Z Geburtshilfe Perinatol 187:293–295, 1983.

122. Hill JA, Devoe LD, Elgammal TA: Central hemodynamic findings associated with cortical blindness in severe preeclampsia. J Reprod Med 30:435–438, 1985.

123. Duke-Elder S: System of Ophthalmology. St Louis, CV Mosby Co, 1971, pp 627, 692, 703, 902.

124. Price J, Marouf L, Heine MW: New angiographic findings in toxemia of pregnancy. Ophthalmology 93(Suppl):125, 1986.

125. Brancato R, Menchini U, Bandello F: Proliferative retinopathy and toxemia of pregnancy. Ann Ophthalmol 19:182–183, 1987.

126. Capoor S, Goble RR, Wheatley T, Casswell AG: White-

centered retinal hemorrhages as an early sign of pre-eclampsia. Am J Ophthalmol 119:804–806, 1995.

127. Weinstein L: Syndrome of hemolysis, elevated liver enzymes, and low platelet count: a severe consequence of hypertension in pregnancy. Am J Obstst Gynecol 142:159–167, 1982.

128. Burke JP, Whyte I, MacEwen CJ: Bilateral serous retinal detachments in the H.E.L.L.P. syndrome. Acta Ophthalmol 67:322–324, 1989.

129. Leff SR, Yarian DL, Masciulli L, et al: Vitreous hemorrhage as a complication of HELLP syndrome. Br J Ophthalmol 74:498, 1990.

130. Levavi H, Neri A, Zoldan J, et al: Pre-eclampsia, "HELLP" syndrome, and postictal cortical blindness. Acta Obstet Gynecol Scand 66:91–92, 1987.

131. Wiebers DO: Ischemic cerebrovascular complications of pregnancy. Arch Neurol 42:1106–1113, 1985.

132. Brown GC, Magargal LE, Shields JA: Retinal arterial obstruction in children and young adults. Ophthalmology 88:18–25, 1981.

133. Greven CM, Slusher MM, Weaver RG: Retinal arterial occlusions in young adults. Am J Ophthalmol 120:776–783, 1995.

134. Acheson JF, Gregson RMC, Merry P, Schullenberg WE: Vaso-occlusive retinopathy in the primary anti-phospholipid antibody syndrome. Eye 5:48–55, 1991.

135. Humayun M, Kattah J, Cupps TR, et al: Papillophlebitis and arteriolar occlusion in a pregnant woman. J Clin Neuroophthalmol 12:226–229, 1992.

136. Blodi BA, Johnson MW, Gass JDM, et al: Purtscher's-like retinopathy after childbirth. Ophthalmology 97:1654–1659, 1990.

137. Nelson ME, Talbot JF, Preston FE: Recurrent multiple branch retinal arteriolar occlusions in a patient with protein C deficiency. Graefes Arch Clin Exp Ophthalmol 227:283–287, 1989.

138. Ayaki M, Yokoyama N, Furukawa Y: Postpartum central retinal artery occlusion simulating Purtscher's retinopathy. Ophthalmologica 209:37–39, 1995.

139. Chew EW, Trope GE, Mitchell BJ: Diurnal intraocular pressure in young adults with central retinal vein occlusion. Ophthalmology 94:1545–1549, 1987.

140. Spitzberg DH: Retinal phlebitis associated with pregnancy. Ann Ophthalmol 14:101–102, 1982.

141. Carpenter F, Kava HL, Plotkin D: The development of total blindness as a complication of pregnancy. Am J Obstet Gynecol 66:641–647, 1953.

142. Cogan D: Ocular involvement in disseminated intravascular coagulopathy. Arch Ophthalmol 93:1–8, 1975.

143. Hoines J, Buettner H: Ocular complications of disseminated intravascular coagulation (DIC) in abruptio placentae. Retina 9:105–109, 1989.

144. Martin VAF: Disseminated intravascular coagulopathy. Trans Ophthalmol Soc U K 98:506–507, 1978.

145. Benson DO, Fitzgibbons JF, Goodnight SH: The visual system in thrombotic thrombocytopenic purpura. Ann Ophthalmol 12:413–417, 1980.

146. Sperry K: Amniotic fluid embolism. JAMA 255:2183–2203, 1986.

147. Chang M, Herbert WNP: Retinal arteriolar occlusions following amniotic fluid embolism. Ophthalmology 91:1634–1637, 1984.

148. Fischbein FI: Ischemic retinopathy following amniotic fluid embolization. Am J Ophthalmol 67:351–357, 1969.

149. Beal MF, Chapman PH: Cortical blindness and homonymous hemianopia in the post partum period. JAMA 244:2085, 1980.

150. Monteiro MLR, Hoyt WF, Imes RK: Puerperal cerebral blindness. Arch Neurol 41:1300–1301, 1984.

151. Duke-Elder S: System of Ophthalmology. St Louis, CV Mosby Co, 1971, p 136.

152. Sommerville-Lange LB: A case of permanent blindness due to toxemia of pregnancy. Br J Ophthalmol 34:431–434, 1950.

153. Cantrill HL, Rodman WP, Ramsay RC: Postpartum *Candida* endophthalmitis. JAMA 143:1163–1165, 1980.

154. Michelson PE, Stark W, Reeser F, Green WR: Endogenous *Candida* endophthalmitis: report of 13 cases and 16 from the literature. Int Ophthalmol Clin 11:125–147, 1971.

155. Haskjold E, Von der Lippe B: Endogenous candida endophthalmitis. Acta Ophthalmol 65:741–744, 1987.

156. Shekleton P, Fidler J, Grinuvade J: A case of benign intracranial hypertension in pregnancy. Br J Obstet Gynaecol 87:345–347, 1980.

157. Salem H, Loux JJ, Smith S, Nichols CW: Evaluation of the toxicologic and teratogenic potentials of sodium fluorescein in the rat. Toxicology 12:143–150, 1979.

158. Halperin LS, Olk RJ, Soubrane G, Coscas G: Safety of fluorescein angiography during pregnancy. Am J Ophthalmol 109:563–566, 1990.

159. Greenberg F, Lewis RA: Safety of fluorescein angiography during pregnancy (correspondence). Am J Ophthalmol 110:323–324, 1990.

160. Mattern J, Mayer PR: Excretion of fluorescein into breast milk. Am J Ophthalmol 109:598–599, 1990.

161. Maguire AM, Bennett J: Fluorescein elimination in human breast milk. Arch Ophthalmol 106:718–719, 1988.

162. Kearns GL, Williams BJ, Timmons OD: Fluorescein phototoxicity in a premature infant. J Pediatr 107:796–798, 1985.

163. Samples JR, Meyer SM: Use of ophthalmic medications in pregnant and nursing women. Am J Ophthalmol 106:616–623, 1988.

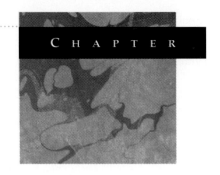

The Rheumatic Retinal Diseases

Rosario Brancato, M.D.

Sandro Vergani, M.D.

Antonio P. Ciardella, M.D.

The rheumatic retinal diseases are a group of sight-threatening inflammatory eye disorders whose etiologies remain obscure. They may occur as a complication of infective, neoplastic, or degenerative disorders; in association with systemic inflammatory diseases (e.g., Behçet's syndrome, sarcoidosis); or as an isolated phenomenon. The ophthalmologic features consist of cells in the vitreous and involvement of retinal vessels: the retinal veins are most commonly affected, and sheathing of the postcapillary venules frequently occurs together with evidence of diffuse capillary leakage on fluorescein angiography. As the retinal capillaries are frequently involved, there is loss of integrity of tight junctions between capillary endothelial cells that results in macular edema and consequently visual loss. In contrast, the retinal arterioles are rarely affected, except in advanced cases, where arteriolar occlusion is characteristically accompanied by multiple retinal vein occlusions.

The pathogenesis of rheumatic retinal diseases has not yet been established, but clinical and experimental data strongly implicate immune mechanisms. The condition may be associated with connective tissue disorders such as systemic lupus erythematosus and Behçet's syndrome, where immune complexes are thought to have a pathogenetic role.[1-6] Circulating immune complexes have also been found in patients in whom retinal vasculitis is the only detectable lesion.[3] Circulating immune complexes, however, might also represent an immune reaction secondary to ocular tissue destruction. A primary role for immune complexes in the pathogenesis of rheumatic retinal diseases is suggested by the evidence obtained in experimental animal models. Furthermore, an increase in vascular permeability, a typical sign of rheumatic retinal diseases, can be reproduced in experimental animals by the direct administration of performed immune complexes. Recent studies suggest a greater relevance of autoimmune rather than immune-complex-mediated pathogenic mechanisms.[1] Experimental models of posterior retinal vasculitis, a retinal vasculitis resembling human disease, develops in animals 9 to 10 days after immunization at a distant site with a retinal autoantigen, usually retinal S antigen. Direct information on the precise mechanisms of autoimmune damage in human rheumatic retinal diseases is difficult to obtain, since most of the material obtained for analysis represents advanced, end-stage disease.

In pathogenic terms it appears that antiretinal autoimmunity is important in both isolated retinal vasculitis and retinal vasculitis accompanying certain systematic inflammatory diseases.

CLINICAL FEATURES OF RETINAL VASCULITIS

The diagnosis of retinal vasculitis is based on the presence of cells in the vitreous in association with involvement of retinal vessels. Fluorescein angiography plays a confirmatory role of the ophthalmoscopic diagnosis and is an indispensable tool for monitoring treatment response. Retinal vasculitis laboratory investigations are unrewarding, as there are few specific tests (HLA typing, angiotensin-converting enzyme [ACE]). In retinal vasculitis vision may be lost in several ways. Usually visual impairment is due to macular damage linked to edema in the active phase, but even after the inflammation has subsided there may be macular and premacular fibrosis.

MANAGEMENT

The appropriate approach to retinal vasculitis will depend on the extent and severity of the inflammatory process, which can range from mild, with no visual loss, to severe, with devastating loss of vision.

In some cases the retinal vasculitis is part of a systemic disorder, the activity of which will also influence treatment. Treatment may be limited to the eye alone or may need to be given systematically.

Visual loss can occur for a variety of reasons, some of which may respond to control of the inflammatory process (vitreitis, macular edema), whereas others will not (macular hole, optic nerve damage).

Features that should prompt direct questioning about sarcoidosis include vitreitis, patchy retinal vascular sheathing, and optic nerve swelling. Similarly, vitreitis, branch vein occlusions, closure and sheathing of postcapillary venules, and choroidal infarcts should raise suspicions of Behçet's disease.

TREATMENT

Patients with active inflammatory disease causing significant visual loss require immunosuppressive treatment. Not all patients with retinal vasculitis have sight-threatening disease; in some cases it can be very mild with peripheral phlebitis and/or a mild vitreitis, with floaters being the sole symptoms.

Sometimes a mild disorder may worsen after a while. Treatment should not be given unless necessary, since its systemic side effects can be worse than the effects of the disorder.

Whether the disease is unilateral or bilateral will also influence treatment. Bilateral sight-threatening disease is usually treated with systemic steroids.

SYSTEMIC STEROIDS

Patients who do not respond to peribulbar injections of steroids and those with bilateral ocular involvement need systemic steroids in doses sufficient to suppress the inflammatory reponse. The doses vary with disease severity, and with age and weight for children under 12 years.

Efficacy of therapy is judged by improvement of the clinical signs, and well as by increase of visual

acuity when its impairment is due to vitreitis, papillitis, and macular edema.

Duration of treatment can vary from months to years. When there is disease in other organs, such as the lung in sarcoidosis, different steroid-reduction regimens may be required, since dose adjustment is then not influenced by ocular involvement alone.

OTHER IMMUNOSUPPRESSIVE DRUGS

When the patients cannot tolerate steroids or when control requires unacceptably high doses, other immunosuppressive agents should be added to the regimen. Cyclosporine is rapidly replacing azathioprine, chlorambucil, and cyclophosphamide as the supplementary agent of choice in patients of all ages, provided they have normal renal function.[11-13]

The cyclosporine dose is controlled mainly by monitoring of serum creatinine. If cyclosporine enables the steroid dose to be lowered, then its introduction has been effective. If not, other immunosuppressive drugs need to be tried.

SPECIFIC CLINICAL ENTITIES

Idiopathic Retinal Vasculitis

The most prevalent findings of this disease are sheathing of peripheral retinal vessels and macular edema (Figs. 42–1 and 42–2). Atrophic pigment epithelial lesions and retinal neovascularization may be observed in these patients. Fluorescein angiography shows in the majority of cases diffuse capillary leakage and capillary closure. Visual acuity is usually conserved.[14,15]

Sarcoidosis

Sarcoidosis is a systemic disease characterized by granulomatous inflammation, the etiology of which is unknown. Retinal venous sheathing and perivascular infiltrates in sarcoidosis are usually "patchy" (Figs. 42–3 and 42–4), but in severe cases can become confluent. Chest x-rays (hilar adenopathy) and raised levels of ACE can lead to the correct diagnosis.[16]

Behçet's Disease

Behçet's disease is a multisystem inflammatory disorder, of unknown etiology, two times more common in men than in women, first described by the Turkish dermatologist Dr. Hulusi Behçet in 1937.[17]

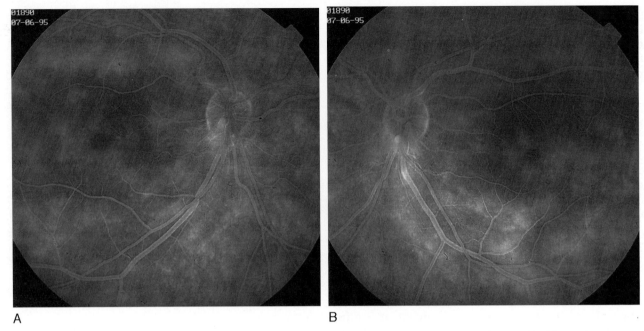

A   B

FIGURE 42–1   *A* and *B*, Fluorescein angiography study of both eyes of a young, otherwise healthy male patient, who was complaining of decreased vision in both eyes. There is cystoid macular edema, localized multifocal periphlebitis, and diffuse leakage of dye from the retinal capillaries.

It represents a frequent cause of retinal vasculitis in Mediterranean countries and in Japan. It was described in males but is increasingly seen also in females. The patients affected are between the ages of 20 and 40 years. The diagnosis is based on the triad of uveitis, oral ulcers, and genital ulcers. The presence of HLA-B5 antigen is frequently associated with ocular involvement.[18] The basic pathologic lesion is an obliterative vasculitis. Biopsies of oral ulcers have shown a neutrophilic infiltration of the ulcer itself and mononuclear cell infiltration of the surrounding tissue, the majority of the cells being CD3+ and CD4+ T lymphocytes and HLA-DR+ cells.[19–21] Interactions between the infil-

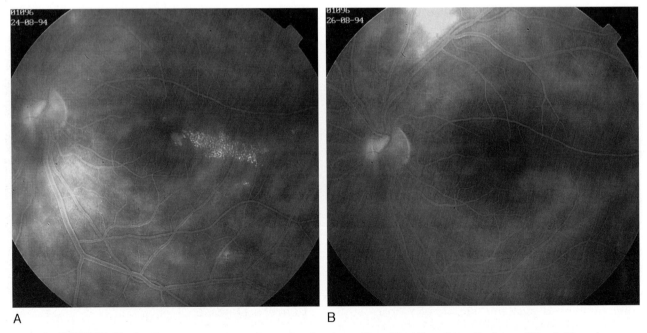

A   B

FIGURE 42–2   Fluorescein angiography study of patient affected by idiopathic retinal vasculitis. *A*, There is marked inflammation of the optic disc, diffuse staining of the retinal vein walls, intraretinal leakage of dye, and lipid deposition in the temporal macula. *B*, Three days after the beginning of high-dose systemic corticosteroid treatment, the angiogram shows an impressive reduction of the macular edema and capillary leakage.

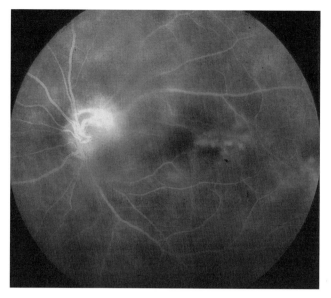

FIGURE 42-3 Fluorescein angiography picture of a patient with sarcoid retinopathy. There is hot disc, periphlebitis, and diffuse intraretinal leakage of dye.

trating cells and the vascular endothelial cells have been suggested to result in the development of occlusive events in Behçet's disease.[22]

Ocular Manifestations

The typical ocular manifestation of Behçet disease is a chronic recurrent uveitis. The first symptoms appear in the third or fourth decade of life. There is always an iritis with inflammatory cells in the anterior chamber (hypopyon is a rare occurrence),

and a vitreitis; the disease is usually bilateral. Fundus examination may reveal the presence of periphlebitis, vein and artery retinal occlusion, white retinal inflammatory infiltrates, neurosensory detachment, and subretinal lipid deposition (Figs. 42-5 through 42-10). The course of Behçet's disease is chronic recurrent, with periods of spontaneous remission and new exacerbation. The prognosis is variable; cases that progress to end-stage disease show optic atrophy and marked reduction of visual acuity.

Treatment

Topical and systemic steroids represent the first treatment choice. Cases that fail to respond to steroid treatment may respond to immunosuppressive drugs such as cyclosporine, azathioprine, chlorambucil, and cyclophosphamide.[11-13,23-25]

Systemic Lupus Erythematosus

Systemic lupus erythematosus (SLE) is a chronic immune disorder characterized by multisystem involvement and clinical exacerbations and remissions. Circulating immune complexes and autoantibodies cause tissue damage and organ dysfunction. Manifestations involving the skin, serosal surfaces, central nervous system (CNS), kidneys, and blood cells are particularly characteristic. Evidence for the autoimmune nature of this disorder lies in the laboratory finding of antinuclear antibodies (ANAs), the demonstration of immune complexes in tissues, and the utilization of complement.

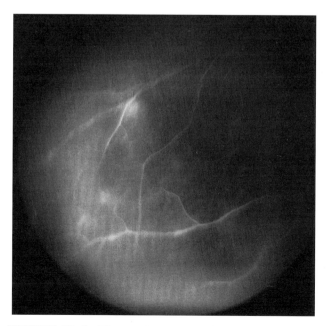

FIGURE 42-4 Fluorescein angiography study of the peripheral fundus in case of biopsy-proven sarcoid retinopathy. There is segmental, multifocal inflammation of the retinal veins.

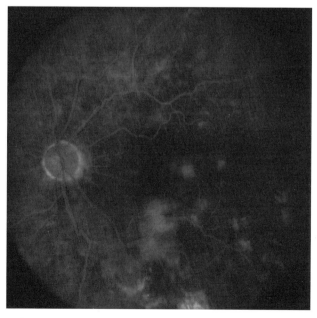

FIGURE 42-5 This angiogram shows a case of active retinal vasculitis in a patient with Behçet's disease: there is diffuse vascular leakage throughout the posterior pole.

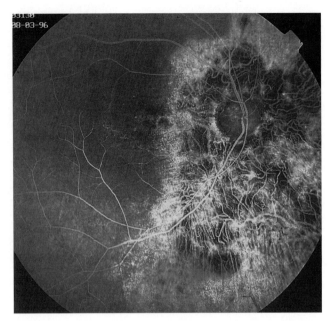

FIGURE 42–6 Fluorescein angiography study of a patient with end-stage Behçet's disease. There is marked attenuation of the retinal vessels, optic atrophy, and marked destruction of the choriocapillaris–RPE layer around the optic disc.

Epidemiology

The overall prevalence of SLE is approximately 15 to 50 cases per 100,000 population. The prevalence in young women of childbearing age is approximately eight to ten times higher than in men. Black women are affected approximately three times as often as white women.[26]

The frequency of occurrence of lupus is higher in the relatives of affected individuals than in the general population, and the disease concordance rate in identical twins approaches 50%.[26]

Etiology

No single cause of lupus has been discovered. Complex interrelationships among environmental factors, genetically determined host immune responses, and hormonal influences probably are critical in the initiation as well the expression of the disease. Twin and genetics studies suggest a genetic predisposition to SLE. Histocompatibility antigens HLA-DR2 and HLA-DR3 are present much more commonly in SLE patients than in controls. Loss of tolerance to autoantigens is central in the pathogenesis of SLE and genetic tendencies toward the development of autoantibodies, B-cell hyperactivity, and T-cell dysfunction are evident in patients with the disease. Viral agents might trigger changes in lymphocyte interactions that would allow disease expression. Since SLE is predominantly a disease of women of childbearing age, hormonal factors are also probably important in modulation of the expression of the disease.[27]

Pathogenesis

All of the clinical features of SLE are manifestations of cellular and humoral immune dysfunction.[28,29]

IMMUNE COMPLEXES. Circulating antigen–antibody immune complexes are deposited in blood vessels and the renal glomerulus, initiating a pathologic response that damages these tissues. These complexes are characteristic features of active disease, and their size, solubility, concentration, and

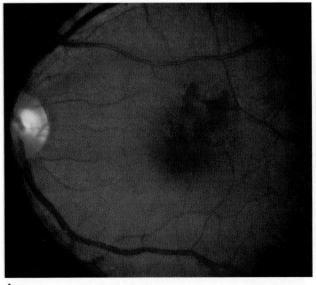

A   B

FIGURE 42–7 Clinical photograph of a patient with Behçet's disease demonstrates retinal vasculitis. *A*, Early lesion. *B*, One month later the ocular inflammation worsened. There is vitreitis, whitish retinal inflammatory infiltrates, and artery and vein sheathing. (From Ryan SJ: Retina, 2nd edition. St Louis, Mosby-Year Book, 1994, with permission. Courtesy of Dr. Douglas A. Jabs.)

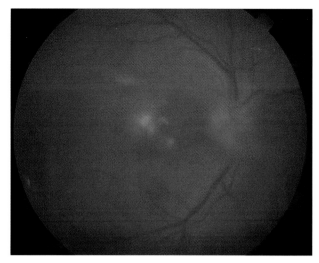

FIGURE 42–8 Clinical photograph of a patient with Behçet's disease showing neurosensory macular detachment and subretinal lipid deposition. (From Yannuzzi LA, Guyer DR, Green WR [eds]: The Retina Atlas. St Louis, Mosby-Year Book, 1995, with permission. Courtesy of Dr. Richard Klein.)

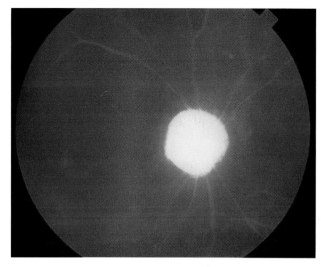

FIGURE 42–10 End-stage Behçet's disease: there is optic atrophy and severe retinal vascular nonperfusion. (From Yannuzzi LA, Guyer DR, Green WR [eds]: The Retina Atlas. St Louis, Mosby-Year Book, 1995, with permission. Courtesy of Dr. Leyla-Suna Atmaca.)

complement-fixing properties as well as vessel hydrostatic forces are important in determining tissue deposition.

RETICULOENDOTHELIAL DYSFUNCTION. Patients with SLE may have impaired ability to clear immune complexes from the circulation due to a dysfunction of the reticuloendothelial system.

LYMPHOCYTE DYSFUNCTION. B-cell hyperactivity, impaired CD8+ cell function, and augmented CD4+ cell activity are present in various combinations in lupus patients, leading to autoantibody

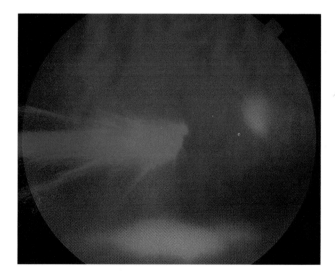

FIGURE 42–9 This patient with Behçet's disease had marked intravitreal inflammation. Note the presence in the anterior vitreous gel of aggregate of inflammatory cells (snowbanks). (From Yannuzzi LA, Guyer DR, Green WR [eds]: The Retina Atlas. St Louis, Mosby-Year Book, 1995, with permission. Courtesy of Dr. Richard Klein.)

production and increased generation of immune complexes.

Pathology

Characteristic microscopic changes in lupus are hematoxylin bodies and fibrinoid necrosis. Hematoxylin bodies are amorphous masses of nuclear material that can be found in connective tissue lesions, they become purple-blue when stained with hematoxylin. Neutrophils that ingest these bodies in vitro are called LE cells. In SLE, immune complexes of DNA, and complement, may stain with eosin (which can also stain fibrin) in vessel wall and connective tissue, demonstrating so-called fibrinoid necrosis.

Inflammatory lesions of capillaries, venules, and arterioles, caused by deposition of immune complexes and variable cellular infiltration, are responsible for much of the tissue destruction and damage seen in SLE. The phospholipid antibody syndrome may be associated with the small-vessel occlusive lesions.[30]

Clinical Features

Fatigue, weight loss, and fever are prominent systemic complaints in this disease.

SKIN. The butterfly rash (i.e., facial erythema over the checks and nose) and the chronic potentially scarring discoid lesions (i.e., coin-shaped lesions with hyperemic margins, central atrophy, and depigmentation) are the most classic skin lesions in SLE.[31]

CNS. Focal or diffuse neurologic disorders occur in approximately 50% of patients. Both generalized manifestations (reactive depression, psychoses, cognitive disturbances) and focal seizure may occur. Magnetic resonance imaging (MRI) scanning reveals CNS lesions in many patients, especially those with focal presentations.[32]

HEART. Symptomatic pericarditis occurs in approximately 20% of SLE patients, myocarditis and coronary vessel vasculitis are less common, but may evolve to congestive heart failure. Nonbacterial endocardial lesions (Libman-Sacks endocarditis) correlate with the presence of phospholipid antibodies; these lesions can be associated with embolic events to the CNS and to the eye.[26]

KIDNEY. Most lupus patients have some clinical and pathologic evidence of renal involvement. Mesangial disease, focal proliferative nephritis, diffuse proliferative nephritis, and membranous glomerulopathy may all be found in lupus patients.[33,34]

Laboratory Findings

COAGULATION PARAMETERS. Antibodies to the phospholipid components of individual clotting factors can interfere with coagulation testing, causing prolongation of the partial thromboplastin time (PTT) not correctable by the addition of normal plasma. Paradoxically, patients with the PTT prolongation (the "lupus anticoagulant") have a higher frequency of thrombosis than bleeding.

SEROLOGIC FINDINGS. Phospholipid antibodies can also cause a false-positive test result for syphilis, more often by interference with reagin (rapid plasma reagin [RPR] or Venereal Disease Research Laboratories [VDRL] testing than with antitreponemal fluorescent treponemal antibody absorption [FTA-ABS]) testing.

IMMUNOLOGIC FINDINGS. Lupus patients commonly have low complement component (C3 and C4) levels as a result of immune complex activation; in many patients falls in serum complement levels parallel disease flare-ups if complement synthesis is unchanged. Hypergammaglobulinemia reflects B-cell hyperactivity. By far the most significant immunologic findings in SLE patients are autoantibodies.

ANAs. Approximately 99% of patients with SLE have ANAs.

Antiphospholipid Antibodies. One third to half of lupus patients exhibit phospholipid antibodies if tested, although the associated clinical syndrome occurs less frequently. Antiphospholipid antibodies can be found by detecting that patients exhibit prolonged PTTs, false-positive syphilis serologies (RPR or VDRL), or positive anticardiolipin test when assayed.

Ocular Manifestations

Chorioretinal involvement in SLE patients may be divided into four groups according to different etiologies and clinical manifestations:

1. Central serous chorioretinopathy.
2. Hypertensive retinopathy
3. Vascular occlusive disease
4. Chloroquine maculopathy.

CENTRAL SEROUS CHORIORETINOPATHY. Renal failure and systemic use of corticosteroids are two risk factors for a severe form of central serous chorioretinopathy (CSC) in lupus patients. While the exact pathogenic mechanism is still unknown, there is evidence in the literature that both renal failure and systemic corticosteroid use may be associated with bullous neurosensory detachment, massive subretinal exudation of fibrin-rich fluid, and fluorescein angiographic evidence of multiple serous detachments of the retinal pigment epithelium[35-40] (Fig. 42–11). In the only pathologic study available, de Venecia[41-42] found subretinal deposits of fibrin in a patient who died of renal failure. Dr. Gass reported the association of systemic steroids and bullous exudative neurosensory detachment.[35] These two risk factors may act separately, or may potentiate each other when they are contemporarily present in the same patient. Renal failure causes an increase in the volume of circulating fluid and consequently increased hydrostatic pressure in the capillary bed; it also may cause proteinuria, depletion of the pool of circulating proteins, and decrease in the oncotic pressure in the capillary bed. These two associated factors (i.e., increased hydrostatic pressure and decreased oncotic pressure) are responsible for transudation of fluid from the capillary bed and tissue edema. The same mechanism at the level of the choriocapillary bed can cause increased transudation of fluids from the choriocapillaris, retinal pigment epithelium (RPE) detachment, and finally mechanical damage to the RPE cells and pinpoint leakage under the neurosensory retina. The mechanism of action of systemic corticosteroids in causing CSC is not yet understood as well. A hypothesis is that the anti-inflammatory action of systemic steroids may impair the healing ability of the RPE cells and facilitate the formation of multiple defects in the RPE layer that ultimately produce pinpoint leakage of fluid under the neurosensory retina.[35]

Treatment. Reduction and, if possible, suspension of the systemic corticosteroid treatment is the first step in treating lupus patients with severe CSC. If there is persistent leakage of fluid under the retina, after interruption of the corticosteroid treatment, laser scatter photocoagulation of the areas of pinpoint leakage may be successful in resolving the neurosensory detachment and improving the vision. The patient must then be followed carefully since there is a high risk of recurrence.

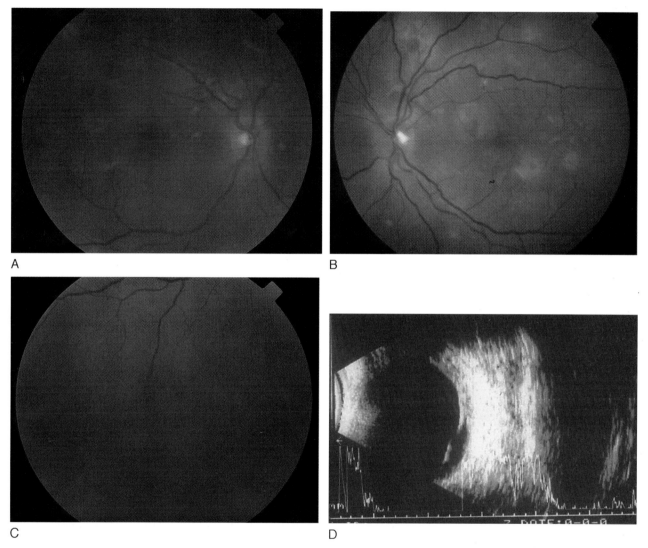

A

B

C

D

FIGURE 42–11 This is a case of a 37-year-old female with SLE for 20 years. She also had hypertension, kidney transplant 7 years before, and was on systemic corticosteroid treatment. An inferior bullous neurosensory detachment was noted in both eyes 1 month before. *A* and *B*, Clinical photograph of the posterior pole of both eyes. Note the presence of multiple detachments of the retinal pigment epithelium, scattered islands of pigmentary atrophy, hyperplasia, subretinal grayish depositions of fibrin, Elschnig's spots, and Zig-freezed lines corresponding to fibrinoid necrosis of the choroid. *C* and *D*, Clinical photograph and ultrasound image of a dependent neurosensory detachment in the inferior periphery of the right eye. *Illustration continued on following page*

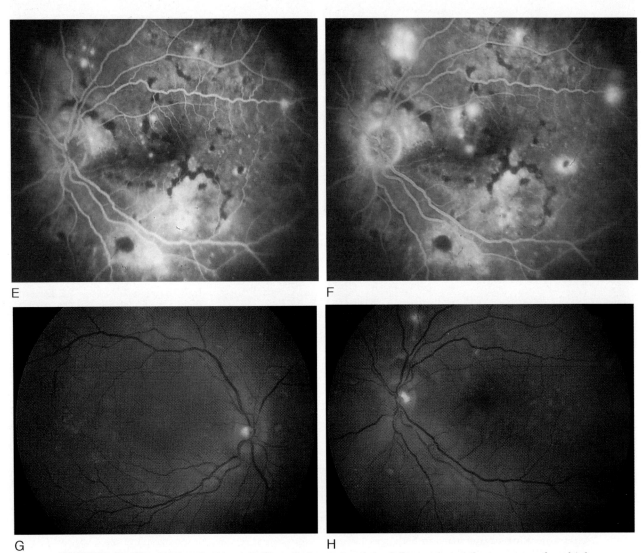

E

F

G

H

FIGURE 42–11 *Continued   E* and *F,* Fluorescein study of the left eye shows the presence of multiple detachments of the retinal pigment epithelium and leakage of dye in the subretinal space in the late phase of the study. *G* and *H,* Two months after scattered laser photocoagulation of the leaking points there is partial resolution of the fibrinous exudation at the posterior pole in both eyes. *Illustration continued on opposite page*

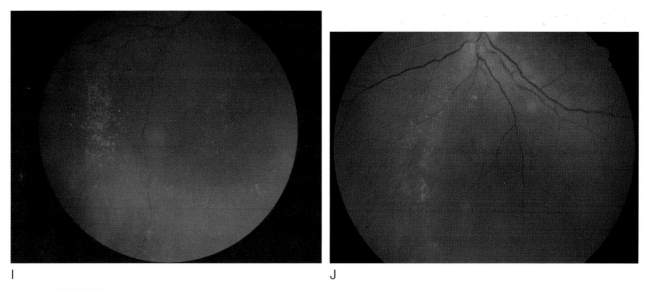

I   J

FIGURE 42–11 *Continued   I* and *J,* There is also partial resolution of the bullous neurosensory detachment. Note the deposition of lipids in the subretinal space caused by the reabsorption of the serous component of the subretinal exudate.

Hypertensive Retinopathy. Lupus patients may have high blood pressure as a consequence of severe renal disease. Hypertensive retinopathy may present with swollen disc, multiple cotton-wool spots, intraretinal hemorrhages, and a macular star of intraretinal lipid deposition. Interestingly, there may also be multiple areas of choroidal infarction, which appear as localized brown reddish areas on ophthalmoscopic examination, and show choriocapillaris nonperfusion on fluorescein angiography.[43–45] These areas of choroidal infarction are called Elschnig's spots, and are usually associated with infarction of the overlying RPE cells, rupture of the external ocular barrier and subretinal transudation of fluid that leads to bullous neurosensory detachment (Figs. 42–11 and 42–12). Patients with SLE may also develop fibrinoid necrosis of the choroid vessels causing macular neurosensory detachment. They may or may not have concomitant hypertension.

Using indocyanine green angiography, we have noted the presence of congested and dilated choroidal vessels in lupus patients. In some cases, the indocyanine dye stains the walls of the large choroidal vessels, suggesting the presence of a choroidal vascular inflammatory component.

Treatment. Medical treatment of hypertensive retinopathy is the first step. When there is persistent neurosensory detachment despite the medical therapy, scatter laser photocoagulation of the areas of RPE damage may be successful in stopping the leakage of fluid, resolving the neurosensory detachment, and improving the vision.

VASCULAR OCCLUSIVE DISEASE. Typically, lupus patients present with an occlusive retinopathy con-

stituted by cotton-wool spots, which are the expression of localized occlusion of retinal arterioles and retinal infarction (Figs. 42–13 and 42–14). These lesions occur in 3 to 29% of cases and are generally found late in the disease.[46,47] Less frequently they experience a more severe form of vascular occlusive disease characterized by central retinal artery occlusion, central retinal vein occlusion, extensive retinal capillary nonperfusion, and choroidal infarction (Figs. 42–15 and 42–16). There is now increasing evidence that the more severe forms of retinal vascular occlusive disease in lupus patients are associated with the presence of circulating autoantibodies, (i.e., lupus anticoagulant and

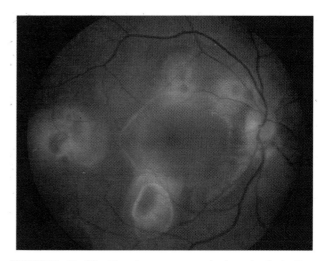

FIGURE 42–12 This lupus patient had multiple bullous neurosensory detachments, subretinal fibrin deposition, and fibrinoid necrosis of the choroid. (From Yannuzzi LA, Guyer DR, Green WR [eds]: The Retina Atlas. St Louis, Mosby-Year Book, 1995, with permission.)

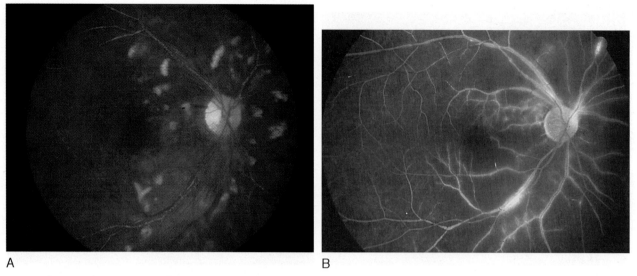

A   B

FIGURE 42–13   *A,* Clinical photograph of a lupus patient that shows the presence of multiple cotton-wool spots, intraretinal hemorrhages, and sheathed retinal vessels. *B,* Fluorescein angiography of the same eye shows capillary nonperfusion, and staining of the inflamed retinal vessels. (From Yannuzzi LA, Guyer DR, Green WR [eds]: The Retina Atlas. St Louis, Mosby-Year Book, 1995, with permission.)

antiphospholipid antibodies).[48-52] A dramatic fundus manifestation of SLE is represented by the presence of combined complete occlusion of the central retinal vein and artery. In this case the ophthalmoscopic picture is quite characteristic: there is diffuse whitening of all the retinal vessels with massive perivascular deposition of inflammatory cells (Fig. 42–17). The white occluded vessels have an appearance of frosted periphlebitis, since they resemble the frosted branches of a tree. Similar fundus appearance is found in an idiopathic retinal disease characterized by a frosted periphlebitis as well, which is called frosted angiitis.[53-55] The same condition may present in patients with positive an-

tiphospholipid antibodies syndrome in the absence of clinical SLE, the so-called primary antiphospholipid antibodies syndrome.[50] Simultaneous involvement of the CNS has been reported to occur more frequently in lupus patients with severe occlusive disease (73%) than in patients without such severe retinal disease (37%).[56] Histopathologic studies have shown immunoglobulin deposition in the walls of occluded vessels.[57]

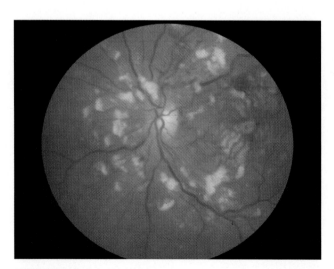

FIGURE 42–14   This patient with SLE had extensive cotton-wool spots. (From Jabs DA, Fine SL, Hochberg MC, et al: Severe retinal vaso-occlusive disease in systemic lupus erythematosus. Arch Ophthalmol 104:558–563, 1986. Copyright 1986 American Medical Association, with permission.)

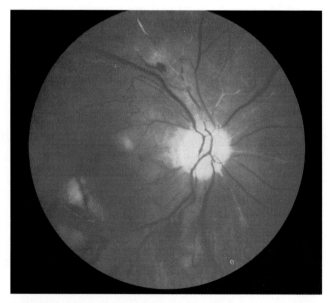

FIGURE 42–15   This lupus patient with positive antiphospholipid antibodies had severe vaso-occlusive disease. Note the presence of diffuse sheathing of the retinal vessels. (From Jabs DA, Fine SL, Hochberg MC, et al: Severe retinal vaso-occlusive disease in systemic lupus erythematosus. Arch Ophthalmol 104: 558–563, 1986. Copyright 1986 American Medical Association, with permission.)

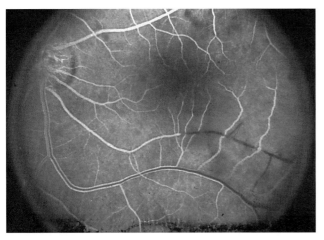

FIGURE 42–16 Fluorescein angiography photograph of a branch retinal artery occlusion in a lupus patient. (From Yannuzzi LA, Guyer DR, Green WR [eds]: The Retina Atlas. St Louis, Mosby-Year Book, 1995, with permission.)

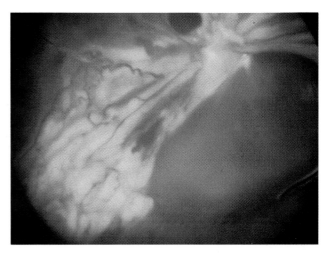

FIGURE 42–18 This lupus patient had diffuse retinal neovascularization, fibrous scarring, and tractional retinal detachment. (From Yannuzzi LA, Guyer DR, Green WR [eds]: The Retina Atlas. St Louis, Mosby-Year Book, 1995, with permission.)

Treatment. There is no known effective treatment for this severe vascular occlusive disease. However, an anticoagulant treatment may be recommended, at least to protect the fellow eye. Since extensive capillary nonperfusion may be complicated by retinal and/or disc neovascularization (Fig. 42–18), there is a rationale for laser treatment of the ischemic retina.

CHLOROQUINE MACULOPATHY. Chloroquine and hydroxychloroquine are often used to treat skin disease and arthritis in patients with SLE. A daily dose of chloroquine in excess of 250 mg, and hydroxychloroquine in excess of 750 mg for a total dose between 100 and 300 g can cause degeneration of

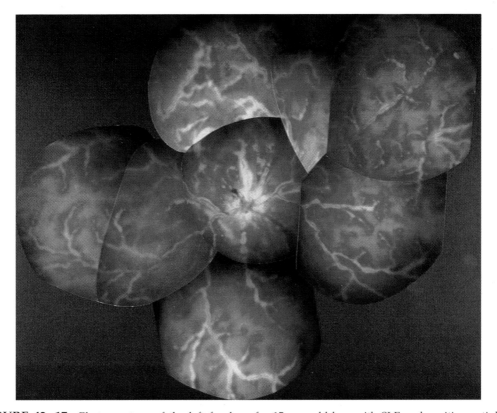

FIGURE 42–17 Photomontage of the left fundus of a 15-year-old boy with SLE and positive antiphospholipid antibodies. There was edematous optic disc, and tortuous retinal veins with a frosted phlebitis appearance. (From Snyers B, Lambert M, Hardy JP: Retinal and choroidal vaso-occlusive disease in systemic lupus erythematosus associated with antiphospholipid antibodies. Retina 10:255–260, 1990, with permission.)

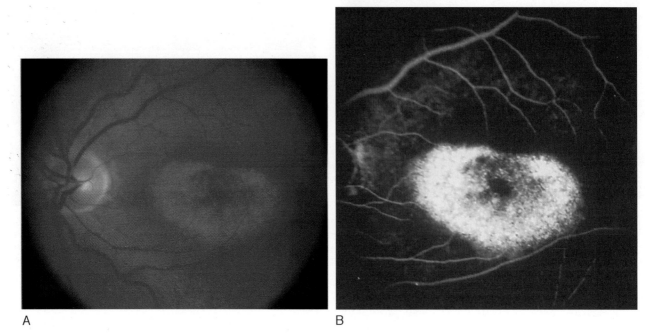

A   B

FIGURE 42–19   *A*, Clinical photograph of a lupus patient with typical bull's-eye maculopathy caused by 20 years of chloroquine treatment. *B*, Fluorescein study of the same eye better reveals the atrophic and pigmentary macular changes. (From Yannuzzi LA, Guyer DR, Green WR [eds]: The Retina Atlas. St Louis, Mosby-Year Book, 1995, with permission.)

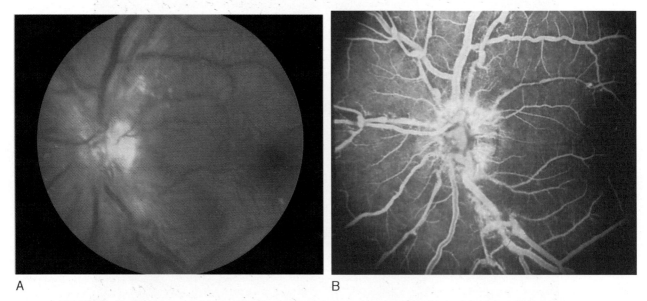

A   B

FIGURE 42–20   A 7-year-old healthy boy with 20/20 vision in both eyes was discovered during a routine eye examination to have peculiar vascular changes in the fundus of both eyes. *A*, Clinical fundus photograph of the left eye that reveals the presence of aneurysmal outpouchings along the retinal arteries, as well as edema and sheathing around the disc. There are also a few hard exudates above the papillomacular bundle. *B*, Fluorescein angiography study of the same eye that shows dye leakage from the optic disc, and from the arterial aneurysm inferotemporally. (From Kincaid J, Schatz H: Bilateral retinal arteritis with multiple aneurysmal dilatations. Retina 3:171–178, 1983, with permission.)

the retinal pigment epithelium and neurosensory retina.[58] Patients typically experience reduced or normal vision, central scotoma, and bull's-eye maculopathy (Fig. 42–19).

Treatment. Since chloroquine may remain in the RPE cells long after cessation of systemic treatment, in most cases once visual loss has occurred it may progress also after the drug has been stopped.[59]

Idiopathic Retinal Vasculitis, Aneurysms, and Neuroretinitis

Idiopathic retinal vasculitis, aneurysms, and neuroretinitis (IRVAN) is an ocular syndrome characterized by retinal artery macroaneurysms, periphlebitis, and optic disc inflammation of unknown etiology. In 1983, Kincaid and Schatz[60] first reported on two patients with bilateral retinal inflammation in which multiple aneurysmal dilatations were a major manifestation, and named the syndrome "bilateral retinal arteritis with multiple aneurysmal dilatations." In 1995, Chang et al[61] reported on ten additional cases and proposed the acronym IRVAN to highlight the salient features of this condition (idiopathic retinal vasculitis, aneurysm, and neuroretinitis). The disease usually manifests itself in the third or fourth decade of life; however, it has been reported in a 7-year-old white boy and in a 9-year-old Latina; there is no sex or race preference. Extensive medical evaluation has failed to reveal any associated systemic manifestations.

Fundus manifestations consist of numerous aneurysmal dilatations typically at and near the bifurcation site of the first and second retinal arteries. Aneurysmal dilatation may also be found on the optic nerve head. Extensive exudation from the aneurysm and intraretinal lipid deposition are usually present. Fluorescein angiography better reveals the presence of retinal and optic disc arterial aneu-

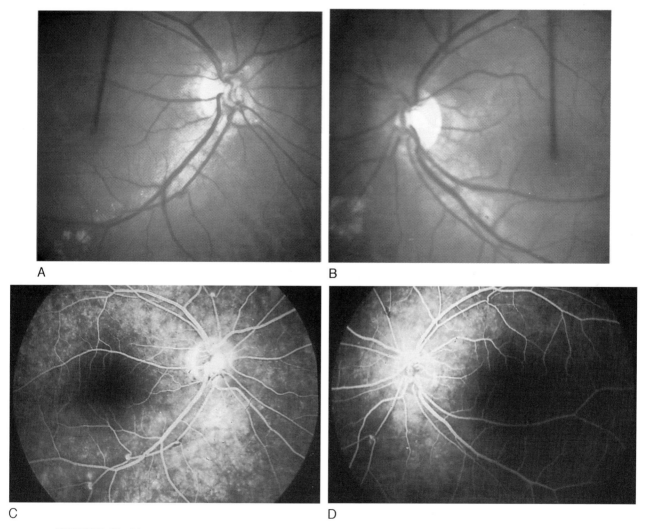

FIGURE 42–21 *A* and *B,* Clinical photograph of both eyes of a 21-year-old healthy asymptomatic Australian male. There are a few arterial aneurysms surrounded by intraretinal lipid deposition. *C* and *D,* Fluorescein study of the same patient better reveals the presence of arterial aneurysms. (Courtesy of Dr. Andrew Chang.)

rysms, and demonstrates inflammatory staining of the retinal veins and arteries as well as of the optic nerve head. While the peripheral retina may be initially unaffected, with the progression of the condition there is retinal arteriole attenuation and eventually capillary nonperfusion, that leads to extensive retinal ischemia (Figs. 42–20 through 42–24).

The course of the disease is variable. Some patients seem to retain good visual acuity, but most show progressive disease with evolution to retinal and disc neovascularization as a consequence of retinal ischemia, vitreous hemorrhage, and neovascular glaucoma. Reduction of visual acuity may be caused by direct lipid exudation in the macula, cys-

toid macular edema, vitreous hemorrhage, or neovascular glaucoma.

We have seen a 40-year-old black female with very advanced disease (Fig. 42–23). She had massive lipid deposition in the macula, extensive retinal capillary dropout, neovascular glaucoma, and non–light-perception vision in one eye. The fellow eye had already received extensive photocoagulation of the ischemic retina and presented diffuse lipid exudation at the posterior pole; visual acuity was 20/100. She had been diagnosed as a case of sarcoid retinopathy on the basis of a borderline ACE level, but fundus examination revealed the presence of the typical retinal aneurysms. Another patient, a 22-year-old asymptomatic female from

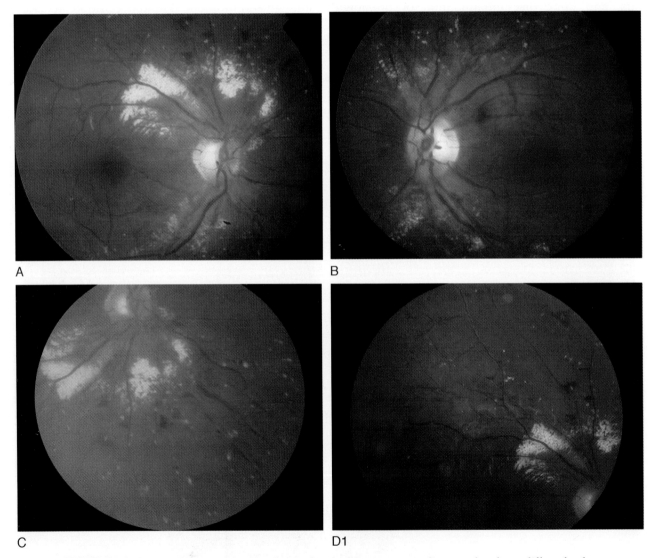

FIGURE 42–22 A 19-year-old healthy female from Afghanistan was discovered to have diffuse fundus changes during a routine eye examination. *A* through *F,* Clinical study of the fundus of both eyes. There are multiple aneurysms at and near the bifurcation site of the retinal arteries and on the optic disc as well. Note also the presence of intraretinal hemorrhages, hard exudates, and capillary nonperfusion in the periphery. *G* through *L,* Fluorescein study of the same patient. *G* and *H,* High-magnification picture of the disc and superotemporal arcade of the left eye that better shows the presence of multiple arterial aneurysms. *Illustration continued on following page*

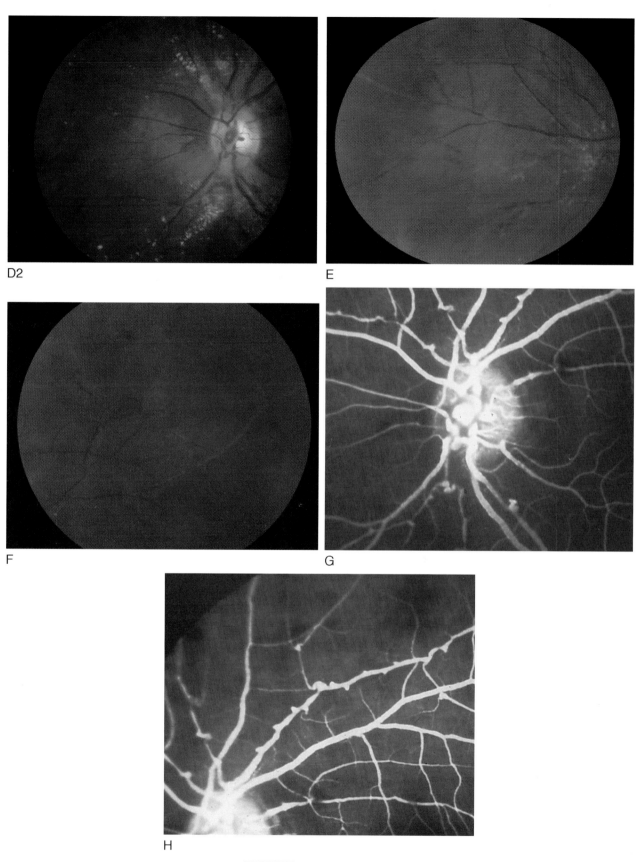

FIGURE 42–22 *Continued.*

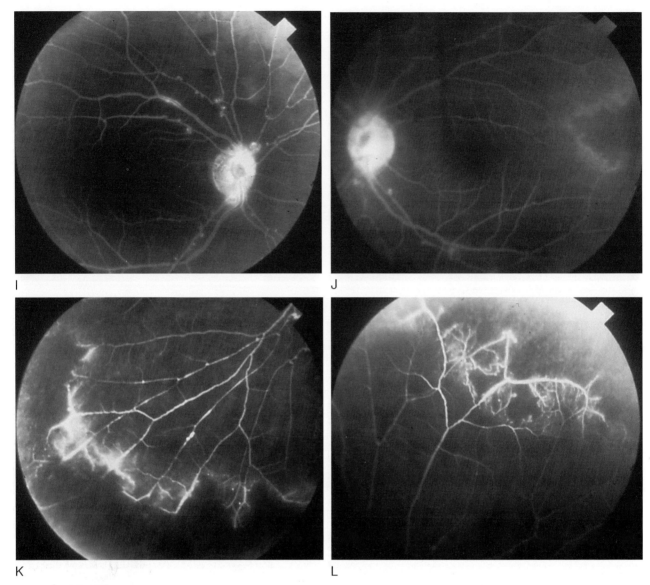

FIGURE 42–22 *Continued   I* and *J*, Late venous phase reveals the presence of leakage of dye from the optic disc and the arterial aneurysms. Note the presence of retinal ischemia in the temporal fundus of the left eye. *K* and *L*, Angiographic pictures of the peripheral fundus reveal the presence of marked capillary dropout and retinal vein anastomosis. There is leakage of dye from the inflamed retinal vessels.

Afghanistan, whom we evaluated for a second opinion, was found by her ophthalmologist during routine examination to have multiple retinal arterial aneurysms and multiple hard exudates at the posterior pole of both eyes. Fluorescein angiography revealed the presence of extensive peripheral capillary nonperfusion, although there was not yet evidence of retinal neovascularization (Fig. 42–22).

Treatment

Since the disease may present a variable course, there is no universally recognized treatment. Some patients have been treated with systemic steroids, but without any positive result. There may be an indication to direct photocoagulation of the leaking aneurysms, when lipid exudation and macular edema cause marked reduction of visual acuity; however, such laser treatment may be complicated by artery occlusion and further visual loss. Dr. Randy presented a case at the Eighth Midwest Ocular Angiography Conference[62] of a 29-year-old man with IRVAN and mild vision reduction in both eyes caused by macular edema. He performed laser photocoagulation along both sides of the retinal aneurysms, without treating directly the aneurysms. Laser treatment was followed by resolution of intraretinal exudation and macular edema, and improvement in the visual acuity. Three years later the patient was still doing very well, without any further retinal exudation (Fig. 42–24).

Extensive retinal capillary nonperfusion may be complicated as in any other situation of retinal ischemia, by secondary neovascularization of the ret-

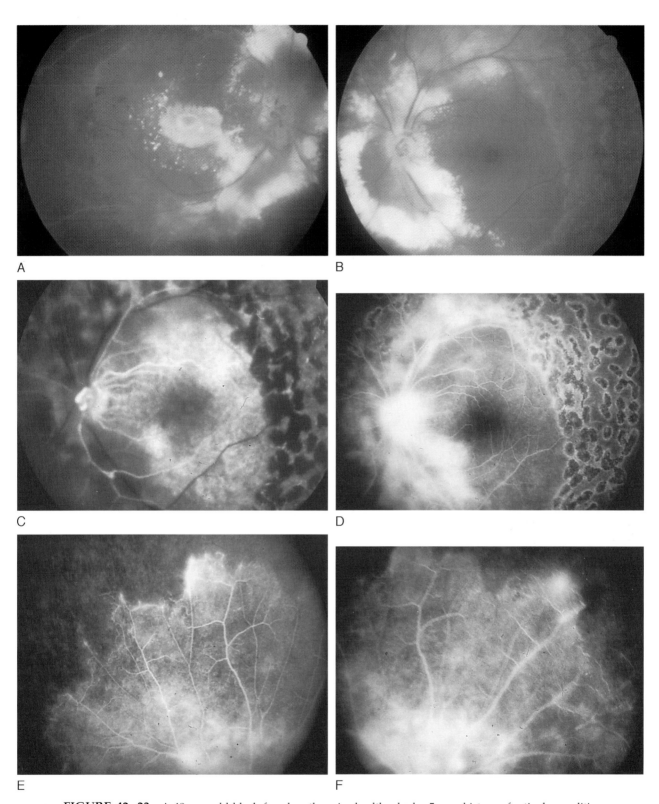

FIGURE 42–23 A 40-year-old black female, otherwise healthy, had a 5-year history of retinal vasculitis. The disease had progressed to neovascular glaucoma and non–light-perception vision in the right eye; the left eye had received panretinal photocoagulation and visual acuity was 20/80. The patient had been diagnosed having sarcoidosis on the basis of a borderline ACE level; tissue biopsy was negative. *A* and *B*, Clinical photographs of the posterior pole of both eyes show massive intraretinal lipid exudation. *C* and *D*, Fluorescein study of the left eye shows multiple retinal aneurysms and late leakage of dye from the optic nerve and the retinal vessels. *E* and *F*, Fluorescein study of the peripheral fundus of the right eye shows extensive retinal ischemia.

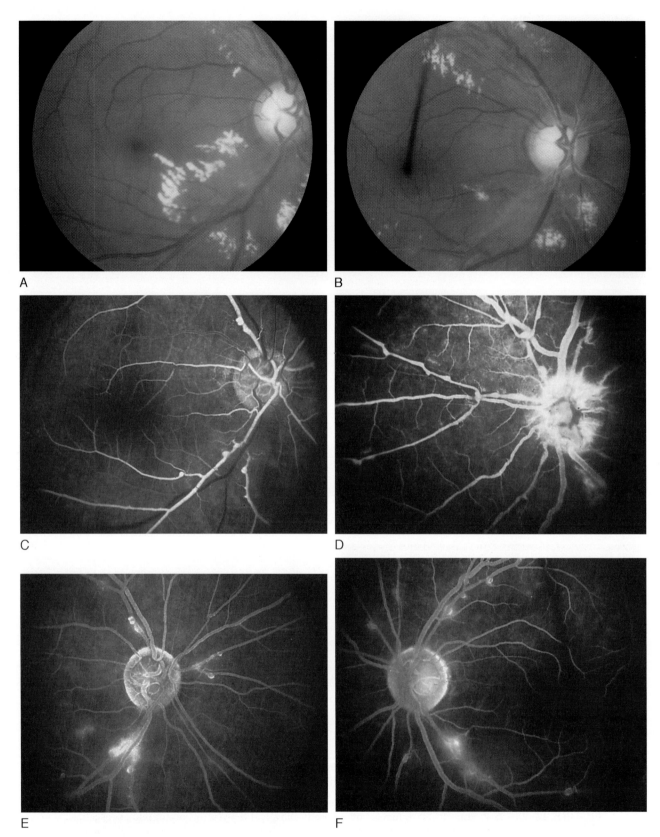

FIGURE 42–24   A 28-year-old male, who was complaining of floaters and mild decrease of vision in both eyes. *A* and *B*, Color photographs of the posterior pole of both eyes demonstrate multiple retinal arterial aneurysms and perivascular lipid exudation. *C* through *F*, Fluorescein study of the same patient show the presence of multiple arterial aneurysms, and leakage of dye from the optic nerve head, and aneurysms as well. *G* and *H*, Three years after laser photocoagulation on both sides of the aneurysmatic dilatations; there is complete resolution of the hard exudates and visual acuity is 20/20 in both eyes. *Illustration continued on opposite page*

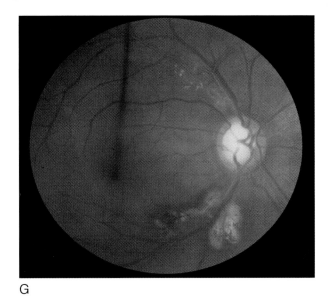

G   H

FIGURE 42–24   *Continued*

ina, disc, and/or angle. Because the limited number of patients described with this condition, there is no available clinical study; however, it appears reasonable to perform laser photocoagulation of the ischemic retina in attempting to prevent the process from evolving towards neovascular complication. Unfortunately, some cases have shown poor response to laser treatment, with progression towards neovascular glaucoma. In the presence of nonclearing vitreous hemorrhage, trans–pars plana vitrectomy is indicated, but also in this case the prognosis is usually poor, with slow progression towards end-stage disease.

In conclusion, this condition is still not well understood, the prognosis is variable, there is no known effective medical treatment, and the role of laser treatment is still controversial.

REFERENCES

1. Aydintug AO, Tokgoz G, D'Cruz DP, et al: Antibodies to endothelial cells in patients with Behçet's disease. Clin Immunol Immunopathol 67:157–162, 1993.
2. Gupta RC, O'Duffy JD, McDuffie FC, et al: Circulating immunocomplexes in Behçet's disease. Clin Exp Immunol 34:213–218, 1978.
3. Kasp E, Whiston R, Dumonde D, et al: Antibody affinity to retinal S antigen in patients with retinal vasculitis. Am J Ophthalmol 113:697–701, 1992.
4. Lehner T: Behçet's syndrome and autoimmunity. Br Med J 1:465–467, 1967.
5. Charteris DG, Champ C, Rosenthal AR, Lightman SL: Behçet's disease: activated T lymphocytes in retinal perivasculitis. Br J Ophthalmol 76:499–501, 1992.
6. Charteris DG, Barton K, McCartney AC, Lightman SL: CD4+ lymphocyte involvement in ocular Behçet's disease. Autoimmunity 12:201–206, 1992.
7. Ishimoto S, Wu GS, Hayashi S: Free radical tissue damages in the anterior segment of the eye in experimental autoimmune uveitis. Invest Ophthalmol Vis Sci 37:630–636, 1996.
8. Nork TM, Mangini NJ, Millecchia LL: Rods and cones contain antigenically distinctive S-antigens. Invest Ophthalmol Vis Sci 34:2918–2925, 1993.
9. Correlation between the physiologic and morphologic changes in experimental autoimmune uveitis induced by peptide G of S-antigen. Invest Ophthalmol Vis Sci 34:1861–1871, 1993.
10. Stanford MR, Robbins J, Kasp E: Passive administration of antibody against retinal S-antigen induces electroretinographic supernormality. Invest Ophthalmol Vis Sci 33:30–35, 1992.
11. Nussenblat RB, Palestine AG, Chan C-C: Cyclosporin A therapy in the treatment of intraocular inflammatory disease resistant to systemic corticosteroids and cytotoxic agents. Am J Ophthalmol 96:275–282, 1983.
12. Muftuoglu AU, Pazarli H, Yurdakul S, et al: Short term cyclosporin A treatment of Behçet's disease. Br J Ophthalmol 71:387–390, 1987.
13. Chavis PS, Antonios SR, Tabbara KF: Cyclosporin effects on optic nerve and retinal vasculitis in Behçet's disease. Doc Ophthalmol 80:133–142, 1992.
14. Graham EM, Stanford MR, et al: A point prevalence study of 150 patients with idiopathic retinal vasculitis: 1. Diagnostic value of ophthalmological features. Br J Ophthalmol 73:714–721, 1989.
15. Kasp E, Graham EM, et al: A point prevalence study of 150 patients with idiopathic retinal vasculitis: 2. Clinical relevance of antiretinal autoimmunity and circulating immune complexes, Br J Ophthalmol 73:722–730, 1989.
16. Forrester JV: Sarcoidosis and inflammatory eye disease. Br J Ophthalmol 76:193–194, 1992.
17. Behçet H: Uber rezidivierende, aophtose durch ein Virus verusachte Geschwure am Mund, an Auge und an den Genitalien. Dermato Wochenschr 105:1152–1157, 1937.
18. Michelson JB, Chisari FV: Behçet's disease. Surv Ophthalmol 26:190–203, 1982.
19. Poulter LW, Lehner T: Immunohistology of oral lesions from patients with recurrent oral ulcers and Behçet's syndrome. Clin Exp Immunol 78:189–195, 1989.
20. Kaneko F, Takahashi Y, Muramatsu Y, et al: Immunological studies on aphthous ulcer and erythema nodosum-like eruptions in Behçet's disease. Br J Dermatol 113:303–312, 1985.
21. Celenligil H, Kansu E, Ruacan S, et al: Characterization of peripheral blood lymphocytes and immunohistological analysis of oral ulcers in Behçet's disease. In O'Duffy JD, Kokmen E (eds): Behçet's Disease. Basic and Clinical Aspects. New York, Marcel Dekker, Inc, 1991, 487–495.

22. Kansu E, Sivri B, Sahin G et al: Endothelial cells dysfunction in Behçet's disease. In O'Duffy JD, Kokmen E (eds): Behçet's Disease. Basic and Clinical Aspects. New York, Marcel Dekker, Inc, 1991, pp. 523–530.

23. Smulders FM, Oostherius JA: Treatment of Behçet's disease with chlorambucil. Ophthalmologica 171:347–352, 1975.

24. Tabbara KF: Chlorambucil in Behçet's disease; a rappraisal. Ophthalmology 90:906–908, 1983.

25. Yazici H, Pazarli H, Barnes CG, et al: A controlled trial of azathioprine in Behçet's syndrome. N Engl J Med 322: 281–285, 1990.

26. Steinberg AD, et al: Systemic lupus erythematosus. NIH Conference (pathogenesis). Ann Intern Med 115:548, 1991.

27. Arnett FC: The genetic basis of lupus erythematosus. In Wallace D, Hahn BH (eds): Dubois' Lupus Erythematosus, 4th edition. Philadelphia, Lea & Febiger, 1992.

28. Nakamura RN, Tan EM: Update on autoantibodies to intracellular antigens in systemic rheumatic diseases. Clin Lab Med 12:1, 1992.

29. Ebling FM, Hahn BH: Pathogenic subsets of antibodies to DNA. Int Rev Immunol 5:79, 1989.

30. Sammaritano LR, Gharavi AE: Antiphospholipid antibody syndrome. Clin Lab Med 12:41, 1992.

31. Callen JP: Treatment of cutaneous lesions in patients with lupus erythematosus. Dermatol Clin 8:355, 1990.

32. Ginzler E, Schorn AK: Outcome and prognosis in systemic lupus erythematosus. Rheum Dis Clin North Am 14:67, 1988.

33. Balow JE, et al: NIH Conference: lupus nephritis (includes treatment). Ann Intern Med 106:79, 1987.

34. Nossent HC, et al: Systemic lupus erythematosus after renal transplantation: patient and graft survival and disease activity. Ann Intern Med 114:183, 1991.

35. Gass JDM, Little HL: Bilateral bullous exudative retinal detachment complicating idiopathic central serous chorioretinopathy during systemic corticosteroid therapy. Ophthalmology 102:737–747, 1995.

36. Eckstein MB, Spalton DJ, Holder G: Visual loss from central serous chorioretinopathy in systemic lupus erythematosus. Br J Ophthalmol 77:607–609, 1993.

37. Gass JDM: Stereoscopic Atlas of Macular Diseases: Diagnosis and Treatment, 4th edition. St Louis, CV Mosby Co, 1997, pp 60–61.

38. Matsuo T, Nakayama T, Koyama T, et al: Multifocal pigment epithelial damages with serous retinal detachment in systemic lupus erythematosus. Ophthalmologica 195:97–102, 1987.

39. Friberg TR, Eller AW: Serous retinal detachment resembling central serous chorioretinopathy following organ transplantation. Graefes Arch Clin Exp Ophthalmol 228: 305–309, 1990.

40. Gass JDM: Bullous retinal detachment and multiple retinal pigment epithelium detachments in patients receiving hemodialysis. Graefes Arch Clin Exp Ophthalmol 230:454–458, 1992.

41. de Venecia G: Fluorescein angiographic smoke stack. Case presentation at Verhoeff Society Meeting, Washington, DC, April 24–25, 1982.

42. Gass JDM: Central serous chorioretinopathy and white subretinal exudation during pregnancy. Arch Ophthalmol 109:677–681, 1991.

43. Carpenter MT, O'Boyle JE, Enzenauer RW, et al: Choroiditis in systemic lupus erythematosus. Am J Ophthalmol 117:535–536, 1994.

44. Diddie K, Aronson AJ, Ernest JT: Chorioretinopathy in a case of systemic lupus erythematosus. Trans American Ophthalmol Soc 75:122–131, 1977.

45. Jabs DA, Hanneken AM, Schachat AP, et al: Choroidopathy in systemic lupus erythematosus. Arch Ophthalmol 106: 230–234, 1988.

46. Gold DH, Morris DA, Henkind P: Ocular findings in systemic lupus erythematosus. Br J Ophthalmol 56:800–804, 1972.

47. Lanham JG, Barrie T, Kohner EM, et al: SLE retinopathy: evaluation by fluorescein angiography. Ann Rheum Dis 41: 473–478, 1982.

48. Pulido JS, Ward LM, Fishman GA, et al: Antiphospholipid antibodies associated with retinal vascular occlusive disease. Retina 7:215–218, 1987.

49. Levine SR, Crofts JW, Lesser GR, et al: Visual symptoms associated with the presence of a lupus anticoagulant. Ophthalmology 95:686–692, 1988.

50. Asherson RA, Merry P, Acheson JF, et al: Antiphospholipid antibodies: a risk factor for occlusive ocular vascular disease in systemic lupus erythematosus and the primary antiphospholipid syndrome. Ann Rheum Dis 48:358–361, 1989.

51. Kleiner RC, Najarian LV, Schatten S, et al: Vaso-occlusive retinopathy associated with anti-phospholipid antibodies (lupus anticoagulant retinopathy). Ophthalmology 96: 896–904, 1989.

52. Snyers B, Lambert M, Hardy JP: Retinal and choroidal vaso-occlusive disease in systemic lupus erythematosus associated with antiphospholipid antibodies. Retina 10: 255–260, 1990.

53. Watanabe Y, Takeda N, Adachi-Usami E: A case of frosted branch angiitis. Br J Ophthalmol 71:553–558, 1987.

54. Kleiner RC, Kaplan HJ, Shakin JL, et al: Acute retinal frosted periphlebitis. Am J Ophthalmol 106:27–34, 1988.

55. Cortina P, Diaz M, Espana E, et al: Acute frosted retinal periphlebitis associated with cytomegalovirus retinitis in a heart transplant patient. Retina 14:463–464, 1994.

56. Jabs DA, Fine SL, Hochberg MC, et al: Severe retinal vaso-occlusive disease in systemic lupus erythematosus. Arch Ophthalmol 104:558–563, 1986.

57. Graham EM, Spalton DJ, Barnard RO, et al: Cerebral and retinal vascular changes in systemic lupus erythematosus. Ophthalmology 92:444–448, 1985.

58. Sassani JW, Brucker AJ, Cobbs W: Progressive chloroquine retinopathy. Ann Ophthalmol 15:19–22,1983.

59. Ehrenfeld M, Nesher R, Merin S: Delayed-onset chloroquine retinopathy. Br J Ophthalmol 70:281–283, 1986.

60. Kincaid J, Schatz H: Bilateral retinal arteritis with multiple aneurysmal dilatations. Retina 3:171–178, 1983.

61. Chang TS, Aylward W, Davis JL, et al: Idiopathic retinal vasculitis, aneurysms, and neuroretinitis. Ophthalmology 102:1089–1097, 1995.

62. Randy N: Eighth Midwest Ocular Angiography Conference. July 31–August 3. Lake Louise, Canada.

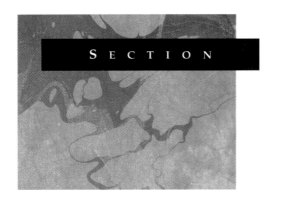

Inflammatory Disorders

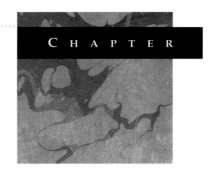

Acute Multifocal Posterior Placoid Pigment Epitheliopathy (AMPPPE)

Donald W. Park, M.D.

Howard Schatz, M.D.

H. Richard McDonald, M.D.

Robert N. Johnson, M.D.

Acute multifocal posterior placoid pigment epitheliopathy (AMPPPE) is an inflammatory syndrome affecting young adults, characterized by multiple, yellow-white, placoid subretinal lesions in the posterior pole. Gass first described the clinical and fluorescein angiographic features of AMPPPE in 1968.[1] Since then, there have been over 40 articles published about AMPPPE, and there is considerable debate over its pathogenesis.

Patients who develop AMPPPE are usually between the ages of 20 and 50, and there is no gender or racial predilection. The disorder is almost always bilateral, with the fellow eye often affected within weeks of the initial attack. Recurrences are rare but have been described.[2] Patients complain of sudden, rapid loss of vision, but a return to 20/30 or better is the norm.[2,3]

CLINICAL PRESENTATION AND ANGIOGRAPHIC FINDINGS

The intense yellow-white placoid lesions of AMPPPE begin in the posterior pole and appear biomicroscopically to be at the level of the retinal pigment epithelium (RPE) or choroid (Fig. 43–1). The lesions are discrete and lobular, with considerable variation in size and shape. The lesions may range from a few to numerous confluent lesions that encompass most of the macula (Fig. 43–2).

Within a few weeks, the acute lesions begin to fade and show retinal pigment epithelial mottling (Figs. 43–1 through 43–4). Concurrent with this healing process is the development of new lesions, both around healed lesions and in new areas of retina (Figs. 43–2 through 43–4).

The fluorescein angiogram of AMPPPE is characteristic. In the acute stages, the lesions show early choroidal hypofluorescence followed by late hyperfluorescence[4–7] (Figs. 43–1 through 43–4). The early hypofluorescence has been interpreted as being due to either blockage of fluorescence by RPE swelling,[1] blockage of fluorescence by inflammatory cells and tissue,[7] or choriocapillaris nonperfusion.[6,8] The late hyperfluorescence is thought to represent diffusion of fluorescein from the choroid into or between damaged RPE cells.[1,2] Healed AMPPPE lesions demonstrate irregularly hyperfluorescent RPE window defects (Figs. 43–2 through 43–5).

New AMPPPE lesions may develop in previously unaffected retina or adjacent to healing lesions (Figs. 43–2 through 43–4). When new, acute lesions develop around healing lesions, the early-phase fluorescein angiograms often show a ring of choroidal hypofluorescence (i.e., acute AMPPPE) surrounding an area of mottled choroidal hyperfluorescence (i.e., healed AMPPPE). This ring pattern is characteristic of AMPPPE (Figs. 43–2 through 43–4).

Recently, indocyanine green (ICG) angiography

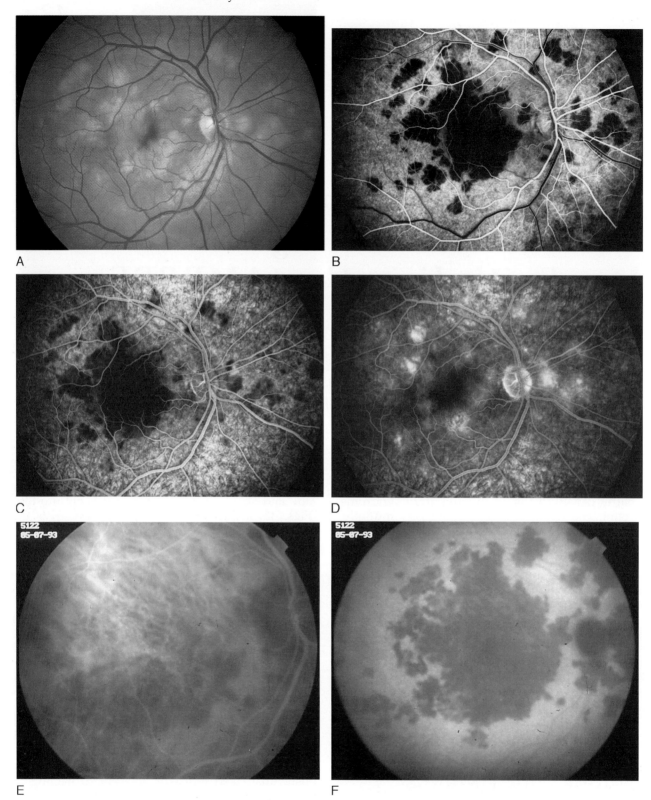

FIGURE 43–1   This 26-year-old white man complained of spots in the center of each eye. He has also had flu-like symptoms, with headaches, myalgias, and fevers for 1 week. His visual acuity measured 20/250 OU. *A*, Ophthalmoscopic photograph, right macula: note the deep, multiple, yellow-white lesions, characteristic of acute AMPPPE. *B*, Early-phase fluorescein angiogram, right macula: the lesions are hypofluorescent. *C*, Mid-phase fluorescein angiogram, right macula: note that the lesions appear smaller and less hypofluorescent. *D*, Late-phase fluorescein angiogram, right macula: the lesions show leakage having become hyperfluorescent and fuzzy. *E*, Early-phase indocyanine green angiogram, right macula: there is choroidal hypofluorescence in the central macula. Some of the larger choroidal vessels are seen within the large zone of hypofluorescence. *F*, Late-phase indocyanine green angiogram, right macula: note the large and small, well-demarcated areas of choroidal hypofluorescence. Eight months later, the vision improved to 20/20 OD and 20/50 OS; the fundi showed healed AMPPPE lesions. *Illustration continued on opposite page*

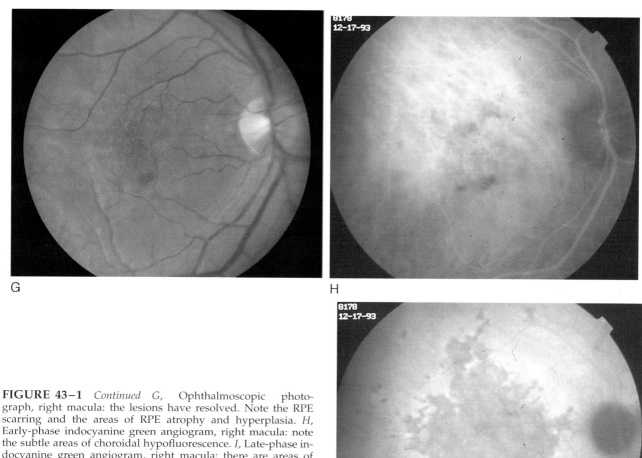

FIGURE 43–1 *Continued* G, Ophthalmoscopic photograph, right macula: the lesions have resolved. Note the RPE scarring and the areas of RPE atrophy and hyperplasia. H, Early-phase indocyanine green angiogram, right macula: note the subtle areas of choroidal hypofluorescence. I, Late-phase indocyanine green angiogram, right macula: there are areas of well-demarcated choroidal hypofluorescence. Compared to 8 months previously (F), the areas of choroidal hypofluorescence are fewer and smaller.

has become clinically available, and there have been several reports on the ICG angiography of AMPPPE.[9,10] ICG is a dye with a peak absorption and fluorescence in the near infrared region of the electromagnetic spectrum.[11,12] Moreover, because ICG is highly protein bound (98%), it is largely confined to the choroidal vasculature. As a result of these properties, ICG angiography permits better visualization of the choroidal vasculature (through overlying RPE) than does fluorescein angiography.

ICG angiography of the acute lesions in AMPPPE shows marked choroidal hypofluorescence in both the early and the late phases of the angiogram[9,10] (Fig. 43–1). In the early phases of the ICG angiogram, large choroidal vessels can be seen in these hypofluorescent areas (Fig. 43–1). In the late phases of the ICG angiogram, the hypofluorescent lesions become well demarcated and irregularly shaped (Fig. 43–1).

The ICG angiography of healed AMPPPE lesions also demonstrates choroidal hypofluorescence in the early and late phases of the angiogram. The hypofluorescent lesions of healed AMPPPE are smaller and less pronounced than the lesions of acute AMPPPE (Fig. 43–1).

VISUAL FIELDS AND ELECTROPHYSIOLOGIC TESTING

Visual field testing has shown variable results. Patients with acute and healed AMPPPE may have paracentral scotomas.[2,13] However, normal visual fields,[14] moderate scotomas,[15] and dense scotomas[14,15] have all been reported in eyes with AMPPPE. These findings most likely result from

Text continued on page 545

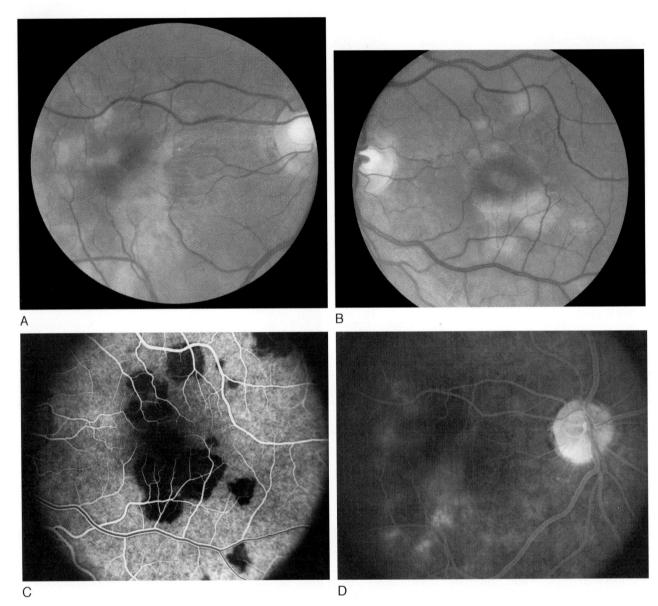

FIGURE 43–2   This 27-year-old white man complained of blurred and distorted vision in each eye. His visual acuity measured 20/25 OD and 20/200 OS. Ophthalmoscopic photograph, right (*A*) and left (*B*) macula: note the yellow-white, acute AMPPPE lesions in each macula. *C*, Mid-phase fluorescein angiogram, left macula: the lesions show choroidal hypofluorescence. Late-phase fluorescein angiogram, right (*D*) and left (*E*) macula: the lesions show leakage with faint, fuzzy, hyperfluorescent staining. One week later, the patient said that the vision in his right eye had markedly declined. His visual acuity measured 20/200 OD and 20/100 OS. *Illustration continued on opposite page*

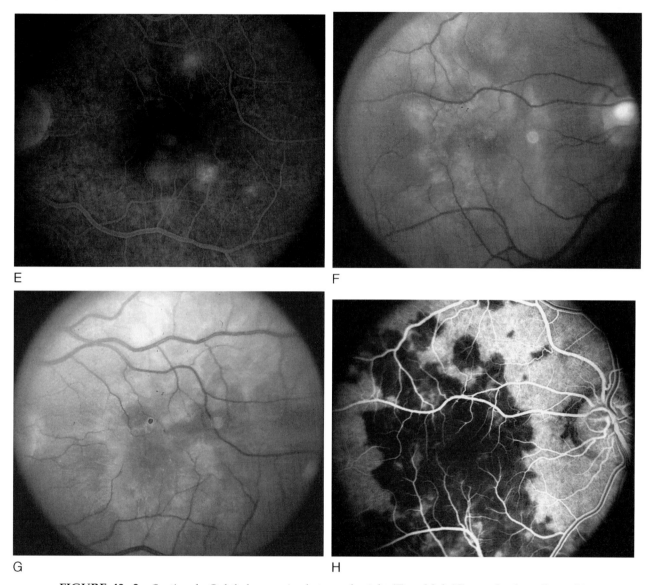

E

F

G

H

FIGURE 43–2 *Continued* Ophthalmoscopic photograph, right (*F*) and left (*G*) macula: the yellow-white lesions have greatly increased, with some contiguous to the old lesions and some in new areas of previously unaffected retina. Early-phase fluorescein angiogram, right (*H*) and left (*I*) macula: note the areas of choroidal hypofluorescence (new, acute lesions) that surround areas of choroidal hyperfluorescence (older, healing lesions). Some of the new areas of choroidal hypofluorescence (acute lesions) are separate from older lesions. *Illustration continued on following page*

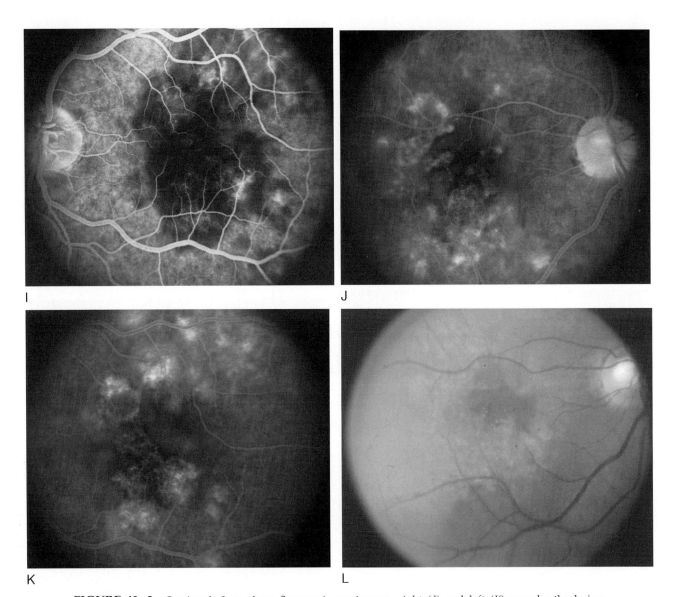

I

J

K

L

FIGURE 43–2 *Continued* Late-phase fluorescein angiogram, right (*J*) and left (*K*) macula: the lesions show leakage. Three months later, his visual acuity measured 20/100 OD and 20/50 OS. Ophthalmoscopic photograph, right (*L*) and left (*M*) macula: each macula shows extensive RPE scarring with hyperplasia and atrophy. *Illustration continued on opposite page*

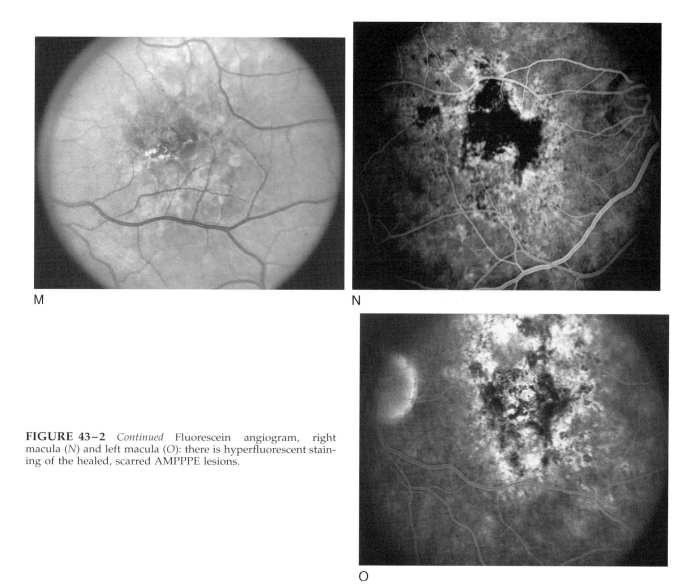

M

N

O

FIGURE 43–2 *Continued* Fluorescein angiogram, right macula (*N*) and left macula (*O*): there is hyperfluorescent staining of the healed, scarred AMPPPE lesions.

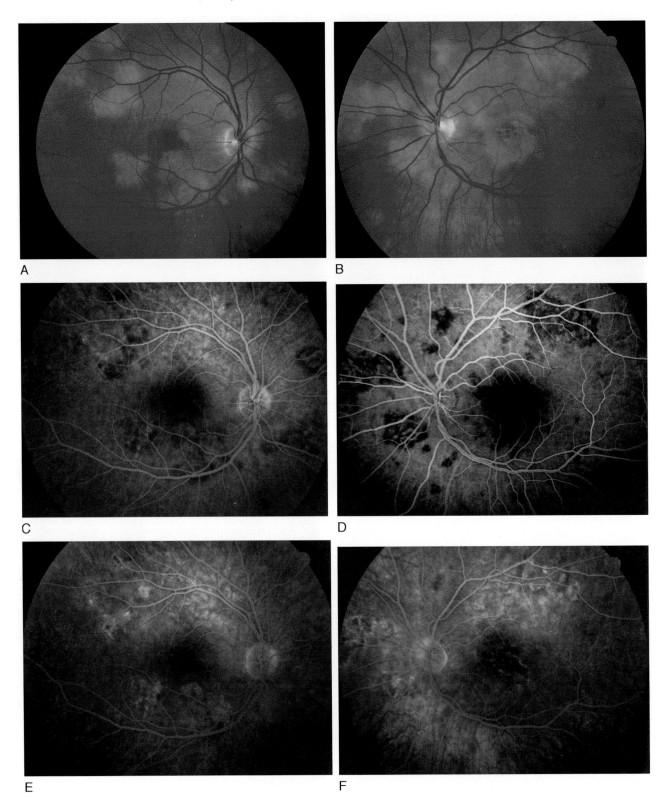

FIGURE 43–3 This 36-year-old man complained of blurred, "blocked," vision in his left eye for a week. His visual acuity measured 20/20 OD and 20/250 OS. Ophthalmoscopic photograph, right (A) and left (B) macula: there are numerous yellow-white lesions in posterior pole. The centers of some of the lesions in the left macula are beginning to heal and show RPE mottling. Fluorescein angiogram, right (C) and left (D) macula: note the areas of irregularly, mottled choroidal hyperfluorescence (healing lesions) surrounded by areas of choroidal hypofluorescence (acute lesions). In some lesions, the areas of choroidal hypofluorescence (more acute lesions) surround the areas of choroidal hyperfluorescent (healing lesions) in a ring-like fashion. Late-phase fluorescein angiogram, right (E) and left (F) macula: there is mild hyperfluorescent staining of the lesions. One month later, his visual acuity measured 20/20 OD and 20/250 OS. *Illustration continued on opposite page*

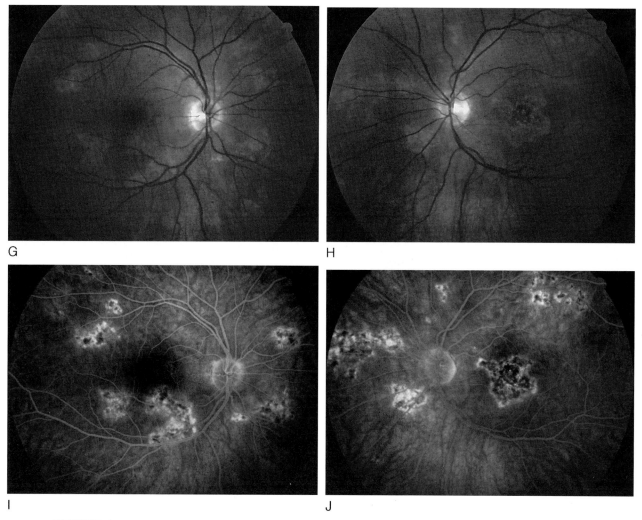

FIGURE 43–3 *Continued* Ophthalmoscopic photographs, right (*G*) and left (*H*) macula: note the RPE mottling and atrophy (i.e., healing lesions) in each macula. Late-phase fluorescein angiogram, right (*I*) and left (*J*) macula: the lesions in each macula stain.

different levels of damage to the overlying RPE and photoreceptor cells. Greater inflammation and damage to these cells increase the likelihood of permanent visual field defects.

The results of electrophysiologic testing in AMPPPE patients also depend on the extent and severity of the disease. The electroretinogram (ERG) and electro-oculogram (EOG) have been reported to be abnormal in some patients[13,16,17] and normal in others.[2,14] Gass,[2] however, reported that most patients with acute AMPPPE seen at the Bascom Palmer Eye Institute have normal ERGs and EOGs.

Abnormalities in dark adaption, color vision, and Stiles-Crawford effect were demonstrated in a patient with AMPPPE.[18] One year after the initial attack, these tests returned to almost normal. Retinal densitometry has also been used to measure cone photopigment kinetics in patients with AMPPPE. In the acute stages of AMPPPE, cone pigment regeneration was found to be slowed, with

variable improvement over time.[19,20] Great variability among patients in the severity of defects and the time to improvement has been noted.[20]

The results of the electrophysiologic testing suggest that there may be widespread damage to the retinal pigment epithelium and the photoreceptors in AMPPPE. The extent of damage, however, varies and depends on the severity of the disease.

OCULAR ASSOCIATIONS

AMPPPE has been described with numerous ocular inflammations. Anterior uveitis,[3,14,21–32] conjunctivitis,[33] episcleritis,[3,26,27,31] marginal thinning of the cornea,[34] subconjunctival hemorrhage,[3] vitreitis,[24,28,31] disc edema,[3,14,31,34–38] retinal hemorrhages,[24,26,35] serous retinal detachments,[3,24,31,39] retinal vasculitis,[3,27,35,40,41] and retinal vascular occlusions[42,43] have all been reported with AMPPPE.

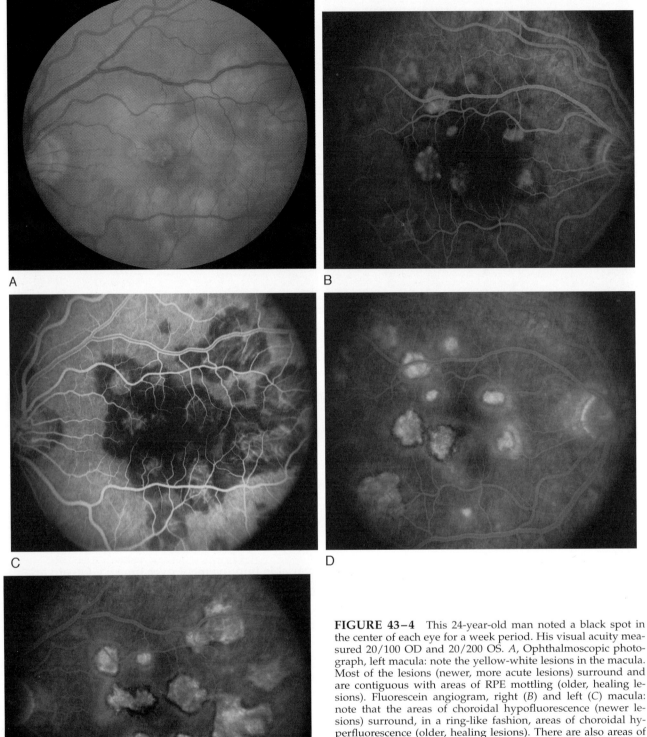

FIGURE 43–4 This 24-year-old man noted a black spot in the center of each eye for a week period. His visual acuity measured 20/100 OD and 20/200 OS. *A*, Ophthalmoscopic photograph, left macula: note the yellow-white lesions in the macula. Most of the lesions (newer, more acute lesions) surround and are contiguous with areas of RPE mottling (older, healing lesions). Fluorescein angiogram, right (*B*) and left (*C*) macula: note that the areas of choroidal hypofluorescence (newer lesions) surround, in a ring-like fashion, areas of choroidal hyperfluorescence (older, healing lesions). There are also areas of choroidal hypofluorescence that are separate from the older healing lesions. Late-phase fluorescein angiogram, right (*D*) and left (*E*) macula: the lesions stain. Note that the older lesions have relatively distinct borders, in contrast to the borders of newer more acute lesions, which appear fuzzy and diffuse.

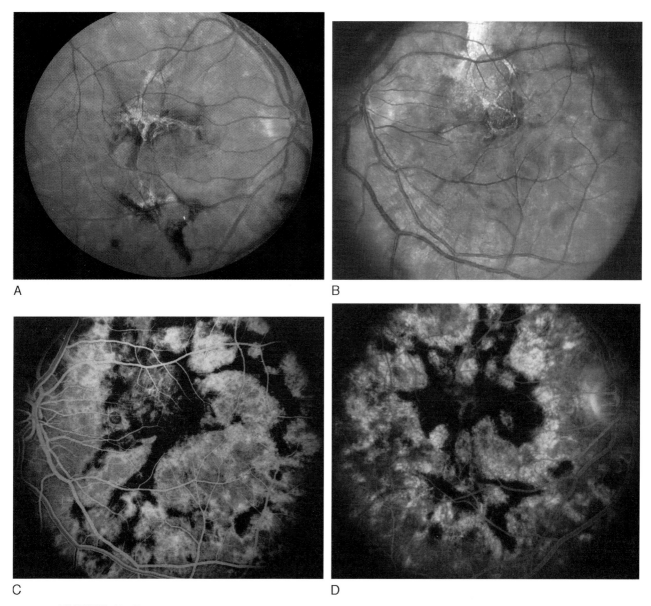

A

B

C

D

FIGURE 43–5   This 14-year-old man noted loss of vision in each eye over a 2-month period. His visual acuity measures 20/200 OU. Ophthalmoscopic photograph, right (A) and left (B) macula: note the extension, pigmented scars in each macula. Fluorescein angiogram, left macula (C) and late-phase fluorescein angiogram, right macula (D): note the areas of choroidal hypofluorescence (blockage of choroidal fluorescence by RPE hyperplasia) surrounded by areas of choroidal hyperfluorescence.

SYSTEMIC ASSOCIATIONS

AMPPPE has also been associated with systemic inflammatory diseases. These include erythema nodosum,[3,30,42,44,45] nephritis,[28,46] transient sensory neural hearing loss,[47] angioedema,[48] sarcoidosis,[49] regional enteritis,[3] and thyroiditis.[34]

In addition, cerebral spinal fluid pleocytosis[14,23,42,50] and cerebral vasculitis[13,24,51–56] have been associated with AMPPPE. Cerebral angiograms have demonstrated focal cerebral vascular narrowing.[13,24,51,53,54] Central nervous system infarcts have been documented on computed tomography (CT) scan.[53] Patients with AMPPPE have experienced ho-

monymous hemianopsias,[13,51,53] ataxia,[52,54] ocular dysmetria,[52] and dysarthria.[54]

ETIOLOGY

Infectious Etiology

Although the etiology of AMPPPE is unknown, some authors have postulated an infectious etiology. Support for this theory comes from the observation that 20 to 50% of patients with AMPPPE experience a prodromal, viral-like illness.[3,14,32,57] Acute AMPPPE has also been associated with adenovirus,[21] *Borellia burgdorferi,*[58,59] schistosomiasis,[60] and tuberculosis.[1,17,61]

Most patients with acute AMPPPE, however, show negative serologic and cerebral spinal fluid testing. Normal or negative laboratory results have been reported for the following in acute AMPPPE: adenovirus,[25,43,46,50,53] blastomycosis,[21] *Borrelia burgdorferi,*[52,53,62] California encephalitis virus,[55] coxsackievirus B5,[24,46] chlamydia,[46] coccidioidomycosis,[21,26] cytomegalovirus,[43,46,53] eastern equine encephalitis virus,[55] *Francisella tularensis,*[46] herpes simplex virus,[21,24,43,46,50] histoplasmosis,[21,25,26,34] human immunodeficiency virus,[46] influenza virus types A and B,[24,25,46,50,53] *Leptospira,*[43] measles,[43,50] mononucleosis,[35] mumps,[24,50] *mycobacterium tuberculosis,*[1,13,21,24,25,49,50,52] *Mycoplasma,*[24,46,50] parainfluenza types 1 and 3,[46,53] respiratory syncytial virus,[46,53] rotavirus,[46] rubella virus,[21] St. Louis encephalitis virus,[55] *Toxoplasma gondii,*[21,26,34,43] *Treponema pallidum,*[13,21,29,52] varicellazoster virus,[21,24,43,46,50] western equine encephalitis virus,[55] and Yersinia.[46] Although AMPPPE may be caused by an infection, it is unlikely that AMPPPE is due to a single infectious agent.

Types of Hypersensitivity Reactions and AMPPPE

Another hypothesis for the pathophysiology of AMPPPE is that AMPPPE represents an allergic or hypersensitivity reaction, of which there are several types. Type I involves IgE antibodies and the release of vasoactive amines to produce an anaphylactic reaction. Type I hypersensitivity is the basis for atopic allergies. Type II hypersensitivity reactions are antibody-dependent, cytotoxic reactions, as seen in hemolytic anemias and blood transfusion reactions. Type III hypersensitivity reactions involve the deposition of antigen–antibody complexes and the activation of complement and neutrophils, which lead to tissue damage; the Arthus reaction and serum sickness are examples of Type III hypersensitivity reactions.[63,64]

Type IV hypersensitivity, or delayed-type hypersensitivity (DTH), derives from activation of sensitized T lymphocytes and is encountered in many allergic reactions to various stimuli, including bacteria, viruses, and fungi.[63,65,66] In Type IV hypersensitivity, it is thought that previously primed T cells release lymphokines that attract and activate macrophages and cytotoxic T cells.[64] Macrophages may give rise to epithelioid cells and giant cells; these may later form granulomas.

Theory of Delayed-Type (IV) Hypersensitivity Reaction

There is strong, indirect evidence that AMPPPE may represent a Type IV, delayed-type hypersensitivity reaction.[8]

Wilson et al[55] reported an autopsy case of a 24-year-old patient with AMPPPE who had developed an associated cerebral vasculitis. The patient died of neurologic complications 1 month later. The autopsy demonstrated a primary thrombo-obliterative vasculitis of the medium-sized arterial branches of the leptomeninges. Histopathologically, the arteritis was segmental, with fibrinoid necrosis within the arterial wall. Surrounding inflammatory cells were comprised of monocytes, lymphocytes, histiocytes, epithelioid cells, and multinucleated giant cells. The inflammation disrupted the internal arterial walls and extended into the vessel lumen, causing thrombosis. The histopathology of this case is consistent with a DTH vasculitis.

AMPPPE has been associated with a host of other diseases that may represent delayed-type hypersensitivities. AMPPPE has been described with erythema nodosum.[3,16,30,42,44,45] The inflammation in erythema nodosum is thought by some to represent a delayed-type hypersensitivity.[67]

Sarcoidosis has been associated with AMPPPE. Dick et al[49] reported a 24-year-old patient with AMPPPE who developed biopsy-proven sarcoidosis 6 weeks later. A renal biopsy revealed an interstitial granulomatous nephritis, with multinucleated giant cells, lymphocytes, and plasma cells. The histopathology of the renal biopsy is consistent with a DTH reaction.

Priluck et al[28] reported leukocytic, granular, epithelial, and hyaline urinary casts in three patients with AMPPPE. These casts resolved simultaneously with the fundus lesions. Leukocytic casts are seen in interstitial nephritis, and the preponderance of T lymphocytes have led investigators[68] to propose a role for DTH in interstitial nephritis. Dick et al's[49] patient with sarcoidosis and AMPPPE also had a type of interstitial nephritis, suggesting that a similar process may have occurred in both patients.

Schistosomiasis has also been associated with AMPPPE. Dickinson et al[60] reported a 17-year-old man who, 6 weeks after returning from Tanzania, developed skin papules simultaneously with fundus lesions characteristic of AMPPPE. Biopsy of the skin lesions revealed *Schistosoma mansoni* ova. Both the skin and fundus lesions resolved after treatment with praziquantel. A delayed-type hypersensitivity reaction is thought to be responsible for the granulomas of schistosomiasis,[69] and a choroidal DTH reaction may have produced AMPPPE in this patient.

Many patients with AMPPPE have had a positive tuberculin skin test.[1,17,61] Up to 50% of patients with tuberculous meningitis have a central nervous system (CNS) arteritis, with the arteritis varying from minor intimal proliferation to an obliterative arteritis.[70] The histopathology of this obliterative arteritis demonstrates lymphocytes, macrophages, and giant cells.[70] This vasculitis is thought to account for the majority of neurologic residua after tuberculous meningitis.[70] Due to the preponderance of mononuclear cells histopathologically,[71,72] this vasculitis is thought to be DTH mediated.[70] The histopathology of DTH-mediated tuberculosis vasculitis is similar to that seen in Wilson's report of AMPPPE and CNS vasculitis.[55]

Another DTH association with AMPPPE may occur in patients who receive vaccinations. Hector[73] reported a 21-year-old who developed chills, headaches, fevers, and blurred vision within 48 hours of receiving a swine vaccine. Five days later, the patient developed fundus lesions characteristic of AMPPPE. AMPPPE has also developed in two patients within 2 weeks of receiving a booster of hepatitis B vaccine.[74] The temporal relationship of the vaccinations and fundus lesions suggest that the vaccine may have induced a hypersensitivity reaction.

Althaus et al[33] reported a 27-year-old man with AMPPPE who, 6 months later, developed an ischemic infarct in the pons. A biopsy of the tibialis anterior muscle 2 weeks later revealed a low-grade inflammation of T cells around arterioles and venules. Perivascular cuffing is characteristically seen in DTH reactions.[64]

Although the histopathology in AMPPPE is unknown, these associations imply that AMPPPE may represent a delayed-type hypersensitivity. AMPPPE most likely represents a nonspecific DTA reaction to various antigenic stimuli.

PATHOPHYSIOLOGY AND EXPLANATION OF ANGIOGRAPHIC FEATURES

Because the fluorescein and ICG angiograms of AMPPPE show choroidal hypofluorescence, the question arises as to what can cause both fluorescein and ICG angiographic hypofluorescence plus a delayed-type hypersensitivity reaction. One explanation is that choroidal fluorescence is obscured by overlying inflammatory material. This idea was proposed by Gass,[1,2] who postulated that the cloudy cytoplasm of the retinal pigment epithelium was responsible for the early hypofluorescence seen on fluorescein angiography. The theory of blockage of choroidal fluorescence by inflammatory cells and inflamed tissue is consistent with a delayed-type hypersensitivity reaction.

The arguments supporting this theory include the variability in the size and shape of the fundus lesions, the failure of the acute lesions to stain with fluorescein from the periphery, and the rapid recovery of vision in AMPPPE.[2] Others, however, suggest that shape and size of the lesions in AMPPPE are consistent with choriocapillaris lobular nonperfusion and that the lesions of AMPPPE represent multiple patches of choriocapillaris ischemia.[75] Other authors have also presented fluorescein angiograms demonstrating peripheral staining of the early hypofluorescent lesions in AMPPPE.[30,39,45] Finally, although the theory of a transient blockage of choroidal fluorescence by RPE edema, inflammatory tissue, or both best explains the prompt recovery of vision in AMPPPE, this theory seems inconsistent with the ICG hypofluorescence of healed AMPPPE lesions, which are no longer actively inflamed.

A second explanation is that choroidal hypofluorescence is caused by a reduction in choroidal vascular filling due to obstructive vasculitis.[6,36,45,75,76] Support for this theory comes from experimental animal models of choroidal vascular occlusion[36,75] and the numerous ocular and systemic vasculitides associated with AMPPPE.[3,24,35,40–42,51,56] Furthermore, the primary thrombo-obliterative vasculitis found in the postmortem study of a patient with AMPPPE[55] would further support the theory of an obstructive vasculitis causing choroidal vascular occlusion. This theory also better explains the ICG hypofluorescence of the healed lesions. Nonetheless, persistent, full choroidal occlusion seems inconsistent with the rapid resolution of the lesions and the prompt recovery of vision in AMPPPE.

It is possible, however, that AMPPPE is due to partial choroidal vascular occlusion. The arteritis in tuberculous meningitis, which is thought to be DTH-mediated, shows varied degrees of vascular occlusion.[70] AMPPPE may also be caused by variable levels of partial choroidal vascular occlusion. It has been shown that, in monkeys, 85% of the total ocular blood flow is to the choroid, and in cats, the oxygen content of choroidal venous blood is 95% of that of arterial blood.[77] In Alm and Bill's[78] feline experiments, oxygen extraction was relatively constant until choroidal blood flow rates fell below 30% of normal. This suggests that the retina needs only a fraction of normal choroidal blood flow to survive. In AMPPPE, choroidal blood flow may be reduced sufficiently to cause ICG choroidal hypofluorescence, yet provide sufficient oxygenation for visual function.

Currently, although it is not possible to disprove either the blockage of fluorescence or the choroidal vascular occlusion theories, the model of partial choroidal vascular occlusion seems consistent with the data.

There is also a possibility that the lesions in AMPPPE represent both choroidal vascular occlusion and blockage of choroidal fluorescence by inflamed tissue and inflammatory cells. Since choroidal blood flow is thought to be the highest in the body,[77,79] it is conceivable that the choriocapillaris filters antigens that initiate a DTH reaction. This reaction may involve both the choroidal vessels and the interstitium, causing hypoperfusion, as well as blockage of fluorescence by inflammatory tissue. In fact, the various diseases associated with AMPPPE are a combination of vasculitides and inflammations of connective tissue. Delayed-type hypersensitivity may cause angiographic hypofluorescence, both by blockage and by choroidal vascular occlusion. Further studies, particularly histopathologic studies, should make the explanations for choroidal

ICG hypofluorescence of acute and healed lesions clear.

DIFFERENTIAL DIAGNOSIS

The differential diagnosis of AMPPPE includes diseases that have multifocal, scattered, deep yellow-white lesions in the posterior pole. These diseases include serpiginous choroiditis; Vogt-Koyanagi-Harada syndrome; multiple evanescent white dot syndrome; multifocal choroiditis; punctate inner choroidopathy; birdshot chorioretinopathy; diffuse unilateral subacute neuroretinitis; sarcoid choroiditis; neoplasms in the choroid; and multifocal choriocapillaris infarcts due to hypertension, systemic lupus erythematosus, toxemia of pregnancy, disseminated intravascular coagulopathy, among other diseases. In most cases, the characteristic biomicroscopic and fluorescein angiographic appearance of AMPPPE is diagnostic. In the early phases of the fluorescein angiogram, most of these diseases will not have the multifocal pattern of early hypofluorescence seen in acute AMPPPE. We will discuss a few of these diseases in greater detail.

The fundus lesions of serpiginous choroiditis and AMPPPE may look similar, especially in advanced, end-stage cases. However, patients with serpiginous choroiditis tend to be older than AMPPPE patients, and there is rarely an antecedent viral-like illness.[80,81] In addition, the fundus lesions of serpiginous choroiditis are usually confluent, start in the peripapillary region, and have active elevated, inflamed margins that extend by pseudopods.[82,83] In contrast, the lesions of AMPPPE spread in a more multifocal fashion. On fluorescein angiography, the acute lesions of serpiginous choroiditis show early central hypofluorescence with a hyperfluorescent border, while the acute lesions of AMPPPE are markedly hypofluorescent. Prolonged active disease, recurrences, and secondary choroidal neovascular membranes are more common in serpiginous choroiditis than in AMPPPE. Some cases, however, have features of each condition and a specific diagnosis is not always possible.

Vogt-Koyanagi-Harada (VKH) syndrome is a systemic inflammatory disease characterized by bilateral panuveitis, optic nerve hyperemia, serous retinal detachments, CNS disease (dysacusis, headaches, meningism), and cutaneous disease (vitiligo, alopecia, poliosis). VKH is seen more commonly in Asians, Hispanics, and American Indians. Although VKH and AMPPPE may occasionally look similar,[36,39,48,84,85] the two entities appear to be distinct. AMPPPE does not have the racial predilections and cutaneous disease of VKH. Also, the two diseases are associated with different HLA types; AMPPPE has been associated with HLA-B7 and HLA-DR2,[5] while VKH has been associated with HLA-DRw53 and HLA-DR4.[84,86] The fluorescein angiogram of VKH shows multiple pinpoint hyperfluorescent dots at the level of the RPE, which leak into the subretinal space; this is markedly different from the early hypofluorescent lesions of acute AMPPPE.

Multiple evanescent white dot syndrome (MEWDS) is a disease of young adults (usually women), with multiple gray-white patches of dots at the level of the RPE, macular granularity, optic nerve edema, an enlarged blind spot on visual field testing, and reduced ERG a-wave and early receptor amplitudes.[87,88] Fluorescein angiography shows early hyperfluorescence of the white dots, often in a wreath-like pattern. MEWDS and AMPPPE can usually be differentiated, based on the distinct fluorescein angiographic and the clinical features of each disease.

PROGNOSIS AND TREATMENT

AMPPPE is usually a self-limiting disease, with rare recurrences. Within several months, most patients return to a visual acuity of 20/40 or better.[3,32,57,89] In Gass'[3] series of 58 eyes with AMPPPE, 97% had a final visual acuity of 20/30 or better. In Wolf et al's[57] series of 53 affected eyes followed for an average of 8 years, 90% achieved a visual acuity of 20/25 or better. In this study, despite excellent final visual acuities, most patients complained of persistent blurred vision, metamorphopsias, and scotomas.

There is a small subset of patients with AMPPPE who have poor final visual acuities.[27,38] In general, these patients have RPE derangements and scars in the central fovea.[32,38]

Because AMPPPE is a self-limiting disease, and most patients have good visual prognoses, they are usually followed without treatment. However, in patients with severe, persistent AMPPPE (with and without CNS involvement) some retinal specialists will prescribe systemic steroids. Although there is some evidence that steroids may have a beneficial effect,[13,53,54] no study has clearly proven the efficacy of steroids in AMPPPE. At present, there is no definitive treatment for severe AMPPPE.

CONCLUSION

AMPPPE is a disease of young adults, characterized by multifocal, yellow-white placoid lesions scattered throughout the posterior pole. The fluorescein angiographic features are characteristic and are useful in differentiating AMPPPE from other diseases. The systemic associations and recent ICG angiographic findings in AMPPPE suggest that partial choroidal vascular occlusion, secondary to a hypersensitivity-mediated obstructive vasculitis, is the cause of AMPPPE. In general, the visual prognosis in AMPPPE tends to be excellent and the disease self-limiting. Future histopathologic studies of eyes with acute AMPPPE may prove valuable in understanding the pathogenesis of this disease and help direct treatment strategies in patients with severe forms of AMPPPE.

Acknowledgments: This work was supported by the Retina Research Fund of St. Mary's Hospital and Medical Center; a grant from the Wayne and Gladys Valley Foundation, Oakland, California; Department of Ophthalmology, California Pacific Medical Center; Heed Ophthalmic Foundation and Department of Ophthalmology, University of Iowa Hospitals and Clinics.

REFERENCES

1. Gass JDM: Acute posterior multifocal placoid pigment epitheliopathy. Arch Ophthalmol 80:177–185, 1968.
2. Gass JDM: Acute posterior multifocal placoid pigment epitheliopathy. In Gass JDM (ed): Stereoscopic Atlas of Macular Diseases. Washington, DC, CV Mosby Co, 1987, pp 504–509.
3. Gass JDM: Acute posterior multifocal placoid pigment epitheliopathy: a long-term follow-up study. In Fine SL, Owens SL (eds): Management of Retinal Vascular and Macular Disorders. Baltimore, Williams & Wilkins, 1983, pp 176–181.
4. Schatz H, Burton TC, Yannuzzi LA, et al: Blocked choroidal fluorescence. In Schatz H, Burton TC, Yannuzzi LA, et al (eds): Interpretation of fundus fluorescein angiography. St Louis, CV Mosby Co, 1978, pp 109–160.
5. Wolf MD, Folk JC, Panknen CA, et al: HLA-B7 and HLA-DR2 antigens and acute posterior multifocal placoid pigment epitheliopathy. Arch Ophthalmol 108:698–700, 1990.
6. Deutman AF, Lion F: Choriocapillaris nonperfusion in acute posterior multifocal placoid pigment epitheliopathy. Am J Ophthalmol 84:652–657, 1977.
7. Schatz H: Other retinal pigment epithelial diseases. Intern Ophthalmol Clin 15(1):181–197, 1975.
8. Park D, Schatz H, McDonald HR, Johnson RN: Acute multifocal posterior placoid pigment epitheliopathy: a theory of pathogenesis. Retina 15:351–352, 1995.
9. Park D, Schatz H, McDonald HR, Johnson RN: Indocyanine green angiography of acute multifocal posterior placoid pigment epitheliopathy. Ophthalmology 102:1877–1883, 1995.
10. Dhaliwal RS, Maguire AM, Flower RW, et al: Acute posterior multifocal placoid pigment epitheliopathy. An Indocyanine green angiographic study. Retina 13:317–325, 1993.
11. Guyer DR, Puliafito CA, Mones JM, et al: Digital indocyanine-green angiography in chorioretinal disorders. Ophthalmology 99:287–291, 1992.
12. Yannuzzi LA, Slakter JS, Sorenson JA, et al. Digital indocyanine green videoangiography and choroidal neovascularization. Retina 12:191–223, 1992.
13. Smith CH, Savino PJ, Beck RW, et al: Acute posterior multifocal placoid pigment epitheliopathy and cerebral vasculitis. Arch Neurol 40:48–50, 1983.
14. Ryan SJ, Maumenee AE: Acute posterior multifocal placoid pigment epitheliopathy. Am J Ophthalmol 74:1066–1074, 1972.
15. Autzen T, Faurschou S: Acute posterior multifocal placoid pigment epitheliopathy. Acta Ophthalmol 64:267–270, 1986.
16. Deutman AF, Oosterhuis JA, Boen-Tan TN, et al: Acute posterior multifocal placoid pigment epitheliopathy: pigment epitheliopathy or choriocapillaritis. Br J Ophthalmol 56:863–874, 1972.
17. Fishman GA, Rabb MF, Kaplan J: Acute posterior multi-
18. Smith VC, Pokorny J, Ernest JT, Starr SJ: Visual function in acute posterior multifocal placoid pigment epitheliopathy. Am J Ophthalmol 85:192–199, 1978.
19. Hansen RM, Fulton AB: Cone pigment in acute posterior multifocal placoid pigment epitheliopathy. Am J Ophthalmol 91:465–468, 1981.
20. Keunen JEE, van Meel GJ, van Norren D, et al: Retinal densitometry in acute posterior multifocal placoid pigment epitheliopathy. Invest Ophthalmol Vis Sci 30:1515–1521, 1989.
21. Azar P, Gohd RS, Waltman D, et al: Acute posterior multifocal placoid pigment epitheliopathy associated with an adenovirus type 5 infection. Am J Ophthalmol 80:1003–1005, 1975.
22. Jenkins RB, Savino PJ, Pilerton AR: Placoid pigment epitheliopathy with swelling of the optic disks. Arch Neurol 29:204–205, 1973.
23. Bullock JD, Flectcher RL: Cerebrospinal fluid abnormalities in acute posterior multifocal placoid pigment epitheliopathy. Am J Ophthalmol 84:45–49, 1977.
24. Holt WS, Regan CD, Trempe C: Acute posterior multifocal placoid pigment epitheliopathy. Am J Ophthalmol 81:403–412, 1976.
25. Fitzpatrick PJ, Robertson DM: Acute posterior multifocal placoid pigment epitheliopathy. Arch Ophthalmol 89:373–376, 1973.
26. Annesley WH, Tomer TL, Shields JA: Multifocal placoid pigment epitheliopathy. Am J Ophthalmol 76:511–518, 1973.
27. Damato BE, Nanjiani M, Foulds WS: Acute posterior multifocal placoid pigment epitheliopathy. A follow up study. Trans Ophthalmol Soc U K 103:517, 1983.
28. Priluck IA, Robertson DM, Buettner H: Acute posterior multifocal placoid pigment epitheliopathy: urinary findings. Arch Ophthalmol 99:1560–1562, 1981.
29. Lowes M: Placoid pigment epitheliopathy presenting as an anterior uveitis. A case report. Acta Ophthalmol 55:800–806, 1977.
30. Van Buskirk EM, Lessell S, Friedman E: Pigmentary epitheliopathy and erythema nodosum. Arch Ophthalmol 85:369–372, 1971.
31. Savino PJ, Weinberg RJ, Yassin JG, et al: Diverse manifestations of acute multifocal placoid pigment epitheliopathy. Am J Ophthalmol 77:659–662, 1974.
32. Williams DF, Mieler WF: Long-term follow-up of acute multifocal posterior placoid pigment epitheliopathy. Br J Ophthalmol 73:985–990, 1989.
33. Althaus C, Unsold R, Figge C, et al: Cerebral complications in acute posterior multifocal placoid pigment epitheliopathy. Ger J Ophthalmol 2:150–154, 1993.
34. Jacklin HN: Acute posterior multifocal placoid pigment epitheliopathy and thyroiditis. Arch Ophthalmol 95:189–194, 1977.
35. Kirkham TH, Ffytche TJ, Sanders MD: Placoid pigment epitheliopathy with retinal vasculitis and papillitis. Br J Ophthalmol 56:875–880, 1972.
36. Young NJA, Bird AC, Sehmi K: Pigment epithelial diseases with abnormal choroidal perfusion. Am J Ophthalmol 90:607–618, 1980.
37. Frohman LP, Klug R, Bielory L, et al: Acute posterior multifocal placoid pigment epitheliopathy with unilateral retinal lesions and bilateral disc edema. Am J Ophthalmol 104:548–550, 1987.
38. Murray SB: Acute posterior multifocal placoid pigment epitheliopathy. Not so benign? Trans Ophthal Soc U K 99:497–500, 1979.
39. Bird AC, Hamilton AM: Placoid pigment epitheliopathy presenting with bilateral serous retinal detachment. Br J Ophthalmol 56:881–886, 1972.
40. Damato BE, Nanjiani M, Foulds WS: Acute posterior multifocal placoid pigment epitheliopathy. Trans Ophthal Soc U K 103:517–522, 1989.
41. Isashiki M, Koide H, Yamashita T, et al: Acute posterior

multifocal placoid pigment epitheliopathy associated with diffuse retinal vasculitis and late haemorrhagic macular detachment. Br J Ophthalmol 70:255–259, 1986.

42. Deutman AF. Acute multifocal ischemic choroidopathy and the choriocapillaris. Int Ophthalmol 6:155–160, 1983.

43. Charteris DG, Khanna V, Dhillon B: Acute posterior multifocal placoid pigment epitheliopathy complicated by central retinal vein occlusion. Br J Ophthalmol 73:765–768, 1989.

44. Lyness AL, Bird AC: Recurrences of acute posterior multifocal placoid pigment epitheliopathy. Am J Ophthalmol 98:203–207, 1984.

45. Laatikainen L, Erkkila H: Clinical and fluorescein angiographic findings of acute multifocal central subretinal inflammation. Acta Ophthalmol 51:645–655, 1973.

46. Laatikainen LT, Immonen I: Acute posterior multifocal placoid pigment epitheliopathy in connection with acute nephritis. Retina 8:122–124, 1988.

47. Clearkin LG, Hung SO: Acute posterior multifocal placoid pigment epitheliopathy associated with transient hearing loss. Trans Ophthalmol Soc U K 103:562–564, 1983.

48. Wright BE, Bird AC, Hamilton AM: Placoid pigment epitheliopathy and Harada's disease. Br J Ophthalmol 62:609–621, 1978.

49. Dick DJ, Newman PK, Richardson J, et al: Acute posterior multifocal placoid pigment epitheliopathy and sarcoidosis. Br J Ophthalmol 72:74–77, 1988.

50. Fishman GA, Baskin M, Jednock N: Spinal fluid pleocytosis in acute posterior multifocal placoid pigment epitheliopathy. Ann Ophthalmol 9:33–36, 1977.

51. Seigelman J, Behren M, Hilal S: Acute posterior multifocal placoid pigment epitheliopathy associated with cerebral vasculitis and homonymous hemianopsia. Am J Ophthalmol 88:919–924, 1979.

52. Kersten DH, Lessell S, Carlow TJ: Acute posterior multifocal placoid pigment epitheliopathy and late-onset meningo-encephalitis. Ophthalmology 94:393–396, 1987.

53. Weinstein JM, Bresnick GH, Bell CL: Acute posterior multifocal placoid pigment epitheliopathy associated with cerebral vasculitis. J Clin Neuroophthalmol 8:195–201, 1988.

54. Stoll G, Reiners K, Schwartz A, et al: Acute posterior multifocal placoid pigment epitheliopathy with cerebral involvement. J Neurol Neurosurg Psychiatry 54:77–79, 1991.

55. Wilson CA, Choromokos EA, Sheppard R: Acute posterior multifocal placoid pigment epitheliopathy and cerebral vasculitis. Arch Ophthalmol 106:796–800, 1988.

56. Hammer ME, Grizzard WS, Travies D: Death associated with acute multifocal placoid pigment epitheliopathy. Arch Ophthalmol 107:170–171, 1989.

57. Wolf MD, Alward WLM, Folk JC: Long-term visual function in acute posterior multifocal placoid pigment epitheliopathy. Arch Ophthalmol 109:800–803, 1991.

58. Bodine SR, Marino J, Camisa TJ, et al: Multifocal choroiditis with evidence of lyme disease. Ann Ophthalmol 24:169–173, 1992.

59. Weigand W. Augenbefunde bei Borreliose-bilateral panuveitis mit exsudativer amatio. Fortschr Ophthalmol 86:659–662, 1989.

60. Dickinson AJ, Rosenthal AR, Nicholson KG: Inflammation of the retinal pigment epithelium: unique presentation of ocular schistosomiasis. Br J Ophthalmol 74:440–442, 1990.

61. Brown M, Eberdt A, Ladas G: Pigment epitheliopathy in a patient with mycobacterial infection. J Pediatr Ophthalmol 10:278–281, 1973.

62. Wolf MD, Folk JC, Nelson JA, Peeples ME: Acute, posterior, multifocal, placoid pigment epitheliopathy and Lyme disease. Arch Ophthalmol 110:750, 1992.

63. Roitt I: Hypersensitivity. In Roitt I (ed): Essential Immunology. Palo Alto, CA, Blackwell Scientific Publications, 1988, pp 193–214.

64. Robbins SL, Cotran RS, Kumar V: Diseases of Immunity. In Robbins SL, Cotran RS, Kumar V (eds): Pathologic Basis of Disease. Philadelphia, WB Saunders Co, 1984, pp 159–213.

65. Green MI, Fields BN: Host response to viruses. In Samter

M, Talmage DW, Frank MM, et al (eds): Immunological Diseases. Boston, Little, Brown & Co, 1988, pp 899–921.

66. Turk JL: Production of delayed hypersensitivity and its manifestations. In Turk JL (ed): Delayed Hypersensitivity. New York, Elsevier/North-Holland Biomedical Press, 1980, pp 13–43.

67. Winkelmann RK, Forstrom L: New Observations in the histopathology of erythema nodosum. J Invest Derm 65:441–446, 1975.

68. Keane WF, Michael AL: Renal disease. In Samter M, Talmage DW, Frank MM, et al (eds): Immunological Diseases. Boston, Little, Brown & Co, 1988, pp 1809–1850.

69. Turk JL: The role of delayed hypersensitivity in granuloma formation. In Turk JL (ed): Delayed Hypersensitivity. New York: Elsevier/North-Holland Biomedical Press; 1980, pp 275–288.

70. Bullock WE: Immunological aspects of mycobacterial infection. In Samter M, Talmage DW, Frank MM, et al (eds): Immunological Diseases. Boston, Little, Brown & Co, 1988, pp 833–861.

71. Doniach I: Changes in the meningeal vessels in acute and chronic (streptomycin-treated) tuberculous meningitis. J Pathol Bacteriol 61:253–259, 1949.

72. Poltera AA: Thrombogenic intracranial vasculitis in tuberculous meningitis. Acta Neurol Belg 77:12–24, 1977.

73. Hector RE: Acute posterior multifocal placoid pigment epitheliopathy. Am J Ophthalmol 86:424–425, 1978.

74. Brezin AP, Massin-Korobelnik P, Boudin M, et al: Acute posterior multifocal placoid pigment epitheliopathy after hepatitis B vaccine. Arch Ophthalmol 113:297–300, 1995.

75. Hayreh SS, Baines JAB: Occlusion of the posterior ciliary artery: II. Chorio-retinal lesions. Br J Ophthalmol 56:736–753, 1972.

76. Hedges TR, Sinclair SH, Gargoudas ES: Evidence for vasculitis in acute posterior multifocal placoid pigment epitheliopathy. Ann Ophthalmol 11:539–542, 1979.

77. Bill A: Blood circulation and fluid dynamics in the eye. Physiol Rev 55:383–417, 1975.

78. Alm A, Bill A: Blood flow and oxygen extraction in the cat uvea at normal and high intraocular pressures. Acta Physiol Scand 80:19–28, 1970.

79. Hayreh SS: Acute choroidal ischaemia. Trans Ophthalmol Soc U K 100:400–407, 1980.

80. Schatz H, Gitter KA, Yannuzzi LA: Inflammation of the pigment epithelium and choriocapillaris. In Yannuzzi LA, Gitter KA, Schatz H (eds): The Macula. Baltimore, Williams & Wilkins, 1979, p 247.

81. Weiss WH, Annesley WH, Shields JA, et al: The clinical course of serpiginous choroidopathy. Am J Ophthalmol 87:133–142, 1979.

82. Schatz H, Maumenee AE, Patz A: Geographic helicoid peripapillary choroidopathy: clinical presentation and fluorescein angiographic findings. Trans Acad Ophthamol & Otolaryngol 78:747–761, 1974.

83. Hardy RA, Schatz H: Macular geographic helicoid choriodopathy. Arch Ophthalmol 105:1237–1242, 1987.

84. Ohno S: Immunological aspects of Behçet's and Vogt-Koyanagi-Harada's diseases. Trans Ophthalmol Soc U K 191:335–341, 1981.

85. Kayazama F, Takahashi H: Acute posterior multifocal placoid pigment epitheliopathy and Harada's disease. Ann Ophthalmol 15:58–62, 1983.

86. Davis JL, Mittal KK, Freidlin V, et al: HLA associations and ancestry in Vogt-Koyanagi-Harada disease and sympathetic ophthalmia. Ophthalmology 97:1137–1142, 1990.

87. Jampol LM, Sieving PA, Pugh D, et al: Multiple evanescent white dot syndrome. I. Clinical findings. Arch Ophthalmol 102:671–674, 1984.

88. Sieving PA, Fishman GA, Jampol LM, Pugh D: Multiple evanescent white dot syndrome. II. Electrophysiology of the photoreceptors during retinal pigment epithelial disease. Arch Ophthalmol 102:675–679, 1984.

89. Lewis RA, Martonyi CL: Acute posterior multifocal placoid pigment epitheliopathy. Arch Ophthalmol 93:235–238, 1975.

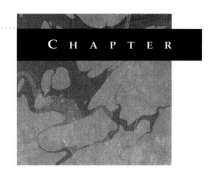

CHAPTER 44

Serpiginous Choroiditis

David Tom, M.D.

Lawrence A. Yannuzzi, M.D.

"... a rare affection often becomes less rare when given an appropriate name."

A. Franceschetti, 1961

Serpiginous choroiditis, because of its rarity and variable presentation, has been described throughout the past half century or more by a great multitude of names. It has been termed geographic helicoid peripapillary choroidopathy,[1,2] geographic choroiditis,[3-8] helicoid peripapillar chorioretinal degeneration,[9,10] geographic choroidopathy,[11,12] serpiginous choroidopathy,[13-17] macular geographic helicoid choroidopathy,[18] and macular serpiginous choroiditis.[19] Helicoid chorioretinal abiotrophy, choroiditis areata, circumpapillary dysgenesis of the pigment epithelium, chorioretinitis striata, helicoid degeneration, and helicoid peripapillary chorioretinal atrophy are a group of disorders whose morphologic description most likely represented variants of the same disease process.[4,8,9,20,21]

This rather rare, chronic, and progressive disease is typically bilateral and represents a pathologic affliction of the retinal pigment epithelium, choriocapillaris, and inner choroid with disruption of the overlying neurosensory retina marked by periods of activity with intervening intervals of quiescence. The active state is characterized by well-demarcated grayish white to yellow lesions at the level of the retinal pigment epithelium and inner choroid, generally but not always beginning at the juxtapapillary region. The lesions can present in or be confined to the macular region, and this form of serpiginous choroiditis is thought to portend a poorer visual prognosis.[18,19] However, the usual hallmark of this disease is relentless extension of prior peripapillary lesions toward the macular and peripheral retina in a helicoid or centrifugal fashion leaving, weeks to months later, a geographical configuration of chorioretinal atrophy, with or without pigmentary disturbances, in its wake. There may exist noncontiguous or skip lesions that may arise independent of previously affected sites.[1,6,11] Less frequently, lesions may extend in a centripetal fashion, spiraling toward the optic disc from the macular or even the far peripheral retina.[16] Given the unpredictability of disease progression, the fovea is never truly safe from eventual involvement. Indeed, it is not usually until the fovea or parafovea region is affected that the patient is aware of having the disease.

CLINICAL CHARACTERISTICS

Age

The typical patient is young to middle aged, with reported ages ranging from 20 to 70[6,16,18,22,23] at initial presentation. There have been reports of patients diagnosed in the middle to late teens.[24,25] Sveinsson reported on an asymptomatic child, age 4, in a family with helicoid peripapillary chorioretinal degeneration.[10]

Sex

There is no male or female predilection, although in some series there appears to be a male preponderance.[1,6,9,16,19,23]

Race

Early studies demonstrated a Caucasian predominance; however, blacks,[16,19] Hispanics,[19] and

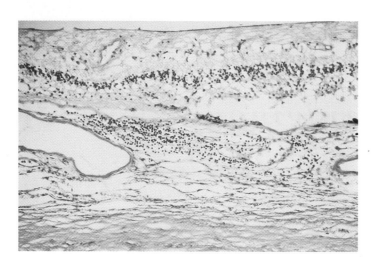

Margin of lesion in serpiginous choroiditis with loss of retinal pigment epithelium and photoreceptor cell layer (*to the left*). Choroidal vein is markedly dilated and an intense lymphocytic infiltrate is present. (From Wu JS, Lewis L, Fine SL, et al: Clinicopathologic findings in a patient with serpiginous choroiditis and treated choroidal neovascularization. Retina 9:292–301, 1989, with permission.)

Asians[26] have subsequently been reported in the literature.

Laterality

The great majority of patients present or eventually develop signs of serpiginous choroiditis in both eyes, usually with asymmetric involvement. If the disease remains unilateral, some authors feel this portends a better visual prognosis.[18]

CLINICAL PRESENTATION

Visual Complaints

The typical patient complains of an abrupt, painless blurring or fogging of vision. A central or paracentral scotoma, either relative or absolute, may also bring the patient into the office. Less commonly, flashes of light,[3,8,23] metamorphopsia,[8,23] or spots[21] may be the presenting symptom. Visual acuity usually ranges from 20/20 to 20/400,[1,18] although visions of finger count to hand motion have been reported on initial presentation.[6,23,27,28]

Ophthalmoscopic and Clinical Features

The acute disease process is manifested by gray, cream to yellow discoloration, with variable degrees of edema, at the level of the retinal pigment epithelium, with a pseudopodal configuration extending in a centrifugal or helicoid manner from the optic disc (Fig. 44–1). Acute lesions begin to fade in the ensuing weeks with development of chorioretinal atrophy and retinal pigment epithelial

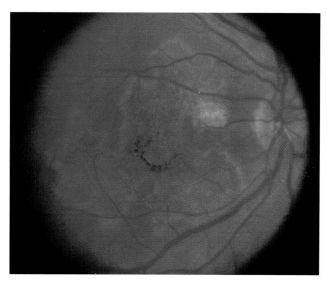

FIGURE 44–2 Subacute stage of serpiginous choroiditis is manifested by the development of chorioretinal atrophy, retinal pigment epithelium migration, and enhanced visibility of the underlying choroidal vasculature.

migration, resulting in a mottled appearance and enhanced visibility of the large choroidal vasculature (Fig. 44–2). Usually at time of presentation, the fundus displays evidence of prior disease with areas of atrophic retinal pigment epithelium, choriocapillaris, and inner choroid with variable retinal pigment epithelium derangement, clumping, and fibrous metaplasia.[1,6,16,29,30] These old, inactive lesions usually, but not always, are contiguous with the new lesion[1,6,11] (Fig. 44–3). Skip or noncontiguous lesions have been reported and may represent new and independent foci of involvement[1,6,11] (Fig. 44–4). Vitreal cells are absent in the majority of cases but may be present, particularly during the active phase, and have been reported in one third

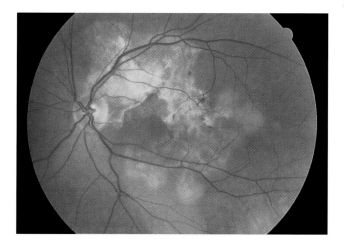

FIGURE 44–1 Pseudopodal extension of prior serpiginous choroiditis lesion. Note the acute creamy yellow macular lesion at the level of the retinal pigment epithelium inferotemporally. These acute lesions are in sharp contrast to the older atrophic areas of affliction in the superior macula. (Courtesy of Stuart L. Fine, M.D.)

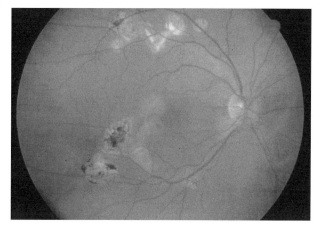

FIGURE 44–3 A new focus of involvement emanating from a prior lesion is seen here in the foveal region. Although most acute lesions are typically contiguous with areas of prior disease, skip lesions may also develop independent of old lesions as demonstrated along the superior temporal arcade. (From Yannuzzi LA, Guyer DR, Green WR [eds]: The Retina Atlas. St Louis, CV Mosby Co, 1995, with permission.)

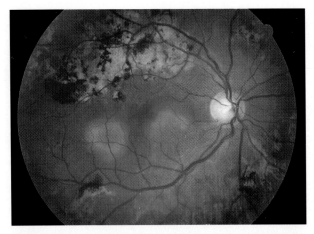

FIGURE 44–4 Acute serpiginous lesions extending into the fovea of a patient with extensive chronic areas of pre-existing disease. Note that new lesions may either arise from areas of previous attack as in the foveal lesion or independently as shown in the temporal parafoveal lesion.

of cases in one series.[6,8,16,25,28,29] The anterior segment examination is generally unremarkable. Rarely, patients may present with signs of inflammation with anterior chamber cells and flare.[3,11,19] Intraocular pressures are usually normal for the age-matched population.

Associated and Unusual Findings
(Table 44–1)

Visual loss may result from active intrinsic destruction by the serpiginous process, resulting chorioretinal atrophy, neurosensory detachment,[1,8,27–29] retinal pigment epithelial detachment,[28] associated cystoid macular edema,[17] or subretinal neovascularization.[8,19,27,29–31] In one study, 26% of serpiginous choroiditis patients followed developed either active choroidal neovascularization or disciform macular scarring.[18,30] Exuberant subretinal neovascularization can even cause subretinal hemorrhage and exudative retinal detachment or lipid exudation

with neurosensory elevation.[8] Neovascularization of the optic nerve head has also been observed.[28,32]

Branch retinal vein occlusion has been documented in a number of cases of serpiginous choroiditis. One was associated with retinal neovascularization[30] and two other cases were thought to have been secondary to a retinal phlebitis.[29,33] A number of investigators have observed an associated inflammatory retinal vascular response in their serpiginous choroiditis patients, characteristically a periphlebitis.[16,23,29,33] Typically, the optic nerve is unaffected. A papillitis with leakage on fluorescein angiography may be rarely noted with active serpiginous choroiditis.[1,25]

Associated Systemic Findings (Table 44–2)

Generally, the serpiginous patient is healthy without systemic disease or antecedent illness. However, a number of associated systemic diseases have been found in patients studied with serpiginous choroiditis.

One of the initial forms of treatment for serpiginous choroiditis was tuberculostatic drugs based on a number of patients with pulmonary tuberculosis earlier in life.[25] Indeed, tuberculosis was assumed to be the causative agent in serpiginous choroiditis by Witmer and Schlaegel in 1952 and 1969, respectively. In one series of nine patients with serpiginous choroiditis, all nine were positive for the tuberculin skin test.[25] Maumenee also felt there was an abnormally high incidence of sensitivity to tuberculin.[20] However, use of antituberculosis therapy often proves ineffective, even when used in combination with systemic steroids.[23,25]

Antecedent respiratory or flu-like illnesses have been observed in some serpiginous choroiditis patients.[25] Maxillary sinusitis has been described,[31] with one patient having a concurrent tooth abscess.[16] One report of serpiginous choroiditis was associated with contralateral adenocystic carcinoma of the orbit and sinus.[31] Two patients with biopsy-proven sarcoidosis were thought to have fundus

TABLE 44–1 Causes of Visual Impairment in Serpiginous Choroiditis

Intrinsic chorioretinal destruction by active disease
Chorioretinal atrophy
Neurosensory detachment
Retinal pigment epithelial detachment*
Subretinal neovascularization
Cystoid macular edema*
Papillitis*
Branch vein occlusion*

* Rare.

TABLE 44–2 Reported Associated Systemic Findings in Serpiginous Choroiditis

Tuberculosis
Respiratory or flu-like illness
Maxillary sinusitis
Adenocystic carcinoma of orbit and sinus
Sarcoidosis
Vitamin A deficiency
Unilateral extrapyramidal dystonia
Transient ischemic attack
Autoimmune thrombocytopenic purpura
Celiac disease
Hypoglycemia

findings consistent with serpiginous choroiditis,[34] although this has not been substantiated in subsequent reports.

A serpiginous choroiditis patient has been described with vitamin A deficiency secondary to gastrointestinal bypass surgery. The patient had associated night blindness that was improved with vitamin A supplementation, without alteration in the course of serpiginous choroiditis.[19]

Neurologic disease has been rarely described in association with serpiginous choroiditis patients. One case report involved a patient with unilateral extrapyramidal dystonia, a nongenetic hemidystonia.[21] Another case described a patient with history of a transient ischemic attack.[23]

Hematologic and serologic testing are generally unrevealing. A patient with autoimmune thrombocytopenic purpura with concomitant celiac disease has been reported.[12]

Hypoglycemia has been described in one patient with severe serpiginous choroiditis with resulting vision in the finger count to hand motion range.[35]

Environmental Exposure

Five of nine patients in one series were exposed to an unusual variety of chemicals including dimethyl sulfoxide, phenol, phenole resins, formaldehyde, asbestos, furene resins, polyethylene, polypropylene, epoxy resins, and polycarbonate.[16] Whether exposure to certain chemical stimuli can affect those genetically predisposed to serpiginous choroiditis is unclear and has not been noted in subsequent studies.

Ancillary Testing

Fluorescein Angiography

The diagnosis of serpiginous choroiditis is typically made by the history of a bilateral, chronic, episodic, and progressive disease process; the classic funduscopic findings; along with the characteristic angiographic study.

Acute lesions are characteristically hypofluorescent in the early phases (Fig. 44–5A). In the middle to late angiogram, the edges of the lesions begin to hyperfluoresce with variable staining of the lesion evolving centrally[29] (Fig. 44–5B). Whether early hypofluorescence represents blockage from the damaged retinal pigment epithelium[11] or nonperfusion of the underlying choriocapillaris,[1,6,29] or both, remains to be elucidated. One observer noticed increased fluorescence within an area of hypofluorescence that was previously lased, resulting in a retinal pigment epithelium window, showing the choroidal flush. This may indicate that the hypofluorescence of an active lesion may be secondary to opacification of the retinal pigment epithelium rather than choroidal vascular closure.[19] Hyperflu-

orescence of the edges of the lesion are thought to represent leakage from adjacent healthy choriocapillaris.[5,25] As the lesion resolves and enters the subacute to chronic stage, there is variable disappearance of the choriocapillaris and retinal pigment epithelium with general preservation of the larger choroidal vessels. Depending on the degree of atrophy of the retinal pigment epithelium and choroid, this may lead to a mottled hyperfluorescent appearance.[25] Prominent pigment hyperplasia may mask the choroidal flush in areas of involvement.[6]

Indocyanine Green Angiography

Recent studies of serpiginous choroiditis during the acute, subacute, and healed states have been analyzed using indocyanine green (ICG) videoangiography.[36] Similar to the fluorescein angiogram, early hypofluorescence followed by late staining of active lesions were observed with acute serpiginous lesions (Fig. 44–6). However, ICG angiography demonstrated active choroidal involvement beyond the boundaries seen by indirect biomicroscopy as well as those delineated by the corresponding fluorescein studies. This may suggest that there exists an expanded ischemic or inflammatory affliction of the choroid underlying the clinically observed lesions.

In the healed state, the ICG and fluorescein both stain in areas of fibrovascular tissue or scarring. Choroidal atrophy is well circumscribed with loss of the choriocapillaris, presumably from localized infarction. Interestingly, there were two patients studied in the healed state displaying multifocal regions of ICG hypofluorescence in isolated areas not seen clinically or demonstrated by fluorescein angiography. Whether this represents occult areas of choroidal hypoperfusion without overt overlying RPE and neurosensory damage or de novo lesions, which may become future active lesions, remains to be seen.

Visual Fields

Visual field studies do not aid in the diagnosis of the disease. The fields generally show relative or absolute scotomata that correspond in size and location to the geographic areas of affliction as seen in the fundus.[1,5] In some cases, the scotomata may become less dense as time passes.[16]

Electrophysiologic Studies

Generally, the electroretinogram (ERG) and electrooculogram (EOG) are normal.[16,29] Some series demonstrated abnormal electrophysiologic testing, particularly in the more advanced serpiginous choroiditis cases. Chisholm et al reported 3 of 26 eyes had abnormal ERG and 8 eyes had reduced levels of the EOG, correlating well with the extent of disease involvement.[6] Laatikainen and Erkkila observed abnormal EOG and normal ERG in affected eyes in their series.[25] It is generally felt that the ab-

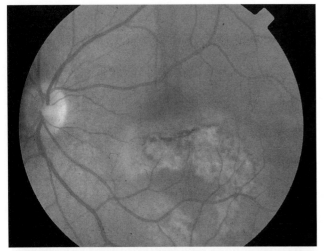

FIGURE 44–5 This 24-year-old patient noted an abrupt visual decline in her left eye. Photography shows acute foveal encroachment, extending from a subacute inferior macula lesion. (Courtesy of Blake Horio, M.D.) *A,* Early fluorescein angiogram demonstrated hypofluorescence of the active serpiginous macula lesion. *B,* Late fluorescein angiogram study shows hyperfluorescence of the edges of the lesions evolving centrally.

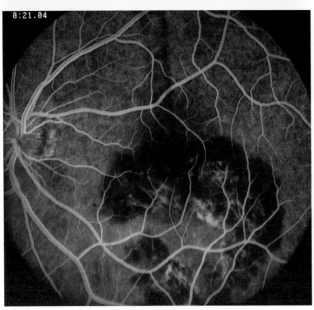

A

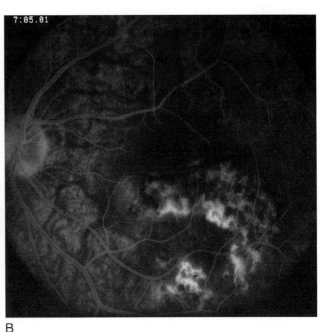

B

normal studies reflect the degree of diseased retina and retinal pigment epithelium rather than a global or widespread degenerative disease. One case report showed a normal global ERG with abnormal focal macular ERG.[5]

Immunologic Studies

Human Leukocyte Antigen (HLA) Typing

To study whether serpiginous choroiditis may be immunologically triggered, HLA typing was performed on a number of patients. Histocompatibility antigen, HLA-B7, was found to occur in 54.5% of serpiginous choroiditis cases compared to 24.3% of controls.[22] HLA-A2 was found in five of six patients in an earlier study.[23]

Immune responsiveness to retinal S antigen was found in 11 patients with serpiginous choroiditis.

When tested in patients with acute posterior multifocal placoid pigment epitheliopathy (APMPPE) and retinitis pigmentosa (RP), there was no significant immune responsiveness detected in these particular subjects. This may reflect the more severe and sustained injury to the photoreceptors and retinal pigment epithelium in serpiginous choroiditis compared to APMPPE and RP.[24]

King et al reported elevated factor VIII–von Willebrand factor antigen levels in eight patients with serpiginous choroiditis. The mean factor VIII–von Willebrand factor activity was 226% compared to an age- and sex-matched control group of 107%. The authors suggested that serpiginous choroiditis may represent an occlusive vascular phenomenon, not unlike other rheumatologic vascular disorders also found with elevated factors, resulting from vascular endothelial damage.[15] Interestingly, these factors were not reduced following systemic steroid treatment.

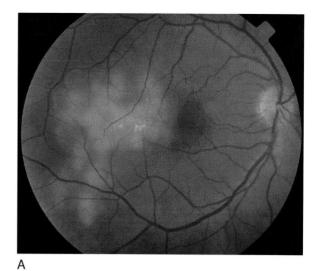

FIGURE 44–6 *A*, Color fundus photography demonstrating acute serpiginous choroiditis lesion. *B*, Indocyanine green (ICG) angiography shows early hypofluorescence of the lesion. Note that the ICG study demonstrates involvement beyond the boundaries seen clinically, as evident in the corresponding color photograph. *C*, Late indocyanine green angiogram reveals hyperfluorescence of the lesion.

A

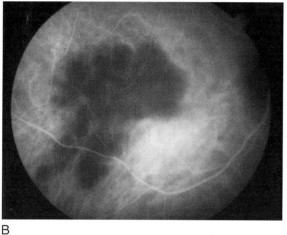

B

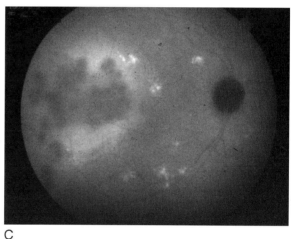

C

NATURAL HISTORY

Serpiginous choroiditis is characteristically a chronic, episodic, bilateral chorioretinal destructive disease with often, but not always, poor visual recovery once the fovea becomes involved. Laatikainen and Erkkila followed 15 serpiginous choroiditis patients aged 20 to 65 years (mean, 35 years) for a period of 1 to 10 years (mean, 5 years). Although initial active lesions lasted a few weeks, there were signs of activity observed in the ensuing 2 to 9 months. Recurrence was seen over a span of 3 months to 4 years later in 8 of 15 patients. Central vision was ultimately lost in 6 of 15 patients, two secondary to subretinal neovascularization.[32] Chisholm et al reported on a long-term follow-up on 20 patients with an average age of 43 (range, 22 to 70 years).[6] The average time between onset of symptoms in the first to second eye was seen to be 5.1 years. They found that visual acuity decreased in only three eyes, which was the result of macular involvement. Weiss et al followed nine patients, average age 46 (range, 22 to 58 years), for a period ranging from 2 to 10 years. Nine of 17 eyes had improved vision even though the foveal or para-

foveal region was eventually involved in 15 of 17 eyes over the follow-up period. One patient had documented disease progression during a 10-year period.[16]

Jampol et al first described three patients with serpiginous choroiditis who subsequently developed subretinal neovascular membranes (SRNVM) with hemorrhaging, lipid exudation, and serous neurosensory detachments.[8] Later, Laatikainen and Erkkila[32] and Blumenkranz et al[30] demonstrated that the development of SRNVM is not as rare as previously thought and may represent a significant minority of serpiginous choroiditis patients with eventual central vision loss.[30,32]

ETIOLOGY AND PATHOGENESIS

Despite extensive study, the etiology of serpiginous choroiditis has remained elusive. Franceschetti in 1962 described 16 patients with a curious helicoid pattern of chorioretinal atrophy, which he termed "helicoid peripapillar chorioretinal degeneration." He further divided this disease entity into a congenital or stationary form and a progressive form, which most likely represents what we now know as serpiginous choroiditis. Although he felt most cases represented a primary hereditary degeneration, he did entertain the notion of a possible inflammatory etiology.[9] Sveinsson reported on a family with helicoid peripapillary chorioretinal degeneration in which 21 family members spanning four generations were examined. Eleven members were found to have helicoidal fundus changes, one as young as 4 years of age. He felt that this represented a congenital hereditary disease transmitted in an autosomal dominant fashion.[10]

Krill and Archer argued that given the slow, relentless, progressive nature of the disease, serpiginous choroiditis likely represented a degenerative rather than inflammatory process.[4] Given that most patients at time of presentation exhibit evidence of prior affliction, it would be difficult to argue against a congenital or hereditary degenerative process. In 1970, Maumenee attempted to make a distinction between choroidal vascular abiotrophy or a degenerative disorder and a similar morphologic picture caused by a choroidal inflammatory disease process. Serpiginous choroiditis, he felt, fell into the inflammatory end of the spectrum and helicoid degeneration the other.[20] More recent studies seem to support an inflammatory hypothesis rather than a degenerative or familial one. It is unclear whether the inflammatory process directly injures the retina–retinal pigment epithelium–choriocapillaris complex or indirectly by a vascular occlusive process. King et al demonstrated elevated factor VIII–von Willebrand factor antigen levels, suggesting vascular endothelial injury from a vascular occlusive phenomenon, perhaps a vasculitis.[15]

Reports of concurrent vitritis,[6,8,16,21,25,28,29] anterior uveitis,[3,11,19] retinal periphlebitis,[16,23,29,33] and papillitis[16,25] support an inflammatory etiology. In 1973, Schatz et al entertained the thought that an infectious mechanism might be a stimulus to the subsequent serpiginous process. Indeed, concomitant or antecedent infectious diseases have been reported, including a flu-like illness,[1,25] maxillary sinusitis,[1,16] tuberculosis,[25] and viral meningitis.[25] Davidorf and Gass (personal communications, 1990) treated two patients with acyclovir with apparent success, suggesting a viral causative agent.[35] However, in one series, nine patients tested negative for a battery of infectious etiologies, including vaccinia virus; herpes simplex virus; herpes zoster virus; cytomegalovirus; adenovirus; influenza A and B; parainfluenza 1, 2, and 3 viruses; respiratory syncytial virus; rubella and rubeola viruses; polio 1, 2, and 3 viruses; and coxsackie A7, A9, and B5 viruses. Toxoplasmosis, ornithosis, and *Mycoplasma pneumoniae* titers were within normal limits.[25]

Work by Wu et al further supported an inflammatory etiology based on their histopathologic study of a postmortem patient with serpiginous choroiditis. Extensive local and diffuse infiltration of the choroid and several retinal venules were seen with lymphocytes. Larger aggregates of lymphocytes were present at the margin of the serpiginous choroiditis lesions with loss of the retinal pigment epithelium and photoreceptor cell layer, suggesting an intense, destructive inflammatory process.[31]

A noninfectious or abnormally enhanced immune response or perhaps even an autoimmune-mediated inflammatory mechanism has been suggested in the pathogenesis of serpiginous choroiditis. Erkkila et al found a statistically significant increase in frequency of HLA-B7 typing in serpiginous choroiditis patients relative to a matched group in a Finnish population.[22] Broekhuyse et al reported pronounced responsiveness to retinal S antigen and opsin, suggesting an autoimmune reactivity to the retinal proteins in serpiginous choroiditis.[24]

Finally, the variable response to anti-inflammatory drugs and lymphocyte suppression with systemic steroids and cytotoxic agents further support that serpiginous choroiditis represents an inflammatory or immunologically mediated disease process.[27,37]

DIFFERENTIAL DIAGNOSIS
(Table 44–3)

A number of dystrophic, ischemic, or infectious inflammatory disorders of the retina, retinal pigment epithelium, or choroid can at certain stages of the disease process mimic serpiginous choroiditis.

APMPPE is foremost in the differential diagnosis of serpiginous choroiditis. APMPPE is an affliction of the retinal pigment epithelium, choriocapillaris, and inner choroid with disruption of the overlying retina first described by Gass in 1968.[38,39] Although its etiology is unclear, more recent studies, including the use of ICG angiography, suggest a vascular occlusive disorder resulting with hypoperfusion of the choroidal vasculature, and subsequent damage to the overlying retinal pigment epithelium and neurosensory retina.[39–41] The age group affected by APMPPE is skewed towards a younger population (mean onset, 26.5 years)[42] than serpiginous choroiditis (mean range of onset, 40 to 45 years), and in one third of cases there is an antecedent viral or flu-like illness in APMPPE.[43] The characteristic findings are multifocal, yellow-white placoid lesions occurring at the level of the retinal pigment epithelium and inner choroid, usually restricted to the posterior pole. Typically, there is rapid resolution with permanent alterations in the retinal pigment epithelium with minimal damage to the choroid and overlying retina and significant improvement in vision weeks after the acute onset of visual disturbance.[38,45] Although recurrence of APMPPE has been reported, the typical patient has a single, self-limiting episode,[46,47] in contradistinction to serpiginous choroiditis. Bilaterality in most instances is the rule, with APMPPE usually affecting both eyes simultaneously, as opposed to serpiginous cho-

TABLE 44–3 Differential Diagnosis of Serpiginous Choroiditis

Acute posterior multifocal placoid pigment epithe-
    liopathy (APMPPE)
Infectious disorders
    Toxoplasmosis
    Presumed ocular histoplasmosis syndrome
        (POHS)
    Tuberculosis
    Syphilis
Inflammatory diseases
    Posterior scleritis
    Multifocal choroiditis
    Sarcoidosis
Degenerative/dystrophic disorders
    Sorsby's pseudo-inflammatory dystrophy
    Central areolar choroidal dystrophy
    Best's disease
    Fundus flavimaculatus
Infiltrative diseases of the choroid
    Non-Hodgkin's lymphoma (reticulum cell
        sarcoma)
    Metastatic tumor
    Choroidal osteoma
Choroidal neovascularization
    Peripapillary subretinal neovascularization
    Idiopathic choroidal neovascularization
    Age-related macular degeneration
    Angioid streaks
    Drusen of optic nerve head
    Pathologic myopia

roiditis in which one eye usually lags behind the other in symptomatology and activity. The fluorescein angiogram is similar in both disorders, with blockage early and hyperfluorescence late. The appearance of fundus lesions is somewhat dissimilar; APMPPE presents with discrete, randomly distributed round to oval placoid lesions, whereas serpiginous choroiditis tends to be contiguous in nature. However, in some cases, serpiginous choroiditis can appear with discrete lesions and APMPPE lesions may interconnect. After resolution, there is typically profound choroidal atrophy and retinal pigment epithelium derangement in serpiginous choroiditis, which is unusual in APMPPE.

The prognosis is generally favorable with APMPPE compared to serpiginous choroiditis, even when lesions affect the foveal region. SRNVM have been reported in both APMPPE and serpiginous choroiditis, but tends to occur more frequently in serpiginous choroiditis.[2,29] Whether APMPPE and serpiginous choroiditis are truly distinct entities or polarized disorders of the spectrum of the same disease process, with serpiginous choroiditis being a more destructive and persistent manifestation, is speculative at this time.

Infectious Disorders

Toxoplasmosis also represents a recurrent retinochoroidal disease, but tends to have a more exuberant inflammatory component with, typically, marked vitritis and direct involvement of the neurosensory retina. As in serpiginous choroiditis, new lesions tend to emanate from prior lesions in toxoplasmosis.

Presumed ocular histoplasmosis syndrome (POHS) presents with punched-out chorioretinal lesions with peripapillary involvement and development of choroidal neovascular membranes. However, the lesions seldom interconnect and are not diffuse in involvement as in serpiginous choroiditis. HLA typing in both disease entities is associated with histocompatibility antigen HLA-B7. Differentiation is based on clinical findings, *Histoplasma capsulatum* skin reaction, and history of residence or travel in histoplasmosis-endemic areas.

Tuberculosis (TB) and syphilis may also mimic serpiginous choroiditis; usually serologic testing and uveitis coexisting in TB and luetic diseases help to differentiate the disorders. Purified protein derivative (PPD) has been shown to be positive in a significant number of earlier serpiginous choroiditis cases.[25]

Inflammatory Conditions of the Choroid

Posterior scleritis, multifocal choroiditis, and sarcoidosis can imitate the fundus findings of serpiginous choroiditis.[2] However, history, ancillary testing such as biopsies, angiotensin-converting enzyme (ACE), chest x-ray, ultrasound, and the presence of significant vitritis or anterior uveitis may help distinguish these entities from serpiginous choroiditis.

Degenerative or Dystrophic Disorders

Sorsby's pseudoinflammatory dystrophy with retinal edema, exudation, hemorrhages, RPE hyperplasia and migration, and occasional development of SRNVM may mimic serpiginous choroiditis.[5] Central areolar choroidal dystrophy, with its sharply delimited round or oval zones of atrophy of the retinal pigment epithelium, and choroid may present in a similar fashion to serpiginous choroiditis.[5] Rarely, Best's disease and fundus flavimaculatus may evolve into a pseudoserpiginous picture. Hereditary patterns with fundus evaluations of family members can help differentiate the dystrophic disorders from serpiginous choroiditis.

Infiltrative Diseases of the Choroid

Non-Hodgkin's lymphoma, metastatic tumor, or choroidal osteoma may present similarly to serpiginous choroiditis at certain stages of their disease process.

Disorders Associated with Choroidal Neovascularization

Peripapillary subretinal neovascularization, idiopathic choroidal neovascularization, age-related macular degeneration, angioid streaks, drusen of the optic nerve head, and pathologic myopia should also be included in the differential diagnosis of serpiginous choroiditis.[2,29]

TREATMENT (Table 44–4)

The relative rarity, natural history of remissions and recurrences, and uncertainty of pathogenesis of serpiginous choroiditis have greatly hindered the search and precluded establishment of definitive treatment modalities. To date, no randomized prospective study has been done to elucidate an effective treatment for serpiginous choroiditis.

Antibiotics and Antivirals

In the early to middle 1970s, many patients with serpiginous choroiditis were treated with various antituberculosis drugs based on increased frequency of a positive Mantoux reaction.[23] Treatment included streptomycin, isoniazid, p-aminosalicylic acid, with or without systemic steroids. In one case, the addition of cytosine arabinoside was made, with questionable results.[25] Other antibiotics have been attempted in serpiginous choroiditis cases, including penicillin and sulfatrimethoprim. Unfortunately, these forms of therapy were found to be ineffective.[25]

Davidorf and Gass (personal communications, 1990) treated two serpiginous choroiditis patients with the antiherpetic drug acyclovir. Both patients appeared to have regression of their lesions after implementation of therapy.[35] Subsequent trials have not been reported in the literature.

Baarsma and Deutman, in 1976, reported on four patients with serpiginous choroiditis who were treated with a combination of corticosteroid, Ledermycin, Complamine, pyrimethamine, and inhalation of carbogen. They felt that restoration in some eyes may or may not have been due to treatment.[5]

The most commonly used therapy for serpiginous choroiditis is corticosteroids. Systemic prednisone (1 mg/kg/day) is typically used, although subtenon injection of retrobulbar steroids (triamcinolone acetonide, 40 mg) is occasionally used, particularly if the fovea is threatened.[18] Most reports to date, however, doubt the efficacy of this mode of treatment in serpiginous choroiditis,[1,3,23,25,48] whereas some authors still feel that steroids may hasten resolution of active serpiginous choroiditis.[6,16,18]

Immunosuppressive Therapy

Cyclosporin A, a T-lymphocyte–suppressing agent, has been found to be effective in experimentally induced uveitis by retinal S antigen, also found elevated in serpiginous choroiditis patients. Its initial use by Laatikainen was reported in 1984 on one patient with recurrent serpiginous choroiditis who failed corticosteroid therapy.[48] No definite response to cyclosporin A was seen. In 1990, Secchi et al treated seven patients with cyclosporin A.[37] Nine of 14 eyes showed significant improvement in visual acuity, with 5 eyes unchanged. Due to the nephrotoxicity of cyclosporin A, the authors advised use only when the macular region of the remaining eye becomes threatened.

Hooper et al, in 1991, reported the use of combination therapy consisting of azathioprine, cyclosporine, and prednisone in five patients with serpiginous choroiditis. They demonstrated rapid remission of active disease in all patients for up to 18 months of follow-up. Two patients relapsed off treatment and responded again when therapy was reinitiated. The appearance of the lesion after resolution with and without treatment was noted to be different. Less destruction of the retinal pigment epithelium and choriocapillaris with reduced retinal pigment epithelium hyperplasia and migration was observed with treatment of triple-therapy immunosuppression. Unlike the use of single-mode immunosuppressive therapy, the simultaneous use of azathioprine, cyclosporine, and prednisone allows reduction of dose, thereby reducing systemic toxicity due to a synergistic effect.[27]

Laser Photocoagulation Therapy

In an attempt to border off the advancement of active serpiginous choroiditis lesions, photocoagulation with laser was reported by Gass[29] and Chisholm et al.[6] Efforts to limit progression towards the fovea were without success.

Laser photocoagulation can, however, be effective when serpiginous choroiditis is complicated by choroidal neovascularization. If the choroidal neovascular membrane is extrafoveal, macular laser ablation can successfully obliterate the membrane with preservation of central vision.[8,31]

Given the treatability of extrafoveal choroidal neovascular membranes, it is important for patients to self-document progression of the disease process with frequent Amsler grid testing.[2]

TABLE 44–4   Treatment Modalities for Serpiginous Choroiditis

Treatment	Mechanism of Action	Effectiveness	Comments
Antituberculosis drugs (streptomycin, isoniazid, p-aminosalicyclic acid)	Synergistic bacteristatic agents against tubercle bacilli.	Not effective	No longer recommended
Acyclovir	Guanosine derivative acting as a herpes-specific thymidase kinase. Inhibits herpes virus DNA polymerase, thereby preventing viral replication.	Anecdotal efficacy	Not extensively tested
Corticosteroids	Suppression of cellular immunity and antibody formation, as well as prostaglandin and leukotriene synthesis. May also cause lysis of T helper cells.	Variable success	Most commonly used form of therapy with questionable value
Cyclosporin A	Immunosuppressive agent that causes clonal deletion of T helper cells. In in vitro studies, cyclosporin A inhibits the production of factors that stimulate T lymphocytic growth.[49]	1. Encouraging results in an open clinical trial. 2. Poor results in an earlier single case report	Possible nephrotoxicity with prolonged use in single-mode therapy
Combination immuno-suppression therapy (azathio-prine, cyclosporin A, prednisone)	Azathioprine (Imuran)—purine analog functioning as a cytotoxic agent that destroys stimulated lymphoid cells. Cellular immunity as well as primary and secondary serum antibody responses are blocked.[49] Mechanisms of cyclosporin A and prednisone as above.	Good results in preliminary small study group	1. Limited trial of five patients 2. Azathioprine may cause bone marrow suppression 3. Triple therapy allows reduced dosing to decrease side effects through synergism
Laser photocoagulation	Thermal destruction.	1. Not effective in containing active lesion 2. Good results for extrafoveal SRNVM	Amsler grid testing recommended for surveillance

REFERENCES

1. Schatz H, Maumenee AE, Patz A: Geographic helicoid peripapillary choroidopathy: clinical presentation and fluorescein angiographic findings. Trans Am Acad Ophthalmol Otolaryngol 78:747–761, 1974.
2. Schatz H, McDonald HR, Johnson RN: Geographic helicoid peripapillary choroidopathy (serpiginous choroiditis). In Schachat AP, Murphy RB (eds): Retina, 2nd edition, Vol 2. St. Louis, CV Mosby Co, 1994.
3. Masi RJ, O'Connor GR, Kimura SJ: Anterior uveitis in geographic or serpiginous choroiditis. Am J Ophthalmol 86: 228–232, 1978.
4. Krill AE, Archer D: Classification of the choroidal atrophies. Am J Ophthalmol 72:562–585, 1971.
5. Baarsma GS, Deutman AF: Serpiginous (geographic) choroiditis. Doc Ophthalmol 2:269–285, 1976.
6. Chisholm IH, Gass JDM, Hutton WL: The late stage of serpiginous (geographic) choroiditis. Am J Ophthalmol 82: 343–351, 1976.
7. Green WR, Wilson DJ: Choroidal neovascularization. Ophthalmology 93:1169–1176, 1986.
8. Jampol LM, Orth D, Daily MJ, Rabb MF: Subretinal neovascularization with geographic (serpiginous) choroiditis. Am J Ophthalmol 88:683–689, 1979.
9. Franceschetti A: A curious affection of the fundus oculi: helicoid peripapillar chorioretinal degeneration. Its relation to pigmentary paravenous chorioretinal degeneration. Doc Ophthalmol 16:81–110, 1962.
10. Sveinsson K: Helicoidal peripapillary chorioretinal degeneration. Acta Ophthalmol 57:69–75, 1979.
11. Hamilton AM, Bird AC: Geographical choroidopathy. Br J Ophthalmol 58:784–797, 1974.
12. Mulder CJJ, Pena AS, Jansen J, Oosterhuis JA: Celiac disease and geographic (serpiginous) choroidopathy with occurrence of thrombocytopenic purpura. Arch Intern Med 143:842, 1983.
13. Hooper PL, Kaplan HJ: Triple agent immunosuppression in serpiginous choroiditis. Ophthalmology 97(Suppl):109, 1990.
14. Hyvarinen L, Maumenee AE, George T, Weinstein GW: Fluorescein angiography of the choriocapillaris. Am J Ophthalmol 67:653–666, 1969.
15. King DG, Grizzard WS, Sever RJ, Espinoza L: Serpiginous choroiditis associated with elevated factor VIII-von Willebrand factor antigen. Retina 10:97–101, 1990.
16. Annesley WH, Shields JA, Tomer T: The clinical course of serpiginous choroiditis. Am J Ophthalmol 87:133–142, 1979.
17. Steinmetz RL, Fitzke FW, Bird AC: Treatment of cystoid macular edema with acetazolamide in a patient with serpiginous choroiditis. Retina 11:412–415, 1991.
18. Hardy RA, Schatz H: Macular geographic helicoid choroidopathy. Arch Ophthalmol 105:1237–1242, 1987.
19. Mansour AM, Jampol LM, Packo KH, Hrisomalos NF: Macular serpiginous choroiditis. Retina 8:125–131, 1988.
20. Maumenee AE: Clinical entities in "uveitis": an approach to the study of intraocular inflammation. Am J Ophthalmol 69:1–27, 1970.
21. Richardson RR, Cooper IS, Smith JL: Serpiginous choroiditis and unilateral extrapyramidal dystonia. Ann Ophthalmol 13:15–19, 1981.
22. Erkkila H, Laatikainen L, Jokinen E: Immunological studies on serpiginous choroiditis. Graefes Arch Clin Exp Ophthalmol 219:131–134, 1982.
23. Laatikainen L, Erkkila H: A follow-up study on serpignous choroiditis. Acta Ophthalmol 59:707–718, 1981.
24. Broekhuyse RM, Herck MV, Pinckers AJLG, et al: Immune responsiveness to retinal S-antigen and opsin in serpiginous choroiditis and other retinal disease. Doc Ophthalmol 69:83–93, 1988.
25. Laatikainen L, Erkkila H: Serpiginous choroiditis. Br J Ophthalmol 58:777–783, 1974.
26. Fujisawa C, Fujiwara H, Hasegawa E: The cases of serpiginous choroiditis. Acta Soc Ophthalmol Jpn 82:135–143, 1978.
27. Hooper PL, Kaplan HJ: Triple agent immunosuppression in serpiginous choroiditis. Ophthalmology 98:944–952, 1991.
28. Wojno T, Meredith TA: Unusual findings in serpiginous choroiditis. Am J Ophthalmol 94:650–655, 1982.
29. Gass D: Diseases causing choroidal exudative and hemorrhagic localized (disciform) detachment of the retina and pigment epithelium. In Stereoscopic Atlas of Macular Diseases, Diagnosis and Treatment, 3rd edition, Vol 1. St Louis, CV Mosby Co, 1987.
30. Blumenkranz MS, Gass DM, Clarkson JG: Atypical serpiginous choroiditis. Arch Ophthalmol 100:1773–1775, 1982.
31. Wu JS, Lewis H, Fine SL, et al: Clinicopathologic findings in a patient with serpiginous choroiditis and treated choroidal neovascularization. Retina 9:292–301, 1989.
32. Laatikainen L, Erkkila H: Subretinal and disc neovascularisation in serpiginous choroiditis. Br J Ophthalmol 66: 326–331, 1982.
33. Friberg T: Serpiginous choroiditis with branch vein occlusion and bilateral periphlebitis. Arch Ophthalmol 106: 585–586, 1988.
34. Edelsten C, Stanford MR, Graham EM: Serpiginous choroiditis: an unusual presentation of ocular sarcoidosis. Br J Ophthalmol 78:70–71, 1994.
35. Brock CJ, Jampol LM: Serpiginous choroiditis. In Albert DM, Jakobiec FA (eds): Principles and Practice of Ophthalmology, Vol 2, Philadelphia, WB Saunders Co, 1994.
36. Giovanni A, Ripa E, Scassellati-Sforolini B, et al: Indocyanine green angiography in serpiginous choroidopathy. Eur J Ophthalmol 6:299–306, 1996.
37. Secchi AG, Tognon MS, Maselli C: Cyclosporine-A in the treatment of serpiginous choroiditis. Int Ophthalmol 14: 395–399, 1990.
38. Gass JDM: Acute posterior multifocal placoid pigment epitheliopathy. Arch Ophthalmol 80:177–185, 1968.
39. Howe LJ, Woon H, Graham EM, et al: Choroidal hypoperfusion in acute posterior multifocal placoid pigment epitheliopathy, an indocyanine green angiography study. Ophthalmology 102:790–798, 1995.
40. Park D, Schatz H, McDonald R, Johnson RN: Indocyanine green angiography of acute multifocal posterior placoid pigment epitheliopathy. Ophthalmology 102:1877–1883, 1995.
41. Dhaliwal RS, Maguire AM, Flower RW, Arribas RW: Acute posterior multifocal placoid pigment epitheliopathy, an indocyanine green angiographic study. Retina 13:317–325, 1993.
42. Jones NP: Acute posterior multifocal placoid pigment epitheliopathy. Br J Ophthalmol 79:384–389, 1995.
43. Ryan S, Maumenee E: Acute posterior multifocal placoid pigment epitheliopathy. Am J Ophthalmol 74:1066–1074, 1972.
44. Savino PJ, Weinberg RJ, Yassin JG, Pilkerton AR: Diverse manifestations of acute posterior multifocal placoid pigment epitheliopathy. Am J Ophthalmol 77:659–662, 1974.
45. Deutman AF, Oosterhuis JA, Boen-Tan NN, Aan De Kerk AL: Acute posterior multifocal placoid pigment epitheliopathy. Br J Ophthalmol 56:863–874, 1972.
46. Lewis RA, Martonyi CL: Acute posterior multifocal placoid pigment epitheliopathy. Arch Ophthalmol 93:235–238, 1975.
47. Lyness AL, Bird AC: Recurrences of acute posterior multifocal placoid pigment epitheliopathy. Am J Ophthalmol 98:203–207, 1984.
48. Laatikainen L, Tarkkanen A: Failure of cyclosporin A in serpiginous choroiditis. J Ocul Ther Surg 3:280–282, 1984.
49. Salmon SE: Drugs and the immune system. In Katzung BG (ed): Basic and Clinical Pharmacology, 3rd edition. East Norwalk, CT, Appleton & Lange, 1987.

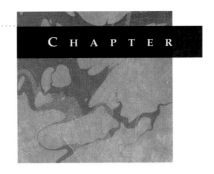

CHAPTER 45

Birdshot Retinochoroidopathy

Jay S. Duker, M.D.

Birdshot retinochoroidopathy is a recently recognized, clinically distinct pattern of posterior segment inflammation of presumed autoimmune etiology. Its course is chronic and remitting, occasionally resulting in significant visual loss due to cystoid macular edema. While quite rare, it has the unique feature of being the human disease most closely linked to a specific HLA type: HLA-A29.

HISTORY, EPIDEMIOLOGY, AND PATHOGENESIS

Ryan and Maumanee[1] initially described birdshot retinochoroidopathy in 1980. They reported a series of 13 patients who shared many of the manifestations of intermediate uveitis except for the lack of "snow banking" on the pars plana. A unique finding that separated these patients from others previously reported, however, was the presence of multiple depigmented spots at the level of the choroid/retinal pigment epithelium. The distribution of the spots throughout the retina reminded the authors of the scatter pattern seen with birdshot from a shotgun, hence the unusual name. Soon afterwards, Gass[2] described an additional 11 patients with the same entity. He referred to it as "vitiliginous chorioretinitis" because of the resemblance of the multiple, deep depigmented choroidal lesions to the characteristic skin depigmentation of vitiligo.

Birdshot retinochoroidopathy is quite rare and as a result accurate population incidences are lacking. Women appear to be affected slightly more commonly than men (60 vs. 40%), consistent with its presumed autoimmune etiology. The onset of birdshot retinochoroidopathy is typically between the fourth and seventh decades, with a median age at diagnosis of 50 years. Nussenblatt and Palestine report a higher incidence in Caucasians of northern European descent.[3]

Nussenblatt et al[4] initially reported that birdshot retinochoroidopathy was closely associated with a specific HLA type: HLA-A29. Subsequent reports suggest that greater than 90% of patients with birdshot retinochoroidopathy will carry this serologic marker.[5-8] This HLA type is typically found in less than 10% of the general population.

Along with this apparent genetic predisposition, patients with birdshot retinochoroidopathy show a positive immune response to interphotoreceptor-binding protein and retinal S antigen.[4,7,8] These findings suggest an inherent autoimmunity to retinal antigens in affected patients.

Birdshot retinochoroidopathy has been rarely associated with systemic findings. Gass[2] was the first to point out the relationship with vitiligo of the skin. Suttorp-Schulten and collaborators[9] reported two patients with suspected ocular Lyme disease in whom birdshot retinochoroidopathy developed. Both patients were HLA-A29 positive. In a series of 11 patients with birdshot retinochoroidopathy, 3 (27%) were found to harbor antibodies to *Borrelia burgdorferi*, the Lyme disease agent. While this association may have been by chance, it is possible that birdshot retinochoroidopathy can be induced by infectious agents. Brod[10] examined a patient with the clinical diagnosis of birdshot retinochoroidopathy who had concurrent biopsy-proven sarcoidosis. HLA-A29 was not present in this woman.

CLINICAL PRESENTATION

The classic lesions of birdshot retinochoroidopathy are choroidal infiltrates.[1,2,11,12] These infiltrates are creamy yellow in color and multiple. The lesions tend to be round to oval shaped or occasionally linear and vary between 500 and 1500 μm in size. They are neither raised nor "punched out" and the overlying retina appears normal. Hemorrhage

565

within the lesions is not seen, although overlying flame retinal hemorrhages can occur. In distribution, they tend to be bilaterally symmetric and preferentially affect the postequatorial retina. Often, but not universally, the macula is spared. The choroidal lesions commonly appear to radiate linearly out from the optic disc following a vascular distribution. Sometimes the spots will coalesce into broader areas of chorioretinal atrophy with depigmentation. Late in the disease course, the posterior fundus can appear quite depigmented ("blond") (Fig. 45–1).

Signs of intraocular inflammation are invariably found in patients with birdshot retinochoroidopathy, although their presence may be subtle and strikingly asymmetric. Vitreous cells develop bilaterally. While the vitritis almost always causes symptoms of floaters, which is the most common reason patients with birdshot retinochoroidopathy seek medical attention, the cellular reaction may not go on to cause significant media opacity. The vitritis may precede the choroidal infiltrates by months to years.[13]

Other signs of chronic intraocular inflammation include retinal venous inflammatory sheathing with associated vascular leakage on fluorescein angiography.[14] Cystoid macular edema (CME) is quite common (approximately half of affected eyes) and is the most common reason for significantly decreased central visual acuity. Disc edema may occur as well and eventually may be replaced by optic disc pallor.

Other late complications include retinal and choroidal neovascularization.[15,16] Rhegmatogenous retinal detachment has also been seen as well as rubeosis irides, epiretinal membranes, cataract, and glaucoma.[7,14]

Externally, eyes with birdshot retinochoroidopathy appear uninjected. There is a low-grade, chronic anterior uveitis with a modest amount of small keratic precipitates in fewer than half of affected eyes. Hypopyon and synechiae are unusual, and if present, should suggest another diagnosis.

Besides floaters due to the intraocular inflammation, patients commonly present with complaints of photopsias, blurred vision, and later, nyctalopia and loss of color vision. Pain and photophobia are not typical complaints. The majority of patients present with good visual acuity (20/40 or better) in at least one eye.

ANCILLARY TESTING

Birdshot retinochoroidopathy is a clinical diagnosis. HLA-A29 testing can help to confirm the diagnosis, but this test is neither 100% sensitive nor 100% specific. Other ancillary tests can assist in determining the extent of the disease and to monitor responses to therapy. None are definitively diagnostic.

Fluorescein angiography is most useful in determining the extent of vascular leakage. It reveals large-vessel perfusion abnormalities in many of the eyes with chronic birdshot retinochoroidopathy. Arterial filling is delayed, especially in eyes with optic atrophy. In contrast, the choroidal filling appears normal. Late in the angiogram, diffuse leakage from the perifoveolar capillaries and the larger veins is common (Fig. 45–2). The lesions of birdshot retinochoroidopathy often do not show abnormal hyper- or hypofluoresence early in fluorescein angiography. Late, the lesions show mild hyperfluoresence. Choroidal, retinal, and optic nerve neovascularization may complicate the course of birdshot retinochoroidopathy. Its appearance on angiography is typical.

Electroretinography (ERG) has been reported to

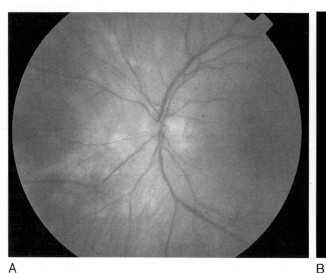
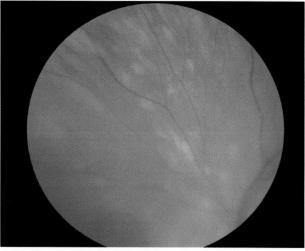

A   B

FIGURE 45–1   *A,* Posterior pole view of the typical appearance of birdshot retinochoroidopathy. *B,* Peripheral view of same patient.

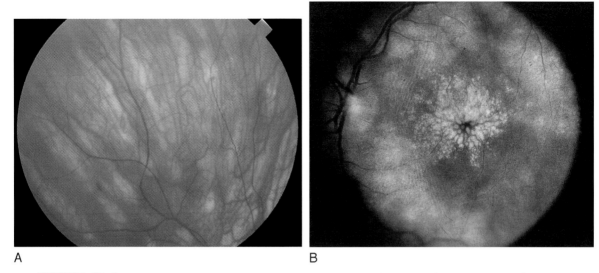

A   B

FIGURE 45–2   *A,* Superior view of a patient with birdshot retinochoroidopathy. *B,* Late-phase fluorescein angiogram showing diffuse leakage and cystoid macular edema.

be variably abnormal in affected eyes, depending on the length of the disease course and the amount of choroidal involvement. In most cases there is a subnormal rod and cone response.[17,18]

DIFFERENTIAL DIAGNOSIS

The differential diagnosis of birdshot retinochoroidopathy includes other entities that produce a chronic mild to moderate bilateral panuveitis with choroidal infiltrates. When the classic birdshot lesions are present with the requisite amount of intraocular inflammation, the diagnosis is usually obvious. More mildly affected eyes or those examined early in the disease course can be very difficult to delineate from these other entities.

As noted in the original descriptions, birdshot retinochoroidopathy may resemble pars planitis (intermediate uveitis). The lack of "snowbanking" in birdshot coupled with the lack of choroidal spots in pars planitis will separate the two entities.

Patients with Harada's disease also have mild to moderate bilateral intraocular inflammation similar to birdshot retinochoroidopathy. Unlike birdshot retinochoroidopathy, Harada's disease must be accompanied by exudative retinal detachment. Upon resolution of the retinal detachments, large areas of chorioretinal atrophy are seen that lack the discrete appearance of birdshot lesions.

Sympathetic uveitis is another chronic intraocular inflammatory condition that has as a manifestation multiple deep, cream-colored inflammatory lesions. Intraocular inflammation is typically more pronounced in sympathetic uveitis and there is a history of invasive ocular surgery or trauma.

Acute posterior multifocal placoid pigment epitheliopathy (APMPPE) and serpiginous choroidopathy can also have deep, cream-colored inflam-

matory lesions with uveitis. Both of these entities tend to affect the posterior pole primarily and their course differs distinctly from birdshot retinochoroidopathy.

Intraocular lymphoma (reticulum cell sarcoma) may manifest an intermediate uveitis-like picture. The choroidal involvement appears different than birdshot retinochoroidopathy, however, and in some cases the retina and choroid will be uninvolved.

TREATMENT AND COURSE

The long-term visual course and best course of therapy for birdshot retinochoroidopathy remain unclear. At present, there is no proven treatment. Based on its presumed inflammatory etiology, corticosteroids have been widely used to treat the inflammatory components of the disease. While corticosteroids remain the mainstay of therapy, most authors report retrospectively no significant improvement or only transient improvement despite their use.[1,3,7,8] Both systemic oral prednisone as well as subtenon injections of corticosteroids have been used.

Patients with birdshot retinochoroidopathy and intact central acuity (20/40 or better) probably require no therapy. Certainly the choroidal lesions themselves do not need to be treated. The major sequelae of retinal vascular leakage resulting in cystoid macular edema and neovascularization may require therapy, however.

Recently, cyclosporin A at both "high" dose (10 mg/kg) and "low" dose (5 mg/kg) has been reported to be effective at controlling the intraocular inflammation and stabilizing the visual acuity in patients with birdshot retinochoroidopathy.[7,19,20] The role of cyclosporin A and the timing of its use remain to be fully evaluated for this condition.

As for the choroidal and/or retinal neovascular complications, no study has been performed to evaluate the role of laser therapy. By extrapolation from other disorders that result in neovascularization of the posterior segment, however, laser therapy is generally recommended for birdshot retinochoroidopathy patients who develop these problems.

REFERENCES

1. Ryan SJ, Maumenee AE: Birdshot retinochoroidopathy. Am J Ophthalmol 89:31–45, 1980.
2. Gass JDM: Vitiliginous chorioretinitis. Arch Ophthalmol 99:1778–1787, 1981.
3. Nussenblatt RB, Palestine AG: Birdshot retinochoroidopathy. In Uveitis. Fundamentals and Clinical Practice. Chicago, Year Book, 1990, p 248–256.
4. Nussenblatt RB, Mittal KK, Ryan S: Birdshot retinochoroidopathy associated with HLA-A29 antigen and immune responsiveness to retinal S-antigen. Am J Ophthalmol 84:147–158, 1982.
5. LeHoang P, Ozdemir N, Benhamou, et al: HLA-A29.2 subtyping associated with birdshot retinochoroidopathy. Am J Ophthalmol 113:33–38, 1992.
6. Priem JA, Kijlistra A, Noens L, et al: HLA typing in birdshot chorioretinopathy. Am J Ophthalmol 105:182–187, 1988.
7. Vitale AT, Rodriguez A, Foster CS: Low-dose cyclosporine therapy in the treatment of birdshot retinochoroidopathy. Ophthalmology 101:822–831, 1994.
8. de Smet MD, Yamamoto JH, Mochizuki M, et al: Cellular immune responses of patients with uveitis to retinal antigens and their fragments. Am J Ophthalmol 110:135–142, 1990.
9. Suttorp-Schulten MSA, Luyendijk L, van Dam AP, et al: Birdshot chorioretinopathy and Lyme borreliosis. Am J Ophthalmol 115:149–153, 1993.
10. Brod R: Presumed sarcoid choroidopathy mimicking birdshot retinochoroidopathy. Am J Ophthalmol 109:357–358, 1990.
11. Priem HA, Osterhuis JA: Clinical manifestations in birdshot retinochoroidopathy. Br J Ophthalmol 72:646–651, 1988.
12. Kaplan HJ, Aaberg TM: Birdshot retinochoroidopathy. Am J Ophthalmol 90:773–782, 1980.
13. Soubrane G, Bokobza R, Coscas G: Late developing lesions in birdshot retinochoroidopathy. Am J Ophthalmol 109:204–210, 1990.
14. Fuerst DJ, Tessler HH, Fishman GA, et al: Birdshot retinochoroidopathy. Arch Ophthalmol 102:214–219, 1984.
15. Brucker AJ, Deglin EA, Bene C, Hoffman ME: Subretinal choroidal neovascularization in Birdshot retinochoroidopathy. Am J Ophthalmol (in press).
16. Soubrane G, Coscas G, Binaghi M, et al: Birdshot retinochoroidopathy and subretinal new vessels. Br J Ophthalmol 67:461–467, 1983.
17. Priem HA, De Rouck A, De Laey JJ, Bird AC: Electrophysiologic studies in birdshot chorioretinopathy. Am J Ophthalmol 106:430–436, 1988.
18. Hirose T, Katsumi O, Pruett RC, et al: Retinal function in birdshot retinochoroidopathy. Acta Ophthalmol 69:327–337, 1991.
19. LeHoang P, Girard B, Deray G, et al: Cyclosporine in the treatment of birdshot retinochoroidopathy. Transplant Proc 20(3 Suppl 4):128–130, 1988.
20. Nussenblatt RB, de Smet MD, Rubin B, et al: A masked, randomized, dose-response study between cyclosporin A and G in the treatment of sight-threatening uveitis of noninfectious origin. Am J Ophthalmol 115:538–591, 1993.

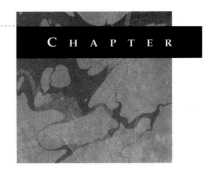

Sympathetic Ophthalmia

Alan H. Friedman, M.D.
Robert Selkin, M.D.

Sympathetic ophthalmia (SO) is a rare disease today.[1] When it does occur, SO usually follows penetrating injury or intraocular surgery. The condition was first recognized by Hippocrates over 2000 years ago, although the first "modern" description was made by Mackenzie, who also appropriately named the disease, in 1830. The first detailed histopathologic description of SO was made by Fuchs in 1905. SO is a cosmopolitan disease. Probably less than 50 cases per year are reported in the United States. In 1890, however, 5% of perforating injuries were associated with the development of SO (Fig. 46–1). As late as 1975, less than 0.1% of perforating injuries were followed by the development of SO. During the period from 1975 to 1980, 0.2% of eyes accessioned in 26 ocular pathology laboratories across the United States showed SO, whereas 1% of eyes accessioned at the AFIP showed SO. Curiously, no cases of SO were reported during the 1967 Arab–Israeli War, although 10% of all casualties were eye injuries.

Sympathetic ophthalmia is more often than not an incurable disease; once acquired, SO does not spontaneously go into remission. Patients have a lifelong association with uveitis. SO following perforating trauma has an incidence of 0.44%, while SO following surgery has an incidence of 0.06%. Both intraocular surgery (such as pars plana vitrectomy, glaucoma filtering surgery, and cataract extraction) and noncontact yttrium-aluminum-garnet (YAG) cyclodestructive procedures have been associated with the development of SO.

Onset occurs in approximately 17% of cases within 1 month; 50% within 3 months; 65% within 6 months; and 90% within the first year after injury. Eight per cent of cases reported in the literature occurred after enucleation of the exciting eye.

The hallmark clinical sign is uveitis in the contralateral eye following penetrating injury or intraocular surgery unless there is some other obvious etiology.[2-4] In the exciting eye, nearly 60% of patients report diminished visual acuity; conjunctival hyperemia occurs in 50% of cases; aqueous cells and flare occur in 50% of cases; keratic precipitates are observed in 30% of cases; cells in the vitreous occur in 25% of cases; posterior synechiae occur in 15%; and cells in Berger's space occur in 10% of cases. Macular and peripapillary edema (Fig. 46–2) are often an early finding and may occur in as many as 20% of all cases. In the sympathizing eye, the earliest symptoms is blurred vision which occurs in 60% and photophobia which occurs in 30 of cases. Blurred vision may be due to decreased amplitude of accommodation. This is an early sign of cyclitis. In the fundus, one can see Dalen-Fuchs (Fig. 46–3) nodules, which are small, discrete yellowish infiltrates that occur at the level of the retinal pigment epithelium.

HISTOPATHOLOGY

The histopathologic findings in sympathetic ophthalmia are typically nonnecrotizing, granulomatous panuveitis (Fig. 46–4). Focal areas of granulomatous inflammation (Fig. 46–5) alternate with areas of mononuclear inflammation and multinucleated giant cells, and epithelioid cells may contain phagocytosed melanin pigment. Dalen-Fuchs nodules collect under an attenuated retinal pigment epithelium (Fig. 46–6). They consist of lymphocytes and epithelioid cells. The choriocapillaris is generally but not always spared of the inflammatory process. The macula area may show a serous separation and the inflammation may extend through the

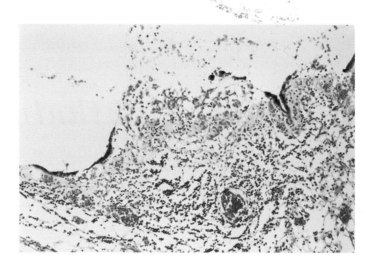

Dalen-Fuchs' nodule in a patient with sympathetic uveitis after pars plana vitrectomy.

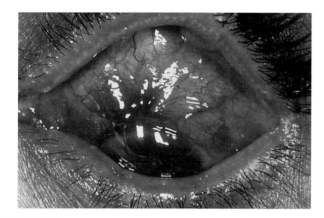

FIGURE 46-1   Clinical photograph shows an area of uveal prolapse superior to the limbus. The pupil is updrawn.

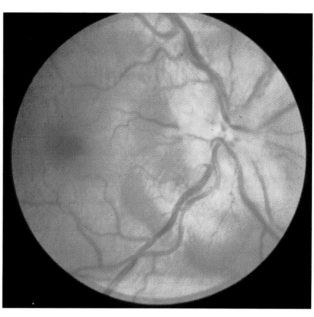

FIGURE 46-2   Clinical photograph showing extensive peripapillary and optic nerve edema.

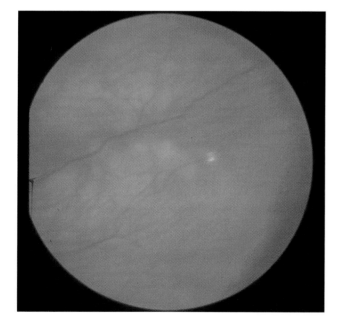

FIGURE 46-3   Clinical photograph showing a Dalen-Fuchs nodule in the midperiphery.

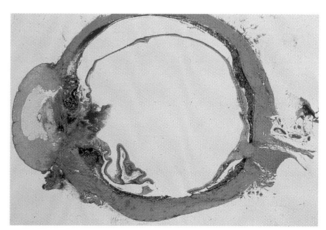

FIGURE 46-4   Photograph of a whole eye section showing the area of primary injury as well as panuveal inflammation.

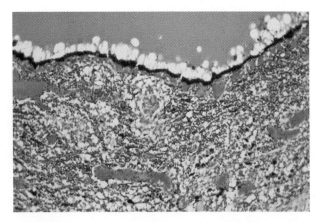

FIGURE 46–5 Photomicrograph shows granulomatous inflammation within the choroid. Note, also, the sparing of the choriocapillaris and the subretinal fluid.

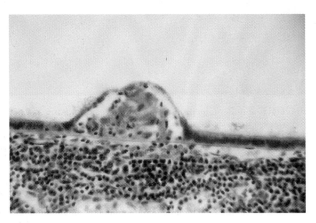

FIGURE 46–6 Photomicrograph of a Dalen-Fuchs nodule. Note the collection of mononuclear cells beneath the attenuated retinal pigment epithelium.

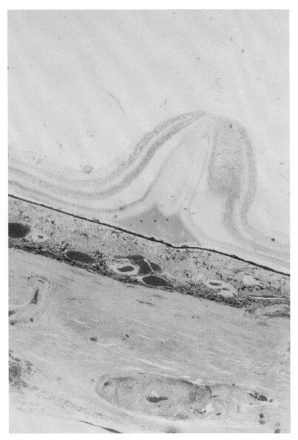

FIGURE 46–7 Photomicrograph showing serous detachment of the sensory retina as well as inflammatory cells surrounding an emissary blood vessel in the sclera.

sclera via the emissaria and form nodules on the episclera (Fig. 46–7).

SEQUELAE

The sequelae of SO are very variable. Secondary glaucoma due to angle closure from peripheral anterior synechiae may necessitate a trabeculectomy with mitomycin. Posterior subcapsular cataract, serous retinal detachments, posterior pole edema, optic neuritis, and secondary optic atrophy are all regularly reported sequelae. We have also seen vitiligo of the skin in both African-American and white patients. In two patients, both white, we noted the development of vitiligo of the retinal pigment epithelium and choroid. In one patient, the condition was arrested by treatment with prednisone, cyclosporine, and azathioprine. The second was totally unresponsive to therapy.

TREATMENT

Sympathetic ophthalmia is generally treated with oral corticosteroids. In some cases when a trial of corticosteroids is unsuccessful, it may be necessary to add cyclosporine or additionally azathioprine. The level of medication may be titrated to control the level of inflammation.

Acknowledgment: This work was supported in part by an unrestricted grant from Fight For Sight, Inc., New York, NY.

REFERENCES

1. Friedman AH, Luntz M, Henley WL. Diagnosis and Management of Uveitis. Baltimore, Williams & Wilkins, 1984.
2. Smith RE, Nozik RM: Uveitis: A Clinical Approach to Diagnosis and Managment. 2nd edition. Baltimore, Williams & Wilkins, 1993, pp 141–143.
3. Nussenblatt RB, Whitcup SM, Palestine AG: Uveitis: Fundamentals and Clinical Procedure. 2nd edition. St Louis, CV Mosby Co, 1996, pp 299–311.
4. Pepose JS, Holland GN, Wilhelmus KR: Ocular Infection and Immunity. St Louis, CV Mosby Co, 1996, pp 723–733.

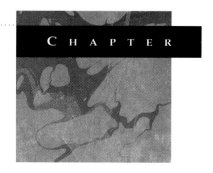

CHAPTER 47

Vogt-Koyanagi-Harada Syndrome

Patrick E. Rubsamen, M.D.

J. Donald M. Gass, M.D.

DEFINITION

Vogt-Koyanagi-Harada syndrome is a bilateral panuveitis associated with exudative retinal detachment. In the past, this syndrome was artificially divided, Vogt-Koyanagi syndrome[1,2] being an anterior inflammatory condition and Harada's disease[3] a posterior uveitis associated with exudative retinal detachment. VKH syndrome now represents a spectrum of disease including both the anterior and posterior manifestations of the condition.[4,5]

ETIOLOGY

The etiology of Vogt-Koyanagi-Harada syndrome is not well understood. The disease appears to be a primary inflammatory condition targeted at melanin-containing cells present in the uveal tract, central nervous system, and skin.[6-8] A T-cell–mediated reaction to ocular antigens seems to be involved.[9-11] This is supported by immunohistochemical studies that have shown class II antigen expression on choroidal melanocytes and the presence of activated T cells in the choroid.[11] Late in the course of the disease there is loss of choroidal melanocytes coupled with infiltration of the choroid with T cells and B cells.[9,10] Although the retina does not appear to be the primary site of injury, a role for humeral immunity has been suggested by the presence of circulating antiretinal autoantibodies.[12] A viral association has been suggested in the past; however, there is no proven infectious cause of the condition.[6]

EPIDEMIOLOGY

The age at onset may range from childhood through later adult life, however the majority of patients will be between their 20s and 40s. The disease has a predilection toward darkly pigmented individuals and patients with Oriental ancestry. A link to Oriental ancestry through the American Indian has been suggested in some patients in the United States.[13-16] Specific HLA associations have been described indicating a probable genetic predisposition to the disease. HLA-DR4, HLA-Drw53, and HLA-DQw3 have been found to be associated with a predilection for VKH syndrome.[15,17,18] Certain HLA gene variations may also play a role in predisposing some patients towards the chronic, relapsing form of the disease.[19] The role of hereditary factors is also supported by the development of VKH syndrome in monozygotic twins.[20]

HISTOPATHOLOGY

Histopathologic evaluation of patients with VKH syndrome has shown an inflammatory reaction presumably targeted at the pigmented cells of the uveal tract. Giant cells with evidence of pigment phagocytosis and loss of choroidal melanocytes have been demonstrated. Previous histopathologic evaluations, during the late phases of the disease, have shown both granulomatous and nongranulomatous infiltration of the uveal tract with predominantly plasma cell infiltration.[5,9] Also in the latter phase of the condition, atrophic changes at the level of the retinal pigment epithelium (RPE) with generalized thinning of the outer segments of the retina are evident.[5,11] Histopathologic examination in the active, early phase of the disease has shown the inflammatory infiltrate to be composed predominantly of activated T cells and macrophages with inflammatory cells in close proximity to choroidal melanocytes.[21] Nondendritic CD 1–positive cells were noted to be present. Inomata has noted a diffuse nongranulomatous inflammatory reaction involving the uveal tract, and has demonstrated subretinal neovascularization in some longstanding cases.[22]

PRESENTING SYMPTOMS

Decreased vision is a common presenting symptom. Although manifestations of the disease may be separated into anterior segment and posterior segment involvement, early in the course of the disease posterior involvement tends to be the predominant feature. Decreased vision is frequently associated with exudative retinal detachment. The condition is usually bilateral, although there may be a delay in onset of visual symptoms between the two eyes. Approximately 80% of patients will present with a bilateral decrease in vision at their first presentation and most will have bilateral involvement within the first 2 weeks.[23] Patients, early on, may also present with complaints of ocular discomfort, but severe ocular pain is not a common complaint.

At the onset of the ocular disease, patients may develop flu-like symptoms such as fever, malaise, headache, and nausea. These systemic manifestations may precede the onset of ocular disease. Neurologic symptoms may include ataxia, confusion, and focal neurologic symptoms.[24] Transient hearing loss and tinnitus may be present.[6,25,26] Audiometric evaluation within the first month of disease confirms the high incidence of hearing loss.[6] These symptoms are felt to be associated with inflammation involving the meninges and inner ear.

Cutaneous findings tend to occur later in the course of the disease. The cutaneous manifestations may include poliosis, vitiligo, madarosis, and alopecia. Late ocular findings include decreased vision and may include ocular pain associated with anterior segment inflammation or elevated intraocular pressure due to secondary glaucoma.

CLINICAL SIGNS

Clinical signs may depend on the point of presentation during the course of the disease. The disease has been previously divided into several stages: a prodromal phase, characterized by systemic symptoms similar to the flu; an ocular phase, where eye findings predominate; and a convalescent or chronic phase, characterized by resolution of ocular

inflammation or persistence of anterior segment disease.[4,6]

Presenting features of the early phase of the disease most typically are manifested by bilateral vitreous inflammation and exudative retinal detachment. Inflammatory cells are present in the vitreous, but many patients do not develop severe vitreous cellular reaction so that it is usually possible to visualize the posterior manifestations of the disease via ophthalmoscopy.

The retinal findings are characteristic and include localized and/or extensive exudative retinal detachment (Fig. 47–1). The exudative detachments usually begin in the posterior segment and are often multifocal with a cloviform appearance.[27] Early in the course of the disease the exudative retinal findings may be manifest simply as retinal striae in the macula due to chorioretinal folds (Fig. 47–2). Extensive near total or total bullous retinal detachment, with fluid that may shift with positioning of the patient, can occur in severe or untreated cases (Fig. 47–3). Retinal detachment is usually bilateral, although a delay of 1 to 2 weeks, and occasionally longer, between the two eyes may occur. Focal, yellow-white lesions that appear to be at the level of the pigment epithelium may be present in some cases (Fig. 47–4). The optic disc, typically, is hyperemic or can develop marked swelling with an appearance similar to optic neuritis (Fig. 47–5).[28]

Once the retinal detachment has resolved, the fundus is characterized by pigmentary alteration. There may be a characteristic generalized depigmentation of the fundus showing the "sunset glow" fundus sign (Fig. 47–6). The pigmentary changes will often be apparent within the first few weeks after resolution of the exudative retinal detachments.[6,25,29] (Fig. 47–7). Irregular areas of marked depigmentation and/or pigment clumping in the macula may develop in some cases (Fig.

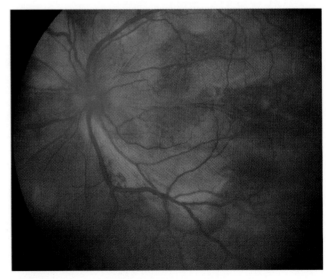

FIGURE 47–1 Multifocal serous retinal detachment with lobulated or cloviform appearance.

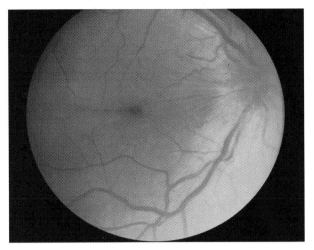

FIGURE 47–2 Chorioretinal folds in the macula with accompanying disc swelling.

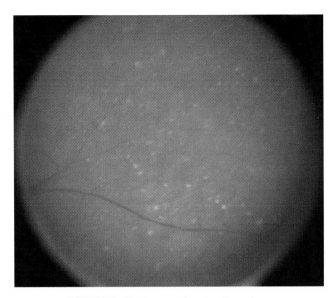

FIGURE 47–4 Peripheral yellow dots.

47–8). Sometimes multifocal atrophic chorioretinal scars may be present that may form a confluent, curvilinear pattern near the equator.[30]

The anterior segment manifestations of the disease may include anterior chamber cell and flare with keratic precipitates present (Fig. 47–9). Cataract and peripheral anterior synechiae formation are typically seen in patients who develop chronic anterior disease. Iris nodules may be seen in these patients as well (Fig. 47–10). Paralimbal vitiligo has been previously described by Sugiura.[6,31] Some patients at initial presentation may develop a shallow anterior chamber or acute angle closure glaucoma associated with marked choroidal inflammation and anterior displacement of the ciliary body.[32–34]

Cutaneous findings (poliosis, madarosis, vitiligo and/or alopecia) occur at some point in approximately one third of patients (Figs. 47–11 through 47–13).[6,23,25,26] The incidence of cutaneous disease

may have decreased with the advent of more aggressive treatment with systemic corticosteroids.[26,35]

DIAGNOSTIC TESTS

Fluorescein angiography will often show very typical findings in VKH syndrome.[29,36–38] Multifocal leaks at the level of the pigment epithelium with pooling of dye in the area of exudative detachments is typically present (Figs. 47–14 and 47–15). There may be patchy areas of delayed choroidal filling present. The patchy choroidal hypofluorescence has

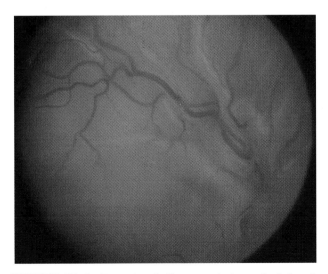

FIGURE 47–3 Extensive, bullous exudative retinal detachment.

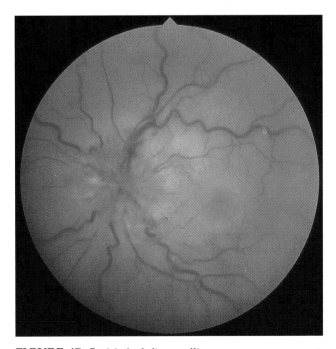

FIGURE 47–5 Marked disc swelling, venous engorgement, and exudative retinal detachment.

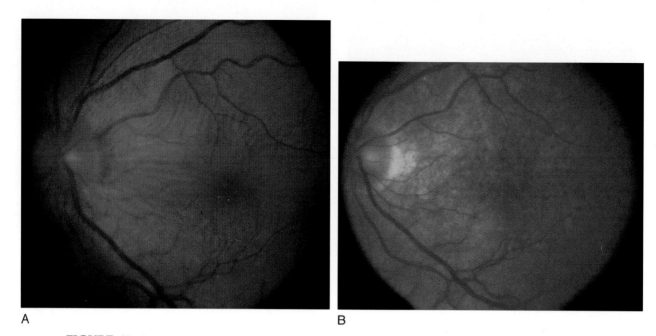

FIGURE 47–6 *A,* Retinal striae secondary to shallow exudative retinal detachment with pigmented fundus as seen on presentation. *B,* "Sunset glow" fundus secondary to pigmentary loss seen 6 months later following resolution of the exudative detachment.

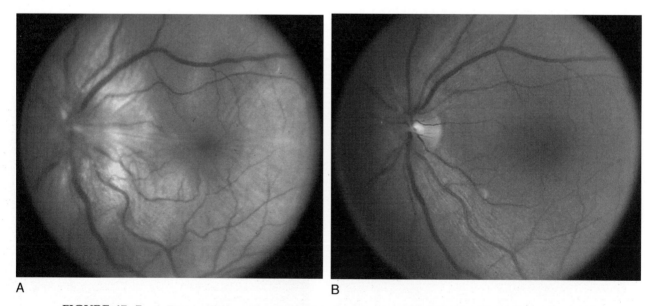

FIGURE 47–7 *A,* Disc swelling and exudative detachment seen on presentation. The patient was treated with systemic corticosteroids (80 mg prednisone per day). *B,* Two weeks following presentation and initiation of treatment resolution of the detachment and disc swelling are evident. Note the early pigmentary mottling present in the macula.

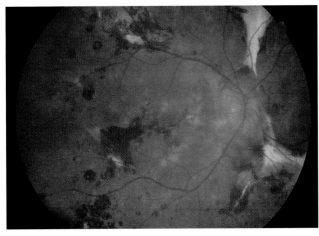

FIGURE 47–8   Marked pigmentary disturbance with subretinal scarring seen in patient with previous extensive exudative retinal detachment (see Fig. 47–3).

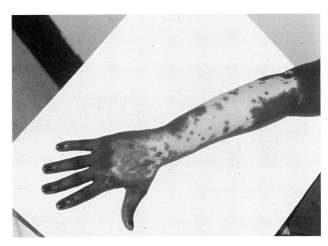

FIGURE 47–11   Vitiligo involving the arm of a patient with VKH syndrome.

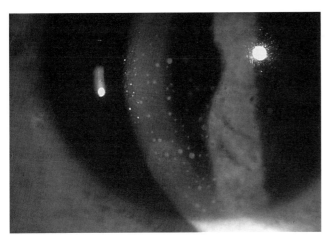

FIGURE 47–9   Large keratic precipitates present on the corneal endothelium.

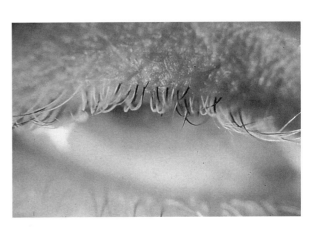

FIGURE 47–12   Poliosis.

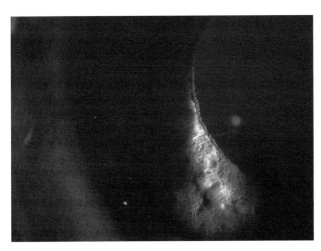

FIGURE 47–10   Iris nodules.

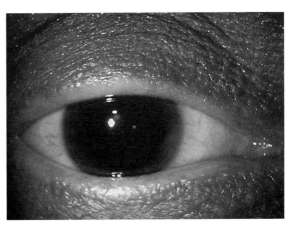

FIGURE 47–13   Madarosis.

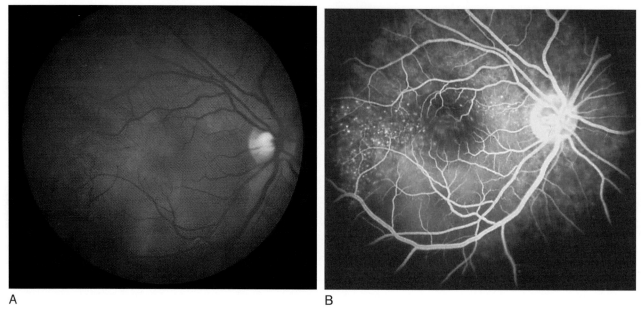

FIGURE 47–14   *A*, Exudative retinal detachment involving the macula in a patient presenting with first episode of VKH syndrome. *B*, Fluorescein angiogram with multifocal pinpoint leaks ("star-in-the-sky" appearance) with blocked background choroidal fluorescence in the inferior macula due to dye accumulation in the subretinal space.

also been documented with indocyanine green videoangiography.[39] There is often staining of the optic disc early in the disease corresponding to disc swelling. The permeability abnormality noted on fluorescein angiography has been shown to be reversible with treatment.[40] Later in the course of the disease, window defects or blocked fluorescence in areas of RPE depigmentation or hyperpigmentation will be evident. Choroidal neovascularization will develop in some cases later in the disease course.[22,41–43]

Diagnostic ultrasound shows diffuse, low-reflective choroidal thickening most evident in the posterior fundus (Fig. 47–16).[44,45] Some other conditions with exudative detachment such as idiopathic uveal effusion syndrome, posterior scleritis, or metastatic carcinoma can be differentiated from VKH, as they tend to show high-reflective choroi-

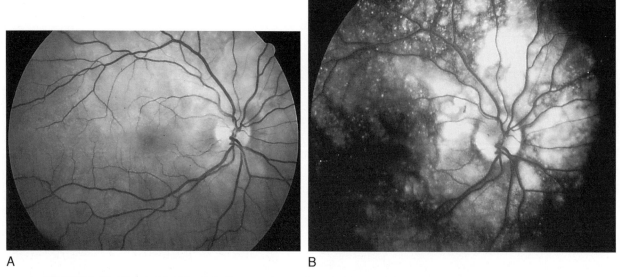

FIGURE 47–15   *A*, Multifocal shallow exudative detachments. *B*, Multiple areas of dye accumulation are present in the later frames of the angiogram demonstrating the extensive nature of the chorioretinal abnormality.

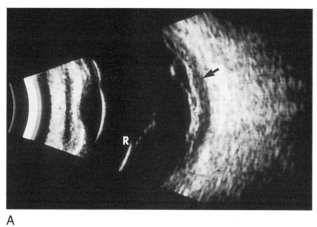
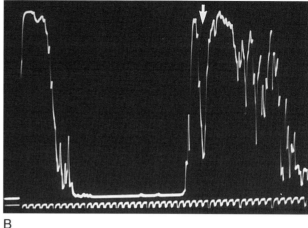

A   B

FIGURE 47–16   *A*, B-scan ultrasound view of the posterior pole shows bullous exudative retinal detachment (R) and diffuse choroidal thickening (*arrow*). *B*, Standardized A-scan in area of attached retina demonstrates low-reflective choroidal thickening (*arrow*).

dal thickening. Overlying exudative retinal detachment will be detectable in those cases with significant detachment. Although optic nerve swelling is a common early feature of VKH syndrome, marked optic nerve swelling on ultrasound is not typical.

Lumbar paracentesis has been used to assist in making the diagnosis of VKH in the past.[6,25,26] Cerebrospinal fluid findings include elevated protein and lymphocyte levels with pleocytosis. The diagnosis of VKH syndrome can often be established based upon clinical findings making the use of a more invasive procedure such as lumbar paracentesis unnecessary in many cases.[23]

Recently, magnetic resonance imaging (MRI) has been used as an adjunct in the diagnosis of Vogt-Koyanagi-Harada syndrome.[46,47] MRI is able to demonstrate choroidal thickening in contrast with the sclera and may help in differentiating diseases that involve both tissues (i.e., posterior scleritis, uveal effusion syndrome). In the active phase of the disease enhancement of the choroid was seen using MRI with contrast media. The choroidal enhancement was seen to diminish following treatment with corticosteroids.

DIFFERENTIAL DIAGNOSIS

The differential diagnosis of VKH syndrome is largely dependent on the time period in the course of the disease at which the patient is initially seen. Beniz et al have noted that, early in the course of the disease, patients may present with an incomplete form of the disease and have emphasized establishing the diagnosis despite this in order to allow timely therapeutic intervention.[48] Early in the disease conditions causing exudative detachment of the retina should be considered.[29] These include idiopathic central serous chorioretinopathy, leukemic infiltration, uveal effusion syndrome, and

sympathetic ophthalmia. In the late phases of the diseases conditions leading to chronic anterior segment inflammation, such as sarcoidosis and Behçet's disease, should be considered in the differential. Sympathetic ophthalmia is a disease that may demonstrate the same clinical findings as VKH syndrome, including cutaneous and ocular manifestations. Sympathetic ophthalmia, however, is nearly always associated with a history of prior intraocular surgery or trauma.

TREATMENT

Treatment of VKH syndrome is targeted at decreasing the intraocular inflammatory reaction. The mainstay of treatment is systemic corticosteroids.[6,25] Oral doses of prednisone between 80 and 100 mg/day typically result in a rapid response.[23] Hayaska et al have recommended the use of oral steroids in the posterior (Harada's) form of the disease.[49] Intravenous pulse treatment may be necessary in more severe cases, particularly when associated with severe anterior inflammation (Vogt-Koyanagi type).[25,49,50] Occasional patients can have spontaneous resolution within weeks without treatment; however, systemic treatment is associated with an improved prognosis. Sarasota et al noted a better visual outcome in patients treated with systemic steroids as compared to patients with topical treatment, but found no difference in outcome between patients treated with oral steroids when compared to pulse therapy.[51]

In the early phase of the disease the inflammatory findings in VKH tend to be very responsive to corticosteroid treatment, often with rapid improvement in vision and resolution of the serous retinal detachments within a couple of weeks of treatment. A common mistake encountered in treatment of this condition, however, is the rapid tapering or discontinuation of steroids after an initial positive response. Patients may develop rebound inflammation in this setting requiring reinitiation of a high steroid dose to obtain a treatment response. Patients should be weaned off steroids slowly after an initial response. We have previously found that the average duration of steroid treatment for the initial episode of the disease is approximately 6 months (range, 2 months to 4 years).

Many patients will develop recurrent inflammation within the first 6 months of disease onset that will require reinitiation of treatment.[6,23] Recurrent retinal detachment is common during this time but does not commonly recur after the first few months of disease. Previously we have found that patients who develop chronic anterior uveitis have a need for a longer duration of steroid treatment (average treatment, 48 months) as compared to patients whose disease remains predominantly posterior (average, 6 months).[23] Timing of onset of treatment may be important. Early treatment seems to result in less long-term inflammation, while premature discontinuation of steroids may result in the onset of chronic uveitis.[49,52] Fujioka found that patients treated within 2 weeks of onset of disease had a mean duration of steroid treatment of approximately 4 months as compared to those patients who had a delay of initiation of steroid treatment (45 months).[53]

In refractory patients, especially those patients that develop chronic anterior uveitis, cyclosporine has been used with some success. This drug may provide an alternative as well in those patients requiring long-term corticosteroids and who have suffered serious steroid-related side effects. Limited series of patients with chronic VKH syndrome have been treated by several investigators with improvement in some cases.[54-57] Doses between 5 and 10 mg/kg of body weight per day have been employed. Hepatic and renal toxicity are reported, but are usually reversible. FK506 is a new immunosuppressive agent that has been evaluated in the treatment of refractory uveitis including VKH syndrome and may provide an alternative for cyclosporine-resistant patients.[58,59] Nonsteroidal anti-inflammatory medications may be useful in place of maintenance systemic steroids in some chronic cases.[60]

PROGNOSIS

Although early reports describe the prognosis as being poor,[4,35] early diagnosis and more aggressive treatment appear to have improved the outcome.[6,13,23,25,26,61] Two thirds or more of eyes with VKH syndrome and undergoing treatment with corticosteroids will maintain visual acuity of 20/40 or better. Twenty per cent or less of eyes will ultimately have visual acuity less than 20/200.[23,26,48] A worse visual prognosis has been noted to be associated with poor vision at presentation and the development of chronic relapsing uveitis or choroidal neovascularization.[23,25]

COMPLICATIONS

A common cause of visual loss in Vogt-Koyanagi-Harada syndrome is pigmentary change or degeneration of the pigment epithelium and retina associated with the posterior segment inflammatory condition.[13] Many patients will develop a generalized depigmentation of the fundus associated with the "sunset glow" sign.[25]

Choroidal neovascularization has been described in patients with VKH syndrome (Fig. 47-17). Neovascularization probably occurs as a response to damage to Bruch's membrane and the retinal pigment epithelium which occurs as a result of the inflammatory reaction near these areas.[22,41,42] Development of this complication is more likely to occur in patients with extensive pigmentary changes and it may be associated with extensive visual loss.[22,23,41-43]

Patients with VKH syndrome may develop either acute or chronic glaucoma. Acute-onset glaucoma may develop early in the course of the disease due to ciliary body swelling and anterior rotation of the lens-iris diaphragm.[32-34] Pupillary block with iris bombéy may also develop due to formation of posterior synechia. Chronic glaucoma predominantly affects those individuals with chronic anterior segment inflammation. Patients may develop open angle glaucoma secondary to inflammation or due to treatment with corticosteroids. Secondary angle closure glaucoma may develop in patients with protracted or severe anterior segment inflammation.[5,62] Patients may respond to medical treatment, but filtering surgery may be necessary. In the setting of chronic inflammation, filtering surgery with antimetabolites such as 5-fluorouracil or mitomycin may be appropriate first-line therapy, possibly resulting in better long-term survival of the filtering bleb and improved intraocular pressure control.[62]

Cystoid macular edema may occur and be a cause of decreased vision in some patients. Rutzen et al noted improved visual acuity and a concomitant decrease in clinically and angiographically documented macular edema in patients with VKH syndrome treated with subtenon triamcinolone injections.[63]

Cataract is a common complication in patients with VKH syndrome and may develop as a result of chronic anterior segment inflammation or long-term corticosteroid use. Successful cataract surgery with implantation of intraocular lenses in the setting of chronic uveitis and VKH syndrome has been reported.[64-66] Patients undergoing cataract surgery should under optimal circumstances have quiescent inflammation for a period of approximately 3

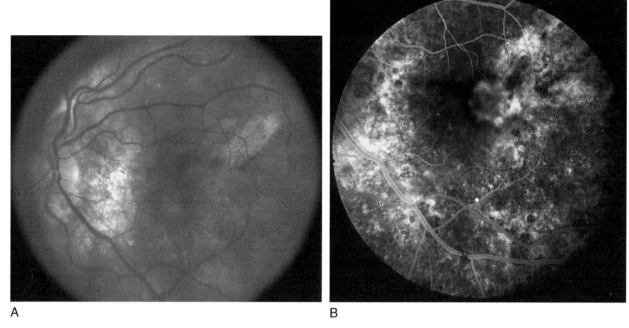

A   B

FIGURE 47-17   *A*, Patient with chronic VKH and macular choroidal neovascular membrane (CNV). Note grayish CNVM with small area of subretinal blood. Extensive pigmentary atrophy and hyperplasia are evident. *B*, Fluorescein angiogram shows area of hyperfluorescence corresponding to area of CNV.

months prior to surgery.[64] Furthermore, preoperative treatment with immunosuppresives may decrease the risk of severe inflammation in the perioperative period. Moorthy et al reported on 19 eyes undergoing cataract extraction in patients with VKH syndrome.[66] The majority of their patients were treated with 40 to 60 mg of prednisone for 1 week preoperatively. Eleven eyes underwent posterior chamber intraocular lens placement at the time of surgery without complication. In eyes with persistent anterior segment inflammation and cataract, a pars plana approach coupled with vitrectomy and without intraocular lens implantation may be the preferred mode of treatment.[66,67]

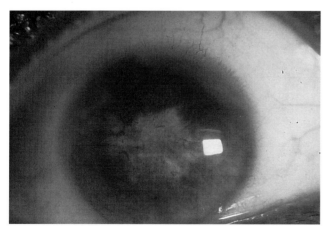

FIGURE 47-18   Dense cataract and posterior synechia in patient with chronic VKH syndrome. Note relative absence of pigment along the limbus in this black patient with paralimbal vitiligo (Sugiura's sign)[31].

Optic atrophy may result from widespread and advanced retinal disease or in association with optic neuropathy. Although optic neuropathy is a relatively infrequent cause of severe visual loss in patients with VKH, it has been reported as the predominant cause of visual loss in some cases.[26,28] Optic disc neovascularization has been found to be associated with chronic uveitis and, although rare, has been reported late in VKH syndrome as well.[68,69]

Anterior segment complications include seclusion of the pupil and band keratopathy. Occasionally, patients will develop severe inflammation resulting in posterior synechia, cataract, and occasionally phthisis bulbi (Fig. 47-18).

Cutaneous changes such as vitiligo and hair loss may occur.[6] The incidence of these findings may have decreased with earlier, more aggressive systemic treatment, although vitiligo develops at some point in at least one quarter of patients.[23,26,35] Permanent neurosensory hearing deficits and other neurologic abnormalities have been reported.[6]

REFERENCES

1. Vogt A: Fruhzeitiges Ergrauen der Zilien und Bemerkungen uber den sogenannten plotzlichen Eintritt dieser Veranderung. Klin Monatsbl Augenheilkd 44:228–242, 1906.
2. Koyanagi Y: Dysakusis, alopecia, und poliosis bei schwerer uveitis nicht traumatischen Ursprungs. Klin Monatsbl Augenheilkd 82:194–211, 1929.
3. Harada Y: Beitrag zur klinischen kenntis von nichteitriger Choroiditis (Choroiditis diffusa acuta). Acta Soc Ophthalmol Jpn 30:356–378, 1926.
4. Cowper AR: Harada's disease and Vogt-Koyanagi syn-

drome: uveoencephalitis. Arch Ophthalmol 45:367–376, 1951.

5. Perry HD, Font RL: Clinical and histopathologic observations in severe Vogt-Koyanagi-Harada syndrome. Am J Ophthalmol 83:242–254, 1977.

6. Sugiura S: Vogt-Koyanagi-Harada disease. Jpn J Ophthalmol 22:9–35, 1978.

7. Hammer H: Cellular hypersensitivity to uveal pigment confirmed by leukocyte migration tests in sympathetic ophthalmitis and the Vogt-Koyanagi-Harada syndrome. Br J Ophthalmol 58:773–776, 1974.

8. Norose K, Yano A, Aosai F, Segawa K: Immunologic analysis of cerebrospinal fluid lymphocytes in Vogt-Koyanagi-Harada disease. Invest Ophthalmol Vis Sci 31:1210–1216, 1990.

9. Chan CC, Palestine AG, Kuwabaraa T, Nussenblatt RB: Immunopathologic study of Vogt-Koyanagi-Harada syndrome. Am J Ophthalmol 105:607–611, 1988.

10. Inomata H, Sakamoto T: Immunohistochemical studies of Vogt-Koyanagi-Harada disease with sunset sky fundus. Curr Eye Res 9:35–40, 1990.

11. Sakamoto T, Murata T, Inomata H: Class II major histocompatibility complex on melanocytes of Vogt-Koyanagi-Harada disease. Arch Ophthalmol 109:1270–1274, 1991.

12. Chan CC, Palestine AG, Nussenblatt RB, et al: Anti-retinal auto-antibodies in Vogt-Koyanagi-Harada syndrome, Behcet's disease, and sympathetic ophthalmia. Ophthalmology 92:1025–1028, 1985.

13. Snyder DA, Tessler HH: Vogt-Koyanagi-Harada syndrome. Am J Ophthalmol 90:69–75, 1980.

14. Nussenblatt RB: Clinical studies of Vogt-Koyanagi-Harada disease at the National Eye Institute, NIH, USA. Jpn J Ophthalmol 32:330–333, 1988.

15. Davis JL, Mittal KK, Freidlin V, et al: HLA associations and ancestry in Vogt-Koyanagi-Harada syndrome and sympathetic ophthalmia. Ophthalmology 97:1137–42, 1990.

16. Martinez JA, Lopez PF, Sternberg P Jr, et al: Vogt-Koyanagi-Harada syndrome in patients with Cherokee ancestry. Am J Ophthalmol 114:615–620, 1992.

17. Zhao M, Jiang Y, Abrahams IW: Association of HLA antigens with Vogt-Koyanagi-Harada syndrome in a Han Chinese population. Arch Ophthalmol 109:368–370, 1991.

18. Zhang XY, Wang XM, Hu TS: Profiling human leukocyte antigens in Vogt-Koyanagi-Harada syndrome. Am J Ophthalmol 113:567–572, 1992.

19. Islam SM, Numaga J, Matsuki K, et al: Influence of HLA-DRB1 gene variation on the clinical course of Vogt-Koyanagi-Harada disease. Invest Ophthalmol Vis Sci 35:752–756, 1994.

20. Itho S, Kurimoto S, Kouno T: Vogt-Koyanagi-Harada disease in monozygotic twins. Int Ophthalmol 16:49–54, 1992.

21. Kahn M, Pepose JS, Green WR, et al: Immunocytologic findings in a case of Vogt-Koyanagi-Harada syndrome. Ophthalmology 100:1191–1198, 1993.

22. Inomata H, Minei M, Taniguchi Y, Hishimura F: Choroidal neovascularization in long standing case of Vogt-Koyanagi-Harada disease. Jpn J Ophthalmol 27:9–26, 1983.

23. Rubsamen PE, Gass JDM: Vogt-Koyanagi-Harada syndrome: clinical course, therapy, and long term visual outcome. Ach Ophthalmol 109:682–687, 1991.

24. Lubin JR, Loewenstein JI, Frederick AR: Vogt-Koyanagi-Harada syndrome with focal neurologic signs. Am J Ophthalmol 91:332–341, 1981.

25. Ohno .S, Minakawas R, Matsuda H: Clinical studies of Vogt-Koyanagi-Harada's disease. Jpn J Ophthalmol 32:334–343, 1988.

26. O'Conner RG: Vogt-Koyanagi-Harada syndrome. Am J Ophthalmol 83:735–740, 1977.

27. Uehara M, Sakisaka H, Ueda S, Yoshioka H: Initial ocular signs in Harada's disease. Folia Ophthalmol Jpn 29:1382–1392, 1978.

28. Lane CM, Jones CA, Bird AC: Optic disc swelling in sympathetic ophthalmitis and Harada's disease. Trans Ophthalmol Soc U K 105:667–673, 1986.

29. Gass JDM (ed): Stereoscopic Atlas of Macular Disease: Diagnosis and Treatment, 3rd edition. St Louis, Mosby-Year Book, 1987, pp 150–153.

30. Chung YM, Yeh TS: Linear streak lesions of the fundus equator associated with Vogt-Koyanagi-Harada syndrome. Am J Ophthalmol 109:745–746, 1990.

31. Friedman AH, Deutsch-Sokol RH: Sugiura's sign: perilimbal vitiligo in the Vogt-Koyanagi-Harada syndrome. Ophthalmology 88:1159–1165, 1981.

32. Hatta M, Kumagaya I, Takeda H, Nomatsu I: Increased ocular tension as initial sign of disease of Harada. Jpn J Clin Ophthalmol 22:141–145, 1968.

33. Shirato S, Hayashi K, Masuda K: Acute angle closure glaucoma as an initial sign of Harada's disease: report of two cases. Jpn J Ophthalmol 24:260–266, 1980.

34. Kimura R, Sakai M, Okabe H: Transient shallow anterior chamber as initial symptom in Harada's syndrome. Arch Ophthalmol 99:1604–1608, 1981.

35. Rosen E: Uveitis with poliosis, vitiligo, alopecia and dysacousia (Vogt-Koyanagi syndrome). Arch Ophthalmol 33:281–292, 1945.

36. Yoshioka H: Fluorescence fundus angiographic findings in early stage of Harada's syndrome. Acta Soc Ophthalmol Jpn 72:2298–2306, 1968.

37. Shimizu K: Harada's, Behcet's, and Vogt-Koyanagi syndromes: are they clinical entities? Trans Am Acad Ophthalmol Otolaryngol 77:281–290, 1973.

38. Kanter PJ, Goldberg MF: Bilateral uveitis with exudative retinal detachment: angiographic appearance. Arch Ophthalmol 91:13–19, 1974.

39. Yuzawa M, Kawamura A, Matsui M: Indocyanine green video-angiographic findings in Harada's disease. Jpn J Ophthalmol 37:456–466, 1993.

40. Masuda K, Tanishima T: Harada's disease: a new therapeutic approach. Jpn J Clin Ophthalmol 23:553–555, 1969.

41. Yoshioka H, Risei F, Kenichi C: Serous and hemorrhagic macular detachment in Harada's syndrome initiated in ocular sign of malignant glaucoma. Folia Ophthalmol Jpn 29:1186–1190, 1975.

42. Ober RR, Smith RE, Ryan SJ: Subretinal neovascularization in the Vogt-Koyanagi-Harada syndrome. Int Ophthalmol 6:225–234, 1983.

43. Moorthy RA, Chong LP, Smith RE, Rao NA: Subretinal neovascular membranes in Vogt-Koyanagi-Harada syndrome. Am J Ophthalmol 116:164–170, 1993.

44. Forster DJ, Green RL, Rao NA: Echographic features of the Vogt-Koyanagi-Harada syndrome. Arch Ophthalmol 108:1421–1426, 1990.

45. Byrne SF, Green RL (eds): Ultrasound of the Eye and Orbit. St Louis, Mosby Year Book, 1992.

46. Johnston CA, Teitelbaum CS: Magnetic resonance imaging in Vogt-Koyanagi-Harada syndrome. Ach Ophthalmol 108:783–784, 1990.

47. Ibanez HE, Grand GM, Meredith TA: Wippold FJ II. Magnetic resonance imaging findings in Vogt-Koyanagi-Harada syndrome. Retina 14:164–168, 1994.

48. Beniz J, Forster DJ, Lean JS, et al: Variations in clinical features of the Vogt-Koyanagi-Harada syndrome. Retina 11:275–280, 1991.

49. Hayaska S, Okabe H, Takahashi J: Systemic corticosteroid treatment in Vogt-Koyanagi-Harada disease. Graefes Arch Clin Exp Ophthalmol 218:9–13, 1982.

50. Kotake S, Ohno S: 'Pulse' methylprednisolone therapy in the treatment of Vogt-Koyanagi-Harada's disease. Jpn J Clin Ophthalmol 38:1053–1058, 1984.

51. Sasamoto Y., Ohno S., Matsuda H: Studies on corticosteroid therapy in Vogt-Koyanagi-Harada disease. Ophthalmologica 201:162–167, 1990.

52. Kawata K, Oka Y: The Vogt-Koyanagi-Harada syndrome: a 14 year review. Jpn J Clin Ophthalmol 31:17–22, 1977.

53. Fujioka T., Fukuda M., Okinami S: A statistic study of Vogt-Koyanagi-Harada syndrome. Acta Soc Ophthalmol Jpn 84:1979–1982, 1980.

54. Nussenblatt RB, Palestine AG, Chan CC: Cyclosporin A therapy in the treatment of intraocular inflammatory dis-

ease resistant to systemic corticosteroids and cytotoxic agents. Am J Ophthalmol 96:275–282, 1983.

55. Harada T, Sugita K, Saito A, Awaya S: Traitement des uveites severes par la ciclosporie A. Ophthalmologica 195: 21–25, 1987.

56. Wakatsuki Y, Kogure M, Takahashi Y, Oguro Y: Combination therapy with cyclosporin a and steroid in severe case of Vogt-Koyanagi-Harada's disease. Jpn J Ophthalmol 32: 358–360, 1988.

57. Wakefield D, McCluskey P, Reece G: Cyclosporin therapy in Vogt-Koyanagi-Harada's disease. Aust N Z J Ophthalmol 18:137–142, 1990.

58. Mochizuki M, Masuda K, Sakane T, et al: A clinical trial of FK506 in refractory uveitis. Am J Ophthalmol 115:763–769, 1993.

59. Ishioka M, Ohno S, Nakamura S, et al: FK506 treatment of noninfectious uveitis. Am J Ophthalmol 118:723–729, 1994.

60. Tsurimaki Y, Shimizu H: An indomethacin treatment for a chronic and complicated Harada's disease. Acta Soc Ophthalmol Jpn 88:70–75, 1984.

61. Moorthy RS, Inomata H, Rao NA: Vogt-Koyanagi-Harada syndrome. Surv Ophthalmol 39:265–292, 1995.

62. Forster DJ, Rao NA, Hill RA, et al: Incidence and manage-

ment of glaucoma in Vogt-Koyanagi-Harada syndrome. Ophthalmology 100:613–618, 1993.

63. Rutzen AR, Ortega-Larrocea G, Frambach D, Rao NA: Macular edema in chronic Vogt-Koyanagi-Harada syndrome. Retina 15:475–479, 1995.

64. Foster CS, Fong LP, Singh G: Cataract surgery and intraocular lens implantation in patients with uveitis. Ophthalmology 96:281–288, 1989.

65. Foster RE, Lowder CY, Meisler DM, Zakov ZN: Extracapsular cataract extraction and posterior chamber intraocular lens implantation in uveitis patients. Ophthalmology 99: 1234–1241, 1992.

66. Moorthy RS, Rajeev B, Smith RE, Rao NA: Incidence and mangement of cataracts in Vogt-Koyanagi-Harada syndrome. Am J Ophthalmol 118:197–204, 1994.

67. Diamond JG, Kaplan HJ: Lensectomy and vitrectomy for complicated cataract secondary to uveitis. Arch Ophthalmol 96:1798–1804, 1978.

68. Shorb SR, Irvine AR, Kimura SJ, Morris BW: Optic disc neovascularization associated with chronic uveitis. Am J Ophthalmol 82:175–178, 1976.

69. To KW, Nadel AJ, Brockhurst RJ: Optic disc neovascularization in association with Vogt-Koyanagi-Harada syndrome. Arch Ophthalmol 108:918–919, 1990.

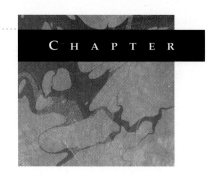

Multiple Evanescent White Dot Syndrome (MEWDS)

Antonio P. Ciardella, M.D.

John A. Sorenson, M.D.

Lawrence A. Yannuzzi, M.D.

In 1984 a new syndrome was independently described by two groups: Jampol and associates in the United States,[1] and Takeda and co-workers in Japan.[2] This syndrome was characterized by the monocular acute onset of temporal or paracentral scotomas accompanied by photopsias associated with multiple white outer retina lesions. The disappearance of the white dots after 4 to 6 weeks suggested the name, multiple evanescent white dot syndrome (MEWDS). Since then, at least 62 patients with MEWDS have been reported in the ophthalmic literature.[1-24]

MEWDS represents a distinct clinical entity based on its demographic, clinical, angiographic, and electrophysiologic findings.

DEMOGRAPHICS

The majority of patients are female (51 of 62 reported cases) with an average age of 27 years (range, 14 to 47 years). No racial predilection has been identified.[1-24]

SYMPTOMS AND CLINICAL FINDINGS

Most patients complain of sudden decrease of vision, often accompanied by dark spots in the periphery of the visual field. Photopsias, described as flickering or shimmering lights, are noted by nearly all patients. Nausea, dizziness, and headaches accompanying the visual symptoms have been reported.[1,3,4] One patient complained of ocular discomfort,[5] and 12 had a preceding "flu-like" illness.[1,4-8]

Visual acuity at the onset of symptoms may range from 20/20 to 20/400 and an afferent pupillary defect is sometimes present. A mild iritis may be noted. Fundus examination reveals characteristic white spots, approximately 100 to 200 μm in size, at the level of the deep retina or the retinal pigment epithelium. The spots are usually more evident in the posterior pole and in the temporal macula, while the fovea is always spared (Figs. 48–1A; 48–2A; 48–3A, C, and D; and 48–4 through 48–6). The spots may fade in one area to reappear in another after several days. A granularity of the retinal pigment epithelium in the foveal area is almost always present (Figs. 48–1A; 48–2A; 48–3A, B, and C; and 48–4 through 48–6). Other findings are mild blurring of the disc margin, isolated areas of perivascular sheathing, and a few vitreous cells in the acute phase of the disease. One patient presented with cotton-wool spots.

VISUAL FIELDS

Visual field findings are variable. The most common is enlargement of the blind spot. Arcuate scotomas, cecocentral scotomas, and central depression[1,4,5,7-17] have also been described. The field loss is usually more than would be expected based on the clinical findings.

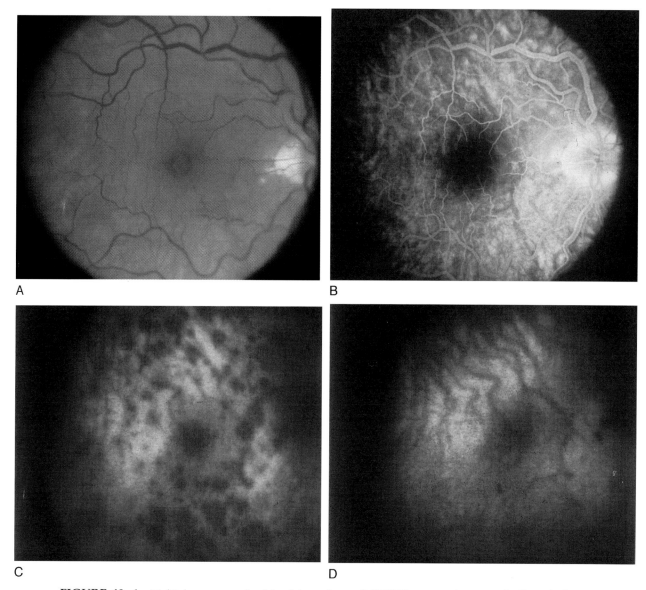

FIGURE 48–1   Multiple evanescent white dot syndrome (MEWDS)—natural course. *A,* Clinical photograph of a patient with recent onset of MEWDS. A few yellowish white dots are evident temporal to the disc. Notice the granular appearance of the RPE in the parafoveal region. *B,* The yellow dots appear hyperfluorescent on fluorescein angiography. The edge of the disc stains with the dye. *C,* Late-phase ICG study shows hypofluorescent dots throughout the posterior pole. *D,* Late-phase ICG study 2 months later reveals almost complete resolution of the hypofluorescent lesions.

ANGIOGRAPHY

Fluorescein angiography reveals early punctate hyperfluorescence often in a wreath-like configuration corresponding to the white dots. The late-phase angiogram reveals the spots and optic nerve head (Figs. 48–1*B;* 48–2*C,* and *D*).[1,18,19] Less common findings are late capillary leakage in the perifoveal area and focal areas of vasculitis.

Indocyanine green (ICG) angiography in the acute phase of MEWDS is characteristic. Unlike the subtle white dots seen clinically or the indistinct punctate hyperfluorescence seen with fluorescein angiography, ICG angiography shows a pattern of hypofluorescent spots throughout the posterior pole and peripheral retina (Fig. 48–1*C*). These hypofluorescent spots appear approximately 10 minutes after the dye injection in the mid ICG phase and persist throughout the remainder of the study. These spots appear larger than the white dots seen clinically, varying in diameter from less than 50 μm to about 500 μm. Many more lesions can easily be identified on ICG angiography than on fundus examination or fluorescein angiography (Fig. 48–1). In a few cases there is also a ring of hypofluorescence surrounding the optic nerve. In these patients a blind spot enlargement on visual field examination is always present. The resolution

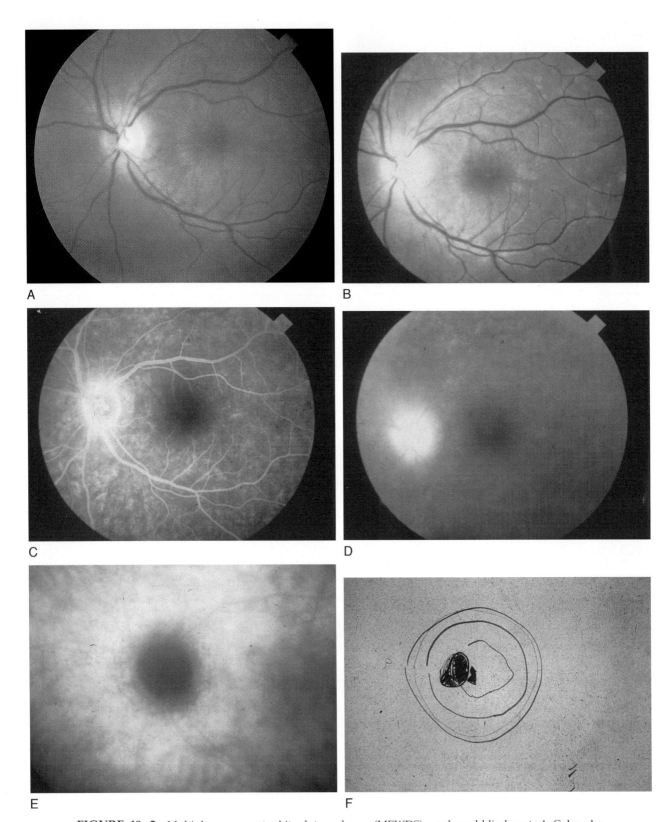

FIGURE 48-2 Multiple evanescent white dot syndrome (MEWDS)—enlarged blind spot. *A,* Color photograph of a patient with acute onset of MEWDS. Only a few yellowish spots are visible temporally. *B,* The spots are more easily visible with a red-free light. *C,* Mid-phase fluorescein angiography demonstrates a few hyperfluorescent spots. The margins of the optic nerve stain with the dye. *D,* Late-phase fluorescein angiography shows marked staining of the optic nerve. *E,* Late-phase ICG study shows a hypofluorescent ring around the optic nerve. *F,* Goldmann visual field demonstrates an enlarged blind spot. *Illustration continued on opposite page*

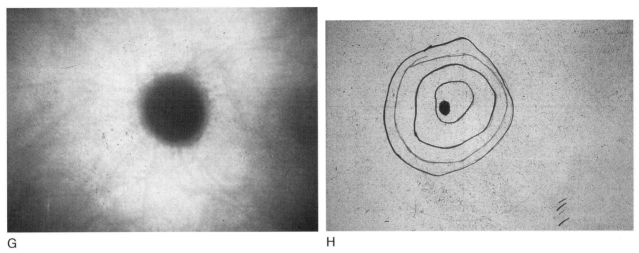

G   H

FIGURE 48–2 *Continued*   *G*, Late-phase ICG study 4 months later demonstrates complete resolution of the hypofluorescent ring around the optic nerve. *H*, Goldmann visual field of the same day shows complete resolution of the enlarged blind spot.

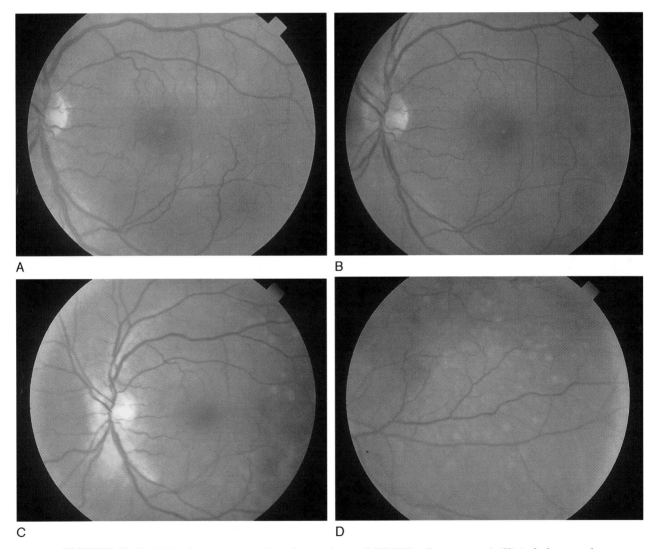

A   B

C   D

FIGURE 48–3   Multiple evanescent white dot syndrome (MEWDS)—Recurrence. *A*, Clinical photograph of a patient with MEWDS. Scattered superficial chorioretinal white dots are visible in the temporal macula. Notice the granular appearence of the fovea. *B*, Four weeks later there was an almost complete resolution of the white dots, while the granular appearance of the fovea persisted. *C* and *D*, Five years later the patient experienced a recurrence in the same eye. A larger number of white dots are visible temporally.

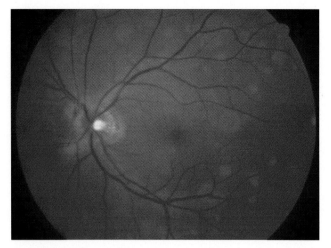

FIGURE 48–4 Multiple evanescent white dot syndrome (MEWDS). Clinical photograph of the left fundus of a patient with MEWDS. Note the presence of widespread and large spots at the posterior pole. Some peripapillary atrophy and pigmentary disturbance is demonstrated in this patient, which may or may not be associated with the overlaying syndrome. (From Yannuzzi LA, Guyer DR, Green WR: The Retina Atlas. St Louis, Mosby Year-Book, 1995, pp 632–638, with permission.)

of the hypofluorescent ring around the optic nerve is accompanied by a normalization of the visual field (Fig. 48–2E, F, and G).

During the convalescent phase, there is resolution of the hypofluorescent spots seen on ICG angiography (Figs. 48–1D and 48–2G) with return of visual function and normalization of the clinical exam.

The hypofluorescent spots may represent inflammatory lesions of the choriocapillaris[15] that could alter the choroidal circulation, diverting choroidal blood flow around these lesions and accounting for the hypofluorescence seen on ICG angiography.[20]

ELECTROPHYSIOLOGY

The electroretinogram (ERG) may be altered during the acute phase of the illness, but it returns to normal with resolution of the disease. The a-wave and early receptor potential amplitudes are decreased.[2,7,10,12,13,19,21] Electro-oculography may be abnormal as well.[2,21,22] Abnormal foveal densitometry has been found in MEWDS both with normal[11] and abnormal[14] ERG findings.

COURSE

The clinical course of MEWDS is usually benign without complication and with full recovery. The majority of patients recover in 3 to 10 weeks. During this period visual acuity usually improves to 20/30 or better and the white spots disappear (Fig. 48–3A and B); however, the foveal granularity usually persists. Sometimes, visual symptoms persist after resolution of the white spots. Visual field defects, photopsia, and dim vision may last for extended periods, even if visual acuity is improved to 20/20. One patient experienced a subfoveal cho-

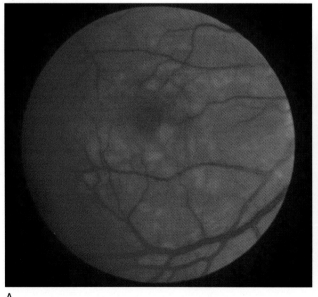

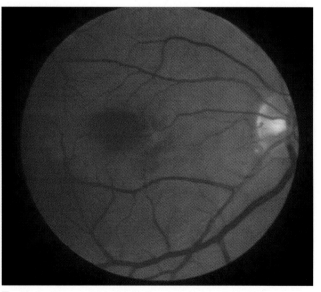

A   B

FIGURE 48–5 Multiple evanescent white dot syndrome (MEWDS). *A,* This patient initially had the characteristic finding of MEWDS with whitish spots and macular granularity. *B,* MEWDS resolved and the patient was later found to have a wedge-shaped reddish macular lesion consistent with acute macular neuroretinopathy (AMN) in the same eye. (From Yannuzzi LA, Guyer DR, Green WR: The Retina Atlas. St Louis, Mosby Year-Book, 1995, pp 632–638, with permission.)

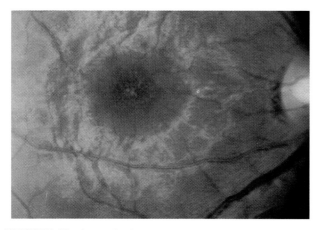

FIGURE 48–6   Multiple evanescent white dot syndrome (MEWDS). High-magnification clinical photograph of a patient with MEWDS that shows the characteristic macular granularity. (From Albert DM, Jakobiec FA: Principles and Practice of Ophthalmology. Philadelphia, WB Saunders, 1994, with permission.)

roidal neovascular membrane approximately 4 months after complete recovery from an episode of MEWDS.[8]

MEWDS is usually unilateral, but 7 of 62 patients reported in the literature have had bilateral involvement.[3,4,9,21–23] In bilateral cases one eye is usually asymptomatic with 20/20 vision or better and only a few white spots peripheral to the arcades. Only five patients have been reported to have a recurrence of MEWDS.[16,23] Aaberg et al first reported two patients with single episodes of recurrence of MEWDS[23]: one patient had a recurrence in the same eye nearly 3 years after the original episode, and the other patient had a recurrence in the fellow eye nearly 4 years after the initial episode. Tsai et al reported three patients with otherwise typical MEWDS who developed multiple recurrences involving both eyes in a period of 5 to 7 years. Despite these recurrences, the patient still retained visual acuity of 20/20 in each eye.[16]

We have seen a patient who experienced a recurrence of MEWDS in the same eye after 5 years (Fig. 48–3).

The etiology of MEWDS is unknown. A viral cause is suspected since the disease has an acute onset and is sometimes preceded by a flu-like illness.[24] Clinically, the white dots appear localized in the RPE and outer retina. The abnormality in the ERG also suggests a dysfunction of the retinal pigment epithelium–photoreceptor complex. The ICG angiography findings suggest an inflammatory disease of the choroid[20] that may alter the choriocapillaris blood flow. Visual field defects, especially blind spot enlargement, are common in MEWDS and suggest involvement of the optic nerve.[9] Recently, studies of the focal ERG in two patients with MEWDS and blind spot enlargement have shown that the amplitude is more reduced in macular ERG than in full-field ERG, indicating that the blind spot enlargement is caused by retinal dysfunction.[13]

DIFFERENTIAL DIAGNOSIS

The diagnosis of MEWDS can usually be made on clinical examination. However, it must be differentiated from other inflammatory disorders of the RPE, choroid, and retina.

Acute posterior multifocal placoid pigment epitheliopathy (APMPPE) causes rapid loss of vision in young patients,[25] but it is usually bilateral. Fundus examination shows multiple, flat gray-white lesions much larger than the spots of MEWDS. These lesions are hypofluorescent in the early fluorescein angiogram and stain late. When the acute phase resolves, the lesions of APMPPE leave a marked alteration of the retinal pigment epithelium.

Acute retinal pigment epitheliitis[26–28] is also characterized by acute loss of vision in a young patient. Discrete clusters of dark spots (localized to the perifoveal region) surrounded by hypopigmented halos are evident. The clinical course is similar for both acute retinal pigment epitheliitis and MEWDS, with complete recovery of vision within 7 to 10 weeks. However, the dark clinical appearance of the spots, the absence of visual field involvement, and the fluoroangiographic aspect of the dots (hypofluorescence surrounded by a hyperfluorescent halo) help in differentiating the two entities.

Birdshot retinochoroidopathy or vitiliginous chorioretinitis presents with multiple depigmented spots at the level of the retinal pigment epithelium-choriocapillaris scattered throughout the fundus.[29,30] Sometimes the white yellowish spots seem to follow the course of the major choroidal vessels. The older age at presentation, chronic course, bilateral involvement, and significant vitreous involvement all help to easily distinguish birdshot choroidopathy from MEWDS.

Several papers have described a group of patients that can probably best be lumped together as cases of multifocal chorioretinitis. They include the following: punctate inner choroidopathy (PIC),[31] multifocal choroiditis and panuveitis,[32] multifocal choroiditis associated with progressive subretinal fibrosis,[33–35] and recurrent multifocal choroiditis.[36] The patients described in these papers are similar. As in MEWDS, they are usually young myopic females who present with acute visual loss in one eye and spots in the fundus. Multifocal chorioretinitis can be chronic and recurrent; although often presenting with unilateral symptoms, findings are usually bilateral. The RPE and inner choroidal spots vary in size but are generally larger than those seen in MEWDS. Papillitis, retinal phlebitis, vitritis, anterior uveitis, cystoid macular edema, and subretinal neovascularization can all be part of the disease process. One or more of these manifestations may predominate in a given patient. Following resolution of the spots in the acute stage, there is some degree of permanent RPE and choroidal damage, which can be atrophic, pigmentary, or cicatricial in nature. Since many disorders may mimic an idiopathic condition, a full medical work-up is needed especially to rule out treatable infections or inflammatory conditions such as syphilis or sarcoidosis. One paper has associated the Epstein-Barr virus with patients having multifocal chorioretinitis[37]; however, another report did not.[38] Calleman[4] reported a 39-year-old woman who presented with headache, photopsias, bilateral reduction of visual acuity, and blind spot enlargement. Fundus appearance was consistent with PIC in one eye and MEWDS in the fellow eye. IgG antibody titer to Epstein-Barr virus capsid antigen was positive. However, it is our feeling that this ubiquitous organism is not likely to be the causative agent in the majority of these cases. It is hoped that more specific serologic testing and ocular tissue analysis will serve to differentiate these disorders into more specific entities in the future. Although these patients may resemble those with MEWDS on presentation, the constellation of physical findings and subsequent course should make it easy to differentiate patients with multifocal chorioretinitis from those with MEWDS.

Ocular toxoplasmosis presenting with the clinical picture of punctate outer retinal toxoplasmosis is another cause of retinochoroiditis that must be differentiated from MEWDS. In this case fundus examination reveals multifocal gray-white lesions at the level of the deep retina and RPE, with little or no overlying vitreous reaction.[39,40] The diagnosis of outer toxoplasmosis is difficult to confirm, but the presence of satellite lesions and positive serologic findings can help to recognize toxoplasmosis as the cause of the inflammation.

Diffuse unilateral subacute neuroretinitis (DUSN) is a clinical syndrome caused by a nematode that can sometimes be visualized in the subretinal space.[42,43] Fundus appearance in the early stage of the disease is characterized by evanescent gray-white lesions at the level of the outer retina and RPE.[40] These lesions usually fade after several days without leaving evident changes in the underlying RPE. A careful exam with a fundus contact lens is often necessary to identify the small nematode, which is usually found near the white deep retinal lesions, has a coiled configuration, and may move when disturbed by light. The diagnosis of DUSN is important to make, since if it is not recognized a chronic course with eventual development of diffuse RPE degeneration, retinal vessel narrowing, optic nerve atrophy, and visual loss may occur.

Acute macular neuroretinopathy (AMN) is another entity that causes loss of vision and paracentral scotoma, sometimes with a typical hourglass appearance, primarily in young patients.[44-46] Fundus examination shows a deep, wedge-shaped reddish discoloration of the retina in the macular area of both eyes. AMN has been related to upper respiratory infections, trauma, and epinephrine injection. The natural course of the disease is usually favorable, with progressive complete recovery of visual acuity. However, paracentral scotomas may persist for more than 1 year. MEWDS and AMN are both characterized by sudden visual loss in a young patient associated with a central defect in the visual field. Two patients have experienced AMN and MEWDS in the same eye, suggesting some similarity in their etiology[19] (Fig. 48–6).

Acute zonal occult outer retinopathy (AZOOR) is characterized by the initial appearance of large peripheral defects in the visual field sometimes contiguous to the blind spot with absence of any evident fundus alteration. The visual field defects are followed by diminished retinal arteriolar diameters, localized chorioretinal atrophy, and bone-spicule pigmentation in the corresponding retinal areas.[47] The alteration in the visual field in absence of any evident fundus lesion may be seen in both MEWDS and AZOOR, but the absence of deep retinal white dots, and the longer clinical course with development of retinal vascular and pigment alteration help in making the diagnosis of AZOOR.

The most difficult diagnostic problem is identifying a case of MEWDS after the chorioretinal spots have faded. At this point in the disease process the presence of an afferent pupillary defect, defective color vision, disc edema, and visual field defects, particularly large blind spots and paracentral scotomas, may suggest primary optic nerve disease. The visual field defects in MEWDS may last for many months following the resolution of the retinal spots. Patients with MEWDS have initially been diagnosed as having optic neuritis or retrobulbar neuritis.[9] Identification of the typical foveal granularity seen in MEWDS or the subtle fluorescein angiographic findings consistent with MEWDS can help in identifying these cases. Testing visual evoked potentials and color vision may also be useful in distinguishing between retinal and optic nerve disease. The acute idiopathic blind spot enlargement (AIBSE) occurs primarily in young females and consists of blind spot enlargement without optic disc edema.[48] This syndrome has features suggesting retinal dysfunction as its cause, including the presence of positive visual symptoms in the region of the scotomas, steep borders of the scotomas, and prolonged recovery time with photostress testing. The patients with AIBSE may represent patients with MEWDS, presenting for examination after the retinal spots have faded.[6,49,50] Some cases of AIBSE, but not all, may be due to MEWDS.

CONCLUSIONS

MEWDS is an inflammatory disease, usually unilateral and more frequent in young females. The presenting symptom is often photopsia, followed by blurring of the vision and defects in the visual field. Fundus examination reveals outer retinal or superficial pigment epithelial white spots, which vary in their size and are usually confined to the posterior pole or midretinal areas. A typical foveal granularity is usually present. Fluorescein angiography shows pinpoint hyperfluorescence corresponding to the white dots and late staining of the disc. ICG angiography shows multiple hypofluorescent spots throughout the fundus. Visual field test typically reveals a scotoma often contiguous to the blind spot.

The natural course is generally benign, with spontaneous disappearance of the lesions and improvement of the visual function in 6 to 8 weeks. However, recurrence cases have been described.

The cause of MEWDS remains unknown and further clinical research is needed to identify the precise pathogenesis.

REFERENCES

1. Jampol LM, Sieving PA, Pugh D, et al: Multiple evanescent white dot syndrome. l. Clinical findings. Arch Ophthalmol 102:671, 1984.
2. Takeda M, Kimura S, Tamiya M: Acute disseminated retinal pigment epitheliopathy. Folia Ophthalmol Jpn 35:2613, 1984.
3. Meyer RJ, Jampol LM: Recurrences and bilaterality in the multiple evanescent white-dot syndrome (Letter). Am J Ophthalmol 101:338, 1986.
4. Callaman D, Gass JDM: Multifocal choroiditis and choroidal neovascularization associated with the multiple evanescent white dot and acute idiopathic blind spot enlargement syndrome. Ophthalmology 99:1678–1685, 1992.
5. Kimmel AS, Folk JC, Thompson HS, et al: The multiple evanescent white-dot syndrome with acute blind spot enlargement (Letter). Am J Ophthalmol 107:425, 1989.
6. Hamed LM, Glaser JSk, Gass JDM, et al: Protracted enlargement of the blind spot in multiple evanescent white dot syndrome. Arch Ophthalmol 107:425, 1989.
7. Slusher MM, Weaver RG: Multiple evanescent white dot syndrome. Retina 8:132, 1988.
8. Wyhinny GJ, Jackson JL, Jampol LM, et al: Subretinal neovascularization following multiple evanescent white-dot syndrome (Case report). Arch Ophthalmol 108:1384, 1990.
9. Dodwell DEG, Jampol LM, Rosenberg M, et al: Optic nerve involvement associated with the multiple evanescent white-dot syndrome. Ophthalmology 97:862, 1990.
10. Nakao K, Isashiki M: Multiple evanescent white dot syndrome. Jpn J Ophthalmol 30:376, 1986.
11. Keunen JEE, van Norren DE: Foveal densitometry in the multiple evanescent white-dot syndrome (Letter). Am J Ophthalmol 105:561, 1988.
12. Sieving PA, Fishman GA, Jampol LM, et al: Multiple evanescent white dot syndrome, II. Electrophysiology of the photoreceptors during retinal pigment epithelial disease. Arch Ophthalmol 102:675, 1984.
13. Horiguchi M, Miyake Y, Nakamura M, Fujii Y: Focal electroretinogram and visual field defect in multiple evanescent white dot syndrome. Br J Ophthalmol 77:452–455, 1993.
14. Van Meel GJ, Keunen JEE, Van Norren D, Van de Kraats J: Scanning laser densitometry in multiple evanescent white dot syndrome. Retina 13:29–35, 1993.
15. Ie D, Glaser BM, Murphy RP, et al: Indocyanine green angiography in multiple evanescent white dot syndrome. Am J Ophthalmol 117:7–12, 1994.
16. Tsai L, Jampol LM, Pollock SC, Olk J: Chronic recurrent multiple evanescent white dot syndrome. Retina 14:160–163, 1994.
17. Jampol LM, Wiredu A: MEWDS, MFC, PIC, AMN, AIBSE, and AZOOR: one disease or many (Editorial). Retina 15:373–378, 1995.
18. Mamalis N, Daily MJ: Multiple evanescent white dot syndrome. A report of eight cases. Ophthalmology 94:1209, 1987.
19. Gass JDM, Hamed LM: Acute macular neuroretinopathy and multiple evanescent white dot syndrome occurring in the same patients. Arch Ophthalmol 107:189, 1989.
20. Obana A, Kusumi M, Yamaguchi M, Miki T: Two cases of multiple evanescent white dot syndrome examined with indocyanine green angiography. Nippon Ganka Gakkai Zasshi 99:244–251, 1995.
21. Jost BF, Olk RJ, McGaughey A: Bilateral symptomatic multiple evanescent white-dot syndrome (Letter). Am J Ophthalmol 101:489, 1986.
22. Laatikainen L, Immomen I: Multiple evanescent white dot syndrome. Graefes Arch Clin Exp Ophthalmol 226:37, 1988.
23. Aaberg TM, Campo RV, Joffe L: Recurrences and bilaterality in the multiple evanescent white-dot syndrome. Am J Ophthalmol 100:489, 1986.
24. Chung Y, Yeh T, Liu J: Increased serum IgM and IgG in the multiple evanescent white-dot syndrome (Letter). Am J Ophthalmol 104:187, 1987.
25. Gass JDM: Acute posterior multifocal placoid pigment epitheliopathy. Arch Ophthalmol 80:177, 1968.
26. Krill AE, Deutman AF: Acute retinal pigment epitheliitis. Ophthalmology 74:193, 1972.
27. Chittum ME, Kalina RE: Acute retinal pigment epitheliitis Ophthalmology 94:1114, 1987.
28. Deutman AF: Acute retinal pigment epitheliitis. Am J Ophthalmol 78:571, 1974.
29. Ryan SJ, Maumenee AE: Birdshot retinochoroidopathy. Ophthalmology 89:31, 1980.
30. Gass JDM: Vitiliginous chorioretinitis. Arch Ophthalmol 99:1778–1787, 1981.
31. Watzke RC, Packer AJ, Folk JC, et al: Punctate inner choroidopathy. Am J Ophthalmol 98:572, 1984.
32. Dreyer RF, Gass JDM: Multifocal choroiditis and panuveitis. A syndrome that mimics ocular histoplasmosis. Arch Ophthalmol 102:1776, 1984.
33. Cantrill HL, Folk JC: Multifocal choroiditis associated with progressive subretinal fibrosis. Am J Ophthalmol 101:170, 1986.
34. Doran RML, Hamilton AM: Disciform macular degeneration in young adults. Trans Ophthalmol Soc UK 102:471, 1982.
35. Palestine AG, Nussenblatt RB, Parven LM, et al: Progressive subretinal fibrosis and uveitis. Br J Ophthalmol 68:667, 1984.
36. Morgan CM, Schatz H: Recurrent multifocal choroiditis. Ophthalmology 93:1138, 1986.
37. Tiedeman JS: Epstein-Barr viral antibodies in multifocal choroiditis and panuveitis. Am J Ophthalmol 103:659, 1987.
38. Sugin S, Spaide R, Yannuzzi L, DeRosa J: Multifocal choroiditis and panuveitis and the Epstein-Barr virus (Poster). Presented at the Association for Research in Vision and Ophthalmology (Annual Meeting). Sarasota, FL, April 1991.
39. Doft BH, Gass JDM: Punctate outer retinal toxoplasmosis. Arch Ophthalmol 103:1332, 1985.
40. Matthews JD, Weiter JJ: Outer retinal toxoplasmosis. Ophthalmology 95:941, 1988.
41. Gass JDM, Scelfo R: Diffuse unilateral subacute neuroretinitis. R Soc Med 71:95, 1978.
42. Gass JDM, Braunstein RA: Further observations concerning the diffuse unilateral neuroretinitis syndrome. Arch Ophthalmol 101:1689, 1983.
43. Kazacos KR, Raymond LA, Kazaces EA, et al: The raccoon ascarid. A probable cause of human ocular larva migrans. Ophthalmology 92:1735, 1985.
44. Bos PJ, Deutman AF: Acute macular neuroretinopathy. Ophthalmology 80:573, 1975.
45. Rush JA: Acute macular neuroretinopathy. Am J Ophthalmol 83:490, 1977.
46. Priluck IA, Buettner H, Robertson DM: Acute macular neuroretinopathy. Am J Ophthalmol 86:775, 1978.

47. Gass JDM: Acute zonal occult outer retinopathy. J Clin Neuroophthalmol 13:79–97, 1993.
48. Fletcher WA, Imes RK, Goodman D, et al: Acute idiopathic blind spot enlargement. A big blind spot syndrome without optic disc edema. Arch Ophthalmol 106:44, 1988.
49. Hamed LM, Schutz NJ, Glaser JS, et al: Acute idiopathic blind spot enlargement without optic disc edema (Letter). Arch Ophthalmol 106:1030, 1988.
50. Singh K, de Frank MP, Shults WT, et al: Acute idiopathic blind spot enlargement. A spectrum of disease. Ophthalmology 98:497–502, 1991.

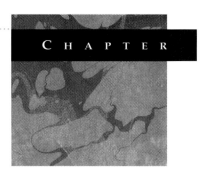

CHAPTER 49

Acute Macular Neuroretinopathy

Robert E. Kalina, M.D.

Acute macular neuroretinopathy (AMN) is among the most rare of all maculopathies. Since initially reported by Bos and Deutman,[1] fewer than 30 cases have been described in the world literature. Remarkably, all but three cases involve young women between the ages of 20 and 30 years. The great majority of cases involve both eyes.

FUNDUS APPEARANCE

Ophthalmoscopy discloses a dramatic appearance characteristic of AMN. Wedge-shaped, red-brown lesions are arranged radially about the center of the macula (Fig. 49–1). These lesions may vary in size from barely detectable to 1.5 mm or more in greatest diameter. The reason for the wedge shape of the lesions and the predilection for the macula is unknown.

Stereo viewing suggests that the lesions of AMN are located in the external neurosensory retina. The retinal pigment epithelium typically appears undisturbed as are the retinal blood vessels.

Why the lesions appear red is unknown. The red appearance of AMN, seen particularly well with red-free light (Fig. 49–2), initially suggests that a thin layer of blood may be responsible. However, fluorescein angiography typically is normal or shows only very slight hypofluorescence corresponding to the lesions, not the dramatically blocked fluorescence that would be expected from blood (Fig. 49–3). A red appearance known as the retinal depression sign occurs following retinal infarction in sickle hemoglobinopathy.[2] The red appearance in the retinal depression sign is an optical illusion caused by light captured within the thinned retina. The macular lesions of AMN do not

appear thinned. A similar appearance has been discussed following resolution of commotio retinae.[3]

NATURAL HISTORY

Most patients with AMN experience the abrupt onset of paracentral scotomata, often with preservation of normal central visual acuity. In several cases, examination soon after the onset of symptoms was said to show macular swelling but, if such swelling exists, it must resolve quickly, since most reports describe only the reddish, wedge-shaped lesions.

Patients with AMN usually are able to outline scotomata on the Amsler grid that correspond exactly to the retinal lesions (Fig. 49–4). Visual function outside the scotomata is subjectively normal. The scotomata typically spare the center of the macula. Rarely, new retinal lesions and scotomata may appear in either the same eye or the fellow eye weeks after initial symptoms.

The red retinal lesions gradually fade and the scotomata become less dense and less distinct. However, both the retinal lesions and the scotomata have been observed to persist for at least 9 years.[4]

LABORATORY TESTING

Patients with AMN have been subjected to a variety of hematologic and radiologic studies that have not produced a unifying hypothesis for causation.

Standard electrophysiologic tests of patients with AMN generally have shown the electroretinogram and electro-oculogram to be normal. However, Sieving and colleagues demonstrated reduction of early retinal receptor potential in a single case of

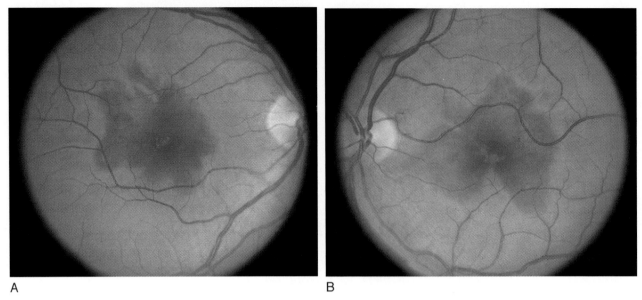

FIGURE 49–1   *A*, Right eye. *B*, Left eye. Red, wedge-shaped lesions surround the center of the macula in a 28-year-old woman 6 weeks after acute hypertension following an intravenous injection of a sympathomimetic.

AMN.[5] Studies of additional patients might confirm their assignment of the pathology to the photoreceptors, also the apparent biomicroscopic location of the red retinal lesions.

ASSOCIATED SYSTEMIC DISORDERS

Many patients with AMN are healthy except for reported associations with oral contraceptive use[6] and viral illness,[7] associations that are so common in the normal population that their significance is difficult to assign. Also, most eyes with AMN show no inflammatory signs that might suggest a viral etiology. Other cases have occurred acutely in temporal relationship to dramatic systemic events that suggest a causal relationship, although the exact mechanism remains obscure. We have seen three young women who developed AMN with persistent paracentral scotomata following acute hypertension caused by intravenous sympathomimetics,[8] and subsequently other reports have appeared in

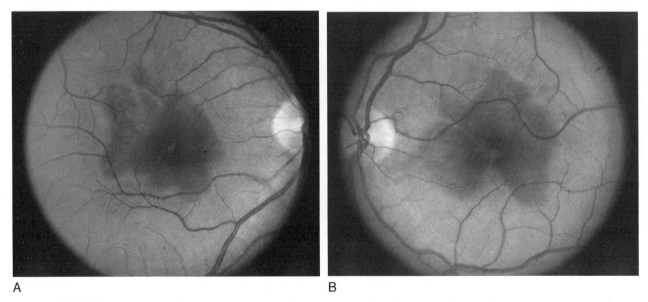

FIGURE 49–2   *A*, Right eye. *B*, Left eye. Red-free photographs of patient in Figure 49–1.

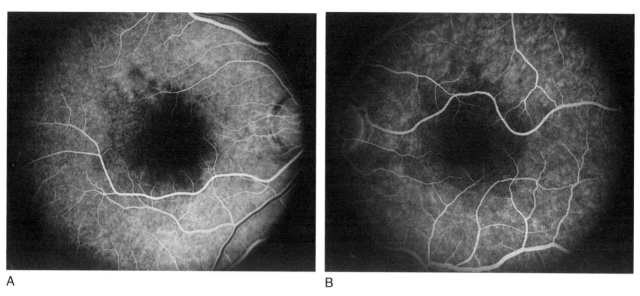

FIGURE 49–3   *A*, Right eye. *B*, Left eye. Fluorescein angiography is normal except for transient faint hypofluorescence roughly corresponding to macular lesions.

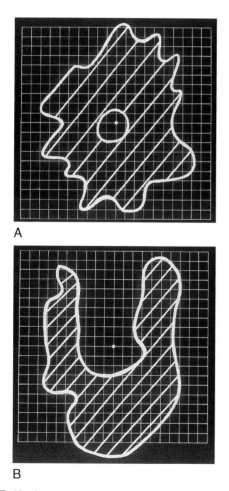

FIGURE 49–4   *A*, Right eye. *B*, Left eye. Scotomata on Amsler grid testing correspond to macular lesions in Figures 49–1 and 49–2.

the literature.[9,10] In addition, we have seen two other young women who developed AMN acutely following adverse reactions to intravenous injection of contrast agent for computed tomography.[11] Both women were treated by intravenous injection of epinephrine, but blood pressure was not recorded immediately. A direct effect of the supplemental adrenergic agents on photoreceptors or other neural cells of the retina has been postulated[8] based on the structural and functional resemblance between the adrenergic receptor protein and rhodopsin discovered through gene sequence analysis.[12] Although the acute onset of symptoms in these cases would also be compatible with a vascular etiology, fluorescein angiography of the retinal and choroidal circulations in our patients appeared normal. We have seen one young woman with macular lesions resembling AMN following recovery from eclampsia.

ASSOCIATED OCULAR DISORDERS

Unilateral AMN has been described in conjunction with multiple evanescent white dot syndrome (MEWDS) occurring in the same eye but not simultaneously in two young women.[13] Both of these eyes demonstrated large blind spots on visual field testing as did one additional unilateral case with AMN alone.[14] Based in part upon these associations, inclusion of AMN in a group of disorders known as acute zonal occult outer retinopathy (AZOOR) has been proposed.[15] Included with AMN would be MEWDS, acute idiopathic blind spot enlargement syndrome (AIBSES), and the pseudo–presumed ocular histoplasmosis syndrome (P-POHS). The limited number of patients studied and the unique features of AMN described earlier in this chapter suggest that to include AMN in such a grouping may be premature.

TREATMENT

As is the case with most obscure ocular disorders of unknown cause, patients have been treated with oral corticosteroids. No evidence exists to suggest that corticosteroid or other treatment is of benefit.

REFERENCES

1. Bos PJ, and Deutman AF: Acute macular neuroretinopathy. Am J Ophthalmol 80:573–584, 1975.
2. Goldbaum MH: Retinal depression sign indicating a small retinal infarct. Am J Ophthalmol 86:45–55, 1978.
3. Campo RV, and Flindall RJ: Traumatic macular atrophy. Ocular Therapy 2:2–7, 1985.
4. Miller MH, Spalton DJ, Fitzke FW, Bird AC: Acute macular neuroretinopathy. Ophthalmology 96:265–269, 1989.
5. Sieving PA, Fishman GA, Salzano T, Rabb MF: Acute mac-ular neuroretinopathy: early receptor potential change suggests photoreceptor pathology. Br J Ophthalmol 68:229–234, 1984.
6. Rush JA: Acute macular neuroretinopathy. Am J Ophthalmol 83:490–494, 1977.
7. Priluck IA, Buettner H, Robertson DM: Acute macular neuroretinopathy. Am J Ophthalmol 86:775–778, 1978.
8. O'Brien DM, Farmer SG, Kalina RE, Leon JA: Acute macular neuroretinopathy following intravenous sympathomimetics. Retina 9:281–286, 1989.
9. Desai UR, Sudhamathi K, Natarajan S: Intravenous epinephrine and acute macular neuroretinopathy (Letter). Arch Ophthalmol 111:1026–1027, 1993.
10. Leys M, Van Slycken S, Koller J, Van de Sompel W: Acute macular neuroretinopathy after shock. Bull Soc Belg Ophtalmol 241:95–104, 1991.
11. Guzak SV, Kalina RE, Chenoweth RG: Acute macular neuroretinopathy following adverse reaction to intravenous contrast media. Retina 3:312–317, 1983.
12. Marx JL: Receptor gene family is growing. Science 238:615–616, 1987.
13. Gass JD, Hamed LM: Acute macular neuroretinopathy and multiple evanescent white dot syndrome occurring in the same patients. Arch Ophthalmol 107:189–193, 1989.
14. Singh K, de Frank MP, Shults WT, Watzke RC: Acute idiopathic blind spot enlargement. A spectrum of disease. Ophthalmology 98:497–502, 1991.
15. Gass JD: Acute zonal occult outer retinopathy. Donders Lecture: The Netherlands Ophthalmological Society, Maastricht, Holland, June 19, 1992. J Clin Neuroophthalmol 13:79–97, 1993.

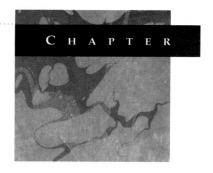

CHAPTER 50

Acute Retinal Pigment Epitheliitis

Benjamin Chang, M.D.

Acute retinal pigment epitheliitis (or Krill's disease), first described in six patients by Krill and Deutman in 1972[1] and in an additional three patients by Deutman in 1974,[2] is a rare, self-limited disorder characterized by acute onset of visual disturbance associated with peculiar macular pigmentary changes. The hallmark of this disease is the characteristic macular lesions consisting of discrete clusters of small, dark gray spots at the level of the retinal pigment epithelium (RPE), each surrounded by a yellow halo-like zone.[1,2] Visual symptoms typically resolve with recovery of vision in the ensuing weeks to months. Although the precise etiology is unknown, it has been postulated that the disorder is an inflammatory condition occurring at the level of the pigment epithelium.[1] Since the first descriptions of this disorder, atypical cases as well as series of patients with similar clinical findings and course have been reported.[3-6]

CLINICAL FINDINGS

Patients with acute retinal pigment epitheliitis are typically healthy young adults without preceding illness or flu-like syndrome who report acute onset of unilateral blurred vision and/or metamorphopsia.[1,2] In most of the cases reported the patient is in the second to fourth decade of life, with no apparent gender predilection. Visual acuity may range from 20/20 to 20/100 at presentation, and most patients will demonstrate central metamorphopsia and/or scotoma on Amsler grid or visual field testing. The natural course is typically benign, with complete to near-complete resolution of visual symptoms, return of visual acuity, and normalization of visual field defects in 6 to 12 weeks without treatment. In two studies, one with eight patients followed for an average of 4.2 years[4] and one with

five patients all followed for over 6 years,[5] all 14 affected eyes of 13 patients recovered 20/20 vision with no recurrence during the follow-up period. Recurrent as well as bilateral cases have been reported, but neither is typical.[1,3,5]

On presentation, the typical macular lesions are generally established, consisting of discrete clusters of hyperpigmented spots at the level of the pigment epithelium, each surrounded by a yellow-white depigmented halo. The optic nerve, retinal vessels, and surrounding retina are normal; retinal edema and subretinal fluid are typically absent. Infrequently, a mild vitreitis may be seen.[5-7] Over time, the dark spots may darken further or fade and become difficult to detect. The surrounding halo may also become less distinct with resolution of the disease.[1-5] Recently, a case of acute retinal pigment epitheliitis in a 25-year-old examined within 3 days of onset of symptoms was reported where the patient was noted to have outer retinal vacuoles that evolved into more typical pigmentary changes on follow-up.[7] These authors hypothesized that the macular pigment epithelial changes may be secondary to a primary inflammation of the outer neurosensory retina.

Typically an isolated event, acute retinal pigment epitheliitis has also been associated with central serous chorioretinopathy (CSCR). In their original paper, Krill and Deutman postulated that the disturbance of the RPE could result in breakdown of the pigment epithelial blood-ocular barrier and lead to subsequent serous fluid leakage.[1] Nine patients with the association between acute retinal pigment epitheliitis and CSCR were noted in a retrospective study.[6] Furthermore, another report clearly documented a case of acute retinal pigment epitheliitis evolving into typical central serous chorioretinopathy.[8] It remains a possibility that retinal pigment epitheliitis plays a role in the pathogenesis of CSCR.

ANGIOGRAPHY

Fluorescein angiography during the acute stages of retinal pigment epitheliitis will generally show variable hyperfluorescence corresponding to the depigmented halo with hypofluorescence of the central dark spot. Specifically, the halo will demonstrate hyperfluorescence, sometimes described as "lacy," consistent with window defect transmission without late leakage or staining.[1,2,4–6] The central hypofluorescence is consistent with blockage from hyperpigmentation. With long-term follow-up, the angiographic findings change very little.[6]

In addition to central visual field and Amsler grid defects mentioned above, other ancillary tests may also be abnormal during the acute process. Color vision abnormalities have been reported in some patients.[1,2] Electroretinography (ERG) and electro-oculography (EOG) were performed on patients in the early reports of this disease. The ERG is typically normal, while the EOG may be abnormal acutely, reverting to normal with clinical resolution of the process.[1,2] Given that the latter measures a mass response electrical potential, it has been suggested that the EOG abnormality implies a more widespread dysfunction at the level of the pigment epithelium in the acute stages than what is clinically detectable on ophthalmoscopy and angiography.

ETIOLOGY

The exact etiology of this entity is unknown. Patients are usually systemically healthy, and the syndrome is not usually heralded by a preceding illness. The prevailing theory holds that it is an inflammatory condition of viral origin, on the basis of its acute onset and benign, self-limited course with recovery, as well as its funduscopic resemblance to rubella retinopathy, although the latter lesions are coarser and more widespread in the fundus. One case reported acute bilateral pigment epitheliitis developing in a woman with fever, chills, and myalgia of unknown origin who had persistent visual symptoms 1 year after onset.[9] A more recent case reported unilateral visual loss and a solitary macular lesion interpreted as acute retinal pigment epitheliitis in an acutely ill young woman found to have hepatitis C.[10] Although these latter two cases are atypical of cases previously reported as acute retinal pigment epitheliitis, they do strengthen the argument of a viral etiology for retinal pigment "epitheliopathy."

DIFFERENTIAL DIAGNOSIS

The differential diagnosis for this disease is limited. The list includes acute macular neuroretinopathy, another rare condition typically afflicting young adults with a flu-like illness with associated visual loss. First described by Bos and Deutman in 1975,

the hallmark of this is the subtle macular finding of dark, reddish brown wedge-shaped or petalloid lesions in the superficial retina.[11] Another macular disease, acute posterior multifocal placoid pigment epitheliopathy (APMPPE),[12] has been mentioned in the differential diagnosis of retinal pigment epitheliitis, but the clinical lesions of APMPPE are distinctly different and it is difficult to confuse the two. Viral retinitides, including rubella, herpes simplex, measles, and cytomegalovirus, can all cause pigmentary changes to develop, but these can usually be differentiated from retinal pigment epitheliitis by more widespread involvement as well as systemic findings of the underlying illness. Pigmentary changes overlying serous pigment epithelial detachments have also been noted to resemble pigment epitheliitis.[6] The most difficult exclusion may be central serous chorioretinopathy, which upon resolution may leave pigment spots and atrophic pigment epithelial zones identical to the lesions of Krill's disease. An important distinction is the absence of serous fluid or fluorescein dye leakage during the acute, symptomatic stage of Krill's disease, as opposed to CSCR, where a serous detachment is nearly always present when the vision is affected.[2]

TREATMENT

Treatment is generally not indicated on account of the self-limited course and favorable outcome. Some cases in the literature had been treated with corticosteroids, but the effect of therapy is difficult to determine given the natural course of recovery without any intervention.[1,8,9]

REFERENCES

1. Krill AE, Deutman AF: Acute retinal pigment epitheliitis. AM J Ophthalmol 74:193–205, 1972.
2. Deutman AF: Acute retinal pigment epitheliitis. Am J Ophthalmol 78:571–578, 1974.
3. Friedman MW: Bilateral recurrent acute retinal pigment epitheliitis. Am J Ophthalmol 79:567–570, 1975.
4. Chittum ME, Kalina RE: Acute retinal pigment epitheliitis. Ophthalmology 94:1114–1119, 1987.
5. Prost M: Long-term observations of patients with acute retinal pigment epitheliitis. Ophthalmologica 199:84–89, 1989.
6. Eifrig DE, Knobloch WH, Moran JA: Retinal pigment epitheliitis. Ann Ophthalmol 9:639–642, 1977.
7. Luttrul JK, Chittum ME: Acute retinal pigment epitheliitis. Am J Ophthalmol 120:389–391, 1995.
8. Piermarocchi S, Corradini R, Midena E, Segato T: Correlation between retinal pigment epitheliitis and central erous chorioretinopathy. Ann Ophthalmol 15:425–428, 1983.
9. Schwartz PL, Rosen DA, Lerner DS, Lichtenfeld PJ: Acute retinal pigment epitheliopathies. Ann Ophthalmol 13:1139–1141, 1981.
10. Quillen DA, Zurlo JJ, Cunningham D, Blankenship GW: Acute retinal pigment epitheliitis and hepatitis C. Am J Ophthalmol 118:120–121, 1994.
11. Bos PJM, Deutman AF: Acute macular neuroretinopathy. Am J Ophthalmol 80:573, 1975.
12. Gass JDM: Acute posterior multifocal placoid pigment epitheliopathy. Am J Ophthalmol 80:177–185, 1968.

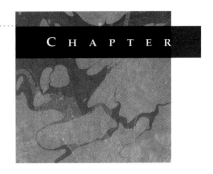

CHAPTER 51

Intermediate Uveitis (Pars Planitis)

David A. Saperstein, M.D.
Antonio Capone, Jr., M.D.
Thomas M. Aaberg, Sr., M.D.

Intermediate uveitis is an idiopathic syndrome consisting of intraocular inflammation centered about the peripheral retina and pars plana. This relatively common inflammatory disease affects otherwise healthy children and young adults and is usually bilateral. It is classically described as painless, having no external inflammation, mild anterior chamber cellular reaction, and a marked exudative response in the peripheral retina and overlying vitreous ("snowbanking"). It is a chronic condition characterized by alternating periods of exacerbation and reduced activity. Vision loss is most commonly due to cystoid macular edema (CME), cataract, and vitreous debris.

The disease was described in the first half of the 20th century by Fuchs[1] and Duke-Elder,[2] but the modern description was written by Schepens[3,4] in 1950. The disease has been given many names, the most common being "pars planitis"[5] and "peripheral uveitis."[6–9] In 1987, the International Uveitis Study Group agreed upon the term "intermediate uveitis."[10]

disease, often painless and indolent, can go undiagnosed for several years, particularly in children.

The age of onset ranges from 5 years to 65 years of age with the mean and median occurring in the third decade of life.[26] Severe cases tend to present at an early age, while older patients generally have a milder form of the disease. Eighty per cent of cases are bilateral,[14,21,27–30] although the majority of cases present asymmetrically, often with symptoms limited to one eye. Most studies reveal no sex predilection[7,14,22,30,31]; however, Althus and Sundmacher reported a 2:1 male/female ratio.[20] It is generally held that there is no racial or geographic predilection,[22,32,33] yet there are few reports of intermediate uveitis in East Asian or African-American patients.[14,28,34,35]

There have been several reports of familial intermediate uveitis.[25,36–38,49] To date no genetic localization has been described. Familial clustering may be due to HLA type producing a primary immunologic suseptibility or a mutation causing a functional defect rendering the affected individuals more susceptible to the disease.

EPIDEMIOLOGY

Intermediate uveitis represents 4 to 16% of all uveitis cases seen in referral practices.[11–19] Althus and Sundmacher[20] reported an incidence of 25% in primary ophthalmology practices. The incidence is 16 to 33% of all uveitis cases presenting among children.[21–25] Ultimately, it is difficult to assess accurately incidence and prevalence data because the

PATHOGENESIS

The etiology of intermediate uveitis is unknown. The inflammatory response present in the vitreous base, peripheral retina, pars plana, and ciliary body suggests an immune system–mediated disease. This general premise is supported by pathologic, serologic, and experimental evidence. Whether the disease is autoimmune, occurs in response to an

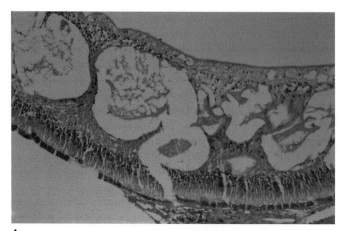

A

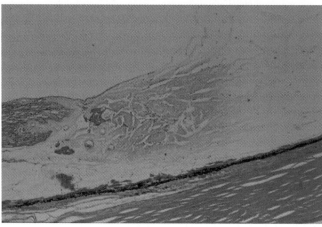

B

A, Extensive cystoid macular edema in eye with intermediate uveitis (pars planitis) of long duration. *B*, Snowbank of intermediate uveitis (pars planitis) consists of collapse and condensed vitreous, with new collagen from fibrous astrocytes from the retina, blood vessels from the retina and minor ciliary epithelial hyperplasia (anterior proliferative vitreoretinopathy). From Paderson JE, Kenyon KR, Green WR, Maumenee AE: Pathology of pars planitis. Am J Ophthalmol 86:762–774, 1978. Copyright 1978, Elsevier Science, with permission.)

infectious antigen, or is a combination of the two is still a matter of debate.

Pathology

The few published histopathologic correlates to intermediate uveitis are in eyes with moderate to chronic disease. Gross pathology reveals dense opacification of the vitreous base, pars plana, and ciliary body predominantly in the inferior portion. Light microscopy of the vitreous base in patients with chronic inflammation reveal collapsed or condensed vitreous infiltrated with blood vessels, lymphocytes, spindle-shaped cells or fibrous astrocytes, and hyperplastic nonpigmented epithelium. This corresponds clinically to the snowbank infiltrate. Fibrovascular membrane formation with lymphocytic infiltrates are seen covering the pars plana and ciliary body.[36,39] Uveal tissue is usually uninvolved[40]; however, focal areas of choroiditis have been reported. Retinal vascular inflammation is primarily perivenous. Both peripheral phlebitis and central papillophlebitis have been reported. The peripheral retinal pigment epithelium (RPE) in chronic cases shows areas of hyperplasia and gliosis.[40]

Electron microscopy of the snowbank regions reveal several venules. It is postulated that the endothelial cells in these venules play a role in the extravasation of lymphocytes into the vitreous cavity. Ablation of the venules and subsequent loss of lymphocytic channels to the area is a proposed theory explaining the therapeutic effect of peripheral cryopexy.[41]

Immunology

Despite many investigations, understanding of the immunology of intermediate uveitis remains elusive. It is widely held that intermediate uveitis, like many other forms of uveitis, is a T-cell–mediated disease. The causative antigen may be native to the immunologically privileged retina or exogenous, such as a virus or bacteria. Experimental autoimmune uveitis (EAU) can be induced in rats immunized with retinal-specific antigens such as S antigen (arrestin) and interphotoreceptor retinoid-binding protein (IRBP). These models have proved successful in assessing treatments and understanding the immunology of uveitis. Although there exist data suggesting a relationship between S antigen and intermediate uveitis, they are not compelling. Lymphocyte stimulation assays in patients affected with intermediate uveitis are elevated in response to S antigen as compared to normals. However, the results of these assays were not statistically different from assays performed in patients suffering from other forms of uveitis, suggesting that this response may be nonspecific.[42]

CLINICAL PRESENTATION

Symptoms

The most common presenting complaint is unilateral painless blurring of vision (to the 20/40 to 20/50 level)[43] accompanied by floaters. More dramatic visual loss can be seen in patients who present with retinal detachment, vitreous hemorrhage, severe or chronic cystoid macular edema, or chronic optic disc edema. Pain, photophobia, and redness about the eye are uncommon; occur most often during the initial episode; and are usually mild. Pain, redness, or photophobia later in the course of the disease should alert the physician to look for other etiologies or associated complications, such as secondary glaucoma.

Signs

Anterior

The conjunctiva and external adnexae are typically not involved, apart from mild conjunctival injection.[33] Children occasionally present with more severe external inflammation and edema. Similarly, corneal epithelium and stroma are usually uninvolved initially. Three to 9% of chronic cases develop band keratopathy.[21,28,32] The corneal endothelium can be normal, have small white keratic precipitates, or develop large pigmented "mutton fat" keratic precipitates.[7,22]

Mild anterior chamber inflammation is common.[3] Rarely, an extensive anterior chamber reaction with organized fibrinous precipitates may be present. The iris initially is uninvolved. Later in the disease iris stromal atrophy with patchy areas of depigmentation and heterochromia can occur.[43,44] Iris neovascularization has also been reported.[45]

The intraocular pressure is usually normal. Gonioscopy may reveal cellular aggregates present in the angle of eyes with or without anterior cellular reactions.[46,47,73] Peripheral anterior and iridolenticular synechiae occur infrequently in intermediate uveitis and are usually associated with severe or chronic anterior segment inflammation.[6,12,45,48] Posterior synechiae are a common complication of extracapsular cataract extraction in these patients. Anterior and posterior synechiae may lead to secondary angle closure glaucoma and pupillary block glaucoma, respectively.

Posterior subcapsular cataracts are very common over the course of the disease. Initially, if present, they are mild. The opacity and incidence increase with the duration of active disease. Focal opacities can occur in the anterior lens epithelium in conjunction with posterior synechiae.[49,50] Zonular dehiscence secondary to chronic inflammation with lenticular subluxation is a rare complication.[51]

Posterior

Vitreous inflammatory infiltrate must be present to make the diagnosis of intermediate uveitis. The cellular reaction can vary from mild to severe, obscuring any view of posterior structures. Early on, the vitreous may have diffuse nonaggregated cells. As the disease progresses, cellular aggregates in conjunction with noncellular vitreous strands and condensations form.[12,46] The infiltrated vitreous liquifies, and partial or complete posterior vitreous separation is common.

Large fibrocellular exudative aggregates of gray-white or yellow material in the inferior vitreous base overlying the pars plana and anterior retina are the classic findings in intermediate uveitis. These may coalesce to form what is commonly referred to as a snowbank (Fig. 51–1). This may extend from the ciliary body to the posterior retina and circumscribe the entire anterior retina and pars plana. Peripheral retinal neovascularization may lead to mild or massive vitreous hemorrhage. The neovascular membranes can grow along the anterior hyaloid face,[9,21,31,45] which can lead to anterior traction retinal detachment secondary to contraction of this anterior vitreous fibrovascular membrane.[52]

CME and its sequelae are the leading causes of significant visual loss in intermediate uveitis. CME is clinically present in 28 to 64% of patients. Angiographic evidence is present in 65 to 79% of patients.[30,48] CME results in blunting of the foveal reflex with cystoid changes in a petaloid pattern emanating from the foveal center. Late in the disease, large thin-walled cysts may progress to inner lamellar or full-thickness macular holes. Chronic CME may lead to cystoid macular degeneration, with rarefaction of the foveal and juxtafoveal retinal pigment epithelium and degeneration of the overlying neurosensory retina, resulting in irreversible vision loss. Epiretinal membrane formation resulting in macular ectopia may occur in the presence or absence of CME.[43]

The retinal vasculature is commonly affected in intermediate uveitis. Focal areas of phlebitis and venous dilatation in the peripheral retina occur early in the disease.[12,31,32,43,48,53] This leads to retinal

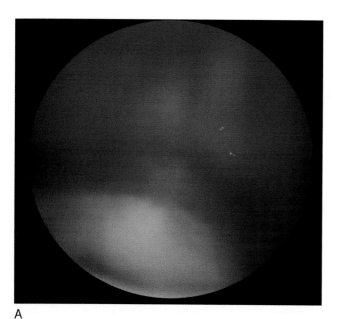

A

FIGURE 51–1 *A*, Scleral depression fundus photograph of a patient with intermediate uveitis recalcitrant to steroid therapy. *B*, Schematic drawing of the same eye highlighting the vitreoretinal infiltrate (snowbank) and the vitreous cellular response. *Illustration continued on opposite page*

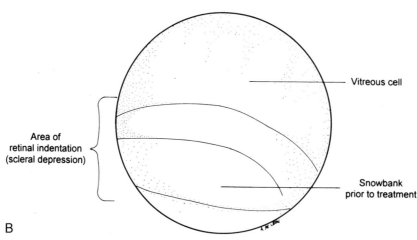

Vitreous cell

Area of
retinal indentation
(scleral depression)

Snowbank
prior to treatment

B

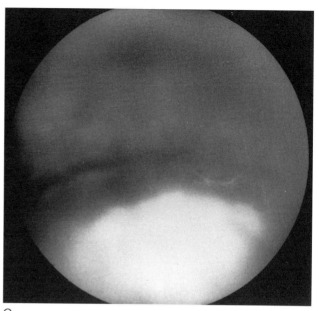

C

FIGURE 51–1 *Continued   C,* Scleral depression late fluorescein angiogram of the same eye. *D,* Schematic of the same photo. Note the diffuse leakage in the snowbank region and the vascular staining. *Illustration continued on following page*

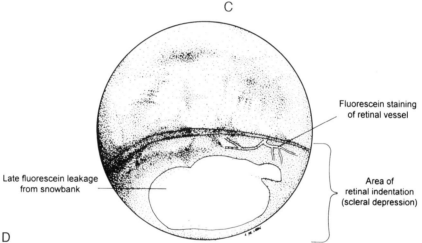

Fluorescein staining of retinal vessel

Late fluorescein leakage from snowbank

Area of retinal indentation (scleral depression)

D

ischemia, microaneurysms, peripheral retinal neovascularization, and optic disc edema.[28,31] Occasionally, the large areas of ischemic retina may appear as a branch or central retinal artery occlusion.[31,48]

Serous, traction, rhegmatogenous, and combined retinal detachments occur in 5% of eyes.[12,14,28,30,32,54] In tertiary retina and uveitis clinics, the incidence of detachment is as high as 15 to 51%.[7,9,48] Recently, Malinowski and colleagues[55] reported an 8.3% rate of retinal detachment in a large tertiary referral center. Serous or exudative detachments occur in response to retinal ischemia and blood retinal barrier compromise. Four types of combined rhegmatogenous/traction retinal detachments were described by Brockhurst and Schepens[9]:

Type 1 detachments occur secondary to small retinal breaks at the ora serrata near areas of exudate. These are low-lying, indolent detachments commonly associated with demarcation lines.

Type 2 detachments occur due to large dialysis-like retinal tears at the posterior edge of areas

of vitreous exudate (snowbank). These are seen in patients with mild chronic intermediate uveitis and are slowly progressive. These may spontaneously resolve if the vitreoretinal exudation occludes the break.

Type 3 detachments occur in patients with severe chronic uveitis associated with retinal neovascularization and extensive circumferential peripheral retinal exudation.

Type 4 detachments occur when neovascularization along the anterior hyaloid face contracts, leading to severe anterior funnel retinal detachments. Such detachments are extremely difficult to repair and usually result in profound loss of vision.

The optic nerve is commonly involved in intermediate uveitis. Disc edema is present in 3 to 20% of eyes.[12,31,48] Optic disc neovascularization occurs in the setting of profound retinal ischemia. Optic atrophy can occur late in the disease as a result of retinal ischemia or secondary glaucoma. Malinowski and colleagues[55] reported in 1992 that optic neu-

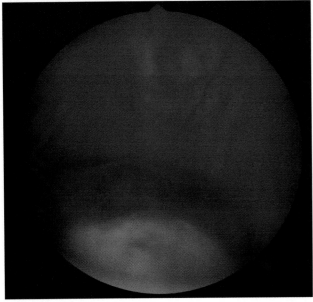

E

FIGURE 51–1 *Continued E*, Scleral depression fundus photograph of the same eye after cryotherapy. Note the less fluffy appearance of the snowbank, one of the cryotherapy scars and the lack of vitreous cell. This is highlighted in the schematic (*F*). *Illustration continued on opposite page*

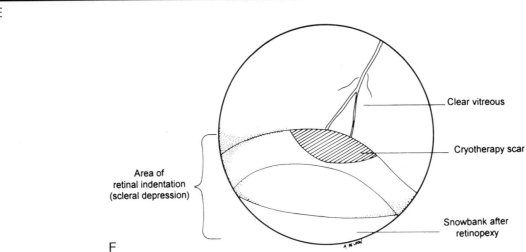

F

ritis develops with or without associated multiple sclerosis in 14.8% of patients with intermediate uveitis. The association of multiple sclerosis (MS) and intermediate uveitis is discussed below.

CLINICAL COURSE AND PROGNOSIS

Several classification schemes have been suggested to describe the clinical course and predict outcomes for intermediate uveitis.[5,7,8,14,22,27,31,56,57] Brockhurst and colleagues[31] classify eyes into four groups: 49% follow a chronic, smoldering course complicated by mild reactivations and remissions; 31% follow a benign course with complete remission and few complications; 15% have severe chronic inflammation complicated by peripheral retinal neovascularization and progressive loss of vision; and 5% of eyes have a dismal course characterized by rapid severe progression with massive exudation, neovascuiari-

zation, and resistance to therapy—the form usually seen in children.[9,12,27] Welch and colleagues[5] split their patients into two groups based on the level of inflammation: 31% had diffuse inflammation and 69% had massive exudation. Kimura and colleagues[31] and Hogan and Smith[14] classified patients on two scales. First on the basis of the level of inflammation at presentation (mild [29 to 43%], moderate [42 to 46%], and severe [11 to 39%]) and second on the basis of clinical course (benign without exacerbations [10%], chronic smoldering without severe exacerbation [59%], and chronic smoldering with one or more severe exacerbations [31%]).

Unfortunately, none of the classifications can accurately predict the course of disease. The sole exception is the rapidly progressive severe disease in children, which has a very poor prognosis. Hogan[58] states that the natural history of the disease has an excellent visual prognosis in 80% of untreated patients. Malinowski and colleagues[55] found that the long-term mean visual acuity outcomes in intermediate uveitis patients followed for an average of

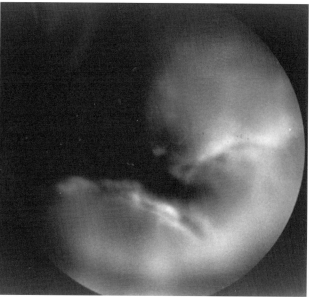

G

FIGURE 51-1 *Continued*   *G*, Scleral depression late fluorescein angiogram of the same eye after cryotherapy treatment. *H*, Schematic representation of the same eye. Note the decrease in leakage from the treated snowbank area and the vascular staining. (All photos are courtesy of Dr. R.G. Josephberg, Yonkers, NY)

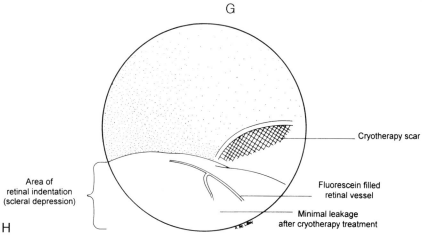

Area of
retinal indentation
(scleral depression)

Cryotherapy scar

Fluorescein filled
retinal vessel

Minimal leakage
after cryotherapy treatment

H

90 months were the same as their presenting visual acuities (20/44 to 20/46). These data suggest that the bulk of intermediate uveitis patients ultimately do well. The most important factor that affects the final visual outcome is the presence of macular involvement. Chronic cystoid macular edema, epiretinal membrane formation, macular retinal detachment, and macular ischemia are all harbingers of poor visual outcome. Malinowski and colleagues[55] report the rates of ocular complications in their series of 108 eyes as follows: visually significant cataracts, 14.8%; chronic cystoid macular edema, 8.3%; retinal detachment, 7.4%; retinal neovascularization with or without associated vitreous hemorrhage, 6.5%; and epiretinal membrane with macular ectopia, 6.5%.

ASSOCIATION WITH MULTIPLE SCLEROSIS

An increased incidence of MS in intermediate uveitis patients has long been noted.[59-61] Patients with

multiple sclerosis can develop intermediate uveitis either prior to or after the onset of their disease. In their long-term series, Malinowski and colleagues[55] reported a 7.4% incidence of well-documented optic neuritis among 54 patients with intermediate uveitis. They also reported the incidence of MS developing in an additional 14.8% of patients. Statistical analysis predicts that there is a 20% chance of developing MS or optic neuritis over a 5-year period in patients with intermediate uveitis. Malinowski and colleagues reported the association of intermediate uveitis and HLA-DR2, a histocompatibility antigen associated with MS.[63,64] This is the first laboratory association between the two diseases.

DIFFERENTIAL DIAGNOSIS

There are no specific tests for intermediate uveitis. The diagnosis is classically made by noting the snowbanks along the anterior vitreous overlying the peripheral retina and pars plana by indirect ophthalmoscopy in young individuals. Many cases of intermediate uveitis present with a mild cellular reaction in the vitreous prior to the formation of snowbanks. Accurate diagnosis becomes more difficult in these cases. The differential diagnosis includes the many causes of vitreous inflammation.

Infectious

Toxocariasis is an important consideration in younger patients with unilateral prominent peripheral inflammation. The diagnosis is made by elevated toxocara antibody titers in the serum.[65] Bilateral posterior uveitis can occur in patients with Lyme disease. The diagnosis is made by serum antibody testing for the infectious agent responsible, *Borrelia burgdorferi*.[66] Infectious retinitis commonly presents with painless vitreous inflammatory infiltrates. In some cases of acute retinal necrosis (ARN) due to herpes simplex or varicella zoster virus, the vitreous inflammatory infiltrate may obscure the retinitis and the disease could be mistaken for intermediate uveitis. The rapid course of ARN distinguishes it from intermediate uveitis. Many other infectious agents can cause a vitreous inflammatory infiltrate, including toxoplasmosis, and bacterial and fungal exogenous and endogenous endophthalmitis.

Idiopathic and Connective Tissue Disease

Sarcoidosis is a common cause of bilateral or unilateral vitreous inflammation. It may present with peripheral phlebitis, cystoid macular edema, and little anterior involvement. The presence of systemic sarcoid manifestations, such as erythema nodosum, conjunctival nodules, swelling of the lacrimal or salivary glands, hilar adenopathy on chest x-ray, or an elevated angiotensin-converting enzyme.[67] Behçet's syndrome is an idiopathic systemic disease that commonly affects Japanese and Mediterranean individuals. The disease is manifest by peripheral necrotizing retinal arteritis and phlebitis. The vasculitis tends to be more severe than that seen with intermediate uveitis; however, vitreous snowbanks do not form. Systemic lupus erythematosus is associated with retinal arteritis and vitreous inflammation. The arteritis usually has a posterior component. Systemic manifestations of Behçet's syndrome include oral/genital aphthous ulcers, arthritis, and skin and central nervous system findings.[68] Eales' disease is an idiopathic bilateral retinal vasculitis that affects both peripheral arteries and veins. The involvement of the arteries in systemic lupus erythematosus, Behçet's, and Eales' diseases is a distinguishing factor when considering intermediate uveitis. As stated earlier, MS can be associated with intermediate uveitis and should

be considered in patients with optic neuritis and/or the history of unexplained episodes of weakness.

Surgical/Trauma

Post–cataract extraction–related CME (Irvine-Gass syndrome) is one of the most common forms of unilateral vitreous inflammation.[69,70] It is characterized by inflammatory cells within the vitreous, CME, and optic nerve edema. There is little or no anterior segment involvement. Anterior chamber and vitreous inflammation can be seen in the setting of recent trauma.

Tumor

Large cell lymphoma (formerly termed "reticulum cell sarcoma") can present as a vitreous infiltrate. Masquerade syndrome, as it is termed, is an important, potentially lethal disease in the differential diagnosis of intermediate uveitis and should be considered in elderly patients with cellular vitreous infiltrates. Retinal, optic nerve, and less frequently choroidal infiltrates are important factors distinguishing this entity from intermediate uveitis.[71]

Ocular

Juvenile rheumatoid arthritis and Fuchs' heterochromic iridocyclitis commonly present with an anterior chamber cellular reaction. With these and other causes of anterior uveitis, spillover into the anterior vitreous is common, but should not be confused with intermediate uveitis. Peripheral retinal detachment/tear can present with the complaint of painless floaters. These may be due to either red blood cells or liberated RPE cells.

Inherited

Bilateral vitreous infiltrates that occur due to systemic autosomal dominant amyloidosis assume a "glass wool" appearance later in the disease.[72]

EVALUATION

Diagnostic testing in patients suspected to have intermediate uveitis is performed primarily to rule out other causes of intraocular inflammation (see Table 51–1). There are no specific tests for intermediate uveitis. The core of laboratory studies includes a complete blood count (myeloproliferative and infectious disease), angiotensin-converting enzyme (sarcoidosis), chest x-ray (sarcoidosis and tuberculosis), tuberculin skin test with anergy panel

TABLE 51–1   Laboratory Work-Up for Intermediate Uveitis Patients

---

Basic work-up
    Complete blood count (CBC) with differential
    Angiotensin-converting enzyme (ACE)
    Tuberculin skin test (PPD) with anergy panel
    FTA-ABS or MHATP
    Chest x-ray
Additional work-up if history or systemic
      symptoms are suggestive
    Antinuclear antibody (ANA)
    Lyme antibody
    Toxocara antibody
    HLA-B27, HLA-DR2

(tuberculosis), and monoclonal antibody–*Treponema pallidum* or fluorescent treponema antibody absorption test (syphilis), and antinuclear antibody (systemic lupus erythematosus and other connective tissue diseases). Immunologic testing for Lyme disease is only performed in patients with an exposure risk to tick bite. Toxocara antibody testing is done in children with a suggestive clinical picture. HLA-B27 typing is not necessary unless one of the intraocular HLA-B27–associated diseases is suspected. HLA-DR2 full typing in patients with a history of MS, optic neuritis, or a previous episode of weakness may help diagnosis. Fluorescein angiography helps in diagnosis and monitoring of CME.

TREATMENT

Treatments for intermediate uveitis are directed towards one or more of the following associated findings: intraocular inflammation, cystoid macular edema, cataract, vitreous opacity, and retinal detachment. Most cases of intermediate uveitis are mild, respond to initial corticosteroid treatment, and have good visual outcomes. Rapidly progressive cases usually result in poor outcomes despite therapeutic intervention. Chronic recurrent and recalcitrant cases are challenging to manage. Complications of the disease and treatment must both be dealt with on an individual basis. The advent of corticosteroids, cryotherapy, vitrectomy, immunosuppressive agents, and laser photocoagulation provide the therapeutic armamentarium from which to choose. Figures 51–2 and 51–3 depict decision trees that provide a guideline suggesting appropriate use of the available therapies, which are discussed in detail below.

Corticosteroids

Since the pathogenesis of intermediate uveitis is unknown, no specific therapy for the disease is known. Most theories suggest an immune-modulated phenomenon. For this reason all treatments focus on suppressing the immune system, either specifically (as in the case of cyclosporine) or generally (as in the case of corticosteroids). Although many immunosuppressive drugs have been tested for their effectiveness in the treatment of intermediate uveitis, topical, peribulbar, or systemic corticosteroids remain the mainstay of treatment.

The effectiveness of topical 1% prednisolone acetate is debatable. While some studies show there is a role for topical therapy in mild cases,[8] others show little or no benefit.[73] If topical steroids are to be effective, the initial frequency of administration should be between 6 and 12 drops per day. Compliance is an important issue with the high-frequency regimen. Complications of topical steroid therapy consist primarily of steroid-induced glaucoma and posterior subcapsular cataract.

Peribulbar injection of long-acting corticosteroids (triamcinolone acetonide) is a highly effective therapy for intermediate uveitis. Reports in the literature cite a two-line increase in visual acuity in approximately 70% of treated eyes,[74–76] and visual acuities of 20/40 or better in 85% of eyes following one or two injections. The recommended dosage for long-acting depot steroid injection is 40 mg triamcinolone acetonide. In conjunction with the long-acting steroid we give a short-acting steroid, 24 mg (1.0 ml) of dexamethasone. In small children, 20 mg of triamcinolone acetonide is effective.[76] Response to steroid injections can vary from rapid dramatic resolution to no response. This phenomenon appears in part to be age related: individuals who respond favorably to injections tend to be younger (average age, 29 years) than those who gained no therapeutic effect (average age, 42 years).[76]

Periocular injections may be delivered to the retroseptal space or the subtenon space. Retroseptal injections can be given transdermally or through a transconjunctival approach. Transdermal injections are made with a 0.5-inch 26-gauge sharp needle in the temporal aspect of the lower lid. The needle is inserted to the hub to ensure that the needle perforates the inferior septum and thus ensure that the steroid is injected to the retroseptal space. In addition to the long- and short-acting steroid, 0.1 ml of 1% or 2% Xylocaine may be injected for pain relief. The disadvantages of this approach include skin depigmentation (particularly in darkly pigmented individuals), secondary preseptal injection of steroid, and discomfort. Advantages of the transdermal route include ease of injection and lower incidence of steroid-induced glaucoma. Prior to the transconjunctival injection, the inferotemporal fornix is anesthetized with 4% topical lidocaine or a tetracaine-soaked pledget. Then the long- and short-acting steroids are injected using a 26- or 27-gauge needle with the bevel aimed toward the globe, through the inferotemporal fornix angled first toward the orbital floor and then posteriorly to ensure placement in the retroseptal space. This

Patient primarily diagnosed with Intermediate Uveitis	**Unilateral disease**	**Mild** Topical Steroids† (if no response - treat as moderate case)	**If no response from injections, they are contraindicated or not tolerated, consider:** 1) Oral Steroids† 2) Cyclosporine† 3) Combined cyclosporine-steroid†	**If no response to oral medications:** **+ Peripheral neovascularization** Cryotherapy or PRP **- Peripheral neovascularization** or **No response to retinopexy** Consider surgery*
		Moderate to Severe Retroseptal steroid injection		
	Bilateral disease	**Mild** Topical Steroids† (If no response treat as a moderate case)	**If no response to maximal oral medications or bilateral steroid injections then consider:**	**+Peripheral neovascularization** Cryotherapy or PRP **- Peripheral neovascularization** or **No response to retinopexy** Consider surgery*
		Moderate to Severe Oral steroids† **If the Oral steroids are contraindicated choose one of the following treatments:** 1) Bilateral retroseptal steroid injection 2) Cyclosporine† 3) Combined Steroid-cyclosporine† **If severe then consider:** Pulsed IV Methyl-prednisilone		

†All patients responding to oral or topical medications should be tapered slowly from medications (see text)

* See Surgical Decision Tree (fig #3)

FIGURE 51–2   A clinical decision tree for extraocular therapy for intermediate uveitis.

offers the advantages of the retroseptal injection with decreased pain and less chance of skin depigmentation. Subtenon injections are usually given through the supertemporal bulbar conjunctiva. The conjunctiva is anesthetized topically as above. While the patient is looking inferonasally, an injection is made with a 26- or 27-gauge 1/2- to 5/8-inch needle with the bevel toward the globe and advanced to the hub of the needle.[76] This method has the advantage of being relatively pain free and delivers the drug to the macular area. The disadvantage of this method is that it requires more patient cooperation than the transdermal approach and patients may be at a higher risk for developing steroid-induced glaucoma.

Oral and Intravenous Steroids

Patients with bilateral disease or recalcitrant unilateral disease can be treated with oral corticosteroids. The recommended dosage is 1 mg/kg (lean body weight) given daily for at least 5 days. The

Intermediate uveitis recalcitrant to other therapies or media opacity in an eye in remission	Visual acuity > 20/60	Observe		
	Visual acuity < 20/60 (Consider surgery*)	Clear Lens		PPV[1,2]
		Visually significant cataract	Active inflammation	PPV+PPL[1,2]
			No active inflammation	
			Opacified vitreous	PPV + PPL[1]
				or
				PPV + ECCE + PCIOL[1]
			Clear Vitreous	PPV + PPL[1]
				or
				ECCE +/- PCIOL[1]

* This chart is only a guideline. The decision to perform surgery is highly individual and based on the physician's experience as well as the needs and desires of the patient.
[1] All surgeries are augmented with perioperative steroids (IV, retroseptal, and/or oral) unless contraindicated. (See text)
[2] Retinal cryopexy or photocoagulation is added intraoperatively when neovascularization is present.

FIGURE 51-3 A surgical decision tree for medically recalcitrant intermediate uveitis.

steroids can be tapered by going to alternate-day therapy and/or reducing the dosage. In many cases, steroids must be tapered slowly over several months and, on occasion, patients must be maintained on steroids for several years. Alternate-day therapy is essential for these patients to lessen steroid-induced complications. In severe cases, both oral and retroseptal steroids may be given in conjunction.[57] For patients with severe disease who respond to but are intolerant of oral steroids, intermittent-pulse intravenous (IV) methylprednisolone therapy (1 to 2 g infused over 1 hour every 6 hours for 2 to 3 days) can effectively induce remission with fewer side effects.

Oral Versus Retroseptal Corticosteroids

The decision of when to give peribulbar injections is made on an individual basis. Generally, injections are not given unless there is a drop in vision, usually associated with cystoid macular edema and/or vitreous debris. Some clinicians will not treat dis-

ease unless the vision drops below 20/40, while others will treat patients with better vision who notice visual decline. Periocular injections are usually given to patients with unilateral disease. Bilateral injections for bilateral ocular disease should also be considered in patients at particularly high risk for oral steroid-induced complications, such as those with peptic ulcer disease, borderline diabetes, diabetes, and pregnancy. Patients who have failed a course of oral steroids should also be considered for periocular injections (unilateral or bilateral).

CRYOTHERAPY AND PANRETINAL PHOTOCOAGULATION

Many patients with unremitting, chronic uveitis recalcitrant to steroid therapy develop neovascularization of the vitreous base. This is usually recognized by the appearance of large-bore vessels in the far periphery extending over the ora serrata, with the neovascularization itself often obscured by local vitreous infiltrate, snowbanking, and the far peripheral location, but can often be seen when performing cryotherapy. Management of neovascularization by either cryotherapy[27,34,45,77] or diathermy[5,45,78,79] has been shown to reduce the exudative response and break the cycle that perpetuates the disease.[80] Recently, panretinal photocoagulation has been shown to be effective in the treatment of peripheral neovascularization.[81]

Cryotherapy is performed under retrobulbar, peribulbar, or subtenon anesthesia in adults and general anesthesia in children. The cryotherapy is applied directly to the areas of exudation using the double freeze-thaw technique. The iceball formed should encompass the entire area of exudate and neovascularization and overlap the uninvolved areas of retina, pars plana, and ciliary body one standard adult cryotip width. If the iceball cannot be seen, then treatment for an equal duration adequate to treat visualized areas should be applied. Retroseptal steroids are injected following the procedure. Marcaine (0.5%) is added if the treatment is performed under general anesthesia. The procedure can be repeated in 3 to 4 months if there is residual disease. Complications secondary to cryotherapy are rare, but include choroidal effusion, retinal detachment, elevated or decreased intraocular pressure, and cataract formation.

The efficacy of peripheral cryopexy has been demonstrated by Devenyi and collaborators.[82] Of 27 patients treated, 78% had complete resolution of uveitis and 19% had a significant decrease in uveitis. The necessity for corticosteroid therapy was eliminated in 90% of patients. Decrease in visual acuity was only seen in 11% of patients.

Panretinal scatter laser photocoagulation (PRP) is the first-line treatment for many ocular diseases complicated by peripheral retinal neovascularization. Park and colleagues[81] recently reported regression of peripheral neovascularization, improvement of CME, and stabilization of vitreous inflammation in ten eyes (six patients) after undergoing PRP alone or in combination with pars plana vitrectomy (PPV). Advantages of PRP over cryotherapy include ease of administration, fewer ocular complications, and less pain. Vitreous opacity may limit the use of laser treatment. PRP appears to be a useful addition to the armamentarium against intermediate uveitis; however, more investigation is necessary before PRP can be recommended as a replacement for cryotherapy.

ANTIMETABOLITE AND IMMUNOSUPPRESSIVE THERAPY

Many antimetabolites and immunosuppressive drugs have been used systemically to treat eyes with intermediate uveitis recalcitrant to other medical therapies. These include methotrexate,[83,84] 6-mercaptopurine,[85] azathioprine,[86] cyclophosphamide,[87,88] and chlorambucil.[89-91] These agents have some therapeutic effect; however, systemic toxicity is generally a limiting factor for these therapies.

Cyclosporine is a potent inhibitor of T-cell function secondary to inhibition of interleukin-2 and interferon γ production. Nussenblatt and Palestine[92] reported the efficacy of cyclosporine in patients who became intolerant or recalcitrant to corticosteroids. Approximately two thirds of the 33 eyes in 17 patients followed long term showed improved vision and decreased vitreous haze. Unfortunately, creatine levels rose in the majority of patients. This has led the authors to amend the dosing regimen, and reportedly now have achieved a high level of successful treatment while minimizing renal toxicity. Therapeutic recommendations for cyclosporine for either initial treatment or when treating patients recalcitrant or intolerant of other therapies in intermediate uveitis is as follows: The initial treatment consists of cyclosporine 5 mg/kg/day with or without prednisone 0.2 to 0.4 mg/kg/day; follow for 4 to 6 weeks. If there is no improvement, increase either cyclosporine to 7 mg/kg/day or prednisone to 0.6 mg/kg/day. The maximum dosage is cyclosporine 7 mg/kg/day with prednisone 0.6 mg/kg/day. Creatine levels must be monitored prior to the initiation of therapy and at 4- to 6-week intervals. Creatinine level increases of 20 to 30% are indications for cessation of therapy. Pre-existing renal disease is a contraindication to cyclosporine treatment.

VITRECTOMY/LENSECTOMY

In patients with significant vitreous opacities either impairing the patient's vision or obscuring the ophthalmologist's view of the periphery, pars plana vitrectomy is an effective treatment for the restoration of vision as well as attenuation of inflammation and the exudative response. Dugel and colleagues[93] reported visual acuity improvement and lessening CME in the majority of 11 eyes operated. In patients with inactive disease suffering from poor vision due to vitreous opacity, the decision to operate is based on the patients estimated visual potential and visual needs. In patients with active disease not responsive to or intolerant of medical therapy, retroseptal steroids, and/or cryotherapy, vitrectomy is becoming a viable, effective alternative. This is particularly true of eyes with significant vitreous opacity or cataract wherein the patient's vision will likely be limited even if the active inflammation is controlled. Vitrectomy also provides a view of the peripheral fundus and, which can be treated at the time of surgery with cryoablation or PRP as described above. General guidelines for vitrectomy include (1) removal of the posterior hyaloid and as much anterior vitreous as possible (obviously limited in phakic patients); (2)

careful inspection of the periphery, looking for neo-vascularization and occult retinal breaks; (3) pre-medication of patients with active disease, with either IV methylprednisolone the day of surgery or preseptal steroid injection up to 3 days to 2 weeks prior to surgery and immediately following the case.

CATARACT

When a visually significant cataract is present and there is vitreous opacity or active disease recalcitrant to other therapies, vitrectomy is combined with either cataract extraction by a limbal approach or pars plana lensectomy. Cataracts in patients with intermediate uveitis are more difficult to remove often due to the presence of preoperative posterior synechiae, fragile iris vessels, and exuberant fibrin formation intraoperatively (as well as postoperatively) within the anterior chamber. The principal advantage of the limbal approach is the ease of insertion of a posterior chamber intraocular lens either during the initial surgery or at some time in the future. The disadvantages are the associated complications, including iris stromal atrophy, iridocapsular synechiae, pupillary block glaucoma, pupillary sphincter sclerosis, hyphema, and intense postoperative inflammation.[94] Therefore, this group of patients should have a peripheral iridectomy to help prevent pupillary block glaucoma. The pars plana approach combined with removing the entire capsule causes less damage to the iris and eliminates the possibility of posterior synechiae, which can lead to pupillary block glaucoma. The disadvantage is that it relegates the patient to aphakia, since we believe sewing in a posterior chamber intraocular lens, placing a lens in the ciliary sulcus, or placing an anterior chamber intraocular lens is contraindicated due to the high likelihood of complications postoperatively from the smoldering inflammation.

SUMMARY

Intermediate uveitis is an idiopathic inflammation of the peripheral retina and pars plana. Many etiologic theories have been postulated, yet none have been compelling. The wide spectrum of clinical presentation may suggest that there are several diseases lumped together under diagnosis of intermediate uveitis. Some cases are coupled with MS. These links may help our understanding of both diseases.

Although the pathophysiology of intermediate uveitis remains unknown, there has been significant therapeutic advances since Schepens' description of the disease.[3,4] Corticosteroids, cryotherapy, anti-inflammatory agents, pars plana vitrectomy, antimetabolites, immunosuppressive agents, and

PRP used alone or in combination therapy can provide more rapid recovery and improved long-term results. Unfortunately, many patients still lose significant vision and have significant morbidity from the treatments as well as the disease. Recalcitrant patients should be treated by or under the guidance of individuals with significant clinical experience, since all therapeutic decisions have potentially serious complications.

REFERENCES

1. Fuchs E: A Textbook of Ophthalmology. Duane A (trans). Philadelphia, JB Lippincott Co, 1908, p 204.
2. Duke-Elder WS: Textbook of Ophthalmology, Vol III, Diseases of the Inner Eye. St. Louis, Mosby Year Book, Inc, 1941, p 2186.
3. Schepens CL: Examination of the ora serrata region: its clinical significance. Acta XVI Concilium Ophthalmologicum (Britannia) 16:1384, 1950.
4. Schepens CL: L'inflammation de la région de l' "ora serrata" et ses sequelles. Bull Mem Soc Franq Ophthalmol 63:113, 1950.
5. Welch RB, Maumenee AE, Whalen HE: Peripheral posterior segment inflammation, vitreous opacities, and edema of the posterior pole. Arch Ophthalmol 64:540, 1960.
6. Brockhurst RJ, Schepens CL, Okamura ID: Uveitis. I. Gonioscopy. Am J Ophthalmol 42:545, 1956.
7. Brockhurst RJ, Schepens CL, Okamura ID: Uveitis. II. Peripheral uveitis. Clinical description and differential diagnosis. Am J Ophthalmol 49:1257, 1960.
8. Brockhurst RJ, Schepens L, Okamura ID: Uveitis. III. Peripheral uveitis. Pathogenesis, etiology and treatment. Am J Ophthalmol 51:19, 1961.
9. Brockhurst RJ, Schepens CL: Uveitis. IV. Peripheral uveitis. The complication of retinal detachment. Arch Ophthalmol 80:747, 1968.
10. Bloch-Michel E, Nussemblast RB: International Uveitis Study Group recommendations for the evaluation of intraocular inflammatory disease. Am J Ophthalmol 103:234, 1987.
11. Nussemblast RB, Palestine AG: Uveitis: Fundamentals and Clinical Practice. Chicago, Yearbook Medical, 1989.
12. Bec P, Arne JL, Phillippot V, et al: Basal uveoretinitis (peripheral uveitis, chronic posterior cyclitis, pars planitis, vitritis, hyaloretinitis) and other inflammations of the peripheral retina (French, English Abstract). Arch Ophthalmol (Paris) 37:169, 1977.
13. Van Metre TE: Role of the allergist in diagnosis and management of patients with uveitis. JAMA 195:105, 1966.
14. Smith RE, Godfrey WA, Kimura SJ: Chronic cyclitis. I. Course and visual prognosis. Trans Am Acad Ophthalmol Otolaryngol 77:760, 1973.
15. Perkins ES, Folk J: Uveitis in London and Iowa. Ophthalmologica 189:36, 1984.
16. Schlaegel TF: Differential diagnosis of uveitis. Ophthalmol Digest 35:34, 1973.
17. Martenet AC: Les cyclitis Chroniques (French, English Abstract). Arch Ophthalmol (Paris) 33:533, 1973.
18. Martenet AC: Importance du test du Kvein dans les recherches etiologigues de l'uveite peripherique. Bull Soc Franc Ophtal 77:604, 1964.
19. Henderly DE, Genstler AJ, Smith RE, Rao NA: Changing patterns of uveitis. Am J Ophthalmol 103:131, 1987.
20. Althus C, Sundmacher R: Intermediate uveitis: epidemiology, age and sex distribution. Dev Ophthalmol 23:15–19, 1992.
21. Hogan MJ, Kimura SJ, O'Connor GR: Peripheral retinitis and chronic cyclitis in children. Trans Ophthalmol Soc UK 85:39, 1965.

22. Schlaegel TF: Ocular Toxoplasmosis and Pars Planitis. New York, Grune & Stratton, 1978.
23. Giles CL: Uveitis in childhood. In Duane T (ed): Clinical Ophthalmology, Vol 4. New York, Harper & Row, 1976.
24. Jutte A, Lemke L, Opitz J: Chronic cyclitis in children. Ophthalmologica 157:169, 1969.
25. Witmer R, Korner G: Uveitis in kindesalter. Ophthalmologica 152:277, 1966.
26. Capone A Jr, Aaberg TM: Intermediate uveitis. In Albert DM, Jakobiec FA (eds): Principles and Practice of Ophthalmology. Philadelphia, WB Saunders Co, 1994.
27. Aaberg TM, Cesarz TJ, Flickinger RR: Treatment of pars planitis. I. Cryotherapy. Surv Ophthalmol 22:120, 1977.
28. Smith RE, Godfrey WA, Kimura SJ: Complications of chronic cyclitis. Am J Ophthalmol 82:277, 1976.
29. Henderly DE, Haymond RS, Rao NA, Smith RE: The significance of pars plana exudate in pars planitis. Am J Ophthalmol 103:669, 1987.
30. Chester GH, Blach RK, Cleary PE: Inflammation in the region of the vitreous base. Pars planitis. Trans Ophthalmol Soc UK 96:151, 1976.
31. Kimura SJ, Hogan MJ: Chronic cyclitis. Arch Ophthalmol 71:193, 1964.
32. Henderly DE, Gentsler AJ, Rao NA, Smith RE: Pars planitis. Trans Ophthalmol Soc UK 105:227, 1985.
33. Smith RE: Pars planitis. In Ryan SJ (ed): Retina, Vol 2. St Louis, CV Mosby Co, 1989.
34. Aaberg TM, Cesarz TJ, Flickinger RR: Treatment of peripheral uveoretinitis by cryotherapy. Am J Ophthalmol 75:685, 1973.
35. Mahlberg PA, Cunha-Vaz JG, Tessler HH: Vitreous fluorophotometry in pars planitis. Am J Ophthalmol 95:189, 1983.
36. Wetzig RP, Chen CC, Nussenblatt RB, et al: Clinical and immunopathological studies of par planitis in a family. Br J Ophthalmol 75:5–10, 1988.
37. Augsburger JJ, Annesley WH Jr, Sergott RC, et al: Familial par planitis. Ann Ophthalmol 13:553–557, 1981.
38. Culbertson WW, Giles CL, West C, Stafford T: Familial pars planitis. Retina 3:179–181, 1983.
39. Eichenbaum JW, Friedman AH, Mamelok AE: A clinical and histopathological review of intermediate uveitis ("par planitis"). Bull NY Acad Med 64:164–174, 1988.
40. Green WR, Kincaid MC, Michels RG, et al: Pars planitis. Trans Ophthalmol Soc UK 101:361–367, 1981.
41. Yoser SL, Forster DJ, Rao NA: Pathology of intermediate uveitis. Dev Ophthalmol 23:60–70, 1992.
42. Davis JL, Chan CC, Nussenblatt RB: Immunology of intermediate uveitis. Dev Ophthalmol 23:71–85, 1992.
43. Maumenee AE: Clinical entities in "uveitis." An approach to the study of intraocular inflammation. XXVI Edward Jackson Memorial Lecture. Am J Ophthalmol 69:1, 1970.
44. Kenyon KR, Pederson JE, Green WR, Maumenee AE: Fibroglial proliferation in pars planitis. Trans Ophthalmol Soc UK 95:391, 1975.
45. Pederson JE, Kenyon KR, Green WR, Maumenee AE: Pathology of pars planitis. Am J Ophthalmol 86:762, 1978.
46. Hogan MJ, Kimura SJ: Cyclitis and peripheral chorioretinitis. Arch Ophthalmol 66:667, 1961.
47. Kravitz D: Study of the anterior angle in anterior segment inflammation of the eye. Am J Ophthalmol 38:622, 1954.
48. Pruett RC, Brockhurst RJ, Letts NF: Fluorescein angiography of peripheral uveitis. Am J Ophthalmol 77:448, 1974.
49. Spencer WH: Lens. In Spencer WH (ed): Ophthalmic Pathology: An Atlas and Textbook, 3rd edition. Philadelphia, WB Saunders Co, 1985.
50. Hooper PL, Rao NA, Smith RE: Cataract extraction in uveitis patients. Serv Ophthalmol 35:120, 1990.
51. Belfort R, Nussenblatt RB, Lottemberg C, et al: Spontaneous lens subluxation in uveitis. Am J Ophthalmol 110:714, 1990.
52. Felder KS, Brockhurst RJ: Neovascular fundus abnormalities in peripheral uveitis. Arch Ophthalmol 100:750, 1982.
53. Finoff WC: Recurrent hemorrhages into the retina and vitreous of young person. Am J Ophthalmol 5:195, 1922.
54. Cantrill HL, Ramsey RC, Knobloch WH, Purple RL: Electro-physiologic changes in chronic pars planitis. Am J Ophthalmol 91:505, 1981.
55. Malinowski SM, Pulido JS, Folk JC: Long-term visual outcome and complications associated with pars planitis. Ophthalmology 100:818, 1992.
56. Kimura SJ, Hogan MJ: Chronic cyclitis. Trans Am Ophthalmol Soc 61:397, 1963.
57. Aaberg TM: Pars planitis. In Fraunfelder FT, Roy FH (eds): Current Ocular Therapy. Philadelphia, WB Saunders Co, 1980.
58. Hogan MJ: Discussion of Gills JP, Buckley CE: Oral cyclophosphamide in the treatment of uveitis. Trans Am Acad Ophthalmol Otolaryngol 74:507, 1970.
59. Breger BC, Leopold IH: The incidence of uveitis in multiple sclerosis. Am J Ophthalmol 62:540–545, 1966.
60. Giles CL: Peripheral uveitis in patients with multiple sclerosis. Am J Ophthalmol 70:17–19, 1970.
61. Nussenblatt RB, Masciulli L, Yarianj DL, Duvoisin R: pars planitis—a demyelinating disease (Letter). Arch Ophthalmol 99:697, 1981.
62. Malinowski SM, Pulido JS, Goeken NE, et al: The association of HLA-B8, B51, DR2, and multiple sclerosis in pars planitis. Ophthalmology 100:1199, 1993.
63. Ogler JJF, Aranson BGW: Immunogenetics of multiple sclerosis. In Panayi GS, David CS (eds): Immunogenetics. London, Butterworth's, 1984, p 177.
64. Calder V, Owen S, Watson C, et al: MS: a localized immune disease of the central nervous system. Immunol Today 10:99–103, 1989.
65. Wilkinson CP, Welch RB: Intraocular Toxocara. Am J Ophthalmol 71:921, 1971.
66. Fujikawa LS: Advances in immunology and uveitis. Ophthalmology 96:1115, 1989.
67. Obenauf CD, Shaw HE, Snydor CF, Clintworth GK: Sarcoidosis and its ophthalmic manifestations. Am J Ophthalmol 86:648, 1978.
68. James DG, Spiteri MA: Behçets disease. Ophthalmology 89:1279, 1982.
69. Irvine SR: A newly defined vitreous syndrome following cataract surgery: interpreted according to recent concepts of the structure of the vitreous: the seventh Francis I. Proctor Lecture. Am J Ophthalmol 36:599, 1953.
70. Gass JDM, Norton EWD: Cystoid macular edema and papilledema following cataract extraction. Arch Ophthalmol 76:646, 1966.
71. Barr CC, Green WR, Payne JW, et al: Intraocular reticulum cell sarcoma: clinicopathologic study of four cases and review of the literature. Surv Ophthalmol 19:224, 1975.
72. Wong VG, McFarlin DE: Primary familial amyloidosis. Arch Ophthalmol 78:208, 1967.
73. Godfrey WA, Smith RE, Kimura SJ: Chronic cyclitis: corticosteroid therapy. Trans Am Ophthalmol Soc 74:178, 1976.
74. Nosik RA: Periocular injection of steroids. Trans Am Acad Ophthalmol Otolaryngol 76:695, 1972.
75. Schlaegel TF, Weber JC: Treatment of pars planitis, II: corticosteroids. Surv Ophthalmol 22:120, 125, 1977.
76. Helm CJ, Holland GN: The effects of posterior subtenon injection of triamcinolone acetonide in patients with intermediate uveitis. Am J Ophthalmol 120:55, 1995.
77. Gills CL: Pediatric intermediate uveitis. J Pediatr Ophthalmol Strabismus 26:136, 1989.
78. Gills JP: Combined medical and surgical therapy for complicated cases of peripheral uveitis. Arch Ophthalmol 79:723, 1968.
79. Cardosa RD, Brockhurst RJ: Perforating diathermy coagulation for retinal angiomas. Arch Ophthalmol 94:1702, 1976.
80. Aaberg TM: The enigma of pars planitis. Am J Ophthalmol 103:828, 1987.
81. Park WE, Mieler WF, Pulido JS: Peripheral scatter photocoagulation for neovascularization associated with pars planitis. Arch Ophthalmol 113:1277, 1995.
82. Devenyi RG, Mieler WF, Lambrou FH, et al: Cryopexy of the vitreous base in the management of peripheral uveitis. Am J Ophthalmol 106:135, 1988.

83. Wong VG, Hersh EM: Methotrexate in the therapy of cyclitis. Trans Am Acad Ophthalmol Otolaryngol 69:279, 1965.
84. Wong VG: Immunosuppressive therapy in ocular inflammatory diseases. Arch Ophthalmol 81:628, 1969.
85. Newell FW, Krill AE, Thomson A: Treatment of uveitis with 6-mercaptopurine. Am J Ophthalmol 61:1250, 1966.
86. Newell FW, Krill AE: Treatment of uveitis with azathioprine (Imuran). Trans Ophthalmol Soc UK 87:499, 1967.
87. Buckley CE, Gills JP: Cyclophosphamide therapy of peripheral uveitis. Arch Intern Med 124:29, 1969.
88. Gills JP, Buckley CE: Oral cyclophosphamide in the treatment of uveitis. Trans Am Acad Ophthalmol Otolaryngol 74:505, 1970.
89. Dinning WJ: Management of chronic uveitis. Trans Ophthalmol Soc UK 96:158, 1976.
90. Godfrey WA, Epstein WV, O'Conner GR, et al: The use of chlorambucil in intractable idiopathic uveitis. Am J Ophthalmol 78:415, 1974.
91. Nozik RA, Godfrey WA, Epstein WV, et al: Immunosuppressive treatment of uveitis. Mod Probl Ophthalmol 16:305, 1976.
92. Nussenblatt RB, Palestine AG: Ciclosporin (Sandimmun) therapy experience in the treatment of pars planitis and present therapeutic guidelines. Dev Ophthalmol 23:177–184, 1992.
93. Dugel PU, Rao NA, Ozler S, et al: Pars plana vitrectomy for intraocular inflammation related to cystoid macular edema unresponsive to corticosteroids: a preliminary study. Ophthalmology 99:1535, 1992.
94. Foster CS: Vitrectomy in the management of uveitis (Editorial). Ophthalmology 95:1111, 1988.

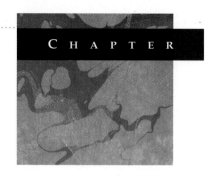

Multifocal Choroiditis, Punctate Inner Choroidopathy, and Other Related Conditions

Jeremiah Brown, Jr., M.D.

James C. Folk, M.D.

Patients with uveitis often present difficult diagnostic and management challenges (Fig. 52–1). There are a number of diseases that cause white lesions in the retina and choroid (Table 52–1). These entities should be considered during the evaluation of each patient. In addition, there are three inflammatory syndromes of unknown etiology that cause multifocal lesions that later scar. These diseases—multifocal choroiditis and panuveitis (MCP), punctate inner choroidopathy (PIC), and the diffuse subretinal fibrosis syndrome (DSF)—have similarities in that (1) they each affect women predominantly, (2) they are characterized by scattered yellow/gray choroidal and retinal pigment epithelial (RPE) lesions that lead to round pigmented chorioretinal scars, and (3) they often cause enlarged blind spots.

MULTIFOCAL CHOROIDITIS WITH PANUVEITIS

Nozik and Dorsch[1] first described two patients who presented with blurred vision, bilateral anterior uveitis, and punched-out chorioretinal scars. Both patients had areas of linear streaks and negative histoplasmin skin tests. Dreyer and Gass presented a series of 28 patients with panuveitis and chorioretinal scars and named the syndrome multifocal choroiditis with panuveitis. Despite the sim-

ilarities with the ocular histoplasmosis syndrome, multifocal choroiditis patients had vitreous cells, typically smaller choroidal lesions, usually negative histoplasmosis skin tests, and were not from areas endemic for histoplasmosis.[2] Morgan and Schatz discussed a series of 11 similar patients and reported success in using corticosteroids to quiet the inflammation and induce regression of choroidal neovascularization (CNV).[3] Reddy et al recently reported on the association of enlargement of the blind spot and the clinical features of a series of 41 patients.[7] The visual prognosis of this group as well as the incidence and treatment of choroidal neovascularization was reported by Brown et al.[8]

Clinical Features

PATIENT CHARACTERISTICS. Patients with multifocal choroiditis and panuveitis are predominantly women, with a reported frequency of 75 to 100%[2,3,7] (Table 52–2). The average age at onset is 30 to 35 years with a range of 9 to 69 years.[2,3,7] There appears to be no racial predilection. Patients usually present with a complaint of blurred vision or scotomata. They may also have photopsias, floaters, mild photophobia, or ocular discomfort. The average refractive error is mildly myopic (−2.00 diopters) with a wide range (−9.00 to +2.50 diopters).[7] Two thirds to three quarters of patients will have

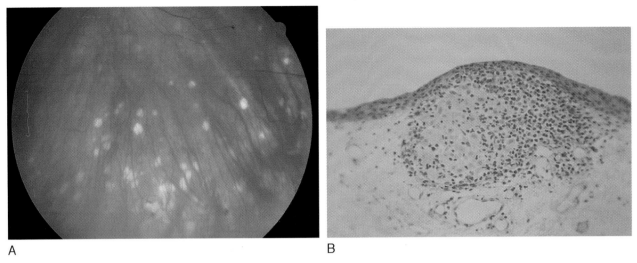

A   B

FIGURE 52-1 *A*, 65-year-old white woman with mild vitreous inflammation and numerous small punched-out chorioretinal scars inferiorly. The patient had a mildly elevated angiotension-converting enzyme and granuloma found on conjunctival biopsy. *B*, Conjunctival biopsy showing granuloma indicating sarcoidosis.

bilateral disease.[2,7] Although the initial visual acuity varies widely, two thirds of the patients will present with visual acuity of 20/50 or better.[8]

Clinical Signs

ANTERIOR SEGMENT. Anterior uveitis may be mild to moderate. Thirty-two per cent of patients in our study had 1 to 3+ anterior chamber cells.[7] Forty-six per cent of patients in Dreyer and Gass's series had anterior uveitis and all had vitreous cells.[2] Vitreous inflammation was found in 76% of patients in our series and was usually mild to moderate in severity.

FUNDUS FINDINGS. Initially, a few to many yellow-gray lesions are seen in the fundus at the level of the retinal pigment epithelium (RPE). Most lesions are 50 to 100 μm in diameter, but may be larger. The lesions are usually round or oval in shape and may be distributed throughout the posterior pole and midperiphery. The majority of lesions will be in the macula or in the nasal quadrant.[7] The lesions may occur singly, in clusters, or in a linear distribution.[1,10] Many patients will have peripapillary lesions, similar to the ocular histoplasmosis syndrome. The acute lesions evolve into atrophic scars with surrounding hyperpigmentation. One third of patients in our series had disc edema or hyperemia at some point in their disease.[7] Some patients develop cystoid macular edema.

It should be noted that some patients with MCP have later been found to have sarcoidosis, despite initial normal angiotensin-converting enzyme levels and normal chest x-rays.[11] These patients often have lesions more typical of sarcoidosis with an inferior predominance. The diagnosis can be made

with conjunctival biopsy demonstrating noncaseating granulomas (Figs. 52–1*A* and *B*).

PERIMETRY. Khorram and co-workers reported enlargement of the blind spot in three patients with MCP.[12] We studied 51 eyes with Goldmann perimetry at various phases of their disease.[7] Enlargement of the blind spot was the most common defect and was found in 47% of eyes. Central and paracentral scotomata were found in 25%. Four eyes had peripheral defects and two eyes had cecocentral scotomata. Twenty-two eyes had full fields. The nasal quadrant of the retina was more likely to be involved than any other quadrant. However, the field defects were larger than could be explained on the basis of visible choroidal lesions alone (Fig. 52–2). The size and depth of the defects appeared to be responsive to steroids in some patients. In most patients, the defect remained, although a few had improvement without treatment.

The etiology of the enlarged blind spots is unknown. One possible explanation involves the distribution of blood supply to the nasal retina. The peripapillary choroid is most often supplied by the medial posterior ciliary artery.[13] This artery usually branches earlier and more acutely from the ophthalmic artery than the lateral posterior ciliary artery(ies), which supply the temporal retina and macula.[14] If MCP is caused by a blood-borne agent, it may have more direct access to the nasal retina. Alternatively, one may consider the topography of the photoreceptors. Curcio and co-workers[15] have demonstrated regional variation in the distribution of photoreceptors. Rod photoreceptors were found to be of highest density in a horizontal ellipse centered in the macula but extending nasal to the optic nerve. Electroretinography (ERG) suggests that the

TABLE 52–1 White Lesions in the Retina and Choroid

Disease	History	Fundus Appearance	Treatment
Infectious			
ARN (HSV, HZV)	Healthy young patients	Geographic areas of white retina with vasculitis	Acyclovir, steroids, laser, vitrectomy
CMV	Immunocompromised, AIDS	Patches of retinitis with hemorrhage	Ganciclovir, foscarnet
PORN (HZV)	AIDS	Deep white retinal lesions in posterior pole; rapidly progressive	Acyclovir, poor prognosis
Disseminated bacterial	Septic, hospitalized	Prominent vitritis	Appropriate antibiotics
Neurosyphilis	Anyone	Diffuse neuroretinitis, vasculitis, chorioretinal infiltrates	Penicillin
Tuberculosis	Previous disease or exposure	Bilateral chronic iridocyclitis, yellow white choroidal lesions	INH, ethambutol rifampin, pyridoxime, pyrazinamide
Candida, Aspergillus	Indwelling catheters	Fluffy white retinitis	Amphotericin, fluconazole
Cryptococcus	Immunocompromised, headache	Multifocal yellow-white lesions	Amphotericin
Histoplasmosis	Ohio/Mississippi river valleys	Multifocal often pigmented lesions, peripapillary atrophy, choroidal neovascularization	Laser for macular CNV, steroids occasionally for choroiditis or neovascularization
Toxoplasmosis	Children, young adults	Focal retinitis, perivasculitis, vitritis	Pyrimethamine, sulfadiazine, prednisone, folinic acid
Pneumocystis carinii choroidopathy	Immunocompromised, AIDS	Multiple bilateral yellow oval or geographic lesions in the posterior pole	Pentamidine, trimethoprim-sulfamethoxazole
Toxocariasis	Young patients	Chronic endophthalmitis, post pole granuloma, peripheral inflammatory mass with retinal traction bands	Thiabendazole, steroids, occasionally vitrectomy
Cysticercosis	Poor hygiene, underdeveloped regions	Dark, mobile, intravitreal mass, severe vitritis if organism dies	Pars plana vitrectomy, praziquantel
DUSN (nematode)	Young, healthy patients	Early, groups of white deep retinal lesions followed by multifocal patches of RPE atrophy, mild constriction of retinal vessels, and optic disc pallor	Thiabendazole, diethylcarbamazine, laser photocoagulation of nematode
Onchocercosis	Travel history to Africa, Central and South America	Anterior uveitis, patchy retinal pigment	Ivermectin
Tumors			
Large cell lymphoma	Elderly	Sub-RPE infiltrates, vitritis	Radiation, chemotherapy
Metastatic	Breast, lung, skin, GI melanoma, prostate	Creamy yellow-white choroidal lesions	Radiation, treat primary

Table continued on opposite page

TABLE 52-1 *Continued*

Disease	History	Fundus Appearance	Treatment
Autoimmune/Idiopathic			
Sarcoidosis	Young, African-American, older white women	Inferior punched-out lesions, vitritis, perivascular sheathing	Corticosteroids
AMPPPE	Young patients	Irregular posterior pole lesions at level of RPE, mild vitritis	None
Serpiginous choroidopathy	Middle-aged women usually	Confluent RPE and inner choroid lesions in jigsaw pattern, radiating out from optic nerve	Corticosteroids
Birdshot choroidopathy	Women, middle aged to older	Hypopigmented lesions swirling outward from optic nerve	Corticosteroids, cyclosporine
MEWDS	Young women	Faint white lesions at the level of the RPE	None

ARN, acute retinal necrosis; HSV, herpes simplex virus; HZV, herpes zoster virus; AIDS, acquired immunodeficiency syndrome; CMV, cytomegalovirus; PORN, progressive outer retinal necrosis; INH, isoniazid; CNV, choroidal neovascularization; DUSN, diffuse unilateral subacute neuroretinitis; AMPPPE, acute multifocal posterior placoid pigment epitheliopathy; RPE, retinal pigment epithelium; MEWDS, multiple evanescent white dot syndrome.

rods may be more severely affected than cones. If the chorioretinal inflammation affects rods more severely, this may explain the large blind spots.

ELECTRORETINOGRAPHY. The degree of abnormality on ERG depends upon the severity of the disease. Dreyer and Gass's study[2] reported a normal or borderline ERG in 16 eyes, a moderately abnormal ERG in five eyes, and a severely reduced ERG in six eyes. We performed electroretinography on ten patients at various points in the course of their disease.[7] Two patients with 20 or fewer lesions per eye had normal ERGs. Five patients with 21 to 50 lesions had rod dysfunction with prolonged cone b-wave implicit times and poor oscillatory potentials. Three patients with greater than 50 lesions had severely affected rod and cone function with very poor oscillatory potentials.

Clinical Course and Treatment

Multifocal choroiditis is bilateral in at least two thirds of patients and recurrences may occur in one or both eyes, singly or simultaneously. Eighty-six per cent of patients (18 of 21) followed 1 year or more demonstrated recurrent inflammation with new symptoms.[7] With recurrences, chorioretinal scars swell with surrounding subretinal fluid. The areas of atrophy may then enlarge, coalesce, and become more pigmented. Angiographically, the

borders of the acute lesions hyperfluoresce and the centers stain gradually and leak late. Old scars appear as window defects with late fading. Pinpoint areas of hyperfluorescence on the initial angiogram, which are not identifiable on clinical examination, may later become recognizable scars during recurrences. Careful correlation with the initial angiogram and fundus photographs demonstrates that in nearly every case, no new lesions occur during these recurrences (Fig. 52–3).

By far, most of the severe visual loss occurs due to CNV, which is found in 32 to 46% of patients.[2,3,8] In our series, 22 of 68 eyes (19 of 41 patients) developed CNV. Often, these were small areas of CNV and in nine patients, the foci of CNV regressed, leaving atrophy or minimal fibrosis. In several patients the CNV appeared to be anterior to the RPE and was partially fed by retinal vessels. In most patients, the CNV evolved from an old choroidal lesion. In several patients, fluorescein angiography revealed a thick hypofluorescent rim, probably due to hyperplastic RPE, completely surrounding the area of neovascularization (Fig. 52–4). Four patients developed multiple areas of CNV including one patient who demonstrated eight separate foci, five of which were within 4 disc areas of the fovea. Four of these five areas of CNV regressed over time. Smaller areas of CNV (<100 μm) were more likely to spontaneously regress than larger CNV (>200 μm).

The pattern of proliferating RPE cells associated with involution with CNV has been previously ob-

TABLE 52–2 Features of Patients with MCP, PIC, and DSF*

Disease	Patients	Mean Age (Years)	Women/Men	Bilateral Disease (No. of Patients)	Mean Follow-up	Mean Final Visual Acuity	EBS	CNV (No. of Patients)	CNV (No. of Eyes)
MCP	41	36	32/9	27	39 months	20/50	47% (24/51)	19/41	22/68 eyes
PIC	16	30	15/1	14	51 months	20/39	41% (9/22)	9/16	12/30 eyes
DSF	5	27	5/0	5	59 months	20/233	20% (2/10)	0/5	0 eyes

* Adapted from Reddy CV, Brown J, Folk JC, et al: Enlargement of the blindspot in chorioretinal inflammatory diseases. Ophthalmology 103:606–616, 1996; and Brown J, Reddy CV, Kimura AE, Folk JC: Long term visual prognosis of multifocal choroiditis, punctate inner choroidopathy and the diffuse subretinal fibrosis syndrome. Ophthalmology 103:1100–1105, 1996, with permission.

MCP, multifocal choroiditis and panuveitis; PIC, punctate inner choroidopathy; DSF, diffuse subretinal fibrosis syndrome; CNV, choroidal neovascularization; EBS, enlarged blind spot on perimetry.

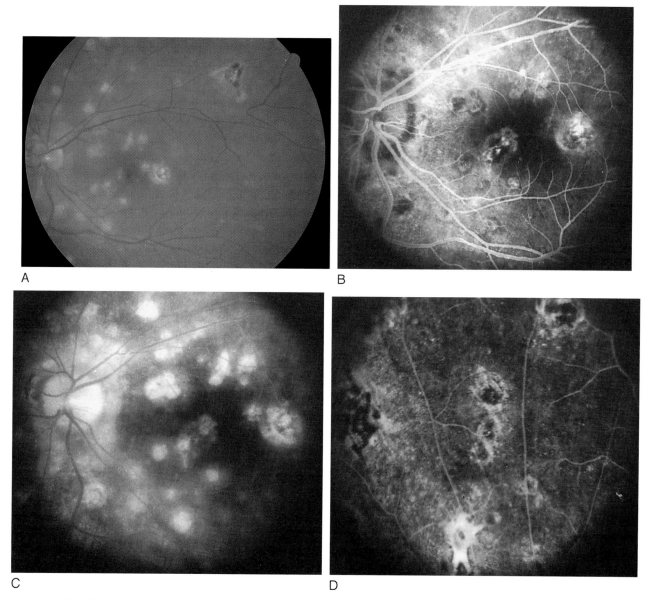

FIGURE 52–2   *A,* Young woman with multifocal choroiditis and a 1-year history of severe visual loss in the left eye. *B,* Early angiogram shows that some of the lesions posteriorly appear to have choroidal neovascularization. *C,* Late in the angiogram other lesions (especially inferior temporal to the disc) are leaking, presumably due to inflammation. *D,* Midphase angiogram superior to the optic nerve head shows larger chorioretinal scars. Notice that the retinal pigment epithelium between the more apparent scars also is abnormal and probably damaged from inflammation. *Illustration continued on following page*

served in a model of experimental choroidal neovascularization.[16] In this model, as the RPE proliferation progressed, subretinal fluid decreased and eventually the neovascularization became inactive as the vessels became enveloped with RPE cells. Inhibitors of neovascularization released by RPE cells may play a role in the regression of CNV.[17]

Steroids and MCP

Corticosteroids do have a role in controlling the inflammation and visual loss in MCP. Morgan and Schatz reported a marked improvement in visual acuity following use of steroids in nine patients.

They also reported one patient who had regression of CNV while on corticosteroids and one patient in which the CNV remained self-limited, yielding a final visual acuity of 20/70. Our group reported on the use of oral and/or subtenon corticosteroids in 17 patients (28 eyes).[8] Sixteen of the 28 eyes (12 patients) had a definite improvement in visual acuity or decreased vitritis concurrent with the use of steroids (Table 52–3). Despite this, 11 of the 28 eyes had a final visual acuity of 20/200 or worse. Of the 15 eyes that improved, 4 eyes (three patients) had CME.

Eight of 11 eyes with visual acuity poorer than 20/200 despite corticosteroid treatment had CNV;

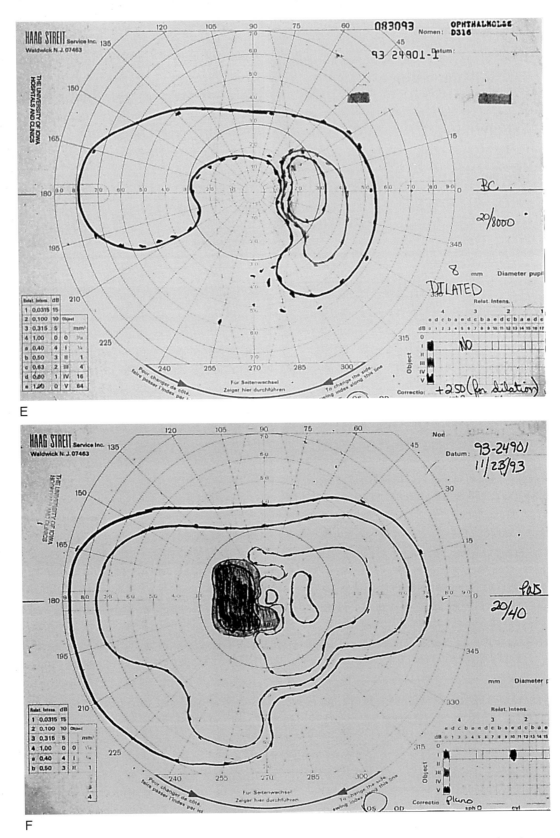

FIGURE 52–2 *Continued* *E*, Severe temporal and inferior visual defect on presentation. Visual acuity was count fingers at 2 feet. *F*, After 3 months of a tapering oral prednisone dose, the visual field has improved and the visual acuity is now 20/40.

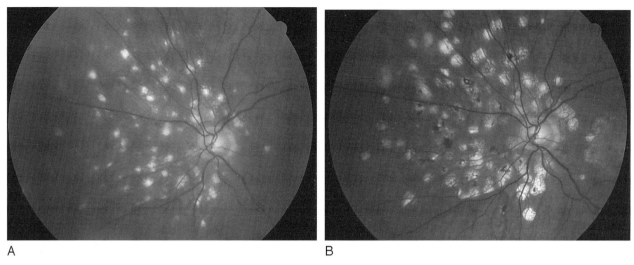

FIGURE 52–3   *A*, Patient with multifocal choroiditis showing nasal preponderance of lesions. *B*, After 4 years of follow-up, the lesions have enlarged and become atrophic, but no new lesions have developed.

however, only five of these eyes (five patients) were on steroids while the CNV was active. In two of these eyes, the CNV was concurrent with active inflammation and regressed as the inflammation regressed during steroid treatment. One of these eyes had recurrence of active CNV once the steroids were stopped. In three of the five eyes, steroids did not improve areas of CNV greater than 200 μm.

Overall, small areas of CNV associated with inflammation were slowed or stopped on steroids. A pigmented ring surrounding the neovascularization membrane was seen both in two patients treated with steroids and in one patient who was not.

Four patients with CME (six eyes) were treated with oral and subtenon corticosteroids. Four of the six eyes had improvement in visual acuity with steroid treatment. Three eyes had a final visual acuity of 20/200 or poorer.

Treatment of MCP with corticosteroids is similar to that used for other forms of uveitis. A high initial dose of prednisone (60 to 80 mg) is followed by a slow taper based on the clinical response. Recurrences during the taper may be supplemented with periocular steroids.

Laser Photocoagulation

Extrafoveal and juxtafoveal CNV regressed nicely with laser photocoagulation in four of four treated eyes (four patients), although late expansion of the laser scar caused visual loss in one of the four.

Visual Prognosis

After a mean follow-up of 39 months, 45 of 68 eyes (66%) had 20/40 or better vision. Thirty-nine of the 41 patients had at least one eye with 20/40 vision. Fourteen of 68 eyes in 12 patients had 20/200 or poorer final visual acuity.[8] Nine of these 14 eyes

had CNV involving the fovea and 3 had cystoid macular edema (Table 52–4). Patients with poor visual outcome were more likely to have bilateral disease and had an average of 36 scars in the macula. All other patients had an average of nine macular lesions.

PUNCTATE INNER CHOROIDOPATHY

Watzke and co-workers described ten healthy myopic women who presented with visual symptoms and yellow lesions in the inner choroid that evolved into pigmented scars.[4] Reddy and colleagues also reported on the clinical features of a series of 16 patients.[7] The long-term visual prognosis of this group was subsequently reported by Brown and co-workers.[8]

Clinical Features

PATIENT CHARACTERISTICS. Patients with PIC are usually young healthy women. These patients report blurred vision, photopsias, and central or paracentral scotomata on presentation. The average refractive error in Watzke's series was −6.50 diopters[4] and −3.67 diopters in our series.[7] There is no history of antecedent illness. Initial visual acuity is usually good, with an average of 20/40[7] (Table 52–2). Decreased visual acuity may be due to choroidal neovascularization or a clustering of lesions under the fovea causing a serous detachment of the retina.

Clinical Signs

ANTERIOR SEGMENT. There is no anterior segment inflammation.

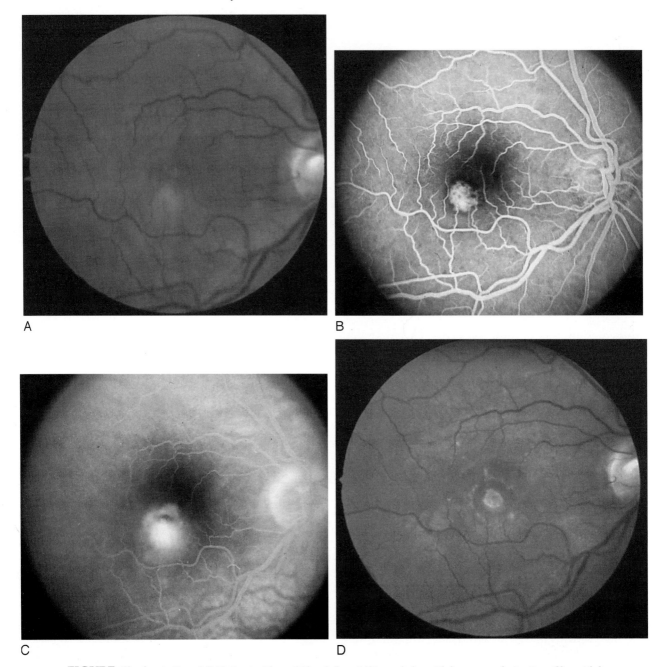

A

B

C

D

FIGURE 52–4   *A, B,* and *C,* Patient with multifocal choroiditis and choroidal neovascularization. Choroidal neovascularization is not surrounded by a hypofluorescent rim and leaks profusely late in the angiogram. *D, E,* and *F,* Just 2 weeks later choroidal neovascularization is now surrounded by prominent hyperpigmented rim that is hypofluorescent on angiography. The neovascular membrane no longer leaks. *Illustration continued on opposite page*

POSTERIOR SEGMENT. The acute lesions tend to be yellow and located at the level of the inner choroid. The lesions range from 50 to 300 μm in diameter, slightly smaller than those found in MCP. There may be overlying subretinal fluid, which is usually minimal (Fig. 52–5). The number of lesions may range from 2 to 6 spots to more than 50. Compared to MCP, more of the lesions are in the posterior pole and fewer in the midperiphery. Five of 30 eyes, however, had a predominance of lesions nasal to the optic nerve head, as often seen in MCP. There

is no vitreous inflammation. Only one patient had recurrent inflammation around the scars.

On fluorescein angiography, the acute lesions are hypofluorescent early and stain late in the study. Old scars appear as transmission defects.

PERIMETRY. Twenty of 30 affected eyes underwent visual field testing using the Goldmann perimeter. Enlargement of the blind spot was found in 41% of eyes, whereas 36% had full fields. Three eyes had central or paracentral scotomata. As in MCP, the

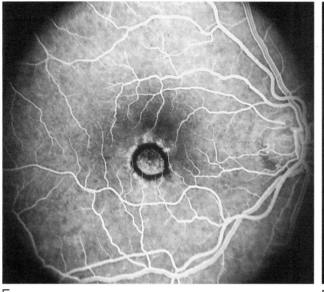
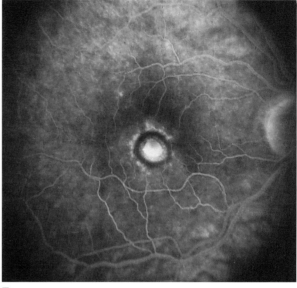

E

F

FIGURE 52–4   *Continued*

enlargement of the blind spot appeared out of pro-portion to the number of lesions visible in the fundus.

ELECTRORETINOGRAPHY. Full-field ERG was within the normal range in seven tested eyes. Three eyes demonstrated asymmetry of the b-wave ampli-tudes, which correlated with a difference in the number of lesions between the eyes.

TABLE 52–3   Use of Corticosteroids*

Disease	Corticosteroid Use	Improvement in Acuity or Decreased Inflammation
MCP	17 patients/28 eyes	11 patients/16 eyes
PIC	5 patients/6 eyes	3 patients/3 eyes
DSF†	5 patients/10 eyes	4 patients/7 eyes

* From Brown J, Reddy CV, Kimura AE, Folk JC: Long term visual prognosis of multifocal choroiditis, punctate inner choroidopathy and the diffuse subretinal fibrosis syndrome. Ophthalmology 103: 1100–1105, 1996, with permission.

† One patient with DSF was treated with cyclosporine and corticosteroid, and one patient was treated with corticosteroid, cyclosporine, and azathiaprine.

MCP, multifocal choroiditis and panuveitis; PIC, punctate inner choroidopathy; DSF, diffuse subretinal fibrosis syndrome.

Clinical Course and Treatment

Most patients with PIC have an excellent visual prognosis. Over a mean follow-up of 51 months, 23 of 30 eyes (77%) retained 20/40 or better visual acu-ity and 6 of 30 eyes (in five patients) had 20/200 or poorer vision.[8] The cause for visual acuity poorer than 20/200 in four of six eyes was CNV.

The acute lesions develop into pale yellow scars over several weeks. The pale yellow lesions de-velop into pigmented scars with atrophy of the ret-ina, choriocapillaris, and choroid over months. The lesions tend to be approximately 500 μm in diam-eter. Cystoid macular edema has not been seen in these patients.

Twelve (nine patients) of 30 eyes (40%) in our study[8] and 5 of 18 eyes (27%) in Watzke's series[4] developed CNV around scars during the follow-up period. In six of our patients, the CNV spontane-ously regressed, leaving the patients with good vi-sion. A hypofluorescent rim surrounding the CNV, perhaps due to hyperplastic RPE, was found on fundus fluorescein angiogram (FFA) in two eyes. The onset of CNV occurred variably throughout the follow-up period; however, most occurred within 1 year of presentation. As in MCP, smaller areas of neovascularization (<100 μm in diameter) were more likely to regress spontaneously than larger ar-eas of neovascularization (>200 μm). One patient had severe visual loss from subfoveal lesions caus-ing atrophy without evident CNV.

Steroids and PIC

Five patients (six eyes) followed in our study were treated with oral or subtenon corticosteroids.[8] Three of the six eyes had a definite improvement in visual

TABLE 52–4 Causes of Visual Acuity Poorer than 20/200 (No. of Eyes/No. of Patients)*

Disease	CNV	CME	Fibrosis/ Scar	RPE Atrophy	Total Eyes/ Total Patients
MCP	11/11	5/4	0	0	68/41
PIC	4/4	0	1/1	1/1	30/16
DSF	0	0	7/5	0	10/5

* From Brown J, Reddy CV, Kimura AE, Folk JC: Long term visual prognosis of multifocal choroiditis, punctate inner choroidopathy and the diffuse subretinal fibrosis syndrome. Ophthalmology 103:1100–1105, 1996, with permission.

CNV, choroidal neovascularization; CME, cystoid macular edema; RPE, retinal pigmented epithelium; MCP, multifocal choroiditis and panuveitis; PIC, punctate inner choroidopathy; DSF, diffuse subretinal fibrosis syndrome.

acuity with the use of steroids (Table 52–3). Two eyes (one patient) were 20/200 or worse due to RPE atrophy and fibrosis. Four of 12 eyes with CNV were treated with steroids. CNV regressed in one eye and persisted in three eyes while on steroids. The CNV was surrounded by a pigmented ring in the one eye in which the CNV regressed. CNV surrounded by a pigmented ring regressed in one patient who was not treated with steroids.

Laser Photocoagulation and Subfoveal Surgery

In our study, two patients with CNV that persisted while on corticosteroids and one patient who was not treated with steroids underwent surgical removal of subfoveal CNV[8] (Fig. 52–6). Each patient had an improvement in visual acuity. Each eye had a final visual acuity of 20/50 or better. Two additional patients had laser photocoagulation of extrafoveal CNV which prevented further visual loss. Each of the photocoagulated eyes has 20/40 or better vision (Table 52–5).

DIFFUSE SUBRETINAL FIBROSIS SYNDROME

In 1982, Doran and Hamilton[9] described four patients who developed subretinal fibrosis following CNV. Palestine and co-workers[5] and later Cantrill and Folk[6] described two series of patients who developed subretinal fibrosis without preceding CNV. Reddy and co-workers reported on the clinical findings in ten eyes.[7]

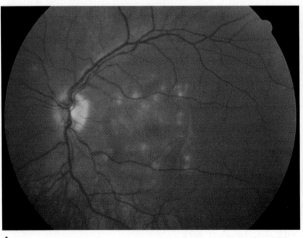
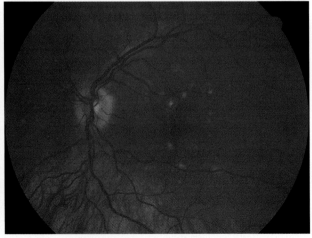

A   B

FIGURE 52–5 *A*, Patient with punctate inner choroidopathy who presented with a serous retinal detachment over a large number of lesions in the posterior pole. *B*, Just four weeks later serous fluid has resolved leaving small punctate scars and a visual acuity of 20/15.

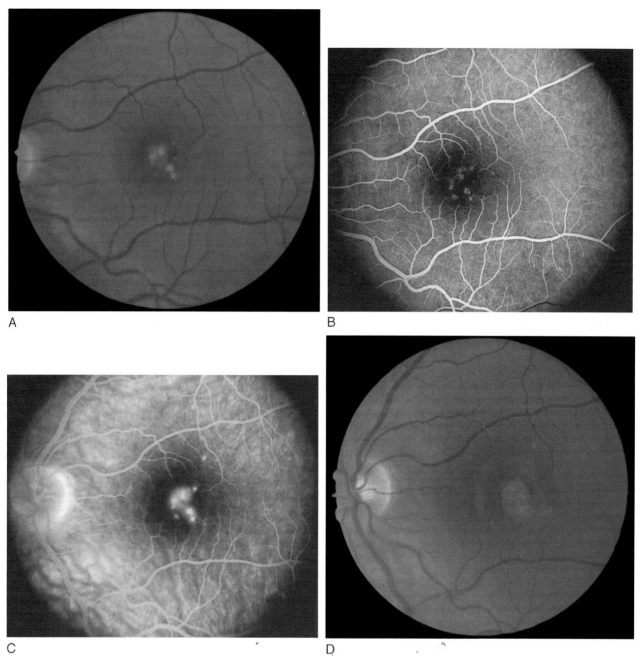

FIGURE 52–6 *A,* Patient with punctate inner choroidopathy and lesions posteriorly. *B* and *C,* Small areas of choroidal neovascularization are present within and around three of the lesions in the fovea. *D* and *E,* Four weeks later choroidal neovascularization has enlarged, resulting in 20/400 vision. *F,* Fundus photograph taken 1 year after subretinal surgery to remove choroidal neovascularization. The patient's vision returned to 20/20. *Illustration continued on following page*

Clinical Features

PATIENT CHARACTERISTICS. All of the patients with the diffuse subretinal fibrosis syndrome (DSF) have been young healthy women with no history of antecedent illness. The ages have ranged from 7 to 58 (Table 52–2). All patients complain of blurred vision or scotomata. In addition some patients report photopsias or floaters. The average refractive error was −1.25 diopters in our study with a range of −7.00 to plano.[7]

Clinical Signs

ANTERIOR SEGMENT. There may be trace to 1+ anterior chamber cell and flare.

POSTERIOR SEGMENT. Many small (100- to 200-μm) lesions are scattered throughout the posterior pole. There is usually a mild vitritis. Over days to weeks, turbid, yellow subretinal fluid may develop. The disease may begin unilaterally or bilaterally, but becomes bilateral in all patients. The lesions are pri-

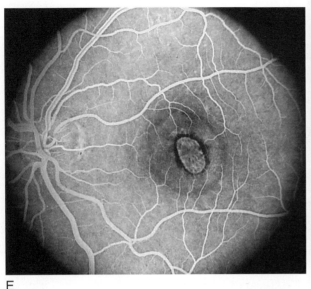

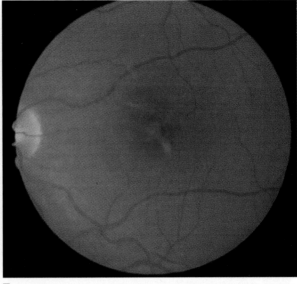

E   F

FIGURE 52–6   *Continued*

marily in the posterior pole. Average initial visual acuity is 20/300.[7]

Fluorescein angiography reveals a diffuse pattern of hyperfluorescence and leakage without a visible network of choroidal neovascular vessels.

PERIMETRY. In our series, 50% of eyes (five of ten) had either central or cecocentral scotomas. Twenty per cent of eyes (two of ten) had enlargement of the blind spot. Field defects correlated with active lesions or scarring.

ELECTRORETINOGRAPHY. Two patients were studied. Both patients had normal full-field ERGs, although asymmetry was present between the eyes

in one patient. This is in contrast with MCP, which has more diffuse damage and a markedly abnormal ERG in cases with severe disease.

Clinical Course and Treatment

Once the yellow lesions coalesce or subretinal fluid is present, white subretinal fibrosis develops soon after. Usually the fibrosis is severe, with broad bands of subretinal tissue and severe visual loss. Recurrences are universal. With each ensuing bout of inflammation, the fibrosis becomes more dense, involving more of the fundus until the disease becomes inactive with severe scarring and visual loss. Ten eyes with a mean follow-up of 59 months demonstrated an average visual acuity of 20/233 (Table 52–2).

Immunosuppressives and DSF

Oral prednisone has a role in controlling inflammation and aiding in the resolution of subretinal fluid (Table 52–3). In our series, five patients were treated with immunosuppressive agents. High-dose oral prednisone alone was successful in two patients who have required lower doses chronically to control their inflammation. Cyclosporine was added and was successful in controlling the inflammation in a third patient who was not controlled with prednisone alone. A fourth patient who did not have visual improvement with prednisone, already had visual loss from severe scarring, which may explain the lack of a response. The final patient has required oral prednisone, cyclosporine, azathioprine, and occasional superior subtenon corticosteroid injections to control inflammation in her re-

TABLE 52–5   Treatment of MCP, PIC, and DSF

Vitritis, CME	Corticosteroids
Extrafoveal CNV > 200 μm	Laser photocoagulation, corticosteroids, observation
Juxtafoveal CNV < 200 μm	Unclear, observation, steroids, laser
Subfoveal CNV	Observation, consider subretinal removal if VA < 20/80 or if lesion enlarging
Subretinal fibrosis syndrome	Corticosteroids, cyclosporine, azathioprine to preserve vision usually in second eye

MCP, multifocal choroiditis and panuveitis; PIC, punctate inner choroidopathy; DSF, diffuse subretinal fibrosis syndrome; CME, cystoidmacular edema; CNV, choroidal neovascularization; VA, visual acuity.

maining eye. Her visual acuity remains 20/20 after cataract extraction. The use of immunosuppressant medications seems to have preserved vision in the second eye (Fig. 52–7). In each patient, the eye that was affected first had the poorer visual acuity.

In DSF, aggressive corticosteroid and other immunosuppressives as needed should be given if one eye has visual loss from scarring and the other eye develops lesions in the posterior pole. Similarly, large yellow mounds beneath the macula is a sign of a poor prognosis and impending fibrosis. Immunosuppression should be tried but may be too late in these patients. Finally, if a patient presents with numerous yellow nodules in the first eye, immediate high-dose oral corticosteroids should be considered. It is true that many of these patients (who probably have PIC) will do very well with little scarring and retain good vision. It is impossible to tell very early in the course of the disease, however, which patients will do well and which will develop severe scarring (at which time immunosuppression will be too late). A short course of prednisone should not harm those patients who would have done well anyway. It may be vision saving, however, in those patients who have the diffuse subretinal fibrosis syndrome. It will become evident quickly which course the patient is taking. The patients who do well develop sharply demarcated atrophic scars (Fig. 52–5). The DSF patient will have recurrent inflammation and swelling around the nodules with yellowish fluid. Review of the literature as well as our experience demonstrate that prednisone frequently is inadequate. Cyclosporine should be added if oral prednisone does not work or controls the inflammation only at high doses. Cyclosporine is useful in lowering the required dose of prednisone needed to control the inflammation.

ETIOLOGY

The etiologies of these syndromes are unknown. Most patients with MCP have negative histoplasmin skin tests. HLA-DR2 has been associated with OHS (76%) but was not seen in patients with MCP (0%).[18] Tiedeman reported an association with Epstein-Barr virus[19]; however, this was not confirmed in another study by Spaide and co-workers.[20] Specific antibodies to herpes viruses were found in aqueous and serum samples in seven patients.[21] It is likely that the lesions of multifocal choroiditis are an immunologically mediated response following exposure to some pathogen. Since new lesions are not seen during recurrences, these events probably are autoimmune-mediated responses to the same antigen or to altered tissue from the original infection. Further work to elucidate the etiology of MCP is needed to define this syndrome more clearly.

The etiology of PIC is unknown. The enlargement of the blind spot suggests that there is more widespread involvement of the retina and choroid than is evident on exam. The positive scotomas and enlargement of the blind spot make it unlikely that this is simply a variant of myopic degeneration. However, the thinning of the retina and choroid in myopes may make more apparent (by causing areas of atrophy) the effects of an inflammatory stimulus that would be subclinical in nonmyopes.

No association with systemic disease has been found for DSF. Histopathology of the diffuse subretinal fibrosis syndrome has been described by Palestine and co-workers.[22] The specimen was a chorioretinal biopsy from a patient in the active phase of the disease. The lesions consisted of choroidal inflammation with predominantly B lymphocytes. Islands of hyperplastic RPE cells were present within zones of fibrosis. Immunohistochemistry studies identified IgG, complement, and fibrin. There was no evidence of antiretinal antibodies. The findings suggested an autoimmune antibody–mediated inflammatory process leading to fibrosis.

DIFFERENT DISEASES/ DIFFERENT HOST RESPONSES

Whether or not each syndrome represents a different disease remains controversial. The syndromes may represent a spectrum of one disease because they all affect primarily young healthy women and manifest with yellow subretinal lesions that lead to scarring.

It is sensible to separate the diseases if doing so provides a more accurate prognosis for our patients, assists their management, or elucidates the pathogenesis of the disease. Those who feel that the conditions should be studied separately point to the different findings and courses of the conditions. Electroretinography demonstrates that MCP is a diffuse disease. Despite the fact that patients with DSF have more severe scarring and poorer prognosis, their inflammation is limited to the posterior pole, which is reflected by normal full-field ERGs. The enlarged blind spots with relatively few apparent scars as seen in MCP are unusual in DSF. Furthermore, despite the fact that the lesions look similar early, patients with DSF have severe subretinal fibrosis, whereas patients with PIC have resolution of their disease without fibrosis.

The host response to the initial inciting pathogen may also play a role. It is interesting that some patients with many lesions in the posterior pole never develop CNV, recurrent inflammation, or significant visual loss, whereas others even with perhaps fewer lesions do suffer severe scarring and visual loss. The differences in clinical courses suggest that the propensity to develop neovascularization or scarring may be related to certain host factors. For example, in the ocular histoplasmosis syndrome, patients with HLA-B7 and HLA-DRw2 have a higher

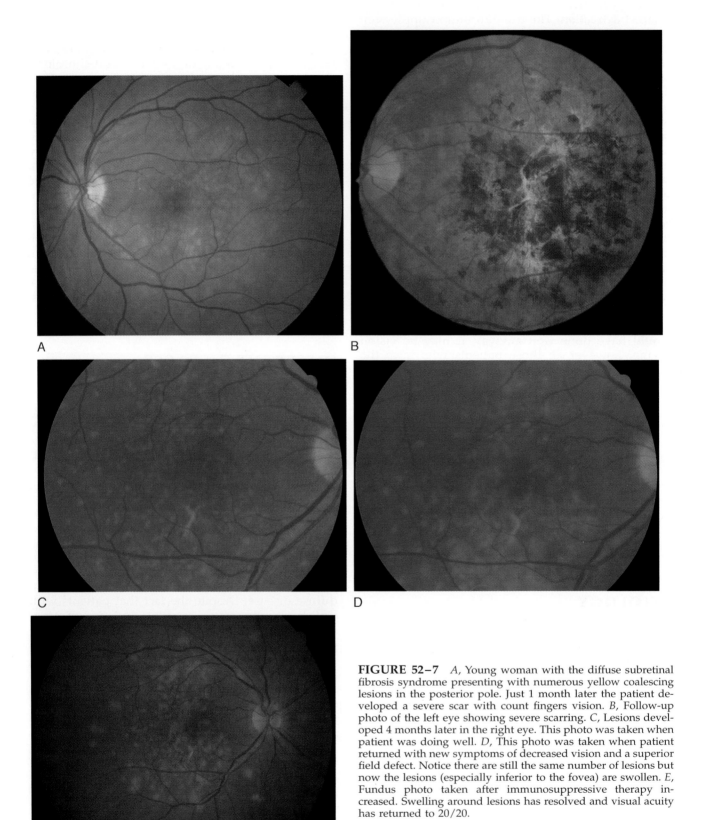

FIGURE 52–7 *A*, Young woman with the diffuse subretinal fibrosis syndrome presenting with numerous yellow coalescing lesions in the posterior pole. Just 1 month later the patient developed a severe scar with count fingers vision. *B*, Follow-up photo of the left eye showing severe scarring. *C*, Lesions developed 4 months later in the right eye. This photo was taken when patient was doing well. *D*, This photo was taken when patient returned with new symptoms of decreased vision and a superior field defect. Notice there are still the same number of lesions but now the lesions (especially inferior to the fovea) are swollen. *E*, Fundus photo taken after immunosuppressive therapy increased. Swelling around lesions has resolved and visual acuity has returned to 20/20.

frequency of disciform scars than those who do not express these histocompatibility antigens.[23-26]

Recurrent inflammation surrounding old scars has also been seen in experimental choroiditis. In the experimental histoplasmic choroiditis model developed by Smith and colleagues, it was found that choroiditis lesions may have lymphocyte infiltrates surrounding scars as long as 10 years following the initial infection.[27-28] In this model, these lesions could be reactivated with antigenic challenge.[29] The lesions of MCP and DSF may be similar in that a primary exposure or infection by one antigen leads to the initial wave of choroiditis lesions. Future reactivations of the lesions may be stimulated by exposures to other cross-reacting antigens or other inflammatory stimuli that affect the altered tissue.

It is reasonable to suspect that the development of progressive choroidal neovascularization or recurrent inflammation causing visual loss in MCP and PIC is related to specific HLA types or other host factors.

SUMMARY

1. Before considering MCP, PIC, or DSF, be sure to rule out potentially more dangerous or treatable causes of multifocal choroidal lesions. Beware of lymphoma in the elderly patient with vitritis and choroidal infiltrates. Investigate possible predisposing factors for a disseminated infection. Do not miss viral retinitis, because it has a poor prognosis if treatment is delayed.

2. Patients with small, punched-out multifocal lesions in the inferior periphery should be evaluated for sarcoidosis. Noncaseating granulomas may be found on conjunctival biopsy.

3. MCP, PIC, and DSF are inflammatory chorioretinal diseases affecting young myopic women, characterized by acute lesions that evolve into round pigmented scars. Patients present with blurred vision, photopsias, or scotomas.

4. Although the visual prognosis is good in most patients with MCP and PIC, nearly half of our patients with MCP (19 of 41) and 9 of 30 of our patients with PIC developed CNV at some time in the course of their disease (Table 52–3). Significant visual loss in PIC and MCP is most often due to CNV (Table 52–4).

5. Patients with MCP may have anterior chamber cell in addition to vitreous inflammation. Recurrent inflammation causes swelling around old lesions and leads to enlarged, coalesced, pigmented, chorioretinal scars.

6. Patients with PIC have smaller lesions, mostly in the posterior pole, with no vitreous inflammation. These patients rarely have recurrence of inflammation around the old scars.

7. Some areas of neovascularization are surrounded by thick hypofluorescent rings on FFA that may represent hyperplastic or proliferating RPE. Many, but not all, of these areas of CNV will regress without treatment.

8. CNV in MCP and PIC may resolve, especially if smaller than 100 μm in diameter. We have not found corticosteroids to significantly induce regression of CNV unless the CNV is small and associated with inflammation. Small areas of neovascularization can be observed or treated with laser photocoagulation if extrafoveal or juxtafoveal. Neovascularization greater than 200 μm in diameter usually does not resolve without treatment and laser photocoagulation should be performed unless the CNV is subfoveal. Subfoveal neovascularization should be observed. If the visual acuity drops or remains poor, then the CNV can be removed surgically and appears to have a good result in these patients (Table 52–5).

9. Corticosteroids may help control vitreous inflammation and cystoid macular edema in some patients with MCP. Attempt to taper the steroids as the inflammation comes under control. If you are not convinced that the steroids are having a beneficial effect, discontinue them or add cyclosporine in severe cases. Steroids are unnecessary in PIC (Table 52–5).

10. In DSF, aggressive corticosteroid and other immunosuppressive treatments should be given if one eye has visual loss from scarring and the other eye develops lesions in the posterior pole. Large yellow mounds beneath the macula are a sign of a poor prognosis and impending fibrosis. Often cyclosporine may be necessary if tapering prednisone results in recurrences or if the patient develops intolerable side effects. Any hope of preserving vision requires prompt use of immunosuppressives with close follow-up (Table 52–5).

REFERENCES

1. Nozik RA, Dorsch W: A new chorioretinopathy associated with anterior uveitis. Am J Ophthalmol 76:758–762, 1973.
2. Dreyer RF, Gass DJ: Multifocal choroiditis and panuveitis. A syndrome that mimics ocular histoplasmosis. Arch Ophthalmol 102:1776–1784, 1984.
3. Morgan CM, Schatz H: Recurrent multifocal choroiditis. Ophthalmology 93:1138–1147, 1986.
4. Watzke RC, Packer AJ, Folk JC, et al: Punctate inner choroidopathy. Am J Ophthalmol 98:572–584, 1984.
5. Palestine AG, Nussenblatt RB, Parver LM, Knox DL: Progressive subretinal fibrosis and uveitis. Br J Ophthalmol 68:667–673, 1984.
6. Cantrill HL, Folk JC: Multifocal choroiditis associated with

progressive subretinal fibrosis. Am J Ophthalmol 101:170–180, 1986.

7. Reddy CV, Brown J, Folk JC, et al: Enlargement of the blindspot in chorioretinal inflammatory diseases. Ophthalmology 103:606–617, 1996.

8. Brown J, Reddy CV, Kimura AE, Folk JC: Long term visual prognosis of multifocal choroiditis, punctate inner choroidopathy and the diffuse subretinal fibrosis syndrome. Ophthalmology 103:1100–1105, 1996.

9. Doran RML, Hamilton AM: Disciform macular degeneration in young adults. Trans Ophthalmol Soc UK 101:471–480, 1982.

10. Spaide RF, Yannuzzi LA, Freund KB: Linear streaks in multifocal choroiditis and panuveitis. Retina 11:229–231, 1991.

11. Hershey JM, Pulido JS, Folberg R, et al: Non-caseating conjunctival granulomas in patients with multifocal choroiditis and panuveitis. Ophthalmology 101:596–601, 1994.

12. Khorram KD, Jampol LM, Rosenberg MA: Blind spot enlargement as a manifestation of multifocal choroiditis. Arch Ophthalmol 109:1403–1407, 1991.

13. Hayreh SS: Segmental nature of the choroidal vasculature. Br J Ophthalmol 59:631–648, 1975.

14. Hayreh SS: The ophthalmic artery: III. Branches. Br J Ophthalmol 46:212–247, 1962.

15. Curcio DA, Sloan KR, Kalina RE, Hendrickson AE: Human photoreceptor topography. J Comp Neurol 292:497–523, 1990.

16. Miller H, Miller B, Ryan SJ: The role of retinal pigment epithelium in the involution of subretinal neovascularization. Invest Ophthalmol Vis Sci 27:1644–1652, 1986.

17. Glaser BM, Campochiaro PA, Davis JL, Jerdan JA: Retinal pigment epithelial cells release inhibitors of neovascularization. Ophthalmology 94:780–784, 1987.

18. Spaide RF, Skerry JE, Yannuzzi, DeRosa JT: Lack of HLA-DR2 specificity in multifocal choroiditis and panuveitis. Br J Ophthalmol 74:536–537, 1990.

19. Tiedeman JS: Epstein-Barr viral antibodies in multifocal choroiditis and panuveitis. Am J Ophthalmol 103:659–663, 1987.

20. Spaide RF, Sugin S, Yannuzzi LA, DeRosa JT: Epstein Barr virus antibodies in multifocal choroiditis and panuveitis. Am J Ophthalmol 112:410–413, 1991.

21. Frau E, Dussaix E, Offret H, Bloch-Michel E: The possible role of herpes simplex virus in multifocal choroiditis and panuveitis. Int Ophthalmol 14:365–369, 1990.

22. Palestine AG, Nussenblatt RB, Chan CC, et al: Histopathology of the subretinal fibrosis and uveitis syndrome. Ophthalmology 92:838–844, 1985.

23. Godfrey WA, Sabates R, Cross DE: Association of presumed ocular histoplasmosis with HLA-B-7. Am J Ophthalmol 85:854–858, 1978.

24. Braley RE, Meredith TA, Aaberg TM, et al: The prevalence of HLA-B7 in presumed ocular histoplasmosis. Am J Ophthalmol 85:859–861, 1978.

25. Meredith TA, Smith RE, Braley RE, et al: The prevalence of HLA-B7 in presumed ocular histoplasmosis in patients with peripheral atrophic scars. Am J Ophthalmol 86:325–328, 1978.

26. Meredith TA, Smith RE, Duquesnoy RJ: Association of HLA-DRw2 antigen with presumed ocular histoplasmosis. Am J Ophthalmol 89:70–76, 1980.

27. Anderson A, Clifford W, Palvolgyi I, et al: Immunopathology of chronic experimental histoplasmic choroiditis in the primate. Invest Ophthalmol Vis Sci 33:1637–1641, 1992.

28. Smith RE, Dunn S, Jester JV: Natural history of experimental histoplasmic choroiditis in the primate. II. Histopathologic features. Invest Ophthalmol Vis Sci 25:810–819, 1984.

29. Palvolgyi I, Anderson A, Rife L, et al: Immunopathology of reactivation of experimental ocular histoplasmosis. Exp Eye Res 57:169–175, 1993.

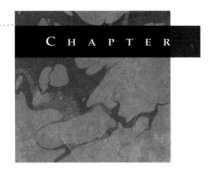

Subretinal Fibrosis and Uveitis Syndrome

Elena Mier-Trotter, M.D.

Robert B. Nussenblatt, M.D.

Subretinal fibrosis and uveitis syndrome is a distinct entity. However, its clinical features can in part be mimicked by other uveitic disorders. In this chapter we will present an overview of this unique entity, followed by a brief outline of the gamut of disorders that should be considered in the differential diagnosis.

The subretinal fibrosis and uveitis syndrome is a type of posterior uveitis characterized by fibrotic-appearing islands which coalesce, leading to the subsequent development of large swathes of subretinal fibrosis. A chronic intraocular inflammatory response is seen as well. However, no systemic or other specific ocular disorders are associated with these changes. This unusual type of uveitis appears to have been first described by Adalbert Fuchs in his 1949 Atlas of ocular fundus.[1] In it he described an "extremely rare" bilateral condition in which there were large areas of connective tissue formation under the retina and leading to a severe drop in visual acuity. In 1984 and 1985 Palestine and associates[2,3] first characterized these patients in the modern literature.

THE ENTITY: CLINICAL MANIFESTATIONS

Most of the patients to date have been young, healthy females between the ages of 12 and 28. The disease has been predominantly seen in African-Americans and has usually been bilateral in presentation.[2-4] However, the entity has been reported to occur in males (personal communication Belfort RJ, MD). The visual acuity (VA) at the time of disease presentation has ranged from 20/20 to counting fingers (CF), depending on whether there is initial macular involvement. The clinical course is variable and recurrences are common; the follow-up time in the literature is about 4 years. During that period of follow-up, all patients have had at least one eye severely handicapped because of the entity.

The ophthalmoscopic appearance of this entity is characterized by whitish yellow "fibrotic"-like subretinal lesions, which progress to form a large sheet of fibrotic looking material[2,4-6] (Fig. 53-1). The lesion can progress to encompass the whole posterior pole, with ultimate loss of vision. However, in some cases the progression may not continue and a steady state may be reached. In some cases the lesion may encircle but not encroach the macula, while in others, though the macula is not directly involved, cystoid macular edema (CME) may result with a subsequent drop in visual acuity.[6] Patients will have a moderate to severe vitreous inflammatory response with low to moderate anterior chamber response.

HISTOPATHOLOGIC AND IMMUNOHISTOPATHOLOGIC FEATURES

Palestine et al[2] and Kim and colleagues[4] evaluated immunohistochemically two eyes from patients with the subretinal fibrosis and uveitis syndrome (Fig. 53-2). These studies demonstrated a marked choroidal infiltrate with a predominance of B cells and plasma cells. CD4+ T cells were also present

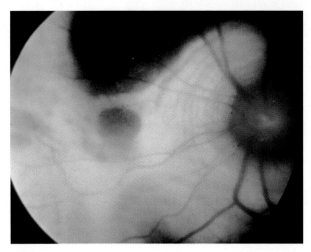

FIGURE 53–1 Extensive subretinal fibrosis involving disc and macular region.

in moderate numbers. One eye[4] showed, in addition, a localized granulomatous lymphocytic infiltrate in the choroid. Complement and IgG deposition were noted at the level of Bruch's membrane. Thick swathes of fibrotic tissue could be seen subretinally. Often this fibrotic tissue will contain islets of cells, mostly retinal pigment epithelium, but sometimes Müller cells.

Is there an explanation for these histologic changes? No evidence for an infection has been seen, and endogenous immunologic alterations are often intoned. The data for this remain sparse. One possible explanation could be that B-cell proliferation and scarring are both due to a shift in T-cell subsets infiltrating into the eye from a Th 1 response to a Th 2 profile. While Th 1 cells are characterized by their production of interferon gamma and interleukin-2 (IL-2), the Th 2 inducer cells have a lymphokine profile rich in interleukin-4 (IL-4), which could stimulate B cells, and transforming growth factor β (TGFβ), a lymphokine associated with scarring and fibrosis.

In addition, in experimentally induced uveoretinitis (EAU) in primates, Fujino and associates[7] observed that B cells were most prominent in the eyes of monkeys that developed subretinal fibrosis. They also conjectured that the expression of intercellular adhesion molecule-1 (ICAM-1) on ocular resident cells of the choroid and retina was necessary for the infiltration and accumulation of inflammatory cells (B cells). Further, Whitcup and colleagues[8] studied six enucleated eyes from patients with uveitis, one of them previously reported by Kim and associates.[4] They found ICAM-1 strongly expressed on the RPE, retinal and choroidal vascular endothelium, and on Müller cells in the retina. Cell adhesion molecules like ICAM-1 are expressed in eyes with posterior uveitis and may be regulated by cytokines such as tumor necrosis factor α (TNF-α).

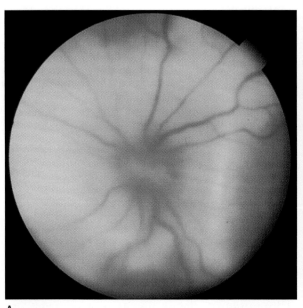

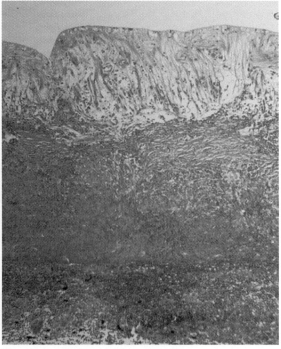

A   B

FIGURE 53–2 *A*, Subretinal fibrosis involving the optic disc of a patient who underwent a chorioretinal biopsy. *B*, Microphotography of the eye with subretinal fibrosis and uveitis syndrome. A thick layer of fibrosis-like tissue is present between the gliotic retina and the heavily inflamed choroid (hematoxylin and eosin, ×100). (Courtesy of Chi-Chao Chan, M.D.)

DIAGNOSTIC TESTS

Laboratory Tests

Laboratory testing does not appear to be contributory. Peripheral blood lymphocytes taken from patients with the subretinal fibrotic and uveitis syndrome showed no in vitro proliferative response to the retinal S antigen.[2]

Fluorescein Angiography

Fluorescein angiography will show predominantly subretinal alterations.[6] In the early phase of the angiogram, one may see multiple areas of blockage of choroidal fluorescence. In the later phase of the angiogram, hyperfluorescence, interpreted as late staining of the lesions without leakage, can be noted.[2]

Electrophysiologic Studies

Most studies report marked alterations in the electroretinogram (ERG), for both rods and cones.[2,3] In the majority of cases, the electro-oculogram (EOG) is markedly diminished as well.

DIFFERENTIAL DIAGNOSIS

For the clinician dealing with ocular inflammations, it is very important to rule out several conditions that could mimic the subretinal fibrosis and uveitis syndrome. The subretinal fibrosis and uveitis syndrome is believed to be unique both in its appearance and its clinical course[2] (Fig. 53–3). Initially, it may be difficult to make the diagnosis of subretinal fibrosis and uveitis syndrome, due to the small size of the patches of subretinal fibrosis. However, most of the lesions in other disorders show considerably more perturbation of the retinal pigment epithelium and rarely are as confluent, deep, and large as are the lesions seen in the subretinal fibrosis with uveitis syndrome. Furthermore, in this entity, there is no overlying detachment as a prerequisite to fibrosis development. These patients do not present with a multitude of "spots" all over the retina. They do not have systemic disease.

The natural course of subretinal fibrosis and uveitis, although not completely understood, may lead in many cases to severe visual handicap.[2-4] Additionally, in subretinal fibrosis and uveitis syndrome the patients did not develop serous or hemorrhagic detachments as in some patients having other syndromes.[9,10] Furthermore, none of the patients with this entity appear to have developed subretinal neovascular membranes.

As mentioned, we believe that the subretinal fi-

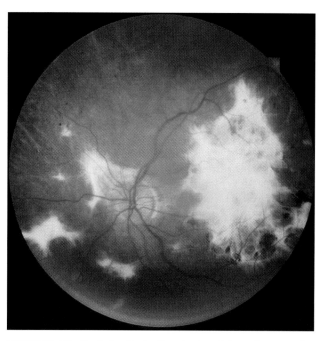

FIGURE 53–3 Subretinal fibrosis involving the macular region.

brosis and uveitis syndrome exists as a distinct entity, as do Cantrill and Folk.[6,9] However, several other uveitic disorders may manifest similar clinical features (Table 53–1). Subretinal fibrosis associated with an intraocular inflammatory response is frequently associated with the gamut of white dot syndromes. White dot syndromes are grouped

TABLE 53–1 Differential Diagnosis of Subretinal Fibrosis and Uveitis Syndrome

White Dot Syndromes
  Multifocal choroiditis associated with progressive subretinal fibrosis
  Multifocal choroiditis and panuveitis
  Punctate inner choroidopathy
  Acute multifocal posterior placoid pigment epitheliopathy
Infectious Conditions
  Tuberculosis
  Syphilis
  Toxoplasmosis
  Fungal infections
  Presumed ocular histoplasmosis syndrome
  Onchocerciasis
Other Conditions
  Sarcoidosis
  Serpiginous choroidopathy
  Birdshot retinochoroidopathy
  Acute retinal pigment epitheliitis
  Acute macular neuroretinopathy
  Sympathetic ophthalmia
  Vogt-Koyanagi-Harada syndrome

together because of their sometimes overlapping features, leading some authors to believe that they represent the broad clinical spectrum of one underlying entity.[6]

Many white dot syndromes may develop subretinal fibrotic changes at some point in their course. Watzke and colleagues[10] reported fibrotic changes in punctate inner choroidopathy, a disorder characterized by small (100 to 500 μm) yellow-white lesions of the inner choroid and pigment epithelium, often with an overlying serous detachment, which healed into atrophic scars, some of them with pigmented borders. Fifty per cent of patients with this disorder developed subretinal neovascular membranes. Cantrill and Folk[9] have reported the association of multifocal choroiditis with progressive subretinal fibrosis. They reported clusters of small (100 to 200 μm) hypopigmented choroidal lesions, some concentrated in the fovea, which healed with the formation of subretinal fibrosis. These lesions later coalesced and enlarged, forming placoid subretinal scars, some with pigmented borders. During the course of the disease, serous and hemorrhagic macular detachments developed in four eyes, with fluorescein angiographic features suggesting subretinal neovascularization. This same phenomenon has been reported recently by other investigators.[11,12]

Many additional ocular inflammatory conditions can develop subretinal fibrosis.[2,6,13] Among these are included infectious disorders such as tuberculosis, syphilis, toxoplasmosis, fungal infections, presumed ocular histoplasmosis syndrome, and onchocerciasis.[14] Many endogenous uveitides will present with white dots of variable sizes and configurations. They can also lead to the development of subretinal fibrosis.[15] Some of these entities include sarcoidosis, serpiginous choroidopathy, birdshot retinochoroidopathy, acute posterior multifocal placoid pigment epitheliopathy, acute retinal pigment epitheliitis, acute macular neuroretinopathy, sympathetic ophthalmia, and the Vogt-Koyanagi-Harada syndrome.[16]

TREATMENT

Therapy is problematic. For the entity of subretinal fibrosis and uveitis syndrome, systemic corticosteroid therapy does not seem to be a particularly effective long-term approach.[2,3,6] While corticosteroids appear to be able to reduce CME in the few patients with this problem, they seem to fail to arrest the course of the subretinal fibrosis. There are anecdotal reports suggesting that some cases have responded to therapy with azathioprine[5] and methotrexate.[7] However, poor results were obtained with cyclophosphamide.[4] Fortunately for some individuals, the progression of the disease can be very slow or stop altogether for unknown reasons. More patients need to be followed in order to have a better understanding of the natural course of this entity.

REFERENCES

1. Fuchs A: Diseases of the Fundus Oculi–Atlas. Philadelphia, The Blakiston Company, 1949, pp 153–156.
2. Palestine AG, Nussenblatt RB, Parver LM, Knox DL: Progressive subretinal fibrosis and uveitis. Br J Ophthalmol 68:667–673, 1984.
3. Palestine AG, Nussenblatt RB, Chan CC, et al: Histopathology of the subretinal fibrosis and uveitis syndrome. Ophthalmology 92:838–844, 1985.
4. Kim MK, Chan CC, Belfort R, et al: Histopathologic and immunohistopathologic features of subretinal fibrosis and uveitis syndrome. Am J Ophthalmol 104:15–23, 1987.
5. Nussenblatt RB: Autoimmune diseases. In Tabbara KF, Nussenblatt RB (eds): Posterior Uveitis, Diagnosis and Management. Massachussets, Butterworth-Heinemann, 1994, pp 99–101.
6. Nussenblatt RB: White-dot syndrome. In Nussenblatt RB, Whitcup SM, Palestine AG (eds): Uveitis. St. Louis, Mosby, 1995, pp 371–384.
7. Fujino Y, Li Q, Chung H, et al: Immunopathology of experimental autoimmune uveoretinitis in primates. Autoimmunity 13:303–309, 1992.
8. Whitcup SM, Chan CC, Li Q, Nussenblatt RB: Expression of cell adhesion molecules in posterior uveitis. Arch Ophthalmol 110:662–666, 1992.
9. Cantrill HL, Folk JC: Multifocal choroiditis associated with progressive subretinal fibrosis. Am J Ophthalmol 101:170–180, 1986.
10. Watzke RC, Packer AJ, Folk JC, et al: Punctate inner choroidopathy. Am J Ophthalmol 98:572–584, 1984.
11. Salvador F, Garcia-Arumi J, Mateo C, et al: Multifocal choroiditis with progressive subretinal fibrosis. Ophthalmologica 208:163–167, 1994.
12. Yamane I, Ishibashi T, Honda T, et al: Multifocal choroiditis associated with progresive subretinal fibrosis. Nippon Ganka Gakkai Zasshi 99:618–623, 1995.
13. Guyer DR, Gragoudas ES: Subretinal fibrosis and uveitis syndrome. In Principles and Practice of Ophthalmology (Retina and Vitreous). Philadelphia, WB Saunders Co, 1994, pp 973–977.
14. Newland HS, White AT, Greene BM, et al: Ocular manifestations of onchocerciasis in a rain forest area of West Africa. Br J Ophthalmol 75:163–169, 1991.
15. BenEzra D, Forrester JV: Fundal white dots: the spectrum of a similar pathological process. Br J Ophthalmol 79:856–860, 1995.
16. Liao HR, Juang C: Formation of pseudodiscs in chronic recurrent Vogt-Koyanagi-Harada syndrome. Can J Ophthalmol 24:280–282, 1989.

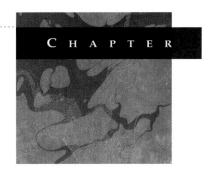

CHAPTER 54

Posterior Scleritis

Alice T. Lyon, M.D.
Lee M. Jampol, M.D.

Posterior scleritis, defined as scleral inflammation primarily posterior to the equator, is an uncommon manifestation of scleritis but is in the differential diagnosis of many more common posterior segment disorders.[1] Isolated posterior scleritis comprises 2 to 12% of all cases of scleritis.[2,3] Women make up the majority, up to 69%, of these patients.[4] Most present in middle age, but posterior scleritis has a wide age range of 8 to 87 years.[5] Posterior scleritis is frequently unilateral but manifests as bilateral disease in 10 to 33% of cases. Bilateral scleritis is most frequently seen in those with underlying systemic inflammatory diseases. In patients with isolated posterior scleritis, about 14 to 60% have an underlying systemic disease.[4,5] For patients with anterior scleritis, this figure is higher. As many as 48% of patients with scleritis have associated systemic vasculitic disease[6] and 33 to 48% have other associated systemic immune-mediated diseases.[1,2,6] Posterior scleritis is recurrent in as many as 43% of patients.[5]

SYMPTOMS

The most common symptoms are decreased vision, and pain and redness. In more severe or extensive cases, there can be additional symptoms resulting from the inflammation of adjoining tissues. These include anterior scleritis, diplopia, and proptosis. Typically, the patient notices decreased vision and is found to have macular involvement including an exudative retinal detachment. The pain is frequently severe and may be felt as orbital (retrobulbar) in quality. Deep, boring pain with periorbital fullness and brow ache are prominent in many patients. Occasionally, pain is absent or is a minor component. The degree of redness and pain present is highly variable, with the more anterior and more fulminant cases presenting with this as a major finding. It is not uncommon for the eye with posterior scleritis to appear white and quiet. In such cases, the diagnosis may be missed.[7]

CLINICAL FINDINGS

Most patients have reduced vision. Vision can range from normal to no light perception depending on the extent of involvement.[5] Often, the anterior segment is quiet. The eye may be exquisitely tender. There is frequently an associated iridocyclitis and there may be anterior scleritis. Sometimes the scleritis is primarily anterior, with a keratouveitis that involves the posterior segment.[6,8] If there is orbital involvement with spread of the inflammation, there can be proptosis, ptosis, periorbital edema, and restricted motility.[9,10] These are more common findings with idiopathic orbital inflammation (pseudotumor).[10]

Dramatic findings may be present on fundus examination. There may be associated vitreous cells in as many as 14 to 75% of cases.[4,11] If the sclera in the peripapillary region is involved or if there is extensive inflammation, the optic nerve may be elevated with an edematous nerve fiber layer. The retinal vessels are usually normal but can be dilated, tortuous, and occasionally focally occluded from vasculitis.[12] There is frequently a prominent exudative retinal detachment and retinal or choroidal folds (Figs. 54–1A through F). The subretinal fluid is usually clear but may be turbid (Figs. 54–1D and E). If the posterior scleritis involves a significant area of the posterior segment, there may be shifting fluid. A focal choroidal thickening, either a reddish or yellow mass, may be present. Ret-

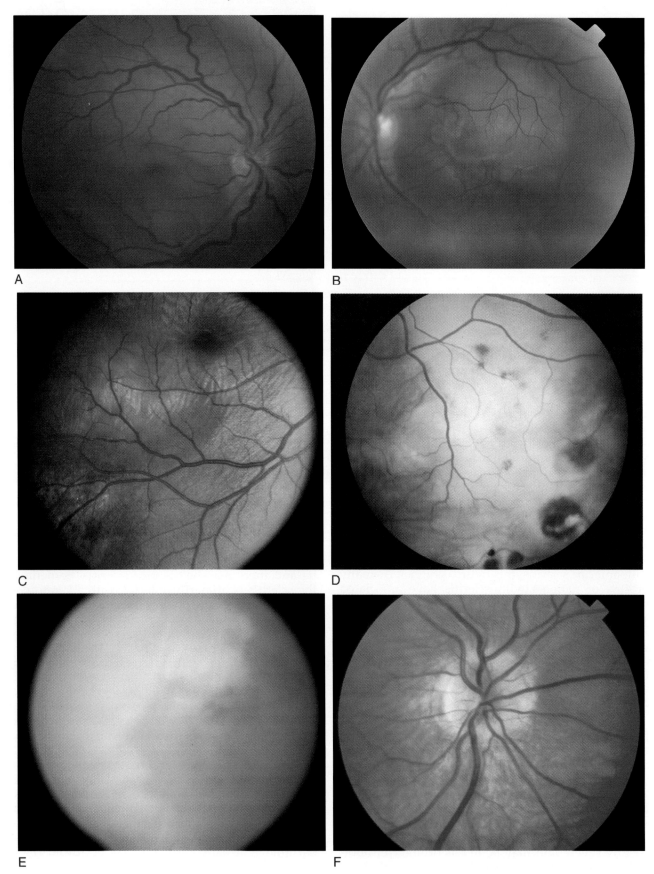

FIGURE 54–1   Exudative retinal detachment involving the macula of a 15-year-old male (*A*), and a 30-year-old male (*B*). (Photographs courtesy of Ann Bidwell, MD and Howard Tessler, MD [*A*] and Robert P. Schroeder, MD [*B*].) Prominent retinal folds in an acute exudative retinal detachment (*C*). Focal vasculitis (*D*) and turbid subretinal fluid in an exudative retinal detachment (*D* and *E*). Peripapillary choroidal folds in a patient with posterior scleritis, left eye (*F*). (Courtesy of Valerie Purvin, M.D.)

TABLE 54–1 Clinical Findings

Decreased vision
Tenderness
Anterior scleritis
Iridocyclitis
Ptosis
Proptosis
Restricted motility
Vitreous cells
Optic nerve edema
Neurosensory retinal detachment
Chorioretinal folds
Retinovascular occlusion
Uveal effusion
Focal choroidal mass
Retinal pigment epithelium detachment
Annular choroidal detachment with or without angle-closure glaucoma

inal pigment epithelium (RPE) detachment,[13] focal choroidal mass,[14–17] and malignant melanoma have been described as common misdiagnoses. Annular choroidal detachments have been reported[18] and can result in angle-closure glaucoma.[19–21] (Table 54–1).

DIFFERENTIAL DIAGNOSES

The findings evoke a long differential diagnosis due to the wide variety of presentations (Table 54–2). Most commonly, idiopathic central serous choroidopathy, choroidal or orbital tumor (primary or metastatic), and uveitis including Vogt-Koyanagi-Harada (VKH) syndrome are considered. In addition, the differential diagnoses of focal choroidal tumor, choroidal folds, exudative retinal detachment, RPE detachment, choroidal detachment, ocular inflammation, and uveitis all include posterior scleritis.

TABLE 54–2 Differential Diagnosis

Idiopathic central serous choroidopathy
Choroidal or orbital tumor (primary or metastatic)
Malignant melanoma
Amelanotic choroidal nevus
Choroidal hemangioma
Benign reactive lymphoid hyperplasia
Scleral buckle[42]
Toxoplasmic scleritis[43]
Vogt-Koyanagi-Harada syndrome
Orbital inflammatory syndrome[44]

TESTING

Fluorescein Angiography

Fluorescein angiography is helpful in the evaluation of these findings. Classically, multiple fine pinpoint leaks at the level of the RPE evolve to fill an overlying neurosensory exudative retinal detachment (Figs. 54–2 and 54–3). There may be optic nerve leakage, vascular staining, and rarely vascular occlusion. Subtle or prominent chorioretinal folds may be present. These findings, however, are not pathognomonic for posterior scleritis. Chorioretinal folds can be seen in the setting of orbital tumors, hyperopia, etc. Many choroidal tumors exhibit pinpoint hyperfluorescence including malignant melanoma, hemangioma, and metastatic tumors. Any disorder associated with uveitis can exhibit disc leakage and venous staining. The fluorescein pattern of VKH syndrome can closely mimic scleritis. VKH is almost invariably bilateral, whereas posterior scleritis may be unilateral.

Indocyanine Green Videoangiography

There have been no reports of indocyanine green (ICG) videoangiography in this disorder. One might expect to see associated hyperfluorescence in the region of posterior scleritis due to the potential breakdown in the integrity of large choroidal vessels.

Ultrasonography

Ultrasonography is very useful in establishing the presence of scleritis. Highly reflective echoes with thickening of the uvea and sclera are usually present. Scleral edema associated with fluid within Tenon's space resulting in an echolucent region just posterior to the sclera results in the classic "T" sign[7,22,23] (Figs. 54–4 and 54–5). This is considered diagnostic of posterior scleritis and is an important test for any patient with possible posterior scleritis. The absence of a choroidal mass is an important feature.

Computed Tomography

Computed tomography (CT) scanning can be helpful in localizing the extent of involvement and may differentiate between infiltrative and inflammatory processes.[24–26] The ill-defined, diffuse scleral thickening may be associated with inflammation of the adjacent periorbital tissues and muscles (Fig. 54–6). This usually enhances with contrast injection. A similar picture can be seen in idiopathic orbital inflammation and it may be difficult to distinguish these two entities.

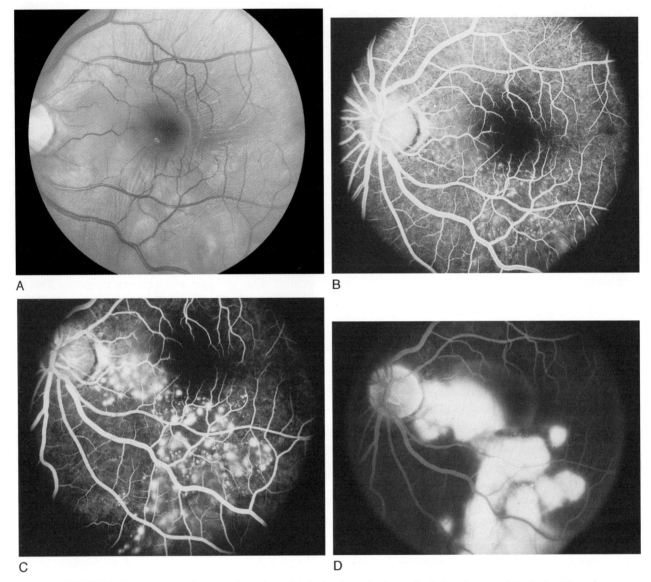

FIGURE 54–2 Color photograph with multiple focal exudative retinal detachments (*A*). Early (*B*) and midphase (*C*) angiography of the same patient with multiple pinpoint leaks at the level of the retinal pigment epithelium. Late angiography (*D*) with filling of the neurosensory retinal detachments.

Magnetic Resonance Imaging

Magnetic resonance imaging (MRI) scanning is often undertaken in cases in which the diagnosis is still difficult or unclear. Pre- and postcontrast-enhanced T1-weighted images with fat suppression techniques can demonstrate distinct enhancement in posterior scleritis. However, uveal melanomas, hemangiomas, and adenomas showed marked enhancement with gadopentetate dimeglumine as well.[25,27] CT scanning is more helpful than MRI in this setting.

SYSTEMIC EVALUATION

Posterior scleritis is an inflammatory disorder of the posterior sclera and adjacent tissues. Histopath-ologic studies of enucleated eyes (mistakenly thought to have malignant melanoma) revealed infiltration of the scleral tissue, vessels, and adjacent choroidal regions with lymphocytes.[28–30] More specifically, Bernauer[30] and associates noted a predominance of T lymphocytes (90%) and a marked perivasculitis with expression of MHC class II molecules.

Scleritis has inflammatory and vasculitic etiologies. Rheumatoid arthritis is reported to be the most common underlying disease, but posterior scleritis can complicate systemic lupus erythematosus, Wegener's granulomatosis, inflammatory bowel disease, sarcoidosis, syphilis, and others (Table 54–3). For this reason, the systemic evaluation usually includes a complete blood count (CBC) with differential, erythrocyte sedimentation rate (ESR), antinuclear antibodies (ANA), antineutro-

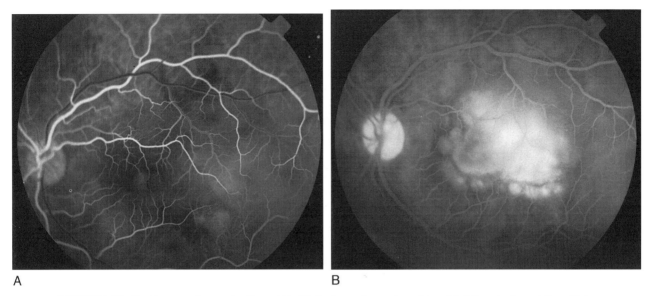

A   B

FIGURE 54–3   Same patient as in Figure 54–1B. Early angiography with mild diffuse leakage (A) and late angiography with filling (B) of the neurosensory retinal detachment.

phil cytoplasmic antibodies (ANCA), angiotensin converting enzyme (ACE), chest x-ray, and sometimes others (Table 54–4). Plain films may help with the diagnosis of arthritis.

TREATMENT

Determining the underlying cause is the key to appropriate and successful treatment. Despite testing, therapy often has to be instituted empirically prior to receiving test results. Usually the response to treatment is immediate and dramatic. Control of this inflammation is frequently approached initially with a nonsteroidal anti-inflammatory agent. A trial of indomethacin 25 to 50 mg orally three to four times a day, with food, induces improvement in

many cases.[31] When remission is obtained, usually in less than 2 weeks, the dose is reduced in half for another 2 weeks. Because of the extensive side effects of oral corticosteroids, an oral nonsteroidal anti-inflammatory agent is tried first. Refractory and recurrent cases frequently require oral corticosteroid therapy with an initial dose of 1 to 1.5 mg/kg orally each morning. This should be given with meals and possibly an accompanying antacid to prevent gastrointestinal ulcers and bleeding. Watson has reported the use of periocular subtenon steroids with good result, without the severe sequelae associated with their use in anterior scleritis and consequently minimizing the associated potential systemic complications. In some cases, indomethacin can be combined with oral corticosteroids, reducing the necessary steroid dose to 0.5 mg/kg.[32]

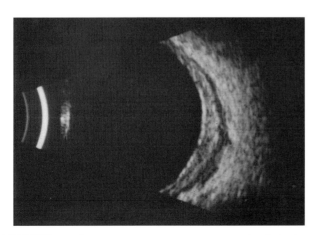

FIGURE 54–4   B-scan echogram with uveoscleral thickening, absence of choroidal mass, and edema in Tenon's space, "T" sign. (Courtesy of Sandra Frazier Byrne.)

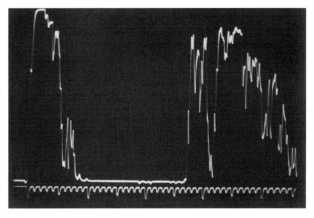

FIGURE 54–5   A-scan echogram with thickened retinochoroidal layers and sclera, and decreased reflectivity with widening of Tenon's space. (Courtesy of Sandra Frazier Byrne.)

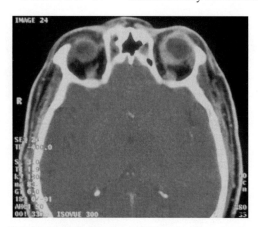

FIGURE 54–6 Computed tomography of thickened posterior sclera in a patient with posterior scleritis, left eye. (Courtesy of Valerie Purvin, M.D.)

The duration of treatment is highly variable. In a patient with an initial prompt, complete resolution, a short course is advisable. This should be withdrawn once the scleritis has become inactive and as tolerated by the patient. In severe cases, and especially those associated with underlying vasculitic or autoimmune diseases, treatment is usually necessary for more prolonged courses and will need to be tapered slowly.

When the inflammation does not respond or remit with the nonsteroidals and/or oral corticosteroids, pulse intravenous methylprednisolone and antimetabolites may be effective. McClusky et al[33] reported the successful use of intravenous methylprednisolone in doses of 1 g three times in the first week followed by 500 mg once or twice weekly as directed by the response. This was used in combination with other agents, including cyclophosphamide 500 mg[34] as necessary to control the inflammation. Complications included elevated serum glucose, psychological disturbances, hypertension, and exacerbation of congestive heart failure.

Either alone or in combination with corticosteroids, the use of cyclophosphamide, cyclosporine, or azathioprine has been described. These patients have more severe underlying disorders and frequently develop more significant complications re-

lated to the scleritis and its treatment. Wakefield and McClusky[35] reported successful cyclosporine use in five of seven cases of necrotizing scleritis. All had failed or developed complications from initial treatment and were started on a dose of 10 mg/kg/day for 2 to 4 weeks. Doses were reduced on a weekly basis until the 5-mg/kg/day level. Corticosteroid use was maintained at the presenting level. Patients were monitored closely for the potential renal, hepatic and lymphoproliferative effects. Hirsutism, tremor, hypertension, and elevated creatinine were seen. The scleritis had a tendency to relapse upon withdrawal of the cyclosporine.

With certain diseases, the scleritis is more refractory to nonsteroidal anti-inflammatory agents and/or corticosteroids. In relapsing polychondritis, the use of azathioprine and cyclophosphamide was required in the majority of patients to control the scleritis.[36] In patients with inflammatory bowel disease and ocular inflammation including scleritis, the combination of nonsteroidal anti-inflammatory agents and corticosteroids was effective in several patients while some required azathioprine as well[37] (Table 54–5).

COMPLICATIONS

The majority of patients with posterior scleritis respond well to the various treatment regimens, although the tendency for relapse is close to 50%

TABLE 54–4 Evaluation

Complete blood count (CBC) with differential
Erythrocyte sedimentation rate (ESR)
Antinuclear antibodies (ANA)
Antineutrophil cytoplasmic antibodies (ANCA)
Angiotensin converting enzyme (ACE)
Chest x-ray
Fluorescein angiography
Ultrasonography
Computed tomography

TABLE 54–3 Systemic Diseases

Rheumatoid arthritis
Systemic lupus erythematosus
Wegener's granulomatosis
Inflammatory bowel disease
Relapsing polychondritis
Procainamide-induced lupus[45]
Psoriatic arthritis[46]

TABLE 54–5 Treatment

Nonsteroidal anti-inflammatory
 Indomethacin 25–50 mg/kg t.i.d.–q.i.d.
Corticosteroid
 Oral 1–1.5 mg/kg/day
 "Pulse" IV methylprednisolone
Azathioprine
Cyclosporine 10 mg/kg/day
Cyclophosphamide (variable)

TABLE 54–6 Complications of
Posterior Scleritis

Recurrence
Visual loss
Uveitis
Cataract
Retinal detachment
Choroidal detachment
Angle-closure glaucoma
Scleral thinning

once medications are withdrawn. Some relapse as a different form of scleritis (e.g., anterior scleritis). This is most prevalent in patients with severe systemic vasculitic diseases. Complications including recurrence of disease, permanent visual loss, glaucoma, cataract, and scleral thinning have been reported[38] (Table 54–6). The visual prognosis is correlated with duration and severity of scleritis, and extent of optic nerve and macular damage. Because posterior scleritis is often elusive to diagnose, treatment is frequently delayed and there is resultant permanent visual loss.[31,32,35–37,39–41]

REFERENCES

1. Watson PG, Hayreh SS: Scleritis and episcleritis. Br J Ophthalmol 60:163–191, 1976.
2. McGavin DDM, Williamson J, Forrester JV, et al: Episcleritis and scleritis. A study of their clinical manifestations and association with rheumatoid arthritis. Br J Ophthalmol 60:192–226, 1976.
3. Waston PG: The diagnosis and management of scleritis. Ophthalmology 87:716–720, 1980.
4. Benson WE: Posterior scleritis. Surv Ophthalmol 32:297, 1988.
5. Calthorpe CM, Watson PG, McCartney AC: Posterior scleritis: a clinical and histological survey. Eye 2(Pt 3):267, 1988.
6. Sainz de la Maza M, Foster CS, Jabbur NS: Scleritis associated with systemic vasculitic diseases. Ophthalmology 102:687, 1995.
7. Benson WE, Shields JA, Tasman W, Crandall AS: Posterior scleritis. A cause of diagnostic confusion. Arch Ophthalmol 97:1482, 1979.
8. Sainz de la Maza M, Foster CS, Tasman W, Crandall AS: Scleritis associated with rheumatoid arthritis and with other systemic immune-mediated diseases. Ophthalmology 101:1281, 1994.
9. Takahashi T, Ikushima K, Arizawa T: Orbital myositis simulating infectious cellulitis: report of two cases. Jpn J Ophthalmol 27:626, 1983.
10. Rootman J, Nugent R: The classification and management of acute orbital pseudotumors. Ophthalmology 89:1040–1048, 1982.
11. Wilhelmus KR, Watson PG, Vasada AR: Uveitis associated with scleritis. Trans Ophthalmol Soc UK 101:351–355, 1981.
12. Frost NA, Sparrow JM, Rosenthal AR: Posterior scleritis with retinal vasculitis and choroidal and retinal infarction. Br J Ophthalmol 78:410, 1994.
13. Berger B, Reeser F: Retinal pigment epithelial detachments in posterior scleritis. Am J Ophthalmol 90:604, 1980.

14. Finger PT, Perry HD, Packer S, et al: Posterior scleritis as an intraocular tumour. Br J Ophthalmol 74:121, 1990.
15. Gedde SJ, Augsburger JJ: Posterior scleritis as a fundus mass. Ophthalmic Surg 25(2):119–121, 1994.
16. Brown GC, Shields JA, Augsburger JJ: Amelanotic choroidal nevi. Ophthalmology 88:1116, 1981.
17. Gupta A, Bansal RK, Bambery P: Posterior scleritis related fundal mass in a patient with rheumatoid arthritis. Scand J Rheumatol 21:254, 1992.
18. Marushak D: Uveal effusion attending scleritis posterior. A case report with A-scan and B-scan echograms. Acta Ophthalmol 60:773, 1982.
19. Quinlan MP, Hitchings RA: Angle-closure glaucoma secondary to posterior scleritis. Br J Ophthalmol 62:330, 1978.
20. Mangouritsas G, Ulbig M: Secondary angle closure glaucoma in posterior scleritis. Klin Monatsbl Augenheilkd 199:40, 1991.
21. Fourman S: Angle-closure glaucoma complicating ciliochoroidal detachment. Ophthalmology 96:646, 1989.
22. Singh G, Guthoff R, Foster CS: Observations on long-term follow-up of posterior scleritis. Am J Ophthalmol 101:570, 1986.
23. Munk P, Nicolle D, Downey D, et al: Posterior scleritis: ultrasound and clinical findings. Can J Ophthalmol 28:177, 1993.
24. Johnson MH, DeFilipp GJ, Zimmerman RA, Savino, PA: Scleral inflammatory disease. Am J Neuroradiol 8:861–865, 1987.
25. Chaques VJ, Lam S, Tessler HH, Mafee MF: Computed tomography and magnetic resonance imaging in the diagnosis of posterior scleritis. Ann Ophthalmol 25(3):89–94, 1993.
26. Trokel SL: Computer tomographic scanning of orbital inflammations. Int Ophthalmol Clin 22(4):81–93, 1982.
27. De Potter P, Flanders AE, et al: The role of fat-suppression technique and gadopentetate dimeglumine in magnetic resonance imaging evaluation of intraocular tumors and simulating lesions. Arch Ophthalmol 113:555, 1995.
28. Young RD, Powell J, Watson PG: Ultrastructural changes in scleral proteoglycans precede destruction of the collagen fibril matrix in necrotizing scleritis. Histopathology 12:75, 1988.
29. Bernauer W, Watson PG, Daicker B, Lightman S: Cells perpetuating the inflammatory response in scleritis. Br J Ophthalmol 78:381, 1994.
30. Bernauer W, Büchi ER, Daicker B: Immunopathological findings in posterior scleritis. Int Ophthalmol 18:229, 1995.
31. Rosenbaum JT, Robertson JE Jr: Recognition of posterior scleritis and its treatment with indomethacin. Retina 13:17, 1993.
32. Mondino BJ, Phinney RB: Treatment of scleritis with combined oral prednisone and indomethacin therapy. Am J Ophthalmol 106:473, 1988.
33. McCluskey P, Wakefield D: Intravenous pulse methylprednisolone in scleritis. Arch Ophthalmol 105:793, 1987.
34. Meyer PA, Watson PG, Franks W, Dubord P: 'Pulsed' immunosuppressive therapy in the treatment of immunologically induced corneal and scleral disease. Eye 1:487–495, 1987.
35. Wakefield D, McCluskey P: Cyclosporin therapy for severe scleritis. Br J Ophthalmol 73:743, 1989.
36. Hoang-Xaun T, Foster CS, Rice BA: Scleritis in relapsing polychondritis. Response to therapy. Ophthalmology 97:892, 1990.
37. Soukiasian SH, Foster CS, Raizman MB: Treatment strategies for scleritis and uveitis associated with inflammatory bowel disease. Am J Ophthalmol 118:601, 1994.
38. Tuft SJ, Watson PG: Progression of scleral disease. Ophthalmology 98:467–471, 1991.
39. McCluskey P, Wakefield D: Current concepts in the management of scleritis. Aust N Z J Ophthalmol 16:169, 1988.
40. Tuft SJ, Fracs PG, Watson FRCS: Progression of scleral disease. Ophthalmology 98:467, 1991.
41. Kalina RE, Mills RP: Observations on long-term follow-up of posterior scleritis. Am J Ophthalmol 102:671, 1986.

42. Bidwell AE, Jampol LM, O'Grady R: Scleritis resembling a scleral buckle. Arch Ophthalmol 111:865, 1993.
43. Schuman JS, Weinberg RS, et al: Toxoplasmic scleritis. Ophthalmology 95:1399, 1988.
44. Kalina PH, Garrity JA, et al: Role of testing for anticytoplasmic autoantibodies in the differential diagnosis of scleritis and orbital pseudotumor. Mayo Clin Proc 65:1110, 1990.
45. Gass DM: Specific choroidal diseases causing disciform macular detachment. In Stereoscopic Atlas of Macular Diseases: Diagnosis and Treatment. St Louis, CV Mosby Co, 1997, 172–180.
46. Turgeon PW, Stamovits TL: Scleritis as the presenting manifestation of procainamide-induced lupus. Ophthalmology 96:68, 1989.

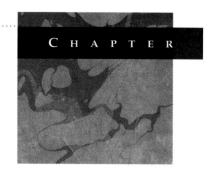

CHAPTER 55

Ocular Sarcoidosis

Antonio P. Ciardella, M.D.
Jason S. Slakter, M.D.

Sarcoidosis may produce granulomas all over the body and then spontaneously disappear without a trace, or may progress to a devastating disease. What are the controlling factors of such a variable response? Is this variability related to different etiologic agents or instead to host characteristics?

Sarcoidosis is characterized by differing presentations, ramifications, and natural course. The lack of knowledge regarding this disease is exemplified by the definition of sarcoidosis formulated at the Seventh International Conference on Sarcoidosis, held in New York in 1976, and still accepted nowadays:

> Sarcoidosis is a multisystem granulomatous disorder of unknown etiology, most commonly affecting young adults and presenting most frequently with bilateral hilar lymphadenopathy, pulmonary infiltration, skin or eye lesions. The diagnosis is established most securely when clinico-radiographic findings are supported by histological evidence of widespread non-caseating epithelioid-cell granulomas in more than one organ system.

HISTORICAL BACKGROUND

The first case of sarcoidosis was described by Jonathan Hutchinson in 1869 at the Blackfriars Hospital for Skin Diseases.[1] Schumaker in 1909 and Bering in 1910 first recognized the iritis as an ocular complication of sarcoidosis. In 1909, the Danish ophthalmologist Heerfordt described uveoparotid fever (Heerfordt's syndrome), which was later identified as a variant of sarcoidosis.[2] Williams and Nickerson, in 1935, first used a suspension from sarcoid tissue in an attempt to induce a skin reaction and they briefly reported the development of a papule at the site of injection in patients with sar-

coidosis. Kveim published a complete account of the histology of this nodule in 1941. Between 1961 and 1964 Louis Siltzbach extensively investigated this test and pioneered its universal application, thus the designation Kveim-Siltzbach test.[3]

EPIDEMIOLOGY

Sarcoidosis has a worldwide distribution but is more frequently described in developed countries. In Sweden, screening x-rays suggested an incidence of 64 per 100,000 population, although autopsy studies indicated the incidence might actually be tenfold higher.[4] In Japan, the incidence was less than 1 per 100,000, and cases were clustered in northern and central Japan.[5] In the United States, the prevalence of the disease is approximately 5 per 100,000 in whites, and 40 per 100,000 in blacks.[6] A similar sixfold increase in the prevalence in the black population has also been reported in South Africa. The disease is uncommon in the Chinese population and American Indians.

Most series from the United States report a 2:1 female/male predominance, whereas some series from Europe have demonstrated an even distribution. Although the majority of cases are diagnosed between the ages of 20 and 40, 10% of cases make their initial presentation after age 60, and the disease is also described in pediatric populations.[4]

Based on most epidemiologic studies, it is apparent that the majority of patients with sarcoidosis are either asymptomatic or have such minor symptoms that medical attention is not sought. Therefore, it has been estimated that 80% of all cases of sarcoid go undetected.[7]

ETIOLOGY

The cause of sarcoidosis remains unknown. Over the years, many infectious organisms and toxic agents have been proposed as the etiology of the disease. There may indeed be a causative transmissible agent in some cases, with mycobacterial tuberculosis the most commonly suggested. In support of this concept, mycobacteria are present more frequently in tissues from sarcoidosis patients than in control tissues. Numerous authors have reported parallel changes in the prevalence of sarcoidosis and tuberculosis in a community.[9,10] In addition, mycobacteria or mycobacteria-like organisms may be cultured from sarcoid tissues in some patients.[11,12] Recently, there have been preliminary reports of the detection of mycobacterial DNA in bronchoalveolar lavage (BAL) fluids from patients with sarcoidosis using the polymerase chain reaction (PCR) technique.[13]

Viruses, *Nocardia*-like organisms, and *Mycoplasma* have also been proposed as potential causative agents.[14] In addition, beryllium may produce a sarcoid-like response. Immunologic derangements, an allergic phenomenon, and genetic predisposition have also been considered possibilities. Some authorities believe that sarcoidosis is, in fact, a syndrome with many causative agents.[14]

PATHOLOGY AND PATHOGENESIS

Sarcoidosis can involve any organ in the body, with the probable exception of the adrenal glands, peritoneum, and pericardium.[14] In a series of necropsy reports of 117 patients with sarcoidosis,[15] the organs involved were widespread, as listed in Table 55–1.

TABLE 55–1 Sarcoidosis in Body Organs

Organ System	Percentage
Lymph nodes	78%
Lungs	77%
Liver	67%
Spleen	50%
Heart	20%
Skin	16%
CNS	8%
Kidney	7%
Eye	6%
Parotid gland	6%
Thyroid gland	4%
Intestine	3%
Stomach	3%
Hypophysis	3%

The basic lesion in sarcoidosis is a noncaseating granuloma made up of compact, radially arranged, epithelioid cells with pale-staining nuclei (former macrophages); a few multinucleated giant cells of the Langhans or foreign body type; and a tiny rim of lymphocytes (Fig. 55–1). Typically, all granulomas are found in the same stage of development. Caseation is absent and sometimes fibrinoid necrosis may be present. Different inclusion bodies have been described in sarcoid granulomas—crystalline bodies,[16] asteroid bodies, and conchoidal bodies of Schaumann—but are also seen in other granulomatous diseases and are therefore not specific for sarcoidosis.[17] Granulomatous vasculitis is frequently found in sarcoidosis and consists of noncaseating granulomas within the intima and media of vessels. These granulomas may compress the lumen and cause obstruction of the vessels, but do not cause necrosis of vessel walls.[18]

The granulomas have a widespread distribution in tissues affected by sarcoidosis. They may resolve spontaneously and completely, leaving no residual scar, or they may cause secondary scarring and fibrosis. Functional impairment is caused by the presence of active granulomas or secondary fibrosis in the involved organ and by the effects of hypercalcemia and hypercalciuria, which may also occur.

Hypercalcemia in sarcoidosis is probably due to increased calcitriol production by the sarcoid granuloma, which increases calcium absorption from the gastrointestinal tract. Patients with sarcoidosis are hypersensitive to vitamin D, and sometimes hypercalcemia is only revealed when patients are exposed to sunlight.[14]

The central finding in sarcoidosis suggesting an altered immune response is the widespread distribution of granulomas.[19–21] Most data suggest that sarcoidosis results from the continuous presentation of antigen by tissue macrophages to T lymphocytes at the site of disease. The modulation of the inflammatory response occurs via a variety of

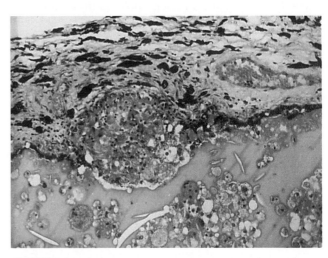

FIGURE 55–1 Biopsy of a conjunctival nodule. A noncaseating sarcoid granuloma is visible in this conjunctival specimen.

cytokines. In most individuals, the inflammatory process resolves without lasting functional sequelae. This may reflect clearance of the inciting antigen, development of humoral or cellular suppressing mechanisms, or a genetic predisposition that limits the immune response. In some patients, however, the inflammatory response is progressive, with the eventual development of fibrosis.[7]

CLINICAL FEATURES

Systemic Manifestations

Patients with sarcoidosis may have generalized complaints, symptoms attributable to extrapulmonary involvement, or findings localized to the respiratory tract. Forty to 50% of patients complain of constitutional symptoms including malaise, weight loss, fevers, sweats, and myalgias.[22-24] Approximately 15 to 30% of patients display signs of peripheral lymphadenopathy, splenomegaly, or hepatic enlargement.[7] Approximately 20% of patients with sarcoidosis are asymptomatic and are picked up on routine chest x-ray.[14]

Involvement of the respiratory tract produces symptoms in 30 to 50% of individuals with sarcoidosis. Characteristic complaints include dyspnea on exertion, chest pain, and nonproductive cough. More importantly, 40 to 70% of patients with sarcoidosis display a reduction in lung volume or diffusion capacity for carbon monoxide. Significant resting hypoxemia is uncommon in sarcoid, though arterial desaturation may occur with exercise.[25-27] In approximately 20% of patients with sarcoidosis, significant reductions in expiratory flow rate, indicating airways obstruction, may be noted on spirometry.[7]

Skin lesions may be found in at least 15% of patients with sarcoid[28] (Fig. 55–2). Lupus pernio, the most classic skin lesion manifested in sarcoidosis, is a violaceous indurated lesion that preferentially involves the ears, lips, and nose. Other common skin lesions include plaques located on the limbs, face, and back in a symmetric distribution; maculopapular eruptions on the face and upper back; subcutaneous nodules (Darier-Roussy lesions) representing dermal and subcutaneous granulomas; and erythema nodosum (found in <10% of American patients), commonly associated with fever, malaise, and polyarthralgia. Human leukocyte antigen HLA-B8 seems to have a strong association with erythema nodosum secondary to sarcoidosis in Caucasians, and its presence augurs a good prognosis.

Central nervous system (CNS) involvement may be seen, with signs of basilar meningitis, psychiatric dysfunction, or a space-occupying lesion.[29-31] CNS involvement occurs in less than 10% of patients. The basilar meningitis may be associated with cranial nerve palsies or hypothalamic/

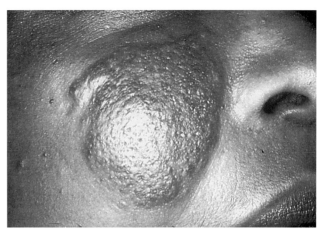

FIGURE 55–2   Skin lesion. A sarcoid nodule is visible on the cheek of this patient. (Courtesy of Dr. Mark Lebwohl.)

pituitary dysfunction. Peripheral neuropathy may also complicate sarcoid.

Cardiac sarcoid is an important and largely undiagnosed complication. Although clinically evident cardiac involvement is rare, autopsy series disclose a 25 to 30% incidence of cardiac involvement.[32-36] Ventricular fibrillation may be the initial presentation of cardiac sarcoid. Other organs that are commonly involved include the upper respiratory tract, bone marrow, spleen, liver, kidneys, musculoskeletal system, endocrine and reproductive system, and exocrine and gastrointestinal system.[14]

Acute sarcoidosis is the most common form of presentation of the disease. It develops suddenly over a period of days or weeks and can be asymptomatic. In about 40% of patients it is associated with erythema nodosum and, in about 25% of patients, constitutional symptoms can be severe, causing serious disability. There is complete resolution of radiographic abnormalities in over 60% of the cases within 1 year and corticosteroids are seldom necessary. Two well-defined acute syndromes have been described:

1. Lofgren's syndrome: comprising erythema nodosum (EN), bilateral hilar lymphadenopathy (BHL), and arthralgia.
2. Heerfordt-Waldenström syndrome: consisting of parotid enlargement, anterior uveitis, facial nerve palsy, and fever.

Chronic sarcoidosis is less common than the acute form of the disease, but it causes permanent functional impairment. It develops insidiously over many months or years and is not associated with constitutional symptoms. The lungs are the organ most commonly involved, and respiratory symptoms such as dry cough and exertional dyspnea are the most common presenting complaints. There is often progressive pulmonary fibrosis and obstruction of the airways.

Ocular Manifestations

A significant number of patients with sarcoidosis seek initial medical examination because of ocular involvement. Considering clinically detectable lesions, Obenauf et al[37] found only hilar lymphadenopathy and pulmonary abnormalities to be more common than ophthalmic manifestations. In their survey of 532 cases of sarcoidosis in the southeastern United States, ocular manifestations were a prominent feature. The first symptoms of the disease involved the eye in 101 patients, and ocular involvement developed during the course of the disease in at least 202 cases. Among the 385 black patients with sarcoidosis, the incidence of ocular involvement was 44.2%, whereas it was 21% in the 143 white patients. A review of sarcoidosis around the world revealed ocular involvement in 11 to 32% of cases.[22] James et al,[38] in a survey of 442 cases, found 27.8% of patients to have ophthalmic manifestations.

In general, the types of ocular abnormalities encountered in sarcoidosis can be classified into three categories (Table 55–2): (1) anterior segment disease, (2) posterior segment disease, and (3) orbital and other disease.

Anterior segment involvement is observed in

about 85% of patients with ocular sarcoidosis. Acute ocular sarcoidosis is generally unilateral, and as the disease becomes chronic, bilateral involvement usually develops. Chronic granulomatous uveitis, characterized by mutton-fat keratatic precipitates (Fig. 55–3), iris nodules, and synechiae, is the most frequent ocular manifestation of sarcoidosis. It occurs in more than half of the patients with ocular disease. Acute iridocyclitis manifests clinically with ciliary injection, aqueous cells, and flare, and sometimes fine keratatic precipitates, but without evidence of chronic inflammation. It is noted in about 15% of patients with ocular sarcoidosis. A common complication of the chronic granulomatous uveitis is cataract, caused both by the chronic inflammation and by treatment with corticosteroids, glaucoma, and band keratopathy (often in association with hypercalcemia).[39]

Conjunctival involvement is also a common feature of sarcoidosis. James et al[38] reported conjunctival involvement in 23.6% of patients with ocular sarcoidosis; Obenauf et al[37] reported conjunctival involvement in 6.9%.

Posterior segment involvement is observed in about 25% of patients with ocular sarcoidosis,[37] and it is the sole manifestation of ocular sarcoidosis in about 5% of cases. The predominant posterior segment manifestations of sarcoidosis are chorioretinitis and retinal periphlebitis.

The choroidal lesions are typically located in the inferior peripheral fundus, and it is unusual for them to appear in the posterior pole. They characteristically appear as patches of creamy yellow choroidal depigmentation (Fig. 55–4), which are later associated with overlying hypo- or hyperpigmentation of the pigment epithelium. Variable-sized yellowish white to waxy chorioretinal nodules have been noted by many authors.[38–41] The chorioretinitis is clinically indistinguishable from that caused by other conditions[40] (Fig. 55–5). Two patterns of chorioretinitis have been observed as the presenting

TABLE 55–2 Incidence of Abnormalities in 202 Patients with Ophthalmic Sarcoidosis*

Abnormalities	No.	%
Anterior segment disease	171	84.7%
Chronic granulomatous uveitis	106	52.5%
Iris nodules	23	11.4%
Acute iritis	30	14.9%
Cataract	17	8.4%
Conjunctival nodules	14	6.9%
Band keratopathy	9	4.5%
Interstitial keratatis	2	1.0%
Posterior segment disease	51	25.3%
Chorioretinitis	22	10.9%
Periphlebitis	21	10.4%
Chorioretinal nodules	11	5.5%
Vitreous cells	6	3.0%
Vitreous hemorrhage	3	1.5%
Retinal neovascularization	3	1.5%
Orbital	53	26.2%
Lacrimal gland	32	15.8%
Optic nerve	15	7.4%
Motility	4	2.0%
Orbital granuloma	2	1.0%

* Modified from Obenauf CD, Shaw HE, Sydnor CF, Klintworth GK: Sarcoidosis and its ophthalmic manifestations. Am J Ophthalmol 86:648–655, 1978, with permission.

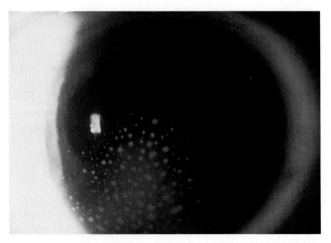

FIGURE 55–3 Anterior segment sarcoidosis. Mutton-fat keratic precipitates are visible in this patient with chronic granulomatous uveitis.

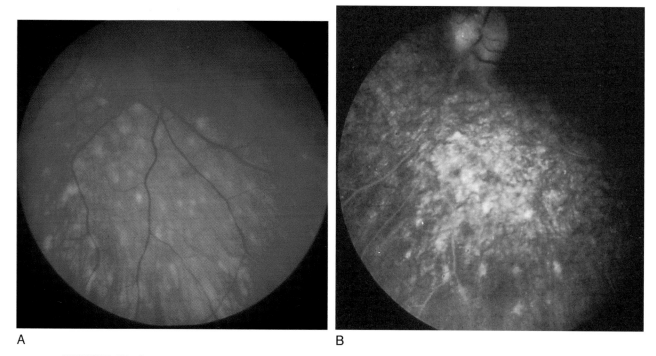

FIGURE 55–4   Sarcoid chorioretinitis. *A*, Clinical photograph of a patient with posterior segment sarcoidosis. Multiple creamy lesions are visible in the inferior peripheral fundus. Note the similarity with the fundus lesions of birdshot choroidopathy. *B*, Late-phase fluorescein angiography of another patient with sarcoid chorioretinitis. Note the hyperfluorescent chorioretinal spots and the staining of the disc.

sign of sarcoidosis.[42] The first is more common and consists of small, discrete white spots in the inferior or nasal periphery, indistinguishable from the lesions of multifocal choroiditis. The second consists of larger, posterior, pale yellow-orange streaks identical to the lesions of birdshot chorioretinopathy (Fig. 55–4).

Retinal periphlebitis, producing the ophthalmoscopic appearance of "candle-wax drippings" in more severe cases, is a hallmark of the disease (Fig. 55–6). This finding, though not pathognomonic, suggests the diagnosis of sarcoidosis. Vitreous opacities were first described by Landers[43] as characteristic grayish white bodies, frequently found in

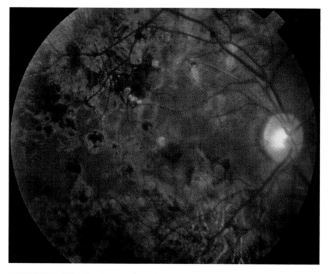

FIGURE 55–5   Sarcoid chorioretinitis—chronic stage. Clinical photograph of a patient with chronic inflammation of the posterior pole. Diffuse areas of hypo- and hyperpigmentation, atrophy, and hypertrophy of the retinal pigment epithelium, are evident throughout the fundus. This end-stage picture mimics that of many chorioretinal inflammatory diseases.

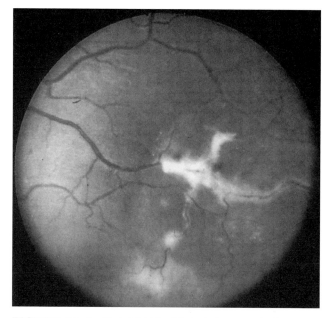

FIGURE 55–6   Periphlebitis. Clinical photograph showing a localized area of retinal periphlebitis. Note the perivascular retinal infiltration accompanied by focal intraretinal hemorrhage.

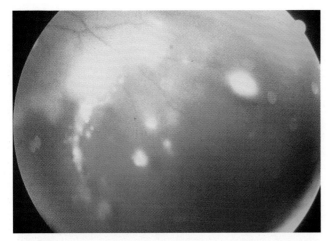

FIGURE 55-7 Vitreous involvement. Vitreous opacities, described in the literature as a "string of pearls," have been reported in as many as 80% of patients with intraocular sarcoid involvement. (Courtesy of Dr. Douglas A. Jabs. From Ryan SJ: Retina, 2nd edition. St. Louis, Mosby-Yearbook, 1994, with permission.)

the inferior vitreous and occurring in chains like a "string of pearls"[41,43] (Fig. 55-7). Cells and opacities in the vitreous have been reported in 30 to 100% of patients with ocular sarcoid.[40,44] Intraretinal hemorrhages, cotton-wool spots, and Roth's spots may also be demonstrated in patients with sarcoidosis (Fig. 55-8).

More unusual presentations of posterior segment involvement in ocular sarcoidosis have been reported. Edelsten et al,[45] for example, described two cases of serpiginous choroiditis as an unusual presentation of ocular sarcoidosis (Fig. 55-9). Ohara et al[46] described a case of sarcoidosis in a pediatric patient with unilateral iridocyclitis, retinal periphlebitis, and severe branch retinal vein occlusion (Fig. 55-10). The ocular lesion suggested sarcoidosis, but routine examinations did not support the clinical diagnosis. Transbronchial lung biopsy demonstrated noncaseating epithelioid granulomas associated with sarcoidosis. With steroid therapy, visual acuity improved from 20/200 to 20/20.

DeRosa et al[47] reported a patient whose initial clinical manifestation of sarcoidosis was a unilateral hemorrhagic retinopathy. The diagnosis of sarcoidosis in this patient was delayed for over a year, principally because of the atypical retinal findings and because repeated chest x-rays and angiotension-converting enzyme (ACE) levels were normal. Enucleation of the eye, performed after complete loss of vision, revealed a large noncaseating granuloma of the ciliary body.

Duker et al[48] described a series of 11 eyes in seven patients, all African-American, with proliferative sarcoid retinopathy (Fig. 55-11). Retinal neovascularization was encountered in all 11 eyes, neovascularization of the optic disc in 2 eyes, and iris neovascularization in 1 eye. In addition, retinal phlebitis was seen in all 11 eyes. In each case, areas of capillary nonperfusion were evident anterior and

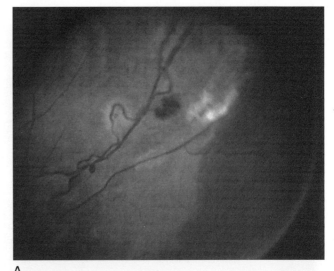

A

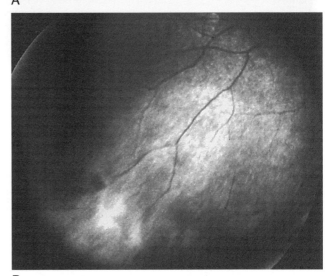

B

FIGURE 55-8 Posterior segment involvement. A and B, Intraretinal hemorrhages, cotton-wool spots (A), and Roth's spots (B) may also be demonstrated in patients with sarcoidosis.

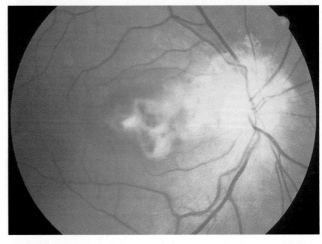

FIGURE 55-9 Posterior segment involvement. Posterior segment lesions may mimic other chorioretinal inflammatory diseases such as serpiginous choroidopathy.

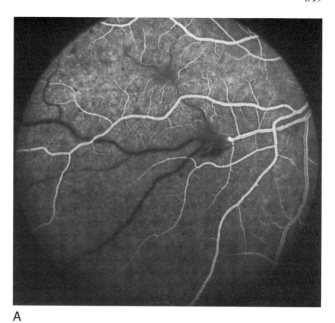

FIGURE 55–10   Branch retinal vein occlusion. *A*, Fluorescein study of a patient with sarcoidosis that shows a branch retinal vein occlusion along the inferotemporal arcade. Note that the obstruction occurs at the site of inflammation rather than at an arteriovenous crossing site. *B*, Wide field montage photo of the same patient demonstrates the peripheral location of the obstruction.

A

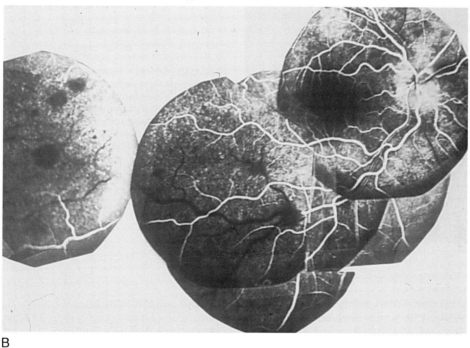

B

adjacent to the new retinal vessels. Retinal vascular nonperfusion in ocular sarcoidosis has been suggested to occur in two ways: (1) venous obstruction due to luminal obliteration by noncaseating granulomata[49–51]; and (2) direct inflammatory invasion of small retinal vessels.[52] In the end stage of the disease traction retinal detachment and diffuse retinal ischemia may result (Fig. 55–12).

Tingey et al[53] described a case of ocular sarcoidosis presenting as a solitary choroidal mass without other signs of intraocular inflammation in a 26-year-old man in whom systemic sarcoidosis was ultimately diagnosed. The mass presented as a slightly elevated, pale yellow choroidal lesion, with overlying subretinal fluid involving the macula.

The vitreous was clear, with no cells or opacities noted. The retinal vessels appeared otherwise normal, with no associated hemorrhages or exudates. The differential diagnosis of a solitary choroidal tumor in the absence of any other intraocular inflammation included solitary choroidal hemangioma, amelanotic melanoma, metastasis, and osseous choristoma. In this patient, the chest x-ray demonstrated bilateral hilar adenopathy, and transbronchial lung biopsy confirmed the diagnosis of sarcoidosis. With steroid therapy the subretinal fluid resolved and the chorioretinal infiltrate flattened, leaving a pale chorioretinal scar without any improvement in visual acuity. Cystoid macular edema (Fig. 55–13) and rhegmatogenous retinal detach-

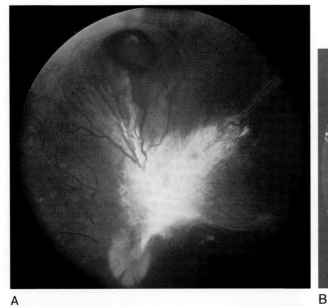

A

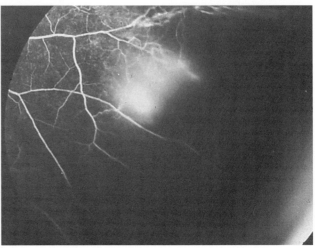

B

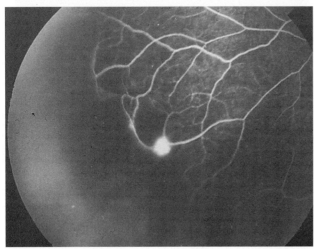

C

FIGURE 55–11   Proliferative sarcoid retinopathy. *A*, Clinical photograph of a patient with proliferative sarcoid retinopathy. Preretinal fibrovascular proliferation, similar to that seen in diabetes, is noted in this patient with sarcoidosis with extensive retinal nonperfusion. *B*, Fluorescein angiography of another patient shows peripheral neovascularization occurring at the margin of extensive retinal ischemia. *C*, Retinal arteriovenous anastomosis is evident posteriorly to the area of retina ischemia. New vessels originate from the anastomosis. Note the similarity with the clinical appearance of sickle cell disease. (Courtesy of Dr. Jay Duker.)

ment (Fig. 55–14) may also complicate posterior segment involvement in ocular sarcoidosis.[39]

It is important to remember that posterior segment sarcoidosis is commonly accompanied by involvement of the central nervous system. In two reviews, the brain was found to be affected in 25[37] and 30%[40] of cases with posterior segment disease. Westlake et al[54] described a case of sarcoidosis involving the optic nerve and hypothalamus in a 20-year-old African-Caribbean woman with a 4-week history of reduced vision in the right eye and a 3-month history of amenorrhea. Funduscopy revealed moderate vitritis and a grossly infiltrated optic disc, with exudation and hemorrhage in the right eye and a normal appearing left fundus. Gadolinium-enhanced magnetic resonance imaging (MRI) of the brain demonstrated asymmetric thickening of the optic chiasm, with infiltration in the region of the hypothalamus, third ventricles, and meninges, and enlargement of the pituitary gland. Menstruation resumed 5 months after the start of

steroid administration, and at the 1-year follow-up, the right visual acuity was 20/30 with marked resolution of the disc swelling. These findings stress the need for a thorough neurologic examination in patients with posterior segment ocular involvement in sarcoidosis.

Optic nerve involvement in sarcoidosis is usually manifested by papilledema secondary to increased intracranial pressure, papillitis (Fig. 55–15), optic neuritis, optic atrophy, and rarely by granulomas of the optic disc[55–59] (Figs. 55–16 and 55–17). When sarcoidosis affects the brain, the intracranial portion of the optic nerve may be involved by the inflammatory reaction (retrobulbar optic neuritis).

An ocular staphyloma has been described by Zeiter et al[60] in a 38-year-old black woman, who presented with severe uveitis and secondary glaucoma. A 9 × 1.5 mm inferior circumlimbal staphyloma, completely covered by conjunctiva, was noted.

Orbital and adnexal structures, primarily the lac-

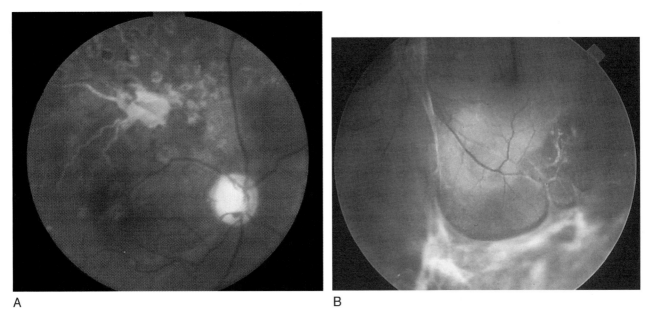

A   B

FIGURE 55–12   Proliferative sarcoid retinopathy. *A*, Clinical photograph of a patient with end-stage sarcoid retinopathy. Chorioretinal scars of retinal photocoagulation are evident superotemporarly. Note the occlusion of the superotemporal artery at the site of localized chorioretinal inflammation. *B*, Clinical photograph of another patient with end-stage disease. Vessel sheathing, artery occlusion, and a band of fibrous tissue extend from the optic nerve to the periphery. (Courtesy of Dr. Jay Duker.)

rimal gland, are affected in 30% of patients with ocular sarcoidosis.[37] Lacrimal gland enlargement is more common in black patients, and its incidence ranges from 6 to 15%.[37,38] Biopsy usually reveals granulomatous inflammation of the involved gland. Lacrimal gland involvement is often bilateral and may be associated with parotid swelling and dacryoadenitis.[37] Patients with lacrimal gland in-

volvement often complain of dry eye. Regression may occur with steroid therapy.

Orbital involvement is a rare cause of unilateral proptosis.[61,62] Obenauf et al[37] found histologically confirmed orbital granulomas in 2 of 202 cases of ocular sarcoidosis. In the same survey, abnormal ocular motility secondary to involvement of the cranial nerves innervating the extraocular muscles

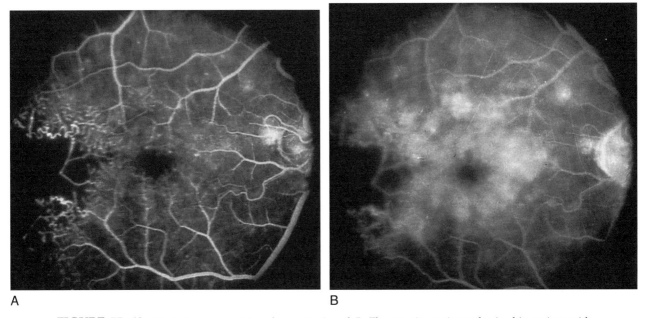

A   B

FIGURE 55–13   Posterior segment involvement. *A* and *B*, Fluorescein angiography in this patient with active sarcoidosis demonstrates temporal macular capillary nonperfusion due to microvascular infarction as well as cystoid macular edema.

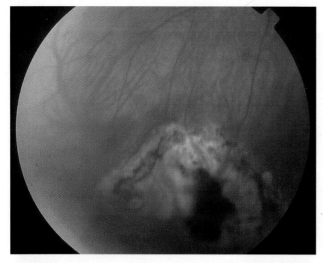

FIGURE 55–14 Posterior segment involvement. Cryopexy scar around a retinal break following vitreoretinal surgical repair for an associated retinal detachment.

was noted in four cases. An isolated third, fourth, or sixth cranial nerve palsy was detected in three patients. One individual had a combined third and fourth nerve palsy.

DIAGNOSIS

Due to the nonspecific nature of ocular findings and the widespread involvement of ocular structures in sarcoidosis, it is often difficult for the ophthalmologist to pin down the precise cause of intraocular inflammation. Given the absence of a specific diagnostic test for this condition, defining ocular sarcoidosis becomes a matter of exclusion. In attempting to make the diagnosis, the first step in evaluation is a search for associated systemic manifestations. A chest x-ray (Fig. 55–18) to identify the presence of hilar adenopathy and for staging the disease is also important (Table 55–3). Once a diagnosis of sarcoidosis is strongly suspected, tissue diagnosis is essential. Biopsy of visible conjunctival nodules, or even normal appearing conjunctival tissue, may yield positive results in up to 30% of cases.[63,64] Biopsy of skin lesion may also be worthwhile. The single test most widely accepted as useful in identifying the histopathologic manifestations of sarcoidosis is a transbronchial lung biopsy, which may yield positive results in as many as 80% of cases.[65,66]

All biopsy material should be cultured for mycobacteria and fungi, and the diagnosis of sarcoidosis cannot be confirmed until specific causes for the noncaseating granuloma have been excluded. Furthermore, noncaseating granulomas are seen in berylliosis, hypersensitivity pneumonias, and many other conditions (Table 55–4). Therefore, to confirm the diagnosis of sarcoidosis, it is important to have at least two tissue sources of granulomatous involvement.[17]

The Kveim-Siltzbach test is primarily of historical interest. Although it may still be used, the antigen is not commercially available, and few centers are still engaged in its production and validation.

Measurement of serum angiotensin-converting

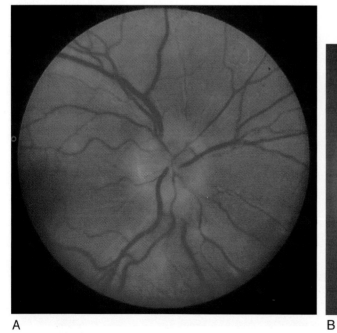
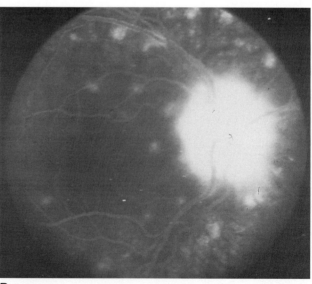

A   B

FIGURE 55–15 Optic nerve involvement. *A*, Clinical photograph of a patient with biopsy-proven sarcoidosis that shows optic disc swelling and faint yellowish chorioretinal spots. *B*, The fluorescein study of the same patient better demonstrates the staining chorioretinal inflammatory lesions as well as the marked hyperfluorescence and staining of the inflamed optic nerve.

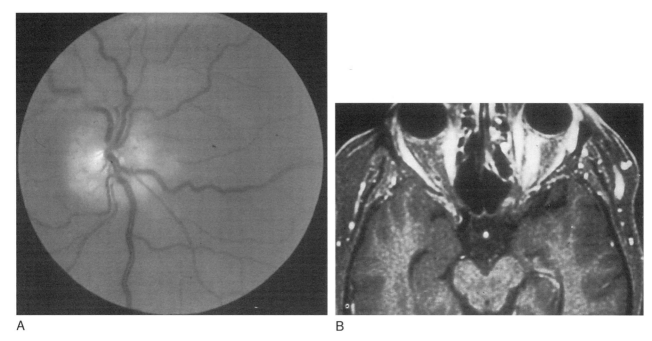

FIGURE 55–16   Optic nerve involvement. *A,* This patient with biopsy-proven sarcoidosis has moderate swelling of the optic nerve head. *B,* MRI scanning revealed granulomatous involvement of the entire orbital portion of the optic nerve. (Courtesy of Dr. Dan Kaufmann.)

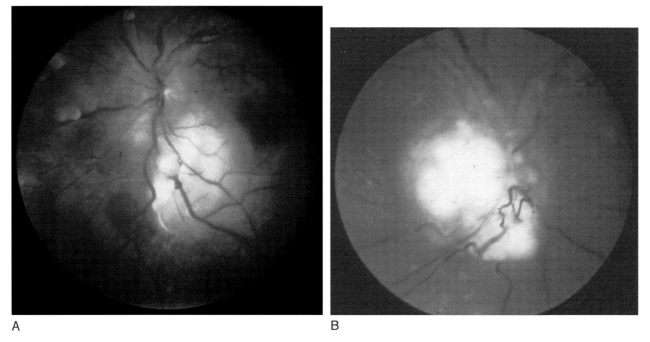

FIGURE 55–17   Optic nerve involvement. *A,* Clinical photograph of the optic nerve of a patient with biopsy-proven sarcoidosis. A large choroidal granuloma is visible inferior to the optic nerve. Note the subretinal hemorrhage and a serous retinal detachment. A retinal vascular anastomosis is evident within the scar and there are a few plaques of inflammatory debris along the inferior vessels. (Courtesy of Dr. Rollins Tindell, Jr.) *B,* Clinical photograph of an optic nerve granuloma in another case of sarcoidosis. Note the candle-wax drippings, which are inflammatory plaques along the venules. An incomplete macular star of exudation is noted in the macula. (Courtesy of Drs. Robert Nussenblat and Douglas A. Jabs. From Ryan SJ: Retina, 2nd edition. St Louis, Mosby-Yearbook, 1994, with permission.)

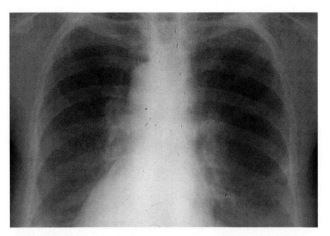

FIGURE 55–18 Systemic sarcoidosis. Chest x-ray of a patient with stage II pulmonary sarcoidosis. Note the hilar lymphadenopathy as well as parenchymal infiltrates.

TABLE 55–4 Causes of Noncaseating Granuloma

Sarcoidosis
Primary biliary cirrhosis
Brucellosis
Tertiary syphilis
Foreign body reaction
Granulomatous arteritis
Hypogammaglobulinemia
Tuberculosis
Leprosy
Fungal infections
Berylliosis
Hypersensitivity pneumonitis
Crohn's disease
Lymphoma

enzyme (SACE) and lysozyme level are the tests most used in the follow-up of sarcoidosis patients. They are both produced by activated macrophages in sarcoid granulomas. Consequently, they reflect the development and number of granulomas. They may be normal in early and acute disease, reflecting the small number of granulomas present at this stage. Overall, SACE is increased in 60% of sarcoidosis patients, and lysozyme in about 40%, but the levels are nonspecific and not helpful in diagnosing sarcoidosis, especially since their serum levels are increased in a number of diseases that are often difficult to distinguish from sarcoidosis (Table 55–5).

TABLE 55–3 Staging of Intrathoracic Sarcoidosis According to the Appearances on the Chest X-Ray at First Presentation

Stage 0:	Normal radiography, found in 3% of patients upon presentation, is represented by a normal chest roentgenogram, though noncaseating granulomas (NCG) may be found on transbronchial biopsy and in other organs. On pulmonary function testing, the diffusing capacity of the lung for carbon monoxide (D_{LCO}) may be low even at this time.
Stage I:	Bilateral hilar lymphadenopathy (BHL), present in 61% of cases. This stage is characterized by BHL, often with right paratracheal nodes, normal lung fields, and NCG on histology in more than 90% of cases.
Stage II:	BHL with pulmonary infiltrates, present in 25.3% of cases.
Stage III:	Pulmonary infiltrates without BHL, present in 9.7% of cases.
Stage IIIB:	Pulmonary fibrosis. It is alternatively referred to as stage IV.

Gallium citrate scans are also used frequently in following the activity of sarcoidosis, though they are nonspecific and therefore of limited use for diagnosis. Gallium uptake is increased in the lungs in sarcoidosis as well as in a variety of disorders including pulmonary tuberculosis, various other interstitial lung diseases, and pulmonary tumors. Gallium is fixed by sarcoid granulomas and is believed to reflect the extent of disease at different sites and the degree of granuloma activity at those sites. Therefore, the value of a gallium scan is in noninvasively assessing the extent and the degree of the inflammatory process, choosing preferential sites for biopsy, and monitoring therapeutic response. A recent report by Power et al[67] suggests that combined SACE determination and gallium scanning can increase the diagnostic specificity for sarcoidosis significantly, to nearly 100%. This testing approach cannot, however, increase the overall sensitivity of identifying sarcoidosis in patients with normal or equivocal chest x-rays.

Cell counts in BAL fluid have been used to assess disease activity. Specifically, high-intensity alveolitis has been defined as lymphocyte counts greater than 28% of total cells in lavage fluid. This high-intensity alveolitis is said to reflect disease activity

TABLE 55–5 Diseases with Increased Serum Angiotensin-Converting Enzyme

Berylliosis
Asbestosis
Gaucher's disease
Hypersensitivity pneumonitis
Miliary tuberculosis
Coccidioidomycosis
Lymphoma
Silicosis
Leprosy
Crohn's disease

and a tendency toward progression of sarcoidosis. Alveolar lymphocytosis is believed to be a direct reflection of this alveolitis. BAL is a useful research tool but has no proven diagnostic role. Lymphocytosis in BAL fluid, and especially an increase in T lymphocytes, is seen in most cases of interstitial lung disease and thus may be useful only as an indicator of disease activity.[68]

Tuberculin testing is negative in 75% of sarcoidosis patients because of the depression of delayed-type hypersensitivity. A positive tuberculin test in a patient with sarcoidosis may suggest concomitant development of tuberculosis.

Changes in serum protein levels, with increased total protein and gamma globulin levels and decreased albumin levels, may be found in active sarcoidosis. Although serum calcium levels and urinary calcium excretion are elevated in a substantial number of patients at some stage, this finding is not of any diagnostic value.

The intraocular lesions more suggestive but not specific for sarcoidosis are mutton-fat keratic precipitates, iris nodules, trabecular meshwork nodules, tent-like peripheral anterior synechiae, "snowball" or "string-of-pearls" vitreous opacities, retinal perivasculitis with candle-wax drippings, and spotty retinochoroidal exudates.

Fluorescein angiography results are similar to other inflammatory diseases of the eye. The fluorescein study may reveal hyperfluorescent chorioretinal spots (Figs. 55–4 and 55–15), leakage and late staining of the retinal vessels, retinal nonperfusion and cystoid macular edema (Figs. 55–10, 55–11, and 55–13), retinal neovascularization (Fig. 55–11), and optic nerve inflammation (Figs. 55–4 and 55–15).

DIFFERENTIAL DIAGNOSIS

Since sarcoidosis has protean manifestations, the differential diagnosis of ocular sarcoidosis includes almost every cause of uveitis. Candle-wax drippings are seen in diffuse unilateral subacute neuroretinitis (DUSN). Sarcoid periphlebitis has features similar to frosted angiitis and must be differentiated from other causes of frosted angiitis, such as systemic lupus erythematosus and cytomegalovirus retinitis. Proliferative sarcoid retinopathy and vitreous hemorrhage must be distinguished from other possible causes of retinal ischemia, such as diabetic retinopathy, central retinal vein occlusion, sickle cell disease, and Behçet's disease.

An optic nerve mass or a solitary choroidal granuloma must be differentiated from other granulomatous diseases, such as tuberculosis and leprosy. A solitary choroidal mass must be also distinguished from a choroidal melanoma or a metastatic choroidal tumor. Papillitis and papilledema may require an extensive work-up for primary optic nerve disease, or compressive lesions of the optic nerve.

Vitritis is an important feature in reticulum cell sarcoma, Whipple's disease, and idiopathic pars planitis. Multifocal choroiditis, punctate inner choroidopathy, presumed ocular histoplasmosis syndrome, and serpiginous choroidopathy share some features with sarcoidosis as well. A fundus picture of birdshot chorioretinopathy, especially in a patient who is HLA-A29–negative, may actually be a manifestation of ocular sarcoidosis.

It is often very difficult to differentiate between sarcoidosis and any of these entities. A complete medical work-up, as mentioned above, and a prolonged follow-up are often necessary to make the exact diagnosis.

TREATMENT

In determining a treatment approach, it must be kept in mind that many patients with acute disease have spontaneous remission with little or no long-term sequelae. In general, the more acute the presentation of the inflammation associated with sarcoidosis, the more likely the patient is to demonstrate spontaneous remission. Intervention is clearly indicated with granulomatous anterior uveitis, involvement of the vitreous with secondary cystoid macular edema or media opacification, secondary glaucoma, proliferative retinopathy, and retinal detachment.

The mainstay of therapy is corticosteroids. Topical application for anterior segment involvement, local injection for mild degrees of posterior segment inflammation, or systemic administration of corticosteroids is quite beneficial. The majority of patients will respond to this form of therapy. Systemic steroid treatment is usually begun with prednisolone 40 mg/day. Higher doses are unnecessary and pulse therapy confers no extra benefit.[63] The dose of prednisolone should be tapered every 2 weeks to about 15 mg/day. If no clinical improvement occurs after 8 weeks of treatment, steroids may be withdrawn, as there is unlikely to be any response after this period. If any improvement is observed, a dose of 10 to 15 mg/day should be maintained for 6 to 8 months or until maximum benefit has been achieved. After this, attempts should be made to gradually reduce the dose to the lowest level in order to keep the disease under control.[69] In case of systemic involvement, simple parameters, such as chest radiographs and pulmonary function tests, can be used to guide clinical judgment.

For acute exudative disease, indomethacin or oxyphenbutazone may be used to enhance the therapeutic effect of steroids. Immunosuppressive agents have been used in aggressive disease with limited results and do not seem to confer any extra advantage over systemic steroid treatment.

General indications for systemic treatment in the

presence of isolated posterior segment ocular inflammation include severe visual loss from macular edema or severe vitritis, optic nerve involvement, choroidal granulomas, and retinal neovascularization. On the other hand, if the vision remains at a level of 20/40 or better and there are no complicating factors, systemic treatment may not be necessary.

In the case of proliferative sarcoid retinopathy, panretinal photocoagulation is usually required to achieve anatomic stabilization in most patients, although the visual prognosis is often poor. Steroid therapy should be used in combination with laser treatment to reduce the associated inflammation.

PROGNOSIS

The overall prognosis in sarcoidosis is good. In approximately 60% of all patients with thoracic sarcoidosis, spontaneous resolution occurs within 2 years. A further 20% of cases resolve with steroid treatment. In 10 to 20%, resolution is unlikely even with steroid treatment, and 50% of those in stage II and 80% of those in stage III have irreversible disease.[70]

The ocular response to steroid therapy in the case of acute sarcoid inflammation of both the anterior and posterior segments is usually good. Steroid therapy is tapered and discontinued as the active inflammation fades. Chronic disease of the anterior segment has a much worse prognosis, may require chronic topical steroid therapy, and may be complicated by glaucoma and cataract formation. Posterior segment disease usually has a better prognosis, but some cases may be complicated by cystoid macular edema, rhegmatogenous retinal detachment, retinal neovascularization, and vitreous hemorrhage. A few cases progress to optic atrophy and diffuse retinal ischemia (Fig. 55–19).

CONCLUSION

In conclusion, understanding ocular sarcoidosis requires a recognition that we are dealing with a widespread multiorgan system disease capable of producing an extensive variety of manifestations, both within and around the eye. Sarcoid should be in the differential diagnosis of any intraocular or adnexal inflammatory condition at initial presentation. It is one of the great mimickers in ophthalmology and may simulate or be associated with a number of other inflammatory diseases. Sarcoidosis may, in fact, not be one disease, but may represent a common inflammatory response to a number of different antigenic stimuli or infectious diseases. Rapid diagnosis and institution of therapy often results in control of the inflammatory process and a positive outcome. Re-evaluation for recurrence of symptoms is required over the long term.

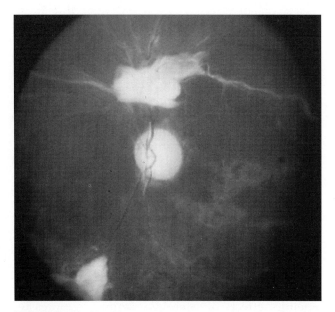

FIGURE 55–19 End-stage ocular sarcoidosis. Extensive sheathing of the vessels with fibrosis may occur in the end stage of ocular sarcoidosis. Note the extensive nonperfusion in this case with optic disc atrophy, fibrous material at the vascular arcades, and retinal epithelium atrophy.

REFERENCES

1. James DG, Timmis B, Barker S, Carstairs S: Radiology in sarcoidosis. Sarcoidosis 6:7–14, 1989.
2. Bruins Sllt WJ: Ziekte van Besnier-Boeck en Febris uveoparotidea (Heerfordt). Ned Tijdschr Geneeskd 80:2859, 1936.
3. Scadding JG, Mitchell DN: Sarcoidosis. 2nd edition. London, Chapman and Hall, 1985, pp 1–71.
4. Teirstein A, Lesser M: Worldwide distribution and epidemiology of sarcoidosis. In Fanburg BL (ed): Sarcoidosis and Other Granulomatous Diseases of the Lung. New York, Marcel Dekker Inc, 1983, pp 101–134.
5. Yamaguchi M, Hosoda Y, Sasaki A, et al: Epidemiological study on sarcoidosis in Japan. Sarcoidosis 6:138–146, 1989.
6. James DG, Neville E, Siltzbach LE, et al: A world view of sarcoidosis. Ann N Y Acad Sci 278:321–332, 1976.
7. Weissler JC: Southwestern internal medicine conference: sarcoidosis: immunology and clinical management. J Med Sci 307:233–245, 1994.
8. Lyons DJ, Fielding JF: What is in a relationship? Sarcoidosis and tuberculosis. Ir Med J 83:76–79, 1990.
9. Bunn DT, Johnston RN: A ten year study of sarcoidosis. Br J Dis Chest 66:45–52, 1972.
10. Brennan NJ, Crean P, Long JP, Fitzgerald MX: High prevalence of familial sarcoidosis in an Irish population. Thorax 39:14–18, 1984.
11. Vanek J, Schwarz J: Demonstration of acid fast rods in sarcoidosis. Am Rev Respir Dis 101:395–400, 1970.
12. Moscovic EA: Sarcoidosis and mycobacterial L forms. Pathol Ann 13:69–164, 1978.
13. Saboor SA, Johnson NMcI, McFadden JJ: Use of polymerase chain reaction and DNA probes in the diagnosis of sarcoidosis and tuberculosis (Abstract). Brtish Thoracic Society summer meeting. Thorax 46:743, 1991.
14. Saboor SA, McI Johnson N: Sarcoidosis. Br J Hosp Med 48: 293–302, 1992.
15. Branson JH, Park JH: Sarcoidosis: hepatic involvement. Ann Intern Med 40:11–45, 1954.

16. Jones Williams W: The nature and origin of Schaumann bodies. J Pathol Bacteriol 79:193–201, 1960.

17. James DG, Lebron REF: Update on sarcoidosis. Bull Intern Med 71:325–335, 1979.

18. Soskel NT, Fox R: Sarcoidosis ...or something like it. South Med J 83:1190–1203, 1990.

19. Mitchell DN, Scadding JG: Sarcoidosis. Am Rev Respir Dis 110:774–802, 1974.

20. Jones-Williams W, Erazmus DA, Valerie-James EM, Davies T: The fine structure of sarcoid and tuberculous granulomas. Postgrad Med J 46:496–500, 1970.

21. Mitchell DN, Scadding JG, Heard BE, Hinson KFW: Sarcoidosis: histopathological definition and clinical diagnosis. J Clin Pathol 30:395–408, 1977.

22. Siltzbach LE, James DG, Neville E, et al: Course and prognosis of sarcoidosis around the world. Am J Med 57:847–852, 1974.

23. Mayock RL, Bertrand P, Morrison CE, Scott JH: Manifestations of sarcoidosis. Analysis of 145 patients, with a review of nine series selected from the literature. Am J Med 35:67–89, 1963.

24. Katara YP, Shaw RA, Campbell PB: Sarcoidosis: an overview II. Clin Notes Respir Dis 20:3, 1982.

25. Sharma OP, Colp C, Williams MH Jr: Pulmonary function studies in patients with bilateral sarcoidosis of hilar lymph nodes. Arch Intern Med 117:436–439, 1966.

26. Athos L, Mohlar JG, Sharma OP: Exercise testing in physiologic assessment of sarcoidosis. Ann N Y Acad Sci 465:491–501, 1986.

27. Sharma OP, Johnson R: Airway obstruction in sarcoidosis: a study of 123 nonsmoking American black patients with sarcoidosis. Chest 94:343–346, 1988.

28. Sharma OP: Cutaneous sarcoidosis: clinical features and management. Chest 61:320–330, 1972.

29. Delaney P: Neurologic manifestations in sarcoidosis. Review of literature with a report of 23 cases. Ann Intern Med 87:336–345, 1987.

30. Sharma OP, Anders A: Neurosarcoidosis: a report of ten patients illustrating some usual and unusual manifestations. Sarcoidosis 2:96–100, 1988.

31. Graham E, James DG: Neurosarcoidosis. Sarcoidosis 5:125–131, 1988.

32. Fleming HA: Sarcoid heart disease. Sarcoidosis 2:20–21, 1985.

33. Flora G, Sharma OP: Myocardial sarcoidosis: a review. Sarcoidosis 2:20–24, 1985.

34. Pehrsson SK, Tornling G: Sarcoidosis associated with complete heart block. Sarcoidosis 2:135–141, 1985.

35. Stewart RE, Graham DM, Godfrey GW, et al: Rapidly progressive heart failure resulting from cardiac sarcoidosis. Am Heart J 115:1324–1326, 1988.

36. Silverman KJ, Hutchins GM, Buckley BH: Cardiac sarcoid: a clinicopathologic study of 84 unselected patients with systemic sarcoidosis. Circulation 58:1204–1215, 1978.

37. Obenauf CD, Shaw HE, Sydnor CF, Klintworth GK: Sarcoidosis and its ophthalmic manifestations. Am J Ophthalmol 86:648–655, 1978.

38. James DG, Anderson R, Langley D, Ainslie D: Ocular sarcoidosis. Br J Ophthalmol 48:461, 1964.

39. Karma A, Huhti E, Poukkula A: Course and outcome of ocular sarcoidosis. Am J Ophthalmol 106:467–472, 1988.

40. Could H, Kaufman HE: Sarcoid of the fundus. Arch Ophthalmol 65:453, 1961.

41. Letocha CE, Shields JA, Goldberg RE: Retinal changes in sarcoidosis. Can J Ophthalmol 10:184, 1975.

42. Vrabec TR, Augsburger JJ, Fischer DH, et al: Taches de Bougie. Ophthalmology 102:1712–1721, 1995.

43. Landers PH: Vitreous lesion observed in Boeck's sarcoid. Am J Ophthalmol 32:1740, 1949.

44. Crick RP: Ocular sarcoidosis. Trans Ophthalmol Soc U K 75:189, 1955.

45. Edelsten C, Stanford MR, Grahm EM: Serpiginous choroiditis: an unusual presentation of ocular sarcoidosis. Br J Ophthalmol 78:70–71, 1994.

46. Ohara K, Okubo A, Sasaki H, Kamata K: Branch retinal vein occlusion in a child with ocular sarcoidosis. Am J Ophthalmol 119:806–807, 1995.

47. DeRosa AJ, Margo CE, Orlick ME: Hemorrhagic retinopathy as the presenting manifestation of sarcoidosis. Retina 15:422–427, 1995.

48. Duker JS, Brown GC, McNamara JA: Proliferative sarcoid retinopathy. Ophthalmology 95:1680–1686, 1988.

49. Madigan JC Jr, Gragoudos ES, Schwartz PL, Lapus JV: Peripheral retinal neovascularization in sarcoidosis and sickle cell anemia. Am J Ophthalmol 83:387–391, 1977.

50. Frank KW, Weiss H: Unusual clinical and histopathological findings in ocular sarcoidosis. Br J Ophthalmol 67:8–16, 1983.

51. Gass JDM, Olson CL: Sarcoidosis with optic nerve and retinal involvement. Arch Ophthalmol 94:945–950, 1976.

52. Spalton DJ, Sanders MD: Fundus changes in histologically confirmed sarcoidosis. Br J Ophthalmol 65:348–358, 1981.

53. Tingey DP, Gonder JR: Ocular sarcoidosis presenting as a solitary choroidal mass. Can J Ophthalmol 27:25–29, 1992.

54. Westlake WH, Heath JD, Spalton DJ: Sarcoidosis involving the optic nerve and the hypothalamus. Arch Ophthalmol 113:669–670, 1995.

55. Brownstein S, Jannotta FS: Sarcoid granulomas of the optic nerve and retina. Can J Ophthalmol 9:372, 1974.

56. Jampol LM, Woodfin W, McLean EB: Optic nerve sarcoidosis. Report of a case. Arch Ophthalmol 87:355, 1972.

57. Kelley JS, Green WR: Sarcoidosis involving the optic nerve head. Arch Ophthalmol 89:476, 1973.

58. Laties AM, Scheie HG: Evolution of multiple small tumors in sarcoid granuloma of optic disk. Am J Ophthalmol 74:60, 1972.

59. Gass JDM, Olson CL: Sarcoidosis with optic nerve and retinal involvement. A clinicopathologic case report. Trans Am Acad Ophthalmol Otolaryngol 77:739, 1973.

60. Zeiter JH, Bhavsar A, McDermott ML, Siegel MJ: Ocular sarcoidosis manifesting as an anterior staphyloma. Am J Ophthalmol 112:345–347, 1991.

61. Henderson JW: Orbital Tumors. Philadelphia, WB Saunders Co, 1973, pp 580–588.

62. Reese AB: Tumors of the Eye, 3rd edition. New York, Harper & Row, 1976, pp 434–466.

63. Khan F, Wessely Z, Chazin SR, Seriff NS: Conjunctival biopsy in sarcoidosis. A simple, safe and specific diagnostic procedure. Ann Ophthalmol 9:671, 1977.

64. Spaide DR, Ward DL: Conjunctival biopsy in the diagnosis of sarcoidosis. Br J Ophthalmol 74:469–471, 1990.

65. DeRemee A: Concise review for primary-care physicians. Sarcoidosis. Mayo Clin Proc 70:177–181, 1995.

66. Ohara K, Okubo A, Kamata K, et al: Transbronchial lung biopsy in the diagnosis of suspected ocular sarcoidosis. Arch Ophthalmol 11:642–644, 1993.

67. Power WJ, Neves RA, Rodriguez A, et al: The value of combined serum angiotensin-converting enzyme and gallium scan in diagnosing ocular sarcoidosis. Ophthalmology 102:2007–2011, 1995.

68. Arnoux A, Danel C, Chretien J: Is bronchoalveolar lavage a mirror of granulomas in the lungs? Sarcoidosis 6:10–11, 1989.

69. Bascom R, Johns CJ: The natural history and management of ocular sarcoidosis. Adv Intern Med 31:213–241, 1986.

70. Moxham J, Costello JF: In Sohuami RL, Moxham J (eds): Textbook of Medicine. London, Churchill Livingstone, 1990, pp 506–511.

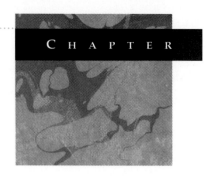

CHAPTER 56

Uveal Effusion

Mark W. Johnson, M.D.

The term "uveal" or "ciliochoroidal effusion" refers to an abnormal accumulation of serous fluid in the outer layer of the ciliary body and choroid. Generally, fluid collects between the delicate connective tissue fibers of the suprachoroidal layer, although in some cases cleavage of these fibers results in a true ciliochoroidal detachment from the sclera.[1] Clinically, the terms "effusion" and "detachment" are used interchangeably. Ciliochoroidal effusion does not refer to a specific entity, but rather to a pathoanatomic condition caused by a variety of ocular and systemic disorders. Because a chronic accumulation of protein-rich fluid in the choroid may result in breakdown of the retinal pigment epithelial fluid barrier, nonrhegmatogenous retinal detachment commonly accompanies ciliochoroidal effusion.

PATHOPHYSIOLOGY

Most cases of ciliochoroidal effusion can be classified into one of the following pathophysiologic categories: (1) hydrodynamic, (2) inflammatory, (3) neoplastic, or (4) associated with abnormal sclera. Despite thorough clinical evaluation, causative factors in occasional patients remain obscure and the effusion defies classification. A brief review of choroidal pathophysiology is helpful in understanding how uveal effusion develops in its various clinical contexts.

In the normal eye, an equilibrium exists between the transmural hydrostatic pressure gradient (difference between intravascular blood pressure and intraocular pressure) and the colloid osmotic pressure gradient of the choroidal capillaries (Fig. 56-1).[2] The osmotic pressure gradient, which draws fluid onto blood vessels and maintains relative dehydration of the suprachoroidal space, depends on a low extravascular colloid (albumin)

concentration.[3] Given the absence of lymphatic channels in the eye, albumin continuously escaping the fenestrated choroidal capillaries into the extravascular space must leave the choroid across the sclera.[4,5] The driving force for this transscleral bulk flow of proteinaceous fluid is the intraocular pressure.[5,6]

It follows from the above that each of the factors listed below alters choroidal fluid dynamics in such a way as to promote the formation of ciliochoroidal effusion. *Ocular hypotony* decreases the driving force for transscleral bulk flow and increases the transmural hydrostatic pressure gradient, both of which facilitate the accumulation of protein and fluid in the supraciliochoroidal space. *Increased uveal venous pressure* causes increased transudation across choroidal capillaries by increasing the transmural hydrostatic pressure gradient. *Inflammation* and other causes of vascular incompetence increase capillary protein permeability, allowing greater leakage of protein into the extravascular space. This effectively reduces the colloid osmotic absorptive force across capillary walls, favoring extravascular fluid retention. And finally, *abnormal scleral composition or thickness* may increase resistance to transscleral protein outflow, causing accumulation of proteinaceous fluid in the suprachoroid. When several factors are present simultaneously, clinical effusion is even more likely to occur. Indeed, production of ciliochoroidal effusion in animal models generally requires two or more pathophysiologic factors working in concert.[2,7,8]

CLINICAL EVALUATION

The past ocular and medical histories often reveal important clues about the cause of a ciliochoroidal effusion. A history of recent ocular surgery (especially glaucoma filtering or scleral buckling proce-

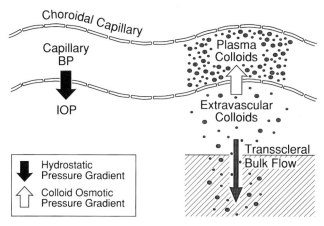

FIGURE 56–1 In normal choroidal capillaries, the transmural hydrostatic pressure gradient is in equilibrium with the colloid osmotic pressure gradient. Colloids escaping the fenestrated capillaries move across the sclera by bulk flow, driven by the intraocular pressure (IOP). (From Biomedical Communications, University of Michigan, with permission.)

dures) or panretinal photocoagulation suggests the probable pathogenesis. Similarly, a history of prior ocular or head trauma should prompt a search for evidence of a cyclodialysis cleft, arteriovenous fistula, or other posttraumatic causes of uveal effusion. Complaints of light flashes or new floaters suggest the possibility of rhegmatogenous retinal detachment with secondary ciliochoroidal detachment. The patient should be questioned regarding symptoms of uveal, scleral, or orbital inflammation to help exclude primary inflammatory causes. In a few patients, clues to the etiology may be found in the medical history, including cardiovascular and renal status; systemic malignancy; or history of human immunodeficiency virus (HIV) infection, connective tissue disease, or myxedema.

The refractive error may be helpful diagnostically in selected patients. An acute myopic shift, resulting from anterior displacement of the lens-iris diaphragm, may be the initial clue to the presence of uveal effusion. Alternatively, high hyperopia suggests an underlying diagnosis of nanophthalmos.

Several anterior segment findings can be helpful in classifying a ciliochoroidal effusion. Dilation of the episcleral veins may be seen in conditions involving increased uveal venous pressure, including cavernous sinus arteriovenous fistulae, Sturge-Weber syndrome, nanophthalmos, and the idiopathic uveal effusion syndrome. In the postoperative or posttraumatic setting, the clinician must exclude a wound leak, filtering bleb, or cyclodialysis cleft as the cause of persistent hypotony precipitating the effusion. Unexplained shallowing or closure of the anterior chamber angle is the physical finding in some cases that initially suggests the presence of an effusion. Finally, significant anterior segment inflammation may suggest a uveitic cause, such as Harada's syndrome, sympathetic ophthalmia, or pars planitis.

Intraocular pressure in eyes with ciliochoroidal effusion may be low, normal, or elevated. In most cases, the intraocular pressure is low, either as a primary or secondary phenomenon. When an obvious cause of decreased intraocular pressure is present (wound leak, filtering bleb, cyclodialysis cleft, rhegmatogenous retinal detachment), the ciliochoroidal effusion probably resulted from preexisting hypotony. Once established, uveal effusion typically perpetuates hypotony by causing ciliary body hyposecretion, increased uveoscleral outflow, or both.[5] The intraocular pressure is typically normal in the idiopathic uveal effusion syndrome and nanophthalmic uveal effusion, presumably owing to diminished uveoscleral outflow through thickened or otherwise abnormal sclera. Some cases of ciliochoroidal effusion present with anterior chamber angle closure and increased intraocular pressure.[9] This is most likely to occur in eyes with impaired venous drainage or inflammation as the primary pathogenic factor, as seen in association with arteriovenous fistula, nanophthalmos, scleral buckling surgery, panretinal photocoagulation, or sclerouveitis.

Ophthalmoscopically, ciliochoroidal detachments are brown-orange, solid-appearing elevations with smooth, convex surfaces (Fig. 56–2). Their serous nature can readily be demonstrated with transillumination of the globe. The solid appearance of choroidal detachments derives from the fact that, unlike rhegmatogenous retinal detachments, they do not undulate appreciably with eye movements. Early or mild effusions generally present as shallow elevations of the pars plana and peripheral choroid; their detection is aided by a clearly visible ora serrata without the use of scleral depression (Fig. 56–3). Larger effusions may be annular or lobular, the characteristic four-lobed configuration resulting from the attachment of the choroid to the sclera at

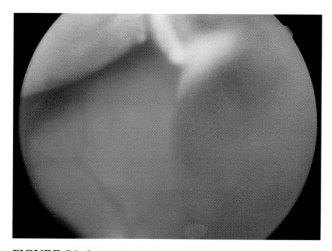

FIGURE 56–2 Multilobed ciliochoroidal effusion, demonstrating characteristic solid-appearing choroidal elevations with smooth, convex surfaces. (From Johnson MW: Ciliochoroidal effusions. In Margo CE, Hamed LF, Mames RN (eds): Diagnostic Problems in Clinical Ophthalmology. Philadelphia, WB Saunders Co, 1994, pp 373–381.)

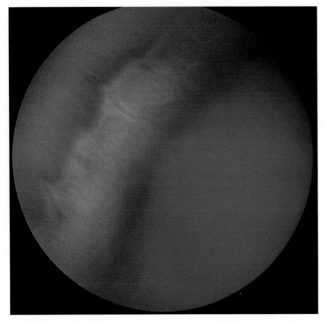

FIGURE 56–3 Mild, annular ciliochoroidal effusion. The ora serrata is visible without scleral depression. (From Johnson MW: Ciliochoroidal effusions. In Margo CE, Hamed LF, Mames RN (eds): Diagnostic Problems in Clinical Ophthalmology. Philadelphia, WB Saunders Co, 1994, pp 373–381.)

the vortex vein ampullae. In all ciliochoroidal effusions there is greater fluid accumulation anteriorly, owing to the anatomy of the connective tissue fibers attaching choroid to the sclera. The anterior connecting fibers are long and tangentially oriented, whereas those in the posterior fundus are short and run more directly from uvea to sclera.[10]

With longstanding ciliochoroidal effusion there is decompensation of the retinal pigment epithelial fluid barrier, with spillover of protein and fluid into the subretinal space resulting in nonrhegmatogenous retinal detachment (Fig. 56–4). As the subretinal protein concentration rises over time, the sub-

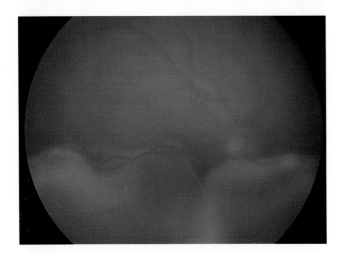

FIGURE 56–4 Gravitationally dependent nonrhegmatogenous retinal detachment in a patient with the idiopathic uveal effusion syndrome.

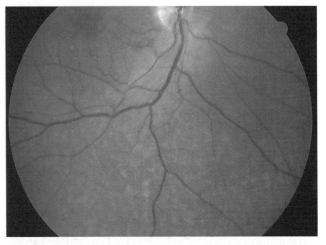

FIGURE 56–5 "Leopard-spot" fundus pigmentation in a patient with a history of the idiopathic uveal effusion syndrome.

retinal fluid becomes heavy and shifts markedly with change in head position. Progressive subretinal fluid accumulation may lead to massive, total retinal detachment. Damage from chronic effusion and secondary retinal detachment may result in widespread depigmentation with multifocal hyperplasia of the retinal pigment epithelium ("leopard spots") (Fig. 56–5).

Because ciliochoroidal effusion may complicate malignant hypertension secondary to renal failure,[11,12] a blood pressure determination should be included in the evaluation of all patients with unexplained effusion.

LABORATORY AND ANCILLARY TESTING

Ophthalmic ultrasound may be helpful in confirming the diagnosis of ciliochoroidal effusion and determining its cause. B-scan echography typically reveals a smooth, thick, dome-shaped membrane with little aftermovement (Fig. 56–6).[13] In contrast to retinal detachment, ciliochoroidal effusion can usually be seen to extend anterior to the ora serrata. Highly bullous ciliochoroidal detachments may extend posteriorly to insert near the edge of, but not directly into, the optic disc. A-scan evaluation demonstrates a thick, 100% spike at tissue sensitivity, which at low sensitivity can often be seen to be double-peaked (Fig. 56–6).[13] High-frequency ultrasound biomicroscopy may demonstrate subtle degrees of supraciliary effusion undetected by B-scan ultrasound and fundus examination.[14] This sensitive imaging modality may prove increasingly useful in defining and treating mechanisms of glaucoma complicating uveal effusions.

Most entities causing ciliochoroidal detachment also produce diffuse thickening of the posterior choroid,[15] which is best appreciated echographi-

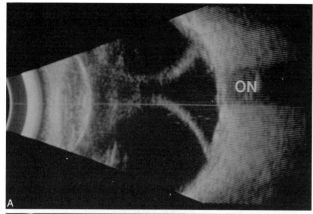

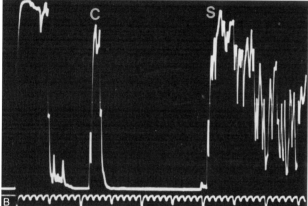

FIGURE 56–6   *A,* Axial B-scan echogram of ciliochoroidal effusion demonstrates smooth, thick, dome-shaped membranes inserting near, but not into, the optic nerve (ON). *B,* Standardized A-scan at tissue sensitivity shows thick, double-peaked retinochoroidal spike (C) with absence of internal echos. S, sclera. (From Johnson MW: Ciliochoroidal effusions. In Margo CE, Hamed LF, Mames RN (eds): Diagnostic Problems in Clinical Ophthalmology. Philadelphia, WB Saunders Co, 1994, pp 373–381.)

cally at low-sensitivity (high-resolution) setting. In general, high-reflective thickening suggests edema, as seen with hypotony, uveitis, posterior scleritis, postoperative effusion, and idiopathic and nanophthalmic effusion. Low-reflective thickening is seen with infiltrative and neoplastic entities such as Harada's syndrome, sympathetic ophthalmia, metastatic tumors, lymphoid infiltrations, and diffuse melanomas.[13]

Although fluorescein angiography has relatively limited diagnostic value in ciliochoroidal effusions, multiple pinpoint fluorescein leaks through the retinal pigment epithelium suggest inflammatory or neoplastic choroidal infiltration as the underlying cause. Neuroradiologic imaging is helpful in confirming the occasional diagnosis of carotid-cavernous or dural arteriovenous fistula.

Other laboratory tests are generally reserved for the systemic evaluation of patients with uveal effusion secondary to uveitis, posterior scleritis, or neoplastic choroidal infiltration. In the absence of inflammatory conditions or suspected neoplasia, laboratory tests for rare associations of ciliocho-

roidal effusion such as myxedema[16] or multiple myeloma[1] are unlikely to be fruitful.

CLASSIFICATION

Given that any disorder producing generalized edema or infiltration of the choroid may result in serous ciliochoroidal elevation, the differential diagnosis of diffuse choroidal thickening is virtually identical to that of ciliochoroidal effusion. The clinical entities that cause these two ocular conditions are most logically categorized by primary pathogenic factor (Table 56–1).[17] As noted above, effusions generally form only when several factors are operating simultaneously.

Hydrodynamic Effusions

Ocular Hypotony

Persistent ocular hypotony from any cause can induce ciliochoroidal effusion, which in turn tends to

TABLE 56–1   Classification of Ciliochoroidal Effusion

Hydrodynamic Factors
  Ocular hypotony
    Wound leak
    Glaucoma filter
    Cyclodialysis cleft
    Penetrating ocular trauma
    Rhegmatogenous retinal detachment
    Ciliary body dysfunction (traction, ischemia)
  Elevated uveal venous pressure
    Arteriovenous fistula
    Sturge-Weber syndrome
    Idiopathic prominent episcleral vessels
    Vortex vein compression by scleral buckle
    Valsalva's maneuver
  Malignant hypertension

Inflammatory Factors
  After trauma or surgery
  After photocoagulation or cryotherapy
  Drug reaction
  Uveitis
  Scleritis
  Orbital cellulitis/pseudotumor

Neoplastic Conditions
  Metastatic carcinoma
  Malignant melanoma
  Lymphoid, leukemic, or melanocytic choroidal
    infiltrations

Secondary to Abnormal Sclera
  Nanophthalmos
  Mucopolysaccharidosis
  Idiopathic uveal effusion syndrome

exacerbate and perpetuate the hypotony. Ciliochoroidal effusion occurring during intraocular surgery probably results from low intraocular pressure combined with other factors such as increased uveal venous pressure and/or increased choroidal vascular permeability.[18-20] When hypotony and uveal effusion follow anterior segment intraocular surgery, careful examination will generally reveal a wound leak or inadvertent filtering bleb.[21,22] Similarly, when unexplained uveal effusion complicates hypotony in any setting, the presence of a cyclodialysis cleft must be excluded by careful gonioscopy. A goniolens with a 2- to 3-mm flange allows the application of suction on the cornea, thereby opening and facilitating visualization of the anterior chamber angle in hypotonous eyes. The effusion typically resolves after closing the wound leak or cyclodialysis cleft. Drainage of suprachoroidal fluid may rarely be needed to help break the hypotony-effusion-hypotony cycle, and systemic corticosteroids are sometimes helpful in reducing inflammation and choroidal vascular permeability.

Transient ciliochoroidal effusion not infrequently follows glaucoma filtering surgery in the early postoperative period and may be accompanied by nonrhegmatogenous retinal detachment (Fig. 56-7).[23] Less commonly, uveal effusion after filtration surgery may be chronic or recurrent,[24] or may occur late after surgery following the reintroduction of aqueous suppressant medication.[25] Ciliochoroidal detachment and flattening of the anterior chamber due to overfiltration often resolves spontaneously or with a glaucoma shell. Suprachoroidal fluid drainage with reformation of the anterior chamber is occasionally necessary in persistent cases.

Penetrating ocular trauma and perforated corneal ulcers commonly combine hypotony with inflammation to precipitate ciliochoroidal detachment. Rhegmatogenous retinal detachment may also result in hypotony and secondary uveal effusion. The presence of large choroidal detachments

may obscure the diagnosis in such cases by hindering the identification of retinal breaks. Other clues, such as retinal hydration lines, nonshifting subretinal fluid, and early proliferative vitreoretinopathy, may be helpful in differentiating primary rhegmatogenous retinal detachment from exudative retinal detachment secondary to ciliochoroidal effusion. Vitrectomy techniques offer significant technical advantages over scleral buckling alone in treating retinal detachment complicated by significant ciliochoroidal effusion.

Various causes of ciliary body dysfunction that result in hypotony may also lead to uveal effusion. Traction on ciliary processes adherent to posterior capsule and lens remnants has been postulated as a mechanism for delayed ciliochoroidal detachment after cataract surgery.[26] Posterior capsulotomy may be curative in such cases. Traction on the ciliary body is also caused by fibrous membrane proliferation in conditions such as uveitis and anterior proliferative vitreoretinopathy. Occasional patients with ocular ischemia due to carotid disease develop uveal effusion that resolves after carotid endarterectomy.

Elevated Uveal Venous Pressure

Carotid-cavernous or dural arteriovenous fistulas may lead to ciliochoroidal effusion and nonrhegmatogenous retinal detachment, presumably on the basis of uveal venous hypertension and increased transudation from choroidal vessels.[27] Signs and symptoms that suggest the underlying diagnosis include headache or orbital pain, exophthalmos, arterialization of conjunctival vessels, chemosis, diplopia, and increased intraocular pressure (Fig. 56-8). A bruit may or may not be audible. When spontaneous uveal effusion is accompanied by such findings, neuroradiologic imaging is indicated. Spontaneous thrombosis of the fistula may occur, leading to resolution of ocular signs and symptoms. In persistent, vision-threatening cases, embolization

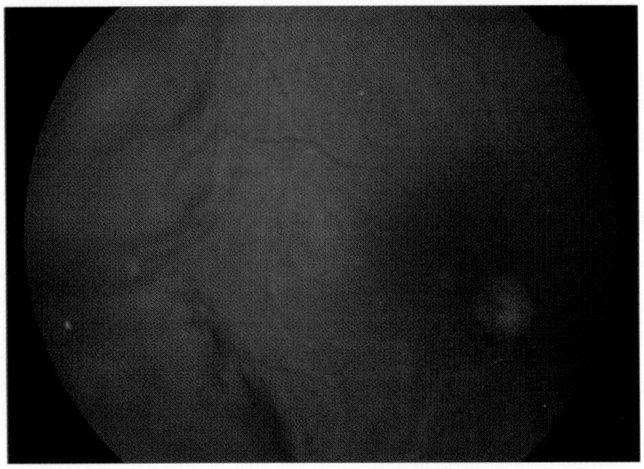

FIGURE 56-7 Diffuse choroidal thickening (note choroidal folds) and peripheral ciliochoroidal detachment following glaucoma filtering surgery.

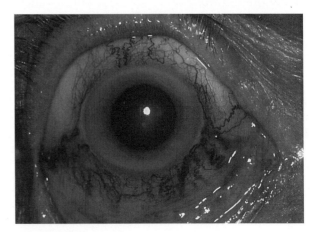

FIGURE 56-8 Arterialization of conjunctival vessels in patient with cavernous sinus arteriovenous fistula.

of the fistula by interventional radiologic techniques may be indicated.

Massive ciliochoroidal detachment may occur during intraocular surgery on patients with unusually prominent episcleral vessels, either idiopathic or associated with the Sturge-Weber syndrome.[18] Elevation of the episcleral venous pressure can be demonstrated in such patients and is assumed to reflect elevated choroidal and ciliary body venous pressure. When the intraocular pressure drops to zero at surgery, a large transmural hydrostatic pressure differential is created in the choriocapillaris, favoring increased filtration of fluid into the extravascular space with rapid development of ciliochoroidal effusion. Prophylactic sclerostomies should be considered during anterior segment surgery in such eyes, as discussed below for nanophthalmos.

Compromise of vortex venous outflow is one of several factors promoting the formation of ciliochoroidal effusion following scleral buckling surgery (Fig. 56–9). Clinical and experimental studies have demonstrated that older age, cryotherapy or diathermy, and intraoperative hypotony after subretinal fluid drainage are additional factors that correlate with the development of postoperative uveal effusion.[7,8,28] Ciliochoroidal effusion in this setting typically appears within several days of surgery and may occasionally be accompanied by vitreous haze and nonrhegmatogenous retinal detachment with shifting subretinal fluid. Although it is generally limited in extent, massive exudative retinal and choroidal detachment with severe ocular pain is occasionally seen within the first 2 weeks postoperatively.[29] Systemic corticosteroids may be helpful in severe cases. If nonpupillary block angle closure complicates the effusion and fails to resolve after 1 week of cycloplegics and topical corticosteroids, argon laser iris retraction may facilitate opening of the angle and prevent synechial closure.[30]

Transient bilateral ciliochoroidal detachments have been reported after several severe and prolonged episodes of emesis.[31] The postulated mechanism is Valsalva-induced elevation of episcleral venous pressure sufficient to increase the filtration rate across the choroidal capillary bed.

Malignant Hypertension

Nonrhegmatogenous retinal detachment and ciliochoroidal effusion, with or without nonpupillary block angle closure, may be seen in the setting of severe renal hypertension[11,12,32] or pregnancy-induced hypertension. It is likely that the pathogenesis of uveal effusions complicating hypertension is multifactorial, with reduced serum oncotic pressure and immune-mediated vascular permeability alterations playing a role in some cases.[32] Histopathologic examination demonstrates inflammation and necrosis of choroidal arterioles and capillaries with disruption of the retinal pigment epithelium. Subretinal and suprachoroidal fluid accumulations resolve as the blood pressure is brought under control.

Inflammatory Effusions

After Trauma or Surgery

Traumatic ciliochoroidal effusion typically occurs in the setting of penetrating ocular injuries, where inflammation is combined with hypotony. Self-limited uveal effusion may also be seen after blunt trauma in the absence of ocular penetration or cyclodialysis.[33,34] When prolonged hypotony and ciliochoroidal effusion follow ocular trauma, the presence of a cyclodialysis cleft must be excluded by meticulous gonioscopy.

Animal studies have demonstrated that accumulation of suprachoroidal fluid is generally not seen with either hypotony or surgical trauma alone.[2] Thus, uveal effusion following intraocular surgery typically occurs when hypotony is combined with compromise of choroidal capillary integrity by surgically induced inflammation and advanced age. Such effusions typically develop within days or weeks after surgery and resolve as the intraocular pressure is normalized and inflammation subsides. Rarely, ciliochoroidal effusion occurs months or years after cataract surgery. Possible mechanisms include low-grade inflammation with increased vascular permeability owing to mechanical irritation by ciliary sulcus-fixated haptics,[35] and traction on ciliary processes adherent to posterior capsule and lens remnants.[26] Systemic steroid therapy may be curative in the absence of ciliary body traction.

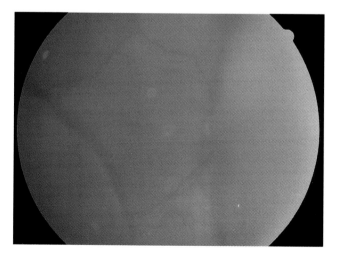

FIGURE 56–9   Large, multilobed choroidal detachments 5 days after an encircling scleral buckle procedure.

After Photocoagulation or Cryotherapy

Thermal injury from panretinal photocoagulation or transscleral cryotherapy increases choroidal vas-

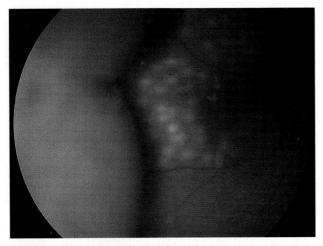

FIGURE 56–10 Ciliochoroidal effusion in eye recently treated with argon laser panretinal photocoagulation.

cular permeability, promoting suprachoroidal fluid accumulation (Fig. 56–10). Ciliochoroidal effusion is more likely to develop with extensive treatment, occurring in as many as two thirds of diabetic eyes receiving standard argon laser panretinal photocoagulation in a single session.[36] Uveal effusion following laser or cryotherapy is generally transient and benign, but may occasionally cause acute angle-closure glaucoma.

Drug Reaction

Acute transient myopia has been reported as a rare, apparently idiosyncratic reaction to various drugs, including sulfonamides and sulfonamide derivatives.[37] Affected patients have generally been young or middle aged and present with acute myopic shift and shallowing of the anterior chamber with or without angle closure. Symptoms and signs resolve within days of stopping the medication. Ciliochoroidal effusion has been documented echographically in such cases,[38] implicating forward rotation of the ciliary body at the scleral spur with anterior displacement of the lens-iris diaphragm as a mechanism for myopia. Increased ciliochoroidal vascular permeability secondary to a hypersensitivity reaction is a plausible explanation for the effusion, particularly since patients typically have a history of taking the responsible drug previously without noticeable side effects.[37]

Uveitis

Conditions that result in uveal inflammation may also produce uveal effusion with nonrhegmatogenous retinal detachment. When signs of uveal effusion are accompanied by vitritis or chorioretinitis, the spectrum of uveitic syndromes must be considered in the differential diagnosis, including Harada's syndrome,[39] sympathetic ophthalmia, pars planitis,[40] syphilis,[41] and toxoplasmosis.[1] The un-

derlying diagnosis is usually determined by a careful history, physical examination, and appropriate serologic testing. Fluorescein angiography may be helpful in detecting choroidal inflammatory infiltration in Harada's syndrome and sympathetic ophthalmia. Anti-inflammatory and/or antimicrobial therapy appropriate for the specific uveitic condition is generally accompanied by resolution of the effusion.

Scleral and Orbital Inflammation

Scleritis must be suspected as the condition underlying ciliochoroidal effusion when the presenting eye is painful and/or red.[42,43] Posterior chorioretinal folds may suggest posterior scleritis even in the absence of ocular pain and hyperemia. Angle-closure glaucoma may develop secondary to a scleritis-induced annular ciliochoroidal detachment.[43] Ultrasound is a sensitive modality for confirming the diagnosis of posterior scleritis. Thickening of the sclera and choroid is seen in association with posterior episcleral edema, an echographic finding that is virtually pathognomonic for this condition.[13] Evaluation for an associated rheumatologic or systemic inflammatory condition is warranted in patients diagnosed with scleritis. This should include testing for HIV, as bilateral uveal effusion with or without evidence of posterior scleritis has been reported as a presenting sign of this infection.[44,45] Treatment of the scleritis with appropriate anti-inflammatory medication generally results in prompt resolution of the uveal effusion.

Ciliochoroidal effusion in an eye previously subjected to scleral buckling surgery must raise suspicion of a buckle infection with secondary scleral inflammation. Adequate treatment for such infections almost always requires removal of the buckle components. Uveal effusion may also accompany orbital inflammation such as pseudotumor or cellulitis, probably as a result of contiguous scleritis or compromise of the vortex venous blood flow.

Neoplastic Effusions

Though uncommon, ciliochoroidal effusion may be seen in eyes with choroidal metastatic tumors or malignant melanoma (Fig. 56–11).[46] In some cases, the secondary choroidal or retinal detachment is so extensive that echography is required to detect the underlying tumor. In other cases, diffuse choroidal thickening is subtle and detected only with echography. Choroidal neoplastic infiltrations that cause uveal thickening, serous retinal detachment, and occasionally ciliochoroidal detachment include leukemia, lymphoma, reactive lymphoid hyperplasia, and paraneoplastic uveal melanocytic proliferation. These entities can generally be differentiated by a careful medical history and systemic evaluation.

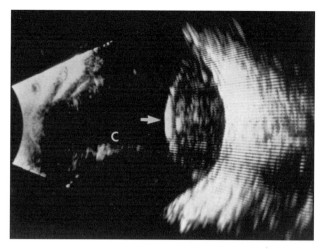

FIGURE 56–11 Presumed metastatic choroidal tumor with associated choroidal effusion in patient with prostatic carcinoma. Notice dome-shaped tumor (*arrow*) with choroidal detachment (C) extending from tumor margin. (From Sneed SR, Byrne SF, Mieler WF, et al: Choroidal detachment associated with malignant choroidal tumors. Ophthalmology 98:963–970, 1991, with permission.)

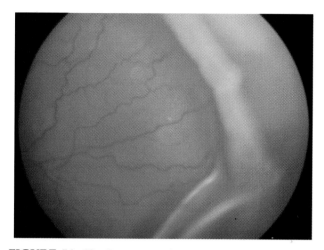

FIGURE 56–12 Spontaneously-occurring peripheral annular ciliochoroidal detachment associated with inferior nonrhegmatogenous retinal detachment in a 36-year-old man with nanophthalmos.

Effusions Secondary to Abnormal Sclera

Nanophthalmos

Nanophthalmos, a pure form of microphthalmia, is a rare disorder in which both eyes are small but unassociated with other ocular or systemic abnormalities. Autosomal dominant and recessive inheritance patterns have been described. Characteristic features include a small eye (axial length generally <20 mm), small corneal diameter, high hyperopia (refractive error +7.00 diopters or greater), shallow anterior chamber, high lens/eye volume ratio, extremely thick sclera, and strong predisposition to develop angle-closure glaucoma.[47]

Ciliochoroidal effusion and nonrhegmatogenous retinal detachment may arise spontaneously and frequently complicate intraocular surgery in nanophthalmic eyes (Fig. 56–12).[47,48] The pathogenesis of uveal effusion in these eyes probably involves increased resistance to both protein movement and venous outflow through the abnormal sclera, which often measures 2.5 mm in thickness.[48] Clinical recognition of such eyes prior to intraocular surgery is critical, given their high complication rate and the efficacy of prophylactic sclerectomy with or without vortex vein decompression.[49,50] In patients with spontaneous nanophthalmic uveal effusion and nonrhegmatogenous retinal detachment, a scleral resection procedure is indicated. As originally described by Brockhurst,[17] this procedure includes decompression of the vortex veins. Simple lamellar sclerectomy and sclerostomy without vortex vein decompression may also be effective.[51]

Mucopolysaccharidosis

Ciliochoroidal effusion with nonrhegmatogenous detachment may occur in patients with systemic mucopolysaccharidoses such as Maroteaux-Lamy syndrome and Hunter's syndrome.[52] In these conditions, deposition of mucopolysaccharide markedly thickens the sclera and interferes with transscleral protein transfer and vortex venous outflow. Although rare, such effusions appear to respond to lamellar sclerectomy and sclerotomy procedures.

Idiopathic Uveal Effusion Syndrome

The idiopathic uveal effusion syndrome is characterized by the insidious onset of ciliochoroidal and secondary retinal detachment in healthy middle-aged men. Other common findings include bilateral involvement, normal-sized eyes, dilation of the episcleral veins, normal intraocular pressure, mild vitreous cells, marked shifting of the subretinal fluid, and leopard-spot pigment epithelial alterations (Fig. 56–13).[53–55] Thickened sclera is present in a majority of patients.[55] Fluorescein angiography highlights the pigment epithelial alterations and typically demonstrates absence of active retinal pigment epithelial leaks (Fig. 56–14). The natural course tends to be prolonged, with remissions and exacerbations leading to a relentless decline in visual function. The diagnosis is based on characteristic clinical findings and exclusion of the other known causes of uveal effusion described in this chapter.

There is increasing evidence that the pathogenesis of this disorder involves the abnormal accumulation of proteoglycan (predominantly dermatan sulphate) in the sclera.[55,56] The proteoglycan deposits and resulting scleral thickening impede the bulk flow of protein across the sclera and inhibit venous drainage through the vortex veins, resulting in the accumulation of protein-rich fluid in the choroid and suprachoroidal space. It is probable that the accumulation of scleral proteoglycan results from a primary defect in scleral fibroblast metabolism and

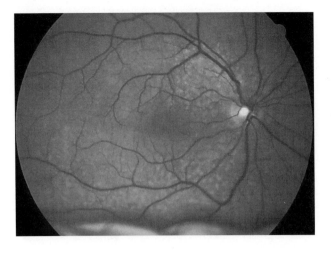

FIGURE 56–13 Idiopathic uveal effusion syndrome. Notice subtle, diffuse yellow leopard-spot pigmentary changes and dependent, nonrhegmatogenous retinal detachment inferiorly. (From Johnson MW: Ciliochoroidal effusions. In Margo CE, Hamed LF, Mames RN (eds): Diagnostic Problems in Clinical Ophthalmology. Philadelphia, WB Saunders Co, 1994, pp 373–381.)

may represent an ocular form of mucopolysaccharidosis.[56] Similar considerations may apply to nanophthalmic eyes, since studies of nanophthalmic sclera have also revealed abnormal proteogylcan synthesis with associated alterations of collagen fibers.[57]

The high success rate of surgical treatment employing quadrantic lamellar sclerectomies without vortex vein decompression further supports the theory that increased resistance to transscleral protein movement plays a primary pathophysiologic role in this disorder.[55,56] Scleral resection typically

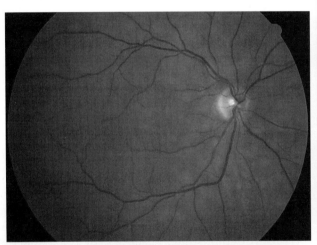

A

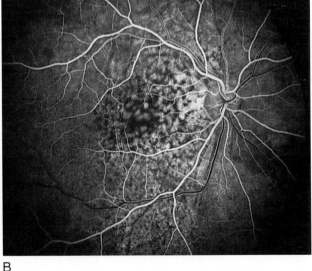

B

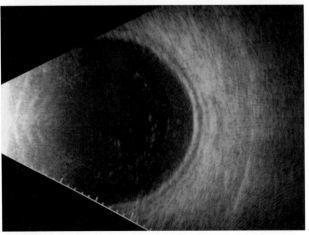

C

FIGURE 56–14 Fundus photograph (*A*) and fluorescein angiogram (*B*) of right eye of 53-year-old man with idiopathic uveal effusion in early stages (before extensive retinal detachment). Note prominent leopard-spot angiographic changes in posterior pole. B-scan echography showed diffuse choroidal thickening (*C*).

results in the prompt disappearance of the ciliocho-roidal detachment and slow resolution of the highly proteinaceous subretinal fluid. In patients with massive nonrhegmatogenous retinal detach-ment, consideration should be given to internal drainage of subretinal fluid at the time of the scler-ectomy procedure, in order to hasten retinal reat-tachment and reduce the degree of irreversible macular damage.[58]

Idiopathic Effusions

In addition to the pathogenic mechanisms dis-cussed above, unidentified factors almost certainly play primary or contributory roles in select cases of ciliochoroidal effusion. It is doubtful that all pa-tients classified as having idiopathic uveal effusion share a common scleral abnormality. It is hoped that further observation and research will identify additional pathophysiologic mechanisms and en-hance our understanding of this enigmatic group of patients.

SIMULATING CONDITIONS

Ciliochoroidal effusion is not infrequently mistaken for malignant melanoma of the choroid. Rarely, a malignant melanoma undetected prior to cataract surgery may simulate a postoperative choroidal de-tachment. Both entities may present in either ring or lobular configurations and be associated with nonrhegmatogenous retinal detachment. Transillu-mination and ultrasonography generally allow clear differentiation between serous choroidal de-tachments and solid choroidal elevations. One should bear in mind, however, that nonpigmented choroidal tumors, similar to ciliochoroidal effusion, may fail to block and may even enhance trans-illumination.

Ciliochoroidal effusion should be differentiated from hemorrhagic choroidal detachment, particu-larly in the postoperative and posttraumatic set-tings. The sudden onset of severe eye pain associ-ated with massive choroidal detachments suggests the diagnosis of delayed postoperative suprachor-roidal hemorrhage. In hemorrhagic choroidal de-tachment, echography reveals multiple low to me-dium reflective echos in the suprachoroidal space. These are absent in serous ciliochoroidal detach-ment. Blockage of transillumination also helps con-firm the presence of blood in the suprachoroidal space.

In a hypotonous eye, scleral infolding may clin-ically simulate ciliochoroidal detachment. In gen-eral, scleral infolding produces indentations that are less uniformly convex and more angular than those seen with ciliochoroidal detachment. When the diagnosis is not apparent clinically, ultrasonog-

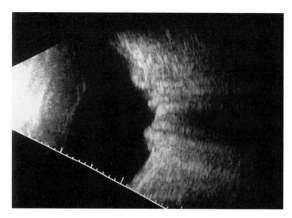

FIGURE 56–15 B-scan echogram of scleral infolding after glaucoma filtration surgery. Note lack of separation between retina-choroid layer and sclera.

raphy readily differentiates these two entities (Fig. 56–15).

Rarely, serous macular detachment may precede the onset of clinically detectable ciliochoroidal ef-fusion in the idiopathic uveal effusion syndrome. Such cases may initially be confused with central serous chorioretinopathy. Fluorescein angiography in the uveal effusion syndrome typically shows an absence of retinal pigment epithelial leaks, in con-trast to the usual case of central serous chorioretin-opathy. Ultrasonography may also help distinguish between these entities by demonstrating diffuse choroidal thickening or shallow serous elevation of the peripheral choroid and ciliary body in cases of uveal effusion.

REFERENCES

1. Green WR: The uveal tract. In Spencer WH (ed): Ophthal-mic Pathology. Philadelphia, WB Saunders Co, 1986, pp 1776–1791.
2. Capper SA, Leopold IH: Mechanism of serous choroidal detachment. Arch Ophthalmol 55:101–113, 1956.
3. Toris CB, Pederson JE, Tsuboi S, et al: Extravascular albu-min concentration of the uvea. Invest Ophthalmol Vis Sci 31:43–53, 1990.
4. Inomata H, Bill A: Exit sites of uveoscleral flow of aqueous humor in cynomolgus monkey eyes. Exp Eye Res 25:113–118, 1977.
5. Brubaker RF, Pederson JE: Ciliochoroidal detachment. Surv Ophthalmol 27:281–289, 1983.
6. Alm A, Bill A: Ocular circulation. In Moses RA, Hart WM Jr (ed): Adler's Physiology of the Eye. Clinical Application. St Louis, CV Mosby Co, 1987, p 199.
7. Hawkins WR, Schepens CL: Choroidal detachment and retinal surgery: a clinical and experimental study. Am J Ophthalmol 62:813–819, 1966.
8. Aaberg TM, Maggiano JM: Choroidal edema associated with retinal detachment repair: experimental and clinical correlation. Mod Probl Ophthalmol 20:6–15, 1979.
9. Fourman S: Angle-closure glaucoma complicating ciliocho-roidal detachment. Ophthalmology 96:646–653, 1989.
10. Moses RA: Detachment of ciliary body—anatomical and physical considerations. Invest Ophthalmol Vis Sci 4:935–941, 1965.
11. Friedman E, Smith TR, Kuwabara T, Beyer CK: Choroidal

vascular patterns in hypertension. Arch Ophthalmol 71: 842–850, 1964.

12. Arora R, Verma L, Kumar A: Renal hypertension presenting as acute angle closure glaucoma. Arch Ophthalmol 109:776, 1991.

13. Green RL, Byrne SF: Diagnostic ophthalmic ultrasound. In Ryan SJ (ed): Retina. St Louis, CV Mosby Co, 1989, pp 225–230.

14. Pavlin CJ, Easterbrook M, Harasiewicz K, Foster FS: An ultrasound biomicroscopic analysis of angle-closure glaucoma secondary to ciliochoroidal effusion in IgA nephropathy. Am J Ophthalmol 116:341–345, 1993.

15. Wing GL, Schepens CL, Trempe CL, Weiter JJ: Serous choroidal detachment and the thickened-choroid sign detected by ultrasongraphy. Am J Ophthalmol 94:499–505, 1982.

16. Richardson J, Walsh M: Uveal effusion as a sign of myxoedema. Br J Ophthalmol 53:557–560, 1969.

17. Brockhurst RJ: Vortex vein decompression for nanophthalmic uveal effusion. Arch Ophthalmol 98:1987–1990, 1980.

18. Bellows AR, Chylack LT, Epstein DL, Hutchinson BT: Choroidal effusion during glaucoma surgery in patients with prominent episcleral vessels. Arch Ophthalmol 97:493–497, 1979.

19. Ruiz RS, Salmonsen PC: Expulsive choroidal effusion: a complication of intraocular surgery. Arch Ophthalmol 94: 69–70, 1976.

20. Swyers EM: Choroidal detachment immediately following cataract extraction. Arch Ophthalmol 88:632–634, 1972.

21. O'Brien CS: Detachment of the choroid after cataract extraction. Arch Ophthalmol 71:527–540, 1935.

22. Bellows AR, Chylack LT, Hutchinson BT: Choroidal detachment: clinical manifestation, therapy and mechanism of formation. Ophthalmology 88:1107–1115, 1981.

23. Lavin M, Franks W, Hitchings RA: Serous retinal detachment following glaucoma filtering surgery. Arch Ophthalmol 108:1553–1555, 1990.

24. Berke SJ, Bellows AR, Shingleton BJ, et al: Chronic and recurrent choroidal detachment after glaucoma filtering surgery. Ophthalmology 94:154–162, 1987.

25. Vela MA, Campbell DG: Hypotony and ciliochoroidal detachment following pharmacologic aqueous suppressant therapy in previously filtered patients. Ophthalmology 92: 50–57, 1985.

26. Magruder GB, Harbin TS: Ciliochoroidal detachment associated with stretched ciliary processes. Am J Ophthalmol 106:357–358, 1989.

27. Harbison JW, Guerry D, Wiesinger H: Dural arteriovenous fistula and spontaneous choroidal detachment: new cause of an old disease. Br J Ophthalmol 62:483–490, 1978.

28. Packer AJ, Maggiano JM, Aaberg TM, et al: Serous choroidal detachment after retinal detachment surgery. Arch Ophthalmol 101:1221–1224, 1983.

29. Topilow HW, Ackerman AL: Massive exudative retinal and choroidal detachment following scleral buckling surgery. Ophthalmology 90:143–147, 1983.

30. Burton TC, Folk JC: Laser iris retraction for angle-closure glaucoma after retinal detachment surgery. Ophthalmology 95:742–748, 1988.

31. Suan EP, Rubsamen PE, Byrne SF: Bilateral ciliochoroidal detachments after Valsalva maneuver. Arch Ophthalmol 111:340, 1993.

32. Wald KJ, Brockhurst RJ, Roth S, Bodine SR: Choroidal effusions in two patients with glomerulonephritis. Ann Ophthalmol 24:64–67, 1992.

33. Dotan S, Oliver M: Shallow anterior chamber and uveal effusion after nonperforating trauma to the eye. Am J Ophthalmol 94:782–784, 1982.

34. Hertz V: Choroidal detachment with notes on scleral de-

pression and pigmented streaks in the retina. Acta Ophthalmol 41:1–96, 1954.

35. Dawidek GMB, Kinsella FM, Pyott A, et al: Delayed ciliochoroidal detachment following intraocular lens implantation. Br J Ophthalmol 75:572–574, 1991.

36. Doft BH, Blakenship GW: Single versus multiple treatment sessions of argon laser panretinal photocoagulation for proliferative diabetic retinopathy. Ophthalmology 89:772–779, 1982.

37. Grant WM, Schuman JS: Toxicology of the eye: effects on the eyes and visual system from chemicals, drugs, metals and minerals, plants, toxins and venoms; also, systemic side effects from eye medications. Springfield, IL, Charles C Thomas, 1993, pp 22–24.

38. Soylev MF, Green RL, Feldon SE: Choroidal effusion as a mechanism for transient myopia induced by hydrochlorothiazide and triamterene. Am J Ophthalmol 120:395–397, 1995.

39. Kimura R, Sakai M, Okabe H: Transient shallow anterior chamber as initial symptom in Harada's syndrome. Arch Ophthalmol 99:1604–1606, 1981.

40. Brockhurst RJ, Schepens CL, Okamura ID: Uveitis: II. Peripheral uveitis: clinical description, complications and differential diagnosis. Am J Ophthalmol 49:1257–1266, 1960.

41. DeLuise VP, Clark SW, Smith JL, Collart P: Syphilitic retinal detachment and uveal effusion. Am J Ophthalmol 94: 757–761, 1982.

42. Sears ML: Choroidal and retinal detachments associated with scleritis. Am J Ophthalmol 58:764–766, 1964.

43. Dodds EM, Lowder CY, Barnhorst DA, et al: Posterior scleritis with annular ciliochoroidal detachment. Am J Ophthalmol 120:677–679, 1995.

44. Ullman S, Wilson RP, Schwartz L: Bilateral angle-closure glaucoma in association with the acquired immune deficiency syndrome. Am J Ophthalmol 101:419–424, 1986.

45. Nash RW, Lindquist TD: Bilateral angle-closure glaucoma associated with uveal effusion: presenting sign of HIV infection. Surv Ophthalmol 36:255–258, 1992.

46. Sneed SR, Byrne SF, Mieler WF, et al: Choroidal detachment associated with malignant choroidal tumors. Ophthalmology 98:963–970, 1991.

47. Singh OS, Simmons RJ, Brockhurst RJ, Trempe CL: Nanophthalmos: a perspective on identification and therapy. Ophthalmology 89:1006–1012, 1982.

48. Brockhurst RJ: Nanophthalmos with uveal effusion. Arch Ophthalmol 93:1289–1299, 1975.

49. Brockhurst RJ: Cataract surgery in nanophthalmic eyes. Arch Ophthalmol 108:965–967, 1990.

50. Jin JC, Anderson DR: Laser and unsutured sclerotomy in nanophthalmos. Am J Ophthalmol 109:575–580, 1990.

51. Allen KM, Meyers SM, Zegarra H: Nanophthalmic uveal effusion. Retina 8:145–147, 1988.

52. Vine AK: Uveal effusion in Hunter's syndrome: evidence that abnormal sclera is responsible for the uveal effusion syndrome. Retina 6:57–60, 1986.

53. Schepens CL, Brockhurst RJ: Uveal effusion: clinical picture. Arch Ophthalmol 70:101–113, 1963.

54. Gass JDM, Jallow S: Idiopathic serous detachment of the choroid, ciliary body, and retina (uveal effusion syndrome). Ophthalmology 89:1018–1032, 1982.

55. Johnson MW, Gass JDM: Surgical management of the idiopathic uveal effusion syndrome. Ophthalmology 97:778–785, 1990.

56. Forrester JV, Lee WR, Kerr PR, Dua HS: The uveal effusion syndrome and trans-scleral flow. Eye 4:354–365, 1990.

57. Yue BY JT, Duvall J, Goldberg MF, et al: Nanophthalmic sclera: morphologic and tissue culture studies. Ophthalmology 93:534–541, 1986.

58. Schneiderman TE, Johnson MW: A new approach to the surgical management of the idiopathic uveal effusion syndrome. Am J Ophthalmol 123:262–263, 1997.

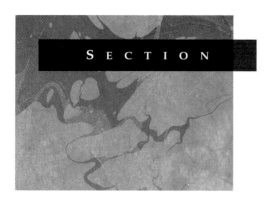

SECTION

V

Infectious Disorders

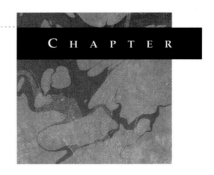

CHAPTER 57

Toxoplasmosis

Ali M. Ramadan, M.D.
Robert B. Nussenblatt, M.D.

Toxoplasmosis is probably the most common protozoal infection of the eye. Nicolle and Manceaux[1] were the first to describe the presence of *Toxoplasma gondii* in the brain of the North African rodent, *Ctenodactylus gundi*, and called the organism *Toxoplasma* because of the arch-shaped appearance of the parasite. But the importance of *Toxoplasma* as a cause of human ocular disease was not recognized until the Czechoslovakian ophthalmologist Jankû[2] described organisms that had the same characteristics in histopathologic sections from an eye of a child. With this discovery, Jankû found the exact etiology for an ocular lesion that used to be considered a congenital coloboma of the macula. Later, Wolf and co-workers[3] succeeded in transmitting the disease into mice via inoculation of the animals with infected human tissue from a child who died of toxoplasmosis.

THE ORGANISM

T. gondii is an obligate intracellular parasite that can infect humans, other mammals, and birds. The organism exists in three forms: tachyzoite (trophozoite), tissue cyst, and oocyst (containing sporozoites). Tachyzoites and tissue cysts are the only forms of the organism found in humans, whereas oocysts are found only in the cat family and are excreted in feces following an enteroepithelial stage of sexual reproduction in the small intestine.

Tachyzoites are oval or crescent shaped and measure 4 to 7 μm in length × 2 to 4 μm in diameter. The tachyzoite is an obligate intracellular form that requires a host cell for growth and, therefore, cannot survive or multiply extracellularly or be maintained in culture medium alone. Tachyzoites can enter cytoplasmic vacuoles in any nucleated mammalian cell. They divide by endodyogeny, an asexual process whereby two daughter cells are formed within one parent cell. Division continues until the cell ruptures, releasing tachyzoites to infect adjacent cells. Intracellular replication and the parasitization of new cells do not slow until an effective immune response develops. Tachyzoites are used in the Sabin-Feldman dye test, the agglutination test, and the fluorescent antibody test; antigens derived from tachyzoites are used in the complement fixation test, the hemagglutination test, and the enzyme-linked immunosorbent assay (ELISA).

Tissue cysts (Fig. 57–1) vary in size from 10 to 100 μm and contain as many as 3000 slowly dividing organisms (bradyzoites); these appear to develop within host cells. Tissue cysts begin to form as early as 1 week after infection. Cysts persist for life in the mammalian host and can be found virtually in any tissue, most commonly myocardium, skeletal muscle, brain, and neural tissue including the retina. Cysts are the pathologic hallmark of chronic (latent) infection and remain clinically silent in immunologically normal hosts. In contrast, cysts provide a ready endogenous source of tachyzoites in patients who become immunosuppressed or who are T-cell deficient as in the acquired immunodeficiency syndrome (AIDS) (Fig. 57–2). In view of the fact that the tissue cyst incorporates elements derived from the host into its wall, it is easily tolerated by the host and no inflammatory reaction is seen around it. Therefore, it remains for years in certain tissues such as the eye or muscles without provoking any immune response. The bradyzoites inside the cyst multiply at a very slow rate, and once the cyst can no longer hold them it ruptures, causing the release of these bradyzoites that convert into tachyzoites and invade contiguous cells. This process is associated with recurrence of retinitis in the host.

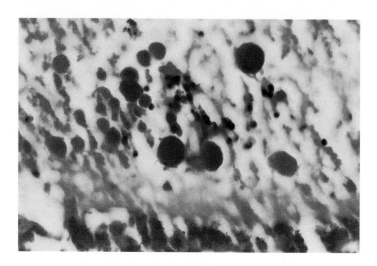

Retina with numerous cysts of *Toxoplasma* organisms in an immunosuppressed woman after renal transplantation.

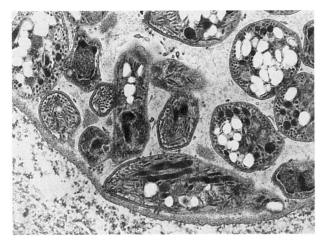

FIGURE 57–1 Electron micrograph showing a large cyst of *Toxoplasma gondii* containing many bradyzoites (magnification × 14,000).

Oocysts are ovoid in shape and measure 10 to 12 μm in diameter and have been found only in members of the cat family. Depending on the form of the organism that infects the cat, oocysts are excreted 3 to 24 days after the initial infection. Millions of oocysts are excreted in the feces of the cat each day for about 2 weeks. Sporogony occurs outside the body, requires 2 to 21 days (depending on the ambient temperature), and results in an infective oocyst. Because ingestion of oocysts may lead to infection, they probably play a major role in the transmission of toxoplasmosis. Oocysts are the most tolerant of the various forms of *T. gondii*. In the extrahost environment, under favorable conditions (warm and moist soil) they may remain infectious for several months to more than a year. However, exposure to boiling water or to dry heat (over 60°C) renders oocysts noninfectious. Oocysts are killed by drying, boiling, and exposure to some strong chemicals, but not to bleach. Oocysts have been isolated from soil and sand frequented by cats,

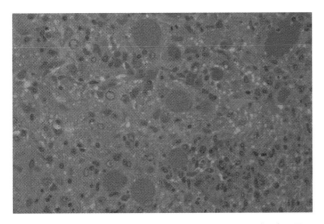

FIGURE 57–2 Photomicrograph showing multiple *Toxoplasma* cysts (*arrows*) and numerous inflammatory cells in the brain tissue of a patient with AIDS (hematoxylin and eosin, × 400).

and outbreaks associated with contaminated water have been reported.

Life Cycle

The protozoan *T. gondii* is found throughout the world in many species of warm-blooded animals. Members of the cat family are its definitive hosts and all other animals, including humans, are intermediate hosts. The organism exists in three forms: tachyzoite (trophozoite), tissue cyst, and oocyst (containing sporozoites). Tachyzoites and tissue cysts are the only forms of the organism found in humans, whereas oocysts are found only in the cat family and are excreted in feces following an enteroepithelial stage of sexual reproduction in the small intestine. In the definitive host, the parasite has both enteroepithelial and extraintestinal cycles, whereas in the intermediate host, it persists only in the extraintestinal cycle.

Toxoplasma are acquired by susceptible cats by ingestion of the flesh of infected birds and rodents containing encysted bradyzoites or by ingestion of oocysts containing infective sporozoites from soil contaminated by feces from other infected cats. In the gastrointestinal tract of the cat, oocysts and tissue cysts are digested by the peptic and intestinal enzymes. The released *Toxoplasma* organisms then invade the mucosal cells of small intestine. Frenkel and co-workers[4] and Hutchison and co-workers[5] showed that the organism undergoes two forms of reproduction in the cat small intestine: an asexual cycle (endodyogeny or schizogony), a process whereby two daughter cells are formed within one parent cell; and a sexual cycle (gametogony) in which a zygote is formed by the union of two gametocytes. This zygote matures in 1 to 4 days into an oocyst. Large quantities of oocysts (up to 10 million per day) are released by rupture of the host cells and are excreted in the feces by the cat for 1 to 3 weeks, beginning 3 to 5 days after ingestion of the *Toxoplasma* cysts or oocysts. Oocysts are not infectious until they undergo sporogony outside the body. Under proper conditions of temperature and moisture they undergo a period of maturation (sporulation), which takes about 1 to 21 days. This process results in the formation of infective oocysts containing viable sporozoites.

When man or other animals (including the cat) eat infected tissues (from any animal) or mature oocysts, the life cycle is completed. In the intermediate host, disruption of the cyst wall or the oocyst by the digestive enzymes liberates viable *T. gondii*, which invade the intestinal epithelium and spread to all host tissue via the bloodstream or lymphatics. In tissues like brain, myocardium, skeletal muscles, or retina, the tachyzoites multiply rapidly by endodyogeny, causing destruction of the host cells. This stage represents the acute phase of the disease. With an intact host immune response, replication of tachyzoites eventually ceases, and most organisms are eliminated. Some, however, will form intracellular tissue cysts containing slowly multiplying organisms (bradyzoites). Because tissue cysts incorporate elements derived from the host into their wall, they can lie dormant in tissues throughout the life of the host.

Epidemiology

Toxoplasma gondii are ubiquitous in nature. It is thought that this organism infects at least 500 million persons worldwide.[6] In the United States, serologic evidence of *T. gondii* infection ranges from 3 to 70% of the adult healthy population.[7,8] Cats, small mammals, and birds serve as the likely natural reservoirs of *T. gondii*, but virtually any animal that has access to and ingests material contaminated by oocysts or cyst-containing tissue can become infected. Cysts can be found, for example, in 10 to 25% of lamb and 25% of pork prepared for human consumption and less so in beef.[9]

The frequency of *Toxoplasma* infection in any population depends on a variety of sociologic, economic, and environmental factors. There is an increasing prevalence of positive serologic reactions with increasing age, with no significant difference between sexes. A screening performed among older people admitted to a district hospital in Oslo showed a prevalence increasing from 23% at the age of 45, to 46% in the age group of 85, indicating an annual incidence of approximately 0.6%.[10] Geographic variations exist: prevalence is lower at higher altitudes, in cold regions, and in hot arid climates.[11,12] These variations could be attributed to the effect of environmental conditions on oocyst survival. Societies where there is an increased consumption of raw and undercooked meat and areas affected by poor sanitation have a high incidence of *Toxoplasma* infection. Outbreaks among families or closed groups may develop after a common source exposure, although there is no evidence of human-to-human transmission other than from a mother to her fetus.

Data on the prevalence of antibodies in pregnant women or women in the childbearing age group for the United States and for other countries are shown in Table 57–1.

Transmission

There are three principal modes of transmission of *T. gondii*: (1) ingestion of oocysts or tissue cysts, (2) maternal transplacental spread, and (3) inadvertent direct administration (Table 57–2). Meat used for human consumption may contain tissue cysts, thus serving as a source of infection when eaten raw or undercooked. Kean and associates[13] reported on an epidemic in medical students following the ingestion of raw hamburger. Tissue cysts may contaminate hands and other households during preparation of infected meat. Oocysts may be ingested with unwashed fruits and vegetables.[14] Uncovered food may also become contaminated with oocysts by insects such as flies or cockroaches. Contaminated raw goat milk has been implicated as a source of *T. gondii* infection.[15,16]

Transmission to the fetus usually occurs when primary *Toxoplasma* infection is acquired during pregnancy. The rate reaches up to 61%.[17] Congenital transmission from immunologically normal women infected prior to pregnancy is extremely rare.[18] Immunocompromised women who are chronically infected have transmitted the infection to their fetuses.

On rare occasions, *T. gondii* has also been transmitted by transplantation of infected organs, especially hearts into seronegative recipients,[19] or by transfusion of whole blood or leukocytes as a result of persistent parasitemia in a normal asymptomatic donor.[18] Transmission may also occur in laboratory

TABLE 57–1 Seroprevalence of *Toxoplasma* Infection in Pregnant Women

Country	Seroprevalence	References
United States	80–90%	35
England	22–23%	194, 195
Finland	20.3%	196
Austria	47%	197
Australia	35%	198
France	84%	199
Denmark	27%	200
Norway	12%	201
Tanzania	35%	202

TABLE 57–2 Modes of Transmission of Toxoplasmosis

Common Causes
Ingestion of tissue cysts in undercooked or raw meat
Ingestion of sporulated oocysts from:
  Unwashed vegetables and fruits
  Handling of contaminated meat
  Uncovered food contaminated by flies or cockroaches
Rare Causes
Transfusion of infected blood into healthy recipient
Transplant of infected organs into healthy recipient
Consumption of contaminated raw goat milk
Inadvertent inoculation of tachyzoites
Inhalation of oocysts

workers by accidental self-inoculation of tachyzoites. Yet another unexpected mode of infection was through the inhalation of sporulated oocysts, described by Teutsch and associates.[20]

Pathogenesis

Tachyzoites have a predilection for neural tissue, which they reach mainly via the bloodstream. Organisms may also reach the eye along the optic nerve, but this is not a common mode of transmission.[21] They establish their focus of infection in the superficial portions of the retina. The lesion induced is a necrotic one that destroys the architecture of the retina. It soon progresses to involve the choroid, so that the disease at this point can certainly be classified as a retinochoroiditis. In immunocompetent hosts tachyzoites stop multiplying and convert into encysted bradyzoites. In view of the fact that the tissue cyst thus formed incorporates elements derived from the host into its wall, it is easily tolerated by the host and no inflammatory reaction is seen around it. Therefore, it remains for years in certain tissues such as the eye or muscles without provoking any immune response. Bradyzoites inside the cyst multiply at a very slow rate, and once the cyst can no longer hold them, it ruptures, causing the release of these bradyzoites that convert into tachyzoites and invade contiguous cells. This process is associated with recurrence of retinitis in the host.

A number of theories have been formulated to explain the pathogenesis of tissue destruction by *Toxoplasma* within ocular tissue. One hypothesis is that when cysts rupture within the retina, the contents are spilled into the surrounding retinal tissue, causing a hypersensitivity reaction and retinochoroiditis.[22,23] An alternative hypothesis is that the recurrent retinochoroiditis may represent an active infection in a predominant manner, but to a lesser extent there is a hypersensitivity response to *Toxoplasma* antigens and possible hypersensitivity to retinal autoantigens.[24-27] Nozik and O'Connor[28] and Newman and co-workers[29] have been unable to induce recurrent inflammatory foci of toxoplasmic retinochoroiditis by inoculating *Toxoplasma* antigens by a number of routes into the rabbit or the monkey.

Another theory suggests that *Toxoplasma* organism releases a toxin that is responsible for the retinochoroidal damage. This theory is supported by the work done on rabbits by Hogan et al.[30] However, the observation noted by Dutton and Hay[31] in their animal experiment that there was no tissue damage around the cysts rules out the possibility of release of toxins. O'Connor has suggested that the retina may be damaged by an "innocent bystander" mechanism whereby active phagocytosis and cell lysis, which accompany inflammatory cell infiltration, result in the release of acid hydrolases and other enzymes that destroy adjacent cells.[32]

In a survey of 40 patients with ocular toxoplasmosis, 16 patients (40%) demonstrated an in vitro proliferative response to the retinal S antigen.[33] Another interesting observation was seen when polymerase chain reaction (PCR) was performed on samples of aqueous humor from 17 Brazilian patients with clinical presentations consistent with ocular toxoplasmosis. The absence of *T. gondii* DNA in the aqueous humor samples of most of the patients supports the concept that proliferation of the parasite might not be the only factor leading to the inflammatory response observed during ocular toxoplasmosis.[34] These findings could indicate that an autoimmune component to the inflammatory disease seen is presumably initiated with destruction of the retina by a parasite and subsequent sensitization to the uveitogenic antigen. The apparent selective photoreceptor damage illustrated in the animal model of Dutton and Hay,[31] where the *Toxoplasma* cyst didn't appear to be the center of the inflammatory attack, argues in favor of an autoimmune component in the disease process.

HUMAN TOXOPLASMOSIS

Human toxoplasmosis can be divided into two broad categories (Table 57–3), acquired and congenital. Congenital infection occurs when the mother's primary infection develops during pregnancy and passes *T. gondii* through the transplacental route to her fetus. Even so, most babies remain unaffected. The acquired infection varies in its course and outcome depending on the immune status of the host. Ocular toxoplasmosis follows either congenital or systemic disease. It occurs in immunodeficient hosts due to human immunodeficiency virus (HIV) infections or other causes, and it can also be either acquired or a reactivation of latent infection (Table 57–2).

Congenital Toxoplasmosis

The rate of fetal infection is related to the stage during which the mother acquires the primary disease.

TABLE 57–3 Human Toxoplasmosis

Congenital
Acquired
Ocular
Congenital
Acquired
In immunocompromised
Congenital
Acquired

If the immunocompetent pregnant woman was infected prior to conception, there is virtually no risk of transmission to the fetus.[17] The incidence of transmission is least early in gestation and greatest later in gestation, and the earlier in gestation the infection is acquired by the fetus, the more likely it is to produce severe fetal manifestations, probably because it occurs during the period of organogenesis. Despite the fact that 70 to 80% of the women of the childbearing age in the United States are at risk for primary infection,[35] the prevalence of acquired toxoplasmosis during pregnancy is approximately 2 to 6 per 1000 women.[7] Once the mother acquires the infection, the fetus is at risk whether the infection in the mother is symptomatic or asymptomatic. The incidence is lowest in the first trimester, about 10 to 20%; 30% during the second trimester, and highest in the third trimester, reaching up to 60%.[36,37] If the infection is acquired during the last weeks before delivery, the rate exceeds 90%.[38]

In contrast, the risk of the fetus developing severe disease is inversely related to gestational age. If maternal infection is acquired early in pregnancy, fetal infection most often results in spontaneous abortion, stillbirth, or severe disease. On the other hand, if maternal infection occurs late in the gestational period, the usual result will be a delivery of an asymptomatic infant with latent infection. This explains why the majority (90%) of newborns with congenital Toxoplasma infection appear normal at birth. Prospective long-term studies indicate that up to 85% of these infants will develop significant sequelae including one or more episodes of active chorioretinitis resulting in blindness or impaired vision.[39–41] In a clinical evaluation of 13 children up to a mean age of 8 years, 11 of the 13 infected children who were asymptomatic at birth suffered several sequelae. The initial manifestation was a retinochoroiditis that appeared at a mean age of 3.7 years.[40]

A wide variety of manifestations of congenital infection occur in the perinatal period. A list of signs and symptoms in a survey of 210 infants is shown in Table 57–4.[42] These range from relatively mild signs, such as small size for gestational age, prematurity, peripheral retinal scars, persistent jaundice, mild thrombocytopenia, and cerebrospinal fluid pleocytosis, to the classic triad of signs consisting of chorioretinitis, hydrocephalus, and cerebral calcifications.

Acquired Toxoplasmosis

Ocular toxoplasmosis in adults and children is usually considered a recurrent manifestation of congenital infection. In 1973, Perkins[43] stated that systemic manifestations in acute acquired toxoplasmosis are rare and that only 2 to 3% of affected patients develop ocular involvement. Perkins based his assumption on certain observations: In spite of

TABLE 57–4   Signs and Symptoms in 210 Infants with Proved Congenital *Toxoplasma* Infection*

Finding	No. Examined	No. Positive (%)
Prematuriy	210	
Birthweight <2500 g		8 (3.8)
Birthweight 2500–3000 g		5 (7.1)
Dysmaturity (intrauterine growth retardation)		13 (6.2)
Icterus	201	20 (10)
Hepatosplenomegaly	210	9 (4.2)
Thrombocytopenic purpura	210	3 (1.4)
Abnormal blood count (anemia, eosinophilia)	102	9 (4.4)
Microcephaly	210	11 (5.2)
Hydrocephaly	210	8 (3.8)
Hypotonia	210	12 (5.7)
Convulsions	210	8 (3.8)
Psychomotor retardation	210	11 (5.2)
Intracranial calcification on x-ray	210	24 (11.4)
Ultrasound	49	5 (10)
Computed tomography of brain	13	11 (84)
Abnormal EEG	191	16 (8.3)
Abnormal CSF	163	56 (34.2)
Microphthalmia	210	6 (2.8)
Strabismus	210	111 (5.2)
Chorioretinitis	210	
Unilateral		34 (16.1)
Bilateral		12 (5.7)

* Data are adapted from a study conducted by Couvreur and colleagues.[42]

the fact that the prevalence of toxoplasmosis tends to increase with age, retinochoroiditis occurs more frequently in the second and third decades than in old age. The other observation that he noted was that patients who manifested ocular signs due to their toxoplasmic infection did not have higher anti–*T. gondii* than individuals without eye disease. Had ocular involvement occurred at the time of initial infection he would have expected to see higher serum antibodies against the parasite in those patients. He also assumed that acquired ocular toxoplasmosis without systemic manifestations of disease should be even less common than ocular disease in patients with symptomatic systemic infections. Similarly, Schlaegel[44] stated that less than 1% of the patients with acute acquired toxoplasmosis develop retinitis and almost every case of ocular disease is probably of congenital origin with late onset.

These traditional "givens" in ophthalmology

have been seriously questioned by the observations and the results of surveys conducted in a small town in southern Brazil. In a survey of 100 normal children, it was observed that 98% of these healthy children between the ages of 10 and 15 years had antibodies to toxoplasmosis. The frequency of retinal scars in the population of this area was 40 per 200 as compared to 1 per 200 in the United States and 6 per 200 in São Paulo, Brazil. In another survey conducted on the population of this town, 184 (17.7%) of 1042 persons examined, were found to have ocular toxoplasmosis, placing the prevalence rate of ocular toxoplasmosis 30 times higher than estimates for this disease in other parts of the world.[45] Reports from other regions of the world speak of different observations. In a study from a Pacific island where 90% of the adult population had been infected with *T. gondii*, no adult had ocular toxoplasmosis.[46]

Of interest was the finding that only 0.9% of young children tested in this region of Erechim, Brazil, had antibodies in their serum to *T. gondii*, further supporting the notion that the ocular lesions were due to postnatal infection. Similar findings were obtained in another prospective study conducted in this region on the newborns up to the age of 5 months; only 0.5 to 0.6% of the cord blood tested revealed anti-*Toxoplasma* antibodies. The other puzzling observation in this region was the familial occurrence of ocular toxoplasmosis in which the mother and several children (nontwins) had retinal lesions. In one case, three generations in the same family were found to have ocular findings.[47] The reason behind this unexceptionally high rate is their habit of eating sausage prepared from raw or poorly cooked pork.

In a recent study, Ronday and co-workers[48] described ocular involvement due to acquired toxoplasmosis in eight patients older than 40 years. All eight patients suffered from unilateral focal chorioretinitis and had no pre-existing retinal scars in either eye. Based on the presence of specific IgM antibodies, rising serum IgG titers in seven of eight patients, and the absence of chorioretinal scars, they believed that their patients suffered from acquired toxoplasmosis.

These studies from southern Brazil and similar reports[49–54] demonstrate that acquired disease is a major mode of transmission of this parasite. However, it is true that results of surveys from other parts of the world may not be consistent with observations seen in Erechim. Even results within the same southern state showed marked difference from results obtained in Erechim. Could these variations be attributed to the presence of different strains of *T. gondii*? Or could it be that a certain population with acquired toxoplasmosis are more susceptible to the development of ocular disease than others? Nevertheless, if what Sibley and Boothroyd[55] reported turns out to be true, that all virulent strains of *T. gondii* are derived from a single clonal lineage, then we can logically assume

that similar mechanisms are at play elsewhere and that acquired disease may be an important mode of transmission.

Clinical Manifestations of Acquired Toxoplasmosis

Only 10 to 20% of cases of acquired toxoplasmosis are symptomatic in adults.[56] The spectrum of acquired toxoplasmosis ranges from subclinical lymphadenopathy to fatal, acute, fulminating disease (Table 57–5). Asymptomatic lymphadenopathy is the most common manifestation. The lymphadenopathy may be localized to a single node or area, or it may be generalized and involve any group of nodes; the cervical nodes are the most commonly enlarged. Lymph nodes will generally be nonsuppurative, discrete, of variable firmness, and nontender.[57] Symptomatic patients may present with a triad of fever, headache, and lymphadenopathy. Fever is usually low grade, but on occasion can be high, rapidly fluctuating, and prolonged. Fatigue can be a prominent feature. A minority of patients may have a sore throat, maculopapular rash, myalgias, arthralgias, urticaria, headaches, or present with hepatosplenomegaly mimicking diseases like Hodgkin's or infectious mononucleosis.[58] Rarely, serious complications may occur with fatal outcome if toxoplasmosis involves the central nervous system (CNS), lungs, or the myocardium.[8,59]

Ocular involvement, mainly in the form of retinochoroiditis, is currently believed to occur in patients with acquired toxoplasmosis. It may sometimes be the initial presentation of the disease or it may be the sole manifestation of the disorder.[49–51,53] The average interval between the onset of systemic symptoms in acquired toxoplasmosis and the development of clinical ocular disease can range from a few days to several years.[53,60]

Toxoplasmosis is a self-limiting infection in im-

TABLE 57–5 Clinical Manifestations of Acquired Toxoplasmosis in Immunocompetent Subjects

Lymphadenopathy
Fever
Headache
Fatigue
Sore throat
Jaundice
Night sweats
Myalgia
Arthralgia
Urticaria
Hepatosplenomegaly
Retinochoroiditis

munocompetent hosts over a period of several weeks, but it can be a prolonged, severely debilitating disorder that may prevent the patient from working many weeks to months. In the immunocompromised host it may result in a fatal outcome.

OCULAR TOXOPLASMOSIS

Ocular toxoplasmosis is probably the most important cause of uveitis in man. Perkins believed that toxoplasmosis accounted for approximately 25% of all cases of uveitis.[61] Schlaegel reported an incidence of 16% of ocular toxoplasmosis on his service.[44] It is the most common cause of posterior uveitis in many studies, accounting for about 25% of all cases of posterior uveitis in the United States. The rate varies in other areas of the world depending on several factors like age, socioeconomic conditions, and eating habits. Toxoplasmosis accounts for over 85% of posterior uveitis cases in certain areas of Southern Brazil, where 17.7% of the population was found to have ocular toxoplasmosis.[45]

Since the *Toxoplasma* organism has a propensity for neural tissue, it is important to keep in mind that the lesion classically begins in the retina in the form of focal necrotizing retinitis, and only with ongoing inflammation will it involve not only multiple layers of the retina but also the choroid (Fig. 57–3).

The lesion is generally bilateral in congenital cases. In one study evidence of bilateral infection was found in 34% of patients with ocular toxoplasmosis.[62] The active lesion can vary in size, but is usually oval or circular and rarely bullous. Acute lesions are soft and cream colored, with indistinct borders; the older lesions are whitish gray, sharply outlined, and marked by accumulation of pigment. Adjacent to the area of active retinitis, one may see hemorrhage, as well as sheathing of the retinal blood vessels (Fig. 57–4). Lesions may be single or multiple (Fig. 57–5). Not uncommonly, reactivation sites will be "satellite" lesions, next to old atrophic ones, indicative of previous toxoplasmic infection. In some large and particularly recalcitrant lesions, the inflammatory exudate that is cast off from the surface of the acute lesion is so dense that clear visualization of the fundus is impossible. In such cases, when the fundus is examined it gives the classic "headlight in the fog" appearance (Fig. 57–6).

With continuing inflammatory disease, the lesion and the overlying vitreous will undergo several changes. The vitreous may contract, and a posterior vitreal detachment is not uncommon. Clumps of inflammatory cells may be seen hanging as balls in the vitreous or precipitate over the detached vitreous face. Further vitreal condensation leads to a "scaffolding" of vitreal strands (Fig. 57–7). Roizenblatt and coauthors[63] refer to the development of vitreous cylinders in toxoplasmosis, a result of con-

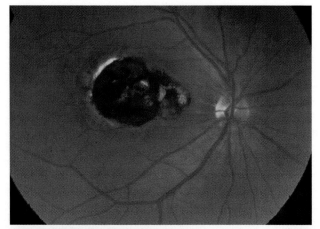
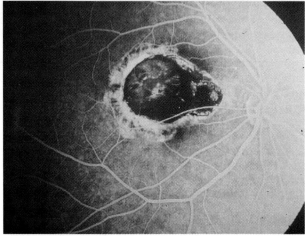

FIGURE 57–3   *A*, A chorioretinal scar is seen in the macular area. Such lesions used to be considered congenital colobomas of the macula before Jankû found the exact etiology. *B*, Central hypofluorescence surrounded by a rim of hyperfluorescence due to late staining of the scar edge.

densation of the collagen fibers. Vitreous condensation will exert persistent traction on the retina. Such retinal traction coupled with atrophic retina may eventually lead to retinal detachment (Fig. 57–8).

Macular edema is almost always present when the acute inflammatory focus is juxtafoveal. It is usually temporary, although cystic changes in the fovea sometimes occur as a result of longstanding edema.[64]

Propensity of the *Toxoplasma* lesions to the macular area may be due to entrapment of free-swimming organisms or parasites containing macrophages in the terminal capillaries of the perifoveal retina. Similar entrapment in the peripapillary capillary network may also explain the frequent occurrence of lesions in the juxtapapillary region. Hogan and associates[62] found that macular lesions were found in 46% of eyes of patients with ocular toxoplasmosis.

Papillitis or optic neuritis due to optic nerve involvement has been seen (Fig. 57–9).[65,66] Some patients presented with severe papillitis, vitreal inflammation, and sector or nerve fiber field defects,

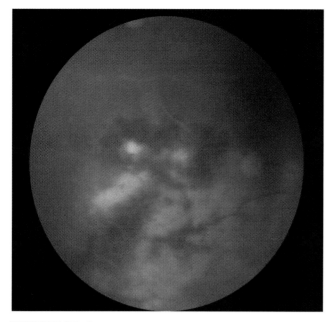

FIGURE 57–4   An acute lesion is seen at the edge of an old one. The acute lesion is soft and cream colored, with indistinct borders. Hemorrhage as well as sheathing of the retinal blood vessels are noticed, whereas the older lesion is seen as whitish gray, sharply outlined, and marked by accumulation of pigment. (Courtesy of Rubens Belfort, Jr., M.D., Brazil.)

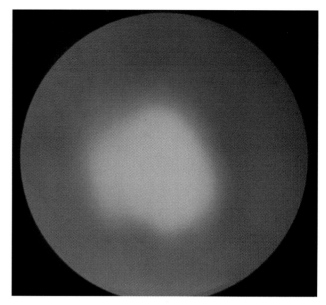

FIGURE 57–6   Dense haze caused by exudate from retinal toxoplasmic lesions showing "headlight-in-the-fog" appearance.

with no apparent retinal foci.[67] The *Toxoplasma* organism was found in the optic nerve of patients at autopsy.[66,68]

The anterior uvea may be the site of severe inflammation characterized by redness of the external eye, cells and protein in the anterior chamber, and small or large keratic precipitate. The inflammation is a hypersensitivity reaction to the *Toxoplasma* antigens.

A curious association between Fuchs' hetero-

chromia and ocular toxoplasmosis was initially made by de Abreu and co-workers.[69] This relationship was further evaluated by La Hey and colleagues,[70] who could not establish a particular relationship between the two entities. However, Schwab[71] suggested that a casual relationship appears to exist between the two entities, at least for a subgroup of patients with Fuchs' heterochromia.

Ocular Complications

The intraocular inflammatory process can play havoc on the ocular tissues (Table 57–6). Macular involvement is common in cases of congenital toxoplasmosis. If chorioretinal scarring occurs in the macular area, the visual function will be damaged beyond repair. Exudative retinal detachment may

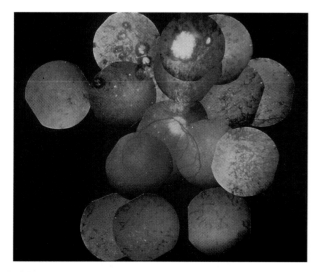

FIGURE 57–5   Multiple satellite lesions along with clumping of pigment are seen in the fundus periphery in a patient with ocular toxoplasmosis. (Courtesy of Rubens Belfort, Jr., M.D., Brazil.)

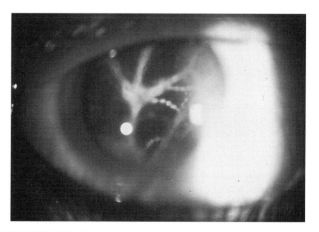

FIGURE 57–7   Scaffolding of vitreal strands in a patient with longstanding ocular toxoplasmic infection.

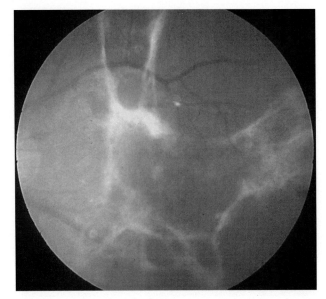

FIGURE 57–8 Vitreous strands like these that are formed as a result of intraocular toxoplasmic infection may eventually lead to retinal detachment because of persistent traction.

TABLE 57–6 Ocular Complications

Macular scars
Macular edema
Retinochoroidal anastomosis
Subretinal neovascularization
Optic disc neovascularization
Retinal hemorrhages
Retinal vein occlusions
Retinal artery occlusions
Optic atrophy
Vitreous condensations
Retinal detachment
Posterior synechia
Secondary glaucoma
Secondary cataract
Strabismus
Scleritis
Visual field defects
Pigmentary retinopathy
Iris atrophy

occur in severe cases.[66] A variety of vascular complications may occur, such as retinochoroidal anastomosis through the damaged Bruch's membrane; subretinal, choroidal, and optic head neovascularization[72–77]; branch retinal artery occlusion[66,78]; retinal vein occlusion[77]; and retinal hemorrhages.[78] Optic atrophy due to papillitis or optic neuritis and nerve fiber bundle field defects are also seen. Posterior synechia, iris atrophy, and secondary glaucoma may be sequelae to spillover of inflammation into the anterior segment of the eye. Other rare complications such as cerebral blindness, oculo-

motor nerve palsies,[79,80] and scleritis (Fig. 57–10) are also encountered.[81]

The Disease in the Immunocompromised Host

In contrast to the benign and self-limited course of infection in the immunocompetent host, systemic and ocular toxoplasmosis in immunocompromised individuals is a fulminant disorder.[82] Patients with HIV-1 infection, and those who are undergoing immunosuppressive therapy for malignancies, organ transplant and autoimmune diseases are at increased risk. The aggressiveness of T. gondii is particularly striking in the CNS, where it is a leading cause of morbidity and mortality. Clinical evidence

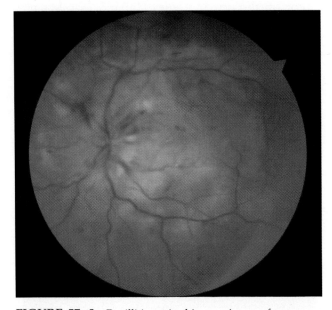

FIGURE 57–9 Papillitis, as in this case, is one of numerous complications that are seen in eyes affected with Toxoplasma infection. (Courtesy of Rubens Belfort, Jr., M.D., Brazil.)

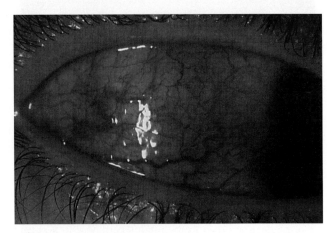

FIGURE 57–10 Scleritis is seen here in an eye that also has posterior uveitis due to toxoplasmosis.

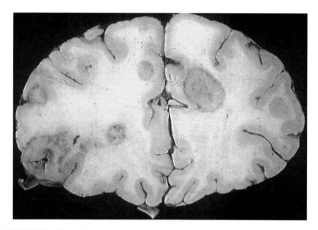

FIGURE 57–11 Cross section of the brain showing several large brain cysts in an AIDS patient who had central nervous system toxoplasmosis.

of neurologic involvement is found in approximately 40% of AIDS patients, and nearly 80% of patients show CNS pathology at autopsy.[83] Cerebral toxoplasmosis (Fig. 57–11) is the most common cause of CNS mass lesions,[84] and along with cryptococcal meningitis is the most common nonviral infection afflicting AIDS patients.[83,85] Discrete mass lesions in the brain due to toxoplasmosis have been observed.[82] Various CNS manifestations have been noticed in the immunocompromised hosts like diffuse encephalopathy, necrotizing encephalitis, altered consciousness, motor and sensory impairment, cognitive impairment and altered consciousness, seizures, and visual disturbances.[83,85]

Ocular toxoplasmosis (Fig. 57–12) is still a relatively uncommon disorder in AIDS patients in the United States. Neurologic involvement due to toxoplasmic infection occurs more frequently than the ocular one. Therefore, the diagnosis of ocular toxoplasmosis in an AIDS patient should initiate the evaluation of possible CNS disease. The ocular lesions resemble the classic picture of necrotizing ret-

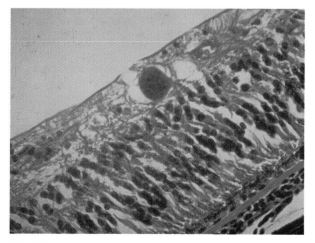

FIGURE 57–12 *Toxoplasma* cyst (*arrow*) is seen in the retina of an AIDS patient who also had ocular toxoplasmosis (hematoxylin & eosin, × 640).

inochoroiditis. Typically, they occur adjacent to retinal vasculature implying that the organisms reach the eye via the bloodstream. Direct extension from the brain via the optic nerve is another possibility. They may be single or multiple, and may occur unilaterally and bilaterally.[66,86–88] The degree of the inflammatory reaction associated with the toxoplasmic retinitis in the vitreous or the anterior chamber depends on the immune profile of the host at that point in time when the reactivation or acquisition of the disease occurs. Prominent inflammatory reaction will be seen if infection occurs when the immune repertoire of the host is still capable of mustering a significant response. Massive areas of retinal necrosis may occur that mimic the acute retinal necrosis syndrome.[89] Very little pigment epithelial reaction is noticed in the eyes of these patients. Vascular sheathing may be present, but bleeding is minimal.

Infection usually produces full-thickness retinal necrosis, but early lesions may be confined to the inner or outer layers.[88] One patient in Holland et al's series had features on histopathological examination that resembled the punctate outer retinal toxoplasmosis described by some authors.[90,91] Rhegmatogenous retinal detachment may be a late complication.

AIDS patients may not mount a significant rise in IgG titers during an acute infection, rendering the titers nondiagnostic in distinguishing between latent and active infection. IgM antibodies are found too inconsistently to be used routinely in diagnosis.[66]

Whether the ocular manifestations of this disease represent reactivation[92–94] or acquired disease[66,88] in the immunosuppressed host is still an unsettled argument among investigators. Those investigators who believe that the lesions are a manifestation of acquired rather than congenital disease base their conclusion on the findings that the areas of retinal necrosis seen in these patients are not associated with pre-existing retinochoroidal scars. None of the cases reported by Holland and associates,[88] and only 1 of the 16 patients reported by Friedman and co-workers[66] had a pre-existing retinochoroidal scar.

Congenital transmission of toxoplasmosis from pregnant women co-infected with *T. gondii* and HIV is increasing in number. Apparently, the incidence of congenital transmission from these mothers appears to be both remarkably and significantly higher than in non–HIV-infected women.[17,95–101] Mitchell et al[95] described four young infants, two of whom were siblings, who were dually infected with HIV and *T. gondii*. Their mothers were similarly co-infected. The mother of the first infant had toxoplasmic encephalitis diagnosed at delivery.

Certain other infectious retinitis entities like cytomegalovirus (CMV) retinitis, acute retinal necrosis (ARN), progressive outer retinal necrosis, and syphilis occur in the immunocompromised subjects with variable frequencies and should be properly differentiated from toxoplasmic retinochoroiditis. The CMV retinitis is the most common infectious disease that occurs in AIDS patients, with toxoplasmosis—according to some authors—in second place.[86] Establishing accurate diagnosis and starting early treatment can go a long way in preserving visual function in these patients.

IMMUNE RESPONSE AND SELF DEFENSES AGAINST *T. GONDII* INFECTION

The high incidence of toxoplasmosis in immunocompromised hosts highlights the important role of the immune response in maintaining the infection with *T. gondii* in a latent form. The bulk of knowledge gathered on the immune defenses against the *T. gondii* infection has been obtained from animal studies. Gazzinelli and co-workers[102] developed an animal model of toxoplasmosis in mice with virus-induced immunodeficiency similar to that observed in AIDS patients. Their idea was to study the reactivation of *T. gondii* in mice infected with LP-BM5 murine leukemia virus.

The major mechanism of resistance against *T. gondii* has been shown to be mediated by T cells[103–106] (Fig. 57–13). CD8+ T lymphocytes appear to confer protection against *T. gondii* through the production of interferon gamma (INF-γ),[107] and/or through lysis of cells infected with *T. gondii*.[108–110] INF-γ induces macrophage activation.[111,112] It is stimulated by p30, and is produced by CD4+, CD8+, and natural killer (NK) cells. CD4+ T lymphocytes were found to be required for the induction of resistance to *T. gondii*.[113] It has been suggested that CD8+ T cells directed against the *Toxoplasma* organism appear during the acute phase of the disease, whereas CD4+ T cells appear with chronicity of the disease.[114]

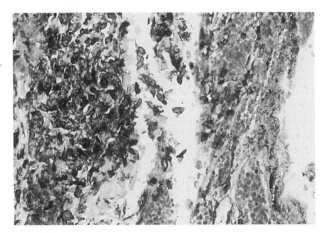

FIGURE 57–13   T-cell infiltration is seen in the retina of an AIDS patient who had ocular *Toxoplasma* infection (CD3 marker, immunoperoxidase, × 400).

The host's response is exceptionally important in the ultimate expression of toxoplasmosis. In animal models, resistance, as measured by survival after challenge with the organism, has been reported to be regulated by at least five genes,[115] one of which is within the region of the H-2 antigen (the equivalent of the major histocompatibility complex [MHC] in human beings).[116] The major surface antigen is p30. The proliferative response of lymphocytes in vitro was much higher in response to purified p22 antigen than p30 antigen.[33] Brown and McLeod[117] have found that class 1 MHC genes, as well as the CD8+ fraction of T cells, determine the cyst number in *Toxoplasma* infection. Others have looked at the effect of cytokines on the multiplication of the *Toxoplasma* organism.

Endogenous tumor necrosis factor-α (TNF-α) appears to play a critical role in the induction of macrophage activity against *T. gondii* mediated by INF-γ.[118] Animal studies have shown that INF-γ induces the production of TNF-α, which in turn, through the production of reactive nitrogen intermediates (RNIs), results in activity against *T. gondii*.[119,120] The in vivo administration of anti–TNF-α antibodies inhibited activity against *T. gondii* mediated by IFN-γ and release of RNIs by murine macrophages.[119]

INF-γ as well as TNF-α and transforming growth factor-β (TGF-β) all appear to play a role in inhibiting multiplication.[121] Gazzinelli and colleagues[122] reported that a reactivation of *T. gondii*, at least in the experimental mouse model, is due to down-regulation of IFN-γ and TNF-α, which leads to decreased macrophage (with a decrease in inducible nitric oxide synthase and macrophage activation gene 1) and glial activation, unrestricted parasite growth, and tissue damage.

Beaman and colleagues[123] reported that interleukin-6 (IL-6) enhanced intracellular reproduction of *T. gondii* and actually reversed the effect of INF-γ–mediated killing. This is of particular note in light of the fact that the retinal pigment epithelium (RPE) produces large amounts of IL-6. IL-2 appears to contribute to resistance against *Toxoplasma* infection. However, it does not seem to exert its action through macrophages.[124]

Recent work has focused on the protective role of IL-12. It has been shown that stimulation of spleen cells from uninfected severe combined immunodeficient (SCID) mice with live *T. gondii* or parasite preparation induced NK cells to produce INF-γ. This activity was found to be dependent on the production of TNF-α and IL-12 by macrophages that induce the NK cells to produce INF-γ.[125,126] Administration of exogenous IL-12 delayed time to death of SCID mice infected with *T. gondii*,[125] whereas administration of anti–IL-12 resulted in earlier mortality.[127] Similarly, administration of monoclonal antibodies to INF-γ and TNF-α to SCID mice infected with *T. gondii* resulted in early mortality.[128] This experiment demonstrated the importance of these cytokines in T-cell–independent resistance to *T. gondii*.

In another experiment, Hunter and associates[129] demonstrated the important role of endogenous IL-12 in mediating resistance to *T. gondii* in immunocompetent mice by illustrating the occurrence of 100% mortality after the administration of anti–IL-12 to these mice. To show the importance of INF-γ and TNF-α, they administered antibodies to these cytokines to the immunocompetent mice. This procedure resulted in abrogation of the protective activity of IL-12.

Although antibodies are usually made, it is the cellular component of the immune system that must be intact for a resolution of the disease process. While immunoglobulins do play a role in facilitating lysis of the extracellular tachyzoites, they are ineffective against the live organisms inside the cells.[130,131]

In an attempt to evaluate why newborn infants seem to have difficulty in clearing the *Toxoplasma* infection, Wilson and Haas[132] evaluated the cellular defenses against *T. gondii* in newborns. They noted that newborn and adult macrophages killed the organism equally, but supernatants from cord blood–derived concanavalin A–stimulated mononuclear cells effectively activated macrophages as compared with supernatants produced from adult blood cells. This difference appears to lie in the CD4+ fraction of the T cells. The cord blood appeared to produce fewer lymphokines capable of activating macrophages, including INF-γ. The authors did not believe that enhanced generation of reactive oxygen intermediates was important in explaining the differences between the adult and the newborn responses, although recent notions would suggest that nitrous oxide and its effects in macrophages may indeed play a very important role. Of interest is that the organism replicates in the macrophages, and this decreased killing in the newborn may then lead to a greater susceptibility.

PATHOLOGY OF OCULAR TOXOPLASMOSIS

Classically, the organisms first lodge in the capillaries of the inner retinal layers. Some authors described cases in which the initial reaction was in the outer retinal layers.[90,91] From the capillary endothelium the parasite extends into adjacent tissues. An intense inflammatory reaction results, with edema and infiltration of polymorphonuclear leukocytes, lymphocytes, plasma cells, mononuclear cells, and in some cases eosinophils. The reaction results in disruption and disorganization of the retinal layers. The inflammatory process almost always extends into the choroid, and Bruch's membrane is destroyed in the process. The choroidal vessels are usually engorged and show perivascular infiltration of lymphocytes, plasma cells, mononuclear cells, and eosinophils. Eventually, the inflammatory process subsides, leaving a pale atrophic scar surrounded by pigmented margins.

DIAGNOSIS

Serologic Studies (Table 57–7)

The definitive diagnosis of ocular toxoplasmosis requires the demonstration of the proliferative form

TABLE 57–7 Guidelines for Interpretation of Results of Serologic Tests for Antibodies Against *Toxoplasma**†

Test	Positive Titer	Titer in Acute Infection	Titer in Chronic Infection
Sabin-Feldman dye test	1:4 Undiluted	≥1:1000	1:4–1:2000
Indirect fluorescent antibody test (IFA)	1:10	≥1:1000	1:4–1:2000
Indirect hemagglutination (IHA)§	1:16	≥1:1000	1:16–1:256
Complement fixation test (CF)	1:4	Varies among laboratories	Negative–1:8
Agglutination test	1:20	1:20–≥1:1000	≤1:12,000–64,000
IFA for IgM antibodies	1:2 Infants‡	≥1:2	Negative
	1:16 Adults	≥1:64	1:20
Enzyme-linked immunosorbent assay (ELISA) for IgM	1.0 Infants	≥1.4	‡
	1.7 Adults	≥1.7	Negative to 3

* Adapted from McCabe RE, Remington JS: Toxoplasmosis. In Warren KS, Mahmoud AAF (eds): Tropical and Geographic Medicine. New York, McGraw-Hill Book Co, 1990, p 314, with permission.
† Values may differ in different laboratories and exceptions to these generalizations may occur.
‡ Unknown at this time.
§ May give false-negative results early in infection. Therefore, IHA should not be used to detect congenital infection or infection during pregnancy.

of *T. gondii* in ocular tissues.[133] *Toxoplasma* retinochoroiditis is, therefore, usually a presumptive diagnosis based on the presence of a compatible lesion in the fundus and positive serologic results for *Toxoplasma* antibodies in the patient's serum. Thus, serologic evidence of the *Toxoplasma* organism becomes a supplementary tool in helping the clinician make the diagnosis. Unfortunately, serologic tests are not flawless for a variety of reasons:

1. The presence of circulating *Toxoplasma* antibodies is not of great importance in view of the fact that many healthy individuals might have been exposed to the *Toxoplasma* infection and have these antibodies resulting in a low specific diagnostic value.
2. The incidence of false-positive results is high.
3. The high titer of anti-*Toxoplasma* IgM antibodies may be transient and easily missed (R. Belfort, personal communication), or high titers of different antibodies may persist for years in normal individuals.
4. Toxoplasmic retinochoroiditis may progress for months in the presence of a stable, low titer.[134]
5. Serologic examination can be used to rule out toxoplasmosis if there are no toxoplasmic antibodies at all by the serologic tests. However, if antibodies are present, one cannot be certain whether they are coincidental or related to the lesion.[134]

This argument about the feasibility of serologic tests is emphasized by the results of a study done by Rothova and co-workers.[135] They noted that even though 100% of their patients with clinically apparent ocular toxoplasmosis revealed IgG antibody positivity, 58% of the control subjects also showed positive results. Therefore, we believe that the diagnosis of ocular toxoplasmosis is very much a clinical one, with serologic findings supportive but not definitive.

Serologic diagnosis of recent primary infection is based on the detection of seroconversion, a marked increase in antibody titers over several weeks, or the presence of IgM antibodies.[136] The most common serologic tests for *Toxoplasma* infection are the Sabin-Feldman dye test (methylene blue dye test), the indirect hemagglutination test (IHA), the indirect fluorescent antibody test (IFA), the complement fixation test (CF), and the ELISA.

Sabin-Feldman Dye Test

The titer is considered positive when more than 50% of the parasites remain unstained. Antibodies appear around 1 week after the infection and reach high titers above 1:1024 in 6 to 8 weeks. The antibody titers start to decline gradually over a period of months to a year. The World Health Organization (WHO) has recommended that titers in the dye test be expressed in international units (IU) per milliliter of serum, compared with an international standard reference serum, which is available on request.[137] The dye test is the reference serologic procedure against which all other methods are evaluated.

Indirect Hemagglutination Test

The IHA test is frequently negative in cases of congenital toxoplasmosis with high dye test titers, and therefore is not recommended for the diagnosis of congenital toxoplasmosis.[17] In addition, because a rise in titer in the IHA test may not be demonstrable for months, it is not satisfactory as a screening method in pregnant women.[138,139] It is, however, an additional test that may be useful in serologic surveys and in the diagnosis of acute acquired infections when the dye test titer has already stabilized and a rising IHA titer may be demonstrated.[17]

Complement Fixing Antibody Test

It has been studied mainly in acquired toxoplasmosis. The special usefulness of the CF test is the demonstration of rising titers when the dye test or IFA test titers are already high and stable.[138,140] A negative CF test turning positive or increasing CF test titers, together with stable high dye test titers, indicate active infection.[17]

Direct Agglutination Test

This test employs whole parasites that have been preserved in formalin. It is very sensitive to IgM antibodies. Nonspecific agglutination (apparently related to naturally occurring IgM *Toxoplasma* agglutinins)[141] has been observed in individuals devoid of antibody in the dye test and conventional IFA test. This test may be used for wide-scale screening of pregnant women[142,143] because it is simple, accurate, inexpensive, and easy to perform.

Conventional Indirect Fluorescent Antibody Test

A positive reaction is detected by the bright yellow-green fluorescence of the organisms when examined by fluorescence microscopy. In general, qualitative agreement with the dye test and the CF and IHA tests has been excellent.[17] Although most workers consider the IFA test to equal the dye test in specificity, it has two distinct disadvantages: (1) false-positive results occur with some sera that contain antinuclear antibodies[144] or the rheumatoid factor and (2) it may demonstrate false-negative reactivity due to competitive inhibition by high levels of *T. gondii*–specific IgG antibodies, which may lead to as many as 40% of the false-negative samples.[145] For this reason, in patients with connective tissue disease, a dye test or ELISA can be performed to document a positive IFA test.

Conventional Enzyme-Linked Immunosorbent Assay

This test has been used successfully to demonstrate IgG, IgM, and IgA antibodies in the pregnant woman, fetus, and newborn.[146,147] Using enzyme-conjugated antibody directed against human IgG[148,149] or against total immunoglobulin,[150-154] the titers correlated very well with titers in the dye, IHA, IFA, and CF tests in some studies[153] but not in others.[154,155]

Enzyme-Linked Immunosorbent Assay for Detection of IgM Antibodies

Because of false-positive results reported with conventional ELISA, a more specific ELISA for the detection of IgM antibodies to *T. gondii* was developed.[156,157] Noat and Remington[157] developed a "double-sandwich" ELISA which they believed was an improvement over the IgM ELISA developed by Camargo and colleagues,[156] particularly in cases where rheumatoid factor was present and in cases with chronic infection. This type of ELISA is more sensitive and more specific than the IgM IFA test for the diagnosis of acute acquired toxoplasmosis and requires about 6 hours for performance.[157]

Western Blot

The protein-blotting technique has been used to detect antigens of *T. gondii* recognized by IgG and IgM antibodies in sera of congenitally infected newborns and their mothers. Patterns of IgG and IgM blots with sera from newborns revealed antigen–antibody reactions (bands) that were not present in the respective blots obtained with sera from their mothers. Ware and colleagues[158] used PCR to identify *Toxoplasma* antigens.

Polymerase Chain Reaction

Ware and colleagues[158] used PCR to identify *Toxoplasma* antigens. Similarly, Grover and colleagues described the usefulness of PCR for rapid diagnosis of congenital *Toxoplasma* infection.[159] In a prospective study of 43 documented cases of acute maternal *Toxoplasma* infection acquired during gestation, PCR correctly identified the presence of *T. gondii* in five of five samples of amniotic fluid from four proven cases of congenital infection and in three of five positive cases from a nonprospective group.

Analysis of Aqueous Humor

Analysis of local antibody production in the aqueous humor is another valuable diagnostic tool.[160] Intraocular synthesis of antibodies is considered to have taken place if the relative amount of *Toxoplasma* antibodies compared to the total immunoglobulin level found in the aqueous exceeds that

measured in a paired serum sample. The quotient of the relative amount of *Toxoplasma* antibodies in the aqueous and serum is named the Goldmann-Witmer coefficient:

$$\frac{\text{antibody titer aqueous}}{\text{total immunoglobulin aqueous}} : \frac{\text{antibody titer in serum}}{\text{total immunoglobulin serum}}$$

Theoretically, a coefficient above 1.0 would indicate a local antibody production within the eye. In view of the variability in the results of the various measurement, an antibody coefficient above 3.0 is considered significant.[160]

Scheiffarth and associates[161] developed an in vivo immunofluorescence by tagging specific anti-*Toxoplasma* antibodies with fluorescein, injected them intravenously, and found that a chorioretinitis could be experimentally induced with this technique. However, much work on this technique is still needed before it can be brought to the human form of the disease.

Serologic Diagnosis of Acquired *Toxoplasma* Infection in the Pregnant Woman

In some countries, like France and Austria, repeated screening of seronegative women is mandatory throughout pregnancy, while most countries have no adopted policy.[38]

The presence of a positive titer (except for the rare false-positive result) in any of the tests mentioned before establishes the diagnosis of *Toxoplasma* infection. Because titers in each of these tests may remain elevated for years, a single high titer does not indicate whether the infection is acute or chronic, nor does it necessarily mean that the clinical findings are due to toxoplasmosis. A negative test indicates no previous infection.

Before a diagnosis of acute *Toxoplasma* infection can be made by means of serologic tests (Table 57–8), it is necessary to demonstrate a rising titer in serial specimens (either conversion from negative to positive titer or a rise from a low to a high titer).[162] Since the majority of cases of acquired *Toxoplasma* infection are subclinical (>80%), the diagnosis relies mainly on the results of serologic tests. The most important fact for the clinician is that any patient with dye test or IFA test titers of higher than 300 IU/ml or 1:1000 and an IgM IFA test titer of 1:80 or higher must be presumed to have recently acquired *Toxoplasma* infection with unless proven otherwise.[17] To ascertain that the IgM titers are not false-positive due to the presence of the "natural IgM antibodies," rheumatoid factor or antinuclear

TABLE 57–8 General Considerations of IgG and IgM Antibody responses to Postnatally Acquired Infection with *Toxoplasma**

Antibodies	Uninfected Individuals	Acute (Recent) Infection	Chronic (Latent) Infection
IgM			
Directed against antigens that cross-react	Present	Present	Present
Directed toward specific *Toxoplasma* antigens	Absent	Present in almost all cases. Period that IgM antibodies are present may vary from a few months. Ability to detect these antibodies depends on serologic technique used.	Most often absent, but IgM antibodies may persist for years in some patients (about 5%). In such cases, titers are almost always low, but in some cases they remain high. Persistence of IgM antibodies is generally associated with low or medium titers of IgG antibodies.
IgG			
Directed toward antigens that cross-react	Absent	Absent (?)	Absent (?)
Directed toward specific *Toxoplasma* antigens	Absent (<2 IU/ml)[†]	Present. Rise from a low titer (≤2 IU/ml) to a high titer (300–6000 IU/ml). In a few asymptomatic patients, titers remain low (100–200 IU/ml). Duration of rise varies with patient and with serologic test used. Depending on serologic techniques, it may take from 2 to 6 months for the IgG antibody titer to reach its peak. This rise in titer is inhibited if patient is treated early in infection.	Present. Stable or slowly decreasing titers (to 2–200 IU/ml). High titers (>300 IU/ml) persist for years in some patients (about 5%). A significant rise in titer is sometimes observed after a normal decrease in titer has occurred (often observed after cessation of treatment).

* From Remington JS, Desmonts G: Toxoplasmosis. In Remington JS, Klein JO (eds): Infectious Disease of the Fetus and the Newborn Infant, 4th edition. Philadelphia, WB Saunders Co, 1990, p 160, with permission.
† Titers are expressed in international units to minimize technical differences that might occur among different laboratories.

antibodies, IgM ELISA may be a more reliable test in these circumstances.[157]

Diagnosis of Fetal Infection

When the diagnosis of post–conceptionally acquired infection is established in a pregnant woman, determining whether or not the fetus has been infected becomes essential for planning what measures are to be taken. If fetal infection is documented prior to 20 weeks' gestation, termination of pregnancy may be considered.

A definitive diagnosis of fetal *T. gondii* infection relies on isolation of the parasite from the fetal blood or amniotic fluid and on serologic examination of fetal serum for evidence of synthesis of specific IgM antibodies.[163] For demonstration of *Toxoplasma*, the sediment from 10 to 30 ml of amniotic fluid and the whole fetal blood clot are injected intraperitoneally into mice. Mice are bled for serologic testing 3 and 6 weeks later; if antibodies are detected, proof of infection must be obtained by examining wet preparations of brain tissue for demonstration of cysts.[163] Major shortcomings of this procedure are that results are not available for at least 3 weeks, and a fetal blood sample is not possible early in pregnancy, so the answer as to whether the fetus is infected may not be available until 24 to 26 weeks' gestation.[164]

Inoculation of amniotic fluid sediment into cell culture offers the opportunity for a more rapid diagnosis: after 4 days of incubation, parasites are identified in monolayers by an indirect immunofluorescence assay.[165] According to the results of Thulliez, tissue culture of amniotic fluid samples is less sensitive than mouse inoculation (53% vs. 73%; n = 53). However, when the cell culture results are considered together with IgM detection in fetal serum, a definitive diagnosis is obtained in 70% of cases within 4 days.[163]

Ultrasonographic examination of the fetus to look for abnormal morphologic signs caused by *Toxoplasma* may provide important information. The sign most frequently noted is cerebral ventricular dilatation that is generally bilateral and symmetrical.[163] However, repeated ultrasonographic assessment of the fetus at regular intervals may be necessary because it has been shown that ventricular dilatation may develop weeks after prenatal diagnosis is made.[166]

A promising new possibility for rapid and sensitive diagnosis of fetal *Toxoplasma* infection in amniotic fluid samples is the PCR test.[159]

Nonspecific tests performed on the fetal blood sample, taken from 20 weeks' gestation, can be indicative of fetal infection[167]; thrombocytopenia, increased levels of total IgM, and gammaglutamyl transferase are the most sensitive. When associated, these abnormal measurements have a high predictive value and justify commencing treatment without waiting for the results of confirmatory tests in cases where the parents wish to continue the pregnancy.[163]

Prenatal diagnosis has been shown to be reliable in a number of centers. Desmonts et al[168] studied 278 women infected with *Toxoplasma* during pregnancy. Termination of pregnancy was requested by the mothers in the nine cases in whom the prenatal diagnosis of congenital toxoplasmosis was established. Among the 209 cases with negative prenatal studies, only one infant was considered to have been infected in utero. In a similar study in Belgium[164] on 49 pregnant women with serologic evidence of maternal toxoplasmosis who underwent prenatal investigation, diagnosis of fetal infection was made in 5 cases. No evidence of congenital infection was noted in the 44 cases in whom *Toxoplasma* infection was ruled out prenatally.

MANAGEMENT OF OCULAR TOXOPLASMOSIS

The primary questions that face every clinician confronted with a case of toxoplasmic retinochoroiditis include: Is treatment warranted? If so, what agents should be used, and for what length of time? For the uveitis group at the National Eye Institute (NEI), the decision to treat would be based on the following criteria:

- A lesion located within the temporal arcades irrespective of size
- A lesion abutting the optic nerve or threatening a large retinal vessel
- A lesion that has induced a large degree of hemorrhage
- A lesion that has induced enough of a vitreal inflammatory response so that the vision has dropped below 20/40 in a previously 20/20 eye, or at least has sustained a 2-line drop from the visual acuity before the acute infection.

A relative indication would be the case of multiple recurrences that developed marked vitreal condensation. Here one might be concerned about the continuation of this process leading to retinal detachment.

The majority of physician members' answers to a questionnaire[169] sent to them by the American Uveitis Society to determine the current treatment practices for ocular toxoplasmosis are consistent with the treatment framework, outlined above, of the uveitis group at the NEI. 75% of the respondents considered any decrease in vision from baseline an indication for treatment.

The currently available drugs do not eliminate tissue cysts in humans and therefore will not prevent recrudescence of latent *Toxoplasma* infection. In light of this fact, the goal of therapy will be to halt the multiplication of the parasite during the active retinochoroiditis and minimize the degree of inflammation and subsequent fibrosis and scarring by using the most potent drugs with least injurious effects.

The enthusiasm of the treating physicians to contain the disease as efficiently as possible with minimum harm to the patient has resulted in several combinations of therapeutic agents. In a prospective multicenter study, Rothova and colleagues[170] used three triple-drug combinations: group 1, pyrimethamine, sulfadiazine, and corticosteroids; group 2, clindamycin, sulfadiazine, and corticosteroids; and group 3, cotrimoxazole (trimethoprim and sulfamethoxazole) and corticosteroids.

Similarly, in a survey[169] of the American Uveitis Society members, eight different antimicrobial agents were combined in 15 different regimens! The combination of pyrimethamine, sulfadiazine, and corticosteroids was used by 32% of clinicians. Clindamycin was used with these three agents (quadruple therapy) by 17%. A combined regimen of sulfadiazine, clindamycin, and corticosteroids was used by 16%. Clindamycin and corticosteroids were used by 6%. All other combinations were used by one respondent each.

As the first drug combination for the treatment of ocular toxoplasmosis, we still use pyrimethamine, sulfadiazine, folinic acid, and ± prednisone (see Table 57–9). Sulfadiazine is given in a dose of 1 g orally four times daily, pyrimethamine in a 50-mg loading dose, then 25 mg orally twice daily, always given concomitantly with folinic acid, 3 to 5 mg three times a week. A baseline analysis of white blood cell count and platelet count followed by weekly counts are obtained for the duration of folinic acid therapy, which we continue for 1 week after stopping pyrimethamine. We generally treat immunocompetent patients for 4 weeks with this regimen. We judiciously add prednisone to the regimen if the lesion is in the posterior pole or threatening the optic nerve head. If the macula or the optic nerve is threatened, we follow the patient very closely, tapering the steroids in such a way that they are stopped before the anti-Toxoplasma therapy is discontinued.

In the study of Rothova et al,[170] the deciding factor on the efficacy of the different combinations was the decrease in the size of the retinal lesion. They found that the triple combination of pyrimethamine was most efficacious, with 52% of the 29 patients treated showing marked decrease (>1/2 disk diameter) in the size of the retinal lesion, compared to 32% of 37 patients and 25% of 8 patients in the second and third groups, respectively.

Several authors[171,172] believe that clindamycin alone or in combination is an effective antimicrobial drug that can cause rapid resolution of the inflamed Toxoplasma lesions and reduce recurrences. Findings in animals showed that clindamycin reached high concentrations in the choroid, vitreous, and retina, and reduced the number of toxoplasmic cysts in rabbits with healed inactive cysts.[173,174]

Opremcak and colleagues[175] used trimethoprim-sulfamethoxazole in the treatment of 16 patients with active ocular toxoplasmosis: alone in 4 patients, in combination with clindamycin in another 4, and in combination with clindamycin and prednisone in 8. They reported that all patients had resolution of the active retinochoroiditis with good gain in visual acuity.

However, it is not feasible to compare the efficacy of therapeutic regimens for ocular toxoplasmosis because it is very difficult, if not impossible, to have two groups with a good number of patients who will have a retinal lesion that has the same size, location, duration, number (if lesions are multiple), number of recurrences, and complications, and the same level of immune competence of the infected patients. Therefore, we believe that talking about efficacy of the commonly used regimens is a matter of personal experience and needs large-scale, well-controlled, multicenter studies.

REVIEW OF THE COMMON ANTIPARASITIC AGENTS AND OTHER DRUGS USED IN THE TREATMENT OF TOXOPLASMOSIS

Pyrimethamine and Sulfonamides

Toxoplasma lack the transmembrane transport systems for physiologic folates and thus synthesize this substance instead. Both pyrimethamine and sulfonamides are inhibitors of folate metabolism and act synergistically when used in combination. The concept of inhibiting two steps in an essential metabolic pathway with separate drugs to produce a supra-additive effect explains the synergistic action of pyrimethamine with sulfonamides. The two steps involved are the utilization of para-aminobenzoic acid (PABA) in the synthesis of dihydropteroic acid, inhibited by sulfonamides, and the reduction of dihydrofolate to tetrahydrofolate, inhibited by pyrimethamine. This results in impaired synthesis of DNA, precluding the replication of the organism.[176] Sulfadiazine is the most common sulfonamide that is used in combination with pyrimethamine.

Excessive doses of pyrimethamine produce a megaloblastic anemia resembling that of folic acid deficiency; this reverses readily on discontinuation of treatment or on administration of leucovorin (folinic acid). In rare cases, this combination may cause skin reactions, such as erythema multiforme, Stevens-Johnson syndrome, and toxic epidermal necrolysis. This combination may be associated with serum sickness–like reactions, urticaria, exfoliative dermatitis, and hepatitis.[176]

Pyrimethamine has been used worldwide against malaria for almost 40 years, and no terato-

TABLE 57–9 Guidelines for the Treatment of Toxoplasmosis

Ocular Toxoplasmosis
Combination of first choice: pyrimethamine + sulfadiazine + leucovorin
  Pyrimethamine (Daraprim), given in a loading dose of 50–75 mg on the first day followed by 25 mg twice daily for 4–6 weeks.
  Sulfadiazine can be given as a 1- to 2-g loading dose, followed by 1 g orally four times a day for 4–6 weeks.
  Folinic acid (leucovorin) 3–5 mg IM or 5–10 mg PO (low absorption rate from gastrointestinal tract) 3 times a week.
Recommendation about this regimen:
  Folic acid–containing vitamins should be stopped during this treatment.
  Take excess of fluids to prevent urinary crystals due to sulfa drugs.
  White blood cell count with differential and a plate cell count should be done at baseline and weekly thereafter.
  Leucovorin should be given for a week after stopping pyrimethamine.
Alternative combination: Clindamycin + Sulfadiazine
  Clindamycin: 300 mg four times PO for 3–4 weeks.
  Sulfadiazine: 2 g as a loading dose, followed by 1 g four times daily for 4 weeks.
Note: corticosteroids may be added to both regimens when visual function is at stake. We give:
  Prednisone 1–1.5 mg/kg/day starting 12–24 hours after initiation of antimicrobial agents and tapering the steroids with the first sign of clinical improvement.
Acquired Toxoplasmosis in Pregnant Women*
  Spiramycin, 1 g every 8 hours daily until fetal infection is settled. If fetal infection is confirmed and pregnancy continued, spiramycin is continued throughout pregnancy plus one of the two regimens:
  Pyrimethamine 25 mg and sulfadoxine 500 mg every 10 days until the end of pregnancy.
                    OR
  Pyrimethamine 50 mg and sulfadiazine 3 g daily for 3 weeks alternating with 3 weeks of daily spiramycin.
  Folinic acid 10–20 mg supplements are administered to the mother during and for 1 week after pyrimethamine therapy.[†]
Congenital Toxoplasmosis in the Infant[†]
The combination of choice: pyrimethamine + sulfadiazine + leucovorin ± corticosteroids.
  Pyrimethamine, in a loading dose of 2 mg/kg/day for 2 days followed by 1 mg/kg/day for 2–6 months, then this dose every Monday, Wednesday, and Friday.
  Sulfadiazine 100 mg/kg/day in two divided doses.
  Leucovorin 10 mg 3 times weekly during and for 1 week after pyrimethamine therapy.
  Corticosteroids have been used when CSF is ≥1 g% and when active chorioretinitis threatens vision. Prednisone is given in a dose of 1 mg/kg/day in two divided doses until resolution of elevated CSF proteins or chorioretinitis improvement.
Active Ocular Disease in Older Children[†]
The treatment of choice: pyrimethamine + sulfadiazine + leucovorin ± corticosteroids.
  Pyrimethamine: Loading dose of 2 mg/kg/day (maximum 50 mg) for 2 days, then maintenance, 1 mg/kg/day (maximum 25 mg) until 1–2 weeks after signs and symptoms have resolved.
  Sulfadiazine: Loading dose of 75 mg/kg, then maintenance, 50 mg/kg every 12 hours until 1–2 weeks after signs and symptoms have resolved.
  Leucovorin: 10–12 mg 3 times weekly until 1 week after discontinuation of pyrimethamine therapy.
  Corticosteroids: The same as in the treatment of congenital infection in infants.
Ocular Toxoplasmosis in Immunocompromised Patients
Managed on the same lines as in immunocompetent subjects except in two points:
  In patients who also have cerebral toxoplasmosis in addition to ocular toxoplasmosis, clindamycin does not cross the blood-brain barrier and therefore its combinations are not recommended.
  Steroids are not used unless extremely indicated.

* Data from Daffos F, Forestier F, Capella-Pavlosky M, et al: Prenatal management of 746 pregnancies at risk for congenital toxoplasmosis. N Engl J Med 318:271–275, 1988.
† Data from Remington JS, McLeod R: Toxoplasmosis. In Remington JS, Klein JO (eds): Infectious Diseases of the Fetus and Newborn Infant, 4th edition. Philadelphia, WB Saunders Co, 1995, p 225.

genic effects have been observed. Based on these data, the WHO in 1978 approved the free use of Fansidar (pyrimethamine 25 mg plus sulfadoxine 500 mg) as malarial prophylaxis in pregnancy.

Clindamycin

The half-life of this antibiotic is about 2.7 hours, and modest accumulation of drug is expected if it is given at 6-hour intervals. Significant concentrations are not attained in the cerebrospinal fluid (CSF), even when the meninges are inflamed, whereas it readily crosses the placental barrier. The reported incidence of diarrhea associated with the administration of the drug ranges from 2 to 20%, with an average of 8%. The most dreadful complication of clindamycin therapy is pseudomembranous colitis caused by a toxin secreted by a strain of Clostridium difficile. It occurs rarely but can be lethal. It can occur during therapy or it may be delayed for several weeks after discontinuation of the offending antibiotic. If significant diarrhea develops during therapy, the drug should be discontinued immediately.[177]

Atovaquone

Atovaquone (Mepron) was used in the treatment of mice infected with several strains of Toxoplasma parasite. Treated mice were sacrificed at 2-week intervals; their examination revealed a steady decline in the number of cysts in their brains compared with untreated control. Furthermore, untreated mice had a high mortality rate, whereas mortality and clinical signs of brain infection were absent in treated ones.[178] Lopez and colleagues[179] reported the successful use of atovaquone in the treatment of ocular toxoplasmosis in a 14-year-old hemophilic boy with AIDS who was unable to continue with the standard anti-Toxoplasma therapy. A new formulation is being used in a study evaluating its use in the treatment of ocular toxoplasmosis in AIDS patients in Brazil. With its in vivo activity against tissue cysts, this agent may become a very potent tool in the management of toxoplasmic encephalitis, particularly in patients with AIDS.

Corticosteroids

The damaging effect of the proliferating T. gondii and the hypersensitivity to Toxoplasma antigens are two important factors in the immunopathogenesis of ocular toxoplasmosis that warrant the use of corticosteroids. However, these agents should be used very judiciously. They act like a double-edged sword. On the one hand, they quell the inflammation, thereby precluding its sequelae including macular edema, vitreous reaction, papillitis and retinal vasculitis that may damage vital structures like macula, maculopapillary bundle, and optic nerve. On the other hand, due to their immunosuppressive effect, they will minimize or totally abrogate the cell-mediated defenses that are keeping the proliferating form of the T. gondii under control, resulting in fulminant infection. Therefore, corticosteroids should only be used (1) in conjunction with other antiparasitic agents (2) and when the retinal lesion is located close to one of the vital ocular structures (3) or in the presence of significant vitreous reaction. Periocular injections of steroids are not recommended because of the fear that they may be associated with severe reaction culminating in loss of useful vision.[180]

Spiramycin

Spiramycin is a macrolide antibiotic used mainly in the treatment of primary acquired Toxoplasma infections during pregnancy. It has an intracellular toxoplasmocidal activity, and is concentrated markedly in the tissues. In placenta its concentration is three to five times higher than the corresponding maternal serum. The drug does not readily cross the blood-brain barrier and therefore does not prevent the development of toxoplasmic encephalitis. The main advantage of spiramycin lies in its complete safely for the pregnant woman, the fetus, and the newborn infant. It has no teratogenic effects. At high doses, however, gastrointestinal distress, such as nausea, vomiting, and diarrhea, has been observed.[38]

Other Modalities of Therapy

Laser treatment has been used on the premise that photocoagulation destroys the organism within the lesion (including tissue cysts) and probably denatures the antigen proteins responsible for the hypersensitivity reaction. It is ideally reserved for lesions that have proved refractory to the standard medical therapy or to patients who are intolerant of systemic treatment.[181]

Ghartey and colleagues[181] treated five patients whose eye lesions were nonresponsive to medical therapy, with laser photocoagulation. Similarly, Spalter and associates[182] treated quiescent lesions in 24 patients with laser photocoagulation in an attempt to prevent recurrences. Theodossiadis and colleages[183] reported the result of laser treatment in 33 eyes (patients) with active toxoplasmic retinochoroiditis followed up for a period of 2 to 9 years, whereas, Fitzgerald[184] used pars plana vitrectomy in the management of four cases of vitreous opacities secondary to presumed toxoplasmosis. To prevent recurrence of retinochoroiditis within the same ocular focus, Steahly[185] used vitrectomy and endolaser photocoagulation in two eyes in which medical treatment failed and vitreous opacification precluded external photocoagulation.

What can be said about photocoagulation and pars plana vitrectomy is that their use may be indicated in situations where the standard medical treatments do not work or toxicities preclude their continued use. The use of photocoagulation for treatment of active lesions should be limited at present given its controversial nature. Higher energy levels may damage the Bruch's membrane. Recurrences cannot be prevented with laser photocoagulation.

TREATMENT WITH PREGNANT WOMEN

When prenatal diagnosis of congenital toxoplasmosis is made in women who wish to continue their pregnancy, theropy reduces the severity of the manifestations of the disease.[167] In France, spiramycin has been used in the treatment of primary toxoplasmosis in pregnant women since 1960 in repeated 3- to 4-week courses throughout pregnancy[38] in a study by Daffos and colleagues[167] on 746 documented cases of maternal *Toxoplasma* infection. Infection was diagnosed antenatally in 39 of 42 fetuses; 24 of the 39 pregnancies were terminated, and 15 were continued. All the mothers were treated with spiramycin 3g/day throughout pregnancy. In the case of the 15 infected fetuses who were carried to term, their mothers were given pyrimethamine with either sulfadiazine or sulfadoxine added to spiramycin started roughly around the 31st week of gestation. No fetal complications of therapy were reported. The combination of prenatal tests, including fetal blood sampling, amniocentesis, and ultrasonography, allowed diagnosis of fetal infection in 39 (93%) of the 42 cases. Of the 15 pregnancies that were continued, four infants had signs of infection at delivery. Peripheral chorioretinitis developed in two of these infants, with no clinical affects up to 18 months of follow-up. The low frequency of fetal infection was attributed to the effect of treatment on these subjects as soon as diagnosis was established. This finding could be indirect evidence of the action of spiramycin on placenta.[167]

All strongly suspected cases of acquired toxoplasmosis in pregnancy ought to be treated. Initially spiramycin should be given until the status of the fetus is definitely settled by amniotic fluid, fetal blood, and ultrasound examination.[38] In proven cases of placental or fetal infection, 3-week courses of pyrimethamine/sulfadiazine alternating with 3-week courses of spiramycin should be given from the beginning of the second trimester. During this treatment, the mother should be carefully monitored for the development of hematologic toxicity. If significant toxicity develops despite treatment with folinic acid, the drug combination is discontinued until the hematologic abnormalities are corrected, and the drug regimen is then restarted.[17] An editorial by *Lancet* in 1983 reported the safety of pyrimethamine in early pregnancy, but as a precaution folinic acid should be added as a supplement.[186]

TREATMENT OF NEWBORN INFANT

Active ocular toxoplasmosis is rare in newborn infants because the ocular lesions would have healed by the time of delivery. Few members of the American Uveitis Society treated newborns with toxoplasmic retinochoroiditis. The treatment of such cases is given until the infant is 1 year old.[169] However, retinochoroiditis in these children will be a manifestation of the systemic infection, and for this reason these infants are generally put on pyrimethamine/sulfadiazine for the first 6 months of life. Thereafter, monthly courses of alternating treatment with spiramycin and with pyrimethamine/sulfadiazine are given for another half a year.[38]

TREATMENT OF IMMUNOCOMPROMISED PATIENTS

Treatment of ocular toxoplasmosis in these patients is carried out roughly along the same lines used for the treatment of the disease in immunocompetent subjects. The retinal lesions respond favorably to treatment with pyrimethamine in combination with sulfadiazine or clindamycin. Of the 14 patients of Friedman and co-workers'[66] series placed on the combination therapy, 13 showed healing of retinal lesions in 4 to 8 weeks. Similar favorable results were reported in other studies.[88] Studies of patients with AIDS who have cerebral toxoplasmosis disclosed a 95% response rate to the combination of pyrimethamine and sulfadiazine therapy.[187] The recurrence rate is high once the treatment is discontinued. Therefore, maintenance therapy must be continued indefinitely in patients with AIDS.

Corticosteroid use in *Toxoplasma* infection in immunocompromised subjects is yet more controversial than in immunocompetent patients for two reasons; the inflammatory reaction associated with toxoplasmosis in these patients is generally minimal, and the already compromised immune status that may be still exerting some control on the multiplication of the tachyzoites will be weakened still further by the steroidal therapy.

PREVENTION

Our understanding of the life cycle of *T. gondii* shows us that by following certain simple measures we can break the cycle of the parasite and prevent its perpetuation. Frenkel[188] formulated the following instructions:

- Feed your cat only dried, canned, or cooked meat.
- Keep your cat from foraging.
- Change litter boxes daily; disinfect them with warm boiling water.
- If pregnant, wear plastic gloves or delegate care of the cat to someone else.
- Use gloves when working in soil contaminated with cat feces.
- Cover children's sand-boxes when not in use.
- Control stray cats.
- Control flies and cockroaches.
- Avoid eating raw meat; heat all meat thoroughly until it changes color.
- Wash your hands before meals and before touching the face.

Foulon,[189] in his illustration of the usefulness of screening tests in curtailing the risks of congenital toxoplasmosis, pointed out that there are two conflicting opinions in terms of proper management of pregnant women. Some authors[190,191] agree about educating women on how to avoid contacting the *Toxoplasma* infection but are not in favor of serologic testing of pregnant women because:

1. Prevalence of toxoplasmosis during pregnancy is rare. Besides, chances of associated damage to the fetus are too small to warrant routine serologic testing.
2. Serologic screening during pregnancy is difficult, costly, and not 100% reliable.
3. To confirm fetal infection requires fetal blood or amniotic samples for cordocentesis and amniocentesis procedures, which can only be done at specialized centers.

On the other hand, others[192] advocate carrying out secondary prevention tests on pregnant women because they believe that:

1. Infection of pregnant women can result in severe fetal morbidity and even death. Besides, up to 50% of patients with latent congenital toxoplasmosis will develop systemic manifestations including recurrent retinochoroiditis that may eventually culminate in stringent impairment of vision.
2. Early recognition of the in utero infection and timely antibiotic treatment during pregnancy reduces the long-term sequelae in the affected child.

We believe that the least we can do is make the teaching of a primary prevention program of toxoplasmosis part of the initial maternity visits to maternity centers. Primary prevention can be very effective in reducing the rate of seroconversion in pregnant women. Foulon and his group[189] assessed the usefulness of primary prevention in 12 consecutive years during which the incidence of congenital toxoplasmosis was studied in 11,286 consecutive pregnant women. The impact of primary prevention was studied by measuring the reduction in seroconversion when hygienic measures were systemically applied. They found that primary prevention reduced the seroconversion rate during pregnancy by 63% ($p = .013$). A survey in maternity hospitals in Paris showed that 29% of women seronegative at delivery were not aware of any preventive measures.[193]

If seroconversion occurs during pregnancy and fetal infection is diagnosed, the option of either termination of pregnancy or antibiotic therapy can be offered to the patient.[189] Serologic testing of pregnant women in countries with low prevalence rates can not be recommended in view of the high cost.

REFERENCES

1. Nicolle C, Manceaux L: Sur une infection à corps de Leishmen (ou organismes voisins) du gondi. C R Seances Soc Biol Fil 147:763–766, 1908.
2. Jankû J: Pathogenesis and pathologic anatomy of coloboma of macula lutea in eye of normal dimensions, and in microphthalmic eye, with parasites in the retina. Cas Lek Cesk 62:1021–1027, 1923.
3. Wolf A, Cowen D, Paige BH: Human toxoplasmosis: occurrence in infants as an encephalomyelitis; verification by transmission to animals. Science 89:226–227, 1939.
4. Frenkel JK, Dubey JP, Miller NL: *Toxoplasma gondii* in cats: fecal stages identified as coccidian oocysts. Science 167:893–896, 1970.
5. Hutchison WM, Dunachie JF: The life cycle of the coccidian parasite *Toxoplasma gondii* in the domestic cat. Trans R Soc Trop Med Hyg 65:380–399, 1971.
6. Kean B: Clinical toxoplasmosis—50 years. Trans R Soc Trop Med Hyg 66:549–567, 1972.
7. Krick JA, Remington JS: Current concepts of parasitology: toxoplasmosis in the adult—an overview. N England J Med 298:550–553, 1978.
8. Beaman MH, McCabe RE, Wong, S-Y, Remington JS: *Toxoplasma gondii*. In Mandell GL, Bennett JE, Dolin R (eds): Principles and Practice of Infectious Diseases. New York, Churchill Livingstone, 1995.
9. Dubey JP: A review of toxoplasmosis in pigs. Vet Parasitol 19:181–223, 1986.
10. Stray-Pedersen B, Lorentzen-Styr A-M: The prevalence of *Toxoplasma* antibodies among 11,736 pregnant women in Norway. Scand J Infect Dis 11:159–165, 1979.
11. Feldman HA, Miller LT: Serological study of toxoplasmosis prevalence. Am J Hyg 64:320–335, 1956.
12. Wallace GD: Serologic and epidemiologic observations on toxoplasmosis on three Pacific atols. Am J Epidemiol 90:103–111, 1969.
13. Kean BH, Kimball AC, Christenson WN: An epidemic of acute toxoplasmosis. JAMA 208:1002–1004, 1969.
14. Frenkel JK: Toxoplasmosis. Pediatr Clin North Am 32:917–931, 1985.
15. Riemann HP, Meyer ME, Theis JH, et al: Toxoplasmosis in an infant fed unpasteurized goat milk. J Pediatr 87:573–576, 1975.
16. Sacks JJ, Roberto RR, Brooks NF: Toxoplasmosis infection associated with raw goat's milk. JAMA 248:1728–1732, 1982.
17. Remington JS, McLeod R, Desmonts G: Toxoplasmosis. In Remington JS, Klein JO (eds): Infectious Diseases of the Fetus and Newborn Infant. Philadelphia, WB Saunders Co, 1995.
18. Siegel SE, Lunde MN, Gelderman AH, et al: Transmission

of toxoplasmosis by leukocyte transfusion. Blood 37: 388–394, 1971.

19. Britt RH, Enzmann DR, Remington JS: Intracranial infection in cardiac transplant recipients. Ann Neurol 9:107–119, 1981.

20. Teutsch SM, Juranek DD, Sulzer A, et al: Epidemic toxoplasmosis associated with infected cats. N Engl J Med 300:695–699, 1979.

21. Berengo A, Frezzotti R: Active neuro-ophthalmic toxoplasmosis: a clinical study on nineteen patients. Adv Ophthalmol 12:265–343, 1962.

22. Frenkel JK: Pathogenesis of toxoplasmosis with a consideration of cyst rupture in *Besonitia* infection. Surv Ophthalmol 6:799–825, 1961.

23. Frenkel JK: Ocular toxoplasmosis. Pathogenesis, diagnosis, and treatment. AMA Arch Ophthalmol 59:260–279, 1958.

24. Tabbara KF: Toxoplasmosis. In Tasman W, Jaeger EA (eds): Duane's Clinical Ophthalmology. Philadelphia, JB Lippincott Co, 1990.

25. O'Connor GR: The influence of hypersensitivity on the pathogenesis of ocular toxoplasmosis. Trans Am Ophthalmol Soc 68:501–547, 1970.

26. Wakefield D, Penny R: Immunology of ocular toxoplasmosis. Aust J Ophthalmol 10:277–281, 1982.

27. O'Connor GR: Manifestations and management of ocular toxoplasmosis. Bull NY Acad Med 50:192–210, 1974.

28. Nozik RA, O'Connor GR: Studies on experimental ocular toxoplasmosis is the rabbit. I. The effect of antigenic stimulation. Arch Ophthalmol 83:724–728, 1970.

29. Newman PE, Ghosheh R, Tabbara KF, et al: The role of hypersensitivity reactions to *Toxoplasma* antigens in experimental ocular toxoplasmosis in nonhuman primates. Am J Ophthalmol 94:159–164, 1982.

30. Hogan MJ, Moschini GB, Zardi O: Effects of *Toxoplasma gondii* toxin on the rabbit eye. Am J Ophthalmol 72:733–742, 1971.

31. Dutton GN, Hay J: Toxoplasmic retinochoroiditis—current concepts of pathogenesis. Trans Ophthalmol Soc UK 103:503–507, 1983.

32. O'Connor GR: Protozoal infections. In Garner A, Klintworth GK (eds): Pathobiology of Ocular Disease. A Dynamic Approach. New York, Marcel Dekker Inc, 1982.

33. Nussenblatt RB, Mittal KK, Fuhrman S, et al: Lymphocyte proliferative responses of patients with ocular toxoplasmosis to parasite and retinal antigens. Am J Ophthalmol 107:632–641, 1989.

34. Brézin AP, Egwuagu CE, Silveira C, et al: Analysis of aqueous humor in ocular toxoplasmosis. N Engl J Med 324:699, 1991.

35. Kimball AC, Kean BH, Fuchs F: Congenital toxoplasmosis: a prospective study of 4,048 obstetric patients. Am J Obstet Gynecol 111:211–218, 1971.

36. Desmonts G, Couvreur J: Congenital toxoplasmosis: a prospective study of 378 pregnancies. N Engl J Med 290:1110–1116, 1974.

37. Wong S-Y, Remington JS: Toxoplasmosis in pregnancy. Clin Infect Dis 18:853–862, 1994.

38. Stray-Pedersen B: Treatment of toxoplasmosis in the pregnant mother and newborn child: Scand J Infect Dis Suppl 84:23–31, 1992.

39. Eichenwald HF: A study of congenital toxoplasmosis: with particular emphasis on clinical manifestations, sequelae and therapy. In Siim JC (ed): Human Toxoplasmosis. Baltimore, Williams & Wilkins, 1959.

40. Wilson CB, Remington JS, Stagno S, Reynolds DW: Development of adverse sequelae in children born with subclinical congenital *Toxoplasma* infection. Pediatrics 66:767–774, 1980.

41. Koppe JG, Loewer-Sieger DM, De Roever-Bonnet M: Results of 20 years follow up of congenital toxoplasmosis. Lancet 1:254–256, 1986.

42. Couvreur J, Desmonts G, Tournier G, Szusterkac M: A study of a homogeneous series of 210 cases of congenital toxoplasmosis in 0 to 11 months detected prospectively. Ann Pediatr (Paris) 31:815–819, 1984.

43. Perkins ES: Ocular toxoplasmosis. Br J Ophthalmol 57:1–17, 1973.

44. Schlaegel TF Jr: Toxoplasmosis. In Duane TD (ed): Clinical Ophthalmology. Hagerstown, MD, Harper & Row, 1976.

45. Glasner PD, Silveira C, Kruszon-Moran D, et al: An unusually high prevalence of ocular toxoplasmosis in southern Brazil. Am J Ophthalmol 114:136–144, 1992.

46. Darrell RW, Pieper S, Kurland LT, Jacobs L: Chorioretinopathy and toxoplasmosis: an epidemiologic study on a south Pacific island. Arch Ophthalmol 71:63–68, 1964.

47. Silveira C, Belfort R Jr, Burnier M Jr, Nussenblatt R: Acquired toxoplasmosis infection as the cause of toxoplasmic retinochoroiditis in families. Am J Ophthalmol 106:362–364, 1988.

48. Ronday MJH, Luyendijk L, Baarsma GS, et al: Presumed acquired ocular toxoplasmosis. Arch Ophthalmol 113:1524–1529, 1995.

49. Michelson JB, Shields JA, McDonald PR, et al: Retinitis secondary to acquired systemic toxoplasmosis with isolation of the parasite. Am J Ophthalmol 86:548–552, 1978.

50. Gump DW, Holden RA: Acquired chorioretinitis due to toxoplasmosis. Ann Intern Med 90:58–60, 1979.

51. Saari M, Vuorre I, Neiminen H, Räisänen S: Acquired toxoplasmic chorioretinitis. Arch Ophthalmol 94:1485–1488, 1976.

52. Stago S, Dykes AC, Amos CS, et al: An outbreak of toxoplasmosis linked to cats. Pediatrics 65:706–712, 1980.

53. Akstein RB, Wilson LA, Teutsch SM: Acquired toxoplasmosis. Ophthalmology 89:1299–1302, 1982.

54. Nussenblatt RB, Belfort R Jr: Ocular toxoplasmosis revisited. JAMA 271:304–307, 1994.

55. Sibley LD, Boothroyd JC: Virulent strains of *Toxoplasma gondii* comprise a single clonal lineage. Nature 359:82–85, 1992.

56. Remington JS: Toxoplasmosis in the adult. Bull NY Acad Med 50:211–227, 1974.

57. McCabe RE, Brooks RG, Dorfman RF, Remington JS: Clinical spectrum in 107 cases of toxoplasmic lymphadenopathy. Rev Infect Dis 9:754–774, 1987.

58. Evans AS: Infectious mononucleosis and related syndromes. Am J Med Sci 276:325–339, 1978.

59. Grant SC, Klein C: *Toxoplasma gondii* encephalitis in an immunocompetent adult: a case report. S Afr Med J 71:585–587, 1987.

60. Masur H, Jones TC, Lempert JA, Cherubini TD: Outbreak of toxoplasmosis in a family and documentation of acquired retinochoroiditis. Am J Med 64:396–402, 1978.

61. Perkins ES: Uveitis and Toxoplasmosis. Boston, Little, Brown & Co, 1961.

62. Hogan MJ, Kimura SJ, O'Connor GR: Ocular toxoplasmosis. Arch Ophthalmol 72:592–600, 1964.

63. Roizenblatt J, Grant S, Foos RY: Vitreous cylinders. Arch Ophthalmol 98:737–739, 1980.

64. Schlaegel TF Jr, Webber JC: The macula in ocular toxoplasmosis. Arch Ophthalmol 102:697–698, 1984.

65. Willerson D Jr, Aaberg TM, Reeser F, Meredith TA: Unusual ocular presentation of acute toxoplasmosis. Br J Ophthalmol 61:693–698, 1977.

66. Gagliuso DJ, Teich SA, Fiedman AH, Orellana J: Ocular Toxoplasmosis in AIDS patients. Trans Am Ophthalmol Soc 88:63–86, 1990.

67. Folk JC, Lobes LA: Presumed toxoplasmic papillitis. Ophthalmology 91:64–67, 1984.

68. Manschot WA, Daamen CBF: Connatal ocular toxoplasmosis. Arch Ophthalmol 74:48–54, 1965.

69. de Abreu MT, Belfort R Jr, Hirata PS: Fuchs' heterochromia cyclitis and ocular toxoplasmosis. Am J Ophthalmol 93:739–744, 1982.

70. La Hey E, Rothova A, Baarsma GS, et al: Fuchs' heterochromia iridocyclitis is not associated with ocular toxoplasmosis. Arch Ophthalmol 110:806–811, 1992.

71. Schwab IR: The epidemiologic association of Fuch's heterochromic irridicyclitis and ocular toxoplasmosis. Am J Ophthalmol 111:356–362, 1991.

72. Gilbert HD: Unusual presentation of acute ocular toxoplasmosis. Albrecht Von Graefes Arch Klin Exp Ophthalmol 215:53–58, 1980.

73. Kayazawa F: Subretinal neovascularization associated with presumed toxoplasmic retinochoroidal scar. Ann Ophthalmol 14:819–812, 1982.

74. Gaynon MW, Boldrey EE, Strahlman ER, Fine SL: Retinal neovascularization and ocular toxoplasmosis. Am J Ophthalmol 98:585–589, 1984.

75. Doft BH: Choroidoretinal vascular anastomosis. Arch Ophthalmol 101:1053–1054, 1983.

76. Fine SL, Owens SL, Haller JA, et al: Choroidal neovascularization as a late complication of ocular toxoplasmosis. Am J Ophthalmol 91:318–322, 1981.

77. Rose GE: Papillitis, retinal neovascularization and recurrent retinal vein occlusion in *Toxoplasma* retinochoroiditis: a case report with uncommon clinical signs. Aust N Z J Ophthalmol 19:155–157, 1991.

78. Braunstein RA, Gass JDM: Branch artery obstruction caused by acute toxoplasmosis. Arch Ophthalmol 98:512, 1980.

79. Wilson WB, Sharpe JA, Deck JH: Cerebral blindness and ocular nerve palsies in toxoplasmosis. Am J Ophthalmol 89:714, 1980.

80. Perry DD, Marritt JC, Greenwood RS, et al: Congenital toxoplasmosis associated with acquired oculomotor nerve (CN III) palsy. J Pediatr Ophthalmol Strabismus 19:265–269, 1982.

81. Schuman JS, Weinberg RS, Ferry AP, Guerry RK: Toxoplasmic scleritis. Ophthalmology 95:1399–1403, 1988.

82. Ruskin J, Remington JS: Toxoplasmosis in the comprised host. Ann Intern Med 84:193–199, 1976.

83. Levy RM, Bredesen DE: Central nervous system dysfunction in acquired immunodeficiency syndrome. J Acquir Immune Defic Syndr 1:41–64, 1988.

84. Levy RM, Rosenbloom S, Perrett LV: Neurodiagnostic findings in AIDS: a review of 200 cases. AJR 147:977–983, 1986.

85. Navia BA, Petito CK, Gold JW, et al: Cerebral toxoplasmosis complicating the acquired immune deficiency syndrome: clinical and neuropathological findings in 27 patients. Ann Neurol 19:224–238, 1986.

86. Cochereau-Massin I, LeHoang P, Lautier-Fau M, et al: Ocular toxoplasmosis in human immunodeficiency virus-infected patients. Am J Ophthalmol 114:130–135, 1992.

87. Grossniklaus HE, Specht CS, Allaire G, Leavitt JA: *Toxoplasma gondii* retinochoroiditis and optic neuritis in acquired immune deficiency syndrome: report of a case. Ophthalmology 97:1342–1346, 1990.

88. Holland GN, Engstrom RE, Glasgow BJ, et al: Ocular toxoplasmosis in patients with the acquired immunodeficiency syndrome. Am J Ophthalmol 106:653–667, 1988.

89. Parke DW II, Font RL: Diffuse toxoplasmic retinochoroiditis in a patient with AIDS. Arch Ophthalmol 104:571–575, 1986.

90. Friedmann CT, Knox DL: Variations in recurrent active toxoplasmic retinochoroiditis. Arch Ophthalmol 81:481–483, 1969.

91. Doft BH, Gass JDM: Punctate outer retinal toxoplasmosis. Arch Ophthalmol 103:1332–1336, 1985.

92. Peacock JE, Folds J, Orringer E, et al: *Toxoplasma gondii* and the compromised host: antibody response in the absence of clinical manifestations of disease. Arch Intern Med 143:1235–1238, 1983.

93. Shepp DH, Hackman RC, Conley FK, et al: *Toxoplasma gondii* reactivation identified by detection of parasitemia in tissue culture. Ann Intern Med 103:218–221, 1985.

94. Remington JS, Anderson SE Jr: Diagnosis and treatment of pneumocytosis and toxoplasmosis in the immunosuppressed host. Transplant Proc 5:1263–1270, 1973.

95. Mitchell CD, Erlich SS, Mastrucci MT, et al: Congenital toxoplasmosis occurring in infants perinatally infected with human immunodeficiency virus 1. Pediatr Infect Dis J 9:512–518, 1990.

96. Cohen-Addad NE, Joshi VV, Sharer LR, et al: Congenital acquired immunodeficiency syndrome and congenital toxoplasmosis: pathologic support for a chronology of events. J Perinatol 8:328–331, 1988.

97. Velin P, DuPont D, Barbot D, et al: Double contamination materno-foetale par le HIV 1 et le Toxoplpasme. Presse Med 20:960, 1991.

98. O'Donohoe JM, Brueton MJ, Holliman RE: Concurrent congenital human immunodeficiency virus infection and toxoplasmosis. Pediatr Infect Dis J 10:627–628, 1991.

99. Taccone A, Fondelli MP, Ferrea G, Marzoli A: An unusual CT presentation of congenital cerebral toxoplasmosis in an 8-month-old boy with AIDS. Pediatr Radiol 22:68–69, 1992.

100. Tovo PA, De Martino M, Gabiano G, et al, and the Italian Register for HIV Infection in Children: Prognostic factors and survival in children with perinatal HIV-1 infection. Lancet 339:1249–1253, 1992.

101. Miller MJ, Remington JS: Toxoplasmosis in infants and children with HIV infection or AIDS. In Pizzo PA, Wilfert CM (eds): Pediatric AIDS: The Challenge of HIV Infection in Infants, Children, and Adolescents. Baltimore, Williams & Wilkins, 1990.

102. Gazzinelli RT, Hartley JW, Fredrickson TN, et al: Opportunistic infections and retrovirus-induced immunodeficiency: studies of acute and chronic infections with *Toxoplasma gondii* in mice infected with LP-BM5 murine leukemia virus. Infect Immun 60:4394–4401, 1992.

103. Wong S-Y, Remington JS: Biology of *Toxoplasma gondii*. AIDS 7:299–316, 1993.

104. Suzuki Y, Remington JS: Dual regulation of resistance against *Toxoplasma gondii* infection by Lyt-2+ and Ly-1+, L3T4+ T cells in mice. J Immunol 140:3943–3946, 1988.

105. Gazzinelli RT, Hakim FT, Hieny S, et al: Synergistic role of CD4+ and CD8+ T lymphocytes in INF-γ Production and protective immunity induced by an attenuated *Toxoplasma gondii* vaccine. J Immunol 146:286–292, 1991.

106. Gazzinelli RT, Xu Y, Hieny S, et al: Simultaneous depletion of CD4+ and CD8+ lymphocytes is required to reactivate chronic infection with *Toxoplasma gondii*. J Immunol 149:175–180, 1992.

107. Suzuki Y, Remington JS: The effect of anti-IFN-gamma antibody on the protective effect of Lyt-2+ immune T cells against toxoplasmosis in mice. J Immunol 144:1954–1956, 1990.

108. Subauste CS, Koniaris AH, Remington JS: Murine CD8+ cytotoxic T lymphocytes lyse *Toxoplasma gondii*–infected cells. J Immunol 147:3955–3959, 1991.

109. Hakim FT, Gazzinelli RT, Denkers E, et al: CD8+ T cells from mice vaccinated with *Toxoplasma gondii* are cytotoxic for parasitic-infected or antigen-pulsed host cells. J Immunol 147:2310–2316, 1991.

110. Yano A, Aosai F, Ohta M, et al: Antigen presentation by *Toxoplasma gondii* infected cells to CD4+ proliferative T cells and CD8+ cytotoxic cells. J Parasitol 75:411–416, 1989.

111. Suzuki Y, Conley FK, Remington JS: Treatment of toxoplasmosis encephalitis in mice with recombinant gamma interferon. Infect Immun 58:3050–3055, 1990.

112. Suzuki Y, Orellana MA, Schreiber RD, Remington JS: Interferon-gamma: the major mediator of resistance against *Toxoplasma gondii*. Science 240:516–518, 1988.

113. Araujo FG: Depletion of L3T4+ (CD4+) T lymphocytes prevents development of resistance to *Toxoplasma gondii* in mice. Infect Immun 59:1614–1619, 1991.

114. Hérion P, Saavedra R: Human T-cell clones as tools for the characterization of the cell-mediated immune response to *Toxoplasma gondii*. Res Immunol 144(1):48–51, 1993.

115. McLeod R, Skamene E, Brown CR, et al: Genetic regulation of early survival and cyst number after peroral *Toxoplasma gondii* infection of A × B/B × A recombinant inbred and B10 congenic mice. J Immunol 143:3031–3034, 1989.

116. McLeod R, Brown C, Mack D: Immunogenetics influence outcome of *Toxoplasma gondii* infection. Res Immunol 144(1):61–65, 1993.

117. Brown CR, McLeod R: Class 1 MHC genes and CD8+ T cells determine cyst number in *Toxoplasma* infection. J Immunolol 145:3438–3441, 1990.
118. Subauste CS, Remington JS: Immunity to *Toxoplasma gondii*. Curr Opin Immunol 5:532–537, 1993.
119. Langermans JAM, van der Hulst MEB, Nibbering PH, van Furth R: Endogenous tumor necrosis factor α is required for enhanced microbial activity against *Toxoplasma gondii* and *Listeria monocytogenes* in recombinant γ interferon-treated mice. Infect Immun 60:5107–5112, 1992.
120. Langermans JAM, Van Der Hulst MEB, Nibbering PH, et al: INF-γ induced L-arginine–dependent toxoplasmastatic activity in murine peritoneal macrophages is mediated by endogenous tumor necrosis factor-α. J Immunol 148:568–574, 1992.
121. Chao CC, Hu S, Gekker G, et al: Effects of cytokines on multiplications of *Toxoplasma gondii* in microglial cells. J Immunol 150:3404–3410, 1993.
122. Gazzinelli RT, Eltoum I, Wynn TA, Sher A: Acute cerebral toxoplasmosis is induced by in vivo neutralization of TNF-alpha and correlates with the down-regulated expression of inducible nitric oxide synthase and other markers of macrophage activation. J Immunol 151:3672–3681, 1993.
123. Beaman MH, Hunter CA, Remington JS: Enhancement of intracellular replication of *Toxoplasma gondii* by IL-6. J Immunol 153:4583–4587, 1994.
124. Sharma SD, Hofflin JM, Remington JS: In vivo recombinant interleukin 2 administration enhances survival against a lethal challenge with *Toxoplasma gondii*. J Immunol 135:4160–4163, 1985.
125. Gazzinelli RT, Hieny S, Wynn TA, et al: Interleukin 12 is required for T lymphocyte-independent induction of interferon-γ by an intracellular parasite and induces resistance in T cell deficient hosts. Proc Natl Acad Sci USA 90:6115–6119, 1993.
126. Sher A, Oswald IP, Hieny S, Gazzinelli RT: *Toxoplasma gondii* induces a T-independent INF-γ response in natural killer cells that requires both adherent accessory cells and tumor necrosis factor-α. J Immunol 150:3982–3989, 1993.
127. Hunter CA, Subauste CS, van Cleave V, Remington JS: Production of gamma interferon by natural killer cells from *Toxoplasma gondii*–injectd SCID mice: regulation by interleukin-10, interleukin-12, and tumor necrosis factor alpha. Infect Immun 62:2818–2824, 1994.
128. Hunter CA, Abrams JS, Beaman MH, Remington JS: Cytokine mRNA in the central nervous system of SCID mice infected with *Toxoplasma gondii*: importance of T cell independent regulation of resistance to *T. gondii*. Infect Immun 61:4038–4044, 1993.
129. Hunter CA, Candolfi E, Subauste C, et al: Studies on the role of interleukin-12 in acute murine toxoplasmosis. Immunology 84:16–20, 1995.
130. Anderson SE Bautista SC, Remington JS: Specific antibody-dependent killing of *Toxoplasma gondii* by normal macrophages. Clin Exp Immunol 26:375–380, 1976.
131. Schreiber RD, Feldman HA: Identification of the activator system for antibody to *Toxoplasma* as a classical complement pathway. J Infect Dis 141:366–369, 1980.
132. Wilson CB, Haas JE: Cellular defenses against *Toxoplasma gondii* in newborns. J Clin Invest 73:1606–1616, 1984.
133. Remington JS, Miller MG, Brownlee I: IgM antibodies in acute toxoplasmosis, II. Prevalence and significance in acquired cases. J Lab Clin Med 71:855–866, 1968.
134. Desmonts G: Definitive serological diagnosis of ocular toxoplasmosis. Arch Ophthalmol 76:839–851, 1966.
135. Rothova A, van Knapen F, Baarsma GS, et al: Serology in ocular toxoplasmosis. Br J Ophthalmol 70:615–622, 1986.
136. Carter AO, Frank JW: Congenital toxoplasmosis: epidemiological features and control. Can Med Assoc J 135:618–623, 1986.
137. World Health Organization: Biological standardization. Twentieth report. WHO Tech Rep Ser 384:1–100, 1968.
138. Welch PC, Masur H, Jones TC, Remington JS: Serologic diagnosis of acute lymphadenopathic toxoplasmosis. J Infect Dis 142:256–264, 1980.
139. Karim KA, Ludlam GB: The relationship and significance of antibody titers as determined by various serological methods in glandular and ocular toxoplasmosis. J Clin Pathol 28:42–49, 1975.
140. Kean BH, Kimball AC: The complement-fixation test in the diagnosis of congenital toxoplasmosis. Am J Dis Child 131:21–28, 1977.
141. Desmonts G, Baufine-Ducrocq H, Couzineau P, Peloux Y: Anticorps toxoplasmiques naturels. Nouv Presse Med 3:1547–1549, 1974.
142. Wilson CB, Remington JS: What can be done to prevent toxoplasmosis? Am J Obstet Gynecol 138:357–363, 1980.
143. Desmonts G, Remington JS: Direct agglutination test for diagnosis of *Toxoplasma* infection: method for increasing sensitivity and specificity. J Clin Microbiol 11:562–568, 1980.
144. Araujo FG, Barnett EV, Gentry LO, Remington JS: False-positive anti *Toxoplasma* fluorescent-antibody tests in patients with antinuclear antibodies. Appl Microbiol 22:270–275, 1971.
145. van Loon AM, van der Logt JTM, Heessen FWA, van der Veen J; Enzyme linked immunosorbent assay that uses labeled antigen for detection of immunoglobulin M and A antibodies in toxoplasmosis: comparison with direct immunoflorescence and double-sandwich enzyme-linked immunosorbent assay. J Clin Microbiol 17:997–1003, 1983.
146. Decoster A, Slizewicz B, Simon J, et al: Platelia-Toxo IgA, a new kit for early diagnosis of congenital toxoplasmosis by detection of anti-P30 immunoglobulin A antibodies. J Clin Microbiol 29:2291–2295, 1991.
147. Stepick-Biek P, Thulliez P, Araujo FG, Remington JS: IgA antibodies for diagnosis of acute congenital and acquired toxoplasmosis. J Infect Dis 162:270–273, 1990.
148. Balsari A, Poli G, Molina V, et al: ELISA for toxoplasma antibody detection: a comparison with other serodiagnostic tests. J Clin Pathol 33:640–643, 1980.
149. van Loon AM, van der Veen J: Enzyme-linked immunosorbent assay for quantitation of *Toxoplamsa* antibodies in human era. J Clin Pathol 33:635–639, 1980.
150. Carlier Y, Bout D, Dessaint JP, et al: Evaluation of the enzyme-linked immunosorbent assay (ELISA) and other serological tests for the diagnosis of toxoplasmosis. Bull WHO 58:99–105, 1980.
151. Denmark JR, Chessum BS: Standardization of enzyme-linked immunosorbent assay (ELISA) and the detection of *Toxoplasma* antibody. Med Lab Sci 35:227–232, 1978.
152. Capron A, Dugimont JC, Fruit J, Bout D: Application of immunoenzyme methods in diagnosis of human parasitic diseases. Ann NY Acad Sci 254:331–334, 1975.
153. Walls KW, Bullock SL, English DK: Use of enzyme-linked immunosorbent assay (ELISA) and its microadaptation for the serodiagnosis of toxoplasmosis. J Clin Microbiol 5:273–277, 1977.
154. Voller A, Bidwell DE, Bartlett A, et al: A microplate enzyme-immunoassay for *Toxoplasma* antibody. J Clin Pathol 29:150–153, 1976.
155. Milatovic D, Braveny I: Enzyme-linked immunosorbent assay for the serodiagnosis of toxoplasmosis. J Clin Pathol 33:841–844, 1980.
156. Camargo ME, Ferreira AW, Mineo JR, et al: Immunoglobulin G and immunoglobulin M enzyme-linked immunosorbent assays and defined toxoplasmosis serological patterns. Infect Immun 21:55–58, 1978.
157. Noat Y, Remington JS: An enzyme-linked immunosorbent assay for detection of IgM antibodies of *Toxoplasma gondii*; use for diagnosis of acute acquired toxoplasmosis. J Infect Dis 142:757–766, 1980.
158. Ware PL, Kasper LH: Strain-specific antigens of *Toxoplasma gondii*. Infect Immun 55:778–783, 1987.
159. Grover CM, Thulliez P, Remington JS, Boothroyd JC: Rapid prenatal diagnosis of congenital *Toxoplasma* infection by using polymerase chain reaction and amniotic fluid. J Clin Microbiol 28:2297–2301, 1990.
160. Kijilstra A, Luyendijk L, Baarsma GS, et al: Aqueous hu-

mor analysis as a diagnostic tool in *Toxoplasma* uveitis. Int Ophthalmol 13:383–386, 1989.

161. Scheiffarth OF, Zrenner E, Disko R, et al: Intraocular in vivo immunofluorescence: a new technique for visualizing structures of the ocular fundus. Invest Ophthalmol Vis Sci 31:272–276, 1990.
162. Remington JS, Gentry LO: Acquired toxoplasmosis infection versus disease. Ann NY Acad Sci 174:1006–1017, 1970.
163. Thulliez P, Daffos F, Forestier F: Diagnosis of *Toxoplasma* infection in the pregnant woman and the unborn child: current problems. Scan J Infect Dis 84(Suppl):18–22, 1992.
164. Foulon W, Naessens A, Mahler T, et al: Prenatal diagnosis of congenital toxoplasmosis. Obstet Gynecol 76:769–772, 1990.
165. Derouin F, Thulliez P, Condolfi E, et al: Early prenatal diagnosis of congenital toxoplasmosis using amniotic fluid samples and tissue culture. Eur J Clin Microbiol 7:423–425, 1988.
166. Hohlfeld P, Daffos F, Thulliez P, et al: Fetal toxoplasmosis: outcome of pregnancy and infant follow-up after in utero treatment. J Pediatr 115:765–769, 1989.
167. Daffos F, Forestier F, Capella-Pavlovsky M, et al: Prenatal management of 746 pregnancies at risk for congenital toxoplasmosis. N Engl J Med 318:271–275, 1988.
168. Desmonts G, Forestier F, Thulliez PH, et al: Prenatal diagnosis of congenital toxoplasmosis. Lancet 1:500–506, 1985.
169. Engstrom RE Jr, Holland GN, Nussenblatt RB, Jabs DA: Current practices in the management of ocular toxoplasmosis. Am J Ophthalmol 111:601–610, 1991.
170. Rothova A, Buitenhuis HJ, Meenken C, et al: Therapy of ocular toxoplasmosis. Int Ophthalmol 13:415–419, 1989.
171. Tabbara KF, O'Connor GR: Treatment of ocular toxoplasmosis with clindamycin and sulfadiazine. Ophthalmology 87:129–134, 1980.
172. Lakhanpal V, Schocket SS, Nirankari V: Clindamycin in the treatment of toxoplasmic retinochoroiditis. Am J Ophthalmol 95:605–613, 1983.
173. Tabbara KF, Dy-Liacco J, Nozik RA, et al: Clindamycin in chronic toxoplasmosis: effects of periocular injection on recoverability of organisms from healed lesions in the rabbit eye. Arch Ophthalmol 97:542–544, 1979.
174. Tabbara KF, O'Connor GR: Ocular tissue absorption of clindamycin phosphate. Arch Ophthalmol 93:1180–1185, 1975.
175. Opremcak EM, Scales DK, Sharpe MR: Trimethoprim-sulfamethoxazole therapy for ocular toxoplasmosis. Ophthalmology 99:920–925, 1992.
176. Webster LT Jr: Drugs used in the chemotherapy of protozoal infections. In Goodman Gilman A, Rall TW, Nies AS, Taylor P (eds): The Pharmacological Basis of Therapeutics. New York, Pergamon Press, 1990.
177. Sande MA, Mandell GL: Antimicrobial agents. In Goodman Gilman A, Rall TW, Nies AS, Taylor P (eds): The Pharmacological Basis of Therapeutics. New York, Pergamon Press, 1990.
178. Araujo FG, Huskinson J, Remington JS: Remarkable in vitro and in vivo activities of the hydroxynaphthoquinone 566C80 against tachyzoites and tissue cysts of *Toxoplasma gondii*. Antimicrob Agents Chemother 35:293–299, 1991.
179. Lopez JS, de Smet MD, Mazur H, et al: Orally administered 566C80 for treatment of ocular toxoplasmosis in a patient with the acquired immunodeficiency syndrome. Am J Ophthalmol 113:331–333, 1992.
180. Sabates R, Pruett RC, Brokhurst RJ: Fulminant ocular toxoplasmosis. Am J Ophthalmol 92:497–503, 1981.

181. Ghartey KN, Brockhurst RJ: Photocoagulation of active toxoplasmic retinochoroiditis. Am J Ophthalmol 89:838–864, 1980.
182. Spalter HF, Campbell CJ, Noyori KS, et al: Prophylactic photocoagulation of recurrent toxoplasmic retinochoroiditis. A preliminary report. Arch Ophthalmol 75:21–24, 1966.
183. Theodossiadis GP, Koutsandrea C, Tzonou A: A comparative study concerning the treatment of active toxoplasic retinochoroiditis with argon laser and medication (follow up of 2–9 years). Ophthalmologica 199:77–83, 1989.
184. Fitzgerald CR: Pars plana vitrectomy for vitreous opacity secondary to presumed toxoplasmosis. Arch Ophthalmol 98:321–323, 1980.
185. Steahly LP: Endolaser photocoagulation of toxoplasmosis. Ann Ophthalmol 20:463–465, 1988.
186. Anonymous (editorial): Pyrimethamine combination in pregnancy. Lancet 29:1005–1007, 1983.
187. Leport C, Raffi F, Matheron S, et al: Treatment of central nervous system toxoplasmosis with pyrimethamine/sulfadiazine combination in 35 patients with the acquired immunodeficiency syndrome. Efficacy of long-term continuous therapy. Am J Med 84:94–100, 1988.
188. Frenkel JK: Breaking the transmission chain of *Toxoplasma*: a program for the prevention of human toxoplasmosis. Bull NY Acad Med 50:228–235, 1974.
189. Foulon W: Congenital toxoplasmosis: is screening desirable? Scand J Infect Dis Suppl 84:11–17, 1992.
190. Frenkel JK: Congenital toxoplasmosis: prevention or palliation. Am J Obstet Gynecol 141:359–361, 1981.
191. Klapper PE, Morris DJ: Screening for viral and protozoal infections in pregnancy. A review. Br J Obstet Gynecol 97:974–983, 1990.
192. Ho-Yen DO, Chatterton JMW: Congenital toxoplasmosis—why and how to screen. Rev Med Microbiol 1:229–235, 1990.
193. Thulliez P: Screening program for congenital toxoplasmosis in France. Scand J Infect Dis Suppl 84:43–45, 1992.
194. Ruoss CF, Bourne GL: Toxoplasmosis in pregnancy. J Obstet Gynaecol Br Commonw 79:1115–1118, 1972.
195. Broadbent EJ, Ross R, Hurley R: Screening for toxoplasmosis in pregnancy. J Clin Pathol 34:659–664, 1981.
196. Koskiniemi M, Lappalainen M, Koskela P, et al: The program for antenal screening of toxoplasmosis in Finland: a prospective cohort study. Scand J Infect Dis Suppl 84:70–74, 1992.
197. Flamm H, Aspöck H: Die Toxoplasmose-überwachung der schwangerschaft in österreich-ergebnisse und probleme. Padiatrie Grenzgeb 20:27–34, 1981.
198. Walpole IR, Hodgen N, Bower C: Congenital toxoplasmosis: a large survey in western Australia. Med J Aust 154(11):720–724, 1991.
199. Desmonts G, Couvreur J: Toxoplasmosis in pregnancy and its transmission to the fetus. Bull NY Acad Med 50:146–159, 1974.
200. Lebech M, Petersen E: Neonatal screening for congenital toxoplasmosis in Denmark: presentation of the design of a prospective study. Scand J Infect Dis Suppl 84:75–79, 1992.
201. Stray-Pedersen B, Pedersen JO, Omland T: Estimation of the incidence of *Toxoplasma* infections among pregnant women from different areas in Norway. Scand J Infect Dis 11:247–252, 1979.
202. Doehring E, Reiter-Owona I, Bauer O, et al: *Toxoplasma gondii* antibodies in pregnant women and their newborns in Dar es Salaam, Tanzania. Am J Trop Med Hyg 52(6):546–548, 1995.

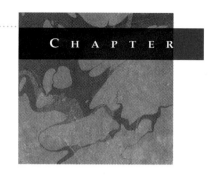

Ocular Toxocariasis

Albert M. Maguire, M.D.

HISTORY

Ocular infestation with the *Toxocara* roundworm was first recognized in eyes enucleated for suspicion of malignancy, infection, or Coats' disease. As the disease entity became better understood, less severe clinical manifestations were recognized and diagnosis became based upon clinical rather than histopathologic findings.[1,2] Nematode endophthalmitis, later identified as *Toxocara canis* infestation, was first reported in a landmark paper by Wilder in 1950.[3] In this clinicopathologic correlation study, Wilder reviewed 46 enucleation specimens in which inflammatory membranes of the vitreous was a prominent histopathologic feature. Eosinophilic abscesses were commonly noted and, in 24 eyes, larvae were found within granulomatous inflammatory masses. Initially, these larvae were incorrectly identified as third-stage hookworm. On later review by Nichols in 1956,[4] they were determined to be second-stage larvae of the roundworm *T. canis*. Retrospective clinical correlation revealed that these eyes had been enucleated from patients presenting with leukokoria and other findings suggestive of retinoblastoma, endophthalmitis, or Coats' disease. Later investigators commented on the anterior location of the inflammatory mass with involvement of the retrolental area, ciliary body, or peripheral retina in eyes with this clinical presentation (Fig. 58–1).[5]

Concurrent with Wilder's work, several reports appeared describing a systemic syndrome in children characterized by eosinophilia and transitory pulmonary infiltrates.[6] In 1952, Beaver and associates[7] identified a *Toxocara* species larva in a liver biopsy specimen from a child with this syndrome, thus establishing *Toxocara* as an etiologic agent. With Nichols' report in 1956 identifying *T. canis* in Wilder's original specimens,[4] a common etiology was demonstrated for the systemic and ocular diseases. The epidemiologic features of *Toxocara* infestation were subsequently characterized including the primary occurrence in the pediatric age group and the association with pica and exposure to dogs.[1,8–12]

Later clinicopathologic correlation studies described other clinical manifestations of ocular *Toxocara* infection. In addition to Wilder's cases of diffuse ocular inflammation (endophthalmitis), descriptions of focal peripheral and posterior pole inflammatory disease appeared. Irvine and associates[13] reported a case of a child presenting with strabismus and decreased vision due to retinal detachment. The eye was enucleated for suspicion of neoplasia and found to have an eosinophilic abscess containing *T. canis* larvae on the inferior pars plana region. Ashton[14] reported four histopathologically confirmed cases of a solitary posterior pole granuloma presenting with diminished vision and/or strabismus. Duguid reviewed the characteristic clinical findings of ocular *Toxocara* presenting with posterior pole granuloma or diffuse endophthalmitis[1,2] and suggested the possibility of clinical diagnosis in selected cases. In a review of 41 cases of ocular *Toxocara* infection, Wilkinson and Welch[5] described the clinical features of the peripheral granuloma form. In this series, which included both presumed and histopathologically confirmed ocular *T. canis* infestation, a peripheral inflammatory mass with secondary tractional changes was found to be the most common clinical presentation. Clinical diagnosis was made in 27 of 28 cases presenting with a focal posterior pole or peripheral granuloma. In contrast, 10 of 11 histopathologic specimens were obtained in cases presenting with the diffuse endophthalmitis form of *Toxocara*, enucleated for suspicion of retinoblastoma.

Several other clinical variants of ocular *Toxocara* have been described and confirmed histopathologically, including isolated vitreous abscess,[14] pars

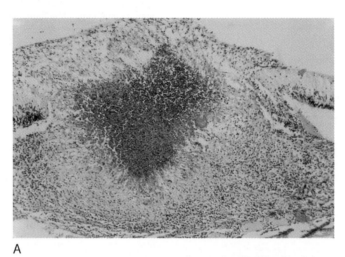

A

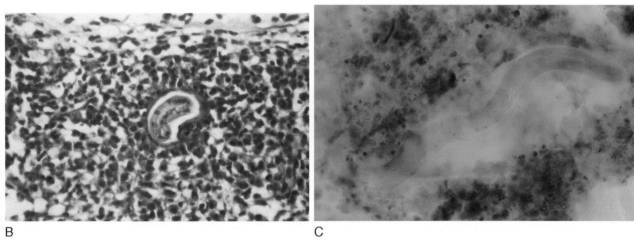

B   C

A, Posterior subretinal inflammatory mass due to *Toxocara canis*. *B*,
Vitreous eosinophilic abscess with second stage larva of *Toxocara
canis*. (From Green WR: Pathology of the vitreous. In Frayer WC
[ed]: Lancaster Course in Ophthalmic Histopathology, Unit 8.
Philadelphia, FA Davis Co, 1981, with permission.) *C*, Second stage
larva of *Toxocara canis* in vitreous specimen from an 18-year-old man
with a 2-month history of ocular inflammatory disease. (From
Maguire AM, Green WR, Michels RG, Erozan YS: Recovery of
intraocular *Toxocara canis* by pars plana vitrectomy. Ophthalmology
97:675–680, 1990, with permission.)

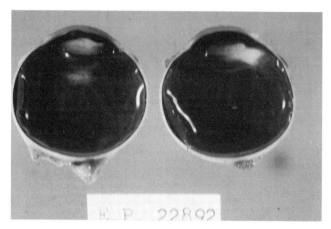

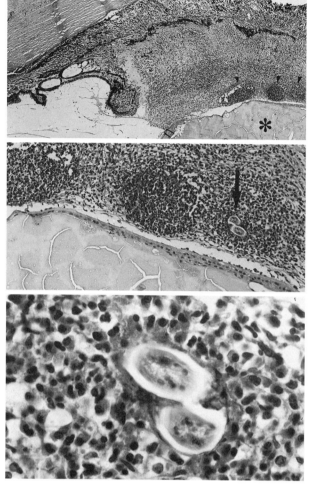

FIGURE 58–1 Nematode endophthalmitis. A 3-year-old child enucleated for suspicion of retinoblastoma. *Left, top,* Gross appearance showing posterior chamber mass. *Right, top,* Fibroinflammatory mass located between the anteriorly displaced iris and lens (*asterisk*) containing multiple eosinophilic abscesses (*arrowheads*) (hematoxylin-eosin, ×35). *Right, middle,* Medium power view revealing a curved larva (*arrow*) surrounded by inflammatory cells (hematoxylin-eosin, ×200). *Right, bottom,* High-power view demonstrating cross section of nematode larva measuring about 22 μm in diameter, consistent with *T. canis* (hematoxylin-eosin, ×900). EP 22892. (From Green WR: Retina. In Spencer WH [ed]: Ophthalmic Pathology: An Atlas and Textbook, Vol 2. Philadelphia, WB Saunders Co, 1985, with permission.)

planitis,[15,16] optic neuritis,[17] and hypopyon uveitis.[18] Clinical manifestations in cases without histopathologic confirmation of *Toxocara* infection include papillitis,[19] motile intraretinal[20,21] and intravitreal larva,[22] keratitis, and iris mass.[23]

PATHOPHYSIOLOGY

Key to the understanding of ocular toxocariasis (OT) is a description of the life cycle of the etiologic agent, the round worm *T. canis* (Fig. 58–2).[11,24] The natural host of *T. canis* is the dog. While *T. canis* can develop into a second-stage larval form in both humans and adult dogs, sexual maturation to egg-producing third-stage larvae occurs only in puppies. During pregnancy of an infected bitch, the second-stage larvae encysted in peripheral tissues resume their migratory behavior. Puppies can then acquire *T. canis* larvae by transplacental, prenatal transmission.[24] Alternatively, postnatal acquisition can occur by ingestion of milk from an infected bitch or by fecal–oral transmission. Transtracheal migration occurs in infected pups and third-stage larvae are coughed up, swallowed, and then ma-

ture to sexually differentiated forms in the small intestine. Adult worms can shed over 200,000 eggs per day. A period of 2 to 3 weeks is required before ova become infective.[25] Within 30 days of birth, puppies shed advanced stage-2 larvae and huge numbers of eggs in the feces.[26] The infection rate in puppies may approach 100%.[27,28] Lactating bitches likewise will shed ova in their feces by the fourth postpartum week.[25,26] Adults become reinfected by the common behavior of licking feces of their puppies.[29] In addition, adult dogs may acquire *T. canis* by ingesting meat of paratenic hosts such as rabbits or mice. *T. canis* infection is highly prevalent in dogs and shows some geographic variation, being more prevalent in southern climates.[12,30,31] Curiously, despite the prevalence of *T. canis* infection, dogs rarely develop ocular disease related to *Toxocara* infestation.

Embryonated eggs are ubiquitous in soil in areas such as playgrounds due to contamination with animal feces.[27,32] *T. canis* ova are quite hardy and may remain viable for months[25] to years[32] under optimal conditions. Prevalence of systemic toxocariasis and of *T. canis* exposure as evidenced by enzyme-linked immunosorbent assay (ELISA) testing appears

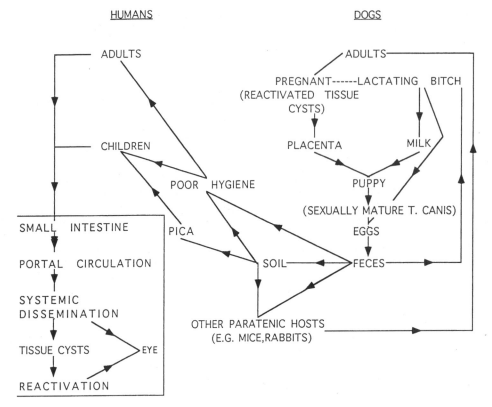

FIGURE 58–2   Transmission of *Toxocara canis*. Acquisition of ocular toxocariasis outlined in box.

greater in the southeastern United States, possibly related to environmental factors that promote survival of infective eggs in the soil.[25]

Human infection occurs by geophagia, oral–fecal transmission, or ingestion of contaminated meat. The organisms mature in the small intestine to become second-stage larvae. Motile second-stage larvae enter the portal circulation and lymphatics and are disseminated throughout the body by hematogenous spread and tissue migration. The larvae burrow through walls of small arterioles to enter target organs and encyst.[24] Further differentiation of *T. canis* to the sexually mature adult form does not occur in humans. Therefore, *T. canis* eggs are not shed in the alimentary tract and examination of stool samples for larvae or eggs is unrewarding.

Clinical manifestations of *T. canis* infestation depend on the parasite burden, site of infection, migratory behavior, and host inflammatory response. Asymptomatic infection with development of delayed hypersensitivity response and serum antibodies to *T. canis* have been observed in children and adults and have been correlated with pica and exposure to dogs.[9,10,12,31,33–36] Subclinical infection presumably relates to infestation with lower numbers of organisms involving noncritical organ sites. Systemic toxocariasis may manifest as a chronic febrile illness with multi–organ system involvement—visceral larva migrans (VLM). Described by Beaver and associates in 1952,[7] the original description of VLM included a syndrome of fever, pul-

monary symptoms, organomegaly, and chronic pronounced eosinophilia in children with a history of pica and exposure to pets. The syndrome has been replicated in institutionalized children by administration of as few as 200 embryonated eggs of *Toxocara*.[37] The degree of peripheral eosinophilia in patients with VLM has been correlated with the level of exposure to *Toxocara* larvae.[12] Although VLM may present a fulminating illness, it is typically a mild, self-limited condition. Despite a common etiologic agent and mode of acquisition, the systemic and ocular forms of toxocariasis are rarely seen within the same individual, either simultaneously or at different points in time. In a study by Brown and co-workers[8] of 245 patients with VLM, only 5% had any indication of ocular involvement. Unlike VLM, systemic findings such as peripheral eosinophilia are infrequently encountered in individuals with OT. In addition, the demographics are different in the two conditions, as the mean age at presentation for patients with VLM is significantly younger than for OT—15 to 30 months[8] versus 7.5[8] to 8.6[9] years.

Ocular Toxocariasis

Acquisition of ocular *Toxocara* infection may occur via lymphatic or hematogenous dissemination during initial systemic infection, after reinfection, or after late reactivation of dormant larvae encysted in peripheral tissues.[25,38] The possibility of late reactivation is supported by both experimental and clinical studies in which viable organisms have been found encysted in peripheral tissues for months to years.[4,11,39] In addition, the later onset of ocular toxocariasis versus systemic VLM is consistent with the possibility of later reactivation of pre-existing encysted larvae.[40]

Larvae enter the eye via the choroidal, ciliary, or retinal arteries. The site of entry may be indicated on histopathologic examination by eosinophilic reaction and scarring of the choroid.[3,41] Occasionally, multiple larvae may invade the eye, as evidenced in histopathologic[3] and clinical[5] studies. Bilateral involvement can occur but is rare.[5] Larvae may exhibit migratory behavior in the eye, moving across the choroid and retina and inciting a scarring response.[42] Wilder[3] reported cases with calcium deposits and bone formation in her original series, but this appears to be an exceptional feature.[1] While it has been argued that inflammation occurs primarily in response to death of the *T. canis* larvae,[22] Nichols[4] noted the presence of live larvae in eosinophilic abscesses from Wilder's original cases. Luxenberg[40] reported a clinical case where he observed a motile intravitreal larva die and disintegrate without inciting a vitreous reaction over a 3-year follow-up period. In an experimental study of *Toxocara* infection in primate eyes, Watzke and co-workers noted that dead larvae often incited little inflammation. They postulated that it is the excretory and secretory products rather than the larva per se that incites an inflammatory response.[39] Infectious larvae may be well tolerated and have been recovered from primate retinas over 1 year[39] and up to 10 years[11] after infection.

Clinical and experimental work have demonstrated the characteristic pathologic findings of eosinophilic inflammatory response in *Toxocara* infestation (Fig. 58–1). The nematode incites an eosinophilic granuloma or abscess in which the larva is enveloped in a central core of eosinophils surrounded by mononuclear cells, histiocytes, epithelioid cells, and occasional giant cells. Vitrectomy aspirates from humans treated for OT may reveal chronic inflammation with a granulomatous component. Eosinophils, though frequent, may not be a prominent feature. Secondary epiretinal membranes with fibrous astrocytes, new collagen, eosinophils, and/or plasma cells may be present.[43]

Injury to ocular structures may occur by a variety of mechanisms. Direct injury may be related to mechanical damage caused by tissue migration of motile larvae, or to toxic injury induced by excretory or secretory products produced by the worm. Damage to ocular structures may also be indirect, related to the degree of host inflammatory response induced by the *T. canis* organism. *T. canis* is capable of inducing a local eosinophilic reaction that may result in toxic injury to the retina.[44] The inflammatory response to individual *Toxocara* organisms may be quite variable in degree, even within the same eye.[39] This reaction appears to determine the extent of ocular injury caused by any one larva.

CLINICAL FEATURES

The average age at presentation of patients with OT is 7.5[8] to 8.6[9] years, with a range of 2 to 30 years.[8] In one ophthalmology practice, OT accounted for 37% of all retinal disease diagnoses in the pediatric age group.[10] Although this condition is predominantly seen in the pediatric population, OT occasionally develops in early adulthood between 16 and 30 years of age, with individual cases up to 50 years reported.[45] Acquisition of toxocariasis infection during adulthood is rare, presumably due to better hygiene and to the infrequency of geophagia in adults. Similarly, the occurrence of toxocariasis is low in young infants because of limited exposure to *Toxocara* at this age.[31] Clusters of cases rarely occur and are presumably related by common exposures.[46,47] Epidemiologic studies have established the risk of contracting ocular *Toxocara* in children who provide a history of pica or recent occupational or recreational exposure to dogs.[1,8–12] Contact with cats or other animals is not associated with the development of OT.

Patients typically present with unilateral decreased vision, strabismus, or leukokoria. A delay between the onset of ocular symptoms and diagnosis of OT is common, averaging over a year in one report.[9] Both eyes are affected with equal frequency.[5] External examination usually demonstrates a white and quiet eye with no discomfort. Characteristic findings on ophthalmologic examination can be categorized as (1) peripheral granuloma, (2) posterior pole granuloma, (3) chronic endophthalmitis, or (4) atypical findings.

A peripheral inflammatory mass in a quiet eye was the most common presentation of intraocular *Toxocara* in the large series reported by Wilkinson and Welch.[5] Decreased vision and strabismus in this form of OT are common, but normal acuity is sometimes encountered. A mild active inflammation may be evident in the anterior or posterior segment. Severe vitreous reaction is uncommon. This form of OT may initially present as an acute, diffuse vitreitis with the peripheral inflammatory mass appearing as the ocular media begins to clear. The inflammatory lesion usually appears as a dense white mass in the ciliary body region associated with epiretinal fibrous membranes and radial retinal folds. A fibrous band with a falciform retinal fold is typically seen between the peripheral granuloma and optic disc (Fig. 58–3). Vitreoretinal and vitreopapillary traction induced by these bands are the most common causes of vision-threatening complications, such as retinal detachment, macular distortion, or optic nerve dysfunction. Ocular damage caused by active inflammation is uncommon in

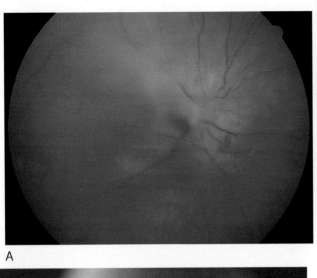

A

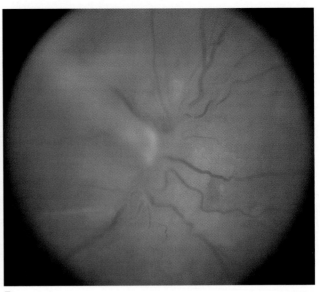

B

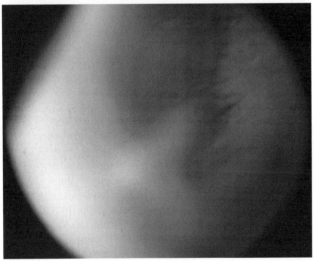

C

FIGURE 58–3   Right eye of a 25-year-old woman with peripheral inflammatory mass from toxocara infection during childhood. *Toxocara* ELISA = 1:256. *A,* Vitreous traction band extending to the disc. Macular area uninvolved. Vision equals 20/300. *B,* Tractional detachment of nasal peripapillary retina. *C,* White, fibrotic mass in the superotemporal pars plana region. Patient later developed a rhegmatogenous retinal detachment in this eye that was successfully repaired with vitreoretinal surgery.

eyes with the peripheral inflammatory mass. Unilateral pars planitis with a diffuse peripheral "snowbank" has been described[15,16] but is uncommon versus the focal peripheral granuloma. In addition, multiple peripheral granulomas are infrequently encountered.[5]

As originally described by Ashton,[14] a discrete inflammatory mass can also occur in the posterior pole region. Patients invariably have decreased vision, amblyopia, or strabismus in a white and quiet eye. Individuals may present during the acute inflammatory phase with an ill-defined posterior pole white lesion with overlying vitreitis that eventually resolves. Often, however, the ocular media are clear and there is minimal inflammation at the time of diagnosis. A discrete white subretinal or intraretinal granuloma with overlying vessels is typically seen. Lesions are usually between $^1/_2$ to 2 disc diameters in size and are located along the temporal aspect of the optic disc (Fig. 58–4). Optic nerve granulo-

mas have been described[17,19] and represent an atypical variant of posterior pole involvement. Fibrotic vitreous bands usually develop with these posterior lesions and may cause tractional complications such as retinal detachment. However, ocular damage results primarily from direct injury to the macula by the nematode and associated abscess. Although these eyes have profound irreversible central visual impairment, they do have a favorable long-term anatomic prognosis.

Patients presenting with the chronic endophthalmitis form of OT are typically younger than those with localized peripheral or posterior pole granulomas.[5] This is consistent with the notion that the localized forms are late, cicatricial manifestations of *Toxocara* infection after resolution of an acute inflammatory phase. In addition to visual loss and strabismus common to patients with focal inflammatory mass, leukokoria is frequently noted in eyes presenting with chronic endophthalmitis. Risk fac-

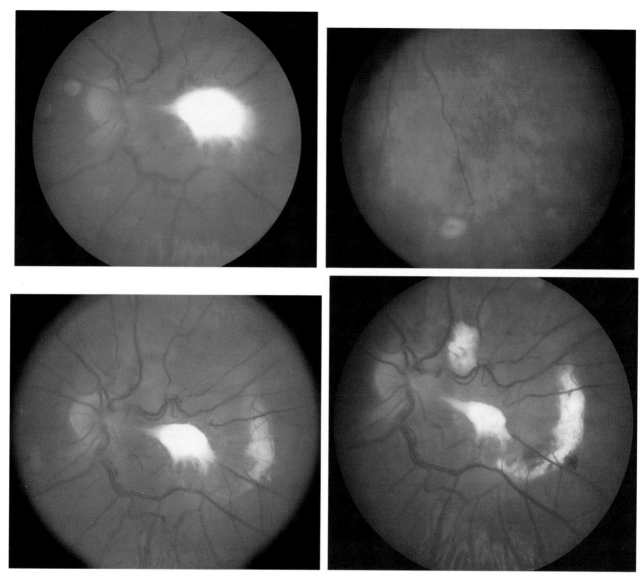

FIGURE 58-4 *Left, top.* Left eye of a 7-year-old child presenting with leukokoria and strabismus. A focal inflammatory mass from *Toxocara* infection is present in the posterior pole. *Right, top.* Lesion in the inferior retina of the same eye. *Left, bottom.* Same eye 15 months later. *Right, bottom,* Six years after initial presentation. Vision equals 20/200. (Courtesy of Dr. Alexander J. Brucker, M.D.)

tors for other forms of exogenous or endogenous endophthalmitis are absent. Externally, these eyes appear quiet despite significant intraocular inflammation. A granulomatous anterior uveitis may be seen along with hypopyon in severe cases. A diffuse, fibrinoid vitreitis is present that obscures view of the posterior fundus. A poorly defined retinal or vitreous abscess may occasionally be visualized. Historically, these eyes were often enucleated for suspicion of retinoblastoma or infectious endophthalmitis. Prognosis in cases with diffuse endophthalmitis depends on the location of the granulomas and the pattern of fibrous membrane organization. Localized inflammatory masses and associated fibrous membranes may develop into typical peripheral or posterior pole forms of ocular OT. Alternatively, widespread vitreous and cyclitic membrane formation may occur.

Atypical presentations of OT have been described, including optic disc granuloma[17]; papillitis[19]; motile intraretinal,[20,21] vitreous,[22] or intracorneal larvae[23]; iris inflammatory mass[23]; and lens involvement.[48] Many of these cases are presumptive based on clinical diagnosis without histopathologic confirmation of *Toxocara* infestation.

DIAGNOSIS

The diagnosis of OT is clinical, based on a combination of history, ophthalmologic examination, and laboratory testing. Morphologic features of peripheral and posterior pole granulomas are characteristic in most instances. In cases with media opacification or advanced cicatricial changes, findings on ophthalmic evaluation may be nonspecific and require ancillary testing to support the diagnosis of OT. Generally, the most helpful noninvasive tests include serum antibody assays and ocular imaging studies.

Historically, many tests have been developed to assess exposure to *T. canis*, including assays of serum for larval antigens or antibodies to *T. canis*, or skin testing for delayed hypersensitivity response.[49] These tests suffered from lack of specificity due to cross-reactivity with other nematode species. The presence of peripheral eosinophilia is a nonspecific finding in individuals with parasitic infection, and is infrequently encountered in patients with OT.[48] A modified ELISA with high specificity for *T. canis* has been developed and has gained widespread acceptance. The serum ELISA is most useful when positive, being a reliable indicator for exposure to *T. canis*. However, a positive test is not diagnostic of ocular *Toxocara* infection per se. Indeed, patients with retinoblastoma may have positive serum ELISA to *T. canis*[47] as an incidental finding of past exposure. Twenty-three per cent of a randomly sampled population of kindergarten children in rural North Carolina had positive ELISAs for *Toxocara* without any clinical indication of systemic or ocular infection.[35] A low or negative serum ELISA for *Toxocara* may be encountered in patients with clinically manifest OT.[41,50,51] Serum titers to *T. canis* in patients with ocular toxocariasis can decrease significantly over time.[50] It has been suggested that any positive titer may be significant if the clinical presentation is compelling. A serum ELISA titer of 1:8 provides both high specificity (90%) and sensitivity (91%) when combined with findings on clinical examination.[47,48] Titers may also be measured from intraocular fluids, and if higher than that simultaneously found in serum, are highly suggestive of primary ocular involvement.[52,53] Because of technical requirements involved in the ELISA assay for *T. canis*, clinical testing is performed at central laboratories, such as the Centers for Disease Control in Atlanta.

Imaging studies are most useful in cases with media opacification in order to delineate posterior segment anatomy and to rule out the presence of intraocular calcification. Ultrasonography may be used to measure axial length to assess for microphthalmia typically seen in persistent hyperplastic primary vitreous (PHPV) versus OT. In cases with diffuse media opacification, ultrasound examination can determine the presence of retinal detachment, mass lesions, and calcification.[54] Computerized axial tomography is exquisitely sensitive at detecting intraocular calcifications, which are more typical for retinoblastoma than OT.

Invasive testing is usually reserved for diagnosis in cases with opaque media where differentiation from retinoblastoma is required. Anterior chamber aspiration for aqueous fluid testing may be considered when the diagnosis is in question. When a hypopyon is aspirated, the presence of eosinophils on cytology is suggestive of OT; conversely, malignant cells may be identified in cases of retinoblastoma.[55] ELISA testing of intraocular fluids may be performed and is highly suggestive of OT when titers are greater than that in serum.[52,53]

Pathology specimens obtained during vitreoretinal surgery[43] or enucleation should be carefully examined for eosinophilic reaction and for *Toxocara* remnants, which may provide definitive diagnosis.

DIFFERENTIAL DIAGNOSIS

The diagnosis of OT is usually straightforward based on findings of the ophthalmic exam. Occasionally, confusion exists with other pediatric conditions causing posterior segment masses, inflammation, or membrane formation (Table 58–1). Symptomatology in these cases is usually nonspecific, with decreased vision, strabismus, or leukokoria. Diseases frequently considered in the differential diagnosis include retinoblastoma, infectious endophthalmitis, posterior uveitis or panuveitis, retinopathy of prematurity (ROP), familial exudative vitreoretinopathy (FEVR), Coats' disease, and PHPV.

Retinoblastoma (RB) is the most common malignant ocular tumor of childhood, and the unilateral, sporadic form is the most important consideration in the differential diagnosis of OT. The mean age of diagnosis for unilateral RB is 23 months, much younger than that for OT—7.5 to 8.6 years.[8,9] On ophthalmic examination, RB is distinguished from ocular toxocariasis by lack of any signs inflammation including anterior segment scarring, secondary cataract, cyclitic membranes, and transvitreal or epiretinal membranes. In RB distortion of posterior segment anatomy by membrane traction is not encountered. In OT, inflammatory masses are rarely seen between the posterior vascular arcades and the retinal periphery. In contrast to retinoblastoma tumors, *Toxocara* granulomas do not increase in size or number. Therefore, depending upon the location of the lesion, a period of observation may be useful in the differential diagnosis.

In eyes with opaque media, ultrasound or computed tomography (CT) scanning may demonstrate calcification typical for retinoblastoma. Conversely, the presence of tractional membranes is highly suggestive of ocular *Toxocara*.[54] Aspiration of intraocular fluids or vitreous for cytology and ELISA testing may be warranted in selected cases.[55]

Differentiation from infectious endophthalmitis is usually straightforward based on history of recent trauma or ocular surgery. Acute onset of painful red eye with external signs of inflammation typical for bacterial endophthalmitis is uncharacteristic in OT. However, delayed, subacute onset with minimal external signs of inflammation can be associated with infection with less virulent bacterial or fungal organisms. Vitreous and/or aqueous sam-

TABLE 58–1 Differential Diagnosis of Ocular Toxocariasis

Condition	Onset	History
Toxocariasis	7.5–8.6 years	Pica/exposure to dogs
Sporadic retinoblastoma	23 months	Negative family history
Infectious endophthalmitis	Any age	Trauma/surgery/sepsis
Toxoplasmosis	Congenital/later reactivation	Normal
Pars planitis	9 years	2:1 male/female
Retinopathy of prematurity	Birth	Premature/low birth weight
PHPV	Birth	Normal
FEVR	Birth	Family history
Coats' disease	Childhood	3:1 male/female

Symptoms/Signs	Laterality
Decreased vision/strabismus/leukokoria	Unilateral
Decreased vision/strabismus/leukokoria	Unilateral
Pain/decreased vision/lid edema	Unilateral/bilateral (endogenous)
Floaters/decreased vision	Unilateral
Floaters/decreased vision	Bilateral (80%)
Leukokoria/strabismus/screening exam	Bilateral (>90% symmetry)
Leukokoria/pediatrician exam	Unilateral (>80%)
Strabismus/decreased vision/leukokoria	Bilateral (asymmetry)
Strabismus/decreased vision/leukokoria	Unilateral (>80%)

Inflammation	Exudation	Membranes/Traction
Present (indolent)	Absent	Present
Masquerade/pseudohypopyon	Absent	Absent
Present (severe/acute)	Absent	Present (resolution phase)
Present (variable intensity)	Absent	Minimal
Present (mild/moderate)	Cystoid edema	Present
Absent	Absent	Present
Absent	Absent	Present (ciliary processes)
Absent	Present	Present
Absent	Present (severe)	Absent

Imaging	Serology
Mass/membranes/traction	Positive toxocara ELISA
Mass/calcium	Negative RB gene
Diffuse infiltrate	Blood cultures/antigen-positive
Diffuse infiltrate	Variable for *T. gondii*
Membranes/pars plana mass	Lyme (rare)
Membranes/traction	Negative
Microphthalmia/fibrovascular stalk	Negative
Membranes/traction	Negative
Subretinal exudate	Negative

PHPV, Persistent hyperplastic primary vitreous; FEVR, familial exudative vitreoretinopathy; ELISA, enzyme-linked immunosorbent assay; RB, retinoblastoma.

pling from microscopic examination and microbiologic studies may provide definitive diagnosis. Endogenous endophthalmitis usually occurs in patients with history of immune deficiency and recent sepsis. Positive cultures from blood or visceral sources are highly suggestive in these cases and rarely need confirmation with examination of intraocular fluids. The differentiation between active toxoplasmosis retinitis and ocular toxocariasis can be difficult if a severe vitreitis is present. The characteristic retinal necrosis caused by active toxoplasmosis might be completely obscured by inflammatory reaction similar to that seen in the chronic endophthalmitis form of ocular toxocariasis. With heavy vitreitis, an ill-defined "headlight-in-the-fog" appearance can be seen with either the active *Toxoplasma gondii* retinal necrosis or *Toxocara* granuloma. Serologic studies for *T. gondii* and *T. canis* may provide useful information in the differential diagnosis. Ultrasonography may demonstrate transvitreal membranes or elevated mass lesion characteristic of *Toxocara*. In both diseases, inflammation will often resolve, revealing the pathogenic fundus lesion. Treatment of inflammation with systemic corticosteroids should be carefully considered, as this may exacerbate retinal infection caused by toxoplasmosis.

Uveitis other than that caused by infection or traumatic etiology rarely results in unilateral disease with features similar to OT. Although OT presenting as unilateral pars planitis has been reported,[15,16] this diffuse pars plana inflammation is unusual in OT. Conversely, unilateral involvement characteristic for OT is atypical for the idiopathic form of pars planitis. Pars planitis is a chronic, recurrent uveitis that is bilateral in greater than 80% of cases and is most typically seen in males in early adulthood. Although differentiation between the two entities may sometimes be difficult on clinical grounds, treatment may not differ, as it will be directed towards active inflammation in either condition.

OT may also present with optic nerve edema or papillitis due to vitreoretinal traction, posterior inflammation, or optic nerve infection.[17,19] Papillitis caused by viral neuroretinitis is not associated with a significant vitreitis or membrane formation. Presence of a typical granuloma should distinguish OT from most other inflammatory conditions.

Pediatric conditions associated with vitreous and epiretinal membrane formation or subretinal fibrosis may pose diagnostic confusion with OT including ROP, FEVR, PHPV, and Coats' disease. Unlike OT, however, these conditions usually present neonatally or early in infancy and lack signs of inflammation or posterior segment inflammatory mass. In addition, characteristic vascular abnormalities are encountered in each of these diseases. ROP is encountered in infants with a history of prematurity and low birth weight. Unlike OT, ROP is a bilateral disease with proliferative vascular changes and membrane formation involving the retinal periphery. Similarly, FEVR is a bilateral condition with characteristic retinal vascular anomalies and membrane formation. FEVR is distinguished by familial inheritance and by the presence of pronounced exudation. PHPV is a congenital condition that is typically unilateral. Microphthalmia is a constant feature. Characteristic morphology includes a fibrovascular stalk from the disc to posterior lens surface and a retrolental fibrovascular mass causing ciliary body traction. Coats' disease is a unilateral condition usually seen in young males. The characteristic fundus lesion is a white, fibrotic subretinal mass in the posterior pole that may be confused with a *Toxocara* granuloma. However, in Coats' disease, typical vascular telangiectasia and lipid exudation are present and epiretinal membrane formation is not seen.

TREATMENT

The most effective treatment of OT is preventative —eliminating the acquisition of the *T. canis* organism.[25] The natural host, sources of contamination, and modes of transmission have been thoroughly elucidated for *Toxocara* infection. Effective preventative measures include aggressive treatment of newborn pups and postparturient bitches with anthelmintic agents,[29] quarantine of animals actively shedding ova, hygienic disposal of contaminated feces, isolation of children at risk from pets, and modification of pica and other unsanitary behaviors in children. Since anthelmintic agents cannot eradicate tissue cysts, adult dogs and pups need to be retreated during each pregnancy when larvae are reactivated and transmission recurs. In addition, education of veterinarians, parents, and children of the health risks associated with *T. canis* infection should be instituted to help interrupt *Toxocara* transmission.[25]

Treatment of ocular toxocariasis depends on the clinical manifestations of the disease. Most cases do not require therapy, as they present without significant inflammation or treatable vitreoretinal pathology. Vitreoretinal surgery has been used effectively to treat complications such as vitreous opacification, epiretinal membrane with macular or optic nerve traction, and retinal detachment.[52,56–61] Favorable functional and anatomic results have been reported with standard vitreoretinal techniques, and stable long-term outcomes have been achieved. It should be recognized that *Toxocara* granulomas may be incorporated into retinal and subretinal tissue (e.g., macular granuloma) and therefore are not amenable to surgical extirpation.[61] Unintentional extraction of *Toxocara* larvae during vitreoretinal surgery has been described but is not considered a therapeutic technique.[43] Visual prognosis after vitreoretinal surgery is often limited by amblyopia common to this pediatric population.[58]

Careful follow-up in conjunction with a pediatric ophthalmologist is recommended for patients at risk for amblyopia.

In cases where motile larvae can be identified on clinical examination, laser photocoagulation may be considered to eradicate infestation and protect against mechanical damage induced by the migrating worm.[21,45,62,63] Heat-induced protein coagulation may potentially prevent antigen release which may cause inflammation.[63]

Medical therapy is directed at inflammation in order to prevent inflammation-induced tissue injury or secondary membrane formation. Local and systemic corticosteroid therapy is useful in managing acute inflammatory reaction.[5,17,20,22,30,64] *T. canis* larvae do not replicate in humans and there is no indication that infestation is exacerbated by corticosteroid-induced immune suppression. Systemic therapy may be indicated in cases with severe vitreitis to reduce vitreous opacification and membrane formation. Anthelmintic agents have been used[5] to kill viable nematodes to prevent injury caused by local tissue destruction by migratory activity or local toxicity. Intraocular penetration of thiabendazole has been demonstrated[65] supporting potential use in treating ocular *Toxocara* infection. It has been suggested that anthelmintic therapy may be undesirable because of inflammation induced by death of the organism. However, clinical and experimental evidence has demonstrated lack of inflammatory response associated with death of *T. canis* larvae and, conversely, severe inflammation with abscess formation with live, motile organisms. Combination therapy with systemic corticosteroids and anthelmintic agents has been used with favorable results.[20] The utility of anthelmintic therapy remains unproven, however.[48]

SUMMARY

Ocular toxocariasis is a common parasitic infestation of childhood causing decreased vision, strabismus, and leukokoria. Frequent posterior segment manifestations include focal inflammatory mass with tractional membranes involving the posterior pole or periphery, or diffuse, chronic endophthalmitis in an otherwise quiet eye. Diagnosis is clinical based on morphology and supportive laboratory and imaging studies. The most important diagnostic consideration is sporadic unilateral retinoblastoma. Treatment is directed at complications related to acute inflammation and membrane traction.

REFERENCES

1. Duguid IM: Features of ocular infestation by *Toxocara*. Br J Ophthalmol 45:789–796, 1961.
2. Duguid IM: Chronic endophthalmitis due to *Toxocara*. Br J Ophthalmol 45:705–717, 1961.
3. Wilder HC: Nematode endophthalmitis. Trans Am Acad Ophthalmol Otolaryngol 55:99–109, 1950.
4. Nichols RL: The etiology of visceral larva migrans. I. Diagnostic morphology of infective second-stage *Toxocara* larvae. J Parasitol 42:349–362, 1956.
5. Wilkinson CP, Welch RB: Intraocular *Toxocara*. Am J Ophthalmol 71:921–930, 1971.
6. Zuelzer WW, Apt L: Disseminated visceral lesions associated with extreme eosinophilia. Am J Dis Child 78:153–181, 1949.
7. Beaver PC, Snyder CH, Carrerra GM, et al: Chronic eosinophilia due to visceral larva migrans: report of three cases. Pediatrics 9:7–19, 1952.
8. Brown DH: Ocular *Toxocara canis* II. Clinical review. J Pediatr Ophthalmol 7:182–191, 1970.
9. Schantz PM, Meyer D, Glickman LT: Clinical, serologic, and epidemiologic characteristics of ocular toxocariasis. Am J Trop Med Hyg 70:1269–1272, 1980.
10. Schantz PM, Weis PE, Pollard ZF, White MC: Risk factors for toxocaral ocular larva migrans: a case-control study. Am J Public Health 70:1269–1272, 1980.
11. Beaver PC: Zoonoses, with particular reference to parasites of veterinary importance. In Soulsby EJL (ed): *Biology of Parasites: Emphasis on Veterinary Parasites*. New York, Academic Press, 1966, 215–227.
12. Glickman LT, Schantz PM: Epidemiology and pathogenesis of zoonotic toxocariasis. Epidemiol Rev 3:230–250, 1981.
13. Irvine WC, Irvine AR Jr: Nematode endophthalmitis: *Toxocara canis*: report of one case. Am J Ophthalmol 47:185–191, 1959.
14. Ashton N: Larval granulomatosis of the retina due to *Toxocara*. Br J Ophthalmol 44:129–148, 1960.
15. Hogan MJ, Kimura SJ, Spencer WH: Visceral larva migrans and peripheral retinitis. JAMA 194:1345–1347, 1965.
16. Greer CH: *Toxocara* infestation of the eye. Trans Ophthalmol Soc Aust 23:90–95, 1963.
17. Bird AC, Smith JL, Curtin VT: Nematode optic neuritis. Am J Ophthalmol 69:72–77, 1970.
18. Smith PM, Greer CH: Unusual presentation of ocular *Toxocara* infestation. Br J Ophthalmol 55:317–320, 1971.
19. Phillips CI, Mackenzie AD: *Toxocara* larva papillitis. Br Med J 1:154–155, 1973.
20. Rubin ML, Kaufman HE, Tierney JP, Lucas HC: An intraretinal nematode (a case report). Trans Am Acad Ophthalmol Otolaryngol 72:855–866, 1968.
21. Sorr EM: Meandering ocular toxocariasis. Retina 4:90–96, 1984.
22. Byers B, Kimura SJ: Uveitis after death of a larva in the vitreous cavity. Am J Ophthalmol 77:63–66, 1974.
23. Baldone JA, Clark WB, Jung RC: Nematode ophthalmitis: Report of two cases. Am J Ophthalmol 57:763–766, 1964.
24. Sprent JFA: The life cycles of nematodes in the family Ascaridea blanchard 1896. J Parasitol 40:608–617, 1954.
25. Schantz P, Glickman LT: Toxocaral visceral larva migrans. N Engl J Med 298:436–439, 1978.
26. Sprent JFA: Post-parturient infection of the bitch with *Toxocara canis*. J Parasitol 47:284, 1961.
27. Slatter DH: Toxocariasis—summary of recent developments. Aust J Ophthalmol 6:143–148, 1978.
28. Mok CH: Visceral larva migrans: a discussion based on review of the literature. Clin Pediatr 7:565–573, 1968.
29. Sprent JFA, English PB: The large round worms of dogs and cats—a public health problem. Aust Vet J 34:161–171, 1958.
30. Schimek RA, Perez WA, Carrera GM: Ophthalmic manifestations of visceral larva migrans. Ann Ophthalmol 11:1387–1390, 1979.
31. Berrocal J: Prevalence of *Toxocara canis* in babies and in adults as determined by the ELISA test. Trans Am Ophthalmol Soc 78:376–413, 1980.
32. Borg OA, Woodruff AW: Prevalence of infective ova of *Toxocara* species in public places. Br Med J 4:470–472, 1973.
33. Woodruff EW, deSavigny DM, Jacobs DE: Study of toxocaral infection in dog breeders. Br J Med 2:1747–1748, 1978.

34. Bass JL, Glickman LT, Eppes BM: Clinically inapparent *Toxocara* infection in children. N Engl J Med 308:723–724, 1983.
35. Ellis GS Jr, Pakalnis VA, Worley G, et al: *Toxocara canis* in infestation: clinical and epidemiological associations with seropositivity in kindergarten children. Ophthalmology 93:1032–1037, 1986.
36. Clemett RS, Williamson HJE, Hidajat RR, et al: Ocular *Toxocara canis* infections: diagnosis by enzyme immunoassay. Aust N Z J Ophthalmol 15:145–150, 1987.
37. Smith MHD, Beaver PC: Persistence and distribution of *Toxocara* larvae in tissues of children and mice. Pediatr 12:491–497, 1953.
38. Sprent JFA: On the migratory behavior of the larvae of the various *Ascaris* species in white mice. I. Distribution of larvae in tissues. J Infect Dis 90:165–176, 1952.
39. Watzke RC, Oaks JA, Folk JC: *Toxocara canis* infection in the eye: correlation of clinical observations with developing pathology in the primate model. Arch Ophthalmol 102:282–291, 1984.
40. Luxenberg MW: An experimental approach to the study of intraocular *Toxocara canis*. Trans Am Ophthalmol Soc 77:542–601, 1979.
41. Kielar RA: *Toxocara canis* endophthalmitis with low ELISA titer. Ann Ophthalmol 15:447–449, 1983.
42. O'Connor PR: Visceral larva migrans of the eye: subretinal tube formation. Arch Ophthalmol 88:526–529, 1972.
43. Maguire AM, Green WR, Michels RG, Erozan YS: Recovery of intraocular *Toxocara canis* by pars plana vitrectomy. Ophthalmology 97:675–680, 1990.
44. Rockey JH, Donnelly JJ, Stromberg BE, Soulsby EJL: Immunopathology of *Toxocara canis* and *Ascaris suum* infections of the eye: the role of the eosinophil. Invest Ophthalmol Vis Sci 18:1172–1184, 1979.
45. Raistrick ER, Hart JCD: Adult toxocaral infection with focal retinal lesion. Br Med J 3:416, 1975.
46. Kirber WM, Nichols CW, Braunstein SN: Unusual presentation of ocular toxocariasis in friends. Ann Ophthalmol 11:573–576, 1979.
47. Pollard ZF, Jarrett WH, Hagler WS, et al: ELISA for diagnosis of ocular toxocariasis. Ophthalmology 86:743–749, 1979.
48. Shields JA: Ocular toxocariasis: a review. Surv Ophthalmol 28:361–381, 1984.
49. Ferguson EC III, Olson LJ: *Toxocara* ocular nematodiasis. Int Ophthalmol Clin 7:583–603, 1967.
50. Searl SS, Moazed K, Albert DM, Marcus LC: Ocular toxocariasis presenting as leukocoria in a patient with low ELISA titer to *Toxocara canis*. Ophthalmology 88:1302–1306, 1981.
51. Pollard ZF: Long-term follow-up in patients with ocular toxocariasis as measured by ELISA titers. Ann Ophthalmol 19:167–169, 1987.
52. Biglan AW, Glickman LT, Lobes LA Jr: Serum and vitreous *Toxocara* antibody in nematode endophthalmitis. Am J Ophthalmol 88:898–901, 1979.
53. Felberg NT, Shields JA, Federman JL: Antibody to *Toxocara canis* in the aqueous humor. Arch Ophthalmol 99:1563–1564, 1981.
54. Kennedy JJ, Defeo E: Ocular toxocariasis demonstrated by ultrasound. Ann Ophthalmol 13:1357–1358, 1981.
55. Shields JA, Lerner HA, Felberg NT: Aqueous cytology and enzymes in nematode endophthalmitis. Am J Ophthalmol 84:319–322, 1977.
56. Triester G, Machemer R: Results of vitrectomy for rare proliferative and hemorrhagic diseases. Am J Ophthalmol 84:394–412, 1977.
57. Hagler WS, Pollard ZF, Jarrett WH, Donnelly EH: Results of surgery for ocular *Toxocara canis*. Ophthalmology 88:1081–1086, 1981.
58. Grand MG, Roper-Hall G: Pars plana vitrectomy for ocular toxocariasis. Retina 1:258–261, 1981.
59. Belmont JB, Irvine A, Benson W, O'Connor GR: Vitrectomy in ocular toxocariasis. Arch Ophthalmol 100:1912–1915, 1982.
60. Rodriquez A: Early pars plana vitrectomy in chronic endopthalmitis of toxocariasis. Graefes Arch Clin Exp Ophthalmol 224:218–220, 1986.
61. Small KW, McCuen BW, deJuan E, Machemer R: Surgical management of retinal traction caused by toxocariasis. Am J Ophthalmol 108:10–14, 1989.
62. Siam A-L: Toxocaral chorio-retinitis. Treatment of early cases with photocoagulation. Br J Ophthalmol 57:700–703, 1973.
63. Fitzgerald CR, Rubin ML: Intraocular parasite destroyed by photocoagulation. Arch Ophthalmol 91:162–164, 1974.
64. Molk R: Treatment of toxocaral optic neuritis. J Clin Neuroophthalmol 2:109–112, 1982.
65. Maguire AM, Zarbin MA, Connor TA, Justin J: Ocular penetration of thiabendazole. Arch Ophthalmol 108:1675, 1990.

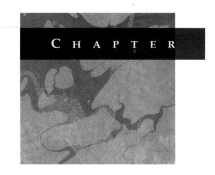

CHAPTER 59

Ocular Cysticercosis

Alan H. Friedman, M.D.

HISTORICAL PERSPECTIVE

Cysticercosis as a recognized entity is well described in antiquity. The first recorded observations of porcine cysticercosis were noted in the Ebers Papyrus (c.1500 BC) in Egypt and in the writings of Hippocrates. The first clinical observation of cysticercus in the eye was noted in 1830 by Soemmering in the anterior chamber. Schott, according to Duke Elder, was the first person to extract the parasite from the anterior chamber of a human eye. The great von Graefe made the first ophthalmologic observation of a cysticercus in the vitreous in 1854 and was the first to remove one from this location.

Infestation by *Cysticercus cellulosae*, the larval form of the pork tapeworm *Taenia solium*, is cosmopolitan although quite rare in Europe and North America. In recent years (1960–70) central nervous system cysticercosis was a recurring problem among gold miners in South Africa. Intraocular and adnexal involvement continues as a public health problem in the West undoubtedly due to the ease of air travel between different areas of the world.[2]

PARASITOLOGY

The phylum Platyhelminthes (or flatworms) contains the class Cestoidea, which is further divided into eight orders. Of the eight orders, the order Cyclophyllidea contains the genus *Taenia*.[3] Three species of *Taenia* are important in the pathogenesis of disease in man. They are *T. solium*, *T. saginata*, and *T. pisiformis*. It is the larval form of the *Taenia solium*, or pork tapeworm, with which we are dealing.

Cysticercosis is the parasitic disease produced by ingestion of ova of *T. solium* from contaminated food or, infrequently, by autoinfection (ingestion of one's own infected feces or by reverse peristalsis).

The adult tapeworm of *T. solium* is found in the upper part of the small intestine. It may measure from 4 to 8 m in length and contain 800 to 1000 segments. The head of the tapeworm is formed by a rostellum composed of a globular scolex about 1 mm in diameter containing a double row of hooklets and four suckers. The narrow neck of the tapeworm is about 5 to 10 cm in length and is connected to the distal nature segments, each measuring 6 × 12 mm and containing 30,000 to 50,000 ova. Segments (proglottides) pass from the bowel in the feces and may rupture in or outside the human stool.

Ova may be imbibed by its intermediate host, the pig, and develop into larvae (oncospheres and metacestodes) that can exist in the parenteral environment, or if the egg is eaten directly by the human host, the worms behave the same as if they were in the intermediate host.[4] The hexacanth (six-toothed) larvae upon emerging from the egg penetrate the intestinal wall and travel via lymphatics and the vascular system to muscles and the central nervous system (CNS).[5] As the larva (or oncosphere) develops it becomes the metacestode or cysticercus. At this stage there is the complete development of an inverted scolex and spiral canal. It is through the spiral canal that the invaginated scolex can evaginate and present on the surface. This process of evagination usually takes place in the small intestine but can be observed in the vitreous.

In the light microscope the cysticercus shows a cystic structure with the scolex either invaginated or evaginated. When the scolex evaginates it appears with its four prominent cup-shaped suckers and a low cushioned rostellum with a double row of hooklets (Fig. 59–1).

The electron microscopic structure of the larvae of cestodes has been studied.[6–8]

Cysticerci may remain viable in intraocular structures for 2 years or more. In the CNS cysticerci may remain viable for 3 to 6 (mean, 4.8) years.[2,9,10]

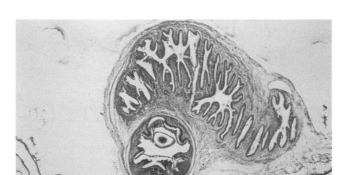

Cyst of *Cysticercus cellulosi* from vitreous with cyst wall, enteric apparatus, solex area, and numerous hooklets. (From Green WR: Pathology of the vitreous. In Frayer WC [ed]: Lancaster Course in Ophthalmic Histopathology, Unit 8. Philadelphia, FA Davis Co, 1981, with permission.)

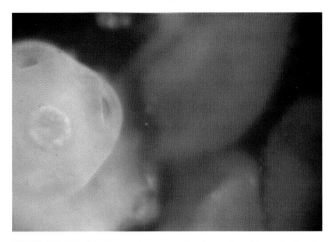

FIGURE 59–1   Gross photograph of a scolex. Note the hooklets on the rostellum. Suckers are present on each of four sides (Toludine blue, ×40).

CLINICAL OBSERVATIONS

Nonocular Cysticercosis

Heavy larval infection may cause muscle pains, weakness, fever or, if the CNS is involved, meningoencephalitis, seizures, intracranial hypertension, and psychic or mental manifestations.[2,9–11] Viable cystic lesions in the CNS (1 to 4 cm × 0.5 to 2 cm) are best visualized by computed tomography (CT) scan or magnetic resonance imaging (MRI) (Fig. 59–2). Calcified cysticerci may be seen on x-ray. A highly sensitive and specific diagnostic immuno-

blot assay is available. It is an enzyme-linked immunoelectrophoresis transfer. Blot assay is performed on serum or cerebrospinal fluid (CSF) at the Centers for Disease Control (CDC).

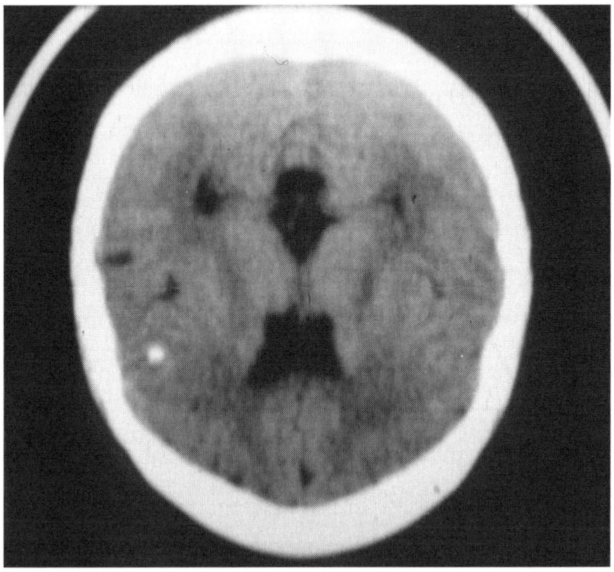

Intraocular and Adnexal Cysticercosis

Of more than 500 cases of ocular cysticercosis collected in several series, about 4% of cases occurred in the orbit or eyelids, 20% occurred in the subconjunctival area, 8% occurred in the anterior segment (the majority are "free" in the anterior chamber; the reminder are attached to the iris or lens capsule, within the lens or cornea; both very rare), and 68% occurred in the posterior segment (41% occurred either subretinal or intraretinally, while 27% occurred in the vitreous).[1]

Cysticercus in the eyelid is usually seen as a painless enlarging mass.[12] Subconjunctival lesions tend to present as somewhat painful, hyperemic epibulbar masses that are sometimes fluctuant. In the anterior chamber, though rare, with about 20 cases reported during the 20th century, cysticerci are seen as the typical cysts, attached to the iris or on occasion to the anterior lens capsule. Usually early discovery of the parasite is associated with minimal anterior uveitis; however, a severe plastic iritis has been observed when the cyst is left untreated.

Cysticercus of the posterior segment is usually seen in the vitreous body[14] (Fig. 59–3) or in the subretinal space (Fig. 59–4).[15,16] The parasite is brought via the posterior ciliary arteries to the subretinal space usually in the region of the posterior pole. The cysts are 3 to 6 disc diameters in size and have

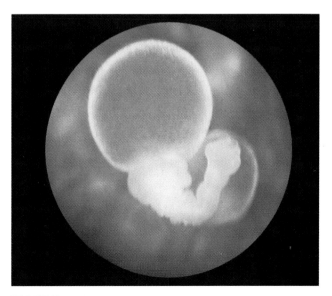

FIGURE 59–2   CT scans show cystic lesion of the brain. (From Friedman AH, Pokorny KS, Suhan J, et al: Electron microscopic observations of intravitreal *Cysticercus cellulosae* [*Taenia solium*]. Ophthalmolgica 1980, with permission. Courtesy of Patricia Cucci, M.D.)

FIGURE 59–3   Clinical photograph showing an evaginated scolex extending from the bladder of a *Cysticercus cellulosae* in the vitreous.

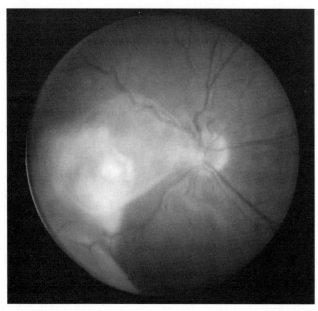

FIGURE 59–4   Clinical photograph of subretinal cysticercus. Note scarring adjacent to parasite. There is an overlying retinal detachment. (From Friedman AH, Pokorny KS, Suhan J, et al: Electron microscopic observations of intravitreal *Cysticercus cellulosae* [*Taenia solium*]. Ophthalmolgica 1980, with permission.)

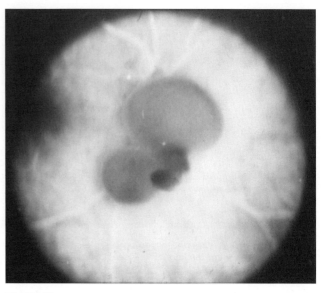

FIGURE 59–6   Intravenous fluorescein angiography fails to enhance cysticerci in the vitreous. (From Friedman AH, Pokorny KS, Suhan J, et al: Electron microscopic observations of intravitreal *Cysticercus cellulosae* [*Taenia solium*]. Ophthalmolgica 1980, with permission.)

an obvious single central scolex. Often, contraction and undulation of the cyst can be seen periodically. Retinal pigment epithelial disturbances, retinal detachment (serous or exudative), retinal edema, intraretinal hemorrhage, and vascular sheathing may be seen. In the later stages of an untreated eye infestation, a severe exudative uveitis can develop and lead to disorganization of the globe.[17]

Cysticerci may traverse the retina and present in the vitreous as quite unmistakable translucent, free-floating cysts. The scolex may be invaginated or evaginated. The cyst itself is quite capable of heaving and undulating movements, which are often accentuated by light.

The cystic nature of the parasite can be confirmed by B-scan ultrasound (Fig. 59–5). Intravenous fluorescein angiography adds little diagnostic assistance to the otherwise striking clinical appearance (Fig. 59–6). Bilateral multifocal intraocular cysticerci have also been described.

HISTOPATHOLOGICAL FINDINGS

Histopathologic examination of eyelid lesions in cysticercosis shows an inflammatory reaction about the cyst wall composed of three distinct layers[12]: an outermost zone formed by dense fibrovascular connective tissue, a middle layer showing large histiocytes intermingled with fibroblasts, and an inner layer containing neutrophils and eosinophils. The scolex with suckers and double row of hooklets is a prominent feature (Fig. 59–7).

Histopathologic examination of enucleated, blind eyes is characterized by the presence of a degenerated, thickened retina detached by subretinal serous exudate.[17] Prominent among cells in the exudate are eosinophils. Cysticerci can be found in sections in the vitreous or in intraretinal or subretinal locations. The parasites may be associated with an intense fibrovascular reaction or may exist as cysts within the retina.

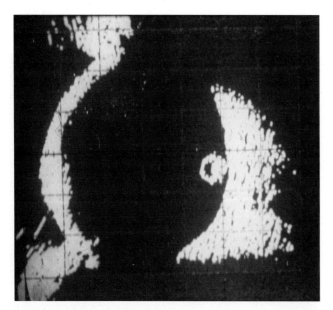

FIGURE 59–5   This B-scan ultrasound shows cystic lesion in the vitreous anterior to the optic nerve head. (From Friedman AH, Pokorny KS, Suhan J, et al: Electron microscopic observations of intravitreal *Cysticercus cellulosae* [*Taenia solium*]. Ophthalmolgica 1980, with permission.)

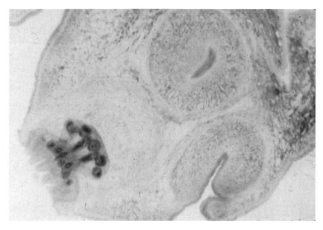

FIGURE 59–7   Light micrograph of scolex displaying suckers at *top* and *middle* and rostellum with double row of hooklets at *upper right*. (From Friedman AH, Pokorny KS, Suhan J, et al: Electron microscopic observations of intravitreal *Cysticercus cellulosae* [*Taenia solium*]. Ophthalmolgica 1980, with permission.)

PROPHYLAXIS AND TREATMENT

Infection may be prevented by thoroughly cooking pork at a minimum of 56°C (133°F) for 5 minutes. Eating properly inspected meats is essential.[18]

Any treatment aimed at eradication of intraocular or adnexal cysticercosis should be directed at surgical removal. Medical treatment, if successful, will only prove to be a Pyrrhic victory, for it will lead to serious intraocular inflammation and eventual loss of the eye. Removal of intravitreal cysticerci by pars plana vitrectomy is straightforward. Subretinal cysticerci can be removed either by a transvitreal or transcleral approach.

Treatment of nonintraocular cysticercosis[9,10] is with a single dose of niclosamide, 2 g given as four tablets (500 mg each) that are chewed one at a time and swallowed with a small amount of water. The dose is titrated for children (1 g for body weight 11 to 34 kg; 1.5 g for body weight >34 kg). As an alternative treatment, praziquantel can be used in a single 10-mg/kg dose. The worm is usually digested, and in time it is passed. The stool should be rechecked in 3 months and 6 months.

Acknowledgment: This work was supported, in part, by an unrestricted grant from Research to Prevent Blindness, Inc, New York, NY.

REFERENCES

1. Duke-Elder S: Cysticercosis, System of Ophthalmology, Vol 15. St Louis, CV Mosby Co, 1978, p 40.
2. Heine HJ, Klintworth GK: Cysticercosis in the aetiology of epilepsy. S Afr J Med 30:32–35, 1965.
3. Freeman RS: Ontogeny of cestodes and its bearing on their phylogeny and systematics. Adv Parasitol 11:481–500, 1973.
4. Voge M: The post-embryonic developmental stages of the cestodes. Adv Parasitol 11:707–726, 1973.
5. Slais J: The morphology and pathogenicity of the bladder worms. Dr W Junk, NV, The Hague, 1970.
6. Lee DL: The structure of the helmuth cuticle. Adv Parasitol 10:347–367, 1972.
7. Hackley DJ: Ultrastructure of the tegument of schistosoma. Adv Parasitol 11:233–245, 1973.
8. Friedman AH, Pokorny KS, Suhan J, et al: Electron microscopic observations of intravitreal *Cysticercus cellulosae* (*Taenia solium*). Ophthalmolgica 180:267–273, 1980.
9. Case Records of the Massachusetts General Hospital: Neurocyticercus, racemose form. N Engl J Med 328:566–573, 1993.
10. Case Records of the Massachusetts General Hospital: Neurocyticerus, racemose form. N Engl J Med 180:267–273, 1993.
11. Pollard ZF: Cysticercosis: an unusual cause of papilledema. Ann Ophthalmol 12:110–112, 1975.
12. Perry HD, Font RL: Cysticercosis of the eyelid. Arch Ophthalmol 96:1255–1257, 1978.
13. Sen DK, Thomas A: Incidence of subconjunctival cysticercosis. Acta Ophthalmol 47:395–399, 1969.
14. Zinn KM, Guillory SL, Friedman AH: Removal of intravitreal cysticerci from the surface of the optic nerve head: a pars plana approach. Arch Ophthalmol 98:714–718, 1980.
15. Bartholomew RS: Subretinal cysticercosis. Am J Ophthalmol 79:670–672, 1975.
16. Topilow HW, Yimoyines DJ, Freeman HW, et al: Bilateral multifocal intraocular cysticercosis. Ophthalmology 88:1166, 1981.
17. Manschot WA: Intraocular cysticercosis. Arch Ophthalmol 80:772–774, 1968.
18. Belding DL: Basic Clinical Parasitology. New York, Appleton-Century-Crofts, 1958, p 240.

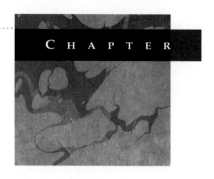

CHAPTER 60

The Retina and Choroid in HIV Infection

Dorothy Nahm Friedberg, M.D., Ph.D.
Monica Lorenzo-Latkany, M.D.

The CMV—a green moon then the world turns
   magenta
My retina
Is a distant planet
A red Mars
From a *Boy's Own* comic
With yellow infection
Bubbling at the corner
I said this looks like a planet
The doctor says—"Oh, I think
It looks like a pizza"

   from *Blue*, the text of a film by Derek Jarman[1]

Over the last 15 years ophthalmologists have become increasingly familiar with the ocular complications of human immunodeficiency virus (HIV) infection. Lesions in the retina and choroid may be the first sign of a disseminated opportunistic infection. Immunocompromised individuals may present diagnostic challenges, both through unusual presentations of known diseases and entirely new disease entities. In the acquired immunodeficiency syndrome (AIDS) changes in patterns of disease are commonplace. Metaphorically speaking, this chapter is a frame in a long movie with lots of villains, few heroes, and an unknown conclusion.

RETINAL AND CHOROIDAL MANIFESTATIONS OF HIV INFECTION

HIV Microvascular Disease

The most common ocular condition in patients infected with HIV is a retinal microvasculopathy also known as AIDS retinopathy. This is a noninfectious microangiopathy affecting the retina and consisting of cotton-wool spots with or without intraretinal hemorrhages.[2] Other characteristics consistent with a microvasculopathy demonstrated on fluorescein angiography include, telangiectatic vessels, microaneurysms, focal areas of nonperfusion, and capillary loss.[2,3] Cotton-wool spots are seen in at least 50 to 70% of patients with AIDS, and occur primarily in the posterior pole.[2] The cotton-wool spots seen in HIV-infected patients are identical to those seen in patients with diabetes mellitus or hypertension.[4] They are discrete areas of retinal opacification appearing as white feathery patches. Cotton-wool spots (Fig. 60–1) and intraretinal hemorrhages (Fig. 60–2) are both evanescent and tend to resolve within a few weeks, rarely causing any symptoms. However, there have been reported cases of ischemic maculopathy[5] and macular edema with lipid star formation corresponding to areas of nerve fiber layer swelling occurring as a result of retinal ischemia.[6] Perivascular sheathing without infectious retinitis is unusual in AIDS patients in the United States, but has been reported in 15% of African patients with AIDS and in 60% of African children with AIDS-related complex.[7]

Ultrastructural studies reveal occluded vessel lumens, swollen endothelial cells, thickened basal laminas, and degenerating pericytes.[5] Retinal trypsin digests have shown that the ratio of endothelial cells to pericytes in AIDS patients without cytomegalovirus (CMV) retinitis is 1.6 compared with 1.1 for controls. In AIDS patients, microaneurysms and attenuated vessels were more commonly found in the peripheral retina when compared to controls.[8] In an autopsy study of 25 consecutive AIDS cases, cotton-wool spots were found in 36% of the eyes. When areas with cotton-wool spots were

HISTOPATHOLOGICAL FEATURES

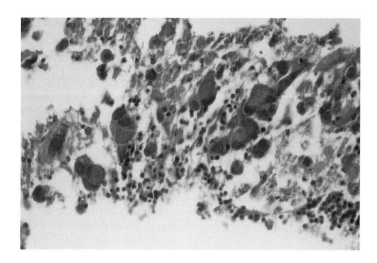

Area of cytomegalovirus retinopathy with neurons that are markedly enlarged by cytoplasmic viral inclusions.

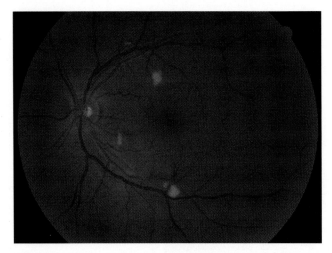

FIGURE 60–1   Multiple retinal cotton-wool spots in the posterior pole of an HIV-infected individual.

studied with immunocytochemistry they were negative for HIV p24 antigen. The authors conclude that if HIV infection of the retinal vascular endothelium is present, it does not lead to detectable p24 antigen in these cells.[9]

There are several theories for the pathogenesis of AIDS microvasculopathy. Immunoperoxidase studies demonstrate the deposition of immunoglobulins along the arteriolar walls, consistent with immune complex disease.[5] Pomerantz and associates have been able to culture HIV in the retina of AIDS patients. Using monoclonal antibodies to HIV proteins they localized the HIV infection to retinal endothelial cells.[10] Engstrom and associates used hemorrheology, the study of deformation and flow properties of cellular and plasmatic components of the blood, to explain the pathogenesis of the HIV microvasculopathy. They found an association between fibrinogen levels and increased red cell aggregation and blood flow sludging, resulting in hypoxia, which leads to the development of a

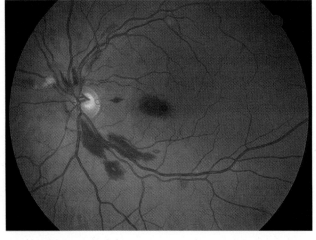

FIGURE 60–2   Retinal hemorrhages in a severely anemic HIV-positive patient.

microvasculopathy. The cause for the increased fibrinogen levels in AIDS patients remains unknown. They did not find an association between circulating immune complex levels and microvasculopathy.[11]

Although cotton-wool spots rarely produce visual disturbances, the lesions are more common in patients with AIDS than in patients with asymptomatic HIV infection.[2,12] A recent study of 453 male patients with HIV confirmed that cotton-wool spots are associated with low CD4 counts. This finding may serve as a nonspecific sign of progression of immunosuppression. Moreover, cotton-wool spots were significantly more common in patients who had acquired HIV through homosexual or bisexual activity compared to intravenous drug use.[13] Although there have been no associations between retinal microangiopathy and the development of AIDS-related retinal infections, cotton-wool spots may contribute to the axonal loss in optic nerves of patients with AIDS.[14] Quiceno and associates found that patients with AIDS had significant impairments in color vision and contrast sensitivity, which can be the result of primary optic neuropathy.[15] Geier and associates found that color contrast deficits are primarily associated with the number of cotton-wool spots.[16]

OCULAR OPPORTUNISTIC INFECTIONS

Cytomegalovirus Retinitis

Virology and Epidemiology

CMV is a DNA virus that is a member of the herpesvirus family. Inclusion-bearing cells characteristic of human CMV were first described pathologically in 1904. Ocular involvement with CMV was first reported in 1947.[17] In the pre-AIDS era CMV rarely caused serious systemic disease, except in children with congenital infection. In the United States there is a 1% incidence, among live births, of intrauterine CMV infection.[18,19] Children born of mothers who have a primary CMV infection during pregnancy may develop a constellation of signs and symptoms that constitute congenital cytomegalic inclusion disease. Only about 10% of congenitally infected newborns are symptomatic, but fatalities may be high.[20] Ocular involvement occurs in about 14% of newborns with congenital cytomegalovirus inclusion disease but does not occur in children in whom infection is acquired perinatally. After age 35 a majority of people have serologic evidence of prior CMV infection.[17] Before the AIDS epidemic, adults who developed clinically significant CMV infection were often iatrogenically immunosuppressed. In these cases the infection generally responded to removal of the causes of immunosuppression, usually medications to hinder transplant rejection.[21,22] Cases of CMV retinitis were very rare during this period.[17,23,24] Since the early 1980s, when AIDS was recognized as a unique disease entity, the number of people affected with CMV retinitis has increased dramatically.

The prevalence of CMV antibody positivity varies geographically from 40 to 100% worldwide.[18] In homosexual men infected with the HIV virus the rate is at least 90%.[25] Current rates of antibody positivity in women in the United States is between 55 and 85%, the greater involvement being in those in lower socioeconomic groups.[19] CMV disease is felt to result from the reactivation of latent virus from a prior infection, so a person's risk of developing CMV depends on their history. To date there are no simple tests to predict which person who is CMV antibody–positive will develop end-organ disease. Studies of antigenemia, antibody response, and CMV polymerase chain reaction (PCR) measurements are underway to see if they will help identify those at highest risk to develop significant CMV infection.[26–29] Mortality from CMV disease has increased; the percentage of patients with AIDS dying from associated CMV infection has increased from 5.2% in 1987 to 9.9% in 1992. This probably reflects improved survival from *Pneumocystis carinii* pneumonia and fungal infections.[30]

Cytomegalovirus is a systemic infection. Although patients may only have signs or symptoms referable to a single organ system, autopsy studies have shown multiple sites are infected that often were unsuspected clinically.[31] With the exception of CMV retinitis, which is diagnosed clinically, tissue biopsy is considered necessary for diagnosis, since the presence of CMV organisms on culture may not indicate significant end-organ disease.

CMV Retinitis in AIDS

CMV retinitis, the most common ocular opportunistic infection in AIDS, affects between 6 and 38% of patients.[32] Although there have been rare cases described in individuals with CD4 counts above 100/mm^3, the majority of patients have CD4 counts under 50/mm^3. In a recently described large trial of patients with newly diagnosed CMV retinitis, the mean CD4 counts were 27 and 29/mm^3.[33] In a prospective study of 132 patients with AIDS and CD4 counts of 200/mm^3 or less, the mean CD4 count in patients with retinitis was 7.4/mm^3; no one with a CD4 count over 50/mm^3 developed retinitis. Twenty per cent of the total group developed retinitis, but 30% of those with CD4 counts under 50/mm^3 did.[34] Low CD8 counts have also been described in patients with retinitis.[35]

Diagnosis of CMV Retinitis

An ophthalmologist may diagnose CMV retinitis when a patient complains of ocular symptoms or during a routine examination in an asymptomatic individual. People vary in their awareness of symp-

toms and may ignore them out of fear of their significance. Patients may not report any symptoms at the time of diagnosis but notice them after they learn of their retinitis. This early increase in symptoms is not usually associated with a worsening of disease, but rather a heightened awareness of visual abnormalities. When symptoms are present they often include floaters, light flashes, and smudged or cloudy vision. Loss of areas of central or peripheral vision are also noted.

In most instances the funduscopic appearance of CMV retinitis allows an experienced observer to make the correct assessment. Biopsy for definitive diagnosis would be too dangerous in most cases of retinal infection. In situations that present diagnostic dilemmas, vitreous aspirates for PCR[36,37] or endoretinal biopsies[38–40] may be required. These procedures should be undertaken only when the risks justify them. Fluorescein angiography, which may show vascular leakage in areas of retinitis, does not usually help in the differential diagnosis of CMV retinitis; documenting lesions by fundus photography is more useful.

CMV retinitis is often accompanied by mild intraocular inflammation. Slit lamp examination reveals fine keratic precipitates on the corneal endothelium as well as anterior chamber and vitreous cells. The inflammation does not usually cause serious visual loss; although patients may complain of floaters, the view of the fundus is rarely obscured. Neither photophobia nor conjunctival injection are commonly seen as part of CMV retinitis.

The appearance of CMV retinitis at presentation is diverse. The classical or fulminant presentation is a hemorrhagic, necrotic retinitis (Fig. 60–3). This type is seen both in the posterior pole and in the periphery. Retinal vessels can be obscured. When hemorrhage is extensive, the necrotic infectious component may be difficult to recognize (Fig. 60–4), and careful follow-up is necessary to make the correct diagnosis. In other instances microangiop-

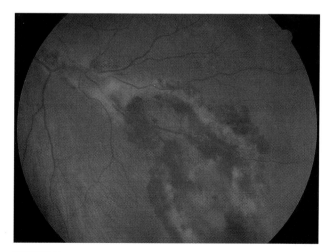

FIGURE 60–3 Classical/fulminant CMV retinitis at diagnosis. Hemorrhage and necrosis are present along the inferotemporal arcade.

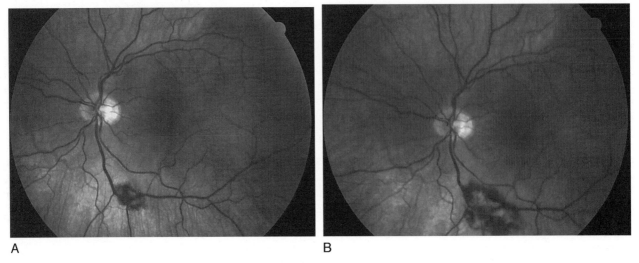

A   B

FIGURE 60–4 *A*, Inferotemporal retinal hemorrhage overlying a CMV lesion in a patient on treatment for CMV colitis. *B*, Patient in *A* 1 week later. The lesion has increased in size and has a clearly necrotic component.

athy may be mistaken for early retinitis (Fig. 60–5). Microangiopathy is rarely symptomatic, or accompanied by inflammation, which is particularly helpful when a puzzling lesion is immediately sight threatening.

Retinitis may also have a more "granular" appearance. Although many feel this is more common in the retinal periphery, it can be seen in early lesions in the posterior pole as well. These granular lesions often have a central atrophic area, which looks like healed retinitis, that is surrounded by a white border with punctate satellite lesions. It may be difficult to delineate the border and to assess retinitis progression in these patients without the careful study of serial retinal photographs (Fig. 60–6). Retinitis can present with a combination of fulminant and granular forms (Fig. 60–7).

A less common presentation is the occurrence of frosted branch angiitis in areas not directly involved with retinitis. These perivascular infiltrates disappear with the treatment of the retinitis[41,42] (Fig. 60–8). A retinal biopsy specimen in one of these cases did not show viral inclusion bodies in the capillary endothelial cells. Immunohistochemical staining failed to show immune complexes or CMV antigen in retinal capillaries.[41] Other unusual vascular abnormalities seen in patients with CMV retinitis include optic disc neovascularization[43] (Fig. 60–9) and branch vein occlusion (Fig. 60–10).

Although retinal detachment is more common in patients with treated CMV retinitis, it can be seen in patients without prior therapy. In two series of patients with CMV retinitis, about 3.4% of eyes were detached at the time of retinitis diagnosis.[44,45]

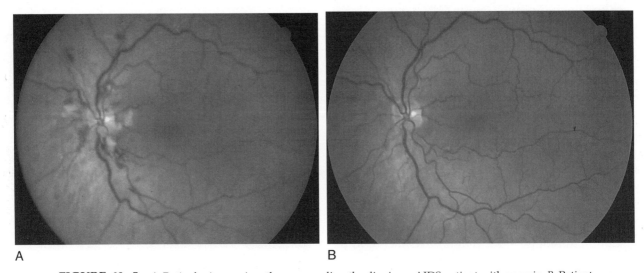

A   B

FIGURE 60–5 *A*, Retinal microangiopathy surrounding the disc in an AIDS patient with anemia. *B*, Patient in *A* 1 month later after anemia has resolved.

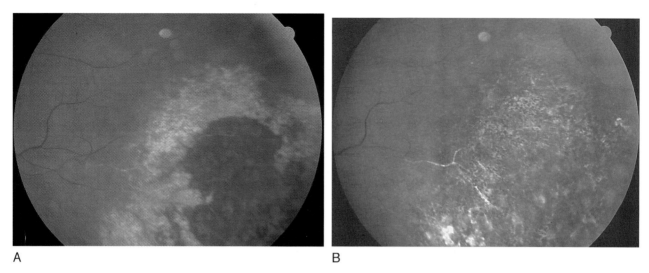

A   B

FIGURE 60–6   *A,* Granular CMV retinitis at diagnosis. The white active border surrounds an atrophic center. *B,* Patient in *A* after treatment. The lesion is completely atrophic. (From Friedman-Kien AE, Cockerell CJ [eds]: Color Atlas of AIDS. Philadelphia, WB Saunders Co, 1996, with permission.)

Surgical repair of the detachment and medical treatment of the retinitis are indicated in these cases (Fig. 60–11).

A small suspicious lesion involving the macula presents a difficult diagnostic dilemma. When a small questionable lesion is in the retinal periphery, one can monitor it untreated without enormous risk of visual loss. This allows time to aid in the diagnosis when the lesion is not obviously infectious. The luxury of observation is lost in situations where the lesion is close to the macula or optic nerve. Here the potential for visual loss is great. If one chooses observation, it must be at short intervals (Fig. 60–12). The occurrence of even small amounts of inflammation in these cases tips the scale toward an infectious rather than a microvascular process.

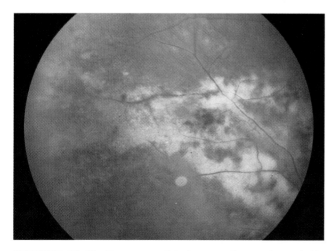

FIGURE 60–7   Concurrent fulminant and granular retinitis at presentation.

Areas of retinitis not directly involving the macula can produce macular edema and transient visual loss.[46] This is one of the rare situations in which therapy can bring about an improvement in visual acuity. That is because visual loss is not due to direct destruction of retinal tissue but is secondary to macular edema (Fig. 60–13).

CMV papillitis can develop either with primary involvement of the optic nerve or through secondary spread from the peripapillary retina. Primary papillitis has a worse visual prognosis[47,48] (Fig. 60–14).

When retinitis presents in a patient on therapy for extraocular CMV, the lesions appear partially treated and symptoms may be blunted. Large areas of the retina may be involved before the patient realizes there is anything wrong. These lesions are similar to the smoldering lesions of slowly progressive retinitis (Fig. 60–15).

PATHOLOGY OF UNTREATED CMV RETINITIS. Untreated retinitis produces a marked retinal necrosis and hemorrhage involving all retinal layers as well as the retinal pigment epithelium. There may be an abrupt transition between healthy and infected retina. Owl's eye cells—enlarged cells with eosinophilic intranuclear inclusions—can be seen; intracytoplasmic inclusions may also be seen. Vessel walls may be thickened. The choroid is minimally involved; however, some mononuclear or polymorphonuclear inflammatory cells can be present. Electron micrographs reveal viral capsids.[49,50]

CMV RETINITIS WITH OTHER OCULAR OPPORTUNISTIC INFECTIONS. Co-infection with CMV and other ocular opportunistic infections has been described both pathologically and clinically. CMV

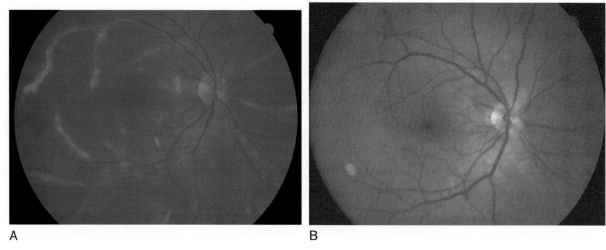

FIGURE 60–8   *A*, Frosted branch angiitis in a patient with a peripheral CMV lesion. *B*, After treatment of CMV retiinitis vessels have returned to normal. (From Friedman-Kien AE, Cockerell CJ [eds]: Color Atlas of AIDS. Philadelphia, WB Saunders Co, 1996, with permission.)

with herpes simplex,[51] HIV,[52] herpes zoster (Fig. 60–16), *Pneumocystis carinii*[53] (Fig. 60–17), and toxoplasmosis[54,55] have been described.

Treatment of CMV Retinitis

In renal transplant patients, retinitis often regresses when exogenous immunosuppressive drugs are withdrawn. Other attempts at treatment in these patients, including laser barricade of lesion borders and adenosine arabinoside, were unsuccessful.[21,22] In the early 1980s, when CMV retinitis was initially described in AIDS patients, there was no known successful therapy. Treatment with acyclovir, vidarabine, interferon alfa, and interleukin-2 did not limit retinitis progression.[56] There has been one report of regression of CMV after zidovudine treatment.[57]

Over the last 10 years there has been tremendous growth in options for the treatment of CMV reti-

nitis. There are currently three approved drugs for the treatment of CMV retinitis and several others that are in various stages of development and may indeed be available at the time of publication. The luxury of choice of medications has strengthened our ability to treat retinitis in the immunosuppressed patient.

SYSTEMIC THERAPY WITH GANCICLOVIR AND FOSCARNET. Ganciclovir [9-(1,3-dihydroxy-2-propoxylmethyl) guanine, or DHPG], was the first intravenous drug approved by the U.S. Food and Drug Administration (FDA) in 1989 for the treatment of CMV retinitis in patients with AIDS. Ganciclovir is a nucleoside analog and relative of acyclovir. It inhibits CMV replication through its triphosphate metabolite by interfering with CMV DNA polymerase. Phosphorylation of ganciclovir occurs more rapidly in CMV-infected cells, probably through viral thymidine kinase. Ganciclovir can also inhibit DNA polymerase in various human cells, such as

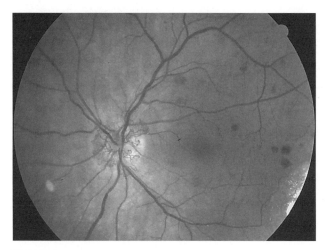

FIGURE 60–9   Optic disc neovascularization in a patient with stable treated CMV retinitis.

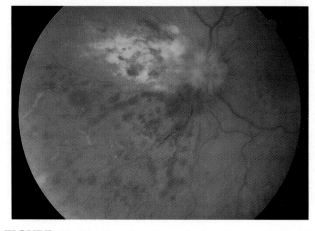

FIGURE 60–10   Branch vein occlusion in a patient with CMV retinitis/papillitis.

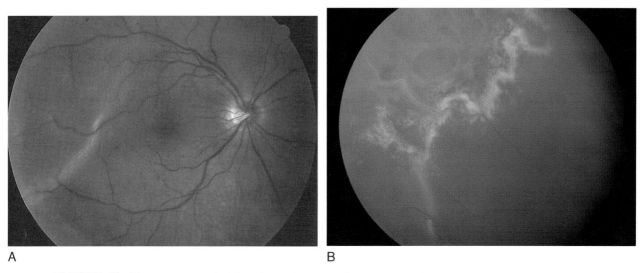

FIGURE 60–11   Posterior pole (*A*) and periphery (*B*) of a patient in whom CMV retinitis presented with a retinal detachment. (From Friedman-Kien AE, Cockerell CJ [eds]: Color Atlas of AIDS. Philadelphia, WB Saunders Co, 1996, with permission.)

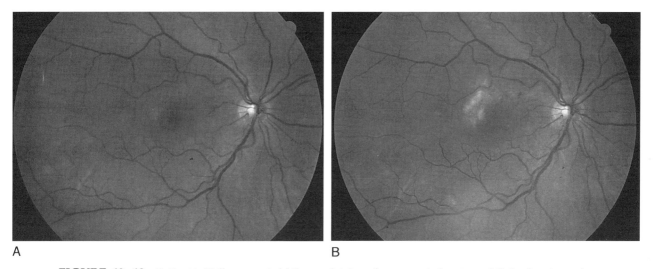

FIGURE 60–12   Patient initially presented (*A*) complaining of a paracentral scotoma. Minimal perivascular whitening was noted and visual acuity was good. Several weeks later (*B*) the lesion looks like CMV retinitis; acuity is still good.

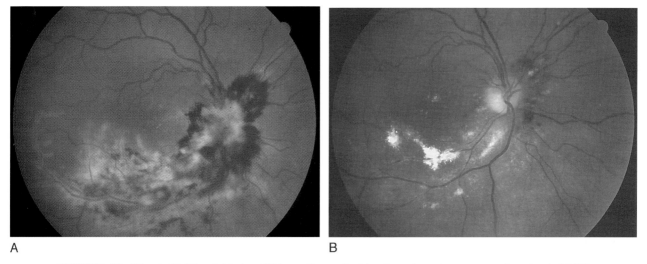

FIGURE 60–13   *A*, CMV retinitis/papillitis at diagnosis. Macular edema is present and acuity is 20/70. *B*, Patient in *A* after 2 months of therapy; vision has returned to 20/25.

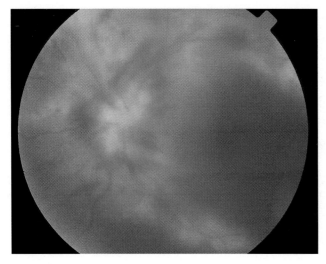

FIGURE 60–14   Primary CMV papillitis with hand movements vision.

the bone marrow, although usually at concentrations higher than are necessary to inhibit viral replication. Ganciclovir is a virustatic drug, and in immunosuppressed patients, must be given continually to be effective. Early studies showed relapse of retinitis occurred quickly after medication was discontinued but progression was delayed if maintenance therapy was used.[58,59] Treatment with ganciclovir decreased the incidence of CMV-positive blood and urine cultures.[58-60]

Pathologic evaluation of patients' eyes with CMV retinitis that have been treated with intravenous ganciclovir show active areas at the margins of scarring. Owl's eye cells can be seen. It is assumed that there are less infectious virions in patients with treated disease.[61,62]

Treatment with intravenous ganciclovir is divided into induction and maintenance phases. In-

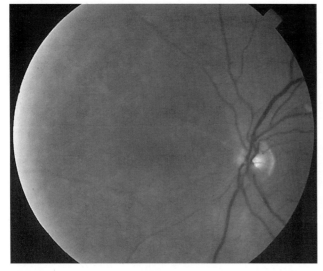

FIGURE 60–15   Subtle granular retinitis with sheathed vessels in the nasal retina of a patient on treatment for CMV colitis.

duction consists of a 2- to 3-week period of infusion of 5 mg/kg of ganciclovir twice daily (total daily dose 10 mg/kg). This dose must be adjusted both for neutropenia and for elevated serum creatinine. Once the retinitis has stabilized, maintenance therapy of 5 mg/kg every day can be initiated. A recent study in patients with relapsed retinitis used a higher dose, 7.5 mg/kg twice a day as induction and 10 mg/kg once a day during maintenance. This regimen was well tolerated.[63]

In 1995 an oral form of ganciclovir was approved both for the maintenance therapy of CMV retinitis and for prophylaxis against development of retinitis. The oral formulation has low bioavailability, which is enhanced when the medication is taken with food. The currently approved dose is 1000 mg taken three times daily. The drug is approved only for maintenance therapy in patients whose retinitis has been stabilized after induction with intravenous anti-CMV medication; the oral formulation is not appropriate for induction therapy.[64] Retinitis progresses more rapidly with oral than with intravenous ganciclovir, so the oral form should be used with great caution in patients where small amounts of progression could have disastrous visual consequences. When patients are initially placed on oral ganciclovir, they should have their retinitis monitored closely to be sure that they respond well to the medication.

Foscarnet (trisodium phosphonoformate) was approved by the FDA in 1991 for treatment of CMV retinitis. Like ganciclovir, it is a virustatic rather than a virucidal drug and, therefore, requires lifelong administration. It selectively inhibits viral DNA polymerase and reverse transcriptase. It requires intravenous administration; an oral formulation has not yet been developed. Like ganciclovir, it is administered in an induction and maintenance regimen. Induction consists of 2 to 3 weeks of a high dose (either 60 mg/kg three times a day or 90 mg/kg twice a day) followed by maintenance therapy of between 90 and 120 mg/kg once a day. Foscarnet requires concomitant hydration and controlled rates of administration usually necessitating the use of a pump.[65-67]

TOXICITIES OF CMV RETINITIS THERAPIES. Both ganciclovir and foscarnet have significant systemic toxicities and, since patients are frequently on multiple medications with overlapping side effects and interactions, management of CMV retinitis requires diligent cooperation between the ophthalmologist and the AIDS-treating physician. It is vital that the ophthalmologist communicate to the internist when a patient's disease is potentially sight threatening so, if systemic medication must be discontinued temporarily, a treatment plan can be developed to preserve vision.

The most common side effect of ganciclovir is neutropenia. An incidence of about 30% has been reported after intravenous administration; but this is less common with oral ganciclovir.[64] If the abso-

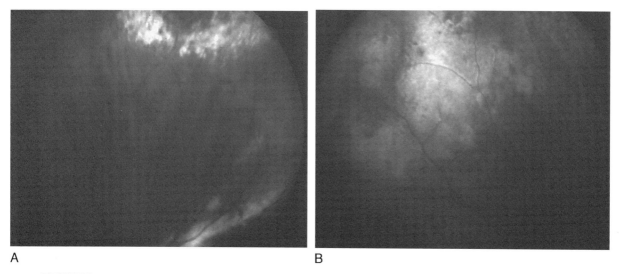

FIGURE 60–16   A, CMV retinitis at presentation in superior periphery OD (3/94). B, Superior temporal periphery of patient in A with lesions of progressive outer retinal necrosis (PORN). CMV is quiescent (9/94).

lute neutrophil count (ANC) goes below 0.50 × 10^9/liter then ganciclovir treatment should be temporarily discontinued. If the ANC is between 0.50 and 1.00 × 10^9/liter, then filgrastim (granulocyte colony-stimulating factor [G-CSF]) can be administered.[68] It is important to monitor the patient's hematologic status during ganciclovir therapy, and concomitant use of any medication known to cause neutropenia must be weighed carefully. Prior to the development of colony stimulating factors and antiretrovirals other than zidovudine (AZT), neutropenia made it difficult to continue anti-HIV therapy while treating CMV retinitis. Anemia can occur with both foscarnet and ganciclovir and erythropoietin treatment can be used to stimulate red cell production.

Nephrotoxicity and disturbances in electrolytes are the most common side effects of foscarnet therapy. Doses must be adjusted for serum creatinine levels and calcium, magnesium, phosphorous, and potassium supplementation may be required.[68] Pa-

tients may have normal serum calcium levels but can experience symptoms of hypocalcemia such as perioral tingling during drug administration. This is because serum ionized calcium may be bound to foscarnet during the infusion. If oral supplementation does not eliminate these symptoms, pretreatment with intravenous calcium may be required. It is vital that the residual calcium be flushed through the catheter prior to foscarnet administration, since otherwise it will precipitate in the catheter, rendering it useless.

Another bothersome side effect of foscarnet is the development of genital ulcers, particularly in uncircumcised men. Hydration as well as copious rinsing of the genitalia after urination will help to avoid this problem. Patients may experience nausea from foscarnet that can sometimes be alleviated by slowing the infusion rate. Pretreatment with an antiemetic is helpful when nausea is infusion related. Initially, seizures were reported with higher frequency in patients on foscarnet.[65] In a recent study there was no difference in the seizure rate in the foscarnet treated and the ganciclovir-treated groups. The presence of central nervous system (CNS) toxoplasmosis was strongly associated with seizures in both groups.[68]

Daily intravenous administration of medication using an indwelling catheter is associated with an increased incidence of sepsis. Catheter-related complications, including sepsis, have been reported in 31% of patients on intravenous ganciclovir, while such complications have been seen in only 10% of patients on oral ganciclovir who may have had catheters for other reasons.[64]

Treatment of CMV retinitis increases survival.[69,70] In 1992, a large multicenter national clinical trial conducted by the Studies of Ocular Complications of AIDS (SOCA) research group compared ganciclovir and foscarnet as treatment for newly diagnosed CMV retinitis. The study was stopped prior

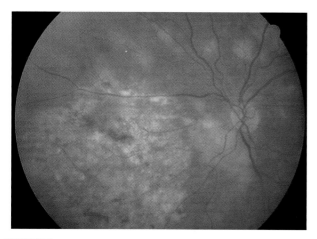

FIGURE 60–17   CMV retinitis (white lesion nasal to the disc) and *Pneumocystis* choroidopathy (multiple yellow lesions).

to completion because of an unexpected and still unexplained differential mortality in the two treatment groups. Patients who were assigned to foscarnet as initial therapy lived a median of 12.5 months, while patients assigned to ganciclovir lived a median of 8.6 months.[33] Initially it was thought that the anti-HIV activity of foscarnet might have been responsible for this, but additional analysis of the data has not supported that hypothesis.[71] It should be noted that both drugs had equal efficacy in delaying progression of CMV retinitis; however, their toxicity profiles were very different. Patients who were initially assigned to foscarnet had a much higher rate of switching to ganciclovir for drug toxicity than did patients assigned to ganciclovir.

It is unusual for retinitis to be treated with a single induction period and lifelong maintenance without the need for periodic reinduction. When evaluated by an independent fundus photography reading center, median time to first retinitis progression was 53 days in the foscarnet-treated group and 47 days in the ganciclovir-treated group. Times to subsequent progressions were even shorter. Strategies for managing relapses with systemic medications have varied. Some favor reinduction with the initial drug, others will switch medications. Several preliminary studies demonstrated significant responses to combination therapy with intravenous foscarnet and intravenous ganciclovir even in patients who had responded poorly to either drug alone[72-74] (Fig. 60–18). A large study of relapsed retinitis conducted by SOCA has confirmed this. The median time to retinitis progression in patients who had at least one relapse was 4.3 months with combination, while it was 1.3 to 2 months with monotherapy. Induction therapy with combination consisted of an induction dose of either foscarnet or ganciclovir combined with a maintenance dose of the other drug. Monotherapy with foscarnet was standard foscarnet induction and maintenance therapy. Monotherapy with ganciclovir used induction doses of between 5 and 7.5 mg/kg twice a day followed by maintenance with 10 mg/kg once a day. This study supports the use of combination over switching therapies for achieving longer times to retinitis progression. Combination therapy with two drugs given intravenously can have a significant negative impact on a patient's quality of life, and this must be considered when making treatment decisions.[63]

Other Therapies

SYSTEMIC. Cidofovir, or (S)-1-[3-hydroxy-2-(phosphonylmethoxy)propyl] cytosine (HPMPC), a nucleotide analog, has recently been approved for the treatment of CMV retinitis. It has a much longer half-life than the currently approved drugs, and experiments have used weekly induction for 2 weeks followed by maintenance treatment every 2 weeks. Even though the medication must be given intravenously, this infrequent dosing regimen avoids the need for an indwelling catheter. Early studies indicate the most serious side effect to be nephrotoxicity.[87] Careful attention to the development of proteinuria as well as adequate hydration and pretreatment with probenecid have reduced the incidence of this complication in subsequent trials.[88]

Early studies suggested human monoclonal anti-CMV antibody (MS-109) delays the progression of CMV retinitis that is being treated by standard antiviral therapies.[89] Randomized clinical trials are underway to evaluate this further.

LOCAL THERAPY WITH GANCICLOVIR AND FOSCARNET. Both ganciclovir and foscarnet have been injected directly into the vitreous either to supplement systemic therapy in patients with disease progression or in those in whom toxicity necessitates cessation of systemic treatment. The eye is a sequestered site, and studies suggest the concentration of intravitreal drug present after intravenous administration may fall below the ID_{50} for certain strains of CMV, resulting in suboptimal treatment.[75] A wide range of doses of ganciclovir have been injected intravitreally with surprising lack of retinal toxicity. Early reports used 200 μg in 0.1 ml, while some current investigators use 500 μg to 2.0 mg for each dose. The only clinically significant side effect of intravitreal injection has been the rare development of endophthalmitis.[76-82] Electroretinographic (ERG) evidence of retinal toxicity was found even with doses as low as 100 μg. There was complete loss of all photopic, scotopic, and flicker responses at doses of 1000 μg, with decreased amplitudes with doses between 100 and 400 μg, but no ERG abnormalities were noted at doses of 25 and 50 μg.[83] Light and electron microscopic studies of retinal samples revealed vacuolization of the outer nuclear layer and the inner segments of the photoreceptors in eyes injected with 100 to 1000 μg of intravitreal ganciclovir. These microscopic findings were also noted in eyes injected with only 25 to 50 μg despite normal ERG responses.

Foscarnet has been used with success at both 1200- and 2400-μg doses.[84-86] Injections are usually given several times a week until retinitis begins to respond and weekly thereafter. Although intravitreal therapy has never been evaluated in a large randomized clinical trial, it has become an accepted part of the threapeutic armamentarium. The need for frequent injections as well as several cases of endophthalmitis have led to the search for a longer lasting method to deliver the drug directly into the eye.

LOCAL THERAPY WITH GANCICLOVIR IMPLANT. Several recent pilot studies as well as controlled studies have evaluated an intravitreal ganciclovir implant device recently approved by the FDA.[90-92] This device is fabricated by enveloping a 6-mg pellet of ganciclovir with 10% polyvinyl alcohol,

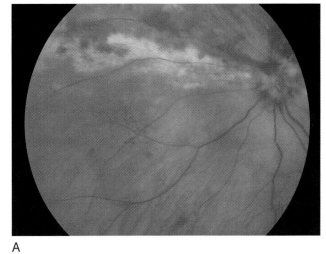

FIGURE 60–18   *A,* Left eye of a patient whose CMV has reactivated on ganciclovir. *B,* Right (*1*) and left (*2*) eyes of patient in *A* after 2 months on foscarnet; OS is quiet and OD is active. *C,* Right (*1*) and left (*2*) eyes of patient in *B* while on a combination of ganciclovir and foscarnet. Retinitis is stable and remained so for many months.

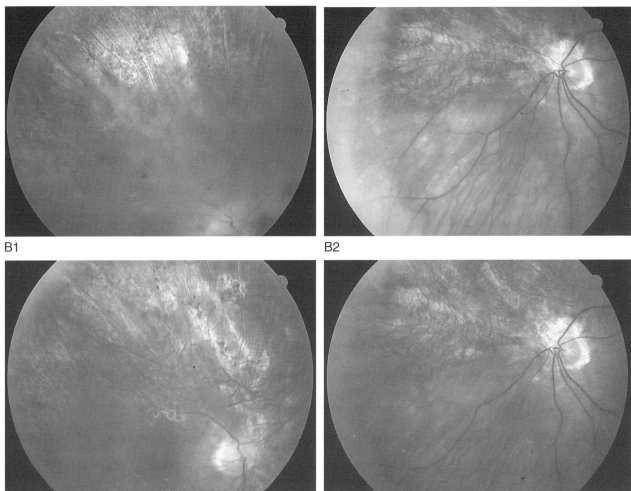

which is then coated, except for the top surface, with ethylene vinyl acetate. The implant is surgically placed in the vitreous cavity through a pars plana incision (Fig. 60–19). This allows the release of 1 μg of ganciclovir per hour into the vitreous. The implant, initially tested in a diverse group of patients with CMV retinitis, showed promise in halting retinitis progression. A randomized study comparing immediate treatment with the device compared to delayed treatment showed that the implant significantly delayed retinitis progression. The median time to progression in the treated group was 226 days. In cases that did progress, analysis of vitreous and residual implant drug lev-

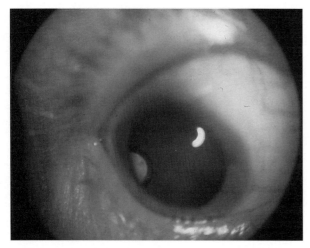

FIGURE 60–19   Postoperative view of ganciclovir implant in place.

els indicated that most cases of progression were related to depletion of active drug rather than resistance.[91]

Several findings temper the enthusiasm for this form of therapy. As has been stated, CMV retinitis is a local, retinal manifestation of systemic CMV infection. Autopsies performed in four patients with the ganciclovir implant in whom there was no suspicion of disseminated CMV infection had significant extraocular CMV infection. Biopsy-proven extraocular CMV was documented in 31% of patients treated with the implant alone. CMV retinitis developed in 67% of previously unaffected eyes of patients who had entered the study with unilateral retinitis. Retinal detachments developed in 18% of patients. Some early detachments may relate to the surgical procedure, although the data did not allow analysis of other factors that might have contributed to this.[91,93]

A pathologic study of seven eyes from five patients who have been treated with the sustained-release ganciclovir implant did not show any toxicity or inflammation related to the device. Light and electron microscopy findings were similar to those reported in cases of treated CMV retinitis.[94]

An ongoing clinical trial comparing intravenous ganciclovir to ganciclovir implant alone to ganciclovir implant plus oral ganciclovir may help us formulate a rational treatment strategy optimal for controlling retinal disease and preventing extraocular CMV as well as spread to the other eye.

Intravitreal injections of cidofovir have also been described. The prime toxicity has been the development of severe ocular hypotony with permanent visual loss. There is a very narrow toxicity/efficacy ratio with this form of treatment, and further work is underway to attempt to determine a safe and effective intraocular dose. As with the intravenous formulation, the intraocular half-life is much longer than other previous intravitreal CMV therapies. Patients' retinitis was controlled with injections every 5 to 6 weeks.[95,96]

A phosphorothioate oligonucleotide, which complements coding sequences in region 2 of the immediate early (IE) transcriptional unit of human CMV, interferes with the production of infectious CMV.[97] Early studies of intravitreally administered drug showing encouraging results in controlling CMV retinitis were complicated by the development of pigmentary retinopathy and complaints of visual field loss in some patients. Current studies with this antisense oligonucleotide are underway to delineate a safe and effective dose regimen for this drug.

PROPHYLAXIS. There is considerable interest in effective prophylaxis for CMV disease. There was some initial enthusiasm about high-dose acyclovir; however, this has not been confirmed in clinical trials.[98] There have been two new studies of oral ganciclovir for CMV prophylaxis with contradictory results. Analysis of the differences in study design explain this. Both evaluated oral ganciclovir at 1000 mg three times daily, both were randomized double-blind and placebo-controlled, and both were limited to patients who had evidence of CMV exposure (either by culture or antibody positivity). One study (CPCRA)[99] enrolled patients who had CD4 counts of $100/mm^3$ or less, while the other (Syntex 1654)[100] enrolled patients with CD4 counts of 50 or less without a prior opportunistic infection or 100 or less with one. The median CD4 counts in the studies were lower in the Syntex study (21 to 23 vs. 33 to $35/mm^3$). In the CPCRA study, which did not find any benefit of oral ganciclovir prophylaxis, patients were not examined for the presence of retinitis at baseline and were only examined by an ophthalmologist if they complained of symptoms suggestive of retinitis.

Syntex 1654 patients were examined at baseline and every 2 months thereafter regardless of ocular symptoms. This study was stopped by the data and safety monitoring board at the first interim analysis because of a very significant reduction in development of retinitis in the treated group. Participants in the CPCRA study were then given the option of crossing over to active drug treatment; about two thirds of the individuals enrolled exercised this option. It is not surprising that the CPCRA study—which enrolled patients with higher CD4 counts, did not evaluate for development of asymptomatic retinitis, and was shorter—did not find results comparable to Syntex 1654.

There is some concern that the widespread use of oral ganciclovir for prophylaxis may induce the development of resistant strains of CMV, making subsequent CMV disease difficult to treat. Early studies do not support this concern (W. L. Drew, personal communication). The ability to identify those most likely to develop CMV retinitis would allow the use of targeted prophylaxis that would limit drug resistance and toxicity.

There is little information about the incidence of retinitis presenting in the absence of symptoms. Recently, in screening for a prevention study, 11.3% of patients were diagnosed with asymptomatic retinitis. It is surprising that four of seven of those diagnosed had sight-threatening disease and three of seven had bilateral disease.[101] There has been no systematic study of the differences in outcome in patients whose retinitis is diagnosed prior to the onset of symptoms. One might speculate that lesions diagnosed early may be smaller and less likely to be bilateral; however, these hypotheses have not been formally evaluated.

Response of Retinitis to Treatment

In order to standardize assessment and description of the response of retinitis to treatment the retina is divided into three zones. Zone 1 includes the retina within 3000 μm of the fovea and 1500 μm from the optic nerve; lesions in this area are considered immediately sight threatening. Zone 2 is defined as the area bounded by the outer limits of zone 1 and an imaginary line drawn through the anterior borders of the ampullae of the vortex veins (the clinical equator). Zone 3 is limited by the outer border of zone 2 and the ora serrata. Lesions in zones 2 and 3 are considered peripheral and not immediately sight threatening[102] (Fig. 60–20). Progression of CMV retinitis is defined as the movement of the border of a CMV lesion by 750 μm along a length of 750 μm or more, or the appearance of a new lesion in either eye that is larger than 25% of the disc area and is separated from old lesions by at least 750 μm.[103] Initial clinical trials of new therapies may compare immediate to deferred treatment for lesions in zones 2 and 3 (not sight threatening). To prevent serious visual consequences it is important to have a narrow tolerance for retinitis movement prior to the initiation of therapy: 750 μm, about one half the diameter of the average optic disc, is easy for clinicians to estimate while examining a patient.

Treated and untreated CMV lesions both progress but at different rates. The location, size, and character of the lesion may affect its progression rate. Anterior progression is more rapid than posterior, and lesions progress at differing rates along the border. Both smaller, presumably early lesions and indolent granular lesions seem to progress more slowly than larger or fulminant edematous ones.[104] Masked photographic reading centers for the interpretation of serial retinal photographs are much quicker than the clinician to suggest that a lesion has progressed.[105] Reasons for this difference are under analysis. It does seem clear that masked reading centers eliminate any possible bias by the clinician, who is usually aware of the treatment assignment in these studies. Photo graders analyze lesion progression separately from lesion activity and may be more willing to confirm progression in cases of minimal border activity. Ophthalmologists should compare photographs from the prior examination, as well as those from earlier in the disease course, when examining patients with retinitis.

In evaluating response to treatment, good-quality retinal photographs encompassing all lesion borders are important. If possible, full-field photographs are even better, as they may reveal early lesions that can be missed on clinical examination. Documentation of lesions in the far periphery, outside of the photographic field, is also important. It is particularly important to assess border movement even in the absence of obvious border activity. Progressive vascular obliteration may be seen in areas of subtle retinitis progression (Fig. 60–21). Sequential visual field testing may also be helpful in monitoring retinitis progression.[105,106] There is a difference between evaluating a patient who is a participant in a clinical trial and making purely clinical decisions about therapy for a patient who is not participating in a trial; the difference between clinical trial end points and clinically significant end points. Movement of 750 μm of a CMV retinitis lesion that is adjacent to the fovea can result in catastrophic visual loss, whereas the same amount of movement in the far retinal periphery in a patient who has multiple life-threatening infections might require a completely different therapeutic approach. They both represent progression of retinitis and would be weighted equally in a clinical trial (Fig. 60–22).

The ideal response to treatment is the appearance of an atrophic retinal scar. These may be pigmented (Fig. 60–23) or have a white appearance[107] (Fig. 60–24). In order to consider a scar inactive, serial retinal photographs showing no border advancement are required. With systemic therapy alone it is unusual for there to be no retinitis progression or relapse. What often occurs over the course of the disease is a series of exacerbations and remissions. Reactivation is not difficult to assess when border margins are clear and new activity is not subtle. Smoldering retinitis, a slow indolent progression with minimal border activity, may be more difficult to assess. When retinitis relapses, a period of reinduction will often produce quies-

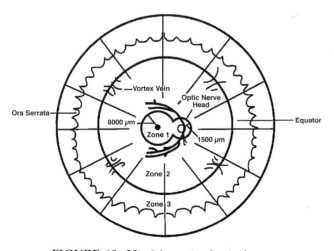

FIGURE 60–20 Schematic of retinal zones.

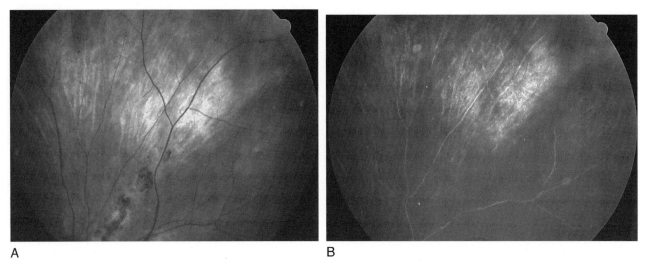

A   B

FIGURE 60–21   Superior temporal retina at presentation (*A*) and 3 months later (*B*). Small area of activity is noted supero-temporal to the disc; this progressed despite therapy. The only evidence of disease progression was the development of the extensive vascular obliteration seen in *B*.

cence. However, after periods of many months large areas of retina may be lost to smoldering retinitis even in the face of vigorous systemic and local treatment.[63,105] (Fig. 60–25).

Local therapy, either with the ganciclovir implant or with intravitreal injections, may decrease smoldering retinitis. In the randomized implant study, retinitis generally became inactive and did not reactivate until the implant was empty.[91] Whether it will be advantageous to develop a program for planned replacement of implants awaits further experience with them. Although current implants are supposed to produce adequate drug levels for 8 months, there is variability between patients. If planned replacement is not contemplated it is important to follow patients closely when ap-

proaching the end of the implant's predicted useful life.[90–92] The optimal method of replacing implants has not been devised.[108] It is important to evaluate the contralateral eye in cases of unilateral retinitis, since there is a significant incidence of development of disease in previously uninvolved eyes[91] (Fig. 60–26).

Retinal Detachments

Besides smoldering retinitis, the other significant complication, particularly of longstanding disease, is the development of retinal detachments.[109–112] Jabs and colleagues described a 50% detachment rate after 1 year. In his study, larger and more anterior lesions were risk factors for the development

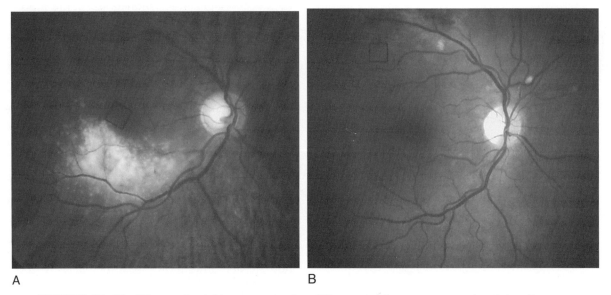

A   B

FIGURE 60–22   750 μm of retinitis progression has different visual consequences when it is adjacent to the macula (*A*) or along the supertemporal arcade (*B*). Small square had sides of 750 μm.

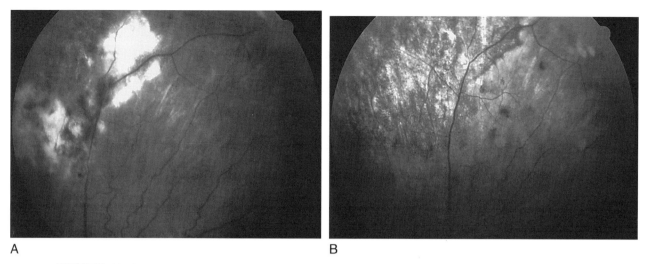

A   B

FIGURE 60–23   Active CMV retinitis (*A*) and the pigmented atrophic scar (*B*) that developed after treatment.

of detachments.[44] Freeman and associates related risk of detachment to extent, zone, and activity of retinitis. Patients with large (>25%) lesions in the periphery (zones 2 and 3) had a higher risk of developing a detachment than those with small zone 1 lesions. The presence of retinitis activity also increased the detachment rate. The 6-month and 1-year detachment rates were 11 and 24%, respectively.[45] Although there are more early retinal detachments with the implant, there does not seem to be an increase in overall detachment rate (B. Kuppermann, personal communication). This may be the result of less lesion activity and slower retinitis progression in patients receiving the implant.

Retinal detachments in patients with CMV retinitis are usually associated with multiple retinal holes in areas of necrotic retina. Small peripheral detachments may be walled off with laser without

progression (Fig. 60–27); however, most detachments eventually require more extensive intervention. Because of the presence of multiple retinal holes and the progressive nature of CMV retinitis, these CMV associated detachments usually require repair with vitrectomy and silicone oil tamponade (Fig. 60–28). Some surgeons also use additional focal endolaser and scleral bucking. Multiple factors such as control of retinitis, cataract development, and optic atrophy influence the final visual acuity of patients after surgery.[113–117] Initially there was some reluctance to repair these detachments because of patients' limited life expectancy. However, patients are living longer and retaining better visual function and one should adopt an aggressive attitude toward repair unless visual potential or intercurrent illnesses dictate otherwise.[114]

Detachment repair with silicone oil is not with-

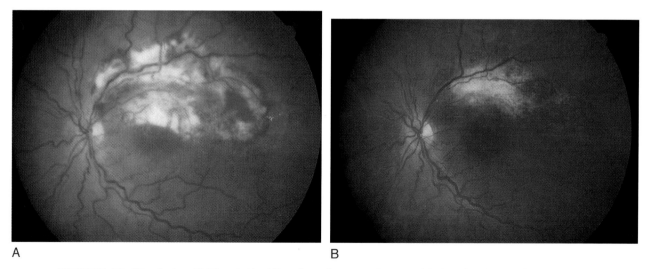

A   B

FIGURE 60–24   Active CMV retinitis (*A*) and a white atrophic scar (*B*) that developed after treatment. Visual acuity improved from 20/200 to 20/30 and has remained stable for almost 3 years. (From Friedman-Kien AE, Cockerell CJ [eds]: Color Atlas of AIDS. Philadelphia, WB Saunders Co, 1996, with permission.)

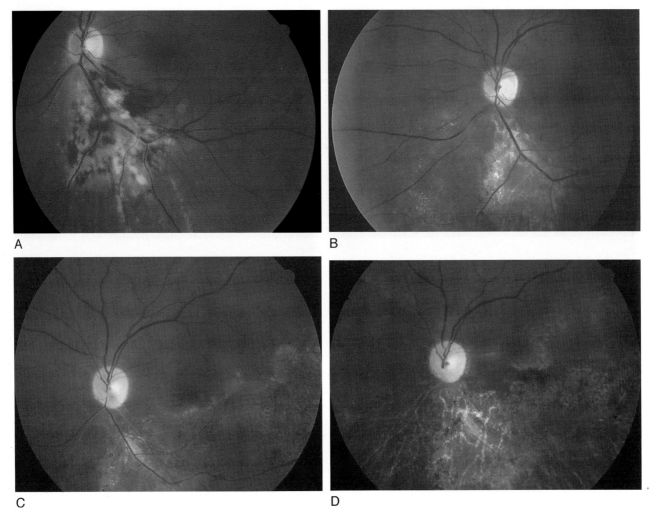

FIGURE 60–25   Smoldering retinitis over a 16-month period that advanced despite aggressive systemic and local therapy. (From Friedman-Kien AE, Cockerell CJ [eds]: Color Atlas of AIDS. Philadelphia, WB Saunders Co, 1996, with permission.)

out complications. After surgery patients have increased hyperopia (mean +5 diopters), which usually necessitates correction with a contact lens to obviate diplopia from anisometropia. Corneal opacification, glaucoma, hypotony, and appearance of emulsified oil in the anterior chamber are rare (Fig. 60–29). Thirty per cent of patients have been reported to develop cataracts after a median time of 192 days postoperatively[114] (Fig. 60–30). Cataract extraction has been done in these patients and some have even placed intraocular lenses (IOLs) in these eyes. IOL calculations require close cooperation with a skilled ultrasonographer as standard formulas are not applicable in these cases.[118]

Visual Prognosis

There is a paucity of information about long-term visual prognosis in patients with CMV retinitis. The percentage of patients with unilateral disease who are treated and develop disease in the previously untreated eye varies widely from study to study.[32,64,68,119] Final visual acuity values are also difficult to assess. One small study showed visual acuity of 20/70 or less in 79% of eyes at a mean of 7.6 months after diagnosis.[119] A larger study showed a decrease to 20/40 or worse vision in about 40% of eyes involved with retinitis and a decrease to 20/100 or worse in about 25% of involved eyes over a 6-month period.[105,106] In another study, about 40% of patients had a deterioration of Snellen acuity over 20 weeks, but less than 10% reported a deterioration in functional vision.[64] Retinal detachment is a cause of significant visual morbidity in patients with retinitis. A large study of treated detachments reported 31% nonambulatory vision in the treated eye at death. The median time to the development of nonambulatory vision was 474 days from surgery.[114] Even with small amounts of vision patients may, with the help of appropriate low-vision aids, accomplish a great deal and retain independence. Referral to agencies who have experience in low vision and in working with patients who are HIV infected is an important part of their care.

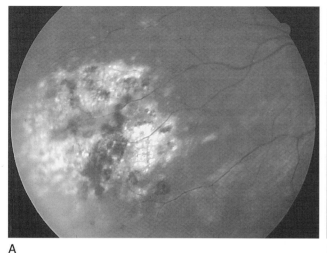

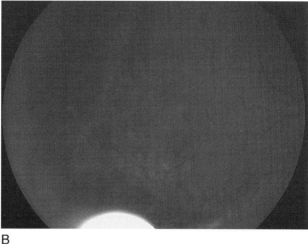

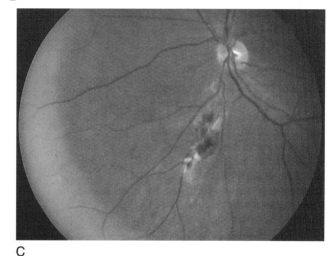

FIGURE 60–26   CMV retinitis OD at diagnosis (*A*) and after placement of a ganciclovir implant (*B*). Note appearance of a new lesion (*C*) that developed in the previously unaffected eye.

Future Trends in CMV Retinitis

Current areas of research interest can be divided into prophylaxis and treatment. An effective, well-tolerated agent to prevent CMV retinitis that would not stimulate the emergence of drug-resistant strains would be welcomed, as would the ability to target prophylaxis to those people most likely to develop retinitis. Successful therapy should limit the progression of lesions and treat both local ocular and systemic aspects of CMV infection. Treatment should be free of noxious side effects and not be so time consuming as to make patients' quality of life dismal. The existence of multiple treatment options that can be tailored to individual patients and can be adjusted over the course of disease will be useful.

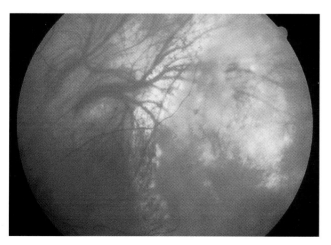

FIGURE 60–27   Retinal detachment walled off by laser. This was stable for many months with 20/20 vision until just prior to death.

OTHER HERPESVIRUS-ASSOCIATED RETINAL INFECTIONS

Acute Retinal Necrosis

The acute retinal necrosis (ARN) syndrome was first described in the Japanese literature 25 years ago.[120] Acute retinal necrosis was first reported in the English literature in 1978.[121] In 1994 the Amer-

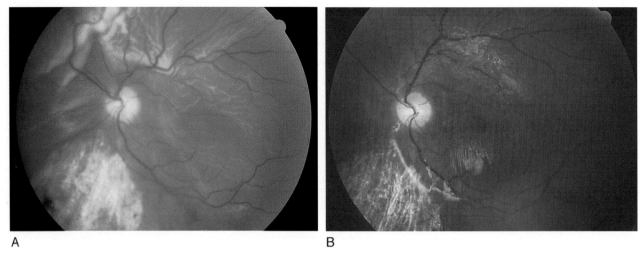

FIGURE 60–28   Retinal detachment pre- (A) and postoperatively (B) in a patient with healed retinitis inferior to the disc. (From Friedman-Kien AE, Cockerell CJ [eds]: Color Atlas of AIDS. Philadelphia, WB Saunders Co, 1996, with permission.)

ican Uveitis Society, finding a lack of agreement on clinical characteristics and imprecision in defining the syndrome, established criteria for diagnosing acute retinal necrosis syndrome. Clinical characteristics that must be seen include: (1) areas of peripheral retinal necrosis with discrete borders (the macula may be involved but in conjunction with peripheral lesions), (2) rapid progression of disease or development of new foci in the absence of antiviral therapy, (3) circumferential spread of the disease, (4) presence of occlusive vasculopathy, and (5) prominent anterior and vitreal inflammation. Supporting characteristics that are not required include optic neuropathy, optic atrophy, scleritis, and pain.[122]

Acute retinal necrosis syndrome had been characteristically described only in otherwise healthy individuals.[123,124] However, since the American Uve-

itis Society based the diagnosis on the clinical appearance and course of the disease only, it is now considered independent of the immunologic status of the host.[122] Although progressive outer retinal necrosis has been described only in AIDS patients and ARN in healthy patients; patients with AIDS can develop either clinical syndrome. Differences in the manifestation of the disease may depend on patients' level of immune dysfunction.[125]

Although the diagnosis of ARN does not depend on the isolation of a pathogen, early electron microscopic studies demonstrated a herpes group virus in all layers of affected retina.[126] Laboratory data including viral cultures, electron microscopic studies, immunocytochemistry, DNA in situ hybridization, and PCR has shown that both herpes simplex virus type 1 and varicella-zoster virus (VZV) are

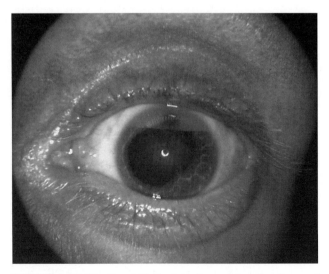

FIGURE 60–29   Emulsified oil in the anterior chamber and anterior capsular plaque on the lens surface in a patient who had had a retinal detachment repair with silicone oil.

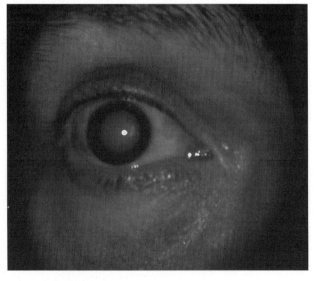

FIGURE 60–30   Mature cataract in a patient who had a retinal detachment repaired with silicone oil.

causative agents in the ARN syndrome.[126-129] The ARN syndrome has also been described secondary to recrudescence of latent herpes simplex virus type 2. Laboratory data successfully identifying which herpes virus is the causative agent in ARN can be performed on ocular tissues using the PCR and the enzyme-linked immunosorbent assay (ELISA) test.[130] Quantitation of antibodies to herpes-group viruses in acute and convalescent serum is not reliable in determining a specific etiologic diagnosis in the ARN syndrome.[131] Although isolation of a pathogen might play a role in designing a proper treatment course, it is irrelevant for the diagnosis of ARN syndrome because the definition is based on the clinical appearance and course of the disease.

In patients with HIV or AIDS, Sellitti et al[132] found that 17% developed acute retinal necrosis after herpes zoster ophthalmicus within 9 months of the appearance of the cutaneous lesions. Even after skin lesions resolve, patients should undergo periodic funduscopic exams and should be instructed to return immediately if they experience any pain, redness, change of vision, or floaters.[132]

Progressive Outer Retinal Necrosis

Progressive outer retinal necrosis (PORN) is a recently described variant of a necrotizing herpetic retinopathy in immunocompromised patients including those with HIV infection. It is thought to be the second most frequent opportunistic retinal infection after CMV retinopathy among North American patients with AIDS.[133,134] Clinical and laboratory evidence suggests that varicella-zoster virus is the causal agent.[125,135] The incidence of varicella-zoster retinitis in severely immunocompromised AIDS patients has been reported to be as high as 2%.[136] Early lesions appear as patchy choroidal and deep retinal lesions occurring in the posterior pole and the retinal periphery.[135] These discrete areas of retinal opacification are usually multiple and can range in size from 50 to several thousand μm in diameter[134] (Fig. 60-31). The retinitis is characterized by primary involvement of the outer retina, with sparing of the inner retina until late in the disease process. It progresses rapidly, resulting in confluent patches of full-thickness necrosis with minimal or no aqueous or vitreal inflammation.[125,137] Retinal vasculopathy is not characteristic of PORN, and when sheathing or occlusions are present it is only in areas with adjacent active retinopathy and occurs late in the disease.[125,134,135,137] A perivascular lucency thought to represent early removal of necrotic debris or edema can result in a pattern of scarring that has a "cracked-mud" appearance[125] (Fig. 60-32). Optic nerve involvement with disc swelling, hyperemia, and optic atrophy, as well as afferent pupillary defects have been reported.[134] Afferent pupillary de-

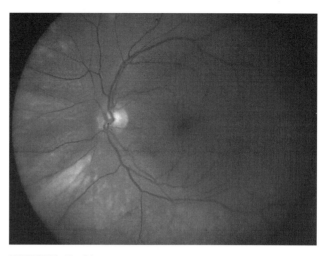

FIGURE 60-31 Progressive outer retinal necrosis (PORN) involving the posterior pole and retinal periphery. A retinal detachment can be seen superotemporally. (From Friedman-Kien AE, Cockerell CJ [eds]: Color Atlas of AIDS. Philadelphia, WB Saunders Co, 1996, with permission.)

fects may be the result of severe unilateral retinal necrosis or may result from unilateral optic neuropathy.

The degree of immunosuppression varies widely among HIV-infected patients, which may account for the variability in the clinical signs of VZV-related retinitis. In contrast to ARN, which can be seen in immunocompetent patients and classically presents with an aqueous or vitreal inflammation, AIDS patients with PORN have little or no inflammatory reaction. The severe immune dysfunction in these patients probably prevents them from mounting an inflammatory response.[137] The incidence of PORN increases in patients with CD4 counts of less than 50 cells/mm³.[136]

Laboratory studies, as well as clinical evidence have implicated a herpes virus, more specifically VZV, as the causative pathogen of PORN. Laboratory data include the detection of VZV antigen

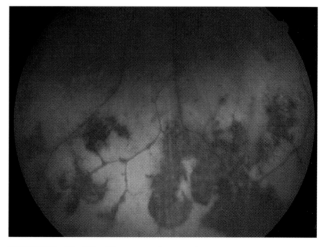

FIGURE 60-32 The retinal periphery in a patient with PORN, note the "cracked mud" appearance.

from a vitreal aspirate, the culture of VZV from chorioretinal specimens, localization of VZV antigen in the outer retina of enucleated specimens by means of immunocytochemistry, as well as the presence of viral capsids, consistent in size and shape with that of herpesviridae, in the outer retina of enucleated specimens.[125] Histologic examination of enucleated specimens revealed that VZV involves the retinal pigment epithelium more than the inner retina.[136] Greven et al[135] were able to show the presence of intranuclear inclusions in choroidal cells from an eye wall biopsy, as well as a positive VZV PCR.[135] In the largest reported series to date, two thirds of the patients had an antecedent history of cutaneous zoster; however, active cutaneous disease at the time of diagnosis of the necrotizing retinitis was uncommon.[134]

Despite the availability of three antiviral drugs (acyclovir, ganciclovir, and foscarnet) with high in vitro activity against herpes viruses, visual outcome is dismal. Engstrom and colleagues who have looked at the largest series thus far and found that two thirds of patients progressed to no light perception (NLP) vision within 1 month of diagnosis, usually from total retinal destruction or retinal detachment (Fig. 60–33). Retinal detachments occurred in 70% of patients within 1 month of diagnosis. There appears to be no relationship between the development of retinal detachments and disease activity or extent of disease at time of diagnosis. Prophylactic laser treatment at a median of 1 week after diagnosis was not beneficial in preventing retinal detachment.[134]

The best treatment regimen for VZV retinopathy in patients with AIDS is not known. Intravenous acyclovir (10 mg/kg every 8 hours) has been used with limited success.[134] Others have used combination therapy with either intravenous (IV) acyclovir (10 to 20 mg/kg every 8 hours) and foscarnet (60 mg/kg every 8 hours) or IV ganciclovir (5 mg/kg every 12 hours) and foscarnet (60 mg/kg every 8 hours).[138] Margolis and associates feel that given

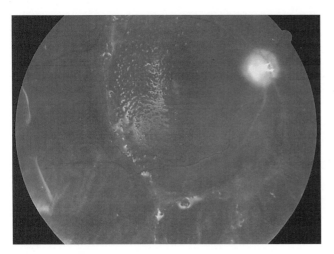

FIGURE 60–33 End-stage PORN with light perception vision, optic atrophy, and residual retinal detachment.

the additive effects of acyclovir and vidarabine against varicella-zoster virus,[139] and the increasing incidence of acyclovir resistance in varicella-zoster virus isolates from patients with AIDS,[140] combination therapy with these two agents (10 mg/kg every 8 hours of IV acyclovir with 10 mg/kg every 8 hours of vidarabine) may be beneficial in the treatment of rapidly progressive VZV retinitis.[125] Recently, there has been a report of using a combination of intravitreal ganciclovir and a new experimental antiviral medication, BV-ara U (sorivudine 40 mg orally every day), to successfully treat a patient with PORN.[141] The treatment was successfully discontinued after 5 months and the patient has had no recurrences for 1 year. The need for a successful antiviral drug against varicella-zoster retinitis is important not only to curtail the devastating ocular effects but also to prevent the increased risk of developing a life-threatening encephalitis in patients with AIDS and varicella-zoster retinitis.[136]

The need for chronic maintenance therapy against opportunistic retinal infections has been well documented in patients with AIDS.[142,143] However, no clear guidelines exist for varicella-zoster retinopathy. If oral acyclovir is to be used for maintenance, it must be remembered that its bioavailability is 15 to 30%.[138] Oral acyclovir (800 mg five times daily) is the most common maintenance regimen used, since this dose is necessary to maintain serum drug levels above the ID50.[144] Johnston and associates[138] recommend the use of IV acyclovir as maintenance, given their experience with recurrences during the administration of oral medications. Despite maintenance therapy, involvement of the second eye is usually not prevented.[138] Recurrences can present either as reactivation of borders from previously quiescent lesions[138] or as the development of new lesions.[134] These two methods of recurrence can be explained by persistence of virus in the retina or recurrent viremia, respectively.

It is important to distinguish progressive outer retinal necrosis from other retinopathies caused by herpesviruses such as acute retinal necrosis and cytomegalovirus retinopathy. In contrast to patients with CMV retinitis, PORN patients exhibit multifocal lesions lacking granular borders and retinal hemorrhages, as well as extremely rapid spread of retinal necrosis. CMV retinitis commonly spreads along the vascular arcades, and at a slower pace. Clinical characteristics of PORN that help differentiate it from ARN include the early involvement of the outer retina, a lack of an occlusive vasculopathy, and minimal or no intraocular inflammation. It is important to differentiate among the three, since treatment options and visual outcomes vary.

Toxoplasmosis

Toxoplasmosis infection is caused by an obligate intracellular protozoan, *Toxoplasma gondii*. The two stages in the life cycle of the protozoan found in humans are the tachyzoites, measuring about 6 μm in length, and cysts measuring up to 200 μm in diameter and possibly containing thousands of bradyzoites.[145] Chorioretinal toxoplasmosis infection is probably the third most common retinal infection in patients with AIDS.[143] In immunocompromised patients, the CNS is the preferred site of infection,[142] with cerebral toxoplasmosis reported in as many as 40% of autopsy cases.[146] Ocular toxoplasmosis is much less common than cerebral toxoplasmosis and accounts for about 1% of AIDS-related retinal infections in the United States.[2] Systemic infection with *T. gondii* is most commonly asymptomatic, and approximately 500 million people worldwide have antibodies to the organism.

The presence of serum IgG antibodies for toxoplasmosis does not necessarily indicate evidence of active ocular infection, but neither does seronegativity exclude the possibility of ocular toxoplasmosis. One of six patients in a large series with CNS involvement were seronegative for IgG antibodies against toxoplasma.[147] Cytopathologic diagnosis of toxoplasmosis organisms from vitrectomy specimens has been reported.[145] Pathologic studies have shown retinal necrosis involving all layers of the retina, with only slight inflammation of the choroid. Trophozoites have been found in the retina and choroid.[142]

Toxoplasmosis in AIDS causes visual impairment if left untreated[148–150]; no case of spontaneous regression has been reported. Holland and colleagues reported a series of eight patients with presumed ocular toxoplasmic retinochoroiditis where no patient had evidence of pre-existing chorioretinal scars and three patients had retinal tears or detachment due to severe retinal necrosis.[142] The absence of pre-existing chorioretinal scars indicates that the majority of AIDS-related cases are not due to reactivations of encysted organisms, as is the case with otherwise healthy hosts. In HIV-infected patients active toxoplasmic lesions are yellow-white, edematous areas of necrotizing retinitis[55] (Fig. 60–34). Lesions have fluffy borders, few scattered intraretinal hemorrhages, and occasional vascular sheathing. Overlying vitreal inflammation ranges from mild to extensive haze that precludes visualization of the fundus. Although the degree of inflammation may be less than in immunocompetent hosts, the inflammatory reaction exceeds that in CMV retinopathy.[143] The lesions can be unilateral or bilateral, single and discrete, multifocal and discrete, or diffuse. Most toxoplasmic lesions in AIDS patients are unifocal and in the posterior pole.[55] Other presentations include miliary toxoplasmic retinitis,[151] and optic neuritis.[149]

Ocular toxoplasmic lesions in an AIDS patient, if left untreated, progress to invade and destroy the whole retina. A survey of regimens used by uveitis specialists in the treatment of ocular toxoplasmosis reveals the lack of a consensus regarding therapy. The current induction therapy of choice for the

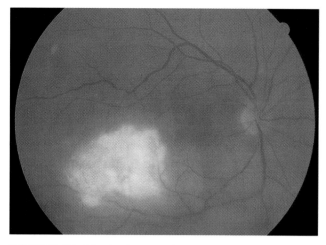

FIGURE 60–34   Ocular toxoplasmosis in an AIDS patient, note absence of retinal pigmentation that is usually seen in immunocompetent individuals.

treatment of ocular toxoplasmosis is the combination of 6 to 8 g/day of sulfadiazine, 50 to 100 mg/day of pyrimethamine, and 10 mg/day of leucovorin until the lesions heal, which usually takes 6 weeks. Adverse reactions to this regimen occur in 20 to 40% of patients with a high rate of relapse upon discontinuation of therapy.[152] Corticosteroids do not appear necessary in that there is little intraretinal inflammation in toxoplasmic lesions in AIDS patients.[142] Maintenance therapy for ocular toxoplasmosis with the combination of pyrimethamine (either 25 or 50 mg/day) and either sulfadiazine or clindamycin resulted in a similar 24-month relapse rate of 20%.

No controlled study of treatment regimens for ocular toxoplasmosis in HIV-infected patients exists, and inferences from the encephalitis trials may be incorrect. Daily therapy with 2 g/day of sulfadiazine and 25 mg/day of pyrimethamine is the suppressive therapy of choice for patients with toxoplasma encephalitis, with an estimated 1-year relapse rate of 6% and without any cases of *P. carinii* reported.[153] Atovaquone, trimethoprim-sulfamethoxazole, pyrimethamine-dapsone, pyrimethamine-azithromycin, and pyrimethamine-clarithomycin have been evaluated in a smaller number of patients.[154] Recently an animal model of ocular toxoplasma has been reported with the ME 49 strain of *T. gondii*, which may prove important in the development of new therapies.[155]

The overall 12-month survival rate in the largest series of HIV-infected patients with ocular toxoplasmosis was 72%.[55] From 29 to 50% of patients with ocular toxoplasmosis have associated CNS involvement, therefore, imaging studies of the brain are recommended.[55,143]

Syphilis

Syphilis, recently re-emerged as a public health problem, has particularly vexing implications in the

HIV-infected population. In the early 1900s syphilis was a leading cause of neurologic disease and a frequent ophthalmologic diagnosis.[156] After the introduction of penicillin the incidence of syphilis decreased dramatically, with less than 10,000 primary and secondary cases reported during the late 1950s. The introduction of "crack" cocaine has contributed to the dramatic increase in the incidence of syphilis since 1985. It is estimated that as few as half of the actual cases of syphilis discovered are ever reported.[157] All patients with active titers and clinical suspicion of syphilis should be encouraged to obtain an HIV test. HIV-infected patients have a disproportionately high incidence of syphilis and syphilitic genital ulcers. As with any genital ulcer that weakens the host's defenses, syphilitic genital ulcers lead to an increased risk of HIV transmission.[158,159] HIV infection may accelerate the course of a concomitant infection with syphilis. There are no well-controlled studies evaluating treatment options for ocular syphilis or concomitant infection of HIV with ocular syphilis.

Treponema pallidum, the causative agent of syphilis, is a member of the family Spirochaetaceae. It is transmitted to an estimated one third of patients through sexual contact, but it can also spread by transfusion of fresh blood or contact with an infected lesion. There are classic stages of syphilis that occur in the immunocompetent host that if untreated usually follow a predictable time course. The stages of syphilis include primary, secondary, tertiary, and neurosyphilis. The latter can occur at any time after the primary stage. Ocular syphilis can be considered equivalent to neurosyphilis.[160]

Although there is no ideal test for syphilis, two different serologic tests are available. The Venereal Disease Research Laboratories (VDRL) or the rapid plasma reagin (RPR) test are often used in screening due to their low cost and high sensitivity. The natural history of titers in untreated syphilis is to reach a peak during secondary syphilis after becoming detectable around the time of primary syphilis. The titers then usually drop to less than a 1:4 dilution in the late latent stage; up to 25% of patients have undetectable VDRL in late stages. There are many infectious and noninfectious conditions, including HIV infection alone, that can give false-positive screening titers.[161] The two commonly employed confirmatory specific treponemal serologic tests are the fluorescent treponemal antibody absorption test (FTA-ABS) and the microhemagglutination test for serologic diagnosis for any stage of syphilis. The serologic diagnosis of syphilis in HIV infection is modified, but it is still unclear how; it may be related to the patient's immunocompetency.[161-163]

Ocular syphilis was estimated to cause 1.1% of uveitis cases from 1970 to 1980.[164] In the largest and most recent retrospective series of 25 patients with ocular syphilis by clinical diagnosis, 68% of patients had uveitis, 12% had either optic neuritis or optic atrophy, 4% had scleritis, and 16% had interstitial keratitis. Serum FTA-ABS was reactive in all patients and serum VDRLs were reactive in 68% of patients. Fifty per cent of patients with a positive serum VDRL that underwent spinal taps had reactive VDRLs in their CSF; two serum VDRL–negative patients had completely normal CSF findings as well.[160]

The recent rise in the number of new cases of syphilis coincides with the AIDS epidemic. There have been several published reports of ocular syphilis in HIV-infected patients.[165-168] The most common manifestations of ocular syphilis in patients with AIDS include severe uveitis, retrobulbar neuritis or optic neuritis, necrotizing retinitis, and vitritis (Figs. 60–35 and 60–36). Not only does syphilis have a more aggressive ocular course in patients with AIDS but nervous system involvement is more frequent in HIV-positive patients.[167,168] A syphilitic necrotizing retinitis with sheathing of retinal vessels and retinal infiltrates with hemorrhages has been described in a patient with AIDS.[165] Gass and associates reported findings of vitritis with large bilateral solitary placoid pale yellowish subretinal lesions with central fading in patients with syphilis and immunosupression. Early-phase fluorescein angiograms showed hypofluorescence in the area of yellow opacification and late-phase angiograms showed staining at the level of the retinal pigment epithelium. There were shallow serous detachments of the overlying retina, a peripheral chorioretinitis, a mild papillitis, and retinal perivasculitis and iritis in some of the patients.[169]

In HIV infection the serologic test may be negative despite presence of ocular syphilis. There have been cases of repeatedly negative serum VDRL in HIV-positive patients including one report of nonreactive serum and CSF-VDRL.[160,167]

Ocular syphilis in HIV-infected patients should

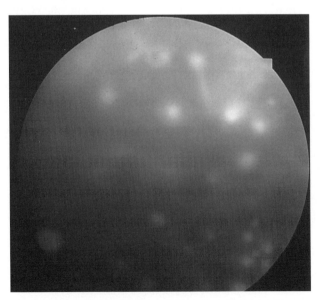

FIGURE 60–35 Syphilitic retinitis in an HIV-positive patient. (From Friedman-Kien AE, Cockerell CJ [eds]: Color Atlas of AIDS. Philadelphia, WB Saunders Co, 1996, with permission.)

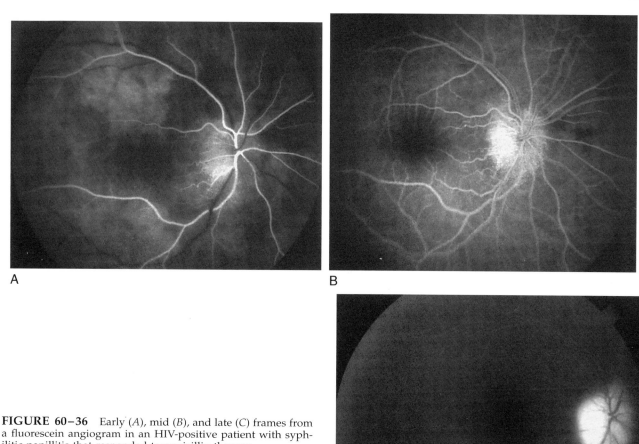

FIGURE 60–36   Early (*A*), mid (*B*), and late (*C*) frames from a fluorescein angiogram in an HIV-positive patient with syphilitic papillitis that responded to penicillin therapy.

be treated aggressively with 2 to 4 million units of aqueous penicillin G every 4 hours intravenously for at least 10 days, followed by 2.4 million units benzathine penicillin G intramuscularly weekly for 3 weeks.[170] Desensitization of patients with penicillin allergy is preferable to treatment with doxycycline.[160] Successful treatment of syphilis should result in the decline of positive titers by 2 dilutions at 6 months.[171] Persistent high VDRL titers may occur despite successful antibiotic treatment, or drop despite unsuccessful treatment in HIV-infected individuals.[156,172] Even high-dose intravenous therapy has been reported as inadequate in preventing serologic and clinical relapse in HIV-infected patients, especially those with secondary syphilis and reactive CSF-VDRL.[173]

Pneumocystis carinii

Pneumocystis carinii pneumonia (PCP) is one of the most common systemic opportunistic infections in

patients with the AIDS. *Pneumocystis carinii* is a unicellular opportunistic protozoan first discovered by Chagas in 1909 and a year later by Carini. The organism exists exclusively in the extracellular space. Its life cycle is divided into three stages: cysts, sporozoites, and trophozoites.

HIV-infected patients rarely develop PCP until their CD4 counts drop below $200/mm^3$.[174] *Pneumocystis carinii* infection most commonly affects the lungs, but extrapulmonary sites of infection include the lymph nodes, spleen, liver, bone marrow, small intestine, pericardium, myocardium, hard palate, periureteral soft tissues, and the choroid. The first report of choroidal *P. carinii* was in 1987, when Macher and colleagues described autopsy findings in an AIDS patient with disseminated pneumocystosis in whom organisms were found in the choroid.[175] In 1989, Rao and colleagues reported the histopathologic findings of an autopsy series of three patients with AIDS who had demonstrated yellow choroidal infiltrates.[176] On gross pathology the choroidal infiltrates corresponded to plaque-like thickened lesions in the choroid, with the larger lesions seen mainly posterior to the equator. Histopathogically, the infiltrates were acellular and eosinophilic, containing vacuolated and frothy material. *P. carinii* organisms were identified using both Gomori's methamine silver stain and electron microscopy. Freeman and colleagues reported a case with bilateral, multifocal, slowly enlarging, round-to-oval lesions at the level of the choroid in the posterior pole and midperiphery. A transcleral choroidal biopsy was performed, and numerous cystic structures characteristic of *P. carinii* were seen within the necrotic choroid using electron microscopy.[177]

A multicenter study of *Pneumocystis* choroidopathy reported on 21 patients with AIDS and presumed *P. carinii* choroidopathy. The lesions are characteristically yellow to pale yellow in color, appear in the choroid, and are found in the posterior pole (Fig. 60–37). They are usually round with irregular borders, and at times progress and become confluent. They range in size from 300 to 3000 μm, increasing in number prior to treatment, and eventually resolving after systemic treatment for *Pneumocystis*. The choroidal infiltrates are not associated with vitreous inflammation. The number of lesions varied from 2 to 50 per eye, and they were bilateral in up to 76% of patients. Fluorescein angiography was significant for early hypofluorescence, with late staining of the lesions. Of the 21 patients, 18 had received inhaled pentamidine as prophylaxis against *Pneumocystis* pneumonia. Although subtle visual field defects were reported, patients usually did not experience visual symptoms or visual loss even when lesions were adjacent to the fovea.[53]

Aerosolized pentamidine was recommended by the Centers for Disease Control in 1989 as one form of prophylaxis for PCP. Aerosolized pentamidine can modify the pulmonary infection, but does not eliminate the systemic spread of the organism.[178] An association between choroidal *Pneumocystis* and

inhaled pentamidine prophylaxis against pulmonary disease has been stressed in the literature.[53,179]

Treatment should be considered in all cases of presumed *P. carinii* choroiditis since its presence implies disseminated *Pneumocystis* infection.[180,181] Treatment of PCP in patients with AIDS consists of trimethoprim-sulfamethoxazole or intravenous pentamidine. The choroidal infiltrates usually resolve within 6 weeks to 4 months after initiation of systemic therapy. Choroidal lesions often fade very slowly and should not be used as the sole marker of therapeutic efficacy.[53] Although treatment is effective in most patients, there is a greater than 60% recurrence rate within 18 months unless prophylactic treatment is instituted[182] (Fig. 60–38). Since the advent of more widespread use of systemic prophylaxis for *Pneumocystis*, there have been fewer cases of *pneumocystis* choroidopathy.

Tuberculosis

The first reported case of ocular tuberculosis was by Maitre-Jan in 1711, and it took over 150 years for Koch to discover the tubercle bacillus and for Julius von Michael to identify the organism in the eye in 1883.[183] Although tuberculosis remains a major cause of morbidity and mortality in third-world countries, in the United States there was a steady decline from 1953 to 1984. However, from 1985 to 1991 the number of cases increased by 18%, with tuberculosis among the HIV-infected population accounting for most of this increase. The incidence of tuberculosis in patients with AIDS is almost 500 times that of the general population.

When a diagnosis of ocular tuberculosis is made, it is most often one involving the uveal tract, either as a chronic anterior uveitis or as disseminated choroiditis.[184] The rich vascular supply of the anterior and posterior uveal tract predispose these areas to tuberculous infection.[185] Choroidal tubercles and tuberculomas are the most common manifestations of ocular tuberculosis. Early choroidal tubercles are round or oval, white, gray-white, or yellow-white, with indefinite borders.[186] They can range in size from 0.5 to 3.0 mm and are usually confined to the posterior pole, but can be seen in the midperipheral fundus (Fig. 60–39). They are usually bilateral and number between one and ten per eye, although cases of 50 to 60 tubercles in each eye have been reported.[187]

Extrapulmonary tuberculosis in patients with HIV infection became an AIDS-defining condition in 1987. Ocular tuberculosis remains an underdiagnosed, or at least an underreported, entity in AIDS patients. In a review of ophthalmic findings in 28 patients with HIV infection, none were found to be the result of tuberculosis; one patient with a Roth's spot was suffering from *Mycobacterium avium-intracellulare* pneumonia.[188] There have been two reported cases of ocular tuberculosis in pa-

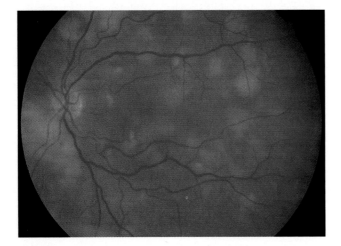

FIGURE 60–37 Multiple lesions of *Pneumocystis* choroidopathy. Visual acuity is excellent even in the presence of parafoveal involvement.

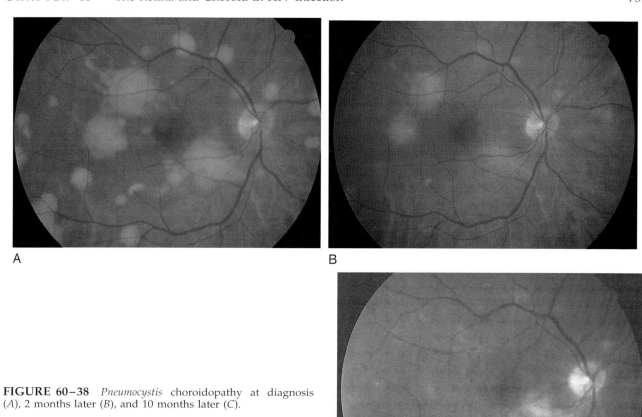

FIGURE 60–38 *Pneumocystis* choroidopathy at diagnosis (*A*), 2 months later (*B*), and 10 months later (*C*).

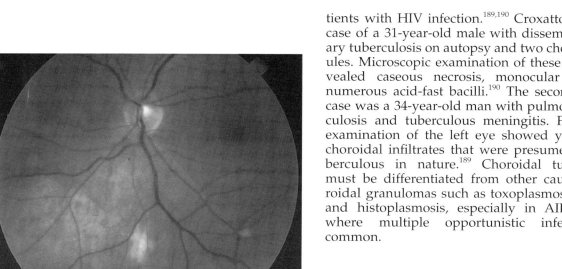

FIGURE 60–39   Tuberculous choroiditis in an HIV-positive patient. (Photograph courtesy of Richard Spaide, M.D.)

tients with HIV infection.[189,190] Croxatto reported a case of a 31-year-old male with disseminated miliary tuberculosis on autopsy and two choroidal nodules. Microscopic examination of these nodules revealed caseous necrosis, monocular cells, and numerous acid-fast bacilli.[190] The second reported case was a 34-year-old man with pulmonary tuberculosis and tuberculous meningitis. Funduscopic examination of the left eye showed yellow-white choroidal infiltrates that were presumed to be tuberculous in nature.[189] Choroidal tuberculomas must be differentiated from other causes of choroidal granulomas such as toxoplasmosis, syphilis, and histoplasmosis, especially in AIDS patients where multiple opportunistic infections are common.

Cryptococcosis

Cryptococcus neoformans, a round to oval encapsulated yeast with a worldwide distribution, is found

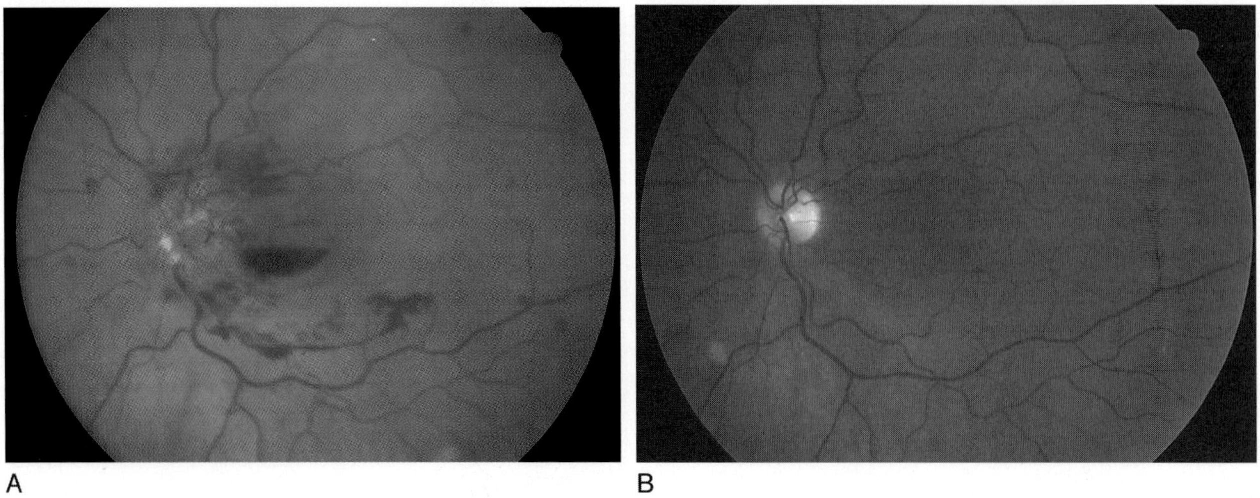

A

B

FIGURE 60–40   Papilledema (*A*) in cryptococcal meningitis that resolved (*B*) after treatment with amphotericin B. Vision remained good. (From Friedman-Kien AE, Cockerell CJ [eds]: Color Atlas of AIDS. Philadelphia, WB Saunders Co, 1996, with permission.)

in high concentrations in pigeon feces. Although infection is acquired through the respiratory tract, it is spread hematogenously and has a predilection for the CNS. The most common manifestation is meningitis or meningoencephalitis.

C. *neoformans* is the most common life-threatening fungal pathogen in patients with AIDS; occurring in 6 to 10% of patients.[191] A recent study of ophthalmic manifestations of cryptococcal infection in 80 HIV-infected patients found papilledema (32.5%) to be the most frequent ocular sign (Fig. 60–40). Visual loss and abducens nerve palsy occurred in 9% of patients and optic atrophy in 2.5%.[192]

Intraocular invasion with *C. neoformans* is less common than the neuro-ophthalmic complications. Retinal and choroidal lesions are usually subclinical and diagnosed at autopsy. Pepose and colleagues found cryptococcal organisms filling capillary lumens in areas adjacent to cotton-wool spots.[5] Choroidal lesions can be yellow-white, multifocal or solitary, and may be associated with optic nerve edema and minimal anterior segment and vitreal inflammation (Fig. 60–41).[193] Sudden bilateral visual loss is a documented complication in AIDS patients with cryptococcal meningitis. Cohen and associates reported a patient with fulminant necrosis of both optic nerves from cryptococcal infection.[194] Optic nerve sheath decompression has been tried with variable success in some patients with chronic papilledema and visual loss.[195]

There are five commonly used systemic antifungal agents in the treatment of AIDS-related cryptococcal infections: IV amphotericin B, flucytosine, ketoconazole, fluconazole, and itraconazole. Prompt institution of IV amphotericin B has proven beneficial in the treatment of cryptococcal chorioretinitis.[196] Initial treatment should be followed by long-term suppressive therapy to prevent relapses.[197]

Miscellaneous Retinal and Choroidal Opportunistic Infections

There are other opportunistic infections less frequently known to cause ocular complications in AIDS patients. *Candida albicans* endophthlamitis is a common complication of disseminated candidiasis. It rarely occurs in AIDS patients. Heinemann and associates presented a case of *Candida albicans* endophthalmitis in a bisexual male with AIDS and no history of drug use. The patient responded to treatment with intravenous amphoterecin B.[198]

A case of *Sporothrix schenckii* endophthalmitis

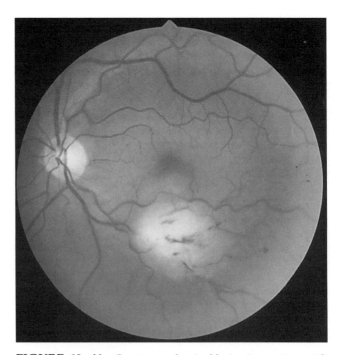

FIGURE 60–41   Cryptococcal retinal lesion in a patient with cryptococcal meningitis.

was reported by Kurosawa and associates in an HIV-infected patient with disseminated cutaneous sporotrichosis. A painful hypopyon uveitis with marked loss of vision developed. Despite treatment with IV amphotericin B, intravitreal kanamycin sulfate and amikacin sulfate, and washout of the anterior chamber, the anterior chamber became completely filled with dense inflammatory material and dense vitreous opacities were apparent on ultrasound. The eye was enucleated and microscopic exams revealed clusters of inflammatory cells on the retinal surface, and vacuolization of the ganglion cells of the inner nuclear layer. Histopathologic examination revealed *S. schenckii* organisms in the anterior and posterior chambers.[199]

Disseminated histoplasmosis is a life-threatening opportunistic infection in AIDS patients. Macher and associates reported a case of an HIV-infected man with disseminated histoplasmosis. Histopathologic and electron microscopic studies using special fungal stains showed numerous budding yeasts in the choroid, retina, and central retinal vein. *Histoplasma capsulatum* was confirmed by immunofluorescent staining.[200]

Specht and associates reported a case of an HIV-infected patient with disseminated histoplasmosis and an ocular complaint of a hazy spot in the vision of his left eye. On funduscopic examination there were creamy white intraretinal and subretinal infiltrates with distinct borders measuring 1/6 to 1/4 disc diameter in size. At autopsy the retina contained multiple white-tan lesions located both superficially and deep without any choroidal thickening. The retinal lesions were seen in a perivascular distribution and contained histoplasma yeasts in all layers. A focal choroiditis was seen near the retinitis. Electron microscopic studies showed oval or spherical *Histoplasma* yeast cells with large eccentric nuclei.[201]

Endogenous bacterial retinitis in two AIDS patients was reported by Davis and associates. Ophthalmoscopic exam revealed discrete patches of retinitis that enlarged slowly over weeks, with accumulation of subretinal fluid and retinal exudate. Histopathologic sections from a retinal biopsy in one patient showed necrotic retina, multiple histiocytes, and encapsulated bacterial forms. Electron microscopy revealed a rigid cell wall structure characteristic of gram-positive bacteria. Both patients had improved vision after treatment with systemic antibiotics.[202]

Uveitis

Iridocyclitis and vitritis in patients with AIDS are usually associated with intraocular opportunistic infection. Farrell and associates describe a case of chronic iridocyclitis and vitritis without any associated opportunistic infection. Treatment with topical and systemic steroids failed to control the in-

flammation, with recurrence when tapering was attempted. An anterior chamber paracentesis was performed with isolation of HIV from the aqueous humor. After treatment with zidovudine was initiated, with tapering of oral steroids, marked improvement of the intraocular inflammation was evident, with complete visual recovery.[203]

MALIGNANCIES

Lymphoma

The non-Hodgkin's lymphomas (NHLs), a heterogeneous group of malignancies, have an increased incidence in HIV-infected patients. While extranodal presentation of NHL in AIDS is common, orbital lymphoma is rare.[204] All cases have been either the small, noncleaved cell or large-cell immunoblastic types. Intraocular lymphoma is rare with no cases identified in a series of 200 AIDS patients and an autopsy evaluation of 25 patients.[2]

Intraocular lymphoma can be primary or secondary. Primary ocular lymphoma usually affects the retina and spares the choroid, while secondary lymphoma usually infiltrates the uvea. Symptoms include rapid onset of visual loss and floaters.[133]

There are four reported cases of intraocular lymphoma in AIDS patients.[205-208] In one patient, large-cell lymphoma presented as confluent yellowish white retinochoroidal infiltrates with perivascular sheathing in the right eye and multiple small, white intraretinal and choroidal infiltrates in the left eye. Cytopathologic diagnosis of the vitreous sample and subsequent examination of the CSF demonstrated the lymphomatous cells. The patient had complete resolution of the infiltrates after whole eye radiation.[205] In a second patient, coexisting intraocular and orbital lymphoma was reported. Biopsy and subsequent enucleation revealed massive retinal necrosis and multiple solid retinal pigment epithelial detachments. Immunophenotyping of the orbital tumor revealed a mixture of both B and T cells.[208] In a third case, large-cell lymphoma was detected both intracerebrally and intraocularly.[206] In a fourth case, an enucleation specimen revealed a B immunoblastic lymphoma with a CD30+ anaplastic large-cell component.[207]

DRUG TOXICITIES

Patients with AIDS are on multiple medications increasing the potential for drug interactions and adverse reactions. Specific retinal and choroidal side effects have been reported with some medications.

Clofazimine

Clofazimine (Lamprene), an iminophenazine dye with antimycobacterial activity previously used in the treatment of dapsone-resistant leprosy, is currently used to treat *Mycobacterium avium* infection in patients with AIDS. It can produce a brownish discoloration of the conjunctiva and brown swirls in the superficial cornea. These changes are without visual compromise and often reversible with discontinuation of the clofazimine.[209,210] There have been two reports of a bull's-eye maculopathy in patients treated with clofazimine. The maculopathy consists of hypopigmented areas with corresponding window defects on fluorescein angiography (Fig. 60–42). The patients had electrophysiologic changes consistent with a generalized retinal degeneration. Patients placed on clofazimine should have periodic funduscopic exams to monitor for macular pigmentary changes.[211,212]

Rifabutin

Rifabutin is a semisynthetic rifamycin used against mycobacterium avium complex (MAC) in AIDS patients. It has been implicated as the causative agent of a hypopyon uveitis. Saran and associates reported acute hypopyon uveitis and bilateral iridocyclitis in seven patients with AIDS being treated with a multidrug therapy for MAC that included rifabutin. All seven patients were on a dosage range of 300 to 600 mg/day. All cases responded to treatment with intense topical corticosteroids, with or without reduction of rifabutin therapy.[213] Jacobs and associates reported a retrospective study of nine patients with AIDS who developed an acute anterior uveitis while being treated with rifabutin for MAC. Five patients initially presented with a

hypopyon, and in three patients hypopyon was bilateral and recurrent. There were no other causes of uveitis identified and in each patient the uveitis resolved without sequelae with treatment with topical corticosteroids alone.[214]

2′,3′-dideoxyinosine (ddI)

2′,3′-dideoxyinosine (ddI) is a purine analog with antiretroviral activity shown to increase CD4 lymphocyte counts and decrease levels of HIV p24 antigen in some patients with AIDS. Retinal lesions and decreased retinal function have been reported in 7% of children with HIV infection treated with high doses of ddI. The retinal lesions first appear as patches of retinal pigment epithelium (RPE) mottling and atrophy in the midperiphery of the fundus and later become circumscribed by a border of RPE hypertrophy. Progression of retinal lesions continued even at lower doses, but ceased after treatment was discontinued. The electroretinogram showed diminished cone mediated responses that worsened during treatment. The Arden ratio on the electro-oculogram was reduced in one patient with severe retinal lesions, but returned to normal after treatment with ddI was discontinued. Gross examination of the enucleated eyes of one of the initially described cases demonstrated multiple 1 to 2 mm round lesions of RPE loss, with areas of RPE hyperpigmentation. Microscopic examination revealed multiple areas of RPE loss with chorioretinal adhesions and partial loss of the choriocapillaris and outer retina up to the inner nuclear layer in the areas of RPE loss. Transmission electron micros-

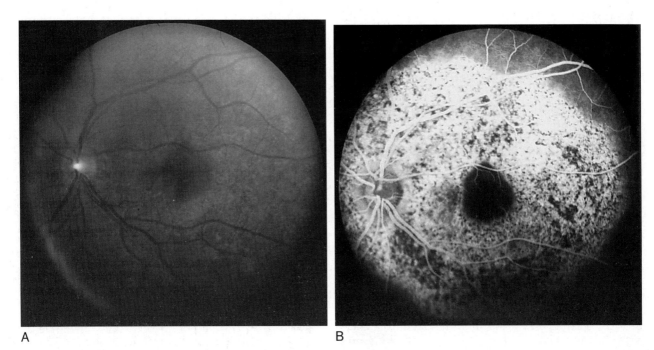

A   B

FIGURE 60–42 Clinical photograph (*A*) and fluorescein angiogram (*B*) of a patient with retinal toxicity from clofazimine.

copy demonstrated enlarged RPE cells with large melanin granules and other RPE cells with reduced number of melanin granules. There was the presence of membranous cytoplasmic inclusion cluster around pigment granules.[215]

Ethambutol

Most cases of ocular toxicity with ethambutol are bilateral and result from a dose related retrobulbar optic neuritis. An axial optic neuritis involves the papillomacular bundle and results in decreased visual acuity, central scotomas, and color vision deficits. The peripheral form occurs with higher doses of ethambutol and results in peripheral visual field defects, with sparing of visual acuity and color vision.[216]

Pretreatment ophthalmologic examinations are not routinely recommended with the exception of patients with pre-existing ocular pathology in which changes in vision after initiation of therapy would be difficult to evaluate. Electrophysiologic tests such as flash and pattern visual-evoked potentials and flash electroretinography may be helpful in early detection of ocular abnormalities.[217]

The current regimen with 15 mg/kg daily has an incidence of ocular toxicity of 0.8%.[218] Symptoms of ocular toxicity usually occur after 2 months of therapy. However, there has been a case report of a patient who developed symptoms after only 2 days of therapy at a dosage of 25 mg/kg daily.[216] Patients should be instructed to discontinue medication once symptoms of ocular toxicity develop. Visual recovery with resolution of visual field defects usually occurs after the drug is stopped, but this may take weeks to months.[219]

SUMMARY

Ocular complications of HIV infection have been described since the beginning of the AIDS epidemic. New and unusual infections, as well as involvement of the eye with AIDS-related malignancies has paralleled these diseases in other organ systems. Diagnosis often requires the close cooperation between ophthalmologists, infectious disease specialists, other AIDS-treating physicians, and pathologists and virologists. The ophthalmologist may be the first to diagnose a systemic opportunistic infection. In certain instances the ophthalmologist may be the first to suspect an underlying HIV infection. Expect the unusual, what you are seeing may be something that no one else has described.

REFERENCES

1. Jarman D: Blue. Woodstock, NY, The Overlook Press, 1993.

2. Jabs D, Green R, Fox R, et al: Ocular Manifestations of Acquired Immune Deficiency Syndrome. Ophthalmology 96(7):1092–1099, 1989.

3. Newsome D, Green W, Miller E, et al: Microvascular aspects of acquired immune deficiency syndrome retinopathy. Am J Ophthalmol 98:590–691, 1984.

4. Mansour A, Jampol L, Longani S, et al: Cotton-wool spots in acquired immunodeficiency syndrome compared with diabetes mellitus, systemic hypertension, and central retinal vein occlusion. Arch Ophthalmol 106:1074–1077, 1988.

5. Pepose JS, Holland GN, Nestor MS, et al: Acquired immune deficiency syndrome: pathogenic mechanisms of ocular disease. Ophthalmology 92:472–484, 1985.

6. Palestine A, Frishberg B: Macular edema in acquired immunodeficiency syndrome-related microvasculopathy. Am J Ophthalmol 111:770–771, 1991.

7. Kestelyn P, Van de Perre P, Rouvroy D, et al: A prospective study of the ophthalmologic findings in the acquired immune deficiency syndrome in Africa. Am J Ophthalmol 100:230–238, 1985.

8. Glasgow B, Weisberger A: A quantitative and cartographic study of retinal microvasculopathy in acquired immunodeficiency syndrome. Am J Ophthalmol 118:46–56, 1994.

9. Farber D, Wiley C, Lynn G, et al: Role of HIV and CMV in the pathogenesis of retinitis and retinal vasculopathy in AIDS patients. Invest Ophthalmol Vis Sci 33:2345–2353, 1992.

10. Pomerantz R, Kuritzkes D, de la Monte S, et al: Infection of the retina by human immunodeficiency virus type 1. N Engl J Med 317:1643–1647, 1987.

11. Engstrom RJ, Holland G, Hardy W, Meisellman H: Hemorheologic abnormalities in patients wih human immunodeficiency virus infection and ophthalmic microvasculopathy. Am J Ophthalmol 109:153–161, 1990.

12. Freeman W, Chen A, Henderly D, et al: Prevalence and significance of acquired immunodeficiency syndrome-related microvasculopathy. Am J Ophthalmol 107:229–235, 1989.

13. Spaide R, Gaissinger A, Podhorzer J: Risk factors for cotton-wool spots and for cytomegalovirus retinitis in patients with human immunodeficiency virus infection. Ophthalmology 102:1860–1864, 1995.

14. Sadun A, Tenhula W, Heller K: Optic nerve pathology associated with AIDS: ultrastructural changes. Sarasota, FL, Association for Research in Vision and Ophthalmology, 1990, p 365.

15. Quiceno J, Capparelli E, Sadun A, et al: Visual dysfunction without retinitis in patients with acquired immunodeficiency syndrome. Am J Ophthalmol 113:8–13, 1992.

16. Geier S, Hammel G, Bogner J, et al: HIV-related ocular microangiopathic syndrome and color contrast sensitivity. Invest Ophthalmol Vis Sci 35:3011–3021, 1994.

17. Boniuk I: The cytomegaloviruses and the eye. Int Ophthalmol Clin 12(2):169–190, 1972.

18. Ho M: Epidemiology of cytomegalovirus infections. Rev Infect Dis 12(Suppl 7):S701–S710, 1990.

19. Stagno S, Whitley R: Herpesvirus infections of pregnancy. N Engl J Med 313:1270–1274, 1985.

20. Alford C, Stango S, Pass R, Britt W: Congenital and perinatal cytomegalovirus infections. Rev Infect Dis 12(Suppl 7):S745–S753, 1990.

21. Pollard RB, Egbert PR, Gallagher JG, Merigan TC: Cytomegalovirus retinitis in immunosuppressed hosts. I. Natural history and effects of treatment with adenine arabinoside. Ann Intern Med 93:655–664, 1980.

22. Egbert PR, Pollard RB, Gallagher JG, Merigan TC: Cytomegalovirus retinitis in immunosuppressed hosts. II. Ocular manifestations. Ann Intern Med 93:664–670, 1980.

23. Carson S, Chatterjee SN: Cytomegalovirus retinitis: two cases occurring after renal transplantation. Ann Ophthalmol 10:275–279, 1978.

24. Nicholson DH: Cytomegalovirus infection of the retina. Int Ophthalmol Clin 15(4):151–162, 1975.

25. Boppana S, Polis M, Kramer A, et al: Virus-specific antibody response to human cytomegalovirus (HCMV) in human immunodeficiency virus type 1-infected persons with HCMV retinitis. J Infect Dis 171:182–185, 1995.
26. Spector S, Merrill R, Wolf D, Dankner W: Detection of human cytomegalovirus in plasma of AIDS patients during acute visceral disease by DNA amplification. J Clin Microbiol 30:2359–2365, 1992.
27. Rasmussen L, Morris S, Wolitz R, et al: Deficiency in antibody response to human cytomegalovirus glycoprotein gH in human immunodeficiency virus-infected patients at risk for cytomegalovirus retinitis. J Infect Dis 170:673–677, 1994.
28. Rasmussen L, Morris S, Zipeto D, et al: Quantitation of human cytomegalovirus DNA from peripheral blood cells of human immunodeficiency virus-infected patients could predict cytomegalovirus retinitis. J Infect Dis 171:177–182, 1995.
29. Drouet E, Boibieux A, Michelson S, et al: Polymerase chain reaction detection of cytomegalovirus DNA in peripheral blood leukocytes as a predictor of cytomegalovirus disease in HIV-infected patients. AIDS 7:665–668, 1993.
30. Selik R, Chu S, Ward J: Trends in infectious diseases and cancers among persons dying of HIV infection in the United States from 1987 to 1992. Ann Intern Med 123:933–936, 1995.
31. Freeman WR, Lerner CW, Mines JA, et al: A prospective study of the ophthalmic findings in the acquired immune deficiency syndrome. Am J Ophthalmol 97:133–142, 1984.
32. Jabs DA, Enger C, Bartlett JG: Cytomegalovirus retinitis and acquired immunodeficiency syndrome. Arch Ophthalmol 107:75–80, 1989.
33. Studies of Ocular Complications of AIDS Research Group in Collaboration with the AIDS Clinical Trials Group. Mortality in patients with the acquired immunodeficiency syndrome treated with either foscarnet or ganciclovir for cytomegalovirus retinitis. N Engl J Med 326:213–220, 1992.
34. Kuppermann BD, Petty JG, Richman DD, et al: Correlation between CD4+ counts and prevalence of cytomegalovirus retinitis and human immunodeficiency virus-related noninfectious retinal vasculopathy in patients with acquired immunodeficiency syndrome. Am J Ophthalmol 115:575–582, 1993.
35. Lowder C, Butler C, Dodds E, et al: CD8+ T lymphocytes and cytomegalovirus retinitis in patients with the acquired immunodeficiency syndrome. Am J Ophthalmol 120:283–290, 1995.
36. McCann J, Margolis T, Wong M, et al: A sensitive and specific polymerase chain reaction-bases assay for the diagnosis of cytomegalovirus retinitis. Am J Ophthalmol 120:219–226, 1995.
37. Mitchell S, Fox J: Aqueous and vitreous humor samples for the diagnosis of cytomegalovirus retinitis. Am J Ophthalmol 120:252, 1995.
38. Martin D, Chi-Chao C, de Smet M, et al: The role of chorioretinal biopsy in the management of posterior uveitis. Ophthalmology 100:705–714, 1992.
39. Schneiderman T, Faber D, Gross J, et al: The agar-albumin sandwich technique for processing retinal biopsy specimens. Am J Ophthalmol 108:567–571, 1989.
40. Freeman W, Wiley C, Gross J, et al: Endoretinal biopsy in immunosuppressed and healthy patients with retinitis. Ophthalmology 96:1559–1565, 1989.
41. Spaide R, Vitale A, Toth I, Oliver J: Frosted branch angiitis associated with cytomegalovirus retinitis. Am J Ophthalmol 113:552–528, 1992.
42. Rabb MF, Jampol LM, Fish RH, et al: Retinal periphlebitis in patients with acquired immunodeficiency syndrome with cytomegalovirus retinitis mimics acute frosted retinal periphlebitis. Arch Ophthalmol 110:1257–1260, 1992.
43. Lee S, Ai E: Disc neovascularization in patients with AIDS and cytomegalovirus retinitis. Retina 11:305–308, 1991.
44. Jabs DA, Engler C, Haller J, de Bustros S: Retinal detachments in patients with cytomegalovirus retinitis. Arch Ophthalmol 109:794–799, 1991.
45. Freeman WR, Friedberg DN, Berry C, et al. Risk factors for development of rhegmatogenous retinal detachment in patients with cytomegalovirus. Am J Ophthalmol 116:713–720, 1993.
46. Gangan P, Besen G, Munguia D, Freeman WR: Macular serous exudation in patients with acquired immunodeficiency syndrome and cytomegalovirus retinitis. Am J Ophthalmol 118:212–219, 1994.
47. Grossniklaus HE, Frank E, Tomsak RL: Cytomegalovirus retinitis and optic neuritis in acquired immune deficiency syndrome. Ophthalmology 94:1601–1604, 1987.
48. Gross JG, Sudan AA, Wiley CA, Freeman WR: Severe visual loss related to isolated peripapillary retinal and optic nerve head cytomegalovirus infection. Am J Ophthalmol 108:691–698, 1989.
49. Neuwirth J, Gutman I, Hofeldt AJ, et al: Cytomegalovirus retinitis in a young homosexual male with acquired immunodeficiency. Ophthalmology 89:805–808, 1982.
50. Bachman DM, Rodrigues MM, Chu FC, et al: Culture-proven cytomegalovirus retinitis in a homosexual man with acquired immunodeficiency syndrome. Ophthalmology 89:797–804, 1982.
51. Pepose JS, Hilborne LH, Cancilla P, Foos RY: Concurrent herpes simplex and cytomegalovirus retinitis and encephalitis in the acquired immune deficiency syndrome (AIDS). Ophthalmology 91:1669–1677, 1984.
52. Skolnik PR, Pomerantz RJ, de la Monte SM, et al: Dual infection of retina with human immunodeficiency virus type 1 and cytomegalovirus. Am J Ophthalmol 107:361–372, 1989.
53. Shami M, Freeman W, Friedberg D, et al: A multicenter study of pneumocystis choroidopathy. Am J Ophthalmol 112:15–22, 1991.
54. Elkins BS, Holland GN, Opremcak M, et al: Ocular toxoplasmosis. Ophthalmology 101:499–507, 1994.
55. Cochereau-Massin I, LeHoang P, Lautier-Frau M, et al: Ocular toxoplasmosis in human immunodeficiency virus-infected patients. Am J Ophthalmol 114:130–135, 1992.
56. Palestine AG, Rodrigues MM, Macher AM, et al: Ophthalmic involvement in acquired immune deficiency syndrome. Ophthalmology 91:1092–1099, 1984.
57. Guyer DR, Jabs DA, Brant AM, et al: Regression of cytomegalovirus retinitis with zidovudine. Arch Ophthalmol 107:868–874, 1989.
58. Palestine AG, Stevens G Jr, Lane HC, et al: Treatment of cytomegalovirus retinitis with dihydroxy propoxymethyl gaunine. Am J Ophthalmol 101:95–101, 1986.
59. Jacobson MA, O'Donnell JJ, Brodie HR, et al: Randomized prospective trial of ganciclovir maintenance therapy for cytomegalovirus retinitis. J Med Virol 25:339–349, 1988.
60. Jabs DA, Newman C, de Bustros S, Polk BF: Treatment of cytomegalovirus retinitis with ganciclovir. Ophthalmology 94:824–830, 1987.
61. Orellana J, Teich SA, Friedman AH, et al: Combined short- and long-term therapy for the treatment of cytomegalovirus retinitis using ganciclovir (BW B759U). Ophthalmology 94:831–838, 1987.
62. Pepose JS, Newman C, Bach MC, et al: Pathological features of cytomegalovirus retinopathy after treatment with the antiviral agent ganciclovir. Ophthalmology 94:414–424, 1987.
63. Studies of Ocular Complications of AIDS Research Group in Collaboration with the AIDS Clinical Trials Group: Combination foscarnet and ganciclovir therapy vs monotherapy for the treatment of relapsed cytomegalovirus retinitis in patients with AIDS. Arch Ophthalmol 114:23–33, 1996.
64. Drew W, Ives D, Lalezari J, et al: Oral ganciclovir as maintenance treatment for cytomegalovirus retinitis in patients with AIDS. N Engl J Med 333:615–620, 1995.
65. Lehoang P, Girard B, Robinet M, et al: Foscarnet in the treatment of cytomegalovirus retinitis in acquired immune deficiency syndrome. Ophthalmology 96:865–874, 1989.

66. Jacobson MA, Causey D, Polsky B, et al: A dose-ranging study of daily maintenance intravenous foscarnet therapy for cytomegalovirus retinitis in AIDS. J Infect Dis 168: 444–448, 1993.

67. Jacobson MA, O'Donnell JJ, Mills J: Foscarnet treatment of cytomegalovirus retinitis patients with acquired immunodeficiency syndrome. Antimicrob Agents Chemother 33:736–741, 1989.

68. Studies of Ocular Complications of AIDS Research Group in Collaboration with the AIDS Clinical Trials Group: Morbidity and toxic effects associated with ganciclovir or foscarnet therapy in a randomized cytomegalovirus retinitis trial. Arch Intern Med 155:65–74, 1995.

69. Henderly DE, Freeman WR, Causey DM, Rao NA: Cytomegalovirus retinitis and response to therapy with ganciclovir. Ophthalmology 94:425–434, 1987.

70. Holland GN, Sison RF, Jatulis DE, et al: Survival of patients with the acquired immune deficiency syndrome after development of cytomegalovirus retinopathy. Ophthalmology 97:204–211, 1990.

71. Studies of Ocular Complications of AIDS Research Group in Collaboration with the AIDS Clinical Trials Group: Antiviral effects of foscarnet and ganciclovir therapy on human immunodeficiency virus p24 antigen in patients with AIDS and cytomegalovirus retinitis. J Infect Dis 172:613–621, 1995.

72. Weinberg DV, Murphy R, Naughton K: Combined daily therapy with intravenous ganciclovir and foscarnet for patients with recurrent cytomegalovirus. Am J Ophthalmol 117:776–782, 1994.

73. Dieterich DT, Poles MA, Lew EA, et al: Concurrent use of ganciclovir and foscarnet to treat cytomegalovirus infection in AIDS patients. J Infect Dis 167:1184–1188, 1992.

74. Kuppermann BD, Flores-Aguilar M, Quiceno JI, et al: Combination ganciclovir and foscarnet in the treatment of clinically resistant cytomegalovirus retinitis in patients with acquired immunodeficiency syndrome. Arch Ophthalmol 111:1359–1366, 1993.

75. Kuppermann BD, Quiceno JI, Flores-Aguilar M, et al: Intravitreal ganciclovir concentration after intravenous administration in AIDS patients with cytomegalovirus retinitis: implications for therapy. J Infect Dis 168(6):1506–1509, 1993.

76. Cantrill HL, Henry K, Melroe H, et al: Treatment of cytomegalovirus retinitis with intravitreal ganciclovir. Ophthalmology 96:367–374, 1988.

77. Heinemann M-H: Long-term intravitreal ganciclovir therapy for cytomegalovirus retinopathy. Arch Ophthalmol 107:1767–1772, 1989.

78. Heinemann M-H: *Staphylococcus epidermidis* endophthalmitis complicating intravitreal antiviral therapy of cytomegalovirus retinitis. Arch Ophthalmol 107:643–644, 1989.

79. Young SH, Morlet N, Heery S, et al: High dose intravitreal ganciclovir in the treatment of cytomegalovirus retinitis. Med J Aust 157(6):370–373, 1992.

80. Ussery FM, Gibson SR, Conklin RH, et al: Intravitreal ganciclovir in the treatment of AIDS-associated cytomegalovirus retinitis. Ophthalmology 95:640–648, 1988.

81. Heery S, Hollows F: High-dose intravitreal gancyclovir for cytomegaloviral (CMV) retinitis. Aust N Z J Ophthalmol 17(4):405–408, 1989.

82. Cribbin K, Orellana J, Lieberman R: Intravitreal ganciclovir in patients resistant to ganciclovir and/or foscarnet. Int Conf AIDS. Amsterdam, 1992, Abstract No PoB 3159.

83. Yoshimuzi M, Lee D, Vinci V, Fajardo S: Ocular toxicity of multiple intravitreal DHPG injections. Graefes Arch Clin Exp Ophthalmol 228:350–355, 1990.

84. Diaz-Llopis M, Chipont E, Sanchez S, et al: Intravitreal foscarnet for cytomegalovirus retinitis in a patient with acquired immunodeficiency syndrome. Am J Ophthalmol 114:742–747, 1992.

85. Diaz-Llopis M, España E, Munoz G, et al: High dose intravitreal foscarnet in the treatment of cytomegalovirus in AIDS. Br J Ophthalmol 78:120–124, 1994.

86. Lieberman RM, Orellana J, Melton RC: Efficacy of intravitreal foscarnet in a patient with AIDS. N Engl J Med 330:868–869, 1994.

87. Polis MA, Baird B, Jaffe HS, et al: A phase I/II dose escalation trial of (S)-1-[3-hydroxy-2-(phosphonylmethoxy)propyl]cytosine (HPMPC) in HIV infected persons with CMV viruria. IXth International Conference on AIDS. Berlin, 1993, p 54, Abstract No WS-B11-5.

88. Lalezari J, Stagg R, Kuppermann B, et al: A phase II/III randomized study of immediate versus deferred intravenous (IV) cidofovir (CDV, HPMPC) for the treatment of peripheral CMV retinitis (CMV-R) in patients with AIDS. Second National Conference on Human Retroviruses Related Infections, 1995, p 170.

89. Tolpin M, Pollard R, Tierney M, et al: Combination therapy of cytomegalovirus (CMV) retinitis with a human monoclonal anti-CMV antibody (SDZ MSL 109) and either ganciclovir (DHPG) or foscarnet (PFA). IXth International Conference on AIDS. Berlin, 1993, p 54, Abstract No WS-B11-2.

90. Sanbourn GE, Anand R, Torti RE, et al: Sustained-release ganciclovir therapy for treatment of cytomegalovirus retinitis. Arch Ophthalmol 110:188–195, 1992.

91. Martin D, Parks D, Mellow S, et al: Treatment of cytomegalovirus retinitis with an intraocular sustained-release ganciclovir implant. Arch Ophthalmol 112:1531–1539, 1994.

92. Anand R, Nightengale S, Fish R, et al: Control of cytomegalovirus retinitis using sustained release of intraocular ganciclovir. Arch Ophthalmol 111:223–227, 1993.

93. Friedberg D: Treatment of cytomegalovirus retinitis with intraocular sustained-release ganciclovir implant (Letter). Arch Ophthalmol 113:1354–1355, 1995.

94. Anand R, Font RL, Fish RH, Nightengale SD: Pathology of cytomegalovirus retinitis treated with sustained release intravitreal ganciclovir. Ophthalmology 100:1032–1039, 1993.

95. Kirsch LS, Arevalo JF, Chavez de la Paz E, et al: Intravitreal cidofovir treatment of cytomegalovirus retinitis in patients with acquired immune deficiency syndrome. Ophthalmology 102:533–543, 1995.

96. Kirsch LS, Arevalo JF, de Clercq E, et al: Phase I/II study of intravitreal cidofovir for the treatment of cytomegalovirus retinitis in patients with acquired immunodeficiency syndrome. Am J Ophthalmol 119:466–476, 1995.

97. Azad RF, Driver VB, Tanaka K, et al: Antiviral activity of a phosphorothioate oligonucleotide complementary to RNA of the human cytomegalovirus major immediate-early region. Antimicrob Agents Chemother 37:1945–1954, 1993.

98. Youle M, Gazzard B, Johnson M, et al: Effects of high-dose oral acyclovir on herpesvirus disease and survival in patients with advanced HIV disease: a double-blind, placebo-controlled study. AIDS 8:641–649, 1994.

99. Brosgart C, Craig C, Hillman D, et al: A randomized placebo controlled trial of the safety and efficacy of oral ganciclovir for prophylaxis of CMV retinitis and gastrointestinal mucosal disease in HIV infected individuals with severe immunosuppression. 35th ICAAC. San Francisco, CA, 1995, p 9, Abstract No LB10.

100. Spector S, McKinley G, Drew W, Stempien M: A randomized double-blind study of the efficacy and safety of oral ganciclovir for the prevention of cytomegalovirus disease in HIV-infected persons. Second National Conference on Human Retroviruses and Related Infections. Washington, DC, 1995, p 56.

101. Baldassano V, Dunn J, Feinberg J, Jabs D: Cytomegalovirus retinitis and low CD4+ T-lymphocyte counts (Letter). N Engl J Med 333:670, 1995.

102. Holland GN, Buhles WC, Mastre B, et al: A controlled retrospective study of ganciclovir treatment for cytomegalovirus retinitis. Arch Ophthalmol 107:1759–1766, 1989.

103. Studies of Ocular Complications of AIDS Research Group in Collaboration with the AIDS Clinical Trials Group: Studies of ocular complications of AIDS foscarnet-ganci-

clovir cytomegalovirus retinitis trial: 1. Rationale, design and methods. Control Clin Trials 13:22–39, 1992.
104. Holland GN, Shuler JD: Progression rates of cytomegalovirus retinopathy in ganciclovir-treated and untreated patients. Arch Ophthalmol 110:1435–1442, 1992.
105. Studies of Ocular Complications of AIDS Research Group in Collaboration with the AIDS Clinical Trials Group: Foscarnet-ganciclovir cytomegalovirus retinitis trial 4. Visual outcomes. Ophthalmology 101:1250–1261, 1994.
106. Bachman DM, Bruni LM, DiGioia RA, et al: Visual field testing in the management of cytomegalovirus retinitis. Ophthalmology 99:1393–1399, 1992.
107. Keefe KS, Freeman WR, Peterson TJ, et al: Atypical healing of cytomegalovirus. Ophthalmology 99:1377–1384, 1991.
108. Morley M, Duker J, Ashton P, Robinson M: Replacing ganciclovir implants. Ophthalmology 102:388–392, 1995.
109. Orellana J, Teich SA, Lieberman RM, et al: Treatment of retinal detachments in patients with the acquired immunodeficiency syndrome. Ophthalmology 98:939–943, 1991.
110. Sidikaro Y, Silver L, Holland GN, Kreiger AE: Rhegmatogenous retinal detachments in patients with AIDS and necrotizing retinal infections. Ophthalmology 98:129–135, 1991.
111. Broughton WL, Cupples HP, Parver LM: Bilateral retinal detachment following cytomegalovirus retinitis. Arch Ophthalmol 96:618–619, 1978.
112. Freeman WR, Henderly DE, Wan WL, et al: Prevalence, pathophysiology, and treatment of rhegmatogenous retinal detachment in treated cytomegalovirus retinitis. Am J Ophthalmol 103:527–536, 1987.
113. Garcia R, Flores-Aguilar M, Quiceno J, et al: Results of rhegmatogenous retinal detachment repair in cytomegalovirus retinitis with and without scleral buckling. Ophthalmology 102:236–245, 1993.
114. Davis J, Serfass M, Lai M-Y, et al: Silicone oil in repair of retinal detachments caused by necrotizing retinitis in HIV infection. Arch Ophthalmol 113:1401–1409, 1995.
115. Dugel PU, Liggett PE, Lee MB, et al: Repair of retinal detachment caused by cytomegalovirus retinitis in patients with the acquired immunodeficiency syndrome. Am J Ophthalmol 112:235–242, 1991.
116. Lim J, Enger C, Haller J, et al: Improved visual results after surgical repair of cytomegalovirus-related retinal detachments. Ophthalmology 101:264–269, 1994.
117. Kuppermann B, Flores-Aguilar M, Quiceno J, et al: A masked prospective evaluation of outcome parameters for cytomegalovirus-related retinal detachment surgery in patients with acquired immunodeficiency syndrome. Ophthalmology 101:46–55, 1994.
118. Stefánsson E, Tiedeman J: Optics of the eye with air or silicone oil. Retina 8:10–19, 1988.
119. Roarty JD, Fisher EJ, Nussbaum JJ: Long-term visual morbidity of cytomegalovirus retinitis in patients with the acquired immune deficiency syndrome. Ophthalmology 100:1685–1688, 1993.
120. Urayama A, Yamada N, Sasaki T, et al: Unilateral acute uveitis with retinal periarteritis and detachment. Jpn J Clin Ophthalmol 25:607, 1971.
121. Young N, Bird A: Bilateral acute retinal necrosis. Br J Ophthalmol 62:581–590, 1978.
122. Holland G, Executive Committee of the American Uveitis Society: Standard diagnostic criteria for the acute retinal necrosis syndrome. Am J Ophthalmol 117:663–667, 1994.
123. Fisher J, Lewis M, Blumenkranz M, et al: The acute retinal necrosis syndrome. Part 1: clinical manifestations. Ophthalmology 89:1309–1316, 1982.
124. Matsuo T, Nakayama T, Koyama T, et al: A proposed mild type of acute retinal necrosis syndrome. Am J Ophthalmol 105(6):579–583, 1988.
125. Margolis T, Lowder C, Holland GN, et al: Varicella-zoster virus retinitis in patients with the acquired immunodeficiency syndrome. Am J Ophthalmol 112:119–131, 1991.
126. Culbertson W, Blumenkranz M, Haines H, et al: The acute

retinal necrosis syndrome. Part 2: Histopathology and etiology. Ophthalmology 89:1317–1325, 1982.
127. Lewis M, Culbertson W, Post M, et al: Herpes simplex virus type 1. A cause of the acute retinal necrosis syndrome. Ophthalmology 96:875–878, 1989.
128. Nishi M, Hanashiro R, Mori S, et al: Polymerase chain reaction for the detection of the varicella-zoster genome in ocular samples from patients with acute retinal necrosis. Am J Ophthalmol 114:603–609, 1992.
129. Rummelt V, Wenkel H, Rummelt C, et al: Detection of varicella zoster virus DNA and viral antigen in the late stage of bilateral acute retinal necrosis syndrome. Arch Ophthalmology 110:1132–1136, 1992.
130. Thompson W, Culbertson W, Smiddy W, et al: Acute retinal necrosis caused by reactivation of herpes simplex virus type 2. Am J Ophthalmol 118(2):205–211, 1994.
131. Pepose J, Flowers B, Stewart J, et al: Herpesvirus antibody levels in the etiologic diagnosis of the acute retinal necrosis syndrome. Am J Ophthalmol 113:248–256, 1992.
132. Sellitti T, Huang A, Schiffman J, Davis J: Association of herpes zoster ophthalmicus with acquired immunodeficiency syndrome with acute retinal necrosis. Am J Ophthalmol 116:297–301, 1993.
133. Dunn J: Other retinal and choroidal manifestations of HIV infection. In Stenson S, Friedberg D (eds): AIDS and the Eye. New Orleans, Contact Lens Association of Ophthalmologists, Inc, 1995.
134. Engstrom R, Holland G, Margolis T, et al: The progressive outer retinal necrosis syndrome. A variant of necrotizing herpetic retinopathy in patients with AIDS. Ophthalmology 101:1488–1502, 1993.
135. Greven C, Ford J, Stanton C, et al: Progressive outer retinal necrosis secondary to varicella zoster virus in acquired immune deficiency syndrome. Retina 15:14–20, 1995.
136. Kuppermann B, Quiceno J, Wiley C, et al: Clinical and histopathologic study of varicella zoster virus retinitis in patients with the acquired immunodeficiency syndrome. Am J Ophthalmol 118:589–600, 1994.
137. Forster D, Dugel P, Frangieh G, et al: Rapidly progressive outer retinal necrosis in the acquired immunodeficiency syndrome. Am J Ophthalmol 110:341–348, 1990.
138. Johnston W, Holland G, Engstrom R, Rimmer S: Recurrence of presumed varicella-zoster virus retinopathy in patients with acquired immunodeficiency syndrome. Am J Ophthalmol 116:42–50, 1993.
139. Biron K, Elion G: Effect of acyclovir combined with other antiherpetic agents on varicella zoster virus in vitro. Am J Med 73:54, 1982.
140. Jacobson M, Berger T, Fikrig S, et al: Acyclovir-resistant varicella zoster virus infection after chronic oral acyclovir therapy in patients with the acquired immunodeficiency syndrome (AIDS). Ann Intern Med 112:187, 1990.
141. Pinnolis M, Foxworthy D, Kemp B: Treatment of progressive outer retinal necrosis with sorivudine. Am J Ophthalmol 119(4):516–517, 1995.
142. Holland G, Engstrom RJ, Glasgow B, et al: Ocular toxoplasmosis in patients with the acquired immunodeficiency syndrome. Am J Ophthalmol 106:653–667, 1988.
143. Holland G: Ocular sequelae. In Broder S, Merigan TJ, Bolognesi D (eds): Textbook of AIDS Medicine. Baltimore: Williams & Wilkins, 1994.
144. Teich S, Cheung T, Friedman A: Systemic antiviral drugs used in ophthalmology. Surv Ophthalmol 37:19–53, 1992.
145. Greven C, Teot L: Cytologic identification of Toxoplasma gondii from vitreous fluid. Arch Ophthalmol 112:1086–1088, 1994.
146. Henin D, Duyckaerts C, Chaunu M-P, et al: Etude neuropathologique de 31 cas de syndrome d'immunodepression acquise. Rev Neurol 143:631, 1987.
147. Porter S, Sande M: Toxoplasmosis of the central nervous system in the acquired immunodeficiency syndrome. N Engl J Med 327:1643–1648, 1992.
148. Heinemann M, Gold J, Maisel J: Bilateral toxoplasma retinochoroiditis in a patient with acquired immune deficiency syndrome. Retina 6:224–227, 1986.

149. Grossniklaus H, Specht C, Allaire G, Leavitt J: *Toxoplasma gondii* retinochoroiditis and optic neuritis in acquired immune deficiency syndrome. Ophthalmology 97:1342–1346, 1990.

150. Park DI, Font R: Diffuse toxoplasmic retinochoroiditis in a patient with AIDS. Arch Ophthalmol 104:571–575, 1986.

151. Berger B, Egwuaugu C, Freeman W, Wiley C: Miliary toxoplasmic retinitis in acquired immunodeficiency syndrome. Arch Ophthalmol 111:373–376, 1993.

152. Luft B, Remington J: AIDS commentary. Toxoplasmic encephalitis. J Infect Dis 157:1–6, 1988.

153. Podzamczer D, Miro J, Bolao F, et al: Twice-weekly maintenance therapy with sulfadiazine-pyrimethamine to prevent recurrent toxoplasmic encephalitis in patients with AIDS. Ann Intern Med 123:175–180, 1995.

154. Kovacs J, and the NIAID-Clinical Center Intramural AIDS Program: Efficacy of atovaquone in treatment of toxoplasmosis in patients with AIDS. Lancet 340:637–638, 1992.

155. Pavesio C, Chiappino M, Gormley P, et al: Acquired retinochoroiditis in hamsters inoculated wtih ME 49 strain toxoplasma. Invest Ophthalmol Vis Sci 36:2166–2175, 1995.

156. Hook EI, Marra C: Acquired syphilis in adults. N Engl J Med 326:1060–1069, 1992.

157. Fleming W, Brown W, Donohue J, Branigin P: National survey of venereal disease treated by physicians in 1968. JAMA 211:1827–1830, 1970.

158. Hook EI: Syphilis and HIV infection. J Infect Dis 160:530–534, 1989.

159. Musher D, Hamill R, Baughn R: Effect of human immunodeficiency virus (HIV) infection on the course of syphilis and on the response to treatment. Ann Intern Med 113:872–881, 1990.

160. Tamesis R, Foster C: Ocular syphilis. Ophthalmology 97:1281–1287, 1990.

161. Hart G: Syphilis tests in diagnostic and therapeutic decision making. Ann Intern Med 104:368–376, 1986.

162. Jurado R, Campbell J, Martin P. Prozone phenomenon in secondary syphilis. Has its time arrived? Arch Intern Med 153:2496–2498, 1993.

163. Augenbraun M, DeHovitz J, Feldman J, et al: Biological false-positive syphilis test results for women infected with human immunodeficiency virus. Clin Infect Dis 19:1040–1044, 1994.

164. Schlaegel TJ, Kao S: A review (1970–1980) of 28 presumptive cases of syphilitic uveitis. Am J Ophthalmol 93:412–414, 1982.

165. Stoumbos V, Klein M: Syphilitic retinitis in a patient with acquired immunodeficiency syndrome-related complex. Am J Ophthalmol 103:103–104, 1987.

166. Passo M, Rosenbaum J: Ocular syphilis in patients with human immunodeficiency virus infection. Am J Ophthalmol 106:1–6, 1988.

167. McLeish W, Pulido J, Holland S, et al: The ocular manifestations of syphilis in the human immunodeficiency virus type 1-infected host. Ophthalmology 97:196–203, 1990.

168. Becerra L, Ksiazek S, Savino P, et al: Syphilitic uveitis in human immunodeficiency virus-infected and noninfected patients. Ophthalmology 96:1727–1730, 1989.

169. Gass J, Braunstein R, Chenoweth R: Acute syphilitic posterior placoid chorioretinitis. Ophthalmology 97:1288–1297, 1990.

170. Berry C, Hootan T, Collier A, Lukehart S: Neurologic relapse after benzathine penicillin therapy for secondary syphilis in a patient with HIV infection. N Engl J Med 316:1587–1589, 1987.

171. Guinan M: Treatment of primary and secondary syphilis: defining failure at the three and six-month follow-up (Editorial). JAMA 257:359–360, 1987.

172. Margo C, Hamed L: Ocular syphilis. Surv Ophthalmol 37:203–220, 1992.

173. Malone J, Wallace M, Hendrick B, et al: Syphilis and neurosyphilis in a human immunodeficiency virus type-1 seropositive population: evidence for frequent serologic relapse after therapy. Am J Med 99:55–63, 1995.

174. Masur H, Michelis M, Greene J, et al: CD4 counts as predictors of opportunistic pneumonias in human immunodeficiency virus (HIV) infection. Ann Intern Med 111:223–231, 1989.

175. Macher A, Bardenstein D, Zimmerman L, et al: *Pneumocystis carinii* choroiditis in a male homosexual with AIDS and disseminated pulmonary and extrapulmonary *P. carinii* infection. N Engl J Med 316:1092, 1987.

176. Rao N, Zimmerman P, Boyer D, et al: A clinical, histopathologic, and electron microscopic study of *Pneumocystis carinii* choroiditis. Am J Ophthalmol 107:218–228, 1989.

177. Freeman W, Gross J, Labelle J, et al: *Pneumocystis carinii* choroidopathy. Arch Ophthalmol 107:863–867, 1989.

178. CDC Update: Guidelines for prophylaxis against *Pneumocystis carinii* pneumonia for persons infected with human immunodeficiency virus. MMWR 38(No S-5):1–9, 1989.

179. Dugel P, Rao N, Forster D, et al: *Pneumocystis carinii* choroiditis after long-term aerosolized pentamidine therapy. Am J Ophthalmol 110:113–117, 1990.

180. Foster R, Lowder C, Meisler D, et al: Presumed *Pneumocystis carinii* choroiditis: unifocal presentation, regression with intravenous pentamidine, and choroiditis recurrence. Ophthalmology 98:1360–1365, 1991.

181. Friedberg D, Greene J, Brook D: Asymptomatic disseminated *Pneumocystis carinii* infection detected by ophthalmoscopy. Lancet 336:1256–1257, 1990.

182. Glatt A, Chingwin K, Landesman S: Treatment of infections associated with human immunodeficiency virus. N Engl J Med 318:1439, 1988.

183. Duke-Elder S, Perkins E: Diseases of the uveal tract. In Duke-Elder S (ed): System of Ophthalmology, Vol. IX. London, Henry Kimpton, 1966.

184. Abrams J, Schlaegel TJ: The role of isoniazid therapeutic test in tuberculous uveitis. Am J Ophthalmol 94:511–515, 1982.

185. Donahue H: Ophthalmic experience in a tuberculosis sanatorium. Am J Ophthalmol 64:742–748, 1967.

186. Olazabal FJ: Choroidal tubercles. JAMA 200:374–377, 1967.

187. Chung Y, Yeh T, Sheu S, Liu J: Macular subretinal neovascularization in choroidal tuberculosis. Ann Ophthalmol 21:225–229, 1989.

188. Humphrey R, Weber J, Marsh R: Ophthalmic findings in a group of ambulatory patients infected by human immunodeficiency virus (HIV): a prospective study. Br J Ophthalmol 71:565–569, 1987.

189. Blodi B, Johnson M, McLeish W, Gass J: Presumed choroidal tuberculosis in human immunodeficiency virus infected host. Am J Ophthalmol 108:605–607, 1989.

190. Croxatto J, Mestre C, Puente S, Gonzalez G: Nonreactive tuberculosis in a patient with acquired immune deficiency syndrome. Am J Ophthalmol 102:659–660, 1986.

191. Saag M: Cryptococcosis and other fungal infections (histoplasmosis, coccidioidomucosis). In Sande M, Volberding P (eds): The Medical Management of AIDS, 4th edition. Philadelphia, WB Saunders Co, 1995.

192. Kestelyn P, Taelman H, Bogaerts J, et al: Ophthalmic manifestations of infections with *Cryptococcus neoformans* in patients with the acquired immunodeficiency syndrome. Am J Ophthalmol 116:721–727, 1993.

193. Denning D, Armstrong R, Fishman M, Stevens D: Endophthalmitis in a patient with disseminated cryptococcosis and AIDS who was treated with itraconazole. Rev Infect Dis 13:1126–1130, 1991.

194. Cohen D, Glasgow B: Bilateral optic nerve cryptococcosis in sudden blindness in patients with acquired immune deficiency syndrome. Ophthalmology 100:1689–1694, 1993.

195. Garrity J, Herman D, Imes R, et al: Optic nerve sheath decompression for visual loss in patients with acquired immunodeficiency syndrome and cryptococcal meningi-

tis with papilledema. Am J Ophthalmol 116:472–478, 1993.

196. Carney M, Combs J, Waschler W: Cryptococcal choroiditis. Retina 10:27–32, 1990.

197. Chuck S, Sande M: Infections with cryptococcal neoformans in the acquired immunodeficiency syndrome. N Engl J Med 321:794–799, 1989.

198. Heinemann M, Bloom A, Horowitz J: *Candida albicans* endophthalmitis in a patient with AIDS. Arch Ophthalmol 105:1172–1173, 1987.

199. Kurosawa A, Pollock S, Collins M, et al: *Sporothrix schenckii* endophthalmitis in a patient with human immunodeficiency virus infection. Arch Ophthalmol 106:376–380, 1988.

200. Macher A, Rodrigues M, Kaplan W, et al: Disseminated bilateral chorioretinitis due to *Histoplasma capsulatum* in a patient with the acquired immunodeficiency syndrome. Ophthalmology 92:1159–1164, 1985.

201. Specht C, Mitchell K, Bauman A, Gupta M: Ocular histoplasmosis with retinitis in a patient with acquired immune deficiency syndrome. Ophthalmology 98:1356–1359, 1991.

202. Davis J, Nussenblatt R, Bachman D, et al: Endogenous bacterial retinitis in AIDS. Am J Ophthalmol 107:613–623, 1989.

203. Farrell P, Heinemann M-H, Roberts C, et al: Response of human immunodeficiency virus-associated uveitis to zidovudine. Am J Ophthalmol 106:7–10, 1988.

204. Reifler D, Warzynski M, Blount W, et al: Orbital lymphoma associated with acquired immune deficiency syndrome (AIDS). Surv Ophthlamol 38:371–380, 1994.

205. Schanzer M, Font R, O'Malley R: Primary ocular malignant lymphoma associated with the acquired immune deficiency syndrome. Ophthalmology 98:88–91, 1991.

206. Stanton C, Sloan BD, Slusher M, Greven C: Acquired immunodeficiency syndrome-related primary intraocular lymphoma. Arch Ophthalmol 110:1614–1617, 1992.

207. Hofman P, Tourneau A, Negre F, et al: Primary uveal B immunoblastic lymphoma in a patient with AIDS. Br J Ophthalmol 76:700–702, 1992.

208. Matzkin D, Slamovits T, Rosenbaum P: Simultaneous Intraocular and orbital non-Hodgkin lymphoma in the acquired immune deficiency syndrome. Ophthalmology 101:850–855, 1994.

209. Negrel A, Chovet M, Baquillon G, Lagadec R: Clofazimine and the eye: preliminary communication. Lepr Rev 55:349–352, 1984.

210. Wallinder P, Gip L, Stempa M: Corneal changes in patients treated with clofazimine. Br J Ophthalmol 60:526–528, 1976.

211. Craythorn J, Swartz M, Creel D: Clofazimine-induced bull's-eye retinopathy. Retina 6:50–52, 1986.

212. Cunningham C, Friedberg D, Carr R: Clofazimine-induced generalized retinal degeneration. Retina 10:131–134, 1990.

213. Saran B, Maguire A, Nichols C, et al: Hypopyon uveitis in patients with acquired immunodeficiency syndrome treated for systemic mycobacterium avium complex infection with rifabutin. Arch Ophthalmol 112:1159–1165, 1994.

214. Jacobs D, Piliero P, Kuperwaser M, et al: Acute uveitis associated with rifabutin use in patients with human immunodeficiency virus infection. Am J Ophthalmol 118:716–722, 1994.

215. Whitcup S, Butler K, Caruso R, et al: Retinal toxicity in human immunodeficiency virus-infected children treated with 2′,3′-dideoxyinosine. Am J Ophthalmol 113:1–7, 1992.

216. Schild H, Fox B: Rapid-onset reversible ocular toxicity from ethambutol therapy. Am J Med 90:404–406, 1991.

217. Dukes M: Drugs used in tuberculosis and leprosy. In Leuenberger P, Meyer H, Baumann H, Sonntag R (eds): Meyer's Side Effects of Drugs. Amsterdam, Elsevier, 1992.

218. AMA: Antimycobacterial drugs. American Medical Association Department of Drugs, Division of Drugs and Technology, 1994. Drug Evaluations Annual.

219. Chatterjee V, Buchanan D, Friedmann A, Green M: Ocular toxicity following ethambutol in standard dosage. Br J Dis Chest 80:288–291, 1986.

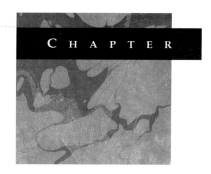

Viral Syndromes

W. Z. Bridges, Jr., M.D.
Paul Sternberg, Jr., M.D.

The acute retinal necrosis (ARN) syndrome and the progressive outer retinal necrosis (PORN) syndrome are two recently described viral syndromes of the retina that have potentially devastating consequences if not diagnosed and treated appropriately. Both syndromes are the result of an infectious retinitis caused by members of the herpesvirus family. They most likely represent different spectrums of the same disease, but there are enough unique characteristics of each syndrome to warrant separate names. The treatment of both syndromes revolves around systemic antiviral medications and the management of subsequent retinal detachment.

ACUTE RETINAL NECROSIS SYNDROME

The acute retinal necrosis syndrome is characterized by the following features: (1) peripheral full-thickness retinitis with well-demarcated borders and rapid circumferential spread, (2) occlusive vasculitis, and (3) prominent vitreitis.[1] Initially, the definition of the ARN syndrome required that the patient be immunocompetent, but recently reported cases in immunocompromised individuals have deleted that requirement for the diagnosis.[2,3] It is now accepted that the etiologic agents responsible for the syndrome are members of the herpesvirus family.[4-7] Prior to the development of specific antiviral therapy, the long-term prognosis was extremely poor. Complex retinal detachments occurred in 75% of eyes, and contributed to a 64% incidence of legal blindness.[8] With the advent of acyclovir, the prognosis has improved; however, retinal detachment continues to be a significant cause of ocular morbidity.

Historically, the first published report of the syndrome has been attributed to Urayama et al in 1971.[9] The syndrome did not appear in the English literature until 1977, when Willerson et al reported two patients with clinical signs consistent with the syndrome.[10] The following year, Young and Bird described a patient with bilateral findings and were the first to coin the term "acute retinal necrosis."[11] The etiology of the syndrome remained a mystery until 1982, when Culbertson and co-workers demonstrated herpesvirus particles within the retina of an enucleated eye.[12] Since that time, almost every member of the herpesvirus family has been implicated as a causative agent.

Epidemiology

The ARN syndrome does not appear to have a racial or gender predilection.[13] The age of onset has a bimodal distribution with peaks occurring at ages 20 and 50. It has been proposed that the bimodal distribution is secondary to the different causative agents within the herpesvirus family and the age at which they are typically manifest systemically. There have been general observations within the literature that the causative agent of the syndrome is herpes simplex virus in younger patients and herpes zoster virus in older patients.[14]

There appears to be an increased susceptibility to the ARN syndrome in patients with specific genetic markers. Human leukocyte antigen (HLA) DQw7 and HLA phenotype Bw62,DR4 were found in increased frequency in patients with ARN as compared to a control population. The significance of this finding in a documented infectious process is unknown. Modulation of the immune response to the initial infection, increased susceptibility to reactivation of latent virus, or increased susceptibility to exogenous herpes infections have all been proposed as potential pathways for genetic influence.[15]

Bilaterality was initially reported to occur in approximately one third of the patients affected with the syndrome.[8] However, more recent reports have shown a much higher incidence of bilaterality. Palay et al found an approximate 70% incidence of bilaterality in patients with untreated disease.[16] Both eyes are rarely affected at the same time. Typically, the fellow eye becomes affected within 2 months of presentation. However, there have been numerous reports of delayed bilateral involvement, with the fellow eye becoming involved as late as 20 to 30 years after the initial presentation.[17–19]

Clinical Features

Symptoms

The majority of patients present with a recent history of hazy, decreased vision. The onset of symptoms is variable but is often insidious in nature. Ocular or periorbital pain is a common complaint.[8,13] The history of previous or concurrent vesicular lesions consistent with primary varicella zoster infection (chickenpox) or herpes zoster dermatitis (shingles) has been reported.[20,21]

Anterior Segment

Conjunctival infection is found in varying degrees. With severe inflammation, episcleritis or scleritis can occur. A moderate anterior uveitis with keratic precipitates is a consistent finding. Both granulomatous and nongramulomatous precipitates have been described (Fig. 61–1). The intraocular pressure is frequently elevated and may serve as an early indicator of herpetic involvement.[8,13,22] The remainder of the anterior segment is normal outside of nonspecific inflammatory changes.

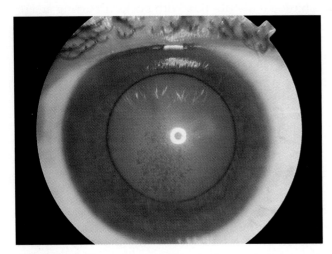

FIGURE 61–1 Anterior segment findings including prominent granulomatous keratic precipitates.

Posterior Segment

The triad of peripheral retinitis, vitreitis, and occlusive vasculitis are mandatory for the diagnosis.[1] The retinitis begins as a whitening of the peripheral retina in multiple patches or broad bands. These lesions represent full-thickness necrosis. There is a sharp demarcation between whitened involved and normal-appearing uninvolved retina (Figs. 61–2 and 61–3). Retinal hemorrhage is not a prominent feature. The patches, or thumbprints, coalesce rapidly within days to weeks. The amount of retinitis usually extends 360 degrees to involve the entire periphery (Figs. 61–4, 61–5, and 61–6). There have been reports of the retinitis limited to only one to two quadrants.[23] This is thought to represent a milder form of the syndrome. Although peripheral coalescence is common, posterior progression is relatively uncommon, with the retinitis often sparing the macular region. The involved retina is thicker than uninvolved and an exudative retinal detachment can occur with active retinitis.[13]

Regression of the active retinitis begins 2 weeks to 1 month subsequent to the initial infection. The areas of retinitis initially become more transparent in perivascular locations. This gives a characteristic "Swiss cheese" appearance to the involved retina. Progressive retinal pigmentation follows this phase, beginning at the posterior border of the lesions. From this point, regression proceeds rapidly.[24]

A moderate to severe vitreitis occurs early in the disease. The vitreitis is initially composed of mononuclear inflammatory cells.[12] As the course of the syndrome progresses, the vitreitis typically worsens. This is thought to be secondary to sloughing of necrotic retina.[25] With time, there is organization of the vitreous with formation of fibrotic bands. These bands play a prominent role in the pathogenesis of subsequent rhegmatogenous retinal detachments.

The vasculitis seen in ARN is occlusive, involving the arterioles primarily.[13] Sheathing and narrowing of the involved vessels are seen in the peripheral retina. Arteriolar occlusion and nonperfusion may be visible in some instances. The vasculitis can involve either the entire retina or only areas with active retinitis. The obliterative nature of the vasculitis is best appreciated by fluorescein angiography (Figs. 61–7 and 61–8).

Some degree of optic nerve involvement occurs in most patients with ARN; however, only a minority will have severe dysfunction that accounts for visual impairment. These patients present with profound visual loss early in the course of their disease. Other indicators of optic nerve dysfunction are present; including a relative afferent pupillary defect, dyschromatopsia, and central visual field loss. Clinically the disc is swollen and hyperemic. Optic nerve enlargement can be documented by computed tomography (CT) scanning. It has been proposed that the etiology of the neuropathy is secondary to direct ischemic necrosis as well as compression from loculated exudate within the optic nerve sheath.[26,27]

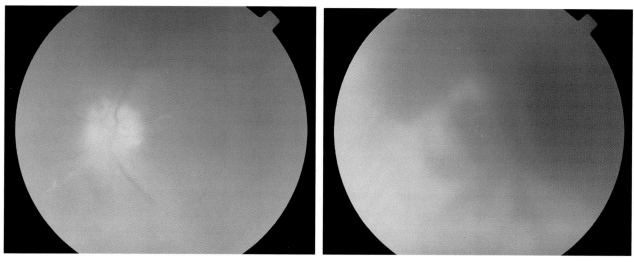

FIGURE 61-2   FIGURE 61-3

FIGURES 61-2 and 61-3   Fundus findings in patient with concomminant HSV encephalitis and the ARN syndrome. There is a hazy view of the posterior pole secondary to the vitritis in Figure 61-2. Examination of the peripheral retina revealed well demarcated areas of retinal whitening consistent with the ARN syndrome.

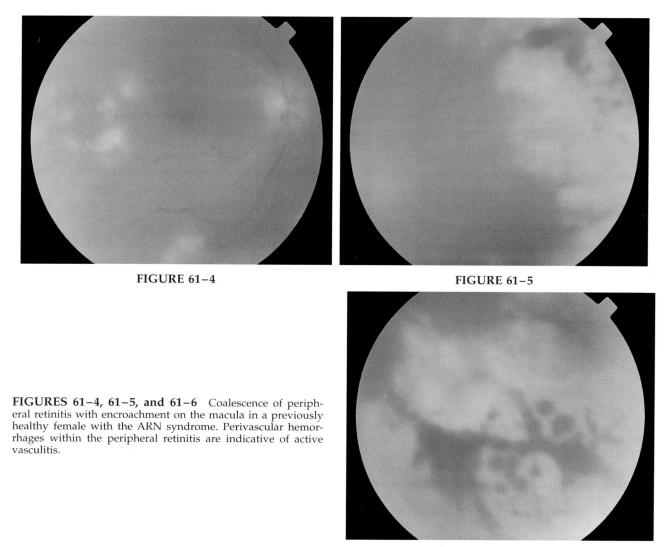

FIGURE 61-4   FIGURE 61-5

FIGURES 61-4, 61-5, and 61-6   Coalescence of peripheral retinitis with encroachment on the macula in a previously healthy female with the ARN syndrome. Perivascular hemorrhages within the peripheral retinitis are indicative of active vasculitis.

FIGURE 61-6

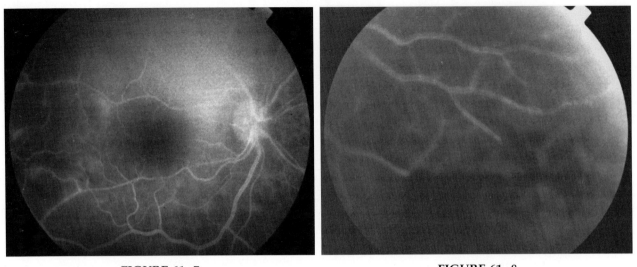

FIGURE 61–7   FIGURE 61–8

FIGURES 61–7 and 61–8   Fluorescein angiogram of the patient in Figures 61–4, 61–5, and 61–6. Perivascular staining of the vessels is present in the temporal macula. In the peripheral retina, there is hypofluorescence secondary to blockage from overlying hemorrhage, as well as evidence of vascular occlusion.

Etiology and Diagnosis

Viral involvement as the etiology of the ARN syndrome was definitively shown in 1982 by Culbertson et al.[12] In an enucleated eye with the characteristic clinical findings of the syndrome, electron microscopy demonstrated viral particles within all layers of the retina. The configuration of these particles was consistent with members of the herpesvirus family. Varicella zoster virus was the first herpes virus to be isolated by culture.[5] Subsequently, herpes simplex virus type 1,[4,25] varicella virus (chickenpox),[6,28] and herpes simplex virus type 2[7] have all been implicated in the syndrome. Cytomegalovirus (CMV) was thought to be the responsible etiology in one case of bilateral ARN[29]; however, the electron microscopic findings were not typical for CMV retinitis and there has not been further evidence of CMV involvement in the recent literature.

The initiation of viral involvement in the syndrome appears to be reactivation of a latent infection involving the varicella zoster virus. Supporting evidence for reactivation includes multiple cases of herpes zoster dermatitis preceding the development of the ARN syndrome.[20,21] It is also well known that the majority of the adult population harbors latent herpesvirus in neural ganglions from which reactivation leads to dermatitis. However, the stimulus that initiates reactivation is a mystery, since the vast majority of patients with the syndrome are healthy and immunocompetent. Whether the virus gains entry to the eye via neural or hematogenous routes after reactivation remains an unanswered question.

Evidence for a neural route exists in multiple animal models that exhibit controlateral retinitis after injection of virus into the ipsilateral anterior chamber.[30] Travel along the optic nerve in a retrograde fashion has been documented in these models.[31] Magnetic resonance imaging (MRI) has also demonstrated enhancement among multiple cranial nerves in a patient who developed ARN subsequent to an episode of contralateral herpes zoster ophthalmicus.[32] Evidence for a hematogenous route includes the high incidence of bilaterality (approximately one third) in the syndrome, which would be unlikely if transmission was via neural pathways. The early multifocal areas of deep retinal whitening are also more consistent with a bloodborne infection. Perhaps the most compelling evidence against a neural route in humans is the absence of viral particles in the optic nerve in histologic studies of enucleated eyes.[5,12,13]

In the cases of the ARN syndrome associated with the remaining members of the herpesvirus family, initiation of the syndrome can be secondary to reactivation or as a sequelae of the concurrent infection. Reactivation of congenital infection appears to be the initiating event in cases of herpes simplex virus type 2–associated ARN.[7] When herpes virus type 1 is involved, the mechanism has been shown either to be secondary to reactivation of a latent infection or as a sequelae of a primary infection.[4,25] ARN syndrome associated with primary varicella virus infection (chickenpox) is a sequelae of the concurrent systemic infection.[6,28]

The ARN syndrome is a clinical diagnosis that is usually made without difficulty. On occasion, the vitreous inflammation can be severe enough to obscure the characteristic peripheral findings. When this occurs, ancillary tests can be very useful to differentiate the syndrome from other inflammatory and infectious disorders (see Table 61–1). Acute and convalescent serum antibody titers have not been helpful in detecting evidence of herpetic in-

TABLE 61–1 Differential Diagnosis for the Acute Retinal Necrosis Syndrome

Behçet's disease
Syphilis
Cytomegalovirus retinitis
Sarcoidosis
Ocular large cell lymphoma
Toxoplasmosis
Candida endophthalmitis

volvement in the syndrome. In a recent review of the literature, only 39% of the cases had a diagnostic increase or decrease in serum antibody levels to herpesvirus upon serial sampling.[33] This disappointing yield is most likely secondary to the inability of a localized infection to affect systemic antibody titers. When intraocular antibody levels are paired with serum levels, the diagnostic yield increases to somewhere between 57[34] and 76%.[33] However, timing of the collection is crucial and samples taken early or late in the disease course may fail to demonstrate adequate antibody levels. The most promising diagnostic test appears to be the polymerase chain reaction (PCR). This highly sensitive test utilizes gene amplification to detect viral DNA from the aqueous humor. It has recently been shown to detect herpesvirus genome in the aqueous humor from three out of four patients with the syndrome.[35] With increased availability, PCR may prove to be the most valuable diagnostic aid with atypical cases.

Histopathology

Light microscopic examination of enucleated eyes with the ARN syndrome has shown involvement of virtually all ocular structures. The cornea shows keratic precipitates consisting of macrophages, lymphocytes, and polymorphonuclear leukocytes located on the endothelium. The iris is infiltrated with plasma cells and eosinophils and can display a prominent perivasculitis in certain areas. Similar chronic inflammatory cells are also present within the trabecular meshwork, ciliary processes, zonules, and pars plana epithelium.[5,12]

The posterior segment shows a full-thickness retinal necrosis in affected areas. Necrotic retina and inflammatory cells spill into the vitreous in areas overlying the necrosis. There is a sharp demarcation between involved and uninvolved retina. The only remaining identifiable retinal structure in areas of necrosis is the skeletal framework of the retinal blood vessels.[5,12,13] Eosinophilic intranuclear and intracytoplasmic inclusions may be identified within the ganglion cell layer and inner nuclear layer of preserved retina. Adjacent retinal pigment

epithelium cells can show similar inclusions.[5,12] Retinal and choroidal vessels show an intense perivascular cellular infiltration consisting of lymphocytes and plasma cells. The endothelial cells of the vessels are swollen and may occlude the lumen. Cellular thrombi may also occlude the lumens of the vessels. The choroid is markedly swollen by cellular infiltration, and may be thickened many times its normal size. There may be zones of granulomatous inflammation noted within the choroid. The optic nerve can be necrotic and infiltrated with plasma cells. The perivascular location of inflammatory cells is also noted within the nerve.[13]

Electron microscopy of affected eyes confirms the presence of extracellular, intracellular, and intranuclear viral particles within all layers of the retina. These viral particles can also be found within the vascular endothelium. Intranuclear particles show a configuration of hexagonal nucleocapsids measuring 80 to 100 nm with a dense central nucleus. Intracytoplasmic particles are fully enveloped and measure 180 to 220 nm in diameter. The above dimensions are consistent with members of the herpesvirus family.[12]

Complications

The most serious and sight-threatening complication of the ARN syndrome is the development of retinal detachment, seen in approximately 75% of eyes with the syndrome.[8] Typically these detachments occur 2 to 3 months after the initial presentation of the syndrome. Organization of the cellular vitreous occurs after regression of the inflammatory stages. This leads to the formation of fibrotic bands within the vitreous that can exert significant tractional forces on the retina. Large retinal holes develop within necrotic retina and at the junction of necrotic and normal retina. The combination of the large retinal holes and tractional vitreous bands leads to complex retinal detachments that are not easily repairable. In addition, the cellular vitreous also contributes to the high incidence of proliferative vitreoretinopathy that is present in most detachments.[36]

Another infrequent complication of the ARN syndrome is the formation of retinal and optic disc neovascularization. Both retinal ischemia and severe intraocular inflammation have been postulated as the causative factors for the neovascularization.[37] The neovascularization has been shown to regress following vitrectomy and panretinal photocoagulation.[37,38]

Treatment

Treatment of the ARN syndrome involves controlling the initial inflammatory/infectious stage and subsequently preventing or repairing the retinal detachments that occur in the cicatricial stage.

Antiviral Therapy

Acyclovir (9-2[2-hydroxyethoxymethyl] guanine; acycloguanosine) is the mainstay of medical treatment for active ARN syndrome. Acyclovir is a nucleoside analog that has potent in vitro activity against herpes simplex virus 1, herpes simplex virus 2, and varicella zoster virus. It selectively targets infected cells only by requiring a virally encoded enzyme, thymidine kinase, to phosphorylate it into an active form, acyclovir monophosphate. After a series of cellular reactions, acyclovir monophosphate is further phosphorylated into acyclovir triphosphate, which is a specific inhibitor of herpesvirus DNA polymerase. The efficacy of intravenous acyclovir in treating ARN syndrome was initially shown by Blumenkranz et al in 1986[24] and has since been confirmed by other studies.[39] In both of the aforementioned studies, acyclovir accelerated regression of pre-existing areas of retinitis and prevented progression of the same lesions. Regression typically began 4 days after initiation of acyclovir therapy and was complete on an average of 33 days after therapy was begun. No new lesions were noted after 48 hours of treatment. Another important benefit of acyclovir therapy is protection of the fellow eye. In untreated eyes with the syndrome, there is an approximate 34% rate of bilaterality.[8] In treated eyes, there is a documented decrease in the incidence of bilateral involvement.[24] One series of patients utilized a survival analysis and showed 87.1% of treated patients to be disease free in the fellow eye at last examination as compared to only 30.4% of untreated patients.[16]

The current recommended dose for initial treatment of the ARN syndrome with intravenous acyclovir is 1500 mg/m^2/day divided into three daily doses. The duration of treatment if 7 to 10 days. Following intravenous therapy, an extended course of oral acyclovir is recommended to protect against reactivation of latent virus. Because the risk of bilateral involvement is greatest in the first 14 weeks, the recommended dose and length of time for oral therapy is 800 mg five times daily for 14 weeks.[16] Prophylaxis longer than 14 weeks is of uncertain value and currently not recommended.

Anti-inflammatory Therapy

Anti-inflammatory therapy, in the form of oral corticosteroids, is beneficial in treating the ARN syndrome for multiple reasons. The most prominent effect of steroids is decreasing the degree of vitreous cellular infiltrate. This should decrease the incidence of vitreous traction band formation, with subsequent decrease in the incidence of retinal detachment formation. With retinal vasculitis playing an important role in the early stages of the syndrome, corticosteriod treatment may help to limit the extent of the vasculitic damage.

Prednisone is the recommended corticosteroid for use in the syndrome. The dose is approximately 1 mg/kg per day given in one daily dose. At least 24 hours of acyclovir therapy should precede the initiation of steriod therapy to prevent the exacerbation of the herpetic infection. Duration of treatment is variable depending on the extent of inflammation and response of treatment.

Antithrombotic Therapy

There is evidence of platelet dysfunction in patients with the ARN syndrome, and this may play a role in the obliterative nature of the vasculitis. One series of cases found platelet hyperaggregation in six of seven patients examined with the syndrome.[40] Treatment with 500 mg/day of aspirin is recommended to reverse the hyperaggregation.

Retinal Detachment Prophylaxis and Treatment

Although acyclovir treatment has been shown to decrease the progression of retinitis, it has no effect on the rate of retinal detachment.[24] Because retinal detachment is the major cause of ocular morbidity in the syndrome, attempts have been made to prevent its occurrence. Clarkson et al were the first to suggest photocoagulation as a form of detachment prophylaxis after noting the difficulty involved in repairing ARN-associated detachments.[36] Since that time, two series of patients have noted favorable outcomes when utilizing peripheral photocoagulation as a form of prohylaxis. Han et al performed laser photocoagulation on five eyes with the ARN syndrome, and all five were attached over a mean follow-up of 15 months.[41] Sternberg et al performed a retrospective review of eyes with the ARN syndrome treated with and without laser photocoagulation.[42] Out of 19 eyes, 12 were photocoagulated and 7 were not. The incidence of retinal detachment in the treated group was 17% as compared to 67% in the untreated group. However, photocoagulation was able to be performed only in eyes with less vitreous opacification, so the more severely involved eyes were selectively placed in the untreated group. These more severely affected eyes may have a higher incidence of retinal detachment regardless of prophylactic treatment.

It is recommended that prophylactic photocoagulation be performed as quickly as possible in patients with the ARN syndrome. The timing of photocoagulation is critical owing to the early occurrence of retinal tears in the syndrome as well as progressive vitreous opacification that may obscure the view posteriorly and prevent placement of photocoagulation.[41] Argon or krypton laser is recommended using 200 to 500-μm spot size. Power is varied to achieve a white retinal burn. Two to three rows of burns should be applied posterior to all areas of involved retina. Additional photocoagulation may have to be applied if the retinitis progresses through the area of prior treatment.[42]

The initial incidence of retinal detachment in the ARN syndrome was established by Fisher et al as 75%.[8] Early attempts at repair utilizing scleral buckling procedures were uniformly unsuccessful. A review of all cases in the literature prior to 1982 revealed a reattachment rate of only 22%.[8] In 1984, Clarkson et al advocated the use of primary vitrectomy procedures in the repair of ARN-associated detachments.[24] Out of 16 eyes with detachments, 10 retinas were reattached at last follow-up. Eight of the ten retinas that were attached received vitreous surgery at some point during their course of treatment. The high incidence of failure associated with primary buckling procedures is thought to be secondary to continued vitreous traction and proliferative vitreoretinopathy.[36] Blumenkranz et al further refined the role of primary vitrectomy in repairing these detachments by utilizing fluid-gas exchange and endolaser without a scleral buckle.[43] They successfully reattached six out of six retinas and achieved a final visual acuity of 20/40 or better in three patients. Directly comparing eyes treated with combined buckling/vitrectomy procedures versus vitrectomy/fluid-gas exchange/endolaser procedures failed to show a statistically significant difference in reattachment rate.[44] However, eyes that underwent conventional buckling/vitrectomy procedures did have an increased incidence of reoperations and postoperative complications. Infusion of intravitreal acyclovir has been advocated by some authors as an adjuvant during the time of surgical repair.[45,46] The intravitreal acyclovir combined with preoperative intravenous acyclovir theoretically increases the concentration of the drug available to the infected cells.

PROGRESSIVE OUTER RETINAL NECROSIS SYNDROME

The PORN syndrome has thus far only been described in patients with the acquired immunodeficiency syndrome (AIDS).[47,48] The syndrome is most likely a forme fruste of the ARN syndrome seen in severely immunocompromised patients, but there does appear to be enough unique clinical characteristics to warrant its own identity. The clinical course of the syndrome is characterized by unrelenting progression of the retinitis, which is typically unresponsive to antiviral treatment.

Epidemiology

The PORN syndrome has thus far only been described in patients that are immunocompromised. The vast majority of the cases are in patients with AIDS. The degree of immunosuppression is typically severe with a median CD4 lymphocyte count of 21 cells/mm^3 in one series.[49] There has been one published report of the syndrome occurring in a patient immunosuppressed secondary to cyclophosphamide and prednisone therapy.[50] However, the clinical signs were not classic for the syndrome, and the case may have represented a variant of another infectious retinitis. Approximately 75% of patients will have only unilateral involvement on presentation, but bilateral involvement eventually occurs in 71% of the same patients.[49]

Clinical Symptoms and Signs

The presenting symptoms for the PORN syndrome include decreased visual acuity and constricted visual fields. Ocular pain is not common. Up to two thirds of patients will give a history of antecedent or concomitant cutaneous zoster infection. The median onset of the syndrome from the development of cutaneous zoster is approximately 2 months.[49]

Anterior Segment

The anterior segment is conspicuously quiet in eyes with the PORN syndrome. There may be a mild anterior chamber reaction, but granulomatous changes are not seen.[47-49] This is in contrast to the ARN syndrome, where a moderate to severe anterior chamber reaction almost universally is present.

Posterior Segment

The posterior pole also shows an absence of a prominent inflammatory reaction. Trace vitreous cells may be present, but in most instances the vitreous cavity is quiet. This most likely is a reflection of the patient's overall severe immunosuppression. Multifocal deep retinal lesions are noted throughout the fundus (Figs. 61–9, 61–10, and 61–11). These lesions are characteristically located only in the outer retina on presentation. They are sharply demarcated and lack the granular borders typically seen in cytomegalovirus retinitis. Approximately one third of the affected eyes can present with the outer retinal lesions present in the macula (Figs. 61–12 and 61–13).[49] Retinal swelling within the macula can give a cherry red spot appearance.[48] The retinal lesions progress rapidly to eventually involve the entire retina. With progression, the retinitis becomes full thickness and the macula is invariably involved. Initial regression of the retinal lesions begins perivascularly, and gives a characteristic "cracked mud" appearance.

The retinal vasculature is normal to minimally involved in the syndrome. The vasculopathy included sheathing or occlusion, but is limited only to areas with active retinitis.[49] Fluorescein angiography shows retinitis limited to the outer retina,

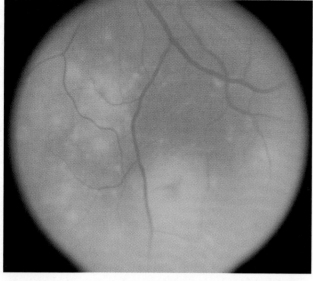

FIGURE 61–9

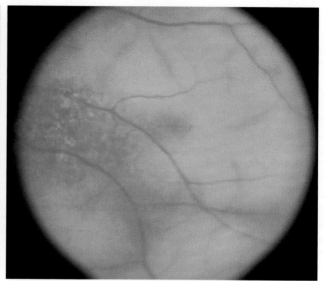

FIGURE 61–10

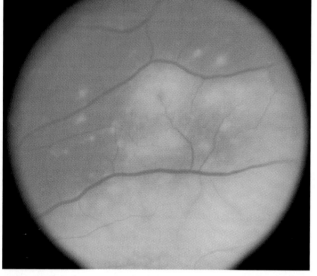

FIGURE 61–11

FIGURES 61–9, 61–10, and 61–11   Multifocal deep retinal infiltrates in a patient with the PORN syndrome.

and confirms the lack of vasculitis (Figs. 61–14 and 61–15).

Optic nerve hyperemia and swelling is seen in a minority of patients. An associated relative afferent pupillary defect is also noted but may be more of an indicator of retinal dysfunction rather than nerve involvement.[49]

Etiology and Diagnosis

Varicella zoster virus has to date been the only virus positively diagnosed as the etiologic agent responsible for the PORN syndrome. Growth of the virus has been documented from an enucleated eye[48] as well as from a retinal biopsy.[49] Other methods of identifying etiologic agents including transmission electron microscopy,[47,49] indirect immunofluorescence,[49] and PCR[47] have also confirmed

varicella zoster virus involvement. More indirect evidence is the high rate of antecedent or concurrent zoster dermatitis in affected patients.

The diagnosis of the PORN syndrome is made clinically and ancillary tests are usually not necessary. The differential diagnosis includes the ARN syndrome, cytomegalovirus retinitis, and toxoplasma retinitis. Differentiating these clinical entities from the PORN syndrome typically is not difficult secondary to the syndrome's characteristic presentation.

Histopathology

Light microscopy of enucleated eyes with the PORN syndrome show normal anterior segments. The retina shows areas of full-thickness necrosis. The necrosis is more marked in the outer nuclear

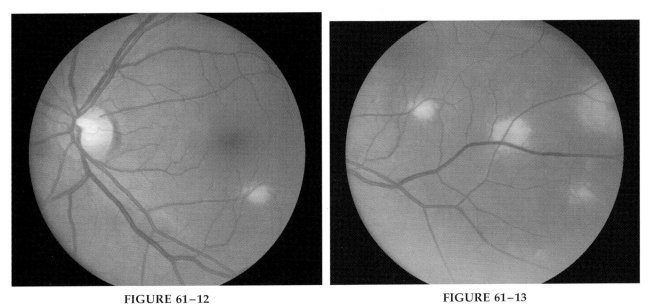

FIGURE 61–12   **FIGURE 61–13**

FIGURES 61–12 and 61–13 Early macular involvement in a patient with the PORN syndrome. (Photo courtesy of Michael J. Diesenhouse, M.D.)

layer. There is choroidal inflammation consisting of lymphocytic cells that can be full thickness or only involve the choriocapillaris. The choroidal inflammation is not spatially related to the retinal inflammation. Lymphocytic infiltration and necrosis of the optic nerve are also present.[48]

Transmission electron microscopy has identified nonenveloped and larger enveloped viral particles within the nuclei of photoreceptors in affected eyes. The nonenveloped particles have a diameter of approximately 80 to 100 nm. The morphology of the viral particles is consistent with the herpesvirus family.[47,48]

Prognosis and Treatment

The overall prognosis of eyes with the PORN syndrome is dismal. Progression of the retinal lesions almost invariably occurs regardless of the antiviral treatment. Antiviral treatment has included intravenous acyclovir, ganciclovir, and combination therapy. Progression of the syndrome occurred in approximately 75% of eyes receiving either intravenous acyclovir or ganciclovir.[49] Combination therapy utilizing both intravenous acyclovir (10 mg/kg every 8 hours) and foscarnet (60 mg/kg every 12 hours) appears to be more promising. Two

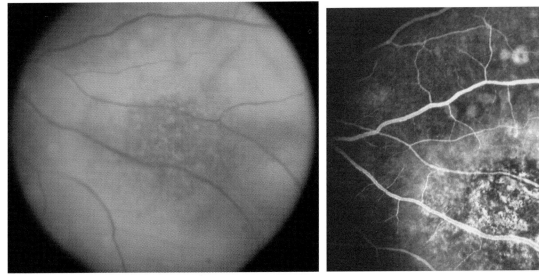

FIGURE 61–14   **FIGURE 61–15**

FIGURES 61–14 and 61–15 Lack of vasculitic changes on fluorescein angiography in the PORN syndrome. Also note the retinitis located in the outer retina.

patients treated with this combination showed slowing or quiescence of disease.[49] Other combinations of antiviral therapy including intravitreal ganciclovir and oral sorivudine[51] as well as intravenous ganciclovir and oral acyclovir have been reported to successfully stop the progression of the syndrome.

Similar to the ARN syndrome, retinal detachments occur in approximately 70% of eyes with the PORN syndrome. However, the tractional component of the detachments and high incidence of proliferative vitreoretinopathy are not seen in the PORN syndrome. This is secondary to the almost nonexistent vitreous reaction in the syndrome. Prophylactic laser photocoagulation does not appear to be helpful in preventing the detachments.[49]

In the largest published series of eyes with the syndrome, 67% achieved a final visual acuity of no light perception (NLP). The median time from diagnosis to NLP was 4 weeks. Final visual acuity was not related to either the extent of disease on presentation, response to treatment, or development of a retinal detachment.[49]

SUMMARY

The ARN and PORN syndromes are recently recognized infectious viral syndromes of the retina caused by members of the herpesvirus family. Although the two syndromes have the same infectious etiology (i.e., herpesvirus family members), their clinical features, including appearance and disease course, are uniquely different. This difference is most likely secondary to the extreme immunosuppression found in patients with the PORN syndrome. Thus, classic presentations of the ARN and PORN syndromes can be thought of as different ends of the spectrum of the same disease. However, their distinction as separate syndromes is of importance for both prognostic and treatment considerations.

Initial treatment for the ARN syndrome has been standardized, and control of the retinitis component of the syndrome can usually be achieved with acyclovir therapy. The major challenge in treatment of the syndrome lies in management of the ensuing retinal detachment. Prophylaxis with laser photocoagulation and newer microsurgical techniques involved in repair of the detachments have improved the eventual outcome of these eyes. However, the syndrome continues to carry a poor prognosis secondary to the high incidence of retinal detachment.

With the advent of the AIDS epidemic, the PORN syndrome only recently has been recognized. Unlike the ARN syndrome, control of the retinitis component of the syndrome has not been achieved successfully with conventional antiviral therapy. The syndrome shows relentless progression and a retinal detachment rate similar to the ARN syndrome. The inability to control the retinitis is either a reflection of the patient's severe immunosuppression or due to the emergence of resistant viral strains. Further experience is treating the syndrome is needed to help find a more successful treatment regimen.

REFERENCES

1. Holland GN: Standard diagnostic criteria for the acute retinal necrosis syndrome. Am J Ophthalmol 117:663–666, 1994.
2. Jabs DA, Schachat AP, Liss R, et al: Presumed varicella zoster retinitis in immunocompromised patients. Retina 7:9–13, 1987.
3. Friberg TR, Jost BF: Acute retinal necrosis in an immunocompromised patient. Am J Ophthalmol 98:515–517, 1982.
4. Lewis LL, Culbertson WW, Post JD, et al: Herpes simplex virus 1 a cause of the acute retinal necrosis syndrome. Ophthalmology 96:875–878, 1989,
5. Culbertson WW, Blumenkranz MS, Pepose JS, et al: Varicella zoster virus is a cause of the acute retinal necrosis syndrome. Ophthalmology 93:559–569, 1986.
6. Culbertson WW, Brod RD, Flynn HW, et al: Chickenpox-associated acute retinal necrosis syndrome. Ophthalmology 98:1641–1646, 1991.
7. Thompson WS, Culbertson WW, Smiddy WE, et al: Acute retinal necrosis caused by reactivation of herpes simplex virus type 2. Am J Ophthalmol 118:205–211, 1994.
8. Fisher JP, Lewis ML, Blumenkranz M, et al: The acute retinal necrosis syndrome. Ophthalmology 89:1309–1316, 1982.
9. Urayama A, Yamada N, Sasaki T: Unilateral acute uveitis with periarteritis and detachment. Jpn J Clin Ophthalmol 25:607–619, 1971.
10. Willerson D Jr, Aaberg TM, Reeser FH: Necrotizing vaso-occlusive retinitis. Am J Ophthalmol 84:209–219, 1977.
11. Young NJA, Bird AC: Bilateral acute retinal necrosis. Br J Ophthalmol 62:581–590, 1978.
12. Culbertson WW, Blumenkranz MS, Haynes H, et al: The acute retinal necrosis syndrome part 2: histopathology and etiology. Ophthalmology 89:1317–1325, 1982.
13. Duker JS, Blumenkranz MS: Diagnosis and management of the acute retinal necrosis syndrome. Surv Ophthalmol 35:327–343, 1991.
14. Nussenblatt RB, Palestine AG: Uveitis: Fundamentals and Clinical Practice. Chicago, Year Book Medical, 1989, p 411.
15. Holland GN, Cornell PJ, Park MS, et al: An association between acute retinal necrosis syndrome and HLA-DQw7 and phenotype Bw62,DR4. Am J Ophthalmol 108:370–374, 1989.
16. Palay DA, Sternberg P Jr, Davis J, et al: Decrease in the risk of bilateral acute retinal necrosis by acyclovir therapy. Am J Ophthalmol 112:250–255, 1991.
17. Rabinovitch T, Nozik RA, Varenhorst, MP: Bilateral acute retinal necrosis syndrome. Am J Ophthalmol 108:735–736, 1989.
18. Martinez J, Lambert HM, Capone A, et al: Delayed bilateral involvement in the acute retinal necrosis syndrome. Am J Ophthalmol 113:103–104, 1992.
19. Falcone PM, Brockhurst RJ: Delayed onset of bilateral acute retinal necrosis syndrome: a 34-year interval. Ann Ophthalmol 25:373–374, 1993.
20. Browning DJ, Blumenkranz MS, Culbertson WW, et al: Association of varicella zoster dermatitis with the acute retinal necrosis syndrome. Ophthalmology 94:602–606, 1987.
21. Yeo JH, Pepose JS, Stewart JS, et al: Acute retinal necrosis syndrome following herpes zoster dermatitis. Ophthalmology 93:1418–1422, 1986.
22. Sternberg P Jr, Knox DL, Finkelstein D, et al: Acute retinal necrosis syndrome. Retina 2:145–151, 1982.
23. Matsuo M, Nakayama T, Koyama T, et al: A proposed mild

type of acute retinal necrosis syndrome. Am J Ophthalmol 105:579–583, 1988.

24. Blumenkranz MS, Culbertson WW, Clarkson JG, Dix R: Treatment of the acute retinal necrosis syndrome with intravenous acyclovir. Ophthalmology 93:296–300, 1986.

25. Duker JS, Nielsen JC, Eagle RC, et al: Rapidly progressive acute retinal necrosis secondary to herpes simplex virus, type 1. Ophthalmology 97:1638–1643, 1990.

26. Sergott RC, Belmont JB, Savino PJ, et al: Optic nerve involvement in the acute retinal necrosis syndrome. Arch Ophthalmol 103:1160–1164, 1985.

27. Sergott RC, Anand R, Belmont JB, et al: Acute retinal necrosis neuropathy. Arch Ophthalmol 107:692–696, 1989.

28. Barondes MJ, Telez F, Siegel A: Acute retinal necrosis after chickenpox in a healthy adult. Ann Ophthalmol 24:335–336, 1992.

29. Rungger-Brandle E, Roux L, Leuenberger PM: Bilateral acute retinal necrosis (barn). Ophthalmology 91:1648–1658, 1984.

30. Whittum JA, McCulley JP, Niederkorn JY, Streilein JW: Ocular disease induced in mice by anterior chamber inoculation of herpes simplex virus. Invest Ophthalmol Vis Sci 30:1065–1073, 1984.

31. Bosem ME, Harris R, Atheron SS: Optic nerve involvement in virus spread in HSV-1 retinitis. Invest Ophthalmol Vis Sci 31:1683–1689, 1990.

32. Farrell TA, Wolf MD, Folk JC, et al: Magnetic resonance imaging in a patient with herpes zoster keratouveitis and contralateral acute retinal necrosis. Am J Ophthalmol 112:735–736, 1991.

33. Pepose JS, Flowers B, Stewart JA, et al: Herpesvirus antibody levels in the etiologic diagnosis of the acute retinal necrosis syndrome. Am J Ophthalmol 113:248–256, 1992.

34. de Boer JH, Luyendijk L, Rothova A, et al: Detection of intraocular antibody production to herpesvirus in acute retinal necrosis syndrome. Am J Ophthalmol 117:201–210, 1994.

35. Nishi M, Hanashiro R, Mori S, et al: Polymerase chain reaction for the detection of the varicella-zoster genome in ocular samples from patients with acute retinal necrosis. Am J Ophthalmol 114:603–609, 1992.

36. Clarkson JG, Blumenkranz MS, Culbertson WW, et al: Retinal detachment following the acute retinal necrosis syndrome. Ophthalmology 91:1665–1668, 1984.

37. Wang C, Kaplan HJ, Waldrep C, Pulliam M: Retinal neovascularization associated with acute retinal necrosis. Retina 3:249–252, 1983.

38. Han DP, Abrams GW, Williams GA: Regression of disc neovascularization by photocoagulation in the acute retinal necrosis syndrome. Retina 8:244–246, 1988.

39. Crapotta JA, Freeman WR, Feldman RM, et al: Visual outcome in acute retinal necrosis. Retina 13:208–213, 1993.

40. Ando F, Kato M, Goto S, et al: Platelet function in bilateral acute retinal necrosis. Am J Ophthalmol 96:27–32, 1983.

41. Han DP, Lewis H, Williams GA, et al: Laser photocoagulation in the acute retinal necrosis syndrome. Arch Ophthalmol 105:1051–1054, 1987.

42. Sternberg P Jr, Han DP, Yeo JH, et al: Photocoagulation to prevent retinal detachment in acute retinal necrosis. Ophthalmology 95:1389–1393, 1988.

43. Blumenkranz M, Clarkson J, Culbertson WW, et al: Vitrectomy for retinal detachment associated with acute retinal necrosis. Am J Ophthalmol 106:426–429, 1988.

44. Blumenkranz M, Clarkson J, Culbertson WW, et al: Visual results and complications after retinal reattachment in the acute retinal necrosis syndrome. Retina 9:170–174, 1989.

45. Peyman GA, Goldberg MF, Uninsky E, et al: Vitrectomy and intravitreal antiviral drug therapy in acute retinal necrosis syndrome. Arch Ophthalmol 102:1618–1621, 1984.

46. Carney MD, Peyman GA, Goldberg MF, et al: Acute retinal necrosis. Retina 6:85–94, 1986.

47. Forster DJ, Dugel PU, Frangieh GT, et al: Rapidly progressive outer retinal necrosis in the acquired immunodeficiency syndrome. Am J Ophthalmol 110:341–348, 1990.

48. Margolis TP, Lowder CY, Holland GN, et al: Varicellazoster virus retinitis in patients with the acquired immunodeficiency syndrome. Am J Ophthalmol 112:119–131, 1991.

49. Engstrom RE, Holland GN, Margolis TP, et al: The progressive outer retinal necrosis syndrome. Ophthalmology 101:1488–1502, 1994.

50. Duker JS, Shakin EP: Rapidly progressive outer retinal necrosis in the acquired immunodeficiency syndrome. Am J Ophthalmol 11:255–256, 1991.

51. Pinnolis MK, Foxworthy D, Kemp B: Treatment of progressive outer retinal necrosis with sorivudine. Am J Ophthalmol 119:516–517, 1995.

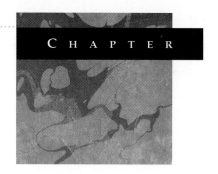

CHAPTER 62

Acute Retinal Necrosis

Mark S. Blumenkranz, M.D.
Gregory Fox, M.D.

Acute retinal necrosis is a fulminant viral infection of the eye caused by members of the herpes hominis family, primarily but not exclusively affecting the posterior segment.[1-7] The American Uveitis Society has proposed specific diagnostic criteria for the designation "acute retinal necrosis," which include peripheral retinal necrosis with discrete borders, rapid progression with circumferential spread in untreated eyes, occlusive vasculopathy with arteriolar involvement, and prominent inflammation in the vitreous and anterior chamber.[8] Additional features commonly encountered in this syndrome include optic neuropathy, granulomatous keratic precipitates, scleritis, and pain.

If untreated, the disease almost invariably leads to blindness through several mechanisms including infectious infiltration of the posterior retina, optic neuropathy, optic atrophy, and, in more than three quarters of patients, late retinal detachment with associated proliferative vitreoretinopathy. Additionally, without treatment, more than two thirds of patients will develop disease in the fellow eye.[1,2,5,6] Treatment is beneficial in this syndrome including intravenous acyclovir for disease amelioration in the involved eye, and prevention in the fellow eye,[9-13] photocoagulation to reduce the risk of retinal detachment in the involved eye,[14] and vitrectomy to repair complex retinal detachment.[12]

Although herpes simplex virus has been demonstrated to be a cause for acute retinal necrosis,[7] it is thought that most cases are caused by reactivation of latent herpes varicella zoster virus.[3,15] In some patients a mild form of acute retinal necrosis may immediately follow the development of chicken pox, which is also caused by herpes varicella zoster virus.[16-18] Acute retinal necrosis has been reported in conjunction with shingles caused by herpes varicella zoster virus as well.[19] A particularly virulent form of retinal necrosis, termed pro-

gressive outer retinal necrosis (PORN), is produced by herpes varicella zoster virus in patients with human immunodeficiency virus (HIV) infection.[20,21] Although an infrequent condition, the incidence of acute retinal necrosis appears to be rising, with a recent estimate of 4.25 per 1 million inhabitants per year noted in Switzerland between January 1990 and March 1993.[22]

CLINICAL FEATURES

Necrotizing Retinitis

The hallmark of the disease is the presence of confluent zones of opaque necrotizing retinitis (Fig. 62–1). Initially the lesions may be subtle, consisting of granular patches or small, round, nummular opacities depending upon the stage of evolution. These generally occur in the equatorial or preequatorial regions and progress in a circumferential as well as posterior direction to form larger confluent patches of wider yellow-white opacities. Depending upon the severity of the disease process and the time of initiation of antiviral therapy, the lesions may be as small as 1 or 2 clock hours, or may completely encircle the retinal periphery over 360 degrees. With treatment and/or time, the lesions regress with the retina becoming markedly atrophic in zones of prior infection, although regaining its normal transparency. The underlying retinal pigment epithelium becomes atrophic as well. The pattern of regression generally occurs at the most posterior extent of the lesions and progresses in an anterior fashion. Patterns of early regression may also be seen adjacent to retinal vessels leading to the so-called paravascular lucencies, or "Swiss cheese" configuration seen in many patients with this condition (Fig. 62–2).

HISTOPATHOLOGICAL FEATURES

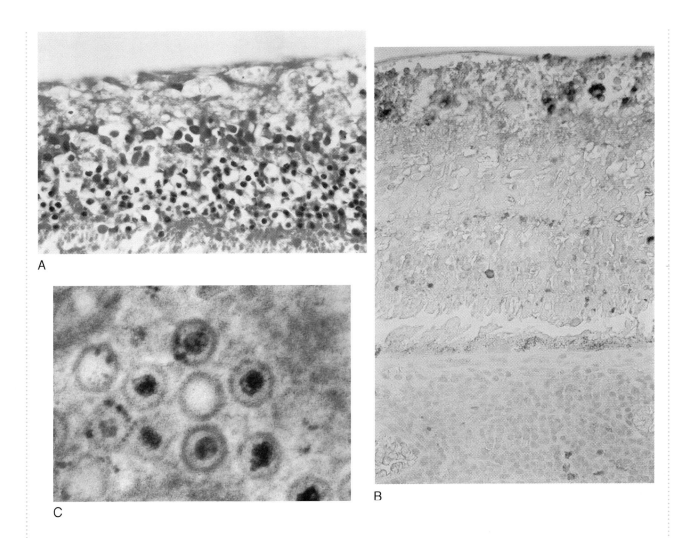

A, Area of early retinal necrosis in a patient with acute retinal necrosis. Some neurons have eosinophilic intranuclear inclusions. (From Gass JDM: Eastern Ophthalmic Pathology Society Meeting, Bermuda, October 1–4, 1981, with permission.) *B,* Area of retina with positive immunoperoxidase staining for herpes zoster in a patient with acute retinal necrosis. (Courtesy of Dr. Jay Pepose.) *C,* Electron microscopic appearance of viral particles in retinal neuron from a patient with acute retinal necrosis. (Courtesy of Dr. Jay Pepose.)

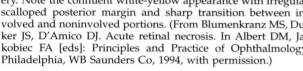

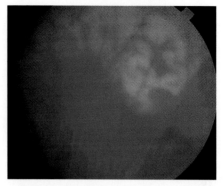

FIGURE 62–1 Typical lesion of ARN involving the periphery. Note the confluent white-yellow appearance with irregular scalloped posterior margin and sharp transition between involved and noninvolved portions. (From Blumenkranz MS, Duker JS, D'Amico DJ. Acute retinal necrosis. In Albert DM, Jakobiec FA [eds]: Principles and Practice of Ophthalmology. Philadelphia, WB Saunders Co, 1994, with permission.)

FIGURE 62–2 Midresolution phase of ARN with development of curvilinear perivascular lucencies within zones of necrosis prior to the development of late pigmentary changes (Swiss cheese appearance). (From Blumenkranz MS, Duker JS, D'Amico DJ. Acute retinal necrosis. In Albert DM, Jakobiec FA [eds]: Principles and Practice of Ophthalmology. Philadelphia, WB Saunders Co, 1994, with permission.)

Retinal Vasculitis

Retinal vasculitis is a prominent feature of this condition, predominantly affecting the arterioles, but to a lesser extent the venules and peripheral retinal capillary beds as well. In fact, the presence of periarteritis rather than periphlebitis and its associated marked intraretinal hemorrhage is one of the features that helps to distinguish acute retinal necrosis from either cytomegalovirus (CMV) retinitis or acute multifocal hemorrhagic retinal vasculitis, which may share other similar features with this condition.[2,23-25] Fluorescein angiography may confirm the presence of zones of peripheral retinal capillary nonperfusion and underlying choroidal vasculitis in addition to involvement of the retinal arterioles.[26] The presence of retinal vasculitis has been confirmed in histopathologic studies in which both large- and small-caliber arterioles demonstrate perivascular cuffing, endothelial cell swelling, and fibrinoid or thrombotic occlusion of the lumina.[3] In addition to retinal vasculitis, patients with acute retinal necrosis demonstrate a conspicuous component of choroidal vasculitis as well, consisting of zones of hypoperfusion or blockage seen in the early frames of fluorescein angiography, and marked thickening, demonstrated both by clinical examination as well as histopathologic examination.

Vitritis

Another feature that separates acute retinal necrosis from other viral infectious of the retina such as CMV, is the presence of prominent vitreitis and anterior granulomatous uveitis. Unlike other forms of anterior and posterior uveitis, acute retinal necrosis may be associated with a rise rather than a decline in the intraocular pressure and the presence of pigmented granulomatous keratitic precipitates (KP) on the corneal endothelial surface. Patients often

complain of pain related to episcleritis and floaters and haze related to vitreous cellular infiltration.[2,7] The vitreous cellular infiltrate is composed of a combination of lymphocytes and plasma cells that are thought to be both responding to intraocular virions, and expressing local antibody.[11,12] High levels of interleukin-6 have also been found.[27] It is thought that the prominent degree of vitreous, cellular, and humoral infiltration leads to secondary cicatrization, which in turn results in the development of large peripheral retinal tears in necrotic retina.

Optic Neuropathy

Optic neuropathy is a frequent component of this condition,[15] and may either be mild, accounting for no significant visual dysfunction, or very severe, even resulting in no light perception vision in the absence of any posterior retinal involvement. The mechanism of vision loss without retinopathy remains somewhat controversial and may reflect either direct viral invasion, or ischemia secondary to vaso-occlusion or nerve sheath compression. Optic nerve sheath decompression has been proposed as one possible therapy, although the benefits of this remain uncertain.[28]

Retinal Detachment

The most serious and frequent complication of acute retinal necrosis is late retinal detachment, which occurs in excess of 75% of untreated eyes, approximately 6 to 12 weeks after the onset of the disease. It is thought that retinal detachment in this condition results as the consequence of two factors: (1) broad zones of peripheral necrotic retina subjected to traction forces by (2) scarred and contracted vitreous membranes. This combination of factors results in the development of large peripheral tears that generally occur at the junction between necrotic and nonnecrotic retina. When retinal detachment does occur in acute retinal necrosis, the prognosis is more unfavorable than in uncomplicated rhegmatogenous retinal detachment because of the multiplicity, large size, and posterior extent of retinal breaks. Retinal detachment is invariably associated with some degree of proliferative vitreoretinopathy.[2,11,12,29,30] Based upon vitreous examination during vitrectomy as well as histopathologic evaluation, it is known that there is extensive growth of pigment epithelial, glial, and fibroblastic membranes on the surface of the retina which are contiguous with organized vitreal membranes (Fig. 62–3). This results in the clinical appearance of fixed or star folds in the peripheral retina in these patients (Fig. 62–4). Although these retinal detachments are amenable to surgical intervention and successful therapy, they require more aggressive operative intervention, often including vitrectomy as well as scleral buckling, extensive membrane removal, and use of long-acting tamponade and endophotocoagulation.[12,29,30]

Other late cicatricial complications of acute retinal necrosis include iris atrophy, cataract, ciliary body fibrosis and hyposecretion, visually significant vitreous opacities, macular pucker, and giant tears of the retinal pigment epithelium.[2,21]

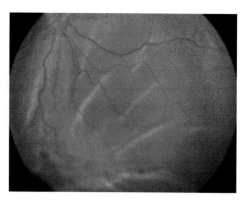

FIGURE 62–4 Retinal folds in stage C2 proliferative vitreoretinopathy associated with ARN. Note the pigmented epiretinal membranes in the lower left corner of this photograph. (From Blumenkranz MS, Duker JS, D'Amico DJ. Acute retinal necrosis. In Albert DM, Jakobiec FA [eds]: Principles and Practice of Ophthalmology. Philadelphia, WB Saunders Co, 1994, with permission.)

disease, and (2) treatment of the late complications, principally retinal detachment.

Acute Phase

Treatment of the acute phase is divided into four components: (1) antiviral therapy, (2) antiinflammatory therapy, (3) antithrombotic therapy, and (4) retinal detachment prophylaxis.

Antiviral Therapy

Intravenous acyclovir is the drug of choice for therapy directed against herpes varicella zoster virus and herpes simplex virus in acute retinal necrosis.[9,13] Both of these infectious agents are generally sensitive to acyclovir, although the herpes simplex virus (0.1 to 1.6 μmol ED_{50}) is more susceptible than herpes zoster varicella virus (3 to 4 μmol ED_{50}). Acyclovir exerts its antiviral activity through the inhibition of viral thymidine kinase and is generally administered at a dose of 1500 mg/m²/day in three divided intravenous doses. The drug is well tolerated by most patients, although it may rarely be associated with central nervous system (CNS) toxicity, urinary calculi, or elevation of creatinine.[3] The approximate duration of intravenous therapy is 7 to 10 days followed by 2 to 4 weeks of oral therapy. In patients in whom intravenous therapy is not possible, oral therapy alone may be considered with acyclovir available in either 200 or 800 mg regimens and daily dosages ranging from 1000 to 4 gm in five equally divided doses.[32] Newer antiviral agents administered by an oral route including famciclovir and valcyclovir may also be effective, although clinical experience with these agents for acute retinal necrosis is limited.[34,35]

THERAPY

Therapy of acute retinal necrosis is divided into two stages: (1) treatment of the acute phase of the

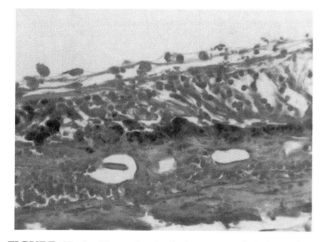

FIGURE 62–3 Zone of retinal pigment epithelial proliferation and migration underlying thinned necrotic peripheral retina. Note the presence of nonpigmented epiretinal membrane on the surface of the necrotic retina. H&E, ×250. (From Blumenkranz MS, Duker JS, D'Amico DJ. Acute retinal necrosis. In Albert DM, Jakobiec FA [eds]: Principles and Practice of Ophthalmology. Philadelphia, WB Saunders Co, 1994, with permission.)

Anti-inflammatory and Antithrombotic Therapy

After 24 to 48 hours of antiviral therapy, anti-inflammatory therapy with prednisone 40 to 60 mg/day is recommended to reduce the severity of intraocular and particularly intravitreal inflammation. Steroids may also have a favorable effect on optic neuropathy in this condition. In addition to steroids and acyclovir, aspirin is administered for its antiplatelet action based upon the demonstration of thrombotic occlusions of retinal and choroidal vessels in acute retinal necrosis syndrome. A dosage of 500 to 650 mg daily is recommended, but more aggressive measures such as heparin and Coumadin do not seem warranted based on the available evidence at this time.

Retinal Detachment Prophylaxis

Because of the high incidence of retinal detachment exceeding 75% of patients who do not receive specific prophylactic therapy, demarcating peripheral laser photocoagulation is recommended if the media are sufficiently clear to permit it. In one study, patients treated with prophylactic laser photocoagulation had a late retinal detachment rate of 17% compared with 66% of patients not receiving photocoagulation. However, the study was not consecutive or randomized and some of the apparent beneficial effect of photocoagulation may have been attributable to lesser disease severity in those eyes permitting photocoagulation contrasted with others.[14]

Treatment of Retinal Detachment

Treatment of retinal detachment associated with proliferative vitreoretinopathy remains problematic. These eyes have multiple retinal breaks occurring at the junction between involved and uninvolved retina, some of which may be large and posteriorly located.[12] As many as 73% may have grade C-1 or greater proliferative vitreoretinopathy.[9,11,12,29,30,32] Scleral buckling alone for retinal detachment associated with acute retinal necrosis is oftentimes unsuccessful, and may be associated with additional complications including ocular fibrin syndrome, choroidal detachment, and ocular hypertension.[29,30] Primary vitrectomy with or without scleral buckling appears to be more effective than scleral buckling alone, and has been associated with favorable anatomic and visual success rates.[12,30,36] In one series a final anatomic success rate of 94% was achieved.[30]

SUMMARY

Acute retinal necrosis is a fulminant viral infection of the eye, primarily involving the retina, pigment epithelium, and choroid with characteristic features and an unfavorable visual prognosis if untreated. Prompt diagnosis and therapy with acyclovir, steroids, aspirin, prophylactic photocoagulation, and vitrectomy if necessary have resulted in an improved prognosis.

REFERENCES

1. Uryama A, Yamada N, Sasaki Y, et al: Unilateral acute uveitis with retinal periarteritis and detachment. Jpn J Clin Ophthalmol 25:607–619, 1971.
2. Fisher JP, Lewis ML, Blumenkranz MS, et al: The ARN syndrome. Part I: Clinical manifestations. Ophthalmology 89:1309–1316, 1982.
3. Culbertson WW, Blumenkranz MS, Haines H, et al: The ARN syndrome, Part 2: Histopathology and etiology. Ophthalmology 89:1317–1325, 1982.
4. Wilkerson D, Aaberg TM, Reeser FH: Necrotizing vaso-occlusive retinitis. Am J Ophthalmol 84:209–219, 1977.
5. Young NJA, Bird AC: Bilateral ARN. Br J Ophthalmol 62:581–590, 1978.
6. Sternberg P, Knox DL, Finkelstein D, et al: Acute retinal necrosis syndrome. Retina 2:145–151, 1982.
7. Lewis ML, Culbertson WW, Post JD, et al: Herpes simplex virus type I. A cause of the ARN syndrome. Ophthalmology 96:875–878, 1989.
8. Holland GN, and the Executive Committee of the American Uveitis Society: Standard diagnostic criteria for the acute retinal necrosis syndrome. Am J Ophthamol 117:663–667, 1994.
9. Blumenkranz MS, Culbertson WW, Clarkson JG, et al: Treatment of the ARN syndrome with intravenous acyclovir. Ophthalmology 93:296–300, 1986.
10. Peyman GA, Morton FG, Uninsky E, et al: Vitrectomy and intravitreal antiviral drug therapy in ARN syndrome. Arch Ophthalmol 102:1618–1621, 1984.
11. Culbertson WW, Clarkson JG, Blumenkranz MS, Lewis ML: Acute retinal necrosis. Am J Ophthalmol 96:683–685, 1983.
12. Blumenkranz MS, Clarkson JG, Culbertson WW, et al: Vitrectomy for retinal detachment associated with ARN. Am J Ophthalmol 106:426–429, 1988.
13. Palay DA, Sternberg P, Davis J, et al: Decrease in the risk of bilateral ARN by acyclovir therapy. Am J Ophthalmol 112:250–255, 1991.
14. Sternberg P, Han DP, Yeo JH, et al: Photocoagulation to prevent retinal detachment in ARN. Ophthalmology 95:1389–1393, 1988.
15. Sergott RC, Belmont JB, Savino PJ, et al: Optic nerve involvement in the ARN syndrome. Arch Ophthalmol 103:1160–1162, 1985.
16. Matsuo T, Ohno A, Matsuo N: Acute retinal necrosis following chickenpox in pregnant woman. Jpn J Ophthalmol 32:70–74, 1988.
17. Culbertson WW, Brod RD, Flynn HW, et al: Chickenpox-associated ARN syndrome. Ophthalmology 98:1641–1646, 1991.
18. Matsuo T, Kuyama M, Matsuo N: Acute retinal necrosis as a novel complication of chickenpox in adults. Br J Ophthalmol 74:443–444, 1990.
19. Browning DJ, Blumenkranz MS, Culbertson WW, et al: Association of varicella-zoster dermatitis with ARN syndrome. Ophthalmology 94:602–606, 1987.
20. Margolis TP, Lowder CY, Holland GN, et al: Varicella-zoster retinitis in patients with the acquired immunodeficiency syndrome. Am J Ophthalmol 112:119–131, 1991.
21. Forster DJ, Dugel PU, Frangieh GT, et al: Rapidly progressive outer retinitis in patients with the acquired immunodeficiency syndrome. Am J Ophthalmol 110:341–348, 1990.
22. Epidemiological characteristics of uveitis in Switzerland. Int Ophthalmol 18:293–298, 1994–1995.

23. Egbert P, Pollard RB, Galligher JG, Merigan T: Cytomegalovirus retinitis in immunosuppressed hosts. Natural history and effects of treatment with adenine arabinoside. Ann Intern Med 93:655–664, 1980.
24. Brown RM, Mendis U: Retinal arteritis complicating herpes zoster ophthalmicus. Br J Ophthalmol 57:344–346, 1973.
25. Blumenkranz MS, Kaplan HJ, Clarkson JG, et al: Acute multifocal hemorrhagic retinal vasculitis. Ophthalmology 95:1663–1672, 1988.
26. Walton R, Byrnes G, Chan C, et al: Flourescein angiography in the progressive outer retinal necrosis syndrome. Retina 16:393–398, 1996.
27. deBoer JH, van Haren MA, de Vries Knoppert WA, et al: Analysis of IL-6 levels in human vitreous fluid obtained from uveitis patients, patients with proliferative intraocular disorders and eye bank eyes. Curr Eye Res 11:181–186, 1992.
28. Sergott RC, Anand R, Belmont JB, et al: Acute retinal necrosis neuropathy. Clinical profile and surgical therapy. Arch Ophthalmol 107:692–696, 1989.
29. Clarkson JG, Blumenkranz MS, Culbertson WW, et al: Retinal detachment following the ARN syndrome. Ophthalmology 91:1665–1668, 1984.
30. Blumenkranz MS, Clarkson J, Culbertson WW, et al: Visual results and complications after retinal reattachment in the ARN syndrome: the influence of operative technique. Retina 9:170–174, 1989.
31. Fox GM, Blumenkranz MS: Giant retinal pigment epithelial tears in acute retinal necrosis. Am J Ophthalmol 116:302–306, 1993.
32. Duker JS, Blumenkranz MS: Diagnosis and management of the ARN syndrome. Surv Ophthalmol 35:327–343, 1991.
33. Laskin OL: Acyclovir. Pharmacology and clinical experience. Arch Intern Med 144:1241–1246, 1984.
34. Perry C, Wagstaff A: Famciclovir; a review of its pharmacologic properties and therapeutic efficacy in herpesvirus infections. Drugs 50:396–415, 1995.
35. Perry C, Faulds D: Valciclovir; a review of its antiviral activity pharmacokinetic properties, and therapuetic efficacy in herpesvirus infections. Drugs 52:754–772, 1996.
36. McDonald HR, Lewis H, Kreiger AE, et al: Surgical management of retinal detachment associated with the ARN syndrome. Br J Ophthalmol 75:455–458, 1991.

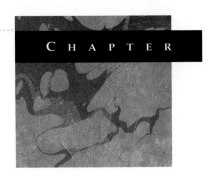

CHAPTER 63

Progressive Outer Retinal Necrosis

David V. Weinberg, M.D.

In 1987 Jabs and co-workers[1] reported presumed herpes varicella-zoster virus (VZV) retinitis in three immunocompromised hosts. Among the three patients, one had the acquired immunodeficiency syndrome (AIDS), cutaneous zoster, and retinitis that was poorly responsive to antiviral therapy. Forster and colleagues described two patients with AIDS and probable VZV retinitis, and coined the name "progressive outer retinal necrosis" (PORN).[2] Several other reports followed, further defining this entity.[3-6]

VZV[7] and herpes simplex virus (HSV)[8] had previously been recognized as causes of acute retinal necrosis (ARN). ARN was first described in healthy patients, but similar cases in patients with suppressed immunity were later described.[1,9] In reviewing the literature of immunosuppressed patients with VZV retinitis, patients with AIDS demonstrate a distinctly attenuated immune response compared to patients with immune suppression from chemotherapy.[1,9,10] The recently defined American Uveitis Society standard diagnostic criteria for ARN[11] includes patients with abnormal immune status, but excludes patients without "a prominent inflammatory reaction in the vitreous and anterior chamber" from a diagnosis of ARN, thereby eliminating many or most patients with AIDS and VZV retinitis. The designation of "PORN" has generally been used to describe patients with AIDS and presumed herpetic retinitis with less inflammation and a more aggressive clinical course than ARN. Engstrom and associates have suggested a set of diagnostic criteria for PORN, and contrasted it with the American Uveitis Association criteria for ARN (Table 63–1).[3]

Although PORN is a newly described entity, it has achieved a status as the second most common opportunistic retinal infection among North American patients with AIDS,[3,6] and as one of the most devastating ocular conditions known to man.

CLINICAL FEATURES

Patients presenting with PORN are infected with the human immunodeficiency virus (HIV), and generally have advanced AIDS, but PORN can occasionally lead to the diagnosis of unrecognized HIV disease. The CD4 lymphocyte count is rarely greater than $100/mm^3$, with a median of $21/mm^3$ in a recent series.[3] A history of an antecedent or ongoing dermatomal zoster eruption is usually elicited, including, but not limited to, herpes zoster ophthalmicus. Other forms of herpetic disease, such as encephalitis[6] may, less commonly, precede PORN. Many patients are being treated or have recently been treated with acyclovir at the time they are diagnosed with PORN.

Most patients present with ocular symptoms, including blurred vision, loss of peripheral or central vision, floaters, and pain. Presenting visual acuity ranges from 20/20 to no light perception (NLP). Infection may be evident in one or both eyes at the time of presentation. The majority of patients presenting with unilateral disease will rapidly develop bilateral involvement.

Involved eyes show no injection or other external signs of inflammation. The anterior chamber and vitreous exhibit no cells or minimal cells by slit lamp examination. Early retinitis appears as clusters of whitish or yellowish punctate areas of retinal opacification, which may appear anywhere in the fundus (Fig. 63–1). Some reports emphasized early posterior pole involvement as a distinguishing feature of varicella-zoster retinitis in patients with

TABLE 63–1 Diagnostic Criteria

Progressive Outer Retinal Necrosis Syndrome	Acute Retinal Necrosis Syndrome
Multifocal lesions characterized by deep retinal opacification without granular borders; there may be areas of confluent opacification	One or more foci of full-thickness retinal necrosis with discrete borders
Lesions located in the peripheral retina with or without macular involvement	Lesions located in the peripheral retina[†]
Extremely rapid progression of lesions	Rapid progression of disease[‡]
No consistent direction of disease spread	Circumferential spread of disease around the peripheral retina
Absence of vascular inflammation	Evidence of occlusive vasculopathy, with arteriolar involvement
Minimal or absent intraocular inflammation	Prominent inflammatory reaction in the vitreous and anterior chamber
Characteristics that support, but are not required, for diagnosis	Characteristics that support, but are not required, for diagnosis
Perivenular clearing of retinal opacification	Optic neuropathy/atrophy Scleritis Pain

* Engstrom RE Jr, Holland GN, Margolis TP, et al: The progressive outer retinal necrosis syndrome. A variant of necrotizing herpetic retinopathy in patients with AIDS. Ophthalmology 101:1488–1502, 1994, with permission.
† Involving the area adjacent to, or outside of, the major temporal vascular arcades.
‡ Progression can be successfully halted in most cases with intravenous acyclovir therapy.

AIDS.[5,6] In a much larger series by Engstrom and colleagues,[3] posterior pole involvement was present at the time of diagnosis in approximately one third of involved eyes, and was usually accompanied by peripheral involvement. The punctate areas become confluent over time as the retinitis spreads in all directions (Figs. 63–2 and 63–3). The advancing edge of retinitis maintains a punctate appearance. There is a tendency for early circumferential involvement of the peripheral retina, accompanied by rapid posterior progression. The impression of "outer retinitis" is based on the smooth, flat appearance of the involved areas, and the mild or absent evidence of vasculitis and hemorrhage. Retinal vasculopathy (sheathing, occlusion) is seen in a minority of patients. Optic nerve edema is rare. Optic atrophy is observed as widespread retina destruction takes place. Friedlander and associates described 3 patients who presented with vision loss due to optic neuropathy days to weeks preceding the development of typical VZV.[12]

As the retina is consumed by the infection, it once again becomes transparent, revealing underlying pigment mottling (Fig. 63–4). The clearing of opacification has a tendency to predominate in a perivascular pattern.

Macular involvement may be present at the time of diagnosis or may occur by posterior progression of more peripheral retinitis. In some patients a very distinctive macular lesion occurs, appearing as perifoveal retinal opacification, with a central lucency, resulting in a "cherry-red spot" (Fig. 63–5).

The rapid pace of spread of the retinitis is one of the most distinguishing features of this disease. In

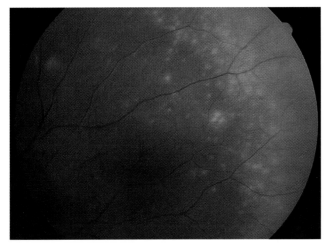

FIGURE 63–1 Multiple areas of retinal opacification in a patient with newly diagnosed PORN. The more peripheral lesions have become confluent. Vitreous cells, vasculitis, and hemorrhage are conspicuously absent.

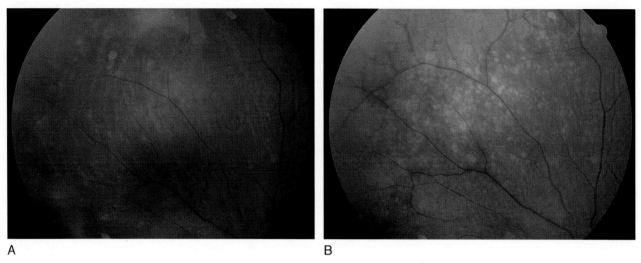

A   B

FIGURE 63–2   *A,* A few punctate opacities are seen in the superonasal quadrant of the left eye of a patient with newly diagnosed PORN. *B,* The same eye 1 week later displays widespread retinal involvement.

the series by Engstrom and associates, visual acuity was NLP in two thirds of eyes within 4 weeks of diagnosis.

As infected areas of retina become necrotic, large necrotic retinal breaks lead to rhegmatogenous retina in the majority of affected eyes, contributing to the overall poor prognosis.

DIFFERENTIAL DIAGNOSIS

PORN has been reported to be the second most common opportunistic retinal infection in patients with AIDS.[3,6] Cytomegalovirus (CMV) retinitis is the most common opportunistic retinal infection in patients with AIDS and shares many features in common with PORN. Patients with CMV retinitis are less likely to have a history of recent cutaneous

zoster infection. Eyes with CMV retinitis usually exhibit some mild inflammatory signs including fine keratic precipitates, aqueous cells, and/or vitreous cells. CMV retinitis usually has a more "rough," edematous, full-thickness appearance than the "smooth," "dry" appearance of PORN. CMV retinitis is more likely to exhibit hemorrhage and vascular sheathing than PORN. Although CMV retinitis is a rapidly progressive infection, it does not compare to the explosive pace of PORN. Measurable expansion of the borders of active CMV retinitis can be documented by careful observation over periods of 1 or 2 weeks. Widespread progression and retinal destruction in PORN is typically observed in a few days (Fig. 63–2).

Although a variant of necrotizing herpetic retinitis, PORN has an appearance, clinical course, response to therapy, and prognosis that differ suffi-

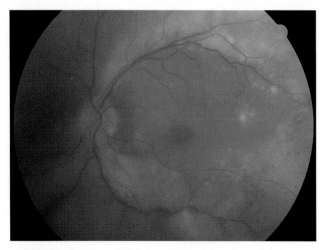

FIGURE 63–3   Near total retinal necrosis in a patient with PORN.

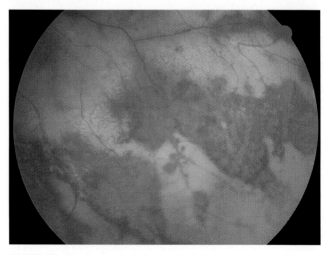

FIGURE 63–4   Partial clearing of retinal opacification revealing retinal atrophy and pigment irregularity.

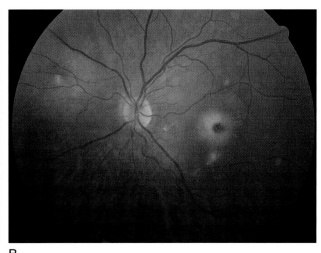

A   B

FIGURE 63-5 Bilateral macular lesions in a patient at the time of PORN diagnosis. Note the perifoveal deep opacification, with a central lucency, creating a "cherry-red spot." There is a separate area of retinitis visible nasal to the left optic nerve.

ciently from ARN that it has been considered a distinct entity. PORN differs sufficiently from ARN that it does not fall within the diagnostic criteria for ARN established by the American Uveitis Society.[11] The diagnostic criteria for PORN and ARN are compared in Table 63-1.

ETIOLOGY

There is sufficient evidence to identify herpes varicella-zoster virus as a cause of PORN. The frequent temporal association between cutaneous zoster or other nonretinal manifestations of VZV infection with PORN provide circumstantial evidence for a causal relationship. Direct evidence of VZV infection has been more difficult to document, partly because of difficulty in obtaining adequate tissue specimens in the wake of such a destructive infection. Some success has been achieved by analyzing tissue and fluid taken at the time of vitrectomy, from chorioretinal biopsy specimens, and from whole, enucleated globes.

Chambers and colleagues found positive immunofluorescence staining for VZV in a retinal biopsy from a patient with AIDS and necrotizing retinitis.[13] In their original description of PORN, Forster and colleagues identified virus particles consistent with a herpes virus by electron microscopy on a retinal biopsy specimen. Polymerase chain reaction (PCR) from a vitreous specimen of the other patient identified DNA from a herpes virus. More specific identification was not successful in either of these patients.[2] Other investigators subsequently identified VZV based on PCR,[3,6,14-16] immunohistochemical staining,[3,5,6,14] and viral culture.[3,5,14] Infection appears to predominate in the outer retina and RPE; however, the end stage is retinal necrosis, leaving only the internal limiting membrane (Fig. 63-6).[6] Evidence for direct infection of the choroid has been inconsistent.[15]

Although VZV appears to be a cause of PORN, it is possible that other viruses not yet identified, such as herpes simplex virus (HSV) may be capable of causing the same clinical syndrome. Concurrent infection with cytomegalovirus and HSV has been found in tissue obtained from eyes diagnosed clinically with CMV retinitis.[17,18]

TREATMENT

Any assessment regarding the efficacy of treatment must be considered in context with the natural history of a disease. In the case of PORN, the course of untreated disease is not known. It is clear that even with antiviral treatment progression is usually swift and the prognosis is very poor. Acyclovir has been the antiviral agent used in the majority of reported cases and would appear to be a logical choice based on the knowledge of VZV as the cause of PORN. Apparent clinical responses to therapy with acyclovir have been reported, but the outcomes have generally been poor. Disappointing results with acyclovir may be due, in part, to viral resistance, since most patients with PORN have previous manifestations of VZV, and previous exposure to acyclovir. Acyclovir-resistant VZV has been recognized in the AIDS patient population.[19-21] Treatment with ganciclovir, foscarnet, and vidarabine has also been reported.[2-6,13,15,22,23] A single case report described successful treatment using intravitreal ganciclovir plus oral sorivudine.[24] Nonrandomized case series have suggested somewhat better outcomes using various combinations of intravenous antivirals, especially ganciclovir and

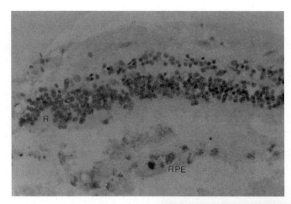
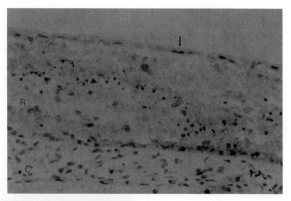
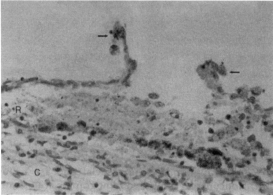

FIGURE 63–6 *Top left,* Low-power micrograph of retina (R). Immunohistochemical staining for zoster antigens (*dark material, arrow*) is concentrated in the outer retina, including the retinal pigment epithelium (RPE). The inner retina appears unperturbed with no evidence of zoster antigen (counterstained with hematoxylin, ×40). *Top right,* Low-power micrograph of retina (R) and choroid (C). Most of the retina is necrotic and there are numerous macrophages present. Immunocytochemical staining for zoster antigens (*dark material, arrow*) shows complete involvement of the retina, except for an intact inner limiting membrane (*arrow*). There is no immunostaining in the choroid (counterstained with hematoxylin, ×40). *Bottom,* Low-power micrograph of the retina (R) and choroid (C). Cells covering the inner-limiting membrane are thick and show focal disruption with pigment epithelial proliferation (*arrows*). Immunocytochemistry demonstrates zoster antigens (*dark material, arrow*) in necrotic retina (counterstained with hematoxylin, ×40). (From Kuppermann BD, Quiceno JI, Wiley C, et al: Clinical and histopathologic study of varicella zoster virus retinitis in patients with acquired immunodeficiency syndrome. Am J Ophthalmol 118:589–600, 1994, with permission.)

foscarnet. Cases of successful treatment with intravenous foscarnet plus intravitreal ganciclovir injections or implant have also been reported.[25]

Like CMV retinitis in patients with AIDS, PORN probably requires chronic maintenance antiviral therapy. Among patients demonstrating control of retinitis on antiviral therapy, relapses have been reported when therapy was withdrawn or reduced.[3,4]

Retinal detachments occur in the majority of eyes with PORN and contribute to the poor visual prognosis. Peripheral laser retinopexy to prevent retinal detachment, or to prevent the posterior progression of peripheral retinal detachment, has been described. Such treatment may delay but probably does not prevent eventual total retinal detachment in most cases.[3,28] Retinal detachment repair using pars plana vitrectomy and silicone oil tamponade has been reported for retinal detachments due to PORN, and is capable of achieving anatomic success and preserving function in eyes that have not been lost to total retinal necrosis.[3,25,28] Contracture of the detached necrotic retina has been observed[25,28] and relaxing retinectomy has been nec-

essary to achieve and maintain reattachment in some cases.[28]

REFERENCES

1. Jabs DA, Schachat AP, Liss R, et al: Presumed varicella zoster retinitis in immunocompromised patients. Retina 7: 9–13, 1987.
2. Forster DJ, Dugel PU, Frangieh GT, et al: Rapidly progressive outer retinal necrosis in the acquired immunodeficiency syndrome. Am J Ophthalmol 110:341–348, 1990.
3. Engstrom RE Jr, Holland GN, Margolis TP, et al: The progressive outer retinal necrosis syndrome. A variant of necrotizing herpetic retinopathy in patients with AIDS. Ophthalmology 101:1488–1502, 1994.
4. Johnston WH, Holland GN, Engstrom RE Jr, Rimmer S: Recurrence of presumed varicella-zoster virus retinopathy in patients with acquired immunodeficiency syndrome. Am J Ophthalmol 116:42–50, 1993.
5. Margolis TP, Lowder CY, Holland GN, et al: Varicella-zoster virus retinitis in patients with the acquired immunodeficiency syndrome. Am J Ophthalmol 112:119–131, 1991.
6. Kuppermann BD, Quiceno JI, Wiley C, et al: Clinical and histopathologic study of varicella zoster virus retinitis in

patients with the acquired immunodeficiency syndrome. Am J Ophthalmol 118:589–600, 1994.

7. Culbertson WW, Blumenkranz MS, Pepose JS, et al: Varicella zoster virus is a cause of the acute retinal necrosis syndrome. Ophthalmology 93:559–569, 1986.

8. Lewis ML, Culbertson WW, Post MJ, et al: Herpes simplex virus type 1. A cause of the acute retinal necrosis syndrome. Ophthalmology 96:875–878, 1989.

9. Friberg TR, Jost BF: Acute retinal necrosis in an immunosuppressed patient. Am J Ophthalmol 98:515–517, 1984.

10. Duker JS, Shakin EP: Rapidly progressive outer retinal necrosis in the acquired immunodeficiency syndrome (Letter). Am J Ophthalmol 111:255–256, 1991.

11. Holland GN, and the Executive Committee of the American Uveitis Society: Standard diagnostic criteria for the acute retinal necrosis syndrome. Am J Ophthalmol 117:663–667, 1994.

12. Friedlander SM, Rahal FM, Ericson L, et al: Optic neuropathy preceding acute retinal necrosis in acquired immunodeficiency syndrome. Arch Ophthalmol 114:1481–1485, 1996.

13. Chambers RB, Derick RJ, Davidorf FH, et al: Varicella-zoster retinitis in human immunodeficiency virus infection. Case report. Arch Ophthalmol 107:960–961, 1989.

14. Hellinger WC, Bolling JP, Smith TF, Campbell RJ: Varicella-zoster virus retinitis in a patient with AIDS-related complex: case report and brief review of the acute retinal necrosis syndrome. Clin Infect Dis 16:208–212, 1993.

15. Greven CM, Ford J, Stanton C, et al: Progressive outer retinal necrosis secondary to varicella zoster virus in acquired immune deficiency syndrome. Retina 15:14–20, 1995.

16. Short GA, Margolis TP, Kuppermann BD, et al: A polymerase chain reaction-based assay for diagnosing varicella-zoster virus retinitis in patients with acquired immunodeficiency syndrome. Am J Ophthalmol 123:157–164, 1997.

17. Pepose JS, Hilborne LH, Pasquale CA, Foos RY: Concurrent herpes simplex and cytomegalovirus retinitis and encephalitis in the acquired immune deficiency syndrome (AIDS). Ophthalmology 91:1669–1677, 1984.

18. Rummelt V, Rummelt C, Jahn G, et al: Triple retinal infection with human immunodeficiency virus type 1, cytomegalovirus, and herpes simplex virus type 1. Light and electron microscopy, immunohistochemistry, and in situ hybridization. Ophthalmology 101:270–279, 1994.

19. Jacobson MA, Berger TG, Fikrig S, et al: Acyclovir-resistant varicella zoster virus infection after chronic oral acyclovir therapy in patients with the acquired immunodeficiency syndrome (AIDS). Ann Intern Med 112:187–191, 1990.

20. Safrin S, Berger TG, Gilson I, et al: Foscarnet therapy in five patients with AIDS and acyclovir-resistant varicella-zoster virus infection. Ann Intern Med 115:19–21, 1991.

21. Pahwa S, Biron K, Lim W, et al: Continuous varicella-zoster infection associated with acyclovir resistance in a child with AIDS. JAMA 260:2879–2882, 1988.

22. Laby DM, Nasrallah FP, Butrus SI, Whitmore PV: Treatment of outer retinal necrosis in AIDS patients. Graefes Arch Clin Exp Ophthalmol 231:271–273, 1993.

23. Friedman SM, Margo CE, Connelly BL: Varicella-zoster virus retinitis as the initial manifestation of the acquired immunodeficiency syndrome (Letter). Am J Ophthalmol 117:536–538, 1994.

24. Pinnolis MK, Foxworthy D, Kemp B: Treatment of progressive outer retinal necrosis with sorivudine. Am J Ophthalmol 119:516–517, 1995.

25. Spaide RF, Martin DF, Teich SA, et al: Successful treatment of progressive outer retinal necrosis syndrome. Retina 16:479–487, 1996.

26. Moorthy RS, Weinberg DV, Teich SA, et al: Management of varicella zoster retinitis in AIDS. Br J Ophthalmol 81:189–194, 1997.

27. Morley MG, Duker JS, Zacks C: Successful treatment of rapidly progressive outer retinal necrosis in the acquired immunodeficiency syndrome (Letter). Am J Ophthalmol 117:264–265, 1994.

28. Weinberg DV, Lyon AT: Repair of retinal detachments due to herpes varicella-zoster virus retinitis in patients with acquired immune deficiency syndrome. Ophthalmology 104:279–282, 1997.

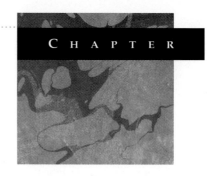

Fungal Diseases

Neil D. Brourman, M.D.
Mark S. Blumenkranz, M.D.

OCULAR CANDIDIASIS

Significant advances in medical technology permitting greater salvage of critically ill patients, an increase in the number and scope of broad-spectrum antibiotics, and an increase in the number of intravenous drug users are thought to have contributed to a rise in the number of cases of endogenous fungal endophthalmitis. Since 1965, more than 100 cases of *Candida* endophthalmitis have been reported.[1,3,7-9,11-15,18,22-24,26,28-32,34-36,39-41,44-46,49,51-57,60-67,69-76] *Candida albicans* is the most common pathogen causing endogenous fungal endophalmitis,[25] but other *Candida* species may produce similar ocular manifestations.[17,64,70,76] In Japan, *Candida* accounts for 90% of the cases of fungal endophthalmitis.[44]

In 1943, Miale[46] first recognized the histologic appearance of *Candida* endophthalmitis in an eye studied 4 years after enucleation. Fifteen years later, Van Buren[80] reported the first case in which the diagnosis was clinically suspected. The patient, who had multiple myeloma and systemic candidiasis, developed an area of retinitis that clinically appeared as a white-centered hemorrhagic infiltrate. The patient died despite treatment with nystatin, and histologic study of the retinal lesion confirmed the presence of yeasts. In 1961, Hoffman and Waubke[40] developed the first experimental model for this disease by injecting *Candida albicans* intravenously into rabbits and mice, thereby producing lesions of *Candida* endophthalmitis that appeared essentially identical to the human lesions.

Clinical Manifestations

Transmission of the Disease

Exogenous infections of *Candida* may occur after intraocular surgery, after penetrating ocular trauma, or as extensions of *Candida* corneal ulcers. Host immunologic suppression is thought to contribute but is not essential for endogenous infection of what is, under normal circumstances, a ubiquitous saprophytic fungus. Prolonged systemic antibiotics, general surgical procedures (especially gastrointestinal), hematologic malignances, poorly controlled diabetes mellitus, indwelling intravenous catheters, prolonged hyperalimentation, and acquired immunodeficiency syndrome (AIDS) can predispose to an opportunistic fungal infection.[4,15,25,32,34,54,56,72] In addition, since 1970, an increased incidence of systemic candidiasis has been noted among intravenous drug abusers.[11,18,21,24,73,75]

Systemic Candidiasis

The diagnosis of disseminated candidiasis remains problematic for the clinician.[26] The protean manifestations of disseminated candidiasis include endophthalmitis, osteomyelitis, arthritis, myocarditis, meningitis, and macronodular skin lesions. Patients with candidiasis may range from profoundly moribund and febrile to asymptomatic and afebrile.

Ocular Candidiasis

OCULAR SYMPTOMS. The clinical manifestations of endogenous candidal infection are variable; they depend on the host's immune status and the clinical stage of the disease. Symptoms include floaters due to vitreitis, painful photophobia due to ciliary spasm, and visual loss.[25,34,73] It should be emphasized that if the patient is moribund and has a central lesion or is fully alert but has lesions located in the periphery of the fundus, extensive disease may be present with no symptoms. In one series of 15

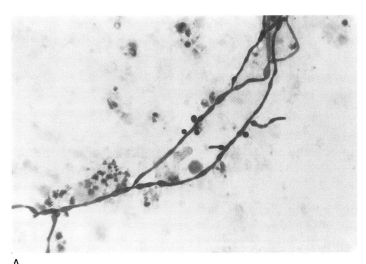

A

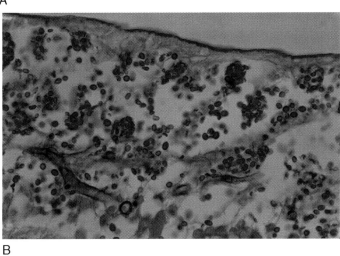

B

A, Pseudohyphae with budding yeast in vitreous specimen from a 27-year-old man who developed endogenous candida enophthalmitis following the use of an elicit intravenous drug. (From Snip RC, Michels RG: Pars plana vitrectomy in the management of endogenous *Candida* endophthalmitis. Am J Ophthalmol 82:699–704, 1976, with permission.) *B*, Cryptococcal organisms in retina of a patient who died from disseminated cryptococcosus. (From Khodadoust AA, Payne JW: Cryptococcal "torulas" retinitis: a clinicopathologic case report. Am J Ophthalmol 67:745–750, 1969. Copyright 1969, Elsevier Science, with permission.)

patients with *Candida* endophthalmitis, 14 had blurred vision and 4 had ocular pain.[25]

RETINITIS AND CHOROIDITIS. The earliest fundus lesion, a focal area of chorioretinitis, appears clinically as a cotton-white fluffy mound. Intravitreal microabscesses containing the organism progress to extend from the retinal lesion into the vitreous cavity as "puff balls" or appear like a "string of pearls"[1,73] (Figs. 64–1 and 64–2). This is in sharp contrast to other causes of retinitis such as toxoplasmosis, herpes simplex, herpes zoster, or cytomegalovirus, which remain confined to the retina and choroid and expand along the plane of the retina rather than into the vitreous. The white retinal lesion is at times surrounded by retinal hemorrhages appearing similar to a Roth's spot. At the time of diagnosis, multiple lesions are found in one half of patients, and two thirds of patients have bilateral lesions.[25] A variable anterior and posterior, granulomatous or nongranulomatous uveitis is usually present, which may progress to severe vitreitis, panuveitis, and ultimately endophthalmitis if left untreated.

OTHER OPHTHALMIC MANIFESTATIONS. Papillitis, scleritis, anterior uveitis, and iris abscess have all been observed.[1,18,25,65] Subretinal neovascularization has been infrequently reported as a late manifestation following the resolution of fungal infections, including *Candida*.[3,8] In some instances this may be successfully treated by photocoagulation.[45] *Candida* is a frequent cause of keratitis and is responsible for as many as 25% of all fungal keratitis cases identified.[46]

Exogenous *Candida Endophthalmitis*

Exogenous fungal endophthalmitis differs in several respects from endogenous fungal endophthal-

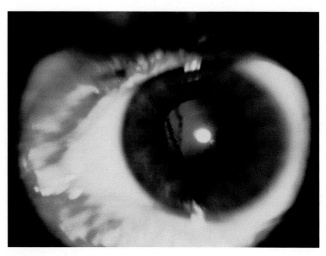

FIGURE 64–2 "String-of-pearls" appearance of candidal microabscesses in vitreous cavity.

mitis. *Candida*, although a common source of endogenous fungal infections, remains a rare cause of exogenous fungal endophthalmitis.[67] Distinctive features of exogenous fungal endophthalmitis are a latent period of weeks to months, in comparison to the much shorter period for bacterial infection.[29,78] Ocular pain is generally less severe in fungal endophthalmitis, and visual acuities at the time of presentation tend to be better than with bacterial infections.[78] The infiltrate in exogenous fungal endophthalmitis tends to remain more localized in the anterior chamber, pupillary space, or anterior vitreous, although diffuse intraocular inflammation can occur in some cases.[67] Endophthalmitis developing from keratitis, regardless of the infecting organism, has a poor visual prognosis, although some successful cases have been reported.[43]

Candida *Endophthalmitis in Children*

Candida endophthalmitis is rare in children. The few reported cases have occurred almost exclusively in premature neonates whose deficient host defense systems and reduced killing ability of leukocytes predispose toward infection.[63] Children with *Candida* endophthalmitis are less likely than adults to have a history of antecedent abdominal surgery.[28] Free-floating vitreous opacities have been reported in some cases.[63]

Endogenous *Candida Endophthalmitis in Intravenous Drug Abusers*

Patients with endogenous *Candida* endophthalmitis associated with intravenous drug abuse frequently have ocular and systemic signs different from those seen in non–drug-abusing patients. Anterior uveitis and extensive vitreous involvement are more common among drug abusers, and these patients may lack the typical retinal lesions,[1] and may not have other systemic features of disseminated can-

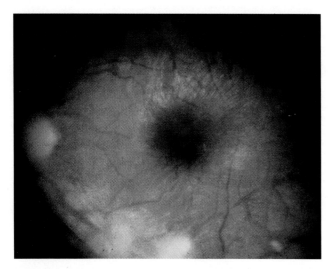

FIGURE 64–1 Typical fundus appearance of candidal retinochoroiditis consisting of fluffy white infiltrate along vascular arcade.

didiasis. Cutaneous manifestations, consisting of deep-seated scalp nodules and pustulosis in hairy zones, appear to be more common among intravenous drug abusers.[24,75]

Candida *in Immunosuppressed Patients*

Patients with severe neutropenia or neutrophilic dysfunction, including those with myelogenous leukemia, may demonstrate multifocal cream- or yellow-colored choroidal lesions, with little or no retinal or vitreal inflammation, similar in appearance to the lesions of ocular lymphoblastic lymphoma. This is invariably associated with multiple deep-seated visceral abscesses and an unfavorable clinical outcome (Fig. 64–3).

Diagnosis

The diagnosis of *Candida* retinitis or endophthalmitis depends largely on the clinical suspicion of a fungal infection. Endogenous fungal infection should be suspected in any immunologically suppressed individual with a white retinal infiltrate, especially if it extends intravitreally accompanied by a variable uveitis. A diagnostic vitrectomy can assist in the management of patients suspected of having *Candida* endophthalmitis, but anterior chamber paracentesis for culture is invariably negative and should be avoided.[7,33,66,74] New techniques for the detection of anti-*Candida* antibody titers, using immunologic analysis of anterior chamber fluid, may help to support the diagnosis of *Candida* endophthalmitis.[51,53] However, these newer techniques have not yet gained wide acceptance.

The diagnosis of disseminated candidiasis can at times be difficult for the clinician.[26,42] Gaines and Remington[30] found that the premortem diagnosis

was made early enough for appropriate treatment in only 15 to 40% of patients. In a large postmortem series of 133 patients, fungal infection was seldom diagnosed antemortem and fungemia was detected in only 18% of the patients.[54] The serologic detection of serum antibodies to *Candida* (cocounterimmunoelectrophoresis, indirect immunofluorescence, precipitation, or monoclonal antibody gold-labeled tests) are neither specific nor sensitive enough to allow accurate diagnosis. False-negative and false-positive rates each approach 50%.[26,60]

Blood, urine, indwelling catheters, or any other potential source of infection should be cultured. However, blood cultures are frequently negative in systemic candidiasis.[11,69] A chest x-ray should be ordered to rule out other infectious diseases. The discovery of a focal, inflammatory, intraocular lesion is strong evidence that exogenous candidemia has progressed to metastatic infection with deep organ involvement.[25] Disseminated candidiasis was found in 78 to 100% of autopsied patients with *Candida* endophthalmitis.[25,36,37,54]

Patients with systemic candidiasis frequently show evidence of ocular dissemination. Griffen et al[36] found that 30% of 82 patients with systemic candidiasis had either clinical or postmortem evidence of *Candida* endophthalmitis. Dupont and Drought[24] found that 39% of 38 heroin addicts treated for systemic candidal infections had ocular manifestations. In the only prospective studies to date, 28 to 37% of patients with *Candida albicans* fungemia developed endophthalmitis.[14,64]

DIFFERENTIAL DIAGNOSIS. The differential diagnosis of *Candida* endophthalmitis includes other causes of chorioretinitis and/or endophthalmitis: toxoplasmosis, cryptococcosis, aspergillosis, histoplasmosis, coccidioidomycosis, blastomycosis, viral retinitis (herpes simplex, herpes zoster, cytomegalovirus), acute retinal necrosis syndrome, and bacterial endophthalmitis. In addition cotton-wool spots can be confused with early *Candida* lesions but unlike candidal lesions remain stable or spontaneously regress.

Histopathology

Pathologically, the primary inflammatory focus is usually found to be in the inner choroid, with fungi later extending from the choroid into the subretinal space and retina.[25,37] In some cases, lesions may appear to be confined to the retina, possibly originating from the deep capillary plexus. The inflammatory reaction to *Candida* is usually a combination of supportive and granulomatous inflammation. With severe inflammation, rupture of the inner limiting membrane may occur.[37] Scattered periodic acid–Schiff (PAS)–positive debris, consisting of tiny globules, may be seen within the inflammatory focus.[25] Identification of the budding yeast forms

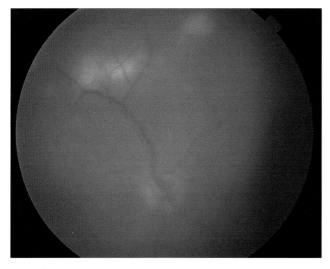

FIGURE 64–3   Multifocal creamy yellow choroidal candidal lesions in patient with disseminated candidiasis, leukopenia, and acute myelogenous leukemia.

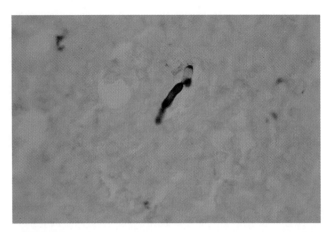

FIGURE 64–4 Candidal organism exhibiting pseudohyphae within vitreous microabscess (Grocott's methemine silver nitrate X 1000). (From Aguilar GL, Blumenkranz MS, Egbert PR, McCulley JP: *Candida* endophthalmitis after intravenous drug abuse. Arch Ophthalmol 97:96–100, 1979, with permission.)

(pseudohyphae) is often difficult (Fig. 64–4), and may be seen in the vitreous.

Chemotherapy

AMPHOTERICIN B. Until recently, amphotericin B, with or without flucytosine, was the most favored and most effective method of treatment for disseminated candidiasis.[7,11] Amphotericin B is a polyene antifungal agent that is fungistatic or fungicidal depending on the concentration of the drug and the resistance of the organism. It binds to and damages the cytoplasmic membrane of susceptible organisms, increases membrane permeability, induces the leakage of cellular constituents, and ultimately causes cell death.[37,56]

Successful treatment of *Candida* endophthalmitis with 5 μg of intravitreal amphotericin B has been the main form of therapeutic intervention. This dose has been shown to be nontoxic in animal studies.[6,41] A normal electroretinogram was recorded in a human eye that previously had 5 μg of amphotericin B injected into the vitreous cavity. Doses greater than 10 μg can cause toxic retinal changes in the rabbit.[6] In animal studies, aphakic eyes showed a more rapid decay of amphotericin levels after a single intravitreal injection compared to phakic eyes, but no appreciable difference in the rate of *Candida* endophthalmitis was noted.[22]

Amphotericin B penetrates the aqueous to some extent after intravenous administration, but it penetrates the vitreous poorly.[35] It is *not* recommended for patients with exogenous (e.g., posttraumatic or postsurgical) fungal endophthalmitis.[5,61] The disadvantages of amphotericin B are its need for intravenous administration and its numerous side effects, including headache, malaise, thrombophlebitis, fever, chills, anorexia, nausea, vomiting, hypokalemia, and hematologic toxicity. Renal dys-

function is the most important and serious toxic effect of amphotericin B.[7,67] Monitoring of amphotericin B toxicity requires measurement of hematocrit, serum potassium, blood urea nitrogen, creatinine, and carbon dioxide values as well as a urinalysis.

The dosage schedules for the intravenous use of amphotericin B have largely been arrived at empirically, depending on host immune factors and the severity of infection, and should be determined in consultation with an infectious disease specialist. Some authors[46] recommend adjusting the dose of amphotericin B by maintaining the patient's serum level between 0.75 and 1.5 μg/ml (pre- and postinfusion levels). Others[10,56] have refuted the value of serum levels and recommend empiric treatment (0.5 to 1 mg/kg/day). Most patients are treated with 1.5 to 2.0 g of amphotericin B for 6 to 12 weeks. Premedication is often needed, such as 25 to 50 mg hydrocortisone sodium succinate added to the infusion bottle; and aspirin, diphenhydramine (Benadryl), or meperidine hydrochloride (Demerol) to control chills and fever. Prochlorperazine (Compazine) is frequently used to control nausea.

Amphotericin has been used in combination with other antifungal medications. Lou et al reported the successful treatment of *Candida* endophthalmitis using amphotericin B and rifampin.[49] Kinyoun[48] and Stern et al[76] reported the successful use of systemic amphotericin B and 5-flucytosine for *Candida* endophthalmitis.

Several other compounds in addition to amphotericin and fluconazole have been employed with variable success.

KETOCONAZOLE. Ketoconazole inhibits the biosynthesis of ergosterol (the main component of the cell membrane of *Candida albicans*) by blocking the C-14 demethylation of lanosterol. Experimental animal studies suggest the efficacy of ketoconazole for candidiasis, but definitive confirmatory clinical trials have not yet been done.[47] Nonrandomized preliminary studies have shown good results with oral ketoconazole for systemic and ocular mycoses.[23] In one study, six of six cases of *Candida* chorioretinitis treated solely with ketoconazole were cured.[24] However, these same investigators recommended amphotericin B with flucytosine as the initial treatment for ocular disease. While the relative indications for antifungal agents remain clinical, experimental studies suggest that the combination of ketoconazole with amphotericin B may be *less* effective than amphotericin B alone.[19,77] Gastrointestinal distress, gynecomastia, oligospermia, and a transient rise in serum liver enzymes may occur in a small percentage of patients treated with ketoconazole.[62]

MICONAZOLE. Miconazole, an imidazole derivative, has largely been replaced by ketoconazole due to the latter's ability to be given orally. Before the introduction of ketoconazole, Blumenkranz and

Stevens[12] had attempted to use miconazole for fungal endophthalmitis in three patients (one with candidiasis). They noted progression of disease in all three with miconazole and improvement after therapy was changed to intravenous amphotericin B. Gallo et al[31] reported the successful combination of miconazole and flucytosine for presumed fungal endophthalmitis in narcotic abusers.

5-FLUCYTOSINE   (5-FLUOROCYTOSINE). 5-Flucytosine is converted to 5-fluorouracil, which inhibits DNA and RNA synthesis. It has excellent absorption from the gastrointestinal tract and good intraocular penetration, and it has been shown to be effective against *C. albicans*.[10,69] However, many strains of *Candida* have been shown to be resistant to this drug. It is recommended that 5-flucytosine be used with amphotericin B because these drugs appear to be synergistic.[48,59,76]

FLUCONAZOLE. A new triazole compound, fluconazole, approved for both oral and parenteral use, is showing great promise for the treatment of oropharyngeal and serious systemic candidal infections[27] and may replace amphotericin B as the drug of first choice for ocular candidiasis. Fluconazole is the only antifungal azole derivative that penetrates into the cerebrospinal fluid (CSF). After a single oral dose of 200 mg of fluconazole, the aqueous humor concentration ranges from 2.7 to 5.4 µg/ml, approximately 80% of the serous concentration.[5] It appears to be as effective as amphotericin B for cryptococcal meningitis.[4] It is more effective than ketoconazole in systemic candidiasis of immunosuppressed as well as normal mice.[68,79] In an animal model, parenterally administered fluconazole penetrated freely into ocular tissue.[71] Topical fluconazole in experimental *C. albicans* keratitis in rabbits penetrated into the cornea and aqueous.[9] Luttrull et al successfully treated patients with endogenous candidal endophthalmitis with oral fluconazole.[50] Akler et al[2] treated six patients and De Palacio et al[21] treated six heroin users with disseminated candidiasis with a combination of oral and systemic fluconazole without need for discontinuations of therapy.

CORTICOSTEROIDS. The role of systemic steroids is controversial. While steroids play a part in preventing late complications of an excessive inflammatory reaction in the eye, the administration of systemic steroids may exacerbate disseminated candidiasis.[7]

Vitrectomy

Pars plana vitrectomy can assist in both the diagnosis of *Candida* endophthalmitis and the management of the infection with intravitreal amphotericin B.[7,33,40,66,74] In experimental studies, vitreous biopsy was used to successfully diagnose *Candida* endophthalmitis in 62% of the cases, while a positive anterior chamber aspiration was rare (1.7%).[39]

Vitrectomy removes both the fungal mass and inflammatory debris and therefore rapidly results in clear media.[41] Caution should be exercised before intravitreal procedures, particularly since rarely cases of *Candida* endophthalmitis may resolve spontaneously,[20] or with parenteral treatment alone.

Clinical Response

The treatment of *Candida* endophthalmitis must be individualized for each patient. The indications for amphotericin B or other antifungal agents, as well as the indications for vitrectomy, remain relative rather than absolute. If a small retinal lesion with minimal vitreous inflammation exists, an aggressive work-up for systemic candidiasis must be performed. If systemic candidiasis is proven, systemic antifungal medication should be employed. The well-known, potentially life-threatening, toxic effects of amphotericin B warrant its use only if clearly dictated by the clinical situation. In most instances, fluconazole appears to give satisfactory results while minimizing potential toxicity.[2,5,21,50] The indications for vitrectomy for ocular candidiasis are (1) diagnosis, (2) for the injection of intravitreal amphotericin B for *Candida* endophthalmitis, or (3) progressive *Candida* chorioretinitis that is not responsive to systemic antifungal therapy and is vision threatening.[21]

The results of treatment for both exogenous and endogenous *Candida* endophthalmitis appear to be superior to bacterial endophthalmitis.[13,29,67,78] In a consecutive series of eight patients with *Candida* endophthalmitis managed with vitrectomy and intravitreal amphotericin B (but without intravenous amphotericin B), 50% achieved a visual acuity of at least 20/50 and 75% achieved a visual acuity of at least 20/200.[13] Similarly, in a consecutive series of 14 patients with *C. parapsilosis* endophthalmitis, 53% achieved visual acuity of at least 20/60 with vitrectomy.[76]

OCULAR COCCIDIOIDOMYCOSIS

Coccidioides immitis is a dimorphic fungus capable of producing ocular disease endemic in the arid and semiarid soils of Central and South America, as well as the southwestern United States including California (particularly the San Joaquin Valley of southeast California), southern Arizona and New Mexico, and southwest Texas. In California, it has been termed San Joaquin fever, valley fever, or desert fever. It can infect both humans and animals, including dogs, cats, horses, and swine.[10,16,43]

Coccidioides immitis exists in two phases of repro-

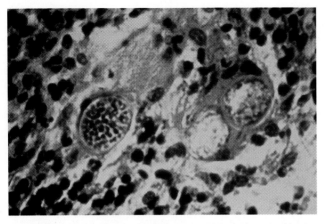

FIGURE 64–5 Photomicrography of coccidioidal spherule containing daughter endospores and thick-walled capsule prior to rupture (hematoxylin-eosin, X 540).

duction. The saprophytic phase resides in soil, its natural habitat, and contains septate hyphae. This phase culminates in the production of thin-walled structures (arthroconidia) that are released into the air and inhaled from airborne dust, thereby initiating infection.

In animal host tissues, the arthroconidia are quickly converted to the parasitic phase. This is characterized by thick-walled spherules, 20 to 100 μm in diameter, which contain numerous endospores. These spherules reproduce asexually in the host, with the daughter endospores contained within the shell of the spherule (Fig. 64–5). These daughter endospores are released by eventual rupture of the spherule wall, and in turn give rise to future generations.

Clinical Manifestations

Transmission of the Disease

Transmission of the disease occurs via inhalation of arthroconidia. Immunosuppressive therapy, especially corticosteroids, is believed to increase the risk of disseminated disease.[5,6,36] The disease is almost four times as frequent in males as in females.[10,43] An association between intraocular coccidioidal endophthalmitis with diabetes mellitus and angioid streaks has been noted in one patient.[5] In most cases, no known predisposing factors are identified.[19]

Systemic Coccidioidomycosis

Primary coccidioidomycosis occurs as a respiratory tract infection. Like histoplasmosis, approximately 60% of the cases are asymptomatic, and 40% have some respiratory or influenza-like symptoms such as cough, fever, malaise, and pleuritic chest pain.[16] The incubation period of the acute respiratory infection is generally about 10 to 14 days. Erythema nodosum is found in 5 to 10% of males and 25% of

females with primary infection, presumably as a hypersensitivity reaction.

Like histoplasmosis, active pulmonary foci of infection usually heal spontaneously.[38] An inactive granulomatous nodule on chest x-ray or a positive skin test to coccidioidin antigen may be the only sign of previous infection. Fewer than 5% of infected patients develop residual chronic pulmonary granulomatous nodules, thin-walled cavities, or miliary pneumonitis. Fewer than 1% of individuals develop disseminated infection, which can spread to the lung, lymph nodes, spleen, skin, subcutaneous tissue, liver, kidney, bone, meninges, adrenal glands, and myocardium.[16,17] The eye is one of the rarest sites of dissemination in coccidioidomycosis.[26,37,40] Disseminated disease usually occurs within weeks following primary pulmonary infection, but, in some cases, it may not occur for up to 1 year.[10]

Ocular Coccidioidomycosis

Ocular coccidiodomycosis may affect either the anterior or posterior segment of the eye. Anterior segment manifestations include phlyctenular conjunctivitis,[39,47] episcleritis, scleritis, or keratoconjunctivitis.[45,46] These manifestations usually occur in association with primary pulmonary infections and are believed to represent self-limiting hypersensitivity responses to the coccidioidal antigen.

Intraocular involvement may occur either anteriorly (as acute or chronic granulomatous iridocyclitis) or posteriorly (as choroiditis, chorioretinitis, or endophthalmitis). The posterior ocular lesions have generally been associated with systemic coccidioidomycosis,[5,7,9,11,13,21] although some cases have been reported in which no other evidence of extrapulmonary disease can be found.[3,5,15,26,33] Most reported cases of ocular coccidioidomycosis have either anterior or posterior involvement; the combination of the two is rare.[5,6]

OCULAR SYMPTOMS. Photophobia and ciliary spasm can occur with anterior segment disease, while decreased vision and photopsia have been reported with posterior segment disease. However, most patients with ocular infection are asymptomatic. Although only few sporadic reports of ocular coccidioidal infection exist, a prospective study of ten consecutive patients with chronic pulmonary disease identified four (all asymptomatic) with posterior segment involvement, suggesting that ocular infection may be more common than is currently believed.[5]

Posterior Segment Disease

Intraocular coccidioidomycosis can cause chorioretinitis, granulomatous iridocyclitis, or progressive endophthalmitis. The spectrum of acute chorioretinitis associated with coccidioidomycosis varies from a large (3 disc diameter) juxtapapillary chorioretinal exudate to the more frequent whitish yellow, metallic, small (0.1 to 0.25 disc diameter) oval, slightly elevated, edematous-appearing chorioretinal lesions scattered throughout the fundus.[6,35,36] With resolution, these lesions tend to shrink, appearing as well-demarcated chorioretinal scars with varying degrees of hyperpigmentation and depigmentation.[34,35,36] Many of these scars seem to have a grayish white gliotic or fibrotic material in their base.

Blumenkranz and Stevens[5] have divided posterior segment involvement into four broad categories:

1. *Diffuse choroiditis.* This is often associated with widely disseminated coccidioidomycosis and carries a poor systemic prognosis (Fig. 64–6).
2. *Large (400 to 1000 μm) elevated juxtapapillary choroidal infiltrates.* These lesions appear to be the most common mode of involvement. Of 16 cases of endogenous coccidioidal endophthalmitis reported prior to 1979, 10 demonstrated this finding, often with associated retinal edema, hemorrhages, and exudates (Fig. 64–7).
3. *Medium sized (150 to 400 μm) spherical opacities at the level of Bruch's membrane and sensory retina.* These lesions appear to represent direct extension from the choroid into the retina. They show a predilection for the macula and posterior pole (Fig. 64–8).
4. *Small peripheral chorioretinal scars (100 to 200 μm) with variable hyperpigmentation and hypopigmentation (Fig. 64–9).* Blumenkranz and Stevens[5] believe that these lesions do not nec-

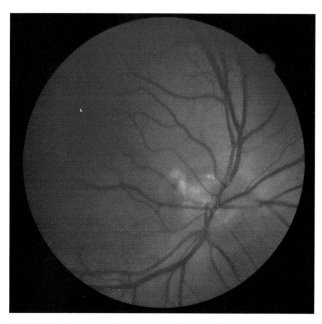

FIGURE 64–7   White juxtapapillary infiltrate, suggestive of cotton-wool spot with slightly elevated margins in patient with chronic pulmonary coccidioidomycosis. (Courtesy of Richard Sogg, M.D.)

essarily represent unequivocal evidence of ocular involvement. However, Rodenbiker et al[37] found that 5 of 54 subjects with documented past infection with *C. immitis* had characteristic inactive peripheral chorioretinal scars, but they found no evidence between the extent of the disease and the presence of scars. They concluded that dissemination of *C. immitis* to the eye occurs more commonly than isolated case reports would indicate.

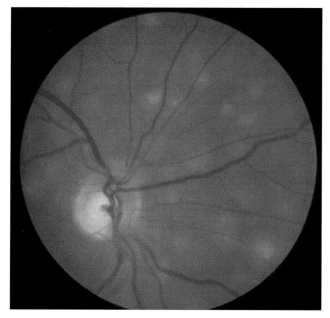

FIGURE 64–6   Multifocal yellow flat choroidal infiltrates in patient with preterminal disseminated coccidioidal choroiditis. (From Little H: Ocular coccidioidomycosis: a clinical ophthalmologic case report. Trans Am Acad Ophthalmol Otolaryngol 76:645–650, 1972, with permission.)

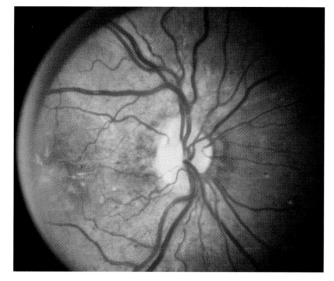

FIGURE 64–8   Fundus in young male with angioid streaks, diabetes mellitus, and chronic pulmonary coccidioidal mycosis demonstrating small round spheroidal opacities in outer retina that faded with successful amphotericin B therapy. (From Blumenkranz MS, Stevens DA: Endogenous coccidioidal endophthalmitis. Ophthalmology 87:974–984, with permission.)

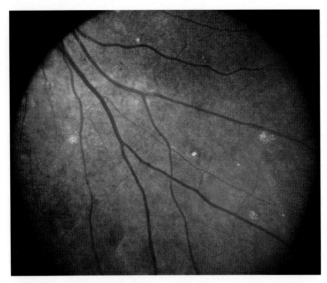

FIGURE 64–9 Small flat scar in periphery of same patient in Figure 64–3 after amphotericin antifungal therapy.

and latex-agglutination test titers rise during the first few weeks after infection, peak at 3 to 6 weeks after infection, and slowly fall over the next 3 months to unrecordable levels. The immunodiffusion test and complement fixation test titers do not become positive until at least 1 month after infection, peak at 2 to 3 months, and remain elevated until late in the disease, which varies depending on the clinical course. The complement fixation test, positive for several months after the primary infection, has more diagnostic value than the immunodiffusion test. Cross-reactivity has been reported in cases of histoplasmosis and blastomycosis, and negative tests have been reported with disseminated ocular infection.[5,31] Papanicolaou and hematoxylin and eosin–stained preparations of anterior chamber fluid or iris tissue may demonstrate intact or disrupted spherules.[33]

Whenever a fungal infection is suspected clinically, the use of skin tests and serologic tests are in no way diagnostic.[45]

Unlike histoplasmosis, macular involvement is uncommon. Only two patients in the English literature with coccidioidomycosis have had macular lesions.[1,26] In contrast to histoplasmosis and candidiasis, documented cases of chorioretinal neovascularization have not been reported.

OTHER OPHTHALMIC MANIFESTATIONS. Eyelid granulomas have been reported only rarely.[25,44] Papilledema, sixth nerve palsy, granulomatous nerve infiltration, and optic atrophy have been reported with central nervous system coccidioidomycosis.[1,34,45] Moorthy et al described three patients with granulomatous iridocyclitis due to coccidioidomycosis, diagnosed by anterior chamber tap. Two of three patients had no evidence of chronic pulmonary or disseminated coccidioidomycosis.[33]

Coccidioidal Endophthalmitis in Children

Golden et al[20] reported the only well-documented case of *C. immitis* chorioretinitis in a 7-week-old infant. The child developed a 1-disc-diameter, juxtapapillary chorioretinal scar during treatment with amphotericin B.

Diagnosis

Skin tests for coccidioidomycosis use a culture filtrate extracted in the laboratory from the saprophytic (i.e., mycelial) phase of the fungus. False-negative skin tests can occur with severe disseminated infections[5,26,34] or in anergic individuals.

Serologic tests include the tube precipitin test, latex agglutination test, immunodiffusion test, and complement fixation test. The tube precipitin test

Histopathology

Five cases have been proven pathologically.[7,11,19,34,45,48] Two of the five showed granulomas in the choroid without lesions in the overlying retina.[11,34] One showed focal destruction of Bruch's membrane by choroidal granulomas, but the overlying retinal pigment epithelium was intact.[48] One showed choroidal granulomas with overlying retinal degeneration, but retinal granulomas or organisms were not found.[7] The fifth showed numerous discrete retinal granulomas with organisms scattered throughout the fundus in a miliary pattern, with choroidal granulomas confined mainly to the middle and large vessel layers.[19] Retinal granulomas do not appear to arise from choroidal granulomas. Rather, both appear to be distinct lesions that arise from hematogenous dissemination.[19]

The granulomatous nodules consist of *C. immitis* organisms, histiocytes, giant cells, plasma cells, and lymphocytes located in either the choroid or the retina.

Differential Diagnosis

The differential diagnosis of coccidioidal choroiditis or retinitis includes syphilis, tuberculosis, sarcoidosis, toxocariasis, cysticercosis, toxoplasmosis, nocardiosis, cryptococcosis, blastomycosis, and other even less common fungal diseases.

Chemotherapy

Amphotericin B is the drug of choice for the treatment of disseminated or progressive pulmonary coccidioidomycosis. Amphotericin B, a polyene antifungal agent, demonstrates activity against all strains of *C. immitis* tested in vitro and in vivo.[12] It damages the cytoplasmic membrane of susceptible organisms, causing increased membrane permeability, leakage of cellular constituents, and ultimately cell death.[24,29]

Although intravenous amphotericin B penetrates the vitreous poorly,[21] it has shown clinical efficacy for intraocular coccidioidomycosis.[4] Oral fluconazole may also be effective, but experience with this agent for coccidioidomycosis is limited.[29] Details of systemic and intraocular amphotericin B therapy are more comprehensively covered in "Ocular Candidiasis," earlier in this chapter.

Miconazole, an imidazole derivative, is a less toxic but possibly less effective alternative to amphotericin B in the treatment of *C. immitis* infections. Preliminary evidence indicates broad antifungal susceptibility to these agents in vitro, and efficacy in vivo in superficial and deep mycoses in both animal models and in humans.[40] In a series of four patients with coccidioidal endophthalmitis, amphotericin B appeared more effective in preventing and reversing intraocular involvement than miconazole, although one patient in this series did develop new ocular lesions during amphotericin B therapy.[5] Other authors[1,14,23,34,45] have also reported progression of intraocular coccidioidomycosis in spite of intravenous amphotericin B.

Ketoconazole, an oral imidazole derivative, has been reported to be effective in the treatment of nonmeningeal coccidioidomycosis. Despite the absence of studies comparing amphotericin B and ketoconazole, their dramatic differences in pharmacology and toxicity rather than their relative efficacy are often the major influences in the selection of initial therapy. A study of 112 patients with progressive nonmeningeal coccidioidomycosis found that a dose of 400 mg daily resulted in a 23% success, while a dose of 800 mg daily resulted in a 32% success.[18] However, ketoconazole has negligible penetration into the central nervous system,[2] and its efficacy for ocular coccidioidal disease is yet to be established.

OCULAR CRYPTOCOCCOSIS

Cryptococcosis is a worldwide infectious disease caused by *Cryptococcus neoformans*, a saprophytic, yeast-like fungus frequently found in animal excreta (especially those of pigeons). As early as 1861,[69] a yeastlike organism causing central nervous system (CNS) disturbance was mentioned in the literature. In 1916, Stoddard and Cutler[54,61] differentiated the pathogenic yeast organism from true yeast and named it *Torula histolytica*, which has subsequently been renamed *Cryptococcus neoformans*. It has become an important human pathogen primarily through its ability to invade the CNS (primarily the brain and meninges). Ocular invasion can also occur.

Clinical Manifestations

Transmission of the Disease

Transmission of the disease occurs via inhalation of the organism into the lungs. Hematogenous dissemination can occur to any organ system but most commonly affects the CNS. The organism is not transmitted from person to person.[43] A predilection for males (80% of the reported cases) has been noted, most likely because of their greater outdoor environmental exposure.[13]

Epidemiologic and immunologic studies have supported the hypothesis that pigeons are reservoirs for human infections.[48,66] The organism is found abundantly in pigeon excreta, and less frequently in other avian excreta, soil, fruit juice, and raw milk.[9,43,47] Pigeon handlers have higher levels of antibodies to cryptococci than nonhandlers.[42,48]

Over 50% of the cases of cryptococcosis have occurred in immunocompromised individuals.[48] Malignant lymphoma, Hodgkin's disease, and other malignant diseases of the reticuloendothelial system impair host defense mechanisms against the organism and increase the likelihood of disseminated disease.[2,18,47,70] *Cryptococcus neoformans* is the most common life-threatening fungal pathogen that infects patients with AIDS.[21] The most common ophthalmic manifestation in a cohort of AIDS patients with cryptococcal infection confirmed by seropositivity were papilledema (32.5%), abducens palsy (9%), and optic atrophy (2.5%).[42] Systemic corticosteroid therapy has also been associated with an increased susceptibility to infection as well as dissemination of *C. neoformans*.[17,28,35] Fatal disseminated cryptococcosis has been reported in a patient treated with systemic steroids for a retinal inflammatory lesion.[50]

Systemic Findings

Pulmonary disease is usually associated with minimal constitutional signs and symptoms. Pulmonary involvement becomes clinically apparent when it causes a pneumonia-like illness, manifested as cough, malaise, chest pain, sputum production, and low-grade fever.[48] Pulmonary infections are usually self-limiting, and diagnosis may be difficult, sometimes requiring biopsy of the affected tissue. Asymptomatic pulmonary infections occur in about one third of the diagnosed cases, and detection usually occurs as a result of roentgenographic examination.[13,48]

Cryptococcal invasion of the CNS can produce symptoms and signs characteristic of meningitis, meningoencephalitis, or a space-occupying lesion. In many instances, the disease clinically appears similar to tuberculosis. Untreated infections of the CNS are generally fatal within 6 months, although chronic infections lasting years can occur.[48] Symptoms of cryptococcosis reflect an increase in intracranial pressure or meningeal irritation. Headache is the most common initial complaint, but lassitude, photophobia, visual blurring, nausea and vomiting, neck stiffness, fever, myalgia, and weakness are all common.

Ocular Cryptococcosis

Neurophthalmic Disease

Ocular complications of cryptococcal meningitis are common, although localization of the fungus itself in the eye is uncommon. At the time of presentation, ocular symptoms are present in 36 to 40% of patients with cryptococcal meningitis.[12,41] Blurred vision is the most common ocular symptom. Papilledema is the most common ophthalmic sign, and untreated, it may progress to cause severe visual loss and optic atrophy.[12,19,30,41,55] Other manifestations include internuclear and supranuclear ophthalmoplegia, nystagmus, sixth nerve palsy, photophobia, and anisocoria.[33,41,46,55] The optic nerve may be directly invaded by cryptococcal organisms,[45] and optic nerve sheath fenestration has been proposed as a potential therapy.[30]

Posterior Segment Disease

In 1944, Cohen[20] reported the first clinical observation of ocular involvement of cryptococcosis in a patient with Hodgkin's disease and bilateral papilledema. Weiss and colleagues,[68] in 1948, were the first to report a case of cryptococcosis with intraocular involvement. Ocular involvement can occur secondary to direct extension of cryptococcal meningitis along the optic nerve, hematogenous spread, or direct inoculation.[67]

Intraocular cryptococcosis can result in choroiditis,[2,6,18,21,25,26] retinitis,[43] endophthalmitis,[36,54,58,64,67] or exudative retinal detachment from an isolated retinal mass.[39,49,57,62,67]

The most frequent manifestation is a focal chorioretinitis that appears initially as a solitary, slightly elevated yellowish white chorioretinal lesion often in a juxtapapillary location with minimal or no associated vitreitis[34,52] (Fig. 64–10). Secondary involvement of the retina resulting in retinal whitening, retinal vasculitis, vitreitis, or rarely panophthalmitis or endophthalmitis. Without treatment, the chorioretinal lesion will continue to progress in size and severity and almost always leads to an exudative retinal detachment, blindness, and frequently enucleation[37,38,57,59,62,67] (Fig. 64–11). Cryptococcal endophthalmitis is much rarer and probably is secondary to direct extension from chorioretinal lesions. The clinical appearance is a diffuse vitreitis with haze and debris and focal, white vitreous exudates that progressively enlarge to involve the entire vitreous.[23,36]

In 1968, Hiles and Font[39] reviewed the 12 previously reported cases of ocular cryptococcosis. They found only nine with histopathologically proven

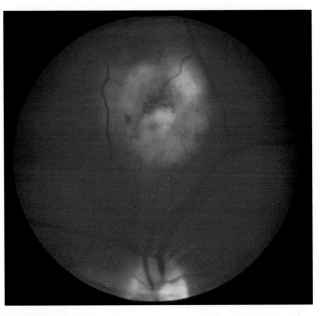

FIGURE 64–10   Solitary cryptococcal choroidal infiltrate in male with exposure to pigeon excrement. (From Shields JA, Wrighty DM, Augsburger JJ, et al. Cryptococcal chorioretinitis. Am J Ophthalmol 89:210–218, 1980. Copyright 1980, Elsevier Science, with permission.)

intraocular infection. They added three additional cases from the Armed Forces Institute of Pathology, to bring the total to 12 documented cases. Between 1968 and 1992, 20 additional cases of ocular cryptococcus have been reported.[25,26,36,39,43,49,57,59,62,64,67] Ten of these patients had chorioretinitis (usually as a large 1- to 4-disc-diameter, solitary chorioretinal whitish mass), six had choroiditis, three had en-

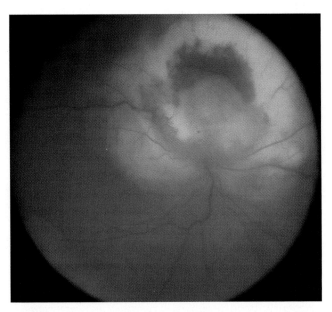

FIGURE 64–11   Enlarged juxtapapillary zone of retinochoroiditis in female with apical pulmonary infiltrate with no history of immunosuppression. Note adjacent exudative retinal detachment and suggestion of retinal neovascularization at apex of lesion.

dophthalmitis, and one had neuroretinitis. Bilateral involvement occurred in approximately one fourth of the cases. At least 75% of patients with ocular cryptococcosis had CNS disease at the time of presentation,[67] although experimental studies in mice suggest that selective involvement of the eye can occur in some cases without systemic disease.[60]

Other Ophthalmic Manifestations

Rarely, "other ocular tissues" may be primarily affected by cryptococci. This can occur as a localized infection, or it can involve the orbit, eyelids, and cornea.[27] Keratitis, iritis, and orbital infection from skin involvement have been rarely reported.[20,27] Doft and Curtin[25] reported combined ocular infection with cytomegalovirus and cryptococcosis in an immunosuppressed patient, and Charles et al described a cryptococcal iris mass in a patient with AIDS diagnosed by paracentesis and finally enucleation.[16]

Diagnosis

Diagnosis of pulmonary cryptococcosis is made with a positive sputum culture along with positive roentgenograms. The radiographic findings vary and include a solitary lesion, diffuse pneumonic infiltration, or cavity lesion.[48]

Diagnosis of cryptococcal meningitis is made by evaluation of the CSF with India ink, blood cultures, CSF cultures, and assay for cryptococcal antigen titers. The cryptococcal antigen in the CSF can be positive in patients with cryptococcal meningitis in patients who have had negative CSF cultures and negative India ink preparations.[6,57] The serum latex agglutination test for detection of antigen is the most sensitive method (99%) of diagnosing cryptococcal meningitis.[17] A titer greater than 1:8 indicates previous or current infection.[55] Similarly, an experimental animal model found the antigen test to be more sensitive than India ink mount or culture in the diagnosis of cryptococcal eye infections.[29] India ink preparations are negative in 50% of cases involving the CNS.[57]

Vitreous aspiration can assist in the diagnosis for cryptococcal endophthalmitis.[39] Vitreous aspiration with membrane filtration and mucin carmine histochemistry[54] have been employed. Fine-needle aspiration of a cryptococcal retinovitreal abscess[37,39] has been an effective method of diagnosis in selected cases.

The differential diagnosis of chorioretinal lesions with associated vitreitis includes other infectious and inflammatory diseases such as tuberculosis, nocardiosis, sarcoidosis, toxoplasmosis, cytomegalovirus, acute retinal necrosis, and other fungal diseases (most notably candidiasis, blastomycosis, and coccidioidomycosis). In addition, metastatic tumors, amelanotic melanomas, large cell lymphomas, and choroidal lymphomas can produce a similar choroidal lesion.

Histopathology

Culture Characteristics

Cryptococcus neoformans is the only pathogenic species of the genus *Cryptococcus* and the only encapsulated yeast capable of invading the human CNS.[41] *Cryptococcus neoformans* is differentiated from other species of cryptococci by its ability to grow well at 37°C, its ability to assimilate different carbohydrates (glucose, mannose, trehalose, xylose, galactose, maltose, sucrose, inositol, dextrin, and starch), its failure to assimilate lactose and potassium nitrate, and its virulence for mice. The diagnosis is aided by the latex slide agglutination test for detecting cryptococcal antigen and the use of hypertonic sucrose media for cultural identification.[35]

The organism is spherical, 4 to 20 μm in diameter, and surrounded by a thick mucinous polysaccharide capsule that does not stain with India ink preparation.[2] The capsule, which is 3 to 7 μm thick, forms a clear halo around the cell. The cell body contains irregular masses or granules. The organism reproduces by budding, does not form true mycelia (hyphae), and grows on an ordinary laboratory aerobic medium such as blood agar or Sabaroud's dextrose agar.

Pathologic examination of involved eyes has disclosed the organism within histocytes as well as free in the extracellular matrix.[38,59] The organism can be found in the choroid, either with[59] or without[2] involvement of the overlying retina. Less commonly, retinal involvement may occur in the absence of uveal involvement.[43]

Chemotherapy

Untreated, cryptococcal meningitis is almost always fatal.[36,43] Since its introduction in 1955, amphotericin B has been the drug of choice for the treatment of disseminated or progressive pulmonary cryptococcosis. For details of amphotericin therapy, see "Ocular Candidiasis," earlier in this chapter.[35,51]

Although intravenous amphotericin B penetrates the vitreous poorly,[34] it has shown clinical efficacy for intraocular cryptococcosis.[5]

Amphotericin B used in association with 5-fluorocytosine improves the outcome and reduces the chance of organism resistance developing in patients with AIDS.[3,5] However, a retrospective study of cryptococcal infections in patients with AIDS concluded that the addition of flucytosine to amphotericin B neither enhanced survival nor prevented relapses.[17]

The maximum serum levels in patients receiving

amphotericin B intravenously in a dosage of 1.2 mg/kg/day are usually no higher than 1.8 μg/ml.[47] This exceeds the minimal inhibitory concentration required for most of the systemic pathogenic fungi, including *C. neoformans*. (The minimal inhibitory concentration of amphotericin B for *C. neoformans* ranges from 0.2 to 0.3 μg/ml). Most patients are treated with 1.5 to 2.0 g of amphotericin B for 6 to 12 weeks, although patients with AIDS often require indefinite suppressive therapy to prevent relapses.[17]

Fluconazole, a new triazole compound, is a recently approved oral or parenteral agent for the treatment of cryptococcal meningitis infections in AIDS patients. Fluconazole is the only antifungal azole derivative that penetrates into the CSF and appears as effective as amphotericin B for cryptococcal meningitis.[1]

INTRAOCULAR BLASTOMYCOSIS

Blastomycosis is a chronic granulomatous fungal infection of humans and lower animals caused by the dimorphic fungus *Blastomyces dermatitidis*. Blastomycosis was first described as a cutaneous disease by Gilchrist in 1894.[13] The eyes may be infected as a result of hematogenous dissemination from a primary pulmonary lesion.[11]

Blastomycosis is most prevalent in the United States, and it has often been termed "North American blastomycosis."[25] It is particularly common in the midwestern states, such as the Ohio and the Mississippi river valleys.[15] It is six times more common in men than in women and is most likely to affect those with outdoor occupations. The majority of patients are 50 years of age or older.

Clinical Manifestations

Transmission of the Disease

Primary infection in humans takes place after inhalation of oval conidia into the lungs. At body temperature, the conidia convert to yeast forms.[10] Outbreaks of the disease have occurred in groups at campsites, and the organism was isolated in the soil during one of these outbreaks.[17,27]

Systemic Findings

The acute primary pulmonary infection often has no symptoms; less commonly, it may cause an influenza or atypical pneumonia syndrome.[22,26] Among the symptomatic patients, at least two clinical types of infections are recognizable. The first, which is quite similar to acute histoplasmosis or coccidioidomycosis, consists of an influenza-like illness, with fever, productive cough, arthralgia, and myalgia. The second type of clinical illness consists of pleuritic chest pain, varying from very severe, to mild pleuritic chest discomfort.[26]

Although acute blastomycotic pneumonia usually resolves spontaneously, progressive forms of disease that involve the lungs, the extrapulmonary organs (most commonly the skin, bones, joints, and prostate gland), or both develop in some patients. Rarely, primary cutaneous blastomycosis results from direct inoculation of the organism by means of a dog bite.

The skin is the most frequent site of dissemination. The most characteristic skin lesion is a large, verrucous ulcer with heaped-up edges.[25] It has sharp serpiginous borders and tends to heal centrally.[31] Extravasation of erythrocytes between the dermis and epidermis may give rise to multiple black dots in subcutaneous skin lesions characteristic of the disease.[3]

Central nervous system blastomycosis occurs in 3 to 10% of the cases, and fewer than 100 cases have been reported.[5,15,31] Patients may have an intracranial abscess, a spinal abscess, or meningitis. Tuberculosis meningitis, meningeal carcinomatosis, and fungal meningitis are the major diagnostic considerations. The absence of pulmonary lesions on chest x-ray does not exclude CNS blastomycosis.[15]

OCULAR BLASTOMYCOSIS. Since Churchill and Stober[9] reported the first case of blastomycosis involving the eye in 1914, only seven cases of intraocular blastomycosis have been reported in the English literature.[2,11,14,18,28,29]

IRIS AND CILIARY BODY GRANULOMAS. Schwartz,[28] in 1931, described the first pathologically proven case of intraocular blastomycosis. The lesion was primarily found in the iris, together with an associated hypopyon, while the choroid remained spared. In 1946, Cassady[7] described a case of intraocular metastatic blastomycosis. Pathologic examination demonstrated that the lesion was located in the iris and ciliary body.

RETINITIS AND CHOROIDITIS. Only six patients have been described with choroidal involvement.[2,11,18,29] Two of these patients also had endophthalmitis, and a third demonstrated bilateral multifocal choroidal lesions.

Sinskey and Anderson[29] reported the pathologic findings in an eye obtained postmortum from a patient who died of miliary blastomycosis. Numerous yellowish white lesions, approximately one eighth–disc-diameter in size, were scattered in the posterior choroid. Microscopic examination of both eyes showed numerous posterior choroidal granulomas, with numerous budding yeast-like organisms consistent with *B. dermatitidis*.

Font et al[11] described a 73-year-old systemically well man who had an enucleation for a painful, blind eye. Histopathologic examination of the eye demonstrated mycotic panophthalmitis caused by

B. dermatitidis, necrosis and detachment of the retina, chronic diffuse granulomatous choroiditis, and episcleral abscess with rupture of the sclera and choroid.

Bond et al[2] reported a case of presumed blastomycosis endophthalmitis in a patient with biopsy-proven sarcoidosis. The patient had a large, pale yellow choroidal lesion in the posterior choroid of his right eye, associated with iritis and vitreitis. Several similar small lesions were present in the choroid of the contralateral eye. Skin cultures, brain and dura biopsies, and lumbar punctures revealed budding yeasts consistent with *B. dermatitidis.* The patient died of hospital-acquired pneumonia. Since a postmortem examination was not performed and since the patient had a history of sarcoidosis, one cannot definitively conclude whether his ocular manifestations were secondary to blastomycosis or sarcoidosis.

Lewis et al[18] described a case of presumed latent blastomycosis in a 36-year-old man who presented 2 months after developing a productive cough and flu-like illness. Fundus examination of the involved left eye demonstrated an oval, yellow, elevated choroidal lesion that measured 1.75 by 2.5 mm, with associated surrounding subretinal fluid. Fluorescein angiography demonstrated early hypofluorescence and late hyperfluorescence of the lesion. A biopsy of an indurated erythematous skin lesion demonstrated a granulomatous inflammatory reaction with yeast organisms characteristic of *B. dermatitidis.* The patient was treated with amphotericin B for a total dose of 2 g. The choroidal lesion and the patient's systemic symptoms rapidly resolved within 2 weeks of starting amphotericin B (Figs. 64–12 and 64–13).

Safneck et al[24] described a pathologically proven

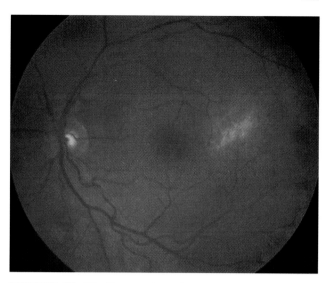

FIGURE 64–13   Same patient after completion of antifungal therapy with resolution of granuloma overlying retinal detachment. (From Lewis H, Aaberg TM, Fary DRB, et al: Latent disseminated blastomycosis with choroidal involvement. Arch Ophthalmol 106:527–530, 1988. Copyright 1988, American Medical Association, with permission.)

case of *B. dermatiditis* endophthalmitis in a 71-year-old woman with night sweats, fevers, and weight loss. She had an enucleation performed for a painful, blind eye. Histologic examination of the eye demonstrated broad-based budding yeasts consistent with *B. dermatitidis* organisms in the anterior chamber, necrosis of the iris and peripheral retina, and a fibrovascular membrane extending from the optic nerve to the ciliary body. A systemic evaluation failed to find evidence of disseminated blastomycosis. She was treated with a 12-week course of amphotericin B and had an uneventful recovery.

OTHER OCULAR MANIFESTATIONS. Studies prior to 1950 reported that eyelid involvement occurs in about 25% of cases.[26] However, recent medical reviews have documented eyelid involvement only rarely[15,23,25] and only infrequent case reports[1] in the ocular literature exist. Keratitis,[33] endophthalmitis,[2,11,24] and orbital involvement[30] have been infrequently reported.

Histopathology

The fungus is dimorphic. Microscopic examination of this growth reveals regular, septate mycelia and conidia formation. In tissues, this fungus characteristically appears as round or oval thick-walled organisms, measuring 8 to 15 μm in diameter, although some cells may be as large as 20 to 30 μm.[15] The cells reproduce in tissues by single budding, and the buds have a broad basal attachment to mother cells. The large size, refractile cell wall, and single broad-based buds serve to differentiate *Blastomyces* from other yeasts. The organisms are read-

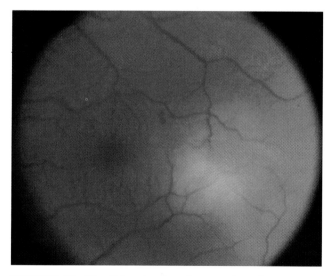

FIGURE 64–12   Color fundus photography of 36-year-old male with choroidal blastomycosis and overlying pale neurosensory detachment. (From Lewis H, Aaberg TM, Fary DRB, et al: Latent disseminated blastomycosis with choroidal involvement. Arch Ophthalmol 106:527–530, 1988. Copyright 1988, American Medical Association, with permission.)

ily visible in ordinary hematoxylin and eosin preparation, although Gomori methenamine silver and PAS may be helpful. The organism grows almost exclusively in the yeast form in vivo, with hyphae only rarely found. Growth at room temperature on Sabouraud's medium is in mycelial (hyphael) form. The tissue form (yeast-like organisms) may be obtained in vitro by incubating cultures at 37°C.[23]

Diagnosis

The differential diagnosis of North American blastomycosis includes entities that can produce a similar choroidal mass: sarcoidosis, posterior scleritis, tuberculosis, cryptococcosis, histoplasmosis, coccidioidomycosis, and primary or metastatic choroidal tumors.

When present, systemic findings suggestive of an influenza type of illness may alert the clinician to blastomycosis, but the systemic findings may be identical to those seen in histoplasmosis and coccidioidomycosis.[26] Definitive diagnosis is made through culture of the organism, frequently from the sputum. Examination of potassium hydroxide–digested fresh sputum may reveal the characteristic budding yeast of B. dermatitidis. The appearance of the chest x-ray is nonspecific and similar to acute histoplasmosis, with multiple soft nodules scattered in both lungs.[8] Skin testing with Blastomyces antigen is unreliable, and cross-reaction with histoplasmosis is common.[5,22] The two available serologic tests—complement fixation and immunodiffusion—are not helpful diagnostic tools in individual cases because of their low sensitivity and specificity.[10,17,22]

A recent study of an outbreak of blastomycosis suggests that an enzyme immunoassay to detect antibody to the A antigen of B. dermatitidis demonstrates a high sensitivity (77%).[17] An assay of the in vitro transformation of lymphocytes in the presence of a Blastomyces alkali- and water-soluble antigen also demonstrates a high sensitivity (81%) of detecting infection. However, the latter test remains investigational.[10]

Treatment

In most patients, acute, epidemic pulmonary blastomycosis is a benign disease with a favorable outcome that does not require antifungal treatment. In an outbreak of 18 patients with blastomycosis, 11 remained asymptomatic, 4 had a mild illness of short duration, and 3 were severely ill.[26] All patients recovered without specific antifungal therapy.

For the past three decades, intravenously administered amphotericin B has been the therapy of choice for blastomycosis. Unfortunately, intravenous amphotericin B is associated with a consid-

erable frequency and variety of toxic manifestations including fever, chills, anorexia, nausea, vomiting, headache, malaise, anemia, hypokalemia, and renal impairment.[19]

Findings from two recent studies indicate that ketoconazole, an oral imidazole antifungal agent, is an effective alternative in immunocompetent patients with mild to moderately severe forms of the disease not involving the CNS. A prospective, randomized, multicenter trial in 80 patients with blastomycosis demonstrated that a high-dose ketoconazole regimen (800 mg/day) was more effective than a low-dose regimen (400 mg/day). The high-dose regimen resulted in a success rate of 100%, compared to 79% in the low-dose group. However, because of the higher frequency of side effects in the high-dose group, the authors recommended that ketoconazole therapy should be begun with the low-dose regimen.[21] In a second prospective study of 44 patients with blastomycosis, a cure rate of 80% was achieved with 400 mg/day ketoconazole.[4] These authors recommend ketoconazole rather than amphotericin B as the initial treatment of blastomycosis that is not overwhelming, and they recommend primary treatment with amphotericin B for severe infections. However, none of their patients had intraocular or CNS disease.

ASPERGILLOSIS AND SPOROTRICHOSIS

Aspergillus is a rare cause of endophthalmitis that occurs primarily in immunocompromised patients. Doft et al reported two cases of endogenous Aspergillus endophthalmitis in drug abusers.[3] In most patients with Aspergillus endophthalmitis, systemic involvement is present. However, in abusers of intravenously administered drugs, systemic involvement is often not present.[3] Aspergillus fumigatus and A. flavus are the two most commonly isolated organisms.[9] More than 20 cases of endogenous Aspergillus endophthalmitis have been reported.[2–4,6,8,9]

The clinical presentation includes anterior uveitis, vitreitis, and fluffy vitreous infiltrates. Symptoms and signs parallel those of candidal endophthalmitis and the two cannot be distinguished clinically. The organism initially causes a slowly progressive whitish yellow choroidal infiltrate that later spreads to involve the retina and vitreous, similar to Candida (Fig. 64–14). Pathologic examination has demonstrated the organism in the retina, choroid, and vitreous (Fig. 64–15). The treatment is comparable to that for candidal endophthalmitis—vitrectomy and intravenous and intravitreal amphotericin B (see Candida treatment above)—although the return of useful vision is thought to be less common and the response to oral fluconazole less well established.[3,9]

Sporotrichosis, a fungal disease caused by the dimorphic fungus Sporotrichum schenckii, is a rare

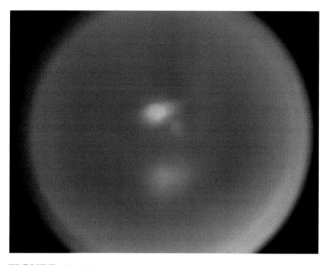

FIGURE 64–14 Severe vitreitis in drug abuse with endogenous *Aspergillus* endophthalmitis documented by culture following vitrectomy. (Courtesy of Bernard Doft, M.D.)

cause of fungal endophthalmitis. Most cases begin as primary cutaneous lesions from inoculation with contaminated soil or vegetable material. Ocular involvement is unusual, and may result from the direct extension from cutaneous lesions of the lids, or less frequently through hematogenous dissemination. Font et al described a 42-year-old man with iritis and retinitis that gradually progressed over several months to involve the entire retina. Enucleation demonstrated the organisms in necrotic retina.[5] Cassady and Foerster described a 50-year-old man with a chronic unilateral uveitis that progressed to endophthalmitis.[1] Enucleation demonstrated massive choroidal and retinal inflammation and numerous dimorphic organisms in the retina. Neither of these patients had signs or symptoms suggestive of disseminated sporotrichosis and neither required systemic antifungal therapy.

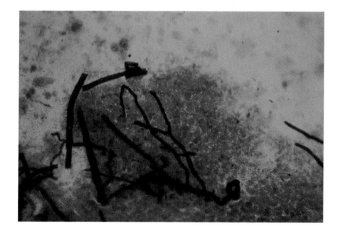

FIGURE 64–15 Branching septate hyphal forms from vitrectomy specimen in patient with *Aspergillus* endophthalmitis (Giemsa, X 430).

REFERENCES

Ocular Candidiasis

1. Aguilar GL, Blumenkranz MS, Egbert PR, McCulley JP: *Candida* endophthalmitis after intravenous drug abuse. Arch Ophthalmol 97:96–100, 1979.
2. Akler ME, Vellend H, McNeely D: Use of fluconazole in the treatment of candidal endophthalmitis. Clin Infect Dis 19:657–664, 1995.
3. Airas KA, Nikoskelainen J: Haematogenous *Candida* endophthalmitis after abdominal surgery. Acta Ophthalmol 65:450–454, 1987.
4. Arndt CAS, Walsh RJ, Lester McCully C, et al: Fluconazole penetration into cerebrospinal fluid: implications for treating fungal infections of the central nervous system. J Infect Dis 157:178–180, 1988.
5. Aust R, Kruse F, Wildfever A, et al: Fluconazole level in aqueous humor after oral drug administration in humans. Ophthalmology 92:829–832, 1995.
6. Axelrod AJ, Peyman GA: Intravitreal amphotericin B treatment of experimental fungal endophthalmitis. Am J Ophthalmol 76:584–588, 1973.
7. Barrie T: The place of elective vitrectomy in the management of patients with *Candida* endophthalmitis. Graefes, Arch Clin Exp Ophthalmol 225:107–113, 1987.
8. Beebe WE, Kirkland C, Price J: A subretinal neovascular membrane as a complication of endogenous *Candida* endophthalmitis. Ann Ophthalmol 19:207–209, 1987.
9. Behrens-Baumann W, Klinge B, Ruchel R: Topical fluconazole for experimental *Candida* keratitis in rabbits. Br J Ophthalmol 74:40–42, 1990.
10. Bennett JE: Chemotherapy of systemic mycosis, Part 1. N Engl J Med 290:30–32, 1974.
11. Bielsa I, Miro JM, Herrero C, et al: Systemic candidiasis in heroin abusers. Int J Dermatol 26:314–319, 197.
12. Blumenkranz MS, Stevens DA: Therapy of endogenous fungal endophthalmitis: miconazole or amphotericin B for coccidioidal and candidal infection. Arch Ophthalmol 98:1216–1220, 1980.
13. Brod RD, Flynn HW Jr, Clarkson JG, et al: Endogenous *Candida* endophthalmitis. Ophthalmology 97:666–674, 1990.
14. Brooks RG: Prospective study of *Candida* endophthalmitis in hospitalized patients with candidemia. Arch Intern Med 149:2226–2228, 1989.
15. Chess J, Kaplan S, Rubinstein A: *Candida* retinitis in bare lymphocyte syndrome. Ophthalmology 93:696–698, 1986.
16. Cogan DG: Immunosuppression and eye disease. First Vail Lecture. Am J Ophthalmol 83:777–788, 1977.
17. Cohen M, Montgomerie JZ: Hematogenous endophthalmitis due to *Candida tropicalis*: Report of two cases and review. Clin Infect Dis 17:270–272, 1993.
18. Collignon PJ, Sorrell T: Disseminated candidiasis. Evidence of a distinctive syndrome in heroin abusers. Br Med J (Clin Res) 287:861–862, 1983.
19. Cosgrove RF, Beezer AE, Miles RJ: In vitro studies of amphotericin B in combination with the imidazole antifungal compounds clotrimazole and miconazole. J Infect Dis 7:757, 1900.
20. Dellon AL, Stark WJ, Chretien PB: Spontaneous resolution of endogenous *Candida* endophthalmitis complicating intravenous hyperalimentation. Am J Ophthalmol 79:648–654, 1975.
21. De Palacio A, Cuetara M, Ferro M, et al: Gluconazole in the management of endophthalmitis in disseminated candidiosis of heroin addicts. Mycoses 36:193–199, 1993.
22. Doft BH, Weiskopf J, Nilsson-Ehle I, et al: Amphotericin clearance in vitrectomized versus nonvitrectomized eyes. Ophthalmology 92:1601–1605, 1985.
23. Drouhet E, Dupont B: Laboratory and clinical assessment of ketoconazole in deep-seated mycosis. Am J Med 74:30–47, 1983.
24. Dupont B, Drouhet E: Cutaneous, ocular, and osteoar-

ticular candidiasis in heroin addicts: new clinical and therapeutic aspects in 38 patients. J Infect Dis 152:577–591, 1985.

25. Edwards JE Jr, Foos RY, Montgomerie JZ, et al: Ocular manifestations of *Candida* septicemia: review of seventy-six cases of hematogenous *Candida* endophthalmitis. Medicine 53:47–75, 1974.
26. Edwards JE, Leher RI, Steihm ER, et al: Severe candidal infections: clinical perspective, immune defense mechanisms, and current concepts of therapy. Ann Intern Med 89:91–106, 1978.
27. FDA Drug Bullet: Fluconazole for fungal infections. Rockville, MD, Department of Health and Human Services, 1990, pp 7–8.
28. Ferry AP: Endogenous *Candida* endophthalmitis in childhood. J Pediatr Ophthalmol 11:189, 1974.
29. Fine BS, Zimmerman LE: Exogenous intraocular fungus infections with particular reference to complications of intraocular surgery. Am J Ophthalmol 48:151–165, 1959.
30. Gaines JD, Remington JS: Diagnosis of deep infection with *Candida*. A study of *Candida precipitins*. Arch Intern Med 132:699–702, 1973.
31. Gallo J, Playgai J, Gregory-Roberts J, et al: Fungal endophthalmitis in narcotic abusers: medical and surgical therapy in 10 patients. Med J Aust 142:386–388, 1985.
32. Getnick RA, Rodrigues MM: Endogenous fungal endophthalmitis in a drug addict. Am J Ophthalmol 77:680–683, 1974.
33. Gilbert CM, Novak MA: Successful treatment of postoperative *Candida* endophthalmitis in an eye with an intraocular lens implant. Am J Ophthalmol 97:593–595, 1984.
34. Graham E, Chignell AH, Eykyn S: *Candida* endophthalmitis: a complication of prolonged intravenous therapy and antibiotic treatment. J Infect Dis 13:167–173, 1986.
35. Green WR, Bennett JE, Goos RD: Ocular penetration of amphotericin B. Arch Ophthalmol 73:769, 1965.
36. Griffin JR, Foos RY, Petit TH: Relationship between *Candida* endophthalmitis, candidemia, and disseminated candidiasis. Concil Ophthalmol 25:661–664, 1976.
37. Griffin JR, Pettit TH, Fishman LS, Foos RY: Blood-borne *Candida* endophthalmitis: a clinical and pathologic study of 21 cases. Arch Ophthalmol 89:450–456, 1973.
38. Hamilton-Miller JM: Fungal steroids and the mode of action of the polyene antibiotic. Adv Appl Microbiol 17:109–134, 1974.
39. Henderson DK, Edwards JE, Ishida K, Guze LB: Experimental hematogenous *Candida* endophthalmitis: diagnostic approaches. Infect Immun 23:858–862, 1979.
40. Hoffmann DH, Waubke TH: Experimentelle untersuchungen zur metastatischen ophthalmie mit der *Candida albicans*. Albrecht Von Graefes Arch Ophthalmol 164:174, 1961.
41. Huang K, Peyman GA, McGetrick J: Vitrectomy in experimental endophthalmitis: part 1—fungal infection. Ophthalmic Surg 10:84–86, 1979.
42. Hughes JM, Remington JS: Systemic candidiasis, a diagnostic challenge. Calif Med 116:8–17, 1972.
43. Insler MS, Urso LF: *Candida* albicans endophthalmitis after penetrating keratoplasy. Am J Ophthalmol 104:57–60, 1987.
44. Ishibashi Y, Hommura S, Watanabe R: Endogenous fungal endophthalmitis in Japan reported from 1974 to 1986. Nippon Ganka Gakkai Zasshi 92:952–958, 1988.
45. Jampol L, Sung J, Walker J, et al: Choroidal neovascularization secondary to *Candida albicans*. Am J Ophthalmol 121:643–649, 1996.
46. Jones BR: Principles in the management of oculomycosis. XXXI Edward Jackson memorial lecture. 79:719–751, 1975.
47. Jones DB: Chemotherapy of experimental endogenous *Candida albicans* endophthalmitis. Trans Am Acad Ophthalmol Soc LXXCVIII:846–895, 1980.
48. Kinyoun JL: Treatment of *Candida* endophthalmitis. Retina 2:215–222, 1982.

49. Lou P, Kazdan J, Bannatyne RM, Cheung R: Successful treatment of *Candida* endophthalmitis with a synergistic combination of amphotericin B and rifampin. Am J Ophthalmol 83:12–15, 1977.
50. Luttrull J, Kubak B, Smith M, et al: Treatment of ocular fungal infections with oral fluconazole. Am J Ophthalmol 199:477–481, 1995.
51. Malecaze F, Bessieres MH, Bec P, et al: Immunological analysis of the aqueous humour in *Candida* endophthalmitis. I: Experimental study. Br J Ophthalmol 72:309–312, 1988.
52. Margo CE, Bombardier T: The diagnostic value of fungal autofluorescence. Surv Ophthalmol 29:374–376, 1985.
53. Mathis A, Malecaze F, Bessieres MH, et al: Immunological analysis of the aqueous humour in *Candida* endophthalmitis. II: clinical study. Br J Ophthalmol 72:313–316, 1988.
54. McDonnell PF, McDonnell JM, Brown RH, et al: Ocular involvement in patients with fungal infections. Ophthalmology 92:706–709, 1985.
55. Medoff G, Kobayashi GS: Strategies in the treatment of systemic fungal agents. N Engl J Med 302:145–155, 1980.
56. Medoff G, Brajtburg J, Kobayashi GS: Antifungal agents useful in therapy of systemic fungal infections. Ann Rev Pharmacol Toxicol 23:303–330, 1983.
57. Miale JB: *Candida albicans* infection confused with tuberculosis. Arch Pathol 35:427–437, 1943.
58. Miller RP, Bates JH: Amphotericin B toxicity: a follow-up report of 53 patients. Ann Intern Med 71:1089–1095, 1969.
59. Montgomerie JZ, Edwards JE Jr, Guze LB: Synergism of amphotericin B and 5-flucytosine for *Candida* species. J Infect Dis 1132:82–86, 1975.
60. Murray IG, Buckley HR, Turner GC: Serologic evidence of *Candida* infection after open-heart surgery. J Med Microbiol 2:463–469, 1969.
61. O'Day DM, Akrabawi PL, Head WS, et al: Laboratory isolation techniques in human and experimental fungal infections. Am J Ophthalmol 87:688–693, 1979.
62. O'Day KM, Heads WS, Robinson RD, et al: Intraocular penetration of topical amphotericin B and natamycin. Curr Eye Res 5:877–882, 1986.
63. Palmer EA: Endogenous *Candida* endophthalmitis in infants. Am J Ophthalmol 89:388–395, 1980.
64. Parke DW II, Jones DB, Gentry LO: Endogenous endophthalmitis among patients with candidemia. Ophthalmology 89:789–796, 1982.
65. Perrault LE Jr, Perrault LD, Bleiman B, Lyons J: Successful treatment of *Candida albicans* endophthalmitis with intravitreal amphotericin B. Arch Ophthalmol 99:1565–1567, 1981.
66. Peyman GA, Vastine DW, Diamond JG: Vitrectomy in exogenous *Candida* endophthalmitis. Graefes Arch Clin Exp Ophthalmol 197:55–59, 1975.
67. Pflugfelder SC, Flynn HW, Zwickey TA, et al: Exogenous fungal endophthalmitis. Ophthalmology 95:19–30, 1988.
68. Richardson K, Brammer KW, Marriott MS, et al: Activity of UK-49,858, a bis-triazole derivate, against experimental infections with *Candida albicans* and *Trichophyton mentagrophytes*. Antimicrob Agents Chemother 27:832–835, 1985.
69. Robertson DM, Riley FC, Hermans PE: Endogenous *Candida* oculomycosis: report of two patients treated with flucytosine. Arch Ophthalmol 91:33–38, 1974.
70. Rosen R, Friedman AH: Successfully treated postoperative *Candida parakrusei* endophthalmitis. Am J Ophthalmol 76:574–577, 1973.
71. Savani DV, Perfect JR, Cobo LM, et al: Penetration of new azole compounds into the eye and efficacy in experimental *Candida* endophthalmitis. Antimicrob Agents Chemother 31:6–10, 1987.
72. Schuman JS, Friedman AH: Retinal manifestations of the acquired immune deficiency syndrome (AIDS): cytomegalovirus, *Candida albicans*, cryptococcus, toxoplasmosis and *Pneumocystis carinii*. Trans Ophthalmol Soc UK 103:177–190, 1983.

73. Servant JB, Dutton GN, Ong-Tone L, et al: Candidal endophthalmitis in Glaswegian heroin addicts: report of an epidemic. Trans Ophthalmol Soc UK 104:297–308, 1985.
74. Snip RC, Michels RG: Pars plana vitrectomy in the management of endogenous *Candida* endophthalmitis. Am J Ophthalmol 82:699–704, 1976.
75. Sorrell TC, Dunlop C, Collignon P, et al: Exogenous ocular candidiasis associated with intravenous heroin abuse. Br J Ophthalmol 68:841–845, 1984.
76. Stern WH, Tamura E, Jacobs RA, et al: Epidemic postsurgical *Candida parapsilosis* endophthalmitis. Clinical findings and management of 15 consecutive cases. Ophthalmology 92:1701–1709, 1985.
77. Sud IJ, Feingold DS: Effect of ketoconazole on the fungicidal action of amphotericin B in *Candida albicans*. Antimicrob Agents Chemother 23:185–187, 1983.
78. Theodore FH: Etiology and diagnosis of fungal postoperative endophthalmitis. Ophthalmology 85:327–340, 1978.
79. Troke PF, Andrews RJ, Brammer KW, et al: Efficacy of UK-49,858 (fluconazole) against *Candida albicans* experimental infections in mice. Antimicrob Agents Chemother 28:815–818, 1985.
80. Van Buren JM: Septic retinitis due to *Candida albicans*. Arch Pathol 65:137–146, 1958.

Ocular Coccidioidomycosis

1. Alexander PB, Coodley EL: Disseminated coccidioidomycosis with intraocular involvement. Am J Ophthalmol 64:283–289, 1967.
2. Ampel NM, Wieden MA, Galgiani JN: Coccidioidomycosis: clinical update. Rev Infect Dis 11:897–911, 1989.
3. Bell R, Font RL: Granulomatous anterior uveitis caused by *Coccidioides immitis*. Am J Ophthalmol 74:93–98, 1972.
4. Bennett JE. Chemotherapy of systemic mycoses. N Engl J Med 1974; 290:30–32.
5. Blumenkranz MS, Stevens DA: Endogenous coccidioidal endophthalmitis. Ophthalmology 87:974–984, 1980.
6. Blumenkranz MS, Stevens DA: Therapy of endogenous fungal endophthalmitis: miconazole or amphotericin B for coccidioidal and candidal infection. Arch Ophthalmol 1980; 98:1216–1220.
7. Boyden BS, Yee DS: Bilateral coccidioidal choroiditis: a clinicopathologic case report. Trans Am Acad Ophthalmol Otolaryngol 75:1006–1010, 1971.
8. Brown WC, Hudson KE, Nesbet AA: Pulmonary coccidioidomycosis associated with Jensen's disease. Am J Ophthalmol 43:965–967, 1957.
9. Brown WC, Kellenberger RE, Judson KE: Granulomatous uveitis associated with disseminated coccidioidomycosis. Am J Ophthalmol 45:102–104, 1958.
10. Bruschi M: Coccidioidomycosis. A Primer. Postgrad Med 30:301–310, 1961.
11. Chandler JW, Kalina RE, Milam DF: Coccidioidal choroiditis following renal transplantation. Am J Ophthalmol 74:1080–1085, 1972.
12. Collins M, Pappagianis D: Uniform susceptibility of various strains of *Coccidioides immitis* to amphotericin B. Antimicrob Agents Chemother 11:1049–1055, 1977.
13. Conan NJ Jr, Hyman GA: Disseminated coccidioidomycosis: treatment with protanemonin. Am J Med 9:408–413, 1950.
14. Coodley EL: Disseminated coccidioidomycosis: diagnosis by liver biopsy. Gastroenterology 53:947–952, 1967.
15. Cutler JE, Binder PS, Paul TO, et al: Metastatic coccidioidal endophthalmitis. Arch Ophthalmol 96:689–691, 1978.
16. Drutz DJ, Cadanzaro A: Coccidioidomycosis. Am Rev Respir Dis 117:559–585, 1978.
17. Forbus WD: A study of 95 cases of disseminated coccidioidomycosis with special reference to the pathogenesis of the disease. Mil Surg 99:633–675, 1946.
18. Galgiani JN, Stevens DA, Graybill JR, et al: Ketoconazole therapy of progressive coccidioidomycosis: comparison of 400 and 800 mg doses and observations at higher doses. Medicine 84:603–610, 1988.
19. Glasgow BJ, Brown HH, Foos RY: Miliary retinitis in coccidioidomycosis. Am J Ophthalmol 104:24–27, 1987.
20. Golden SE, Morgan CM, Bartley DL, et al: Disseminated coccidioidomycosis with chorioretinitis in early infancy. Pediatr Infect Dis 5:272–274, 1986.
21. Green WR, Bennett JE, Goos RD. Ocular penetration of amphotericin B. Arch Ophthal 73:769, 1965.
22. Green WR, Bennett JE: Coccidioidomycosis: report of a case with clinical evidence of ocular involvement. Arch Ophthalmol 77:337–340, 1967.
23. Haegle AJ, Evans DJ, Larwood TR: Primary endophthalmic coccidioidomycosis. In Ajello L (ed): Coccidioidomycosis. Tucson, AZ, University of Arizona Press, 1967, pp 37–39.
24. Hamilton-Miller JM. Fungal steroids and the mode of action of the polyene antibiotic. Adv Appl Microbiol 1974; 17:109–134.
25. Irvine AR Jr: Coccidioidal granuloma of lid. Trans Am Acad Ophthalmol Otolaryngol 72:751–754, 1968.
26. Lamer L, Paquin F, Lorange G, et al: Macular coccidioidomycosis. Can J Ophthalmol 17:121–123, 1982.
27. Levitt JM: Ocular manifestations in coccidioidomycosis. Am J Ophthalmol 31:1626–1628, 1948.
28. Lovenkin LG: Coccidioidomycosis: report of a case with intraocular involvement. Am J Ophthalmol 34:621–623, 1951.
29. Luttrull JK, Wan WL, Kubak BM, et al: Treatment of ocular fungal infectious with oral gluconazole. Am J Ophthalmol 119:477–481, 1995.
30. Medoff G, Kobayashi GS. Strategies in the treatment of systemic fungal agents. N Engl J Med 1980; 302:145–155.
31. Michelson JB, Belmont JB, Higginbottom P: Juxtapapillary choroiditis associated with chronic meningitis due to *Coccidioides immitis*. Ann Ophthalmol 15:666–668, 1983.
32. Miller RP, Bates JH. Amphotericin B toxicity: a follow-up report of 53 patients. Ann Intern Med 1969; 71:1089–1095.
33. Moorthy RS, Rao NA, Sidikaro F, et al: Coccidioidomycosis iridocyclitis. Ophthalmology 101:1923–1928, 1994.
34. Olivarria R, Fajardo LJ: Ophthalmic coccidioidomycosis: case report and review. Arch Pathol 92:191–195, 1971.
35. Pettit TH, Learn RN, Foos RY: Intraocular coccidioidomycosis. Arch Ophthalmol 77:655–671, 1967.
36. Rainin EA, Little JL: Ocular coccidioidomycosis: a clinicopathologic case report. Trans Am Acad Ophthalmol Otolaryngol 76:645–651, 1972.
37. Rodenbiker HT, Ganley JP, Galgiani JN, et al: Prevalence of chorioretinal scars associated with coccidioidomycosis. Arch Ophthalmol 99:71–75, 1981.
38. Rodenbiker HT, Ganley JP: Ocular coccidioidomycosis. Surv Ophthalmol 24:263–289, 1980.
39. Rutala PJ, Smith JW: Coccidioidomycosis in potentially compromised hosts: the effect of immunosuppressive therapy in dissemination. Am J Med Sci 275:283–295, 1978.
40. Skipworth GB, Bergin JJ, Williams RM: Coccidioidal granulomas of skin and conjunctiva treated with intravenous amphotericin B: report of a case. Arch Dermatol 82:605–608, 1960.
41. Smith CE: Epidemiology of acute coccidioidomycosis with erythema nodosum. Am J Public Health 30:600–611, 1940.
42. Stein HF: Disseminated coccidioidomycosis. Dis Chest 36:136–145, 1959.
43. Stevens DA: Coccidioidomycosis and the indications for chemotherapy. Drugs 26:334–336, 1983.
44. Trowbridge DH: Ocular manifestations of coccidioidomycosis. Trans Pac Coast Otoophthalmol Soc 33:229–246, 1952.
45. Tygeson P: Observation on non-tuberculous phlyctenular keratoconjunctivitis. Trans Am Acad Ophthalmol Otolaryngol 58:128–132, 1954.
46. Wood TR: Ocular coccidioidomycos: report of a case presenting as Parinaus's oculoglandular syndrome. Am J Ophthalmol 64(Suppl):587–590, 1967.

47. Zakka KA, Foos RY, Brown WJ: Intraocular coccidioidomycosis. Surv Ophthalmol 22:313–321, 1978.

Ocular Cryptococcosis

1. Arndt CAS, Walsh RJ, Lester McCully C, et al: Fluconazole penetration into cerebrospinal fluid: implications for treating fungal infections of the central nervous system. J Infect Dis 157:178–180, 1988.
2. Avendano J, Tanishima T, Kuwabara T: Ocular cryptococcosis. Am J Ophthalmol 86:110–113, 1978.
3. Bennett JE, Sismukes WE, Duma RJ, et al: A comparison of amphotericin B alone and combined with flucytosine in the treatment of cryptococcal meningitis. N Engl J Med 301:126–131, 1979.
4. Bennett JE. Chemotherapy of systemic mycosis, Part 1. N Engl J Med 290:30–32, 1974.
5. Bennett JE: Flucytosine. Ann Intern Med 86:319–322, 1977.
6. Beyt BE: Diagnosis of cryptococcal endophthalmitis. Am J Clin Pathol 79:272, 1983.
7. Beyt BE, Waltman SR: Cryptococcal endophthalmitis after corneal transplantation. N Engl J Med 298:825–826, 1978.
8. Birkmann LW, Bennett DR: Meningoencephalitis following enucleation for cryptococcal endophthalmitis. Ann Neurol 4:476–477, 1979.
9. Bisseru B, Bajaj A, Carruthers RH, Chhabra HN: Pulmonary and bilateral retinochoroidal cryptococcosis. Br J Ophthalmol 67:157–161, 1983.
10. Blackie JD, Danta G, Sorrell T, Collignon P: Ophthalmological complications of cryptococcal meningitis. Clin Exp Neurol 21:263–270, 1985.
11. Blackie JD, Danta G, Sorrell T, Collignon P: Ophthalmological complications of cryptococcal meningitis. Clin Exp Neurol 21:263–270, 1985.
12. Cameron ME, Harrison A: Ocular cryptococcosis in Australia, with a report of two further cases. Med J Aust 1:935–938, 1970.
13. Campbell GD: Primary pulmonary cryptococcosis. Am Rev Respir Dis 94:236, 1966.
14. Chapman-Smith JS, Parr DH, Say PJ: Ocular cryptococcosis in New Zealand. NZ Med J 91:291–293, 1980.
15. Chapman-Smith JS: Cryptococcal chorioretinitis: a case report. Br J Ophthalmol 61:411–413, 1977.
16. Charles NC, Boxrud C, Small E: Cryptococcosis of the anterior segment in acquired immune deficiency syndrome. Ophthalmology 99:813–816, 1992.
17. Chuck SL, Sande MA: Infection with Cryptococcus neoformans in the acquired immunodeficiency syndrome. N Engl J Med 321:794–799, 1989.
18. Church WH, Palace J, Dick DJ, et al: Cryptococcal choridoretinitis and immunodeficiency. Postgrad Med J 63:969–971, 1987.
19. Cohen DB, Glasgow BJ: Bilateral optic nerve cryptococcosis in sudden blindness in patients with acquired immune deficiency syndrome. Ophthalmology 100:1689–1694, 1993.
20. Cohen M: Binocular papilledema in a case of torulosis associated with Hodgkin's disease. Arch Ophthalmol 32:477–479, 1944.
21. Condon PI, Terry SI, Falconer H: Cryptococcal eye disease. Doc Ophthalmol 44:49–56, 1977.
22. Cowley EP, Grekin EP, Curtis AC: Torulosis: A review of the cutaneous and adjoining mucous membrane manifestations. J Invest Dermatol 14:327, 1950.
23. Crump JR, Elner S, Elner V, et al: Cryptococcal endophthalmitis: case report and review. Clin Infect Dis 14:1069–1073, 1992.
24. Dismukes WE: Cryptococcal meningitis in patients with AIDS. J Infect Dis 157:624–628, 1988.
25. Doft BH, Curtin VT: Combined ocular infection with cytomegalovirus and cryptococcosis. Arch Ophthalmol 100:1800–1803, 1982.
26. Ehrhorn J, Grosse G, Staib F, et al: Introkulare cryptococcose. Klin Monatsbl Augenheilkd 168:577–583, 1976.
27. Francois J, Rysselaere M: Cryptococcosis. In Oculomycoses. Springfield, IL, Charles C Thomas, 1972, pp 316–326.
28. Friedenwald JS, Wilder HC, Maumenee AE, et al: Ophthalmic Pathology: An Atlas and Textbook. Philadelphia, WB Saunders Co, 1952, p 152.
29. Fujita NK, Hukkanen J, Edwards JE Jr: Experimental hematogenous endophthalmitis due to Cryptococcus neoformans. Invest Ophthalmol Vis Sci 24:368–375, 1983.
30. Garritt JA, Herman O, Imes R, et al: Optic nerve decompression for visual loss in patients with acquired immune deficiency syndrome and cryptococcal meningitis with papilledema. Am J Ophthalmol 116:472–478, 1993.
31. Gill WD: Torula mycosis in man with special reference to involvement of the upper respiratory tract. Trans Am Laryngol Rhinol Otolaryngol Soc 40:247, 1934.
32. Goldstein E, Rambo ON: Cryptococcal infection following steroid therapy. Ann Intern Med 56:114, 1962.
33. Gonyea EF, Heilman KM: Neuro-ophthalmic aspects of central nervous system cryptococcosis. Arch Ophthalmol 87:164–168, 1972.
34. Green WR, Bennett JE, Goos RD: Ocular penetration of amphotericin B. Arch Ophthalmol 73:769, 1965.
35. Grieco MH, Freilich DB, Louria DB: Diagnosis of cryptococcal uveitis with hypertonic media. Am J Ophthalmol 72:171–174, 1971.
36. Hamilton-Miller JM: Fungal steroids and the mode of action of the polyene antibiotic. Adv Appl Microbiol 17:109–134, 1974.
37. Hendedrly DF, Liggett PE, Rao NA: Cryptococcal chorioretinitis and endophthalmitis. Retina 7:75–79, 1987.
38. Hester D, Kylstra J, Eifrig D: Isolated ocular crypto in an immunocompetent patient. Ophthalmic Surg 23:29–31, 1992.
39. Hiles DA, Font RL: Bilateral intraocular cryptococcosis with unilateral spontaneous regression. Am J Ophthalmol 65:98–108, 1968.
40. Hiss PW, Shields JA, Augsburger JJ: Solitary retinovitreal abscess as the initial manifestation of cryptococcosis. Ophthalmology 95:162–165, 1988.
41. Jones DB: Chemotherapy of experimental endogenous Candida albicans endophthalmitis. Trans Am Ophthalmol Soc LXXVIII:846–895, 1980.
42. Kestelyn P, Taelman H, Bogaerts J, et al: Ophthalmic manifestations of infections with Cryptococcus neoformans in patients with acquired immunodeficiency syndrome. Am J Ophthalmol 116:721–727, 1993.
43. Koudadoust AA, Payne JW: Cryptococcal (torular) retinitis: a clinicopathologic case report. Am J Ophthalmol 67:745–750, 1969.
44. Kumar RK, Lykke WJ: Disseminated cryptococcosis with ocular involvement. Aust NZ J Med 9:444–447, 1979.
45. Kupfer C, McCrane E: A possible case of decreased vision in cryptococcal meningitis. Invest Ophthalmol 13:801–804, 1974.
46. Lesser RL, Simon RM, Leon H, et al: Cryptococcal meningitis and internal ophthalmoplegia. Am J Ophthalmol 87:682–687, 1979.
47. Littman JL. Cryptococcosis (torulosis): current concepts and therapy. Am J Med 27:976–998, 1959.
48. Littman JL, Walter JE: Cryptococcosis: current status. Am J Med 45:922–932, 1968.
49. Malton ML, Rinkoff JS, Doft BS, et al: Cryptococcal endophthalmitis and meningitis associated with acute psychosis and exudative retinal detachment. Am J Ophthalmol 104:438–439, 1987.
50. Medoff G, Kobayashi GS: Strategies in the treatment of systemic fungal agents. N Engl J Med 302:145–155, 1980.
51. Medoff G, Brajtburg J, Kobayashi GS: Antifungal agents useful in therapy of systemic fungal infections. Ann Rev Pharmacol Toxicol 23:303–330, 1983.
52. Miller RP, Bates JH: Amphotericin B toxicity: a follow-up report of 53 patients. Ann Intern Med 71:1089–1095, 1969.
53. Morinelli EN, Dugel P, Roffenburgh L, et al: Infectious multifocal choroiditis in patients with acquired immune

deficiency syndrome. Ophthalmology 100:1014–1021, 1993.

54. O'Dowd GJ, Frable WJ: Cryptococcal endophthalmitis: diagnostic vitreous aspiration cytology. Am J Clin Pathol 79:382–385, 1983.

55. Okun E, Butler WT: Ophthalmologic complications of cryptococcal meningitis. Arch Ophthalmol 71:52–57, 1964.

56. Schulman JS, Friedman AH: Retinal manifestations of the acquired immune deficiency syndrome (AIDS): cytomegalovirus, *Candida albicans*, cryptococcus, toxoplasmosis and *Pneumocystis carinii.* Trans Ophthalmol Soc UK 103:177–190, 1983.

57. Schulman JS, Leveque C, Coats M, et al: Fatal disseminated cryptococcosis following intraocular involvement. Br J Ophthalmol 72:171–175, 1988.

58. Sciortino AK, McHaffie RA, Alliband GT, et al: Cryptococcosis. Arch Intern Med 102:450–454, 1958.

59. Shields JA, Wrighty DM, Augsburger JJ, et al: Cryptococcal chorioretinitis. Am J Ophthalmol 89:210–218, 1980.

60. Staib F, Mishra SK, Grosse G, et al: Ocular cryptococcosis—experimental and clinical observations. Z Bakteriol 237:378–394, 1977.

61. Stoddard JL, Cutler EC: Torula infection in man. Monograph 6. Rockefeller Institute for Medical Research, 1916.

62. Stone SP, Bendig J, Hakim J, et al: Cryptococcal meningitis presenting as uveitis. Br J Ophthalmol 72:167–170, 1988.

63. Turner PP: A case of cryptococcosis with choroidal torulomata. East Afr Med J 36:220–223, 1959.

64. Vogiatzis KV, Makley TA, Werling K: Cryptococcosis in a phthisical eye. Ann Ophthalmol 13:433–435, 1981.

65. Wager HE, Calhoun FP Jr: Torula uveitis. Trans Am Acad Ophthalmol 58:61–67, 1954.

66. Walter JE, Atchison RW: Epidemiologic and immunological studies of *Cryptococcus neoformans.* J Bacteriol 92:82, 1966.

67. Weiss RF, Everett ED, Sprouse R, et al: Endogenous cryptococcal endophthalmitis. South Med J 74:482–483, 1981.

68. Weiss C, Perry IH, Shevky MC: Infection of the human eye with *Cryptococcus neoformans.* Arch Ophthalmol 39:739, 1948.

69. Zenker: Encephalitis mit Pilzentwickelung im Gehirn, Jahresb. d. Gesellsch. f. Natur- u. Heilk. in Dresden, 1861–1862, 51.

70. Zimmerman LE, Rappaport H: Occurrence of cryptococcosis in patients with malignant disease of the reticuloendothelial system. Am J Clin Pathol 24:1050, 1954.

Intraocular Blastomycosis

1. Barr CC, Gamel JW: Blastomycosis of the eyelid. Arch Ophthalmol 104:96–97, 1986.

2. Bond WI, Sanders CV, Joffe L, et al: Presumed blastomycosis endophthalmitis. Ann Ophthalmol 14:1183–1188, 1982.

3. Bongiorn FJ, Leavell UW, Wirtschafter JD: The black dot sign and North American cutaneous blastomycosis. Am J Ophthalmol 78:145–147, 1974.

4. Bradsher RW, Rice DC, Abernathy RS: Ketoconazole therapy for endemic blastomycosis. Ann Intern Med 103:872–879, 1985.

5. Buechner HA, Clawson CM: Blastomycosis of the central nervous system. II. A report of nine cases from the Veterans Administration Cooperative Study. Am Rev Respir Dis 95:820–826, 1967.

6. Buechner HA, Seabury JH, Campbell CC, et al: The current status of serologic, immunologic and skin tests in the diagnosis of pulmonary mycoses. Chest 63:259–270, 1973.

7. Cassady JV: Uveal blastomycosis. Arch Ophthalmol 35:84–97, 1946.

8. Christoforidis AJ: Radiologic manifestations of histoplasmosis. Am J Roentgenol Radium Ther Nucl Med 109:478–490, 1970.

9. Churchill F, Stober AM: A case of systemic blastomycosis. Arch Intern Med 13:568–574, 1914.

10. Dismukes WE: Blastomycosis: leave it to beaver. N Engl J Med 314:575–577, 1986.

11. Font RL, Spaulding AG, Green WR: Endogenous mycotic panophthalmitis caused by *Blastomyces dermatitidis.* Report of a case and a review of the literature. Arch Ophthalmol 77:217–222, 1967.

12. Gilchrist TC: A case of blastomycotic dermatitis in man. Johns Hopkins Hosp Rep 1:269–283, 1896.

13. Gilchrist TC: Protozoan dermatitis. J Cutan Genet Dis 12:496–499, 1894.

14. Gottlieb JL, McAllister IL, Guttman, et al: Choroidal blastomycosis. A report of two cases. Retina 15:248–252, 1995.

15. Gonyea EF: The spectrum of primary blastomycotic meningitis: a review of central nervous system blastomycosis. Ann Neurol 3:26–39, 1978.

16. Katzenstein ALA: Mycobacterial infections and fungal and protozoal disease. In Thurlbeck WM (ed): Pathology of the Lung. New York, Thieme, 1988, pp 221–246.

17. Klein BS, Vergeront JM, Weeks RJ, et al: Isolation of *Blastomyces dermatitidis* in soil associated with a large outbreak of blastomycosis in Wisconsin. N Engl J Med 314:529–534, 1986.

18. Lewis H, Aaberg TM, Fary DRB, et al: Latent disseminated blastomycosis with choroidal involvement. Arch Ophthalmol 106:527–530, 1988.

19. Medoff G, Kobayashi GS: Strategies in the treatment of systemic fungal agents. N Engl J Med 302:145–155, 1980.

20. Nouira R, Denquezli M, Skhiri S, et al: Cutaneopulmonary bastomycosis. Ann Dermatol Venereol 121:180–182, 1994.

21. National Institute of Allergy and Infectious Diseases Mycoses Study Group: Treatment of blastomycosis and histoplasmosis with ketoconazole: results of a prospective randomized clinical trial. Ann Intern Med 103:861–872, 1985.

22. Recht LD, Phillips JR, Eckman MR, et al: Self-limited blastomycosis: a report of thirteen cases. Am Rev Respir Dis 119:1109–1112, 1979.

23. Rodrigues MM, Laibson P, Kaplan W: Exogenous mycotic keratitis caused by *Blastomyces dermatitidis.* Am J Ophthalmol 75:782–789, 1973.

24. Safneck JR, Hogg GR, Napier LB: Endophthalmitis due to *Blastomyces dermatitidis*: case report and review of the literature. Ophthalmology 97:212–216, 1990.

25. Sarosi GA, Davies SF: Blastomycosis. Am Rev Respir Dis 120:911–938, 1979.

26. Sarosi GA, Hammerman KJ, Tosh FE, Kronenberg RS: Clinical features of acute pulmonary blastomycosis. N Engl J Med 290:540–543, 1974.

27. Sarosi GA, Seerstock DS: Isolation of *Blastomyces dermatitidis* from pigeon manure. Am Rev Respir Dis 114:1179–1183, 1976.

28. Schwartz VJ: Intraocular blastomycosis. Arch Opthalmol 5:581–589, 1931.

29. Sinskey RM, Anderson WB: Miliary blastomycosis with metastatic spread to posterior uvea of both eyes. Arch Ophthalmol 54:602–604, 1955.

30. Vida L, Moel SA: Systemic North American blastomycosis with orbital involvement. Am J Ophthalmol 77:240–242, 1974.

31. Witorsch P, Utz JP: North American blastomycosis: a study of 40 patients. Medicine 47:169–200, 1968.

Aspergillosis and Sporotrichosis

1. Cassady JR, Foerster HC: *Sporotrichum schenckii* endophthalmitis. Arch Ophthalmol 85:71–74, 1971.

2. Demicco DD, Reichman RC, Violette J, et al: Disseminated aspergillosis presenting with endophthalmitis. A case report and a review of the literature. Cancer 53:1995–2001, 1984.

3. Doft BH, Clarkson JG, Rebell G, Forster RK: Endogenous *Aspergillus* endophthalmitis in drug abusers. Arch Ophthalmol 98:859–862, 1980.

4. Elliott JH, O'Day DM, Gutaw GS, et al: Mycotic endophthalmitis in drug abusers. Am J Ophthalmol 88:66–72, 1979.
5. Font RL: Granulomatous necrotizing retinochoroiditis caused by *Sporotrichum schenkii*. Report of a case including immunofluorescence and electron microscopical studies. Arch Ophthalmol 94:1513–1519, 1976.
6. Johns KJ, O'Day KM, Feman S: Chorioretinitis in the contralateral eye of a patient with *Acanthamoeba* keratitis. Ophthalmology 95:635–638, 1988.
7. Marines HM, Osato MS, Font RL: The value of calcofluor white in the diagnosis of mycotic and *Acanthamoeba* infections of the eye and ocular adnexa. Ophthalmology 94:23–26, 1987.
8. Naidoff MA, Green WR: Endogenous *Aspergillus* endophthalmitis occurring after kidney transplant. Am J Ophthalmol 79:502–509, 1975.
9. Roney P, Barr CC, Chun CH, et al: Endogenous *Aspergillus* endophthalmitis. Rev Infect Dis 8:955–958, 1986.
10. Wash TJ, Orth DH, Shapiro CM, et al: Metastatic fungal chorioretinitis developing during *Trichosporon* sepsis. Ophthalmology 89:152–156, 1982.

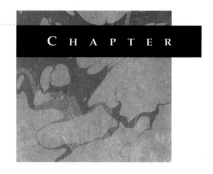

Ocular Syphilis

Allen C. Ho, M.D.

Syphilis, a sexually transmitted disease caused by the spirochete *Treponema pallidum*, has been a known ophthalmic pathogen since early descriptions by Hutchinson and Baeder in the 19th century and has been clearly described as a systemic disease since the 15th century.[1-3] Subsequent reports have highlighted the wide variability of manifestations and have emphasized the lack of pathognomonic signs of ocular syphilis. Indeed, syphilis should be included in the differential diagnosis of any ocular inflammatory condition.

With the introduction of penicillin in the 1940s, syphilis became a treatable disease and its incidence decreased. In the 1960s the annual incidence of new cases, 10 per 100,000, had reached a plateau. In spite of specific therapy, however, recent national incidence rates of syphilis have been alarming. Since the second half of the 1980s, the United States has been inflicted with a syphilis epidemic.[4,5] The current syphilis epidemic began in 1986 when a 75% increase in new cases to 20 per 100,000 was the highest single-year increase since 1949.[6] Recent trends note substantial increases in urban centers, lower socioeconomic groups, and individuals who engage in high-risk sexual or drug abuse behavior.[4,7] The reasons for the current epidemic are probably multifactorial, including a rising incidence of human immunodeficiency virus (HIV) infection; a lack of education among the afflicted; the ineffectiveness of spectinomycin (a recommended therapy for penicillin-resistant gonorrhea) to eradicate *Treponema pallidum*; and an unfamiliarity with a disease among physicians now that 40 years have passed since penicillin has altered the natural history, progression, and clinical presentations of syphilis.[8,9]

Although the current incidence of ocular syphilis is not known, ophthalmologists will continue to be challenged by these patients. The key to diagnosis of syphilitic eye disease is a high index of suspicion and a familiarity with its protean clinical manifestations and mimickry.

CONGENITAL SYPHILIS

Congenital syphilis accounted for less than $^1/_{10}$ of 1% of reported syphilis in 1991.[4] Newborns typically exhibit chronic rhinitis and papulomacular rashes. Surviving infants resolve these systemic manifestations, enter a latent phase that is characteristic of congenital and acquired syphilitic infections, and then develop signs of late congenital syphilis. Hutchinson's classic triad includes interstitial keratitis (Fig. 65–1), sensorineural deafness, and notched incisors (Fig. 65–2).[1] Maternal–fetal infection also results in a variable patterns of uveitis, "salt-and-pepper" retinal pigment epithelium (RPE) changes (peripheral involvement is more characteristic) (Figs. 65–3 and 65–4), and isolated spots of RPE hyperpigmentation with surrounding halos of depigmentation. Other systemic findings include saber shins, saddle nose deformities, and chronic periostitis.[9]

NATURAL HISTORY OF ACQUIRED SYSTEMIC DISEASE

The natural history of acquired systemic syphilis is divided into three clinical stages.[10] *Treponema pallidum* is transmitted through mucuous membranes or open skin-to-skin contact in acquired syphilis. Typically, a 3-week incubation period ensues. The primary stage is characterized by a painless indurated genital chancre at the site of inoculation and regional adenopathy. Secondary syphilis will ensue 6 to 8 weeks after the chancre.[10,11] Hematogenous spread of *Treponema pallidum* causes maculopapular skin lesions, typically on the palms and soles of the patient.[10,12] There may be constitutional symptoms such as fever, joint pain, headache, and loss of appetite during secondary syphilis.[10] Most mucocu-

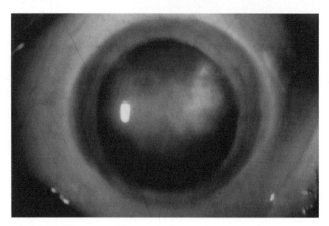

FIGURE 65–1   Interstitial keratitis (inactive) in a patient with congenital syphilis.

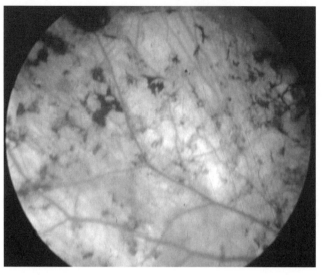

FIGURE 65–3   Peripheral "pseudo-retinitis pigmentosa" pigmentary retinopathy in a patient with congenital syphilis.

taneous lesions spontaneously resolve, and approximately 20 to 25% of patients will develop relapses involving anogenital and oral lesions. The remainder of the patients enter a latent asymptomatic phase of disease. Approximately 15 to 25% of the cases progress to tertiary syphilis with associated neurosyphilis, cardiovascular syphilis, and gummata (nodular indolent granulomas).[8,11,12] Classically, most ocular findings have been associated with hematogenous spread, that is, the secondary form of the disease. Others believe ocular involvement to be strongly suggestive of central nervous system (CNS) involvement and therefore synonymous with neurosyphilis or tertiary syphilis.[13] Although ocular syphilis most commonly presents during secondary and tertiary stages of systemic disease, the disease and its sequelae may present during any stage, active or latent.

OCULAR MANIFESTATIONS OF ACQUIRED SYPHILIS

Syphilis may affect any ocular tissue or the ocular adnexa.[8,14] In general, the infection may manifest as

either a *granulomatous mass lesion* (gummata of secondary or tertiary syphilis) or as an *inflammatory condition* (any stage). In the penicillin era, gummata are decidedly uncommon and *uveitis is the most common ophthalmic manifestation of syphilis*[13,15] (Table 65–1). Although the incidence of ocular manifestations in systemic syphilis is unknown, many authors have attempted to determine the percentage of all patients with uveitis who have a syphilitic etiology. Classically, syphilitic anterior uveitis is a granulomatous reaction with mutton fat keratic precipitates. The anterior reaction may be mild or severe with hypopyon. Early reports prior to 1925 noted the highest incidence of syphilis among patients with uveitis (19 to 70%).[14,16,17] Later, in 1982, Schlagel and Kao reported a 1.1% incidence of

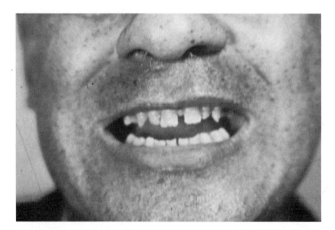

FIGURE 65–2   Hutchinson's teeth of congenital syphilis. Note the abnormal dentition and notched incisors. (Courtesy of Norman Medow, M.D.)

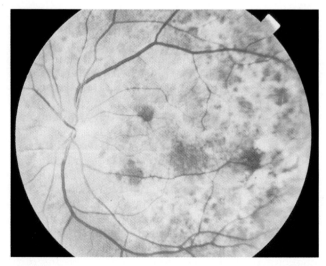

FIGURE 65–4   Pigmentary retinopathy in a patient with congenital syphilis. Note patchy hyperpigmentation and hypopigmentation of the fundus. (Courtesy of Norman Medow, M.D.)

TABLE 65–1 Most Common Ocular Manifestations of Acquired Syphilis

Uveitis, anterior and/or posterior
Chorioretinitis, diffuse or localized form
Retinal vasculitis

TABLE 65–2 Vitreoretinal Manifestations of Acquired Syphilis

Chorioretinitis, diffuse or placoid
Retinitis
Retinal vasculitis
Retinal perivaculitis
Central retinal vascular occlusion, arterial or venous
Branch retinal vascular occlusion, arterial or venous
Vitritis
Serous retinal detachment
Uveal effusion
Pseudoretinitis pigmentosa
Retinal pigment epithelial detachment
Choroidal neovascular membrane
Macular or retinal edema
Cystoid macular edema
Macular stellate figure
Retinal necrosis

syphilitic uveitis during the years 1970 through 1980.[10] They found an equal incidence of anterior versus posterior uveitis. In a 5-year experience (1983 through 1989) at the uveitis service at the Massachusetts Eye & Ear Infirmary, 25 of 1020 new patients (2.5%) had presumptive syphilitic eye disease. Seventeen of these 25 patients (68%) had either anterior, posterior, intermediate, or panuveitis.[13]

A multitude of common as well as rather uncommon anterior segment manifestations of ocular syphilis have been reported: conjunctivitis of any severity or response (nodular, diffuse, ulcerated), eyelid or conjunctival chancres, episcleritis, scleritis, interstitial keratitis (usually deeper corneal involvement with congenital infection), iris papules or nodules (acutely red lesions that may progress to yellow-brown or hypopigmented iris lesions), iridoschisis associated with congenital syphilis, marginal keratitis, localized corneal amyloidosis, as well as lens subluxation or dislocation.[11–14,18–24]

The ocular adnexal structures may also be involved: eyelid papulomacular rash and loss of eye lashes (madaurosis) are associated with the systemic rash and patchy alopecia of secondary syphilis. Luetic tarsitis and chronic blepharitis may mimic preseptal cellulitis with a thickened, hyperemic eyelid.[48] Periostitis of the upper orbital rim with constant pain exacerbated by direct pressure and eye movement has been reported. Many of these reports describe a delay in proper diagnosis and treatment because a syphilitic etiology was not initially considered.[48] Once again, a high clinical index of suspicion in anterior segment, external, and ocular adnexal disease is important in the diagnosis of this treatable yet underdiagnosed condition.

The most common posterior segment manifestations of acquired syphilis (Table 65–2) are chorioretinitis and retinal vasculitis (Fig. 65–5) (central rather than peripheral involvement is characteristic but not absolute in acquired syphilis).[8,11] Two forms of syphilitic chorioretinitis are generally recognized.[11,25–27] The first form is a diffuse bilateral chorioretinitis that exhibits multiple gray-yellow, inflammatory chorioretinal lesions with associated vitreitis, retinal vasculitis, retinal edema, and shallow subretinal fluid accumulation. This diffuse form typically occurs during secondary syphilis. The second form is a localized large, solitary, placoid, pale yellow, subretinal bilateral lesion that typically affects the region of the optic disc or macula

(Figs. 65–6 through 65–8).[25] Shallow serous retinal detachment, peripheral chorioretinitis, mild papillitis, retinal vasculitis, and vitritis are common associated findings. Overlying vitreitis may obscure clear visualization of the lesion and has been reported to mimic reticulum cell sarcoma.[13,25] The localized form is thought to occur in late stages of systemic syphilis and may be associated with asymptomatic infection.[11,25] Gass et al[25] state that the biomicroscopic and angiographic findings of the localized form of syphilitic chorioretinitis may be the most specific findings described in secondary syphilis to date.[25]

A wide variety of less common posterior segment clinical manifestations of ocular syphilis reflect the host's response to posterior segment inflammation such as chorioretinitis and retinal vasculitis. Halperin et al[28] note that choroidal neovascularization, retinal vasculitis, retinal perivasculitis and associated arterial or venous occlusion, central retinal artery or vein occlusion, pseudoretinitis pigmentosa, macular stellate figure, retinal or macular edema, cystoid macular edema, macular pseudohypopyon, neuroretinitis, retinal detachment, uveal effusion, retinal necrosis, optic neuritis, optic perineuritis, and disc edema have all previously been described.[11,26–48] Unexplained posterior segment inflammation must prompt a consideration of luetic disease.

Neuro-ophthalmic involvement of ocular syphilis most commonly affects the optic nerve.[49] The optic nerve appearance and function may vary from clinically inapparent retrobulbar optic neuritis, to mild hyperemia and normal visual acuity to, less commonly, end-stage optic atrophy. Late neurosyphilis patients may present with irregular, unequal, and poorly reactive pupils. These Argyll

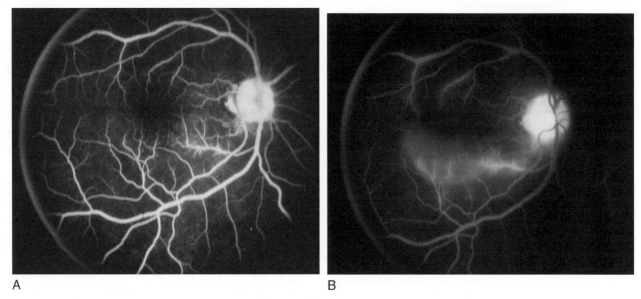

A   B

FIGURE 65–5   *A,* Syphilitic retinal phlebitis and papillitis. Fluorescein angiography demonstrates retinal venous staining and leakage as well as some, *B,* staining of the optic disc.

Robertson pupils classically respond better to an accomodative target than to light. Other cranial nerve involvement, including the third, fourth, fifth, sixth, and seventh, may be observed with syphilitic infection of the central and peripheral nervous systems.[8] Eighth nerve involvement is more typical of congenital than acquired syphilis.[8,49]

SYPHILIS AND HIV INFECTION

Concurrent HIV and syphilitic infection may lead to a more aggressive and recalcitrant course of systemic and ocular syphilitic disease.[25,50–56] Ophthalmologists must recognize that *ocular syphilis may be the presenting sign of HIV infection and neurosyphilis.*[55]

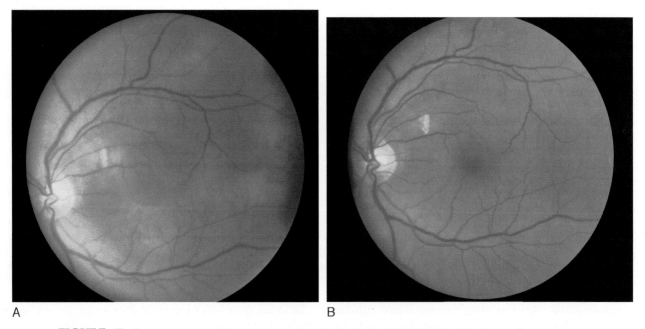

A   B

FIGURE 65–6   *A,* Acute syphilitic posterior placoid chorioretinitis (ASPPC). Note the confluent macular placoid choroidal and outer retinal inflammatory lesion. *B,* Resolved ASPPC after intravenous penicillin. (From Gass JDM, Braustein RA, Chenoweth RG: Acute syphilitic posterior placoid chorioretinitis. Ophthalmology 97:1288–1297, 1990, with permission.)

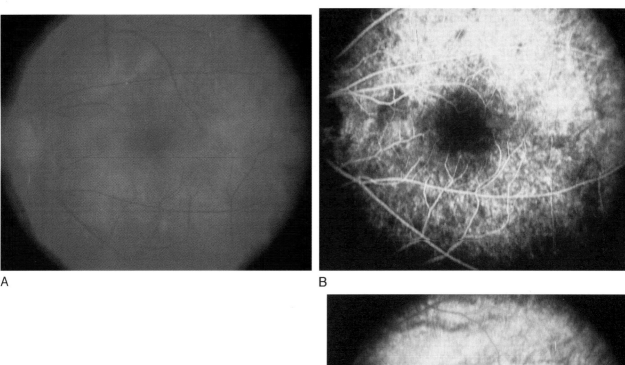

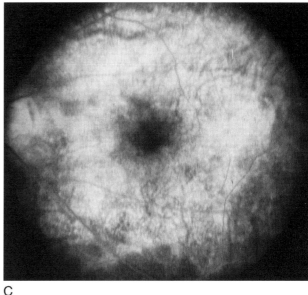

C

FIGURE 65–7 *A*, Acute syphilitic posterior placoid chorio-retinitis (ASPPC). The lesion is at the level of the outer retina and the retinal pigment epithelium and demonstrates some granularity at the edges of the lesion. *B* and *C*, The fluorescein angiogram reveals mottled hyperfluorescence during the transit phase and then late hyperfluorescence. (Courtesy of George Williams, M.D.)

Johns et al have stated that concurrent syphilis and HIV infection may alter the natural history of systemic syphilis by "increasing the propensity of the disease to progress to neurosyphilis, decreasing the latency before the onset of neurosyphilis, increasing the severity of the manifestations of neurosyphilis, or rendering the standard therapy for primary and secondary syphilis inadequate."[50] Similarly, other authors have noted more aggressive ocular syphilis in HIV-infected patients.[25,51,53–55] Becerra et al noted that 12 of 17 HIV-positive patients with luetic uveitis had abnormal spinal fluid analyses.[53] In 1990, McLeish et al reported their initial experience in treating ocular syphilis in HIV-1–infected hosts and concluded that current regimens accepted for the treatment of neurosyphilis appeared to be adequate for the treatment of ocular syphilis in these patients (median follow-up, 6 months).[55] Recently, Halperin has reported a case of presumptive syphilitic neuroretinitis with negative serologic testing due to

HIV infection. This patient responded to high-dose intravenous penicillin.[56]

DIAGNOSIS, SEROLOGIC TESTING, AND CEREBROSPINAL FLUID ANALYSIS

Treponema pallidum is thin, elongated, coiled bacterium and a member of the family Spirochaetaceae. Other pathogenic treponemes of this family include the genera *Borrelia* and *Leptospira*; accordingly, syphilis and Lyme disease share many ocular and systemic manifestations. The treponemes are classified by their different abilities to cause disease in humans.[2]

There are two classes of serologic tests to detect antibodies to *T. pallidum* infection. The fluorescent treponemal antibody absorption test (FTA-ABS)

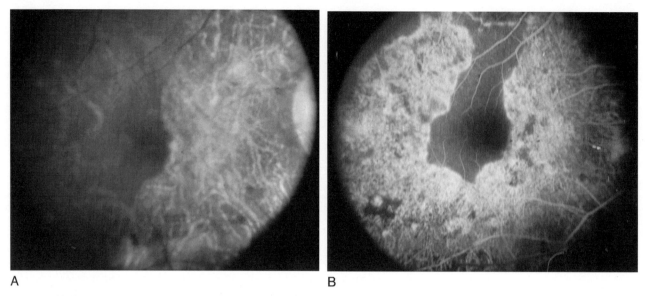

FIGURE 65–8   *A*, Pigmentary retinopathy in a patient with resolved acquired syphilitic retinitis. *B*, Note the extensive retinal pigment epithelial disturbance highlighted on fluorescein angiography. Vision is 20/40.

and the microhemagglutination assay–*Treponema pallidum* (MHA-TP) are specific for antitreponemal antibodies. FTA-ABS titers typically remain elevated for life. Thus, this is a useful test for prior infection. In contrast, the Venereal Disease Research Laboratories (VDRL) and the rapid plasma reagin (RPR) are nonspecific serologic cardiolipin flocculation tests for *T. pallidum* infection. The nonspecific serology tests reflect disease activity and therefore may also be used to monitor therapy. Results of RPR and VDRL tests can vary by one serial dilution on repeated testing and therefore significant changes in titers are at least fourfold.[2] Biologic false-positive results may occur from a variety of infectious and noninfectious diseases including but not limited to Lyme disease (*Borrelia burgdorferi*), leprosy, HIV, viral hepatitis, tuberculosis, bacterial endocarditis, chronic liver disease, pregnancy, and systemic lupus erythematosus.[2]

Serologic false-negative results may occur, particularly during certain stages of syphilis and in certain patient populations. During primary syphilis, 20 to 30% of infected patients may have negative VDRL or RPR results and 15 to 35% have negative FTA-ABS or MHA-TP.[8,58] In late syphilis, 2 to 5% of patients will be seronegative to both specific and nonspecific tests and approximately 25% of untreated patients will become nonreactive to VDRL testing alone.[2,8,58] Patients with concurrent HIV infection and CD4 cell counts less than 200/mm³ may be seronegative to all serologic tests for syphilis.[8,55] Therefore, one should consider empiric antibiotic therapy for patients with compelling systemic and ocular manifestations of syphilis but seronegative testing.

Matjucha and Katz note that lumbar puncture and cerebrospinal fluid (CSF) VDRL assay may be useful in determining disease activity in patients with positive FTA-ABS.[8] Although controversial, some believe that all patients with anterior uveitis, the most common manifestation of ocular syphilis, require CSF analysis. While the indications for lumbar puncture and cerebrospinal fluid analysis in patients with ocular syphilis remain unclear, optic disc involvement and posterior segment manifestations are compelling reasons to perform the procedure. Between 22 to 70% of patients with active neurosyphilis demonstrate positive CSF-VDRL.[54] Positive CSF-VDRL titers reflect active disease and therefore would require systemic high-dose antibiotic therapy.[8]

Musher et al recommend CSF assays on all HIV-infected patients with ocular syphilis to detect asymptomatic neurosyphilis.[55] The corollary to this recommendation is that all patients with neurosyphilis should be tested for concurrent HIV infection. Patients with ocular syphilis may or may not have neurosyphilis. Patients with ocular syphilis and HIV-1 infection are more likely to have an aggressive progression to neurosyphilis or may already have concurrent neurosyphilis.

THERAPY

The principal goals of therapy are to resolve active manifestations of syphilis, prevent late sequelae, and prevent transmission of the disease. Penicillin remains the standard of therapy for syphilis with or without concurrent HIV infection (Table 65–3). Guidelines for the treatment of ophthalmic syphilis are still not entirely clear and some authorities recommend treatment for possible neurosyphilis, especially with concurrent HIV infection.[20,53,55] Treatment of HIV-positive ocular syphilis with in-

TABLE 65–3 Recommended Antibiotic Therapy for Syphilis*†

Concurrent HIV infection

12–24 million units of daily aqueous crystalline intravenous PCN G for 10–14 days followed by 2.4 million units of intramuscular benzathine PCN G for 3 weeks

No HIV infection

Congenital syphilis: PCN G 100,000–150,000 units/kg daily IM or IV for 10–14 days or PCN G procaine 50,000 units/kg IM daily for 10–14 days.

Primary or secondary syphilis: PCN G 2.4 million units IM, one dose; for PCN-allergic patients, doxycycline 100 mg PO bid or tetracycline 500 mg PO qid for 14 days

Late latent syphilis (>1 year) or syphilis of unknown duration: PCN G 2.4 million units IM weekly, 3 weeks; for PCN-allergic patients, doxycycline 100 mg PO bid or tetracycline 500 mg PO qid for 28 days

Tertiary syphilis including neurosyphilis: as per concurrent HIV infection

Sexual exposure: PCN G 2.4 million units IM, one dose; for PCN-allergic patients, doxycycline 100 mg PO bid or tetracycline 500 mg PO qid for 14 days

* Data from Berry CD, Hooton TM, Collier AC, Lukehart SA: Neurologic relapse after benzathine penicillin therapy for secondary syphilis in a patient with HIV infection. N Engl J Med 316:1587–1589, 1987, with permission.

† These are guidelines and therapy may be modified by an infectious disease specialist, especially in concurrent HIV and syphilis infection when treatment courses may be longer. Some authorities recommend intravenous antibiotic therapy for all cases of intraocular syphilis.

tramuscular benzathine penicillin (primary and secondary syphilis regimen) may be inadequate; therefore, a regimen of 12 to 24 million units of daily aqueous crystalline intravenous penicillin G (10 to 14 days) followed by 2.4 million units of weekly intramuscular benzathine penicillin G (3 weeks) has been recommended by several sources.[13,59] Recommendations from the Centers for Disease Control in managing HIV-1 and neurosyphilis include (1) an appropriate clinical response to therapy, (2) serial monthly serum reagin titers for the first 3 months and at 6 month intervals thereafter, and (3) a two-dilution decrease in titer by 6 months.[60]

In patients without HIV infection, therapy is di-

rected by clinical ophthalmic and systemic response to treatment, and follow-up serologic testing. We recommend a regimen of 12 to 24 million units of daily aqueous crystalline intravenous penicillin G (10 to 14 days) for patients with intraocular syphilis. For penicillin-allergic patients, use of intravenous doxycycline, chloramphenicol, and ceftriaxone has been reported.[61–63] Close interaction with an infectious disease specialist will optimize patient care and follow-up for infected individuals.

SUMMARY

The current syphilis epidemic will confront ophthalmologists with patients afflicted by a wide variety of ophthalmic manifestations. Uveitis, retinal vasculitis, and chorioretinitis, the most common clinical presentations of *Treponema pallidum* infection, are imminently treatable if timely diagnosis is confirmed. The key to diagnosis of ocular syphilis is a high clinical index of suspicion and an overall familiarity with its patterns of inflammation and mimickry. Concurrent HIV infection may dictate a more aggressive natural history of disease and therefore demands more aggressive therapy and closer patient follow-up. Ocular manifestations of syphilis may be a marker for neurosyphilis as well as HIV infection. Therefore, intravenous antibiotic therapy should be considered.

Acknowledgments: The authors would like to acknowledge Dr. Robert Braunstein, Dr. R.G. Chenoweth, Dr. J. Donald M. Gass, Dr. Norman B. Medow, and Dr. John Sorenson and Wills Eye Hospital for clinical photographs.

REFERENCES

1. Hutchinson J: Congenital syphilis. Ophthalmic Hosp Rep 1:191–198, 1858.
2. Hook EW III, Marra CM: Acquired Syphilis in Adults. N Engl J Med 16:1060–1069, 1992.
3. Sidler-Huguenin: Uber die hereditar-syphilitischen Augenhintergrundsveranderungen, nebst einigen allgemeinen Bemerkungen uber Augenkrankungen bei angeborener Lues. Beitr Augenheilkd 51:1, 1904.
4. Centers for Disease Control: MMWR 40(19):314–323, 1991.
5. Webster LA, Rolfs RT, Nakashima AK: Regional and temporal trends in the surveillence of syphilis. MMWR CDC Surveillence Summaries 40(3):29–33, 1991.
6. Rolfs RT, Nakashima AK: Epidemiology of primary and secondary syphilis in the United States, 1981–9. JAMA 264:1432–1437, 1990.
7. Fichtner RR, Aral SO, Blount JH, et al: Syphilis in the United States. 1967–1979. Sex Transm Dis 10:77, 1983.
8. Matjucha ICA, Katz B: The neuro-ophthalmology of spirochetal infections. In Katz B (ed): Neuro-ophthalmology in Systemic Disease. Philadelphia, WB Saunders Co, 1992, pp 549–565.
9. Tramont ED: *Treponema pallidum* (syphilis). In Mandell GL, Douglas RG Jr, Bennett JE (eds): Principle and Practice of Infectious Diseases, 3rd edition, Vol 2. New York, Churchill Livingstone, 1990, pp 1794–1808.

10. Holmes KK: Syphilis. In Petersdorf RG, Adams RD, Braunwald E, et al (eds): Harrison's Principles of Internal Medicine, 10th edition. New York, McGraw Hill, 1983, pp 1034–1045.

11. de Souza EC, Jalkh AE, Trempe CL, et al: Unusual central chorioretinitis as the first manifestation of early secondary syphilis. Am J Ophthalmol 105:271–276, 1988.

12. Schlagel TF Jr, Kao SF: A review (1970–1980) of 28 presumptive cases of syphilitic uveitis. Am J Ophthalmol 93:412–414, 1982.

13. Tamesis RR, Foster CS: Ocular syphilis. Ophthalmology 97:1281–1287, 1990.

14. Schulman JA, Peyman GA: Syphilitic gummatous iridocyclitis. Ann Ophthalmol 21:333–336, 1989.

15. Duke-Elder S: System of Ophthalmology, Vol 9. St Louis, CV Mosby Co, 1966, pp 292–321.

16. Irons EE, Brown EVL: The etiology of iritis. JAMA 81:1770–1776, 1923.

17. Bruns HD: Syphilis and iritis. Arch Ophthalmol 54:462–465, 1925.

18. McCarron MJ, Albert DM: Iridocyclitis and an iris mass associated with secondary syphilis. Ophthalmology 10:1264–1268, 1984.

19. Spoor TC, Wynn P, Hartel WC, Bryan CS: Ocular syphilis: acute and chronic. J Clin Neuroophthalmol 3:197–203, 1983.

20. Walsh F, Hoyt A: Syphilis in the cornea and sclera. In Clinical Neuro-Ophthalmology, 3rd edition, Vol. 2. Baltimore, Williams & Wilkins Co, 1969, pp 1562–1572.

21. Wilhelmus KR, Yokoyama CM: Syphilitic episcleritis and scleritis. Am J Ophthalmol 104:595–597, 1987.

22. Pearson PA, Amrien JM, Baldwin LB, Smith TJ: Iridoschisis associated with syphilitic interstitial keratitis. Am J Ophthalmol 107:88–89, 1989.

23. Martinez JA, Sutphin JE: Syphilitic interstitial keratitis masquerading as staphylococcal marginal keratitis. Am J Ophthalmol 107:431–432, 1989.

24. Hill JC, Maske R, Bowen RM: Secondary localized amyloidosis of the cornea associated with tertiary syphilis. Cornea 9(2):98–101, 1990.

25. Gass JDM, Braunstein RA, Chenoweth RG: Acute syphilitic posterior placoid chorioretinitis. Ophthalmology 97:1288–1297, 1990.

26. Morgan CM, Webb RM, O'Connor GR: Atypical syphilitic chorioretinitis and vasculitis. Retina 4:225, 1984.

27. Kranias G, Schneider D, Raymond LA: A case of syphilitic uveitis. Am J Ophthalmol 91:261, 1981.

28. Halperin LS, Lewis H, Blumenkranz M, et al: Choroidal neovascular membrane and other chorioretinal complications of acquired syphilis. Am J Ophthalmol 108:554–562, 1989.

29. Saari M: Disciform detachment of the macula. Acta Ophthalmol 56:510, 1978.

30. Crouch ER Jr, Goldberg MF: Retinal periarteritis secondary to syphilis. Arch Ophthalmol 93:384–387, 1975.

31. Savir H, Kurz O: Fluorescein angiography in syphilitic retinal vasculitis. Ann Ophthalmol 8:713, 1976.

32. Smith JL: Acute blindness in early syphilis. Arch Ophthalmol 90:256, 1973.

33. Lobes LA, Folk JC: Syphilitic phlebitis simulating branch vein occlusion. Ann Ophthalmol 13:825, 1981.

34. Volpi U: Pseudo-retinitis pigmentosa caused by acquired syphilis. Ann Ottalmol Clin Ocul 92:408, 1966.

35. Blodi RC, Harvouet F: Syphilitic chorioretinitis. Arch Ophthalmol 79:294, 1968.

36. Skalka HW: Asymetric retinitis pigmentosa, luetic retinopathy and the question of unilateral retinitis pigmentosa. Acta Ophthalmol 576:351, 1979.

37. Fewell AG: Unilateral neuroretinitis of syphilitic origin with a striate figure at the macula. Arch Ophthalmol 8:615, 1932.

38. Martin NF, Fitzgerald CR: Cystoid macular edema as the primary sign of neurosyphilis. Am J Ophthalmol 88:28–31, 1979.

39. Verhoeff FA: A case of syphilitic retinochoroiditis juxtapapillaris with microscopic examination. Arch Ophthalmol 45:352, 1916.

40. Folk JC, Weingeist TA, Corbett JJ, et al: Syphilitic neuroretinitis. Am J Ophthalmol 95:480, 1983.

41. Arruga J, Valentines J, Mauri, et al: Neuroretinitis in acquired syphilis. Ophthalmology 92:262, 1985.

42. Veldman E, Bos PJM: Neuroretinitis in secondary syphilis. Doc Ophthalmol 64:23–29, 1986.

43. Deluise VP, Clark SW, Smith JL, Collart P: Syphilitic retinal detachment and uveal effusion. Am J Ophthalmol 94:757, 1982.

44. Graveson GS: Syphilitic optic neuritis. J Neurol Neurosurg Psychiatry 13:216, 1950.

45. Lorentzen SE: Syphilitic optic neuritis. A case report. Acta Ophthalmol 45:769, 1967.

46. Toshniwal P: Optic perineuritis with secondary syphilis. J Clin Neuroophthalmol 7:6–10, 1987.

47. Rush JA, Ryan EJ: Syphilitic optic perineuritis. Am J Ophthalmol 91:404–406, 1981.

48. Ouano DP, Brucker AJ, Saran BR: Macular pseudohypopyon from secondary syphilis. Am J Ophthalmol 119:372–374, 1995.

49. Walsh RB, Hoyt WF: Syphilis. In Clinical Neuro-Ophthalmology, 3rd edition, Vol. 2. Baltimore, Williams & Wilkins Co, 1969, pp 1547–1548.

50. Johns DR, Tierney M, Felsenstein D: Alteration in the natural history of neurosyphilis by concurrent infection with the human immunodeficiency virus. N Engl J Med 316:1569–1572, 1987.

51. Musher DM, Hammell RJ, Baughn RE: Effect of human immunodeficiency virus on the course of syphilis and the response to treatment. Ann Intern Med 113:872–881, 1990.

52. Passo MS, Rosenbaum JT: Ocular syphilis in patients with human immunodeficiency virus infection. Am J Ophthalmol 106:1–6, 1988.

53. Becerra LI, Ksiazek SM, Savino PJ, et al: Syphilitic uveitis in human immunodeficiency virus-infected and noninfected patients. Ophthalmology 96:1727–1730, 1989.

54. Levy JH, Liss RA, Maguire AM: Neurosyphilis and ocular syphilis in patients with concurrent human immunodeficiency virus infection. Retina 9:175–180, 1989.

55. McLeish WM, Pulido JS, Holland S, et al: The ocular manifestations of syphilis in the human immunodeficiency virus type 1-infected host. Ophthalmology 97:196–203, 1990.

56. Halperin LS: Neuroretinitis due to seronegative syphilis associated with human immunodeficiency virus. J Clin Neuroophthalmol 12:171–172, 1992.

57. Paris-Hamelin A: Syphilis serology in 1991. J Clin Neuroophthalmol 11:144–151, 1991.

58. Tramont EC: *Treponema pallidum* (syphilis). In Mandell GL, Douglas RG Jr, bennett JE (eds): Principles and Practice of Infectious Diseases, 3rd edition, Vol. 2. New York, Churchill Livingstone, 1990, pp 1827–1828.

59. Berry CD, Hooton TM, Collier AC, Lukehart SA: Neurologic relapse after benzathine penicillin therapy for secondary syphilis in a patient with HIV infection. N Engl J Med 316:1587–1589, 1987.

60. Centers for Disease Control: Recommendations for diagnosing and treating syphilis in HIV-infected patients. MMWR 37:600–602, 607–608, 1988.

61. Tramont EC: The case against benzathine penicillin as the treatment for neurosyphilis. In Smith JL (ed): Neuro-ophthalmology update. New York, Masson. 1977, pp 325–328, 1977.

62. Johnson RC, Bey RF, Wolgamot SJ: Comparison of the activities of ceftriaxone and penicillin G against experimentally induced syphilis in rabbits. Antimicrob Agents Chemother 21:984–989, 1982.

63. Hook EW III, Baker-Zander SA, Moskovitz BL, et al: Ceftriaxone therapy for asymptomatic neurosyphilis. Case report and Western blot analysis of serum and cerebrospinal fluid IgG response to therapy. Sex Transm Dis 13(Suppl 3):185–188, 1986.

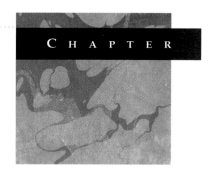

Tuberculosis

Samir C. Patel, M.D.

Sander Dubovy, M.D.

Tuberculosis is a disease of worldwide prevalence. It is caused by *Mycobacterium tuberculosis*, an acid-fast-staining, obligate aerobe.[1] In the United States, between 1953 and 1984, reported cases of tuberculosis steadily declined from approximately 84,000 to 24,000. However, since 1984, the rate of the disease has increased approximately 16% over the subsequent 5 years.[2] This resurgence is probably attributable to an increase in the human immunodeficiency virus (HIV)–infected population, increased numbers of immigrants from countries with a high prevalence of tuberculosis, and perhaps, the elimination of public health programs directed towards reducing tuberculosis.[3,4]

PATHOGENESIS

The primary infection is initiated upon inhalation of infected airborne droplets originating from patients with pulmonary tuberculosis. These small particles (1 to 5 μm) usually lodge in the terminal air spaces of the lower and middle lung lobes. The alveolar macrophages engulf the mycobacterial inoculum, and owing to the lack of a protective immune response, intracellular organisms continue to replicate and cause the macrophages to rupture. The bacilli gain access to the regional lymph nodes via the lymphatic channels and eventually metastasize to distant organs by hematogenous dissemination. Protective immunity typically develops within 2 to 10 weeks, characterized by the development of a granulomatous response and eventual necrosis and/or calcification of the initial and metastatic foci of infection. This primary infectious process is usually subclinical in the immunocompetent population.[3,5]

The majority of immunocompetent patients do not develop clinically active disease but reflect a state of dormancy induced by the acquired immunity. Approximately 5% develop clinically active disease within the first 2 years. An additional 5% develop reactivated disease many years later. HIV-infected patients develop tuberculosis at an approximate rate of 8% per year.[3] Patients with silicosis, a history of intravenous drug abuse, renal allografts and systemic immunosuppression as well as diabetics, alcoholics, occupants of homeless shelters, and urban immigrants are also at a higher risk of developing tuberculosis.[6–9]

In some cases, during the primary infection or reactivation phase, a rampant hematogenous dissemination results in miliary tuberculosis. This is a potentially life-threatening situation characterized by multisystem involvement and millet seed radiographic findings. This radiographic pattern may take 4 to 6 weeks to develop, often delaying diagnosis. Typical intraocular findings may aid in the early diagnosis of this condition.[1,10,11]

HIV-infected patients exhibit a relative cell-mediated dysfunction predisposing them to tuberculosis. In addition, this altered immunity results in an increased rate of miliary infiltration, relative lack of classic pulmonary disease manifestation (i.e., cavitary lesions), earlier progression from infection to clinical disease, and a higher rate of extrapulmonary disease.[4,10] Tuberculosis in an HIV-infected patient is an acquired immunodeficiency syndrome (AIDS) defining disease.[4,12]

OCULAR MANIFESTATIONS

Ocular tuberculosis is rare, affecting 1.4% of patients with active disease.[13,14] Intraocular and periocular involvement from tuberculous infection may result from the primary infection, secondary hematogenous dissemination, or contagious spread, or may be a result of an immune reaction to the tuberculous antigen. In general, intraocular manifestations are considered to evolve from hematogenous spread, whereas primary or direct infection may cause infection of the conjunctiva and cornea.[11]

A wide spectrum of ocular findings have been reported to occur as a single entity or in variable combinations. These include scleritis (with or without perforation),[15] exudative mass in the anterior chamber,[16] acute or chronic iritis (with or without nodules),[17] ciliary body granuloma,[4] peripheral uveitis,[18] choroidal tubercles,[11,19-23] subretinal abscess,[16] retinal vasculitis,[24] retinal mass,[25] subretinal neovascularization,[26] central vein occlusion, endophthalmitis,[27] and panophthalmitis.[11,28,29]

Conjunctival disease may present as a nodular or ulcerated lesion with regional lymphadenopathy.[30] Direct inoculation,[31] spread from adjacent sinus disease, and hematologic spread have been implicated as possible mechanisms. Corneal involvement may occur from adjacent tissue spread of disease affecting uvea or sclera. Manifestations include interstitial keratitis, ulceration, and occasionally corneal perforation. Scleral infection commonly presents as a focal necrotizing anterior scleritis with ulceration. Phlyctenules may affect the conjunctiva or cornea. They are thought to result from delayed hypersensitivity to the tuberculous protein.[32]

Tuberculosis as a cause of uveitis has been decreasing over the past 50 years.[11,33,34] In 1941, 80% of granulomatous uveitis was thought to be of tuberculous origin, decreasing to 20% in 1960.[35] It has been postulated that stricter diagnostic criteria, emergence and recognition of other uveitic syndromes, and decrease in systemic tuberculosis (until 1984) are responsible for this trend.[11]

Anterior uveal syndromes commonly occur in the form of chronic granulomatous iridocyclitis, multiple iris nodules (miliary tuberculosis) and, occasionally, as acute anterior iritis. Choroidal disease is the most common manifestation of intraocular tuberculosis, reflecting the hematologic embolization of the bacilli. The variability in presentation is

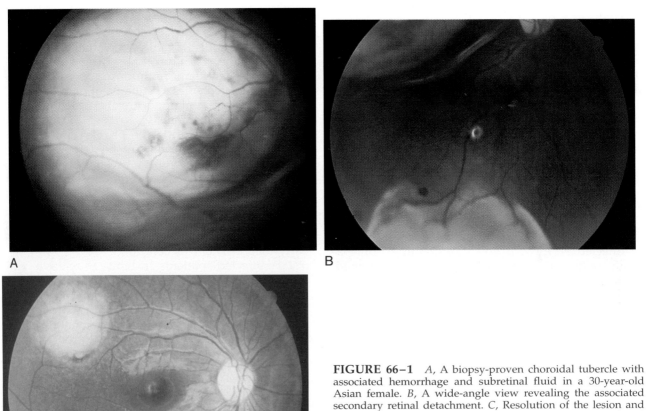

A

B

C

FIGURE 66–1 A, A biopsy-proven choroidal tubercle with associated hemorrhage and subretinal fluid in a 30-year-old Asian female. B, A wide-angle view revealing the associated secondary retinal detachment. C, Resolution of the lesion and subretinal fluid after treatment. (A through C courtesy of Carl D. Regillo, M.D. and Jerry Shields, M.D.)

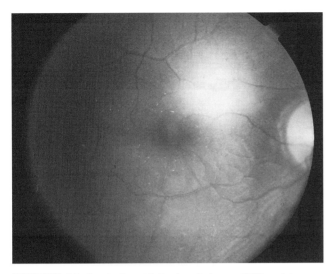

FIGURE 66–2   A choroidal tubercle in an HIV-positive patient with a history of intravenous drug abuse and miliary tuberculosis. Refractile particles represent talc emboli.

due to differences in the virulence of the organism, host resistance, and presence or absence of host immunity.[4,19,20,22,23,26]

Choroidal tubercles are polymorphic lesions that present as single or multiple, oval gray-white or yellow-white lesions with indefinite borders[11,19,20–23,36] (Figs. 66–1 through 66–3). They are initially flat but may become elevated with time. They range in size from 1 to several disc diameters and exhibit a variable amount of pigmentation. Associated findings include serous retinal detachment (Fig. 66–1B), exudation, vitritis, and papillitis. The anterior segment is usually unre-

markable. There has been one case report of macular subretinal neovascularization presenting with choroidal tubercles.[26]

The findings on fluorescein angiography are variable.[11,19,20,37] There may be areas of early blocked fluorescence corresponding to tuberculous nodules that become hyperfluorescent in the late phase of the angiogram.[11,38] The fluorescein angiogram may also demonstrate early hyperfluorescence of the tuberculoma with late staining[11,19] (Fig. 66–3B). Ultrasound findings are also variable.[11,18] B-scan ultrasonography has typically shown a solid elevated mass with an absent scleral echo due to the absorption by inflammatory cells. A-scan ultrasonography may demonstrate spikes of low internal reflectivity.[11,19] Choroidal tubercles are frequently observed in the miliary form of tuberculosis. They have also been reported in conjunction with pulmonary tuberculosis or inactive disease.[19,20]

The differential diagnosis of choroidal tubercles is dependent upon size, multiplicity, and elevation of the tubercle. One should exclude sarcoid granuloma, syphilis, uveal melanoma, choroidal hemangioma, metastatic disease, large cell lymphoma, and various multifocal chorioretinopathies.[4] In patients with AIDS,[39] additional considerations include choroidal pneumocystosis, Candida chorioretinitis, cryptococcosis, and Nocardia choroidal infiltration.

A subretinal abscess is a relatively rare manifestation and may present as an ill-defined, yellow subretinal mass. It may remain localized to the subretinal space or may break out into the vitreous cavity causing severe inflammation.[16] Associated findings may reveal variable amounts of exudation,

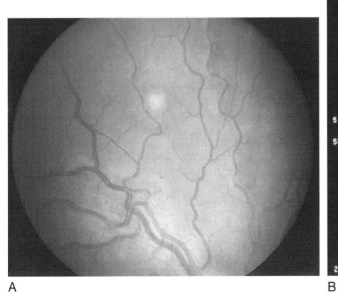

A

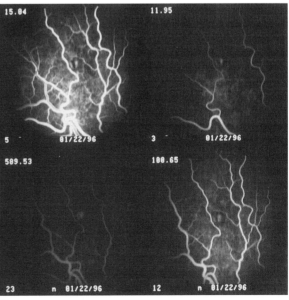

B

FIGURE 66–3   A, Presumed choroidal tuberculous lesion in a patient with active pulmonary tuberculosis. B, Fluorescein angiogram reveals early hyperfluorescence and late staining in this case.

hemorrhage, and secondary retinal detachment. The differential diagnosis includes toxoplasmosis, toxocariasis, fungal disease, *Nocardia* organisms,[40] and large cell lymphoma.

Scattered reports of retinal periphlebitis due to direct tuberculous infection have been presented in patients with active systemic disease and variable anterior segment inflammation. These lesions have shown a good response to antituberculous chemotherapy. Other forms of retinal involvement such as retinitis and retinal masses are extremely rare.[24,25]

Retinal periphlebitis is also encountered in connection with Eales' disease.[41,42] This is a controversial topic referring to a syndrome occurring typically in healthy males from India or Pakistan, with tuberculoprotein hypersensitivity during their third or fourth decade. It is a diagnosis of exclusion and is characterized by peripheral retinal capillary nonperfusion, arteriovenous shunts, segmental aneurysms, retinal neovascularization, and recurrent vitreous hemorrhages. The majority of evidence supports an immune-mediated mechanism of retinal phlebitis in these patients.

DIAGNOSIS

Diagnosis of tuberculosis involving the conjunctiva, sclera, and eyelids may be secured by obtaining a biopsy of the involved tissue. Histopathologic analysis usually reveals caseating granulomas with Langerhans' giant cells and acid-fast bacilli.

Intraocular tuberculosis is usually a clinical diagnosis requiring analysis of the characteristic lesion, epidemiologic factors, presence of active systemic disease, systemic skin testing, and often a therapeutic trial. In general, a presumptive diagnosis of intraocular tuberculosis is made when a patient with a characteristic lesion has proven active systemic disease. Typical chest x-ray findings; sputum analysis; biopsy of the liver, lymph nodes, and bone marrow; stool for acid-fast smear; and cultures of blood, urine, cerebrospinal, and pleural fluid may be employed to establish the presence of active systemic disease.[4] A direct smear and culture from intraocular fluid or tissue may be required for a definitive diagnosis, particularly in countries endemic for tuberculosis.[16,43]

Skin testing is commonly utilized to establish exposure to *M. tuberculosis*. The test is based on an antigenic response of the individual to autoclaved components of the organism.[44] A standard dose of 5 tuberculin units is injected intradermally and the amount of induration is measured in 48 to 72 hours. Test interpretation depends on the prevalence of infection in the patient's community and risk factors for tuberculosis. The Centers for Disease Control (CDC) considers reaction of 5 mm or more to be positive in very-high-risk individuals (i.e., HIV patients, patients with abnormal chest x-rays), 10 mm or more to be positive in high-risk individuals (i.e.,

foreign born individuals, members of low socioeconomic backgrounds), and 15 mm or more to be positive in individuals with no risk factors.[45]

A positive skin test without active systemic disease is usually insufficient to make a presumptive diagnosis of intraocular tuberculosis.[4,46] In this case the diagnosis may be based on the presence of a characteristic intraocular lesion, lack of response to nontuberculous medication, and a positive response to antituberculous therapeutic trial. Intraocular fluid/tissue sample may be considered for definitive diagnosis.

TREATMENT

Extrapulmonary tuberculosis, including ocular tuberculosis, is usually treated similarly to pulmonary disease. There has been a recent increase in multidrug-resistant tuberculosis that has coincided with the increased incidence of the disease. The CDC has addressed this issue, and current guidelines recommend that all patients with newly diagnosed tuberculosis be placed on a four-drug regimen of isoniazid, rifampin, pyrazinamide, and either streptomycin or ethambutol. Treatment usually lasts 6 to 9 months, and should be coordinated with a knowledgeable specialist.[47] Systemic steroids should not be used in ocular tuberculosis, as their use has been associated with a lengthened disease course and an increased rate of recurrence. Topical cycloplegics and steroids may be used adjunctively.

DRUG TOXICITY

Given the low incidence of ocular findings among patients with systemic tuberculosis, one is more likely to encounter ocular toxicity from tuberculous therapy. Ethambutol,[48,49] isoniazid,[50,51] and streptomycin[52] have all been reported to be associated with optic neuropathy. Ethambutol-induced optic neuropathy may present with anterior papillitis or retrobulbar neuritis and may cause central or peripheral visual loss. Toxicity is dose dependent, with an incidence of 0 to 15% with presently used regimens. Management requires cessation of ethambutol use and improvement usually occurs in 1 to 6 weeks.[53] Isoniazid optic neuritis may also present with anterior or retrobulbar forms, with or without the commonly seen peripheral neuropathy. Treatment should be discontinued if signs of toxicity appear. Pyridoxine has been used to treat isoniazid-associated peripheral neuropathy, and some have advocated its use for prophylaxis and treatment of optic neuritis.[54] Streptomycin has been reported to cause retrobulbar optic neuritis, however, the evidence is not nearly as strong as for the agents described above.[51,52]

REFERENCES

1. Daniel TM: Tuberculosis. In Isselbacher KJ, Braunwald E, Wilson JD, et al (eds): Harrison's Principles of Internal Medicine, 13th edition. New York, McGraw-Hill, 1994.
2. Barnes PF, Bloch AB, Davidson PT, Snider DE Jr: Tuberculosis in patients with human immunodeficiency virus infection. N Engl J Med 324:1644–1650, 1991.
3. Waxman S, Gang M, Goldfrank L: Tuberculosis in the HIV-infected patient. Emerg Med Clin North Am 13:179–198, 1995.
4. Dunn JP, Helm CJ, Davidson PT: Tuberculosis. In Pepose JS, Holland GN, Wilhelmus KR (eds): Ocular Infection & Immunity. St Louis, CV Mosby Co, 1996.
5. Weissler JC: Southwestern internal medical conference: tuberculosis-immunopathogenesis and therapy. Am J Med Sci 305:52–65, 1993.
6. Brudney K, Dobkin J: Resurgent tuberculosis in New York City: human immunodeficiency virus, homelessness, and the decline of tuberculosis control programs. Am Rev Respir Dis 144:745–749, 1991.
7. Centers for Disease Control: Tuberculosis among foreign-born persons entering the United States: recommendations of the advisory committee for elimination of tuberculosis. MMWR 39(RR-18):1–21, 1990.
8. Centers for Disease Control: Tuberculosis among homeless shelter residents. MMWR 40:869–877, 1991.
9. Mansour AM: Renal allograft tuberculosis. Tubercle 71:147–148, 1990.
10. Trucksis M, Baker AS: Mycobacterial diseases: tuberculosis and leprosy. In Albert DM, Jakobiec FA (eds): Principles and Practice of Ophthalmology, Vol 5. Philadelphia, WB Saunders Co, 1994.
11. Helm CJ, Holland GN: Ocular tuberculosis. Surv Ophthalmol 38:229–256, 1993.
12. Centers for Disease Control: 1993 revised classification system for HIV infection and expanded surveillance case definition for AIDS among adolescents and adults. MMWR 41(RR-17):1–19, 1992.
13. Donahue H: Ophthalmologic experience in a tuberculosis sanatorium. Am J Ophthal 64:742–748, 1967.
14. Pfeiffer RL, Lewen RM, Yin H: Tuberculosis. In Pepose JS, Holland GN, Wilhelmus KR (eds): Ocular Infection & Immunity. St Louis, CV Mosby Co, 1996.
15. Nanda M, Pflugfelder SC, Holland S: Mycobacterium tuberculosis scleritis. Am J Ophthalmol.
16. Biswas J, Madhavan HN, Gopal L, Badrinath SS: Intraocular tuberculosis: clinicopathologic study of five cases. Retina 15:461–468, 1995.
17. Asensi F, Otero MC, Perez-Tamarid D, et al: Tuberculosis iridocyclitis in a three-year-old girl. Clin Pediatr 30:605–606, 1991.
18. Psilas K, Aspiotis M, Petroutsos, G, et al: Anti-tuberculosis therapy in the treatment of peripheral uveitis. Ann Ophthalmol 23:254–258, 1991.
19. Jabbour NM, Faris B, Trempe CL: A case of pulmonary tuberculosis presenting with a choroidal tuberculoma. Ophthalmology 92:884–887, 1985.
20. Cangemi FE, Friedman AH, Josephberg R: Tuberculoma of the choroid. Ophthalmology 87:252–258, 1980 .
21. Massaro D, Katz S, Sachs M: Choroidal tubercles: a clue to hematogenous tuberculosis. Ann Intern Med 231–241, 1964.
22. Illingworth RS, Wright T: Tubercles of the choroid. Br Med J 2:365–3658, 1948.
23. Olazabal F Jr: Choroidal tubercles: a neglected sign. JAMA 200:374–377, 1967.
24. Rosen PH, Spalton DJ, Graham EM: Intraocular tuberculosis. Eye 4:486–492, 1990.
25. Saini JS, Mukherjee AK, Nadkarni: Primary tuberculosis of the retina. Br J Ophthalmol 70:533–535, 1986.
26. Chung YM, Yeh TH, Sheu SJ, Liu JH: Macular subretinal neovascularization in choroidal tuberculosis. Ann Ophthalmol 21:225–229, 1989.
27. Dvorak-Theobald G: Acute tuberculosis endophthalmitis: report of a case. Am J Ophthalmol 45:403, 1958.
28. Darrell RW: Acute tuberculosis panophthalmitis. Arch Ophthalmol 78:51–54, 1967.
29. Menezo JL, Martinez-Costa R, Marin F, et al: Tuberculous panophthalmitis associated with drug abuse. Int Ophthalmol 10:235–240, 1987.
30. Anhalt EF, Zavell S, Chang G, Byron HM: Conjunctival tuberculosis. Am J Ophthalmol 50:265–269, 1960.
31. Chandler AC, Locatcher-Khorago D: Primary tuberculosis of the conjunctiva. Arch Ophthalmol 71:202–205, 1964.
32. Gibson WS: The etiology of phlyctenular conjunctivitis. Am J Dis Child 15:81–115, 1918.
33. Schlaegel TF Jr, O'Connor GR: Metastatic nonsuppurative uveitis. Int Ophthalmol Clin 17:87–108, 1977.
34. Henderly DE, Genstler AJ, Smith RE, Rao NA: Changing patterns of uveitis. Am J Ophthalmol 103:131–136, 1987.
35. Woods AC: Modern concepts of the etiology of uveitis. Am J Ophthalmol 50:1170–1187, 1960.
36. Gur S, Silverstone BZ, Zylberman R, Berson D: Chorioretinitis and extrapulmonary tuberculosis. Ann Ophthalmol 19:112–115, 1987.
37. Santoni G, Fiore C, Lupidi G, Galuppo I: tuberculose miliare choroidienne: etude angiofluorographique. Ophthalmologica 184:6–12, 1982.
38. Lyon CE, Grimson BS, Peiffer RL, Merritt JC: Clinicopathological correlation of a solitary choroidal tuberculoma. Ophthalmology 92:845–850, 1985.
39. Morinelli EN, Dugel RU, Riffenburgh R, Rao NA: Infectious multifocal choroiditis in patients with acquired immune deficiency syndrome. Ophthalmology 100:1014–1021, 1993.
40. Gregor RJ, Chong CA, Augsburger JJ, et al: Endogenous Nocardia asteroides subretinal abscess diagnosed by transvitreal fine needle aspiration biopsy. Retina 9:118–121, 1989.
41. Dastur DK, Singhal BS: Eales' disease with neurological involvement. II. Pathology and pathogenesis. J Neurol Sci 27:323–345, 1976.
42. Elliot AJ: 30-year observation of patients with Eales' disease. Am J Ophthalmol 80:404–408, 1975.
43. Barondes MJ, Sponsel WE, Stevens TS, Plotnik RD: Tuberculous choroiditis diagnosed by chorioretinal endobiopsy. Am J Ophthalmol 112:460–461, 1991.
44. Reichman LB: Tuberculin skin testing. Chest 76:764–770, 1979.
45. American Thoracic Society and Centers for Disease Control: Diagnostic standards and classification of tuberculosis. Am Rev Respir Dis 142:725-735, 1990.
46. Rosenbaum JT, Wernick R: The utility of routine screening of patients with uveitis for systemic lupus erythematosus or tuberculosis: a bayesian analysis. Arch Ophthalmol 108:1291–1293, 1990.
47. Centers for Disease Control: Initial therapy for TB in the era of multidrug resistance: recommendations of the advisory council for the elimination of TB. MMWR 42:1–80, 1993.
48. Carr RE, Henkind P: Ocular manifestations of ethambutol. Arch Ophthalmol 67:566–571, 1962.
49. Leibolt JE: The ocular toxicity of ethanbutol and its relationship to dose. Ann N Y Acad Sci 135:904–909. 1966.
50. Keeping JA, Searle CWA: Optic neuritis following isoniazid therapy. Lancet 2:278, 1955.
51. Sutton PH, Beattie PH: Optic atrophy after administration of isoniazid with P.A.S. Lancet 1:650–651, 1955.
52. Sykowski P: Streptomycin causing retrobulbar optic neuritis. Am J Ophthalmol 34:1446, 1951.
53. Chatterjee VKK, Buchanan DR, Friedman AI, Green M: Ocular toxicity following ethambutol in standard dosage. Br J Dis Chest 80:288-291, 1989.
54. Kass I, Mandel W, Cohen H, Dressler SH: Isoniazid as cause of optic neuritis and atrophy. JAMA 164:1740–1743, 1957.

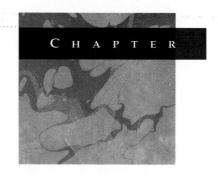

CHAPTER *67*

Diffuse Unilateral Subacute Neuroretinitis

Jason S. Slakter, M.D.
Antonio P. Ciardella, M.D.

Diffuse unilateral subacute neuroretinitis (DUSN) is a syndrome caused by a nematode that moves around in the subretinal space. It was first described as a distinct clinical entity by Gass and Scelfo in 1978,[1] characterized by unilateral visual loss with vitreous inflammation, optic disc swelling, and retinitis, associated with recurrent crops of gray-white lesions affecting the outer retina. In the late stage of DUSN, there is progressive visual loss, optic nerve atrophy, attenuation of the retinal vessels, and development of focal or diffuse atrophic changes in the retinal pigment epithelium.

EPIDEMIOLOGY

DUSN is prevalent in the southeastern United States, Caribbean area, and probably Latin America. Recently it has been described in two Brazilian[2] patients and in one German[3] patient. DUSN typically affects patients in the second and third decades of life (age range, 8 to 65),[4,5] with males affected more frequently than females. It often has an insidious onset, with 18 of 37 patients in one study presenting with advanced visual loss secondary to the late stages of the disease.[4]

ETIOLOGY

The precise identification of the nematode responsible for DUSN remains controversial. While numerous case reports had described the presence of a viable nematode moving in the subretinal space in patients with a clinical picture of DUSN,[6-9] it

was Gass and Braunstein[5] who first characterized the nature and distribution of these organisms. They found that the nematodes ranged in size from 400 to 2000 μm, with a diameter of no greater than 1/20 of the length. These organisms moved by a coiling and uncoiling motion and sometimes slithering in a snake-like fashion. In addition, a geographic relationship has been noted with respect to the size of the nematodes. Patients presenting in the southeastern United States and Caribbean were noted to have organisms ranging from 400 to 1000 μm in size, while organisms ranging from 1500 to 2000 μm in length were noted in the northern Midwest.

Gass and Braunstein[5] postulated that at least two different nematodes were responsible for the DUSN syndrome due to this geographic variation. The smaller of the two was proposed to be *Ancylostoma caninum*, a common hookworm parasite of dogs, which is a frequent cause of cutaneous larval migrans in the southeastern United States. Its infective third-stage larva measures approximately 650 μm, and it can survive in host tissues for years without changing size or shape.

Kazakos and co-workers[10,11] have suggested that the larger one was *Baylisascaris procyonis*, an intestinal round worm of lower carnivores (raccoons and squirrels). This organism grows from an initial size of 300 μm to a maximal size of 2000 μm, which correlates well with the range of length of the nematode observed clinically in human DUSN.[10] The *B. procyonis* is a common cause of ocular larval migrans in North America associated with central nervous system infections.[12,13] In support of this hypothesis, Kazakos et al point out that a number of patients specifically described exposure to raccoons and other potential host animals prior to the onset of DUSN.[10] On the other hand, Gass has pointed out that in 100 cases of DUSN at the Bascom Palmer Eye Institute, few of these patients reported any exposure to raccoons or other possibly infected carnivores.[14] In addition, patients did not manifest any signs of central nervous system involvement, which would make *B. procyonis* highly unlikely as a cause for DUSN, at least in their population.

Other authors have suggested *Toxocara canis*[9,15] as a possible cause of DUSN, but the lack of serologic evidence in most of the patients with DUSN and the small size of the infective second-stage larval form of *T. canis* makes it an unlikely causative agent in most patients with DUSN. However, in a case

with the clinical appearance of DUSN a motile nematode was aspirated from the subretinal space after trans–pars plana vitrectomy and retinotomy. Morphology of the nematode was consistent with a third-stage toxocara larva[16] (Fig. 67–1). In those other few cases where biopsy specimens of the intraocular nematode from human DUSN are available, the precise classification of the organism has been impossible due to the inherent difficulties of morphologic identification of nematode species. The various biopsy specimens have been characterized as being consistent with a diagnosis of *Baylisascaris* or *Ancylostoma*, but in no case has specific identification of an organism been made.[14,17]

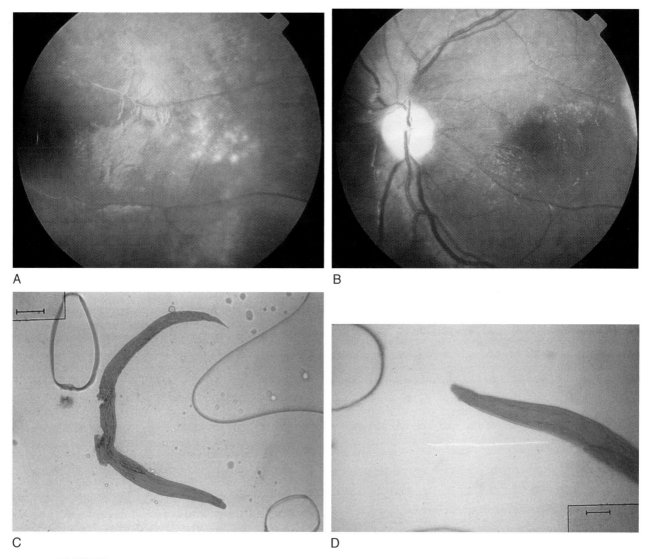

FIGURE 67–1   Diffuse unilateral subacute neuroretinitis (DUSN). Surgical removal of the subretinal nematode. *A*, Clinical photograph of the left eye of a 9-year-old Brazilian male who was discovered to have decreased vision to the level of counting fingers at 2 m during a routine eye examination. Notice the retinal arteriolas narrowing, and the active yellow-white deep retinal dots clustered in the temporal macula. The worm is barely visible in a coiled configuration. A trans–pars plana vitrectomy was performed and the nematode aspirated through a retinotomy. *B*, Postoperative appearance of the same eye 3 months after surgery. Retinal arteriolas narrowing, optic atrophy, and an epiretinal membrane emanating from the retinotomy scar are evident. *C*, Photograph of the entire nematode after surgical removal. *D*, High-power view of the proximal end of the nematode. Morphologic features were typical for *Toxocara canis*.

PATHOGENESIS

There is now mounting evidence that DUSN is a multietiologic syndrome caused by different species of nematodes, and perhaps other helminths. It is likely that different tissue-migratory nematodes could generate similar changes resulting in DUSN. Larval secretory-excretory products, including various enzymes and metabolic wastes produced by nematode larvae, could cause localized toxic effects and/or stimulate an inflammatory response, especially one mediated by eosinophils.[5,18,19] Toxic eosinophil granule proteins, released locally in response to nematode larval secretory-excretory products, may also damage ocular tissues, leading or contributing to DUSN.[18,19] Histopathology from a patient with DUSN revealed a nongranulomatous vitritis and retinitis as well as retinal and optic nerve perivasculitis.[1] There was extensive degeneration of the peripheral retina with mild posterior retinal degeneration. Mild optic atrophy, retinal pigment epithelium degeneration, and a low-grade nongranulomatous choroiditis were also appreciated. There was no eosinophilic infiltration noted in the retina or choroid.

The pathogenesis of DUSN appears to be a local effect on the outer retina secondary to by-products of the intraocular nematode.[1,14] These are manifested by the clinically apparent gray-white lesions. In addition, there is a more diffuse toxic reaction, affecting both the inner and outer retinal tissue. In the later stages of the disease, this diffuse toxic reaction progresses to involve the ganglion cells, and secondary arteriolar narrowing occurs.[14]

CLINICAL FEATURES

The clinical features of DUSN may be divided into early and late manifestations. In the early stage, patients may complain of floaters associated with mild to moderate visual loss, with visual acuity ranging from 20/30 to 20/200.[4] Occasionally they may notice paracentral or central scotoma, and in some cases these scotomata are specifically described as being transient or mobile.[4] They may also complain of ocular discomfort. An afferent pupillary defect may be noted. Anterior segment examination may be normal or occasionally conjunctival injection, ciliary flush, anterior chamber cells and flare, fine keratitic precipitates, and hypopyon may be present. Posterior segment examination invariably reveals mild to moderate vitritis,[14] optic disc swelling, and narrowing of the retinal arterioles.

The most characteristic feature of this syndrome is the presence of multiple, focal gray-white lesions of the deep retina or retinal pigment epithelium (Figs. 67–2 and 67–3). They vary in size from 0.25 to 1 disc diameter and tend to cluster in the macular region or in the temporal juxtamacular region.[4] With careful observation, a motile worm, located in

the subretinal space, may be noted near these lesions (Figs. 67–2 and 67–3). As mentioned, the nematodes vary in length from 400 to 2000 μm.[5,14] They appear smooth in outline, tapered on both ends, and often assume an S-shaped or coiled configuration. They may be noted to move under direct observation, particularly when exposed to bright light. A white glistening sheen is noted over the region (Figs. 67–3 and 67–4).

The active evanescent white lesions, which are probably caused by substances left by the nematode in its wake, fade within a period of days as the nematode moves elsewhere in the eye, only to recur in an adjacent site over the ensuing weeks. Frequently, the lesions resolve without any ophthalmoscopic or angiographic evidence of damage. More commonly, however, minor changes in the retinal pigment epithelium are observed. Less than 1% of these lesions are of sufficient intensity to cause a visible chorioretinal scar, which may simulate that seen in the presumed ocular histoplasmosis syndrome (POHS).[20]

Other less frequently encountered clinical signs include focal retinal and subretinal hemorrhages, perivenous exudates and sheathing, localized serous detachments of the neurosensory retina, and neovascularization.[4] Retinal striae radiating from the macular region associated with active lesions have been described.[1]

If the nematode is not recognized and photocoagulated, it may survive in the subretinal space for 4 years or longer, resulting in the progression of the disease to the late stages. The late manifestations of DUSN are characterized by a dense central or paracentral scotoma, severe visual acuity loss (<20/400), and a positive afferent pupillary defect on the involved side.[4,14] Ophthalmoscopic examination reveals focal as well as diffuse retinal pigment epithelium depigmentation and mottling, most typically noted in the paramacular region, sparing the center of the macula in a majority of patients. There is generalized narrowing of the retinal arterioles and marked optic disc pallor (Figs. 67–1, 67–4, and 67–5). Subretinal neovascularization or organized disciform scars may be noted.[14] Peripapillary arteriolar sheathing has also been described.

While a close correlation between the degree of optic atrophy and retinal arteriolar narrowing is appreciated, these changes do not correlate well with the severity of visual loss.[1,4,5,14] The marked loss of visual acuity is typically accompanied by minimal changes in the macular area and is presumably the result of toxic dysfunction of the retina and optic nerve induced by the nematode.

DIAGNOSIS

A thorough clinical examination is important in looking for the cluster of active, gray-white outer retinal lesions. If they are present, the nematode

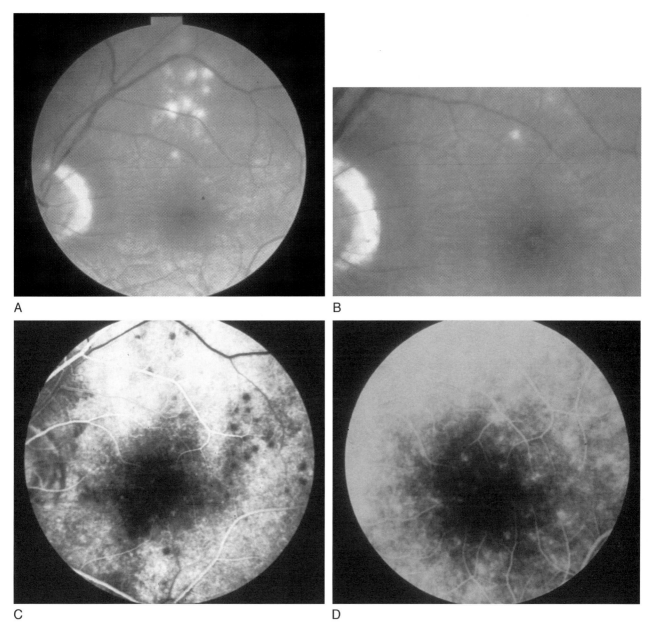

FIGURE 67–2   Acute stage of DUSN. *A*, Clinical photograph of a patient with recent blurring of vision in his left eye. Multiple deep white dots are visible in the superior macular area. *B*, High magnification of the same eye shows the nematode in the subretinal space, just superior to the fovea. The nematode appears in an S-shaped configuration with tapered ends. A deep white retinal lesion is visible superiorly. *C*, Early-phase fluorescein angiogram shows early hypofluorescence of the white dots. *D*, Late-phase fluorescein study reveals staining of these retinal lesions.

will usually be found biomicroscopically in their vicinity. In the absence of these lesions, a tedious search of the entire fundus using a three-mirror or a wide-angle contact lens is necessary to locate the worm.

Fluorescein angiography in the early stages of the disease reveals leakage from the optic nerve head capillaries as well as some generalized paravenous leakage.[4] There are minimal changes in the retinal pigment epithelium, most notably some mild window defect. The clinically apparent gray-white lesions exhibit early hypofluorescence and

late staining and hyperfluorescence consistent with an inflammatory focus (Fig. 67–2), similar to that seen with acute multifocal posterior placoid pigment epitheliopathy (AMPPPE).[4,5,14] Cystoid macular edema has been described in several patients.[4] In the later stages of the disease, diffuse areas of focal hyperfluorescence secondary to retinal pigment epithelial loss in the paramacular region are noted. The relative sparing of the central macula is manifested by only a mild degree of mottled hyperfluorescence in this region.[1,4] In the more severely affected patients, patchy choroidal filling in

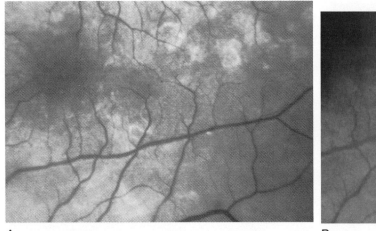

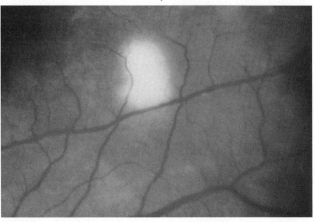

A   B

FIGURE 67–3   Laser photocoagulation of DUSN. *A*, High-magnification clinical photograph demonstrating a yellow-white subretinal nematode in the inferotemporal macula. Notice the coiled configuration and the tapered ends. A few white dots and a diffuse glistening reflex are visible in the same area. *B*, High-magnification clinical photograph of the same area immediately after laser photocoagulation of the subretinal nematode. A white discoloration of the retina is obtained to ensure the death of the nematode.

the early phases of the angiogram associated with a delay in the appearance of dye in the retinal arterioles and an increased arteriolar to venous circulation time is noted.[1] This retinal perfusion delay is well correlated with the degree of optic atrophy and arteriolar narrowing noted clinically. Unfortunately, no angiographic abnormalities specifically associated with the mobile subretinal nematode have been described. With the development of subretinal neovascularization and disciform scars, typical angiographic changes will be seen.[5]

The electroretinogram (ERG) may be normal in the very early stages of the disease.[4] As multiple sites of the retinal pigment epithelium and outer retina become involved, however, a moderate to severe decrease in the ERG may be noted. The b-wave is affected more than the a-wave and in the later stages may be completely extinguished.[14] The ERG is normal in the unaffected eye. The electrooculogram is abnormal in approximately 50% of the patients, particularly in the late phases of the disease.[4] Paracentral and central visual field changes have been described.[6]

Serologic studies, including enzyme-linked immunosorbent assay (ELISA) for *Toxocara canis* and Western blot analysis for *Baylisascaris procyonis* have been performed, but appear to be of limited usefulness in making the diagnosis of DUSN.[5,21] Recently, Goldberg et al[22] reported one patient with DUSN who was seropositive for *Baylisascaris procyonis* infection on Western blot analysis. No serologic test is currently available for *Ancylostoma*.

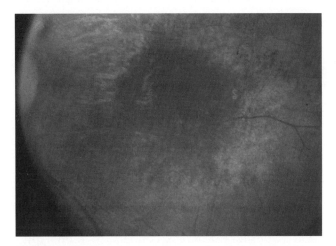

FIGURE 67–4   Chronic late stage of DUSN. Fundus photograph of a young male with a 1-year history of progressive severe decrease in vision in his left eye. A small motile subretinal nematode is visible temporally. A white glistening reflex is evident over the entire posterior pole. Note also the narrowing of the retinal vessels.

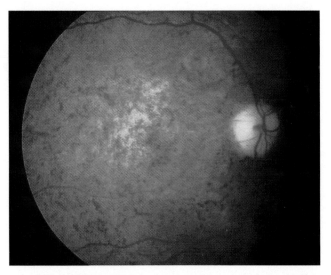

FIGURE 67–5   Chronic stage of DUSN. Clinical photograph of a chronic case of DUSN. Diffuse pigmentary retinal alteration, arteriolar narrowing, and optic nerve pallor are evident.

Analysis of stool for ova and parasites and hematologic evaluation for eosinophilia have been uniformly negative as well.[14]

NATURAL COURSE AND TREATMENT

The natural course of untreated DUSN involves multiple recurrent episodes of diffuse and focal inflammation of the retina and retinal pigment epithelium with secondary progressive visual loss.[1,4,5,14] The recurrent crops of evanescent graywhite lesions fade and then recur, with resultant gradual destruction of the retinal pigment epithelium and outer retina. Subsequent loss of ganglion cells and retinal arteriolar narrowing is associated with optic atrophy and loss of central vision (Fig. 67–5). Patients may exhibit an insidious loss of vision or may present with a more rapid deterioration of vision associated with multiple severe episodes of retinitis and vitritis.[1] Matsumoto et al[23] reported one case of DUSN complicated by an epiretinal membrane and traction retinal detachment. At the time of the surgery the membrane was noted to be transretinal, passing through a full-thickness retinal defect into the subretinal space.

While the use of antihelmintic agents in initial therapeutic trials was unsuccessful,[5] more recent experience by Gass et al[24] suggests that, particularly in those patients with moderately severe vitreous inflammation, thiabendazole may pass the inner retinal barrier and be efficacious in killing the nematode. The recommended dosage for these patients is a regimen of oral thiabendazole, 22 mg/kg twice a day for 2 to 4 successive days. The recommended maximum daily dose is 3 g. The signs of positive response to treatment have been classified into three stages. Six to 8 days after treatment there is fading of the retinitis lesions and appearance of a new, single focus of retinitis (presumably representing the reaction to the dead nematode). At 4 weeks after treatment, decreased vitritis and a focal chorioretinal scar at the site of the nematode is observed. By 6 months after treatment, inactivity and the absence of new lesions should be noted. Because of the gastrointestinal and other potential side effects of thiabendazole, the same authors are planning a trial of irvemectin, a drug with minimal side effects, in patients with DUSN and in whom the nematode is not found.

The use of corticosteroids was initially suggested in treating patient with DUSN. Early temporary improvement with oral corticosteroid administration, however, is followed by recurrence of symptoms and progressive loss of vision.[4] At the present time, photocoagulation of the nematode with laser is the treatment of choice for patients with DUSN. Patients typically show subsequent stabilization or improvement of visual acuity following photocoagulation of the nematode. In fact, direct laser pho-

tocoagulation has been effective in destroying the worm and halting the progression of the disease[5,9,14,17] (Fig. 67–3). No significant intraocular inflammation has been associated with this treatment, although incomplete destruction of the nematode antigens may potentially initiate an inflammatory response. In the only case treated by our group, a mild transient uveitis occurred following photocoagulation of the organism. The nematode in this case was within an exudative detachment of the macula, making it technically difficult to destroy completely. Survival and liberation of the nematode's cell wall antigen was presumed to be the mechanism of postlaser transient uveitis.

As no recovery of visual function has been noticed once severe retinal pigment epithelial or optic nerve changes have occurred, early treatment of the subretinal nematode is recommended in order to prevent these late manifestations of the disease.

DIFFERENTIAL DIAGNOSIS

DUSN may mimic a wide variety of chorioretinal diseases.[14] Any disease manifesting unilateral papillitis, papilledema, retrobulbar neuritis, and/or vitritis should be included in the differential diagnosis. When DUSN patients have an associated perivasculitis with severe perivenous involvement, retinal sarcoidosis should be considered. Outer retinal and retinal pigment epithelial disorders including multifocal choroiditis with panuveitis, AMPPPE, serpiginous choroidopathy, multiple evanescent white dot syndrome, Behçet's disease, toxoplasmosis, ocular histoplasmosis syndrome, and retinitis pigmentosa should be considered. A unilateral optic atrophy secondary to retrobulbar or intracranial lesions should be considered when patients present in the late stages of the disease. While many of these diseases are untreatable, DUSN is a condition in which prompt identification and destruction of the infecting nematode can result in the cessation of symptoms and the preservation of good visual acuity.

REFERENCES

1. Gass JDM, Scelfo R: Diffuse unilateral subacute neuroretinitis. J R Soc Med 71:95–111, 1978.
2. Cunha de Souza E, Lustosa da Cunha S, Gass JDM: Diffuse unilateral subacute neuroretinitis in South America. Arch Ophthalmol 110:1261–1263, 1992.
3. Kuchle M, Knorr HL, Medenblik-Frysch S, et al: Diffuse unilateral neuroretinitis syndrome in a German most likely caused by the racoon roundworm, Baylisascaris procyonis. Graefes Arch Clin Exp Ophthalmol 231:48–51, 1993.
4. Gass JDM, Gilbert WR, Guerry RK, Scelfo R: Diffuse unilateral subacute neuroretinitis. Ophthalmology 85:521–545, 1978.
5. Gass JDM, Braunstein RA: Further observation concerning the diffuse unilateral subacute neuroretinitis syndrome. Arch Ophthalmol 101:1689–1697, 1983.
6. Rubin ML, Kaufman HE, Tierney JP, Lucas HC: An intra-

retinal nematode (a case report). Trans Am Acad Ophthalmol Otolaryngol 72:855–866, 1968.

7. Parsons HE: Nematode chorioretinitis: report of a case with photographs of a viable worm. Arch Ophthalmol 47:799–800, 1952.

8. Price JA, Wadsworth JAC: An intraretinal worm: report of a case of macular retinopathy caused by invasion of the retina by a worm. Arch Ophthalmol 83:768–770, 1970.

9. Raymond LA, Guitierriz Y, Strong LE, et al: Living retinal nematode (filarial-like) destroyed with photocoagulation. Ophthalmology 85:944–949, 1978.

10. Kazacos KR, Vestre WA, Kazakos EA, Raymond LA: Diffuse unilateral neuroretinitis syndrome: probable cause. Arch Ophthalmol 102:967–968, 1984.

11. Kazakos KR, Raymond LA, Kazakos EA, Vestre WA: The racoon ascarid: a probable cause of human ocular larval migraines. Ophthalmology 92:1735–1744, 1985.

12. Huff DS, Neafie RC, Binder MJ, et al: The first fatal Baylisascaris infection in humans: an infant with eosinophilic meningoencephalitis. Pediatr Pathol 2:345–352, 1984.

13. Fox AS, Kazakos KR, Gould NS, et al: Fatal eosinophilic meningoencephalitis and visceral larval migranes caused by the racoon ascarid Baylisascaris procyonis. N Engl J Med 312:1619–1623, 1985.

14. Gass JDM: Stereoscopic Atlas of Macular Disease: Diagnosis and Treatment, 3rd edition. CV Mosby Co, St Louis, 1983, pp 470–479, 510–511.

15. Maguire AM, Zarbin MA, Conner TB, Justin J: Ocular penetration of thiabendazole. Arch Ophthalmol 108:1675, 1990.

16. Cunha de Souza E, Nakashima Y: Diffuse unilateral subacute neuroretinitis. Report of transvitreal surgical removal of a subretinal nematode. Ophthalmology 102:1183–1186, 1995.

17. Williams GA, Aaberg TM, Dudley SS: Perimacular photocoagulation of presumed Baylisascaris procyonis in diffuse unilateral subacute neuroretinitis. In Gitter K, Schatz H, Yannuzzi LA (eds): Laser Photocoagulation of Retinal Diseases. San Francisco, Pacific University Press, 1988.

18. Rockey JH, Donnelly JJ, Stromberg BE, Soulsby EJL: Immunopathology of Toxocara canis and Ascaris suum infections of the eye: the role of the eosinophil. Invest Ophthalmol Vis Sci 18:1172–1184, 1979.

19. Hamann KJ, Kephart GM, Kazakos KR, Gleich GJ: Immunofluorescent localization of eosinophil granule major basic protein in fatal human cases of Baylisascaris procyonis infection. Am J Trop Med Hyg 40:291–297, 1989.

20. Gass JDM, Olsen KR: Diffuse unilateral subacute neuroretinitis. In Ryan S, Lewis HL (eds): Retina, 2nd edition. St Louis, CV Mosby Co, 1993, pp 1643–1649.

21. Brown DH: Ocular Toxocara canis. Part II. Clinical Review. J Pediatr Ophthalmol 7:182–191, 1970.

22. Goldberg MA, Kazakos KR, Boyce WM, et al: Diffuse unilateral subacute neuroretinitis: morphometric, serologic, and epidemiologic support for Baylisascaris as a causative agent. Ophthalmology 100:1695–1701, 1993.

23. Matsumoto BT, Adelberg DA, Del Priore LV: Transretinal membrane formation in diffuse unilateral subacute neuroretinitis. Retina 15:146–149, 1995.

24. Gass JDM, Callanan DG, Bowman CB: Oral therapy in diffuse unilateral subacute neuroretinitis. Arch Ophthalmol 110:675–680, 1992.

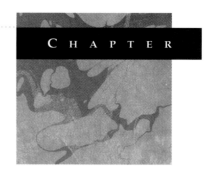

CHAPTER 68

Myiasis

Antonio P. Ciardella, M.D.

David R. Guyer, M.D.

Lawrence A. Yannuzzi, M.D.

OPHTHALMOMYIASIS

Myiasis is the invasion of living vertebrates by larvae of certain Diptera. It can be classified according to the site of larval invasion. Ocular involvement may be external to the globe (ophthalmomyiasis externa) or within the globe (ophthalmomyiasis interna). Intraocular invasion of the posterior segment (ophthalmomyiasis interna posterior) by the larval forms of some flies that belong to the order Diptera is uncommon, rarer still is the finding of a larva suspended within the vitreous. The larvae responsible for human infestation are usually obligatory parasites; that is, they need to live in the host tissue to complete their vital cycle.

The fly associated with internal ophthalmomyiasis has been identified as the parasite fly of rodents, *Cuterebra*.[1,2] The usual hosts for these parasites include rabbits, rats, squirrels, field mice, and chipmunks.

The eggs or the larval form of the fly are deposited on human corneal or conjunctival surface by an adult fly, by another vector such as a mosquito, or by the patient's hands. Once on the external surface of the eye, the larva is able to pass through the sclera and to reach the anterior chamber, the vitreous (Fig. 68–1), and the subretinal space (Figs. 68–2 and 68–3),[3–10] sometimes causing a subconjunctival hemorrhage at the site of entrance.[1] This larva is usually white or semitranslucent, segmented, and tapered at both ends. In the subretinal space, the larva is able to grow from an initial length of 1 mm to an average of 3 to 5 mm before dying, or in some cases as much as 15 mm; the oxygen tension under the retina can in fact support the life of the organism for awhile.[1] Instead, when the larva enters the vitreous, it usually dies due to an ab-sence of nutrients. The death of the larva is followed by an inflammatory response that may vary from a local vitritis to an intense endophthalmitis.

After entering the subretinal space, the larva migrates in a random manner around the entire fundus leaving crisscrossing atrophic tracks in the retinal pigment epithelium (RPE), and pigmented lumps, which are considered pathognomonic of posterior internal ophthalmomyiasis.[2–4] These are more clearly visible on fluorescein angiography study (Figs. 68–2 and 68–3). The nature of the pigmented clumps remains unknown, but they may represent reactive hyperplasia of RPE cells at sites of subretinal hemorrhages, or possibly mark sites of penetration through the choroid. Alternatively, they may result from damage to the RPE due to the movement, feeding, or toxins produced by the maggot, or by a combination of these factors.[1]

Clinical manifestations secondary to the intraocular invasion of the larva may vary widely. The eye may remain largely asymptomatic,[3,5,6] or symptoms may be confined to those of mild uveitis or vitritis.[2,7] More severe cases may be complicated by subretinal (Fig. 68–2) or vitreous hemorrhage,[8] retinal detachment,[8,9] and optic atrophy.[9] There also may be intermittent or persistent ocular pain,[2] conjunctivitis,[7] and periorbital edema.[7] Only rarely are both eyes affected. In more favorable cases the maggot may leave the eye without causing any symptoms, despite the diffuse damage to the RPE.

The presence of diffuse alteration of the RPE with numerous, confluent, linear, and arcuate atrophic tracks should always suggest the possibility of ophthalmomyiasis. Fluorescein angiography better reveals the peculiar pattern of the RPE tracks.

Other organisms may migrate and move around in the subretinal space, such as the nematode re-

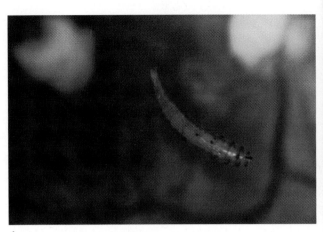
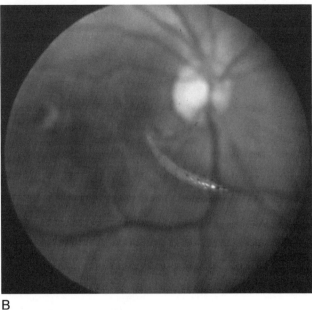

A   B

FIGURE 68–1   Ophthalmomyiasis. *A*, fly larva was noted in the vitreous cavity in this patient. *B*, One year later the larva appeared stable. (Courtesy of Kenneth G. Julian, C.R.A., F.O.P.S. From Yannuzzi LA, Guyer DR, Green WR: The Retina Atlas. St Louis, Mosby Year-Book, 1995, pp 584–598, with permission.)

sponsible for diffuse unilateral subacute neuroretinitis (DUSN), the *Alaria mesocercaria* trematode and other worms; however, none of them are capable of producing such a widespread pattern of atrophic tracks in the RPE. A white linear or arcuate atrophic track may also be found in the equator area both in multifocal chorioretinitis and in presumed ocular histoplasmosis syndrome (POHS). The definitive clinical diagnosis of ophthalmomyiasis can only be made with the identification of the organism in the subretinal space.

In the presence of active intraocular inflammation, the treatment of choice is corticosteroid therapy, via either systemic or local administration. If inflammation cannot be controlled, surgical removal of the larva is indicated. When there is no active inflammation and the maggot is identified under the retina, the ophthalmologist may choose careful follow-up or may destroy the maggot. Laser photocoagulation of the subretinal maggot is the treatment of choice. If the larva is located in the vitreous it may be removed by pars plana vitrectomy. The destruction of the larva usually does not induce an inflammatory response.[3,10]

INTRAOCULAR GNATHOSTOMIASIS

Gnathostomiasis is a disease caused by the migration and metabolites of larvae of the gnathostoma species.[11–13] Gnathostoma is classified as a Nematoda; subclass Secernentea. Nematodae are elongated, cylindrical, unsegmented worms.[12] *Gnathostoma* is characterized by a distinct head bulb, which

is covered by four rows of hooks (Fig. 68–4); the third-stage larva is about 4 to 6 mm long, and 0.5 mm wide[12] (Figs. 68–4 through 68–7). Although several species of *Gnathostoma* have been reported,[11] most human infection is due to *Gnathostoma spinigerum. Gnathostoma spinigerum* was first found to be responsible for human infection by Levinsen[14] in 1890 in the breast abscess of a woman living in what is now Thailand. The disease is prevalent in Southeast Asia, Indonesia, the Philippines, China, and Japan.[15]

The life cycle of the organism is quite complex. During the three larval stages, the parasite lives first in freshwater, then successively in two intermediate hosts. The first intermediate host is the *Cyclops*, a genus of minute crustacean, in which the second-stage larvae develop. Cold-blooded vertebrates, such as freshwater fish and frogs, ingest the infected *Cyclops* and become the second intermediate host. The common definitive host of *G. spinigerum* include wild and domestic felines and dogs, which become infected by ingestion of a second intermediate host. *G. spinigerum* reaches maturity in definitive hosts, located in the walls of their stomach, and pass eggs in the feces. Eggs develop and hatch about 1 week after entering fresh water. Free-swimming, first-stage larvae emerge and die unless ingested by one of several species of *Cyclops* within 2 or 3 days, and the life cycle is completed.[11–13]

Humans are unusual hosts for *Gnathostoma*. Generally, they become infected by eating a second intermediate host. The third-stage larvae can migrate in human tissues, but they cannot reach maturity. For this reason, humans are not considered to be infective even when harboring worms. The most

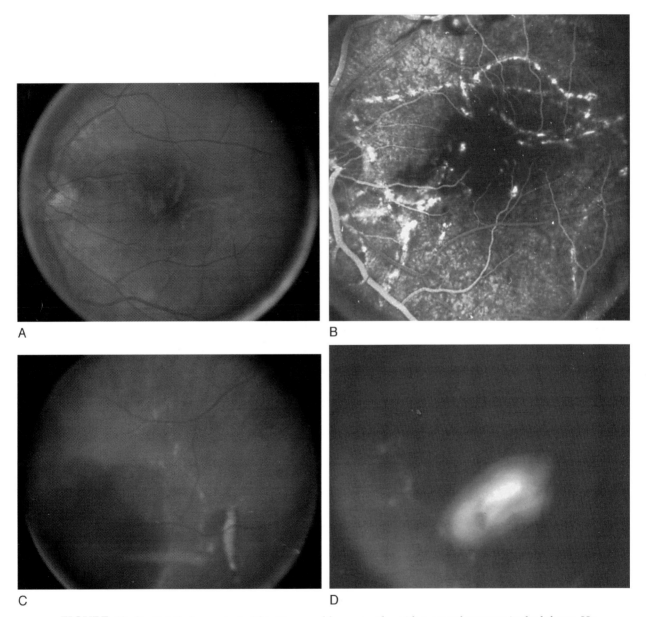

A

B

C

D

FIGURE 68–2 Ophthalmomyiasis. This 21-year-old man awoke with a central scotoma in the left eye. He had just completed an around-the-world cruise, including a stop in Ceylon, where he went deer hunting. *A*, Fundus examination of the posterior pole reveals macular hemorrhage, retinal edema, and yellowish tracks, which represent linear atrophy of the pigment epithelium. *B*, Fluorescein study of the same patient better delineates numerous atrophic tracks at the posterior pole, but no leak was present in the macular area. *C*, Clinical photograph of the inferonasal fundus. The worm was located near a patch of subretinal hemorrhage. Note the presence of atrophic tracks between the worm and the hemorrhage. *D*, Direct laser photocoagulation resulted in death of the organism. (From Fritzgerald CR, Rubin ML: Intraocular parasite destroyed by laser photocoagulation: a case report. Arch Ophthalmol 91:162–164, 1974. Copyright 1974, American Medical Association, with permission.)

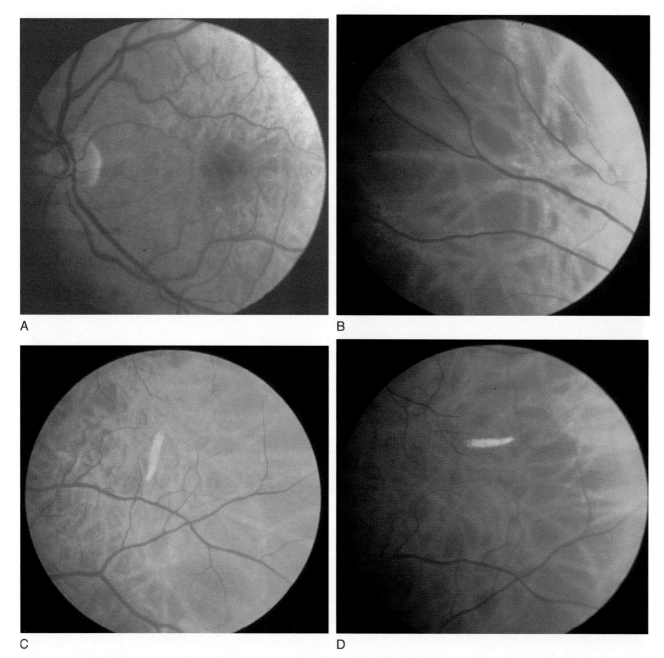

A

B

C

D

FIGURE 68–3   Ophthalmomyiasis. Atrophic tracks are noted in this patient at the posterior pole (A), and in the periphery (B). A motile maggot can be demonstrated in the midperiphery (C). It was able to move towards the fovea in a few minutes (D). Fluorescein study of the same patient shows the unusual pattern of cross-hatched or "railroad" tracks in the RPE (E and F). (Courtesy of Dr. Miriam Ridley. From Yannuzzi LA, Guyer DR, Green WR: The Retina Atlas. St Louis, Mosby Year-Book, 1995, pp 584–598, with permission.)
Illustration continued on opposite page

common sites of infection in humans are the skin and mucous membranes. Particularly worrisome is the involvement of the central nervous system, because of the potential fatal prognosis in such cases.[16]

Ocular gnathostomiasis is a rare condition. Sen and Ghose[17] described the first case of ocular involvement in 1945, and since then, no more than a dozen well-documented cases have been reported,[17–25] three of which are from the United States.[22,23,25]

The route by which the worm gains access to the eye is not clear. It has been postulated that *G. spinigerum* may gain access to the eye through the retina and choroid, causing subretinal hemorrhages,[22] retinal scars,[17,21] and tears.[22] The worm has been found alive in all reported cases[17–25]: in eight patients in the anterior chamber[17–22,24] (Fig. 68–5), and in two in the vitreous[23,25] (Figs. 68–4, 68–6, and 68–7). Symptoms may vary from the subjective perception of an actively moving filament in the visual field,[25] to a severe uveitis with signs of inflamma-

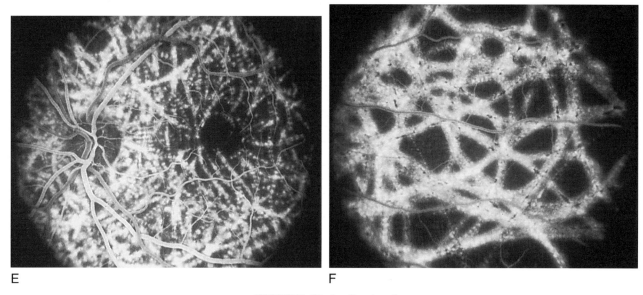

E   F

FIGURE 68–3 *Continued*

tion in both the anterior and posterior segment: marked conjunctival hyperemia and ciliary flush, hypopyon in the anterior chamber, keratic precipitates, vitritis, periphlebitis, retinal exudates, and inflammation of the optic nerve.[21] At the site of penetration of the organism in the eye, a subretinal hemorrhage,[22] a retinal scar,[17,21] or tear[22] may be noted.

In attempting to make a diagnosis, the direct visualization of the motile organism within the eye is necessary. A complete blood count with differential determination may be in the normal range or show an eosinophilia.[22,25] A systemic examination to search for other larvae seems unnecessary in the absence of specific symptoms. Generally, gnathostomiasis is associated with only one larva, and since the organisms do not reproduce in humans, stool for parasitic examination is negative.[25] In cases with associated central nervous system involvement, neurologic signs are usually present. In these cases computed tomography or magnetic resonance imaging may reveal evidence of hemorrhages.

Differential diagnosis includes any other form of uveitis involving both the anterior and posterior segments, particularly when the inflammation is related to the intraocular invasion by other living worms.

At the moment there is no effective medical therapy for ocular gnathostomiasis in humans. The definitive treatment for intraocular gnathostomiasis remains surgical removal of the worm.[25] It is preferable to remove the entire worm with a suction device, rather than crushing it with forceps or with a vitreous cutter, since microscopic fragments of the larva left in the eye could induce an inflammatory response.

The final prognosis is generally favorable, with definitive remission of the inflammation and complete recovery of visual acuity. However, two cases have been complicated by retinal detachment.[22,23]

INTRAOCULAR ANGIOSTRONGYLIASIS

Angiostrongylus cantonensis is the most common cause of eosinophilic meningitis in Southeast Asia.[26,27] Adult worms live in the small pulmonary arterioles of rats, where ova hatch to the first-stage larva; then the larvae migrate to the bronchi and esophagus, and pass in the feces. Snails, slugs, and crustaceans are intermediate hosts. When rats eat these organisms, third-stage infective larvae enter their circulation and infect the heart, lungs, brain, and spinal cord. Then, larvae migrate out of the vessels to infect the nervous tissue, develop into the fourth- and fifth-stage larva in the brain, and enter the venous circulation again. Then they return to the heart, and mature to an adult worm in the rat's pulmonary arteries.[26,27] Humans are facultative hosts; the route of infection is by eating raw food, such as *Pila* snails, African snails, fish, and crustaceans. In addition, contaminated vegetables or water may be sources of human infection, in which larvae migrate through the circulation to the brain, subarachnoid space, and eye.[26–28] The fifth-stage larva is about 10 to 25 mm long, and 0.2 to 0.3 mm wide.

The possible routes of ocular and orbital invasion are as follows[27]:

1. During the earlier stage of arterial migration, some of the small third-stage larvae may enter the arteries that go to the eye, rather than to the brain, and develop into fourth- and fifth-stage larvae in the anterior chamber.
2. After developing to the fifth stage in brain tis-

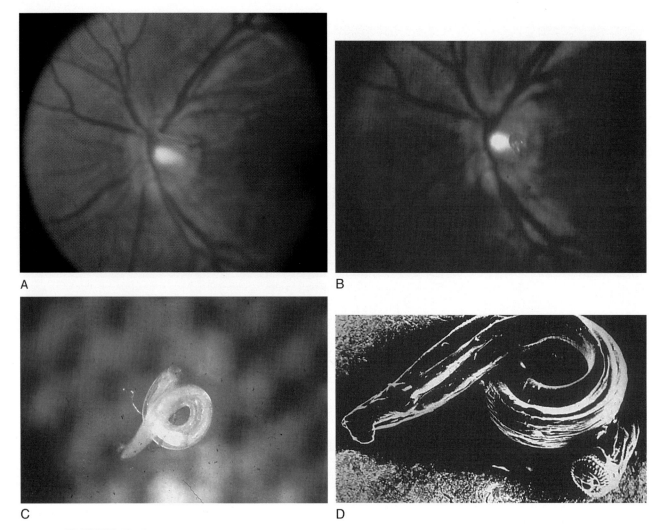

FIGURE 68–4 Gnathostomiasis. A 29-year-old woman complained of an actively moving filament in her central field of vision in the left eye. The patient was born and raised in Lebanon, but had moved to the United States 3 years earlier. She had also traveled to Africa and Mexico 4 years and 2 months, respectively, before the onset of the visual symptoms. She denied any associated systemic complaints. *A* and *B*, Clinical photograph of the left eye shows the living worm in the vitreous chamber, over the disc. The worm is extended (*A*), and coiled (*B*). *C*, The worm was alive after removal from the eye, and moved slowly in a saline solution. It measured approximately 1.5 mm in length, and had a knob-like structure at the cephalic end. *D*, Scanning electron microscopic study of the *G. spinigerum* with a segmented head bulb (*bottom right*).
Illustration continued on opposite page

sue, the larvae may enter the retinal arteries, or the vortex veins, and migrate to the eye.

3. Fifth-stage larvae may migrate along the surface of the brain, traverse the optic nerve, migrate between the optic nerve itself and the nerve sheath, and enter the eye through the cribriform plate.

In a large review of 484 cases of eosinophilic meningitis most likely caused by *A. cantonensis*, unilateral optic disc swelling, probably due to a secondary optic neuritis, was noted in 12% of cases.[26] It was believed to be caused by injury to the optic nerve during the migration of the worm.

In the literature there are several reports of intraocular invasion by *A. cantonensis*: it has been found in the anterior chamber[29–31] (Fig. 68–8), vitreous chamber[27] (Fig. 68–9), and subretinal space[28] (Fig. 68–10).

Clinical manifestations of eosinophilic meningitis caused by angiostrongyliasis include headache, meningitis, nausea, vomiting, paresthesia, cranial nerve palsies, seizures, paralysis, and lethargy.[26]

Ocular manifestations include exophthalmus, lid swelling, inflammation of the anterior and posterior segments, decreased vision, and subjective perception of a moving object in the visual field.[27]

Corticosteroid treatment may be useful in controlling the inflammation, but identification and removal of the worm are always necessary for definitive treatment. When the worm is located in the anterior chamber, it can be easily removed through

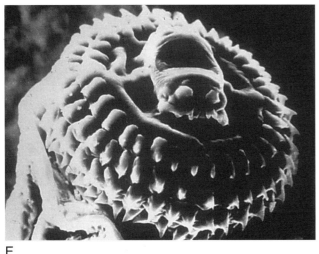
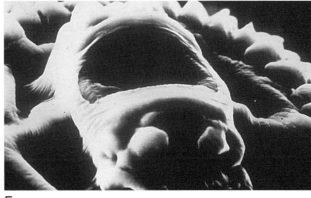

E   F

FIGURE 68–4   *Continued*   *E*, Higher power view of the head bulb, with four rows of hooklets. The mouth is located at the center of the head bulb and has two lips with sensory papillae. *F*, Higher power view of the mouth and lips of the parasite. Each lip has a pair of sensory papillae. (From Funata M, Custis P, De La Cruz Z, et al: Intraocular gnathostomiasis. Retina 13: 240–244, 1993, with permission.)

a limbal incision.[29–31] If it is located in the vitreous space, 12 hours of prone positioning of the patient may be sufficient to induce gravitation of the worm into the anterior chamber.[27] If it is in the subretinal space, it is usually necessary to remove the worm through a sclerotomy,[28] or to perform a pars plana vitrectomy and a retinotomy to reach the subretinal space.

INTRAOCULAR ASCARIDIOSIS

Porrocaecum and *Hexameter* are roundworms that belong to genera of the class Nematoda, in the subfamily Ascaridinae. The adult worm is found in the stomach or intestine of carnivorous reptiles, birds,

and mammals. It produces thick-shelled eggs that are unembryonated when passed in the feces. The eggs in soil or water develop a larval stage that is infective when digested by an intermediate host, such as a shrew, mouse, mole, gopher, or rat. After development in the tissues of the intermediate host, the larva infects the final host. Mature larvae have thick lateral cords, paired excretory glands, an expansive intestine with large granular cells, and numerous tall celomyarian somatic muscles (Fig. 68–11). The larvae are about 9 mm long and 0.5 mm wide.

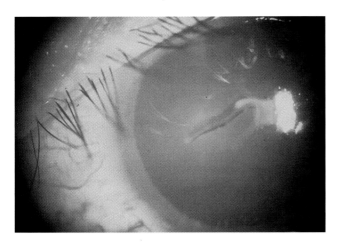
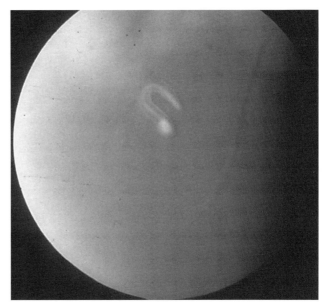

FIGURE 68–5   Gnathostomiasis. *Gnathostoma spinigerum* in the anterior chamber. (Courtesy of Dr. Prut Hanutsaha. From Yannuzzi LA, Guyer DR, Green WR: The Retina Atlas. St Louis, Mosby Year-Book, 1995, pp 584–598, with permission.)

FIGURE 68–6   Gnathostomiasis. *Gnathostoma spinigerum* in the vitreous, over the retina. (Courtesy of Dr. Prut Hanutsaha. From Yannuzzi LA, Guyer DR, Green WR: The Retina Atlas. St Louis, Mosby Year-Book, 1995, pp 584–598, with permission.)

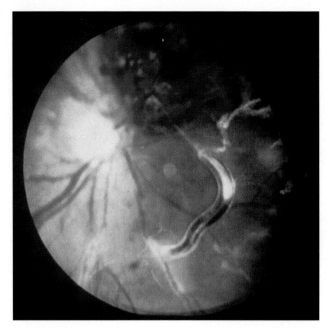

FIGURE 68–7 Gnathostomiasis. Another case of intravitreal gnathostomiasis shows the worm, blood, and waste material. (Courtesy of Dr. Charles Mango. From Yannuzzi LA, Guyer DR, Green WR: The Retina Atlas. St Louis, Mosby Year-Book, 1995, pp 584–598, with permission.)

Humans are unusual hosts, and may become infected by eating raw food or drinking water contaminated with the egg-bearing feces of a carnivorous final host.[32]

In the literature there is only one case of intraocular infection with a large worm belonging to either the *Porrocaecum* or *Hexametra* species.[32] In this case the worm was removed from the eye through a pars plana vitrectomy and retinotomy (Fig. 68–11).

OCULAR ONCHOCERCIASIS

The microfilaria *Onchocerca volvulus* is responsible for endemic human infection in some areas of central Africa. Microfilariae are usually found in high number in the skin and eye of infected individuals. A mean of 120 microfilariae per milligram of skin of the buttock was found in a group of 140 patients from the Sudan savanna.[33] In the same study microfilariae were seen in the cornea, anterior chamber, and vitreous, respectively, in 95.75, 85.7, and 33.6% of the patients. Microfilariae have also been found in the retina, both in living subjects[34] and in histopathologic studies[35-38] of patients with onchocerciasis.

Hissette[39] (1932), Bryant[40] (1935), and Ridley[41] (1945) first described ocular fundus changes in central Africa, which consisted of atrophy of the retinal pigment epithelium and choroid, and they suggested that there was an association between these lesions and infection with *O. volvulus*. Subse-

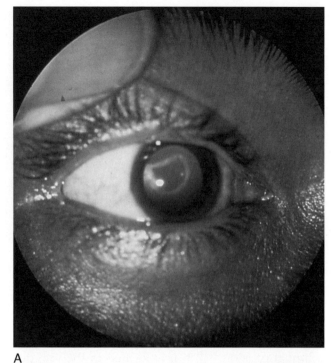

A

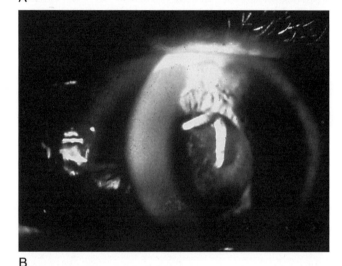

B

FIGURE 68–8 Ocular Angiostrongyliasis. *A* and *B*, These two cases revealed *A. cantonensis* in the anterior chamber. (Courtesy of Prut Hanutsaha, M.D.)

quently, other epidemiologic studies[33,42] supported the association between microfilariae infection and atrophic fundus changes. Optic neuritis and optic atrophy were also found in some patients with onchocerciasis.[33]

Clinically this syndrome simulates tapetoretinal dystrophy. Patients complain of visual field loss and poor night vision. Fundus examination reveals the presence of diffuse atrophy of the retinal pigment epithelium and choriocapillaris, together with isolated clumps of hyperpigmentation. These lesions are more frequently seen at the posterior pole (Figs. 68–12, and 68–13) and temporal to the fovea, but in more advanced cases they may involve the

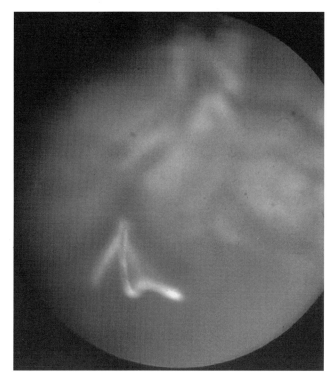

FIGURE 68–9 Ocular Angiostrongyliasis. *A. cantonensis* is seen floating in the vitreous space, over the optic nerve head. (Courtesy of Prut Hanutsaha, M.D.)

entire fundus (Fig. 68–14). Other observed lesions include (1) well-defined areas of subretinal fibrosis with widespread atrophy of the retinal pigment epithelium and choroid, (2) hyperpigmentation of the retinal pigment epithelium that may be widespread and that may simulate the appearance of a pigmentary retinopathy (pseudoretinitis pigmentosa),

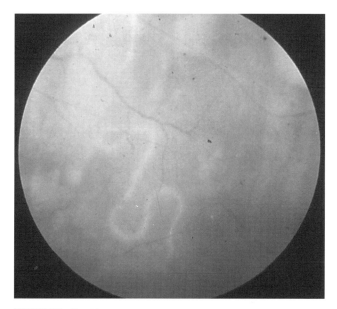

FIGURE 68–10 Ocular angiostrongyliasis. *A. cantonensis* appears as an actively mobile, white roundworm, under the retinal vessels. (Courtesy of Prut Hanutsaha, M.D.)

(3) pale ill-defined choroidal lesions that are probably choroidal granulomas, (4) severe uveitis with cell reaction in the anterior and vitreous chamber and secondary cystoid macular edema, (5) peripapillary chorioretinal atrophy or hyperpigmentation, and (6) optic nerve atrophy (Fig. 68–12) and optic nerve swelling.

Fluorescein angiography is useful to better delineate the extension of areas of retinal pigment epithelium and choriocapillaris atrophy, dilatation of the superficial capillaries of the optic disc and peripapillary retina, leakage of dye from the inflamed optic nerve, and localized areas of periphlebitis in some cases of marked intraocular inflammation.

The mechanism of ocular damage in patients with onchocerciasis is not yet completely understood. The fact that microfilariae have been found in the retina and choroid of eyes with diffuse fundus alterations (Fig. 68–15) is not sufficient to establish a direct relationship between onchocerciasis and ocular disease. However, there is strong epidemiologic evidence that *O. volvulus* is responsible for severe chorioretinal and optic nerve atrophy, at least in areas where onchocerciasis is endemic.[33]

Given the peculiar appearance of the fundus, and the subjective symptoms of visual field loss and night blindness, this syndrome must be differentiated from retinitis pigmentosa and hypovitaminosis A. This last condition must always be excluded in patients with night blindness and atrophic fundus changes, since it may be endemic in the same geographic areas where onchocerciasis is present, and it is treated with adequate dietary supplementation.

Microfilaricide drugs used in the treatment of patients infected with *O. volvulus* include diethylcarbamazine citrate (DEC-C) and suramin.[43] However, both of these drugs cause severe systemic reactions and ocular side effects such as an increase in the area of chorioretinal atrophy, optic disc inflammation, and visual field loss.

ALARIA MESOCERCARIA

Alaria species are diplostomatid trematodes that live as adults in the small intestine of carnivorous mammals. Their life cycle involves a succession of three hosts: the first intermediate host is a snail, the second intermediate one is a tadpole or frog, and the third and definitive host is a carnivore.[44,45] An unencysted, migratory larva, the mesocercarida, develops in the frog, and is infective to the carnivore upon ingestion.

Some animals, such as bullfrogs, snakes, alligators, birds, and mammals (including rodents, raccoons, and opossums), are paratenic or transport hosts; that is, they become infected with mesocercariae by ingesting these larvae in infected tadpoles or frogs. Then the mesocercariae reinvade the

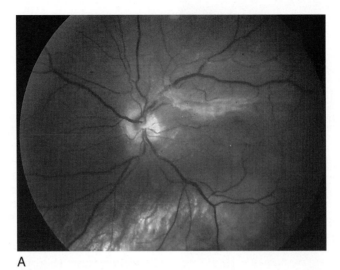

A

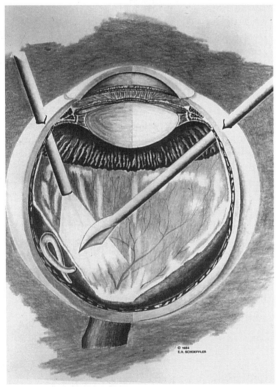

B

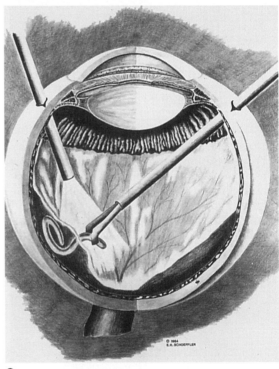

C

FIGURE 68–11 A 27-year-old white American man presented complaining of a 3-week history of decreased vision in his left eye. Visual acuity in the left eye was light perception. Slit lamp examination of the left eye demonstrated 2+ flare and cells in the anterior chamber, and 4+ white cells in the posterior vitreous. There was a total retinal detachment as well. The right eye was normal. It was thought that a retinal hole must be the causative agent and the patient was taken to the operating room, where drainage of the subretinal fluid was accomplished to improve visualization. At that time ophthalmoscopic examination revealed a large white, round, subretinal band, that extended from the ora to the optic nerve and caused a tenting of the retina. Stimulated by the light, the strand began to move and a subretinal worm was recognized. It was decided to freeze the worm with a cryoprobe, and to perform a pars plana vitrectomy and remove the worm through a retinotomy. After the operation the patient's vitreous remained clear and his retina was attached, but he subsequently developed a macular pucker, which required a second vitrectomy with membrane peeling. After the surgery his visual acuity improved to 20/80. Histologic studies of the worm were performed. *A*, This clinical photograph shows the white subretinal worm inferior to the optic nerve. The nematode is curled on itself at each end. *B* and *C*, Drawing of the nematode being removed from the subretinal space. A retinotomy was created to reach the subretinal space (*B*), and the nematode was grasped with vitreous forceps (*C*). *Illustration continued on opposite page*

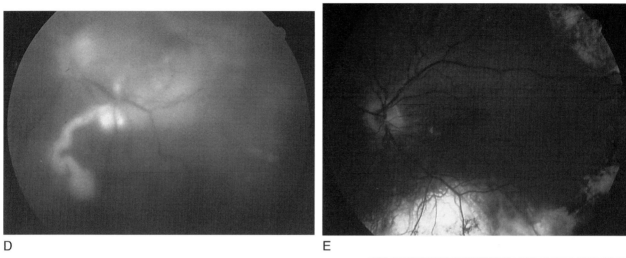

D

E

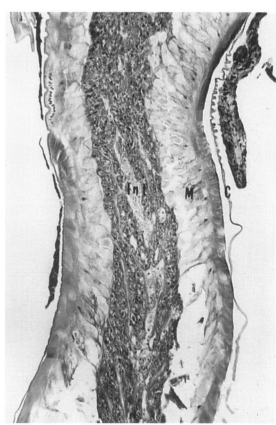

F

FIGURE 68–11 *Continued   D*, Clinical photograph after removal of the subretinal worm. There was chorioretinal scarring inferiorly and a macular pucker. *E*, Fundus photograph after removal of preretinal membrane showing a smooth macular area. *F*, Frontal section of the larva showing intestine (Int), somatic muscles (M), and cuticle (C). *Illustration continued on following page*

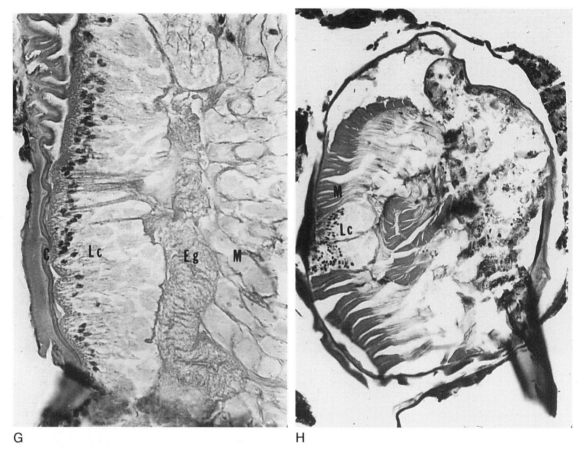

G   H

FIGURE 68–11 *Continued* *G*, Frontal section of larva showing cuticle (C), lateral chord (Lc), excretory gland (Eg), and somatic muscles (M). *H*, Transverse section of the larva showing somatic muscle (M) and lateral chord (Lc). (From Goodart RA, Riekhof FT, Beaver PC: Subretinal nematode. An unusual etiology for uveitis and retinal detachment. Retina 5:87–90, 1985, with permission.)

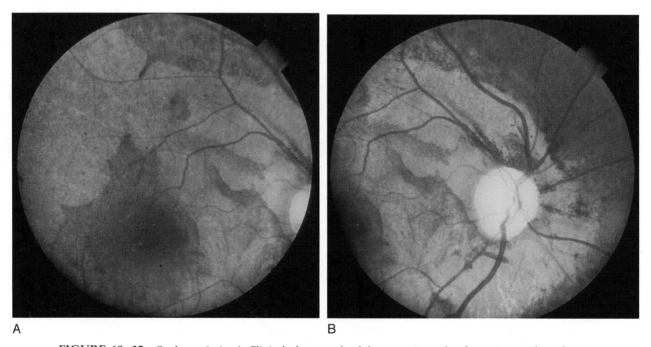

A   B

FIGURE 68–12 Onchocerciasis. *A*, Clinical photograph of the posterior pole of a patient with onchocerciasis. There is extensive chorioretinal atrophy. *B*, Clinical photograph of the optic nerve of the same patient reveals optic atrophy and vascular attenuation. (Courtesy of Dr. Robert Murphy. From Yannuzzi LA, Guyer DR, Green WR: The Retina Atlas. St Louis, Mosby Year-Book, 1995, pp 584–598, with permission.)

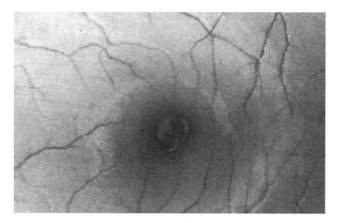

FIGURE 68–13 Onchocerciasis. High-magnification clinical photograph demonstrates the presence of atrophic changes of the macula in a patient with onchocerciasis. (Courtesy of Dr. Robert Murphy. From Yannuzzi LA, Guyer DR, Green WR: The Retina Atlas. St Louis, Mosby Year-Book, 1995, pp 584–598, with permission.)

somatic tissues, and remain as mesocercariae, which are capable of new infection.[44–50]

Humans become infected by eating intermediate or paratenic hosts containing mesocercariae. The most common route of human infection is by eating inadequately cooked frogs' legs, with subsequent migration of the mesocercariae to various internal tissues, including the eye.[44,47,49] Another possibility is via the direct penetration of the mesocercaria into the eye, once it has been accidentally transferred to the conjunctiva by a patient who is handling raw frogs' legs. This route is supported by experimental evidence of direct entrance of mesocercaria in the rabbit eye.[49]

Alaria species identified in North America include *A. americana*, *A. marcianae*, and *A. arisaemoides*, occurring primarily in canids and felids, and *A. mustelae* in mustelids.[44,45,50] *A. mesocercaria* measures about 500 μm long and 200 μm wide; its shape is typical of a trematode (tapered anteriorly, and wider and rounded posteriorly); and it moves by retracting and rounding up, extending, and bending.

There have been five published cases of human infection with *A. mesocercaria*.[47–49,51,52] Shea et al[47] reported a 29-year-old woman from Ontario who probably became infected by direct penetration of the mesocercaria into the eye after accidental transfer to the conjunctiva while the patient was handling and preparing raw frogs' legs for cooking. Beaver et al[48] reported a skin infection of a man in Louisiana. Freeman et al[49,51] reported a case of a fatal human infection in a 24-year-old man from Ontario. In this case, autopsy revealed several thousand mesocercariae in the patients viscera. A large bullfrog captured near his farm had about 4000 mesocercariae, the majority of which were in the musculature of the hindlegs, which is the preferred site for concentration of these larvae in frogs.[49] McDonald et al[52] reported two cases of ocular infection in two Asian men from the San Francisco area. For both of these patients the probable source of infection was ingestion of undercooked frogs' legs containing *A. mesocercaria* in local restaurants. Byers and Kimura[53] reported a case of uveitis after the death of an unidentified larva (probably *A. me-*

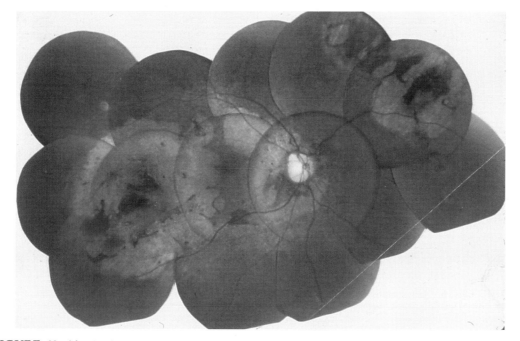

FIGURE 68–14 Onchocerciasis. Extensive chorioretinal atrophy is noted throughout the fundus in this patient. (Courtesy of Dr. Robert Murphy. From Yannuzzi LA, Guyer DR, Green WR: The Retina Atlas. St Louis, Mosby Year-Book, 1995, pp 584–598, with permission.)

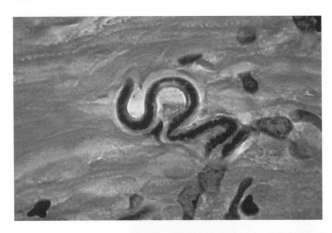

FIGURE 68–15 Onchocerciasis. Histopathologic examination of another case reveals the microfilaria. (Courtesy of Dr. Robert Murphy. From Yannuzzi LA, Guyer DR, Green WR: The Retina Atlas. St. Louis, Mosby Year-Book, 1995, pp 584–598, with permission.)

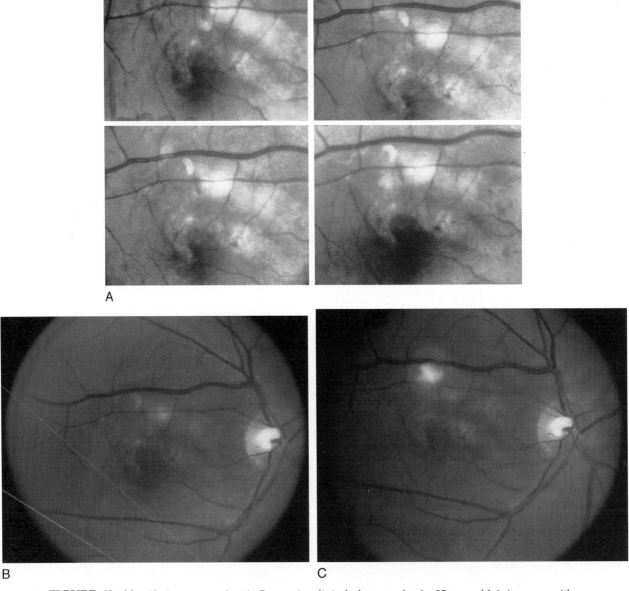

FIGURE 68–16 *Alaria mesocercariae.* *A,* Composite clinical photograph of a 35-year-old Asian man with a 3-year history of decreased vision in his right eye. This patient had a subretinal worm, which was able to migrate into the subretinal space, and to change shape and position (*arrowheads*). *B,* Wider field color photograph of the same patient shows the subretinal *A. mesocercaria* (*arrowhead*), pigment epithelial scarring, and retinitis in the superior macula. *C,* Clinical photograph of the same patient after successful photocoagulation of the worm. (Courtesy of Dr. H. Richard McDonald. From McDonald HR, Kazacos KR, Schatx H, Johnson RN: Two cases of intraocular infection with *Alaria mesocercariae* [Trematodes]. Am J Ophthalmol 117:447, 1994, with permission.)

socercaria) in the vitreous cavity of a 17-year-old boy from San Francisco.

Intraocular infection by *A. mesocercaria* usually resembles a chronic posterior uveitis. Patients complain of a long-lasting, sometimes intermittent decrease in vision, visual field defects, and floaters. Fundus examination may reveal signs of vasculitis, multiple foci of gray-white outer retinitis, pigmentary retinal changes, papillitis, intraretinal hemorrhages, and later optic atrophy. When the mesocercaria is present in the vitreous cavity, it may cause vitreous inflammation and secondary cystoid macular edema. Fundus examination may reveal a small white-yellow circular or ovoid mass under the retina, which moves by retracting and extending (Fig. 68–16).

Systemic or periocular injections of corticosteroids are beneficial in decreasing intraocular inflammation. Thiabendazole has proven to be of some utility against intraocular nematodes,[53,54] but has no activity against trematodes. Once the subretinal worm has been identified, direct laser photocoagulation of the worm is the treatment of choice, if it is located away from the macula[3,10,47,52,55–59] (Fig. 68–16). Vitrectomy to remove subretinal or intravitreal worms has also been reported to be an effective treatment.[1,32,52,60–63]

The differential diagnosis includes other forms of intraocular larva migrans, such as diffuse unilateral subacute neuroretinitis; myiasis; gnathostomiasis; onchocerciasis; and other causes of posterior chronic uveitis including syphilis, tuberculosis, sarcoidosis, Behçet's disease, and Lyme disease. The identification of the larva of *A. mesocercaria* is necessary for definitive diagnosis.

REFERENCES

1. Custis PH, Pakalnis WA, Klintworth GK, et al: Posterior internal ophthalmomyiasis, identification of a surgically removed cuterebra larva by scanning electron microscopy. Ophthalmology 90:1583, 1983.
2. Dixon JM, Winkler CH, Nelson JH: Ophthalmomyiasis interna caused by the cuterebra larva. Trans Am Ophthalmol Soc 67:110, 1969.
3. Fritzgerald CR, Rubin ML: Intraocular parasite destroyed by photocoagulation. Arch Ophthalmol 91:162, 1974.
4. Gass JDM, Lewis RA: Subretinal tracks in ophthalmomyiasis. Arch Ophthalmol 94:1500, 1976.
5. Slusher M, Holland W, Weaver R, et al: Ophthalmomyasis interna posterior, subretinal tracks and intraocular larvae. Arch Ophthalmol 97:885, 1979.
6. Steahly L, Peterson C: Ophthalmomyiasis. Ann Ophthalmol 14:137, 1982.
7. O'Brien CS, Allen JH: Ophthalmomyiasis interna anterior. Report of hypoderma larva in anterior chamber. Am J Ophthalmol 22:996, 1939.
8. Edwards KM, Meredith TA, Hagler WS, et al: Ophthalmomyasis interna causing visual loss. Am J Ophthalmol 97:605–610, 1984.
9. DeBoe M: Dipterous larva passing from the optic nerve into the vitreous chamber. Arch Ophthalmol 10:824, 1933.
10. Forman AR, Cruess AF, Benson WE: Ophthalmomyiasis treated by argon laser photocoagulation. Retina 4:163, 1984.
11. Kean BH, Sun T, Ellsworth RM: Color Atlas and Text of Ophthalmic Parasitology. New York, Igaku-Shoin, 1991, pp 151–156.
12. Zaman V: Atlas of Medical Parasitology. Sidney, ADIS Press, 1979, pp 195–221.
13. Chitwood BG, Chitwood MBH: Introduction to Nematology, Baltimore, University Park Press, 1950, pp 284–285.
14. Manson-Bahr P: Manson's Tropical Diseases, 16th edition. London, Cassell, 1966, p 945.
15. Belding DL: Basic Clinical Parasitology. New York, Appleton-Century-Crofts, 1958, p 213.
16. Punyagupta S, Bunnag T, Juttijudata P: Eosinophilic meningitis in Thailand: clinical and epidemiological characteristics of 162 patients with myeloencephalitis probably caused by gnathostoma. J Neurol Sci 96:241–256, 1990.
17. Sen K, Ghose N: Ocular gnathostomiasis. Br J Ophthalmol 29:618, 1945.
18. Witemberg G, Jacoby J, Steckelmacher S: A case of ocular gnathostomiasis. Ophthalmologica 119:114–122, 1950.
19. Gyi K: Intraocular gnathostomiasis. Br J Ophthalmol 44:42–45, 1960.
20. Khin T: Intraocular gnathostomiasis. Br J Ophthalmol 52:57–60, 1968.
21. Choudhury AR: Ocular gnathostomiasis. Am J Ophthalmol 70:276–278, 1970.
22. Tudor RC, Blair E: *Gnathostoma spinigerum*: an unusual cause of ocular nematodiasis in the Western hemisphere. Am J Ophthalmol 72:185–190, 1971.
23. Bathrick ME, Mango CA, Mueller JF: Intraocular gnathostomiasis. Ophthalmology 88:1293–1295, 1981.
24. Kittiponghansa S, Prabriputaloong A, Pariyanonda S, et al: Intracameral gnathostomiasis: a cause of anterior uveitis and secondary glaucoma. Br J Ophthalmol 71:618–622, 1987.
25. Funata M, Custis P, De La Cruz Z, et al: Intraocular gnathostomiasis. Retina 13:240–244, 1993.
26. Punyagupta S, Juttijudata P, Bunnag T: Eosinophilic meningitis in Thailand. 1. Clinical studies of 484 typical cases probably caused by *Angiostrongylus cantonensis*. Am J Trop Med 20:815, 1971.
27. Kanchanaranya C, Punyagupta S: Case of ocular angiostrongyliasis associated with eosinophilic meningitis. Am J Ophthalmol 71:931–934, 1971.
28. Kanchanaranya C, Prechanond A, Punyagupta S: Removal of living worm in retinal *Angiostrongylus cantonensis*. Am J Ophthalmol 74:456–458, 1972.
29. Prommindaroj K, Leelawongs N, Pradatsundarasar A: Human angiostrongyliasis of the eye in Bangkok. Am J Trop Med Hyg 11:759, 1962.
30. Ketsuwan P, Pradatsundarasar A: Second case of ocular angiostrongyliasis in Thailand. Am J Trop Med Hyg 15:50, 1966.
31. Ketsuwan P, Pradatsundarasar A: Third case of ocular angiostrongyliasis in Thailand. J Med Assoc Thai 48:799, 1965.
32. Goodart RA, Riekhof FT, Beaver PC: Subretinal nematode. An unusual etiology for uveitis and retinal detachment. Retina 5:87–90, 1985.
33. Bird AC, Anderson J, Fuglsang H: Morphology of posterior segment lesions of the eye in patients with onchocerciasis. Br J Ophthalmol 60:2–20, 1076.
34. Murphy RP, Taylor H, Greene BM: Chorioretinal damage in onchocerciasis. Am J Ophthalmol 98:519–521, 1984.
35. Rodger FC, Chir M: The pathogenesis and pathology of ocular onchocerciasis. Am J Ophthalmol 49:327, 1960.
36. Paul EV, Zimmerman LE: Some observations on the ocular pathology of onchocerciasis. Hum Pathol 1:581, 1970.
37. Neumann E, Gunders E: Pathogenesis of the posterior segment lesion of ocular onchocerciasis. Am J Ophthalmol 75:82, 1973.
38. Anderson J, Font RL: Ocular onchocerciasis. In Binford CH, Connor DH, Ash JE (eds): Pathology of Tropical and Extraordinary Disease. Washington, DC, Armed Forces Institute of Parasitology, 1976, pp 373–381.
39. Hissette J: Ann Soc Belg Med Trop 12:433, 1932.

40. Bryant J: Trans R Soc Trop Med Hyg 28;523, 1935.
41. Ridley H: Brit J Ophthalmol Monogr (Suppl) 10, 1945.
42. Anderson J, Fuglsang H: Ocular onchocerciasis. Trop Dis Bull 74:257–272, 1977.
43. Bird AC, El-Sheikh H, Anderson J, Fuglsang H: Changes in visual function and in the posterior segment of the eye during treatment of onchocerciasis with diethylcarbamazine citrate. Br J Ophthalmol 64:191–200, 1980.
44. Pearson JC: Studies on the life cycles and morphology of the larval stages of *Alaria arisaemoides*, Augustine and Uribe, 1927, and *Alaria canis*, La Rue and Fallis, 1936 (Trematoda: Diplostomidae). Can J Zool 34:295, 1956.
45. Johnson AD: Life history of *Alaria marcianae* (La Rue, 1917, Walton, 1949 (Trematoda: Diplostomidae). J Parasitol 54: 324, 1968.
46. Shoop WL, Corkum KC: Epidemiology of *Alaria marcianae* mesocercariae in Louisiana. J Parasitol 67:928, 1981.
47. Shea M, Maberley AL, Walters J, et al: Intraretinal larval trematode. Trans Am Acad Ophthalmol Otolaryngol 77: 784, 1973.
48. Beaver PC, Little MD, Tucker CF, Reed JR: Mesocercaria in the skin of a man in Louisiana. Am J Trop Med Hyg 26: 422, 1977.
49. Freeman RS, Stuart PF, Cullen SJ, et al: Fatal human infection with mesocercariae of the trematode *Alaria americana*. Am J Trop Med Hyg 25:803, 1976.
50. Johnson AD: *Alaria mustelae*. Description of mesocercariae and key to related species. Trans Am Microsci Soc 89:250, 1970.
51. Fernandes BJ, Cooper JD, Cullen JB, et al: Systemic infection with *Alaria americana* (Trematoda). Can Med Assoc J 115:1111, 1976.
52. McDonald HR, Kazacos KR, Schatx H, Johnson RN: Two cases of intraocular infection with *Alaria mesocercaria* (Trematoda). Am J Ophthalmol 117:447–455, 1994.
53. Byers B, Kimura SJ: Uveitis after death of a larva in the vitreous cavity. Am J Ophthalmol 77:63, 1974.
54. Gass JD, Callanan DG, Bowman CB: Oral therapy in diffuse unilateral subacute neuroretinitis. Arch Ophthalmol 110:675, 1992.
55. Gass JD, Braunstein RA: Further observations concerning the diffuse unilateral subacute neuroretinitis syndrome. Arch Ophthalmol 101:1689, 1983.
56. Gass JD: Stereoscopic Atlas of Macular Diseases. Diagnosis and Treatment, 3rd edition, Vol 2. St Louis, CV Mosby Co, 1987, pp 470–475.
57. Olsen KR, Gass JDM: Diffuse unilateral subacute neuroretinitis. In Ryan SJ (ed): Retina, Vol 5. St Louis, CV Mosby Co, 1989, pp 655–661.
58. Goldberg MA, Kazacos KR, Boyce WM, et al: Diffuse unilateral subacute neuroretinitis in California. Morphologic, serologic, and epidemiologic support for *Baysilascaris* as a causative agent. Ophthalmology 100:1695, 1993.
59. Williams GA, Aaberg TM, Dudley SS: Perimacular photocoagulation of presumed *Basylisascaris procyonis* in diffuse unilateral subacute neuroretinitis. In Gitter KA, Schatz H, Yannuzzi LA, McDonald HR (eds): Laser Photocoagulation of Retinal Disease. San Francisco, Pacific Medical Press, 1988, pp 275–280.
60. Shields JA: Ocular toxocariasis. A review. Surv Ophthalmol 28:361, 1984.
61. Hutton WL, Vaiser A, Synder WB: Pars plana vitrectomy for removal of intravitreous *Cysticercus*. Am J Ophthalmol 81:571, 1976.
62. Rapoza PA, Michels RG, Semeraro RJ, Green WR: Vitrectomy for excision of intraocular larva (hypoderma species). Retina 6:99, 1986.
63. Gjotterberg M, Ingemansson SO: Intraocular infestation by the reindeer warble fly larva. An unusual indication for acute vitrectomy. Br J Ophthalmol 72:420, 1988.

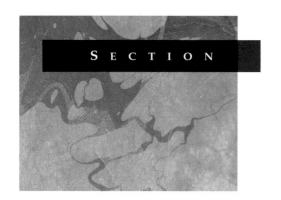

Traumatic Disorders

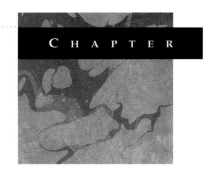

CHAPTER *69*

Posterior Segment Manifestations of Blunt Trauma

Eric A. Postel, M.D.
William F. Mieler, M.D.

Ocular trauma is a leading cause of visual impairment in the United States,[1] and levies a tremendous penalty in both direct and indirect costs.[2] Males are approximately nine times more often affected than females[2-8] and most victims are under the age of 40.[2,4,5,7,8] The effects of blunt trauma are more commonly encountered than those of penetrating injury.[2-4]

Blunt ocular trauma may result from direct injury to the eye or adjacent structures, or from injury to remote parts of the body. Its manifestations are protean and often reflect damage to multiple structures within the eye (Table 69–1). In addition, blunt trauma can cause rupture of the globe, which may be suggested by the presence of severe intraocular or periocular hemorrhage associated with visual acuity of light perception or worse, media opacification, abnormal chamber depth, or a low intraocular pressure.[9]

Discrete entities have been described where examination has revealed primary involvement of specific anatomic layers.[10] No treatment exists for many of these conditions, but early recognition and diagnosis may allow prevention of debilitating sequelae.[11]

DIRECT OCULAR OR PERIOCULAR INJURY

Traumatic Retinal Tears, Detachments, and Dialyses

Blunt ocular trauma causes from 10 to 19%[12-14] of all phakic detachments. Several studies have shown

that traumatic retinal detachment is more common among males than females, and typically occurs in younger patients than nontraumatic retinal detachment.[13-15] Goffstein and Burton[14] examined 586 primary phakic retinal detachments and found the mean age to be 28 years, compared with 53 years in the nontrauma group. Seventy-eight per cent of traumatic detachments occurred in males, compared to 48% of nontraumatic detachments. In addition, they suggested that myopic eyes are predisposed to retinal detachment following blunt trauma.

Retinal dialysis is the most common abnormality leading to retinal detachment after ocular contusion, and occurs most often in the inferotemporal quadrant.[14,16] Goffstein and Burton[14] and Tasman[16] reported that inferotemporal dialyses accounted for 31 to 54% of traumatic retinal detachments. Superior or superonasal dialyses caused 22 to 38% of retinal detachments. Cox,[15] however, found superonasal dialyses to be more common than inferotemporal dialyses, occurring in 38 and 27% of 143 affected eyes, respectively.

Johnston[17] reported retinal detachment occurring in 84% of patients who suffered retinal breaks due to ocular contusion. Sixty-four per cent of these retinal detachments were due to dialyses, which were most common inferotemporally. The retinal break or detachment was diagnosed within 24 hours of injury in 31% of these cases, while 64% were identified within 6 weeks. Surgical intervention successfully reattached 96% of these retinas. Other studies have shown a similar latent interval between the contusion and the identification of retinal tears or detachment.[14-16]

The mechanism of retinal dialysis formation

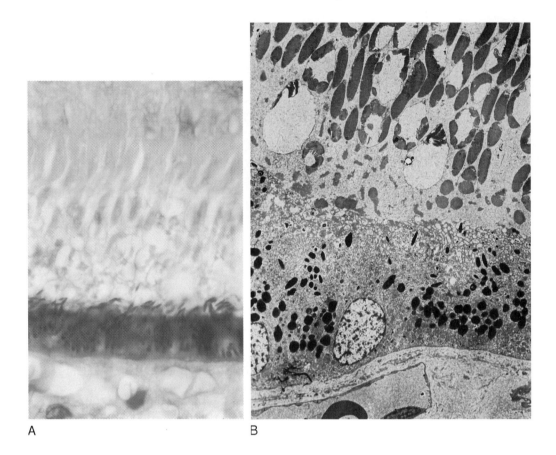

A, Swelling and disruption of photoreceptor outer segments in acute traumatic retinopathy (Berlin's edema) (commotio retinae). B, Ultrastructural appearance of photoreceptor outer segment swelling and disruption in acute commotio retinae. (A and B From Mansour AM, Green WR, Hogge C: Histopathology of commotio retinae. Retina 12:24–28, 1992, with permission.)

TABLE 69-1 Blunt Trauma

Direct
    Retinal tear/dialysis/detachment
    Macular hole
    Chorioretinitis sclopeteria
    Choroidal rupture
    Commotio retinae
    Contusion/tear of RPE
    Optic nerve evulsion

Indirect
    Shaken baby syndrome
    Terson's syndrome
    Purtscher's retinopathy
    Fat embolism syndrome
    Valsalva retinopathy
    Whiplash retinopathy
    Bungee-jumping retinopathy

RPE, retinal pigment epithelium.

seems clear. Ocular contusion produces a forceful anteroposterior compression of the globe, with a resultant lateral expansion of the equatorial region and disinsertion or tearing of the retina.[11,18] Weidenthal and Schepens[18] confirmed this by firing BBs into the corneas of mounted pig eyes. Nasal dialyses were frequently identified, and their occurrence could be reduced by limiting equatorial expansion.

Cox[15] found avulsion of the vitreous base in 26% of patients and considered it pathognomonic for traumatic retinal detachment. In addition, 36% of patients developed retinal holes in areas with no apparent vitreous attachment. These were equally divided between small, round, atrophic breaks and large irregular holes with ragged edges, and were most common in the inferotemporal quadrant. Goffstein and Burton[14] found giant retinal tears in 16% of cases, retinal flap tears with adherent vitreous in 11%, and tears in areas of lattice degeneration in 8%. Large, radial tears extending from the optic nerve, and giant retinal tears have also been reported to occur in a boxer.[19] Giovinazzo et al[20] and others[21] reported multiple eye injuries occurring in boxers, including retinal tears in 24%. Sixteen per cent of these were horseshoe tears, and 8% were operculated tears. Multiple tears were found in more than 50% of these eyes.[20]

Establishing a causal relationship between ocular trauma and delayed retinal detachment may be difficult. Clues to the traumatic etiology include: (1) unilateral pathology, (2) giant retinal tears or dialyses, (3) age less than 40 years, (4) latent interval from trauma to detachment of less than 2 years, and (5) objective evidence of trauma.[10,14]

Retinal tears caused by ocular contusion may be treated with cryopexy or photocoagulation. Retinal detachments and dialyses are treated with scleral buckling, pneumatic retinopexy, or vitrectomy.[10] The overall anatomic success rate for repair of retinal detachment is similar for detachments due to blunt trauma and nontraumatic detachments,[22,23] although it may be lower in the presence of irregular posterior tears or giant retinal tears (Fig. 69-1).

Special mention must be made of recent reports of air bag-related ocular injuries,[24-30] particularly retinal detachment. Although air bags save lives and reduce morbidity,[31] serious eye injuries including retinal dialysis,[25] retinal detachment,[25,26] and choroidal rupture[27] have been reported.

Macular Holes

Macular edema, cysts, and holes may occur after blunt trauma, sometimes in association with commotio retinae, subretinal hemorrhage, choroidal rupture, or whiplash separation of the vitreous from the retina.[32] Macular holes (Fig. 69-2) have been found in up to 6% of eyes after contusion injury.[15] In addition, indirect injury such as a lightning strike has been reported to cause macular holes, macular edema,[33] retinal folds, and electrooculogram (EOG) abnormalities.[34] These holes are rarely an isolated cause of rhegmatogenous retinal detachment,[11] so the presence of a retinal detachment in these cases should alert the examiner to the possibility of coexisting pathology. The treatment of full-thickness macular holes may involve vitrectomy, membrane stripping, gas tamponade, and biologic mediators; however, success rates for repair of traumatic macular holes have not been reported.

Chorioretinitis Sclopeteria

Chorioretinitis sclopeteria is a term introduced to describe the rare finding of traumatic chorioretinal

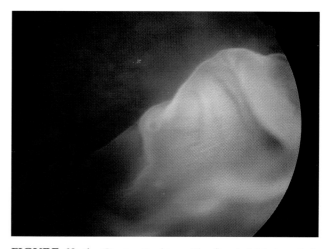

FIGURE 69-1 Giant retinal tear. The flap is folded posteriorly and the outer retinal surface is visible.

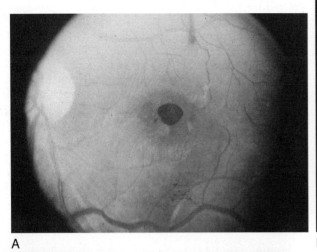

A

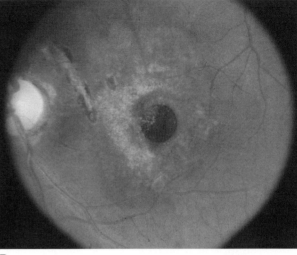

B

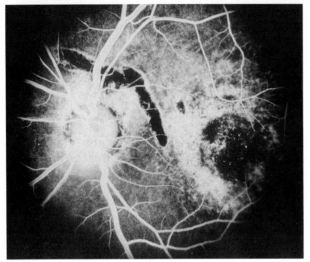

C

FIGURE 69–2   Traumatic macular hole. *A,* A small, central, full-thickness retinal defect exists shortly after blunt injury. Areas of commotio retinae are also visible. *B,* Late appearance of a traumatic macular hole, with surrounding pigmentary irregularity. The optic nerve is pale and a choroidal rupture is present. *C,* Fluorescein angiography shown in case *B* showing irregular hyperfluorescence corresponding to RPE disturbance. No choroidal neovascularization is evident in the region of the choroidal rupture.

rupture resulting from a nonpenetrating, high-velocity injury to the globe (Fig. 69–3).[35–37] Vitreous hemorrhage may accompany sclopeteria.[10] Martin et al[37] described eight eyes in which direct or tangential, nonpenetrating, high-velocity injury resulted in chorioretinal rupture. In all cases, the chorioretinal rupture corresponded to the external impact site. Seven of the eight eyes were managed by observation only, and none of those eyes developed a retinal detachment during the first 6 months of observation. Two eyes eventually developed retinal detachments, but both were felt to be due to tears distant from the site of chorioretinal rupture.

Visual acuity may be normal with sclopeteria, although extensive fibrosis and scarring may develop in the injured area. In the series noted above,[37] final visual acuity was 20/20 or better in four eyes. Vision was reduced in the other eyes due to presumed foveal trauma, development of a macular hole, traumatic optic neuropathy, vitreous hemorrhage, and retinal detachment.

The pathogenesis of sclopeteria is related to the relative differences in tensile strength of the retina, choroid, sclera, and posterior hyaloid.[37] With rapid deformation of the globe, the induced tensile stresses cause rupture of the choroid and retina, while the more elastic posterior hyaloid remains intact. The choroid and retina then retract as a single unit, exposing the underlying sclera. Fluid does not enter the subretinal space because the choroid and retina remain apposed, and because the posterior hyaloid remains intact over the rupture site. In addition, most patients in this series were young and therefore had a formed vitreous, which might lower the risk of retinal detachment.

Choroidal Rupture

Choroidal rupture can occur after blunt injury to the globe and represents a less severe element within the spectrum of injury that includes chorioretinitis sclopeteria. The mechanism of choroidal

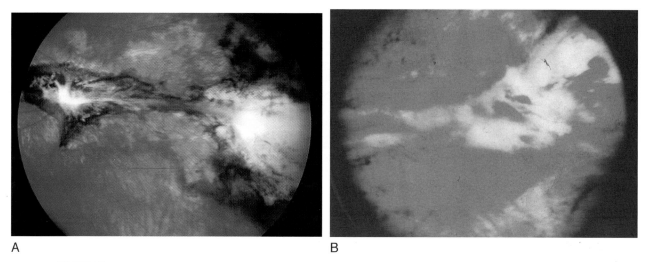

FIGURE 69–3 Chorioretinitis sclopeteria. *A*, Acute appearance, with preretinal and vitreous hemorrhage overlying the retinochoroidal defect. No retinal detachment was present. *B*, Late appearance with pigmentary hypertrophy and fibrosis. The retina remained attached.

rupture is primarily mechanical,[38] although a vascular disturbance and pressure necrosis have also been suggested.[39] Like sclopeteria, it is due to abrupt deformation of the globe. It has been classified as either a direct or indirect[10,40] tearing of the choroid, retinal pigment epithelium (RPE), and Bruch's membrane. A direct choroidal rupture occurs anteriorly at the site of impact and is typically oriented parallel to the ora serrata. Indirect choroidal ruptures are located posteriorly, and are crescentic and concentric with the optic disc (Fig. 69–4).[10] Choroidal ruptures are often obscured by subretinal or vitreous hemorrhage acutely, and may be accompanied by commotio retinae[41] or subretinal fluid. If the fovea is involved, visual acuity may be commensurately affected.

Aguilar and Green[40] describe a spectrum of findings in 47 cases of choroidal rupture. Fibroblastic activity is usually present 6 to 14 days after injury, and a well-developed scar is usually formed by 3 to 4 weeks. RPE hyperplasia was common at the margins of the healed lesions, and in four eyes exuberant scar formation occurred with extension through the retina and into the vitreous cavity. Choroidal neovascularization was consistently present during the healing process, but in most cases regressed spontaneously. In two cases, choroidal neovascularization extended into the vitreous cavity, and subretinal pigment epithelial neovascularization persisted in one case.

Chorioretinal anastomosis,[42] optic nerve pallor,[43] and subretinal neovascularization[10,44,45] have all been reported to occur after choroidal rupture. In addition, visual field defects such as baring of the

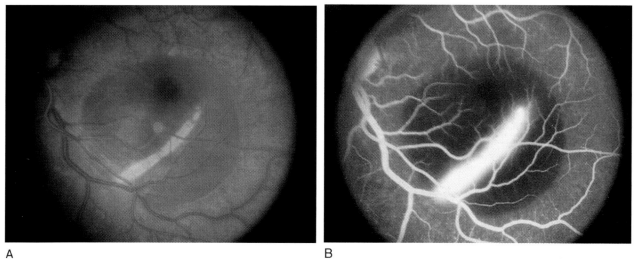

FIGURE 69–4 Choroidal rupture. *A*, Shortly after injury, there may be subretinal fluid associated with choroidal rupture. *B*, Fluorescein angiography showing hyperfluorescence of rupture. No choroidal neovascular membrane is present.

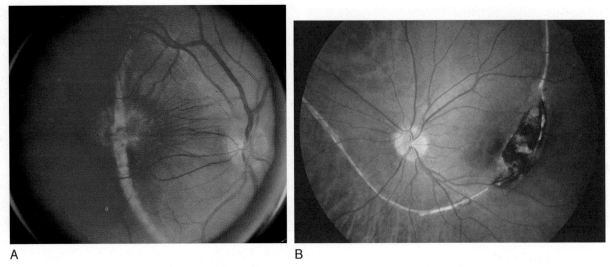

A   B

FIGURE 69–5 Choroidal rupture. *A,* Choroidal rupture concentric to the disc, that traverses the fovea. There is fibrosis and contraction, causing retinal striae nasal to the fovea. *B,* Wide-field view of extensive choroidal rupture that bisected the fovea. There is marked pigmentary disturbance in the foveal region.

blind spot, central or pericentral scotomata, and generalized constriction have all been associated with indirect choroidal rupture.[43,44]

Final visual acuity may vary after choroidal rupture, and can be severely affected if the fovea is involved (Fig. 69–5). Wood and Richardson[46] reported 17 of 30 eyes regaining 20/40 vision after choroidal rupture. Late development of subretinal neovascularization is the major cause of delayed loss of vision after choroidal rupture,[11] although pigmentary retinopathy and inner retinal damage may also occur.[46] Subretinal neovascularization occurs in 5 to 25% of cases of indirect choroidal rupture.[44,45] These membranes can occur within months or many years after the injury,[41] and may be associated with a serous or hemorrhagic detachment of the macula.[41,47] Photocoagulation of these membranes may be successful in select cases.[47]

Commotio Retinae

Commotio retinae (Berlin's edema) was first described in 1873,[48] and is characterized by transient whitening or opacification at the level of the deep sensory retina.[10] The disturbance may be confined to the macula or may involve extensive areas of the peripheral retina, and may be associated with choroidal rupture, and subretinal, retinal, and/or preretinal hemorrhage (Fig. 69–6).[49] The retinal whitening in the macula may clear completely with restoration of normal vision. However, permanent visual impairment may be associated with a normal-appearing macula, or there may be development of pigmentary disruption (Fig. 69–7), or partial- or full-thickness macular holes.[49] Fine granular changes in the retina associated with pockets

of vitreous liquefaction have also been noted after resolution of commotio retinae.[11]

Berlin suggested that the retinal opacity was due to extracellular edema.[48] Others have identified fluid-filled spaces in the outer retinal layers,[50] intracellular edema of retinal glial cells,[51] and disruption of photoreceptor outer segments.[52] Sipperly et al[53] studied experimentally induced commotio retinae in owl monkeys. Funduscopic examination revealed retinal opacification 4 to 12 hours after injury in 7 of 12 eyes with commotio retinae. Fluorescein angiography revealed no leakage of dye acutely. Histologic examination revealed disruption of the photoreceptor outer segments immediately after injury. No major extracellular edema was seen. Twenty-one hours after injury, photoreceptor inner

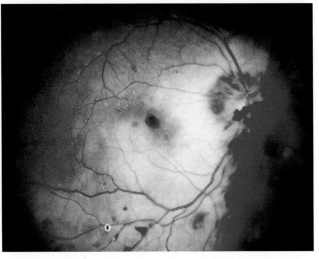

FIGURE 69–6 Commotio retinae. Appearance shortly after injury with profound retinal whitening; a prominent cherry-red spot; and intraretinal, preretinal, and vitreous hemorrhage.

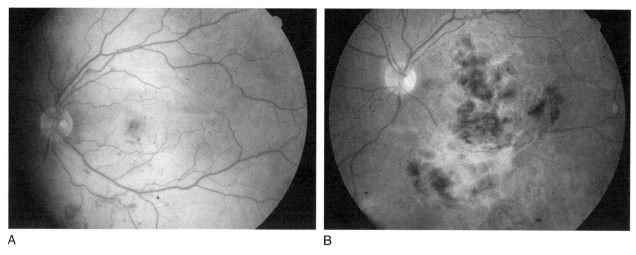

A   B

FIGURE 69–7 Commotio retinae. *A*, Acute appearance with retinal whitening involving primarily the posterior pole. There is a cherry-red spot present. *B*, Late pigmentary changes and fibrosis after resolution of commotio retinae.

segments had severe degeneration of their mitochondria, and the RPE was actively phagocytizing the disrupted outer segments. RPE cells had begun to migrate among the outer segment fragments and into the outer retina 48 hours after injury. Eventually multiple layers of RPE cells developed on Bruch's membrane and in severely affected areas the photoreceptor outer segments were absent and the inner segments were directly opposed to the pigment epithelium. Generalized thinning of the outer plexiform and the outer nuclear layers followed.

Mansour et al[54] examined a freshly enucleated human eye and found marked disruption of the photoreceptor outer segments and their accumulation in the subretinal space, and damage to the adjacent RPE. Pulido and Blair[55] performed fluorescein angiography and vitreous fluorophotometry on ten patients with commotio retinae and were unable to demonstrate any disruption of the blood-retinal barrier. Fundus reflection densitometry revealed impaired photopigment kinetics in two patients with commotio retinae, a finding supporting the histopathologic data on commotio retinae.[56]

The treatment of commotio retinae is observation. When the macula is involved, final visual acuity may be impaired.

Contusion and Tears of the Retinal Pigment Epithelium

Blunt ocular trauma may cause tearing or contusion of the RPE (Fig. 69–8), with subsequent RPE cell edema and overlying serous retinal detachment.[41,57] Friberg[57] reported a cream-colored discoloration of the posterior pole and a macular hole occurring after blunt injury. Fluorescein angiography showed gradual staining of the RPE and a hyperfluorescent spot corresponding to the macular hole without se-

rous retinal or pigment epithelial elevation. Eventually pigment clumping and RPE atrophy ensued, and fluorescein angiography 5 months after injury revealed only window defects.

Contusion and tearing of the RPE represent variations in the spectrum of injury that includes commotio retinae, choroidal rupture, and sclopeteria. Blight and Hart[52] found transient intracellular edema in the RPE and photoreceptor outer segment disruption after experimentally induced blunt trauma. If the injury is severe, leakage of serous fluid into the subretinal space may occur.[10,41]

Levin et al[58] reported RPE tears occurring in two patients after blunt trauma. Neither patient had a pre-existing RPE detachment. They hypothesized that acute tangential stresses on and around the posterior pole are responsible for such tears, and

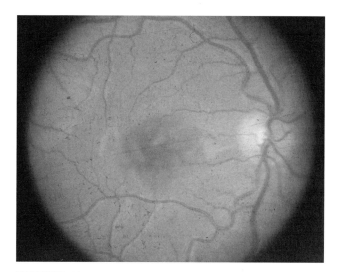

FIGURE 69–8 RPE contusion. Subtle areas of subretinal whitening in the macula of a patient with RPE contusion. The findings are typically much less pronounced than those of commotio retinae.

that this force must be too weak to cause rupture of both the RPE and Bruch's membrane.

Like commotio retinae, vision may be severely affected if the injury involves the macula. There is no specific treatment for this condition.

Optic Nerve Evulsion

Evulsion of the optic nerve is a rare and visually devastating event. It was first described by Salzmann in 1903,[59] and early reports involved severe concussive or penetrating orbital injuries during wartime,[60,61] although it may occur after more minor injuries.[62] Several mechanisms for optic nerve evulsion have been proposed,[60,63] and all suggest a tear at the lamina cribrosa with disruption of the axons at that point. Peripapillary retinal evulsion has been seen in association with optic nerve evulsion, and is presumably due to severe anterior displacement and abduction of the globe.[64]

Optic nerve evulsion typically results in immediate, profound loss of vision. The evulsion may be partial,[62,65] in which case some visual function may be retained, or it may be complete,[66] resulting in loss of light perception. Examination reveals hemorrhage overlying the optic nerve head region with varying amounts of intraocular hemorrhage when the evulsion is complete (Fig. 69–9). A partial evulsion may be difficult to identify initially, and may simulate the appearance of an optic pit.[62] Fluorescein angiography may demonstrate absent,[64] partial,[65] or complete[62] filling of the retinal vasculature, presumably via communication with the choroidal vasculature.[66] Computed tomography or magnetic resonance imaging usually demonstrates an apparently intact optic nerve sheath. Fibroglial proliferation eventually fills the cavity left by the evulsion.[10]

INDIRECT OCULAR INJURY

Shaken Baby Syndrome

Thirty to 40% of abused children will have ophthalmoscopic evidence of injury.[67–69] Violent shaking, direct ocular or head trauma, chest injuries, and choking can result in a multitude of anterior and posterior segment manifestations. The most common and consistent finding, however, is retinal hemorrhage,[67–69] which may occur in 65 to 89% of cases and involve all layers of the retina.[70] Eisenbry[71] reported that 64% of abused children less than 3 years old had retinal hemorrhages in contrast to 3% with retinal hemorrhages after accidental head injuries. Diffuse retinal hemorrhages, perimacular folds,[72] cotton-wool spots, papilledema, and venous engorgement may be present,[69,73] and the appearance of the fundus may simulate Purtscher's retinopathy, Terson's syndrome, or central retinal vein occlusion (Fig. 69–10).[10] Vitreous hemorrhage, retinal detachment, retinoschisis, and chorioretinal atrophy may also be present.[70,74]

In most cases there is intracranial hemorrhage or contusion.[10] Retinal hemorrhages may precede the development of intracranial hemorrhage,[75] and may be the first sign of nonaccidental injury. Wilkinson et al[76] found an association between subhyaloid hemorrhage greater than 2 disc areas in size, vitreous hemorrhage, or diffuse hemorrhage involving the peripapillary and peripheral retina to be associated with a high initial neurologic score. They suggest that the likelihood of severe neurologic injury seems to be higher in this group than in those without these characteristics.

The ophthalmologist plays an important role in diagnosing child abuse, and must be aware of the legal implications of this role. Following recognition, treatment may include repair of retinal de-

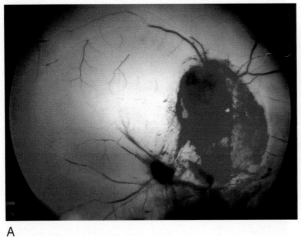
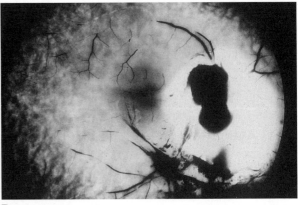

A   B

FIGURE 69–9   Optic nerve evulsion. A blow to the forehead caused an optic nerve evulsion in this patient. *A*, Acute appearance, with marked retinal ischemia caused by nonperfusion of retinal vasculature. Hemorrhage overlies the evulsed nerve. *B*, Fluorescein angiography demonstrating lack of retinal perfusion, though the choroidal circulation remains intact.

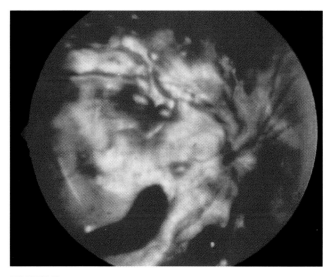

FIGURE 69–10   Shaken baby syndrome. In the right eye there is marked retinal, preretinal, and vitreous hemorrhage; cotton-wool spots; a swollen optic disc; and venous engorgement.

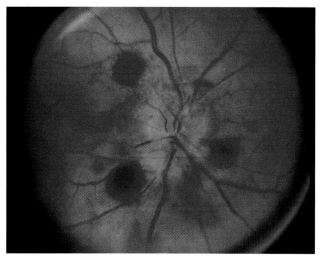

FIGURE 69–11   Terson's syndrome. Multiple areas of preretinal and mild vitreous hemorrhage are present. Intracranial hemorrhage was also present.

tachment and vitrectomy for nonclearing vitreous hemorrhage.[10]

Terson's Syndrome

Vitreous hemorrhage occurring in association with subarachnoid hemorrhage was first described by Litten in 1881,[77] and then by Terson in 1900.[78] About 20% of patients suffering either spontaneous or posttraumatic subarachnoid or subdural hemorrhages develop intraocular hemorrhages usually confined to the juxtapapillary and macular areas (Fig. 69–11).[79,80] Hemorrhage usually occurs beneath the internal limiting membrane, but may break through into the vitreous cavity. The most common sequela of Terson's syndrome is epiretinal membrane formation, which occurs in up to 78% of eyes.[81] Perimacular retinal folds,[82] similar to those seen in the shaken baby syndrome, and retinal detachment[83,84] have been associated with Terson's syndrome.

The pathogenesis of Terson's syndrome is unknown. Early work[85] suggested that the hemorrhage dissected from the subarachnoid space through the optic nerve sheath and into the eye. However, the lack of a direct communication between the subarachnoid space and vitreous of a normal eye, and the observation that hemorrhage is not always contiguous with the optic nerve, make this explanation unlikely.[10]

A more likely explanation was proposed by Terson,[78] who suggested that intraocular hemorrhage was due to the rupture of peripapillary and epipapillary capillaries when increased intracranial pressure caused elevated venous pressure. Miller and Cuttino[86] suggested that compression of the central retinal vein increases the venous pressure in Terson's syndrome.

Shultz et al[81] found that 25 of 30 eyes recovered visual acuity of 20/50 or better within 2 years. An equal number of patients received vitrectomy or were treated conservatively, and there was no difference in final visual acuity between the two groups. Visual recovery was hastened by vitrectomy and it has been proposed for visually immature infants and adults with bilateral[81] or nonclearing[87] hemorrhages.

Purtscher's Retinopathy

Following severe compression injury to the head or trunk, multiple patches of superficial retinal whitening and retinal hemorrhages surrounding the optic nerve head may develop (Fig. 69–12).[88] A similar retinopathy has been associated with pancreatitis,[89] chronic renal failure,[90] cardiac aneurysm,[91] childbirth,[92] and connective tissue disorders.[88] Fluorescein angiography reveals leakage of dye from the retinal vasculature, perivenous staining, retinal and optic disc edema, and impairment of retinal arteriolar and capillary perfusion.[10,93] Resolution of the retinopathy can take several months or more, and may be associated with permanent visual loss due to pigment epithelial changes and optic atrophy.[93]

The pathogenesis of Purtscher's retinopathy is unclear. Theories include air embolism,[93] fat embolism,[94] complement-induced granulocyte aggregation,[95] and leukoembolism.[92] Lesions similar to Purtscher's retinopathy have been produced by the infusion of glass beads into the common carotid artery[96] and fibrin clots into the ophthalmic artery.[97] Some of these theories are supported by the observation that severe trauma and acute pancreatitis activate the complement system.[10]

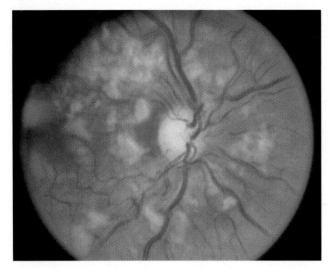

FIGURE 69–12 Purtscher's retinopathy. There is marked retinal whitening involving the posterior pole. A similar appearance may be seen in other conditions (see text).

There is no known treatment for Purtscher's retinopathy.

Fat Embolism Syndrome

The fat embolism syndrome (FES) is recognized in about 5% of patients after fracture of long bones.[10] It affects multiple organ systems and may be fatal in 20% of cases.[98] Retinal manifestations include successive crops of cotton-wool spots and small blot hemorrhages,[99] and central retinal artery obstruction,[100] and may be seen in 50 to 60% of patients with FES.[101] Chuang et al[102] examined 100 patients with long-bone or pelvic fractures and found cotton-wool spots and retinal hemorrhages in four individuals, none of whom were suspected of FES

prior to their examination. This suggests that retinal examination for patients at risk may identify subclinical FES, although with rapid rehabilitation from injury this syndrome is rarely seen. The visual prognosis for patients with FES is generally good, but permanent paracentral scotomas may occur.[102]

Valsalva Retinopathy

A sudden rise in intra-abdominal or intrathoracic pressure against a closed glottis (Valsalva's maneuver) may cause a rapid increase in venous pressure with spontaneous rupture of superficial retinal capillaries.[103,104] Affected patients may suffer visual loss during or after activities such as heavy lifting, straining at stool, coughing, vomiting, and sexual stimulation.[105]

Typical fundus findings include a well-circumscribed, round or dumbbell-shaped, bright red mound of blood beneath the internal limiting membrane in or near the central macular area (Fig. 69–13).[103] A fluid level may develop, and as the hemorrhage clears, visual acuity typically returns to normal.[10] Dense premacular hemorrhage can limit final visual acuity, however. The neodymium: yttrium-aluminum-garnet (Nd:YAG) laser may be used to puncture the posterior hyaloid and drain the blood in some cases.[106]

Similar lesions may occur without any discernible history of excessive activity or Valsalva's maneuver,[107,108] and may be associated with familial retinal arteriolar tortuosity.[10,109] As in classic Valsalva retinopathy, vision usually returns to normal.

Whiplash Retinopathy

Whiplash retinopathy consists of a history of traumatic flexion-extension of the head and neck with-

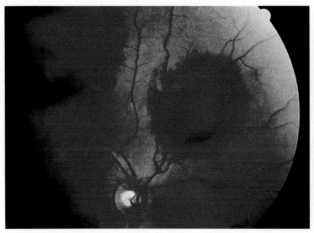
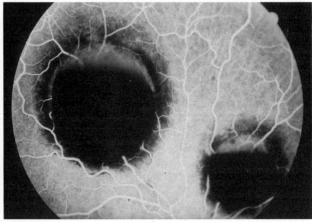

A   B

FIGURE 69–13 Valsalva retinopathy. *A*, Multiple areas of preretinal hemorrhage showing fluid levels. *B*, Fluorescein angiography of *A*, showing blockage of fluorescence by preretinal hemorrhage, and the fluid level present in each area of hemorrhage.

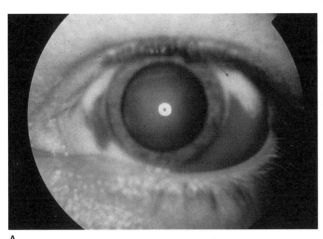 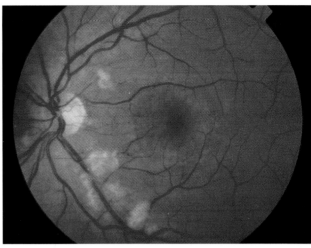

A   B

FIGURE 69-14   Bungee-jumping retinopathy. *A,* External appearance of the left eye of a young man after bungee jumping, with subconjunctival hemorrhage. *B,* Fundus appearance of bungee-jumping retinopathy, showing areas of retinal whitening. (Courtesy of C. F. Blodi, M.D., Des Moines, IA.)

out direct eye injury,[32] and is therefore similar to the shaken baby syndrome, although it is generally less pronounced. There is an immediate mild reduction in visual acuity in one or both eyes, usually to no worse than 20/30, and the development of a gray swelling in the fovea associated with the formation of a 50- to 100-μm foveolar pit. The retinal opacity and visual disturbance are transient, but the pit and its whitish border remain.[110] Identical lesions may be seen after blunt ocular trauma, solar retinopathy,[111] and bungee jumping.[112] Other abnormalities have been associated with whiplash injuries, such as decreased convergence and accommodation, decreased stereoacuity, extraocular muscle paresis, and posterior vitreous detachment.[113] There is no known treatment.

Bungee Jumping

Bungee jumping may produce a Purtscher's-like retinopathy (Fig. 69-14) and result in RPE mottling and permanent scotomata.[114] Swelling may also be seen in the macular region similar to acute macular neuroretinopathy. These changes presumably occur due to the acceleration-deceleration forces involved in bungee jumping. There is no known treatment.

CONCLUSION

A variety of local, as well as systemic, injuries may cause posterior segment abnormalities. Vision may be unaffected, mildly affected, or profoundly impaired. The effects of trauma may be immediate or delayed, and for most conditions there is no specific treatment. Familiarity with the posterior segment manifestations of blunt ocular trauma and distant

trauma may allow more accurate prognostication, and, perhaps, prevention or limitation of some damaging sequelae.

Blunt ocular trauma levies tremendous costs on society, and remains one of the most common causes of visual loss in this country. Clearly, more effort is required to educate and prevent blunt ocular injury from occurring.

REFERENCES

1. Sternberg P Jr: Trauma: principles and techniques of treatment. In Ryan SJ (ed): Retina, Vol. 3. St Louis, CV Mosby Co, 1994.
2. Schein OD, Hibberd PL, Shingleton BJ, et al: The spectrum and burden of ocular injury. Ophthalmology 95:300–305, 1988.
3. LaRoche GR, McIntyre L, Schertzer RM: Epidemiology of severe eye injuries in childhood. Ophthalmology 95:1604–1607, 1988.
4. Liggett PE, Pince KJ, Barlow W, et al: Ocular trauma in an urban population: review of 1132 cases. Ophthalmology 97:581–584, 1990.
5. Karlson TA, Klein BEK: The incidence of acute hospital-treated eye injuries. Arch Ophthalmol 104:1473–1476, 1986.
6. Strahlman E, Elman M, Daub E, Baker S: Causes of pediatric eye injuries: a population-based study. Arch Ophthalmol 108:603–606, 1990.
7. Appiah AP: The nature, causes, and visual outcome of ocular trauma requiring posterior segment surgery at a county hospital. Ann Ophthalmol 23:430–433, 1991.
8. Atmaca LS, Yilmaz M: Changes in the fundus caused by blunt ocular trauma. Ann Ophthalmol 25:447–452, 1993.
9. Klystra JA, Lamkin JC, Runyan DK: Clinical predictors of scleral rupture after blunt ocular trauma. Am J Ophthalmol 115:530–535, 1993.
10. Williams DF, Mieler WF, Williams GA: Posterior segment manifestations of ocular trauma. Retina 10(Suppl 1):S35–S44, 1990.
11. Dugel PU, Ober RR: Vitreoretinal manifestations of blunt ocular trauma. In Ryan SJ (ed): Retina, Vol. 3. St Louis, CV Mosby Co, 1994.

12. Dumas JJ: Retinal detachment following contusion of the eye. Int Ophthalmol Clin 7:19–38, 1967.
13. Schepens CL, Marden D: Data on the natural history of retinal detachment. Further characterization of certain unilateral nontraumatic cases. Am J Ophthalmol 61:213–226, 1966.
14. Goffstein R, Burton TC: Differing traumatic from nontraumatic retinal detachment. Ophthalmology 89:361–369, 1982.
15. Cox MS, Schepens CL, Freeman HM: Retinal detachment due to ocular contusion. Arch Ophthalmol 76:678–685, 1966.
16. Tasman W: Peripheral retinal changes following blunt trauma. Trans Am Ophthalmol Soc 70:190–198, 1972.
17. Johnston PB: Traumatic retinal detachment. Br J Ophthalmol 75:18–21, 1991.
18. Weidenthal DT, Schepens CL: Peripheral fundus changes associated with ocular contusion. Am J Ophthalmol 62:465–477, 1966.
19. Carter JB, Parke DW: Unusual retinal tears in an amateur boxer. Arch Opthalmol 105:1138, 1987.
20. Giovinazzo VJ, Yannuzzi LA, Sorenson JA, et al: The ocular complications of boxing. Ophthalmology 94:587–596, 1987.
21. Wedrich A, Velikay M, Binder S, et al: Ocular findings in asymptomatic amateur boxers. Retina 13:114–119, 1993.
22. Burton TC: Preoperative factors influencing anatomic success rates following retinal detachment surgery. Trans Am Acad Ophthalmol Otolaryngol 83:499–505, 1977.
23. Michels RG: Results of retinal reattachment surgery. In Retinal Detachment. St Louis, CV Mosby Co, 1990.
24. Kuhn F, Morris R, Witherspoon CD, et al: Air bag: friend or foe? Arch Ophthalmol 111:1333–1334, 1993.
25. Whitacre MM, Pilchard WA: Air bag injury producing retinal dialysis and detachment. Arch Ophthalmol 111:1320, 1993.
26. Han DP: Retinal detachment caused by air bag injury. Arch Ophthalmol 111:1317–1318, 1993.
27. Rosenblatt MA, Freilich B, Kirsch D: Air bag-associated ocular injury. Arch Ophthalmol 111:1318, 1993.
28. Lesher MP, Durrie DS, Stiles MC: Corneal edema, hyphema, and angle recession after air bag inflation. Arch Ophthalmol 111:1320–1322, 1993.
29. Driver PJ, Cashwell LF, Yeatts RP: Airbag-associated bilateral hyphemas and angle recession. Am J Ophthalmol 118:250–251, 1994.
30. Scott IU, John GR, Stark WJ: Airbag-associated ocular injury and periorbital fractures. Arch Ophthalmol 111:25, 1993.
31. Huelke DF, Moore JL, Ostrom M: Air bag injuries and occupant protection. J Trauma 33:894–898, 1992.
32. Gass JDM: Stereoscopic Atlas of Macular Diseases: Diagnosis and Treatment, 3rd edition. St Louis, CV Mosby Co, 1987, p 556.
33. Handa JT, Jaffe GJ: Lightning maculopathy: a case report. Retina 14:169–172, 1994.
34. Lagreze WDA, Bomer TG, Aiello LP: Lightning-induced ocular injury. Arch Opthalmol 113:1076–1077, 1995.
35. Goldzieher W: Beitrag zur Pathologie der orbitalen Schussverletzungen. Z Augenheilkd 6:277, 1901.
36. Richards RD, West CE, Meisels AA: Chorioretinitis sclopeteria. Am J Opthalmol 66:852–860, 1968.
37. Martin DF, Awh CC, McCuen BW, et al: Treatment and pathogenesis of traumatic chorioretinal rupture (sclopeteria). Am J Ophthalmol 117:190–200, 1994.
38. Duke-Elder WS: Textbook of Ophthalmology, Vol 6. St Louis, CV Mosby Co, 1954, pp 5829–5837.
39. Siegrist MH: Traumatische Ruptur von Ciliararterien. Klin U Med Inst der Schweie 3:554, 1895.
40. Aguilar JP, Green WR: Choroidal rupture: a histopathologic study of 47 cases. Retina 4:269–275, 1984.
41. Gass JDM: Stereoscopic Atlas of Macular Diseases: Diagnosis and Treatment, 3rd edition. St Louis, CV Mosby Co, 1987, p 170.
42. Goldberg MF: Chorioretinal vascular anastomoses after blunt trauma to the eye. Am J Ophthalmol 82:892–895, 1976.
43. Glazer LC, Han DP, Gottlieb MS: Choroidal rupture and optic atrophy. Br J Opthalmol 77:33–35, 1993.
44. Wyszynski RE, Grossniklaus HE, Frank KE: Indirect choroidal rupture secondary to blunt ocular trauma: a review of eight eyes. Retina 8:237–243, 1988.
45. Wood CM, Richardson J: Chorioretinal neovascular membranes complicating contusional eye injuries with indirect choroidal ruptures. Br J Ophthalmol 74:93–96, 1990.
46. Wood CM, Richardson J: Indirect choroidal ruptures: aetiological factors, patterns of ocular damage, and final visual outcome. Br J Ophthalmol 74:208–211, 1990.
47. Fuller B, Gitter KA: Traumatic choroidal rupture with late serous detachment of the macula: report of successful argon laser treatment. Arch Ophthalmol 89:354–355, 1973.
48. Berlin R: Zur sogenannten commotio retinae. Klin Monatsbl Augenheilkd 1:42–78, 1873.
49. Gass JDM: Stereoscopic Atlas of Macular Diseases: Diagnosis and Treatment, 3rd edition. St Louis, CV Mosby Co, 1987, p 552.
50. Yanoff M, Fine B: Ocular Pathology. Hagerstown, MD, Harper & Row, 1975, p 153.
51. Hart JCD, Blight R: Electrophysiological and pathological investigation of concussional injury. Trans Ophthalmol Soc UK 95:326–334, 1975.
52. Blight R, Hart JCD: Structural changes in the outer retinal layers following blunt mechanical non-perforating trauma to the globe: an experimental study. Br J Ophthalmol 61:573–587, 1977.
53. Sipperly JO, Quigley HA, Gass JDM: Traumatic retinopathy in primates: the explanation of commotio retinae. Arch Ophthalmol 96:2267–2273, 1978.
54. Mansour AM, Green WR, Hogge C: Histopathology of commotio retinae. Retina 12:24–28, 1992.
55. Pulido JS, Blair NP: The blood-retinal barrier in Berlin's edema. Retina 7:233–236, 1987.
56. Liem AT, Keunen JEE, Van Norren D: Reversible cone photoreceptor injury in commotio retinae of the macula. Retina 15:58–61, 1995.
57. Friberg TR: Traumatic retinal pigment epithelial edema. Am J Ophthalmol 88:18–21, 1979.
58. Levin LA, Seddon JM, Topping T: Retinal pigment epithelial tears associated with trauma. Am J Ophthalmol 112:396–400, 1991.
59. Salzmann M: Die Ausrissing des Sehnersen (avulsio nervi optica). Z Augenheilkd 9:489, 1903.
60. Lister W: Some concussion changes met with in military practice. Br J Ophthalmol 8:305–318, 1924.
61. Caiger MH: Ocular injuries resulting from the war. Trans Ophthalmol Soc UK 61:54–73, 1941.
62. Park JH, Frenkel M, Dobbie JG, Choromokos E: Evulsion of the optic nerve. Am J Ophthalmol 72:969–971, 1971.
63. Stanton-Cook L: Injury simulating congenital anomaly. Br J Ophthalmol 37:188–189, 1953.
64. Williams DF, Williams GA, Abrams GW, et al: Evulsion of the retina associated with optic nerve evulsion. Am J Ophthalmol 104:5–9, 1987.
65. Hart JCD, Pilley SFJ: Partial evulsion of the optic nerve: fluorescein angiographic study. Br J Ophthalmol 54:781–785, 1970.
66. Hillman JS, Myska V, Nissim S: Complete avulsion of the optic nerve: a clinical, angiographic, and electrodiagnostic study. Br J Ophthalmol 59:503–509, 1975.
67. Friendly DS: Ocular manifestations of physical child abuse. Trans Am Acad Ophthalmol Otolaryngol 75:318–332, 1971.
68. Jensen AD, Smith RE, Olson MI: Ocular clues to child abuse. J Pediatr Ophthalmol Strabismus 8:270–272, 1971.
69. Harley RD: Ocular manifestations of child abuse. J Pediatr Ophthalmol Strabismus 17:5–13, 1980.
70. Kaur B, Taylor D: Fundus hemorrhages in infancy. Surv Ophthalmol 37:1–17, 1992.
71. Eisenbry AB: Retinal hemorrhage in the battered child. Child Brain 5:40–44, 1979.

72. Massicotte SJ, Folberg R, Torczynski E, et al: Vitreoretinal traction and perimacular retinal folds in the eyes of deliberately traumatized children. Ophthalmology 98:1124–1127, 1991.
73. Gass JDM: Stereoscopic Atlas of Macular Diseases: Diagnosis and Treatment, 3rd edition. St Louis, CV Mosby Co, 1987, p 562.
74. Harcourt B, Hopkins D: Permanent chorioretinal lesions in childhood of suspected traumatic origin. Trans Ophthalmol Soc UK 93:199–205, 1973.
75. Giangiacomo J, Khan JA, Levine C, Thompson VM: Sequential cranial computed tomography in infants with retinal hemorrhages. Ophthalmology 95:295–299, 1988.
76. Wilkinson WS, Han DP, Rappley MD, Owings CL: Retinal hemorrhage predicts neurologic injury in the shaken baby syndrome. Arch Ophthalmol 107:1472–1474, 1989.
77. Litten M: Über einige vom allgemein-klinischen Standpunkt aus interessante Augenveranderungen. Berl Klin Wochnschr 18:23–27, 1881.
78. Terson A: De l'hemorrhagie dans la corps vitre au cours de l'hemorragie cerebrale. Clin Ophthalmol 6:309, 1900.
79. Shaw HE Jr, Landers MB III, Sydnor CF: The significance of intraocular hemorrhages due to subarachnoid hemorrhage. Ann Ophthalmol 9:1403–1405, 1977.
80. Gass JDM: Stereoscopic Atlas of Macular Diseases: Diagnosis and Treatment, 3rd edition. St Louis, CV Mosby Co, 1987, p. 560.
81. Schultz PN, Sobol WM, Weingeist TA: Long-term visual outcome in Terson syndrome. Ophthalmology 98:1814–1819, 1991.
82. Keithahn MAZ, Bennett SR, Cameron D, Mieler WF: Retinal folds in Terson syndrome. Ophthalmology 100:1187–1190, 1993.
83. McRae M, Teasell RW, Canny C: Bilateral retinal detachments associated with Terson's syndrome. Retina 14:467–469, 1994.
84. Velikay M, Datlinger P, Stolba U, et al: Retinal detachment with severe proliferative vitreoretinopathy in Terson syndrome. Ophthalmology 101:35–37, 1994.
85. Daubler FH, Marlow SB: A case of hemorrhage into the optic nerve sheaths as a direct extension from a diffuse intrameningeal hemorrhage caused by rupture of aneurysms of a cerebral artery. Arch Ophthalmol 46:553–556, 1917.
86. Miller AJ, Cuttino JT: On the mechanism of massive preretinal hemorrhage following rupture of a congenital medial-defect intracranial aneurysm. Am J Ophthalmol 31:15–24, 1948.
87. Clarkson JG, Flynn HW Jr, Daily MJ: Vitrectomy in Terson's syndrome. Am J Ophthalmol 90:549–552, 1980.
88. Gass JDM: Stereoscopic Atlas of Macular Diseases: Diagnosis and Treatment, 3rd edition. St Louis, CV Mosby Co, 1987, p 558.
89. Sanders RJ, Brown GC, Brown A, Gerner EW: Purtscher's retinopathy preceding acute pancreatitis. Ann Ophthalmol 24:19–21, 1992.
90. Stoumbos VD, Klein ML, Goodman S: Purtscher's-like retinopathy in chronic renal failure. Ophthalmology 99:1833–1839, 1992.
91. Kozlowski JM, Peters AL: Purtscher's-like retinopathy associated with a cardiac aneurysm. Arch Ophthalmol 110:880–881, 1992.
92. Blodi BA, Johnson MW, Gass JDM, et al: Purtscher's-like retinopathy after childbirth. Ophthalmology 97:1654–1659, 1990.
93. Burton TC: Unilateral Purtscher's retinopathy. Ophthalmology 87:1096–1105, 1980.
94. Inkeles DK, Walsh JB: Retinal fat emboli as a sequela to acute pancreatitis. Am J Ophthalmol 80:935–938, 1975.
95. Jacob HS, Craddock PR, Hammerschmidt DE, Moldow CF: Complement-induced granulocyte aggregation: an unsuspected mechanism of disease. N Engl J Med 302:789–794, 1980.
96. Ashton N, Henkind P: Experimental occlusion of retinal arterioles (using graded ballotini). Br J Ophthalmol 49:225–234, 1965.
97. Behrens-Baumann W, Scheurer G, Schroer H: Pathogenesis of Purtscher's retinopathy: an experimental study. Graefes Arch Clin Exp Ophthalmol 230:286–291, 1992.
98. Beck JP, Collins JA: Theoretical and clinical aspects of posttraumatic fat embolism syndrome. In Calandruccio RA (ed): American Academy of Orthopaedic Surgeons Instruction Course Lectures, Vol 22. St Louis, CV Mosby Co, 1973, pp 38–87.
99. Blake J: Ocular embolism. Trans Ophthalmol Soc UK 95:88–93, 1975.
100. Evans JJ: Cerebral fat embolism with recovery and involvement of the central retinal artery. Br J Ophthalmol 24:613–616, 1940.
101. Adams CBT: The retinal manifestations of fat embolism. Br J Accident Surg 2:221–224, 1971.
102. Chuang EL, Miller FS, Kalina RE: Retinal lesions following long bone fractures. Ophthalmology 92:370–374, 1985.
103. Gass JDM: Stereoscopic Atlas of Macular Diseases: Diagnosis and Treatment, 3rd edition. St Louis, CV Mosby Co, 1987, p 564.
104. Duane TD: Valsalva hemorrhagic retinopathy. Trans Am Ophthalmol Soc 70:298–313, 1972.
105. Friberg TR, Braunstein RA, Bressler NM: Sudden visual loss associated with sexual activity. Arch Ophthalmol 111:738–742, 1995.
106. Tassignon MJ, Stempels N, Mulders LV: Retrohyaloid premacular hemorrhage treated by Q-switched Nd-YAG laser. Graefes Arch Clin Exp Ophthalmol 227:440–442, 1989.
107. Pruett RC, Carvalho AC, Trempe CL: Microhemorrhagic maculopathy. Arch Ophthalmol 99:425–432, 1981.
108. Pitta CG, Steinert RF, Gragoudas ES, Regan CD: Small unilateral foveal hemorrhages in young adults. Am J Ophthalmol 89:96–102, 1980.
109. Goldberg MF, Pollock IP, Green WR: Familial retinal arteriolar tortuosity with retinal hemorrhage. Ophthalmology 73:183–191, 1972.
110. Kelley JS, Hoover RE, George T: Whiplash maculopathy. Arch Ophthalmol 96:834–835, 1978.
111. Gass JDM: Stereoscopic Atlas of Macular Diseases: Diagnosis and Treatment, 3rd edition. St Louis, CV Mosby Co, 1987, p 570.
112. Blodi CF, Heilskov TW: Retinal injuries following bungee jumping. Presented at the Macula Society 16th Annual Meeting, Naples, FL, 1993.
113. Burke JP, Orton HP, Strachan IM, et al: Whiplash and its effect on the visual system. Graefes Arch Clin Exp Ophthalmol 230:335–339, 1992.
114. Rice TA, Weidenthal DT, Zgrabik M: Retinal injury from bungee jumping presented at the Retina Society 25th Annual Scientific Meeting, New York, NY, 1992.

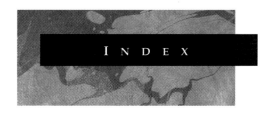

INDEX

Note: Page numbers in *italics* refer to illustrations; page numbers followed by t refer to tables.

Abducens palsy, from cryptococcosis, 781
Abetalipoproteinemia, angioid streaks in, 170t
  manifestations of, 169t
  retinitis pigmentosa and, 906, *907*
Acetaminophen, retinal folds from, 265
Acetazolamide, for cystoid macular edema, 247t
Achromatopsia, congenital, 942, *943*, 943t, *944*
Acquired immunodeficiency syndrome (AIDS). See *Human immunodeficiency virus (HIV) infection.*
Acute idiopathic blind spot enlargement (AIBSE), 590
  acute macular neuroretinopathy and, 595
  choroiditis and, 143
Acute lymphocytic leukemia, 1194–1195
  diagnosis of, 1496
Acute macular neuroretinopathy, 593–596. See also *Macular neuroretinopathy, acute.*
Acute multifocal posterior placoid pigment epitheliopathy, 535–551
  clinical presentation of, 537, 539
  differential diagnosis of, 550, 567, 589, 598
    from DUSN, 809, 811
    from intraocular lymphomas, 1207
    from serpiginous choroiditis, 558, 560
  electrophysiologic testing in, 539, 545
  etiology of, 547–549
  fluorescein angiography of, 537, *538–547*, 539, 549–550
  hypersensitivity reactions and, 548
    delayed-type, 548–549
  hypofluorescence in, 35, 537, *538–546*
  indocyanine green angiography of, 537, 539, *539*
  infections and, 547–548
  ocular associations with, 545
  pathophysiology of, 549–550
  prognosis for, 550
  systemic associations with, 547
  treatment of, 550
  visual fields in, 539, 545
  white ocular lesions in, 617t
Acute myelogenous leukemia, 1195
Acute retinal necrosis. See *Chorioretinitis, sclopetaria.*
Acute retinal necrosis (ARN) syndrome, 749–755, 760–764. See also *Progressive outer retinal necrosis (PORN).*
  anterior segment in, 750, *750*
  anti-inflammatory therapy for, 754, 764
  antithrombotic therapy for, 754, 764
  antiviral therapy for, 754, 763

Acute retinal necrosis (ARN) syndrome (*Continued*)
  characteristics of, 749
  clinical features of, 750, 760–763
  complications of, 753
  diagnosis of, 752–753
  differential diagnosis of, 752–753, 753t, 762, 763
    from cryptococcosis, 783
    from intermediate uveitis, 606
    from progressive outer retinal necrosis, 766, 767t, 769
    from toxoplasmosis, 681–682
  epidemiology of, 749–750
  etiology of, 752–753
  histopathological features of, 753, 761
  in HIV infected, 731–732, 734, 1483–1484
  laser photocoagulation for, 754–755
  necrotizing retinitis in, 760, *762*
  optic neuropathy in, 762
  posterior segment in, 750, *751, 752*
  retinal detachments in, 749, 753, 762–763, *763*, 1483–1484
    prophylaxis for, 754–755, 764
  retinal vasculitis in, 762
  scleral buckling for, 755, 763, 764
  treatment of, 753–755, 763–764
  vitrectomy for, 755
  vitritis in, 762
  white ocular lesions in, 616t
Acute zonal occult outer retinopathy (AZOOR), acute macular neuroretinopathy and, 595
  differential diagnosis of, from MEWDS, 590
Acyclovir, for acute retinal necrosis, 750, 763
  for cytomegalovirus prophylaxis, 726
  for progressive outer retinal necrosis, 757–758
  for serpiginous choroiditis, 562, 563
  for varicella-zoster virus, 734, 769–770
    resistance to, 769
Adenocarcinoma, of retinal pigment epithelium, 1120–1122
  clinical features of, 1120, *1121*
  diagnosis of, 1120–1121, *1121, 1122*
  differential diagnosis of, from combined hamartoma of retina and RPE, 1128
    from uveal melanoma, 1075t, 1079, *1079*
  histopathological features of, 1120, *1121*
  management of, 1121–1122, *1122*
Adenoma, of retinal pigment epithelium, 1120–1122
  clinical features of, 1120, *1121*
  diagnosis of, 1120–1121, *1121, 1122*

Adenoma (*Continued*)
  differential diagnosis of, from combined hamartoma of retina and RPE, 1128
    from uveal melanoma, 1075t, 1079, *1079*
  histopathological features of, 1120, *1121*
  management of, 1121–1122, *1122*
Adenoviruses, acute multifocal posterior placoid pigment epitheliopathy and, 547–548
Adult T-cell leukemia/lymphoma, intraocular involvement in, 1212
Afferent pupillary defect, in optic nerve melanocytoma, 1188
  in traumatic injuries, 1376
Age-related extramacular degeneration, differential diagnosis of, from uveal melanoma, 1075t, 1080, *1080*
Age-related macular degeneration (AMD). See *Macular degeneration, age-related.*
Age-related maculopathy (ARM). See *Maculopathy, age-related.*
Aging, cobblestone degeneration in, 17–18
  cystic degeneration of retina in, 14–15, *15*
  ocular changes with, 10–18
  of ganglion cells, 11
  of macula, 10–11
  of RPE, 11–14
  retinoschisis in, 15–17, *16*
AIDS. See *Human immunodeficiency virus (HIV) infection.*
Air travel, contraindicated, after intraocular gas use, 1328
Air-bag related ocular injuries, 833
Air-gas exchange, in vitrectomy, 1310–1311
Alagille syndrome, 931
  chorioretinal folds in, 263, 931
Åland Island eye disease, 935t, 936
Alaria mesocercaria, 821, 825, *826*, 827
  differential diagnosis of, *814*
Albinism, ocular, salt-and-pepper retinopathy in, 964t
  retinitis pigmentosa and, 905t
Alport's syndrome, 930
  Coats' disease and, 393
  retinal pisciform flecks in, 930, *931*
Alzheimer's disease, ganglion cell aging in, 11
Amacrine cells, 8
Amaurosis fugax, central retinal artery obstruction and, 271
  in ocular ischemic syndrome, 373
Amikacin, for endophthalmitis, 1390, 1402, 1468, 1468t

Aminocaproic acid, for hyphema, 1379
Aminoglycoside toxicity, differential diagnosis of, from central retinal artery/vein occlusion, 280, 280t
4-Aminoquinoline retinopathy, differential diagnosis of, from retinitis pigmentosa, 910–911, *912*
AMN. See *Macular neuroretinopathy, acute.*
Amniotic fluid embolism, in pregnancy, 509
Amphotericin B, adverse effects of, 777
    for blastomycosis, 786
    for candidiasis, 776
    for coccidioidomycosis, 780–781
    for cryptococcosis, 740, 783–784
    for endophthalmitis, 1473, 1474
AMPPPE. See *Acute multifocal posterior placoid pigment epitheliopathy.*
Amsler grid, for age-related macular degeneration, 96
Amyloidosis, differential diagnosis of, intermediate uveitis, 606
Ancylostoma caninum, 806, 807
Anemia, retinopathy of, differential diagnosis of, from bone marrow transplantation retinopathy, 494
Anesthesia, for vitrectomy, 1300–1301
Angioedema, acute multifocal posterior placoid pigment epitheliopathy and, 547
Angiogenesis, 122
    biology of, 122–123
Angioid streaks, 142, *142, 143*, 163–175
    choroidal neovascularization and, 142, *166, 171, 172, 173, 175*
        treatment results for, 1452, *1453*
    clinical signs of, 165–167
    complications of, 173
    differential diagnosis of, from age-related macular degeneration, 96
        from serpiginous choroiditis, 562
    evolution of, 173
    fluorescein angiography in, *165, 166, 167*
    fundus examination in, 165, *166, 167*
    histopathological features of, 163, 164
    in abetalipoproteinemia, 170t
    in Ehlers-Danlos disease, 169t
    in hereditary spherocytosis, 169t
    in Paget's disease, 163, 169t, 173
    in pseudoxanthoma elasticum, 168, 169t, 170–173
    in sickle cell retinopathy, 142, *142*, 163, 169t, 173, 445, *445*
    in thalassemia, 169t
    indocyanine green angiography in, 166, *167*, 168
    management and treatment of, *171*, 174–175, *175*
    natural history of, 174
    posttraumatic Bruch's membrane ruptures and, *163, 165, 173*, 174
    risk factors for, 174
    surgery for, 142
    symptoms of, 165, *165*
    systemic diseases associated with, 167–173, 169t–170t
Angiomatosis retinae (von Hippel's lesion). See also *von Hippel-Lindau disease.*
    differential diagnosis of, from Coats' disease, 394
Angiostatin, 124
Angiostrongyliasis, intraocular, 817–819, *820–821*

Angiostrongylus cantonensis, 817
Angiotensin II, hypertensive optic neuropathy and, 368
Angiotrophic large cell lymphoma (ALCL), intraocular involvement in, 1212
Angle pick, for subretinal surgery, 132, *133*
Anterior chamber associated immune deviation (ACAID), cystoid macular edema and, 246
Anterior hyaloidal fibrovascular proliferation, postoperative, 1315
Anterior ischemic optic neuropathy, cilioretinal artery occlusion and, 281
    differential diagnosis of, from Leber's idiopathic optic neuroretinitis, 887
    radiation retinopathy and, 481
Anterior segment changes, in bone marrow transplantation, 488, 489t
Antiangiogenic therapy, for choroidal neovascularization, 122–124
Antibiotics. See also individual drugs.
    for endophthalmitis, intraocular, 1467–1468, 1468t
        periocular, 1468t, 1470–1471
        prophylactic, 1474–1475
        systemic, 1468t, 1470
        topical, 1468t, 1471
        with and without vitrectomy, 1469, 1469t
    ocular disorders from, 864
Antibody testing, vitrectomy samples for, 1487–1488, 1491
Anticardiolipin antibody (ACA), ocular manifestations of, 465
Anticoagulant therapy, for central retinal vein occlusion, 295
Antifibrinolytic agents, for retinal artery occlusion, 278
Antifungal agents. See specific agents and infections.
Antihelminthic agents. See also individual agents.
    for toxocariasis, 707
Anti-inflammatory drugs, for acute retinal necrosis, 750, 764
    nonsteroidal, for cystoid macular edema, 245, 248
        for posterior scleritis, 640
Antimetabolite agents, for intermediate uveitis, 610
Antioxidants, for age-related macular degeneration, 89–91, 848
    protective effect of, 844, 847, 848
Antiphospholipid-protein antibodies (APA), in SLE, 520
    ocular manifestations of, 464–465, *466–467*
Antithrombin III deficiency, 465
Antithrombotic therapy, for acute retinal necrosis, 750, 764
Antituberculous drugs, 804
    for serpiginous choroiditis, 556, 562, 563t
APA syndrome, ocular manifestations of, 464–465, *466–467*
APC resistance, 460. See also *Protein C, resistance to activated.*
Aphakia, retinal detachment and, 1233–1234, 1244
Aqueous humor analysis, for toxoplasmosis, 683t, 685
Arachidonic acid, cystoid macular edema and, 246

Area centralis, of retina, 3
Argon laser, 62
Argon laser photocoagulation. See *Laser photocoagulation.*
Argon laser photocoagulators, 64
Argon-krypton laser photocoagulators, 64
Argyll-Robertson pupils, 795–796
ARN. See *Acute retinal necrosis (ARN).*
Arterial hypertension. See *Hypertension.*
Arteriohepatic dysplasia (Alagille syndrome), 931
    chorioretinal folds in, 263, 931
Arterioles, hypertension and, 347
    retinal, 8
Arteriosclerosis, hypertension and, 347
Ascaridiosis, intraocular, 819–820, *822–824*
Aspergillosis, 786–787
    differential diagnosis of, from candidiasis, 775
    white ocular lesions in, 616t
Aspergillus, endophthalmitis from, 1473–1474
Aspergillus flavus, 786
Aspergillus fumigatus, 786
Aspiration biopsy, fine needle. See *Fine needle aspiration biopsy.*
Asteroid hyalinosis, B-scan ultrasonography of, 50, *50*
Astrocyte-like cells, 8
Astrocytes, 8
Astrocytic hamartoma, 1182–1183
    calcifications in, 1183, *1184, 1185*
    clinical features of, 1182, *1183*
    diagnosis of, 1182–1183, *1184, 1185*
    fluorescein angiography of, 1183, *1184*
    histopathological features of, 1182, *1183, 1184*
    management of, 1183
    ultrasonography of, 1183, *1185*
Atherosclerosis of carotid artery, ocular ischemic syndrome from, 372
Atovaquone, for toxoplasmosis, 689t, 690
Atrophic macular degeneration, 79. See also *Drusen.*
Atrophic maculopathy with hereditary ataxia, bull's eye maculopathy in, 1033t, 1034
Autofluorescence, 36
Autoimmune diseases, 514–533. See also *Rheumatic retinal diseases.*
Autosomal dominant crystalline dystrophy, differential diagnosis of, from Bietti's crystalline dystrophy, 1045
Aversion response, as defense mechanism, 844
Azathioprine, for intermediate uveitis, 610
    for posterior scleritis, 640
    for serpiginous choroiditis, 562
    immunosuppression from, intraocular lymphomas and, 1204

Bacillus, endophthalmitis from, 1390, 1401, 1473
Bacterial infections. See also individual bacteria.
    diagnostic vitrectomy of, 1492–1495
    endophthalmitis from. See also *Endophthalmitis.*
    differential diagnosis of, from candidiasis, 775

Bacterial infections (*Continued*)
  retinitis from, in HIV infection, 741
Balloon buckles, for break localization, 1292, *1294*
  for retinal detachment, 1288–1296
    complications of, 1293
    history of, 1288
    indications for, 1291–1293, *1291–1295*
    pathophysiology of, 1288, *1289*
    results of, 1293, 1296t
    technique of, 1288–1289, *1290*
Band keratitis, in uveitis, 601–604
Bardet-Biedl syndrome, retinitis pigmentosa and, 905
Bartonella henselae, 887
Basal lamina, deposits in, 11–12, *12*, 83, 85
  of RPE, 4
Basal linear deposits, 12, *13*, 83, 85
Basic fibroblast growth factor, choroidal neovascularization and, 123
Bassen-Kornzweig syndrome, retinitis pigmentosa and, 906, *907*
Batten-Mayou disease, bull's eye maculopathy in, 1030, 1033t
  retinitis pigmentosa and, 905–906
Baylisascaris procyonis, 806, 807
BB pellet injuries, 1373, 1376, 1386, 1403
Behçet's disease, 514, 515–517, *517–519*
  differential diagnosis of, from DUSN, 811
    from intermediate uveitis, 606
    from Vogt-Koyanagi-Harada syndrome, 579
  ocular manifestations of, 517, *517–519*
  treatment of, 517
Benign concentric maculopathy, 1025–1035
  color vision in, 1028
  dark adaptation in, 1028
  differential diagnosis of, 1028, 1030–1031, 1033t, 1034
    from atrophic maculopathy with hereditary ataxia, 1033t, 1034
    from central areolar choroidal dystrophy, 1031, 1033t, 1034
    from central areolar pigment epithelial dystrophy, 1031, 1033t
    from chloroquine retinopathy, 1028, 1033t
    from clofazimine retinopathy, 1030, 1033t
    from cone dystrophy, 1030, 1033t
    from dominant drusen, 1031, 1033t
    from dominant slowly progressive macular dystrophy, 1033t, 1034
    from fenestrated sheen macular dystrophy, 1033t, 1034
    from foveomacular pigment epithelial dystrophy, 1034
    from Hallervorden-Spatz syndrome, 1033t, 1034
    from hydroxychloroquine retinopathy, 1030, 1033t
    from Leber's congenital amaurosis, 1033t, 1034
    from pattern dystrophy, 1031, 1033t
    from retinitis pigmentosa, 1031, 1033t
    from Spielmeyer-Vogt (Batten-Mayou) disease, 1030, 1033t
    from Stargardt's disease, 1030–1031, 1033t
    from trichorrhexis nodosa bull's eye, 1033t, 1034

Benign concentric maculopathy (*Continued*)
    from unilateral acute idiopathic maculopathy, 1033t, 1034
  electrophysiology in, 1028
  family pedigree in, 1025, *1026*
  fluorescein angiography of, 1026–1027, *1028–1030*
  history of, 1025
  indocyanine green angiography of, 1027, *1031*
  mode of inheritance of, 1028
  ophthalmoscopic features of, 1026, *1026, 1027*
  pathogenesis of, 1028
  retinal function tests in, 1027–1028, 1032t
  symptoms of, 1026
  visual acuity in, 1027
  visual field in, 1028
Benign reactive lymphoid hyperplasia (BRHL), intraocular, 1214–1215
  diagnosis of, 1215
  differential diagnosis of, 1214, 1214t
Benzoporphyrin derivative-monoacid (BPD-MA), 74
  for choroidal neovascularization, in AMD, 118
Berlin's edema. See *Commotio retinae.*
Best's disease, 989–1004
  associated ocular findings in, 997
  choroidal neovascularization in, 147–148
  differential diagnosis of, *993, 995, 998, 999, 1001, 1002, 1003*
    from central areolar choroidal dystrophy, 956t
    from pattern dystrophy of RPE, 1006
    from serpiginous choroiditis, 561
  electrophysiology of, 997
  epidemiology of, 991
  fluorescein angiography of, *992, 995, 996*, 996–997, *1000*
  genetics of, 989, 991, *991*
  histopathological features of, 990, 1000–1002
  hypofluorescence in, 33
  macular holes and, 223
  management of, 1002, 1004
  natural history of, 991
  ophthalmoscopic findings in, 991–996, *994–1002*
  pattern dystrophy of RPE and, 1007, *1011*
  visual acuity in, 991, *992*
  vitelliform lesions of, 991, *992, 993, 994–996, 998–1000, 1002, 1002*
Betadine solution, in pneumatic retinopexy, 1278
  in vitrectomy, 1301
Bicarbonate, for intraocular irrigation, 1301–1302
Bietti's crystalline dystrophy, 951t, 974–975, 1037–1048
  biomicroscopic findings in, 1038–1039, *1040*
  clinical course of, 974–975
  clinical features of, 974, *975*
  clinical manifestations of, *1038*, 1038–1039, *1039*
  diagnosis of, 1039, 1042–1043
  differential diagnosis of, 1043–1046
    from autosomal dominant crystalline dystrophy, 1045
    from canthaxanthine deposits, 1044
    from cystinosis, 1044

Bietti's crystalline dystrophy (*Continued*)
    from gyrate atrophy, 1045
    from idiopathic juxtafoveolar retinal telangiectasis, 1045
    from oxalosis, 1044
    from Sjögren-Larsson syndrome, 1044–1045
    from talc emboli, 1044
    from tamoxifen retinopathy, 1044
  diffuse type of, 1039
  electrophysiology of, 1043
  epidemiology of, 1037
  etiology and pathogenesis of, 1046, 1048
  fluorescein angiography of, *1038*, 1042, *1042*
  histopathological features of, 975, 1045–1046, *1045–1048*
  history of, 1037
  localized (regional) type of, 1039
  ophthalmoscopic findings in, 1039, *1040–1042*
Bifocal chorioretinal atrophy, hereditary progressive, 975–976
Bilateral pseudoretinitis pigmentosa, 908t, 909–917
Biomicroscopy, in age-related macular degeneration, 96
Biopsies, fine needle aspiration. See *Fine needle aspiration biopsy.*
  in sarcoidosis, 652, *654*, 654t
  vitreous, 1489–1501. See also *Vitrectomy, diagnostic.*
    diluted, 1491, 1491t
    undiluted, 1491, 1491t
Bipolar cells, 7–8
Birdshot retinochoroidopathy, 565–568
  clinical presentation of, 565–566, *566*, 647
  differential diagnosis of, 567
    from AMPPPE, 550
    from intraocular lymphomas, 1207
    from MEWDS, 589
    from sarcoidosis, 655
  electroretinography of, 566–567
  epidemiology of, 565
  fluorescein angiography of, 566, *567*
  history of, 565
  pathogenesis of, 565
  treatment and course of, 567–568
  white ocular lesions in, 617t
Black sunburst, in sickle cell retinopathy, 441–442, *442, 443*
Blastomyces dermatitidis, 784
Blastomycosis, 784–786
  clinical manifestations of, 784–785
  diagnosis of, 786
  differential diagnosis of, from candidiasis, 775
    from coccidioidomycosis, 780
    from cryptococcosis, 783
  histopathological features of, 785–786
  ocular, 784–785, *785*
  systemic manifestations of, 784
  transmission of, 784
  treatment of, 786
Blepharitis, from syphilis, 795
Blessing-Iwanoff cysts, 15, *15*
Blink response, as defense mechanism, 844
Blocked fluorescence, causes of, 31t, 32
Blood flow, autoregulation of, 346–347
  breakdown of, *346*, 346–347
Blood removal, in vitrectomy, 1311
Blood-ocular barrier, 5, 8, 347
  breakdown of, in cystoid macular edema, 242

Blood-ocular barrier (*Continued*)
  choroid lack of, 347
  optic nerve head lack of, 347
Blood-retinal barrier, 347
  at RPE level, 347
  breakdown of, proliferative vitreoret-
      inopathy and, 1350, 1351
    traumatic, 1374
  in retinal blood vessels, 347
Bone marrow transplantation, anterior
      segment changes in, 489t
  for leukemia, 1202
  ophthalmic complications of, 489t
  posterior segment changes in, 488,
      489t
  radiation retinopathy and, 479
  retinopathy of, 488–496
    clinical features of, 491–492, *492*
    differential diagnosis of, 493–494,
        494t
    epidemiology of, 489–491
    etiology of, 489–491
    fluorescein angiography of, 492–493,
        493
    history of, 488
    pathology of, 493
    prevention of, 495–496
    prognosis for, 494–495, *495*
    risk factors for, 489, 489t
    treatment of, 494–495
Brachytherapy, for choroidal neovascu-
      larization, *128*
  for retinoblastoma, 1146, *1147*
Branch retinal artery occlusion, 277, *278*
  differential diagnosis of, from radiation
      retinopathy, 483
    from syphilis, 795
    from toxoplasmosis, 680
  in protein C deficiency, 462
  in sickle cell retinopathy, 442, *444*
Branch retinal vein occlusion, 308–315
  acute phase of, 308, *310*
  chronic phase of, 308, 310, *310*
  complications of, 310–312
  diagnosis of, 308–310
  differential diagnosis of, from parafo-
      veal telangiectasis, 400, 405
    from postsurgical cystoid macular
        edema, 242–243
    from radiation retinopathy, 483
  fluorescein angiography of, *310*, 310–
      311, *311*, *312*
  from cytomegalovirus, 718, *720*
  from syphilis, 795
  histopathological features of, 309
  in pregnancy, 508
  in serpiginous choroiditis, 556
  iris neovascularization from, 312
  laser management of, 312–314, *314*
    bypass, 315
    for macular edema, 312–314
    for retinal neovascularization, 314,
        314
  macular edema from, 308
    ischemic, *311*, 311–312
    laser management of, 312–314
    perfused, 310–311, *311*
  medical management of, 315
  of hemiretinal vein, 314
  retinal neovascularization from, 312,
      312, *313*
    laser management of, 314, *314*
  traction retinal detachment from, 312
Breast carcinoma, choroidal metastasis
      and, 1104, 1105, 1107, 1108

Bruch's membrane, 3, 4, 83
  aging of, 11
  breaks in, and CNV, 94, *95*, 137, 140,
      142, 144, 145, 196
    angioid streaks and, *164*, *173*, 174
  coccidioidomycosis in, 779, *779*
  diffuse thickening of, 12, *13*
  histoplasmosis and, 138
  staining of, in fluorescein angiography,
      31
  uveal melanoma breaking through,
      1067, *1068*, 1069
B-scan ultrasonography, contact, 47–54,
      69. See also under specific
      disorders.
    clinical, 49–54
    gray scale in, 49
    of asteroid hyalinosis, 50, *50*
    of chorioretinal folds, 257–258
    of choroidal detachment, 52, *52*
    of choroidal malignant melanoma,
        52, 52–53
    of cysticercosis, 712, *712*
    of globe shape, 54, *54*
    of intraocular foreign body, 53–54
    of lens, 49, *49*
    of metastatic tumors, 53, *53*
    of ocular calcification, 53
    of posterior vitreoretinal interface,
        50, *50*
    of retinal detachment, *51*, 51–52
      traction, 51–52, *52*
    of retinal tears, 50, *51*
    of retinoschisis, 51, *51*
    of trauma, 53–54, *54*
    of tumors, *52*, 52–53
    of vitreous opacities, 49–50, *50*
    real time in, 48
    three-dimensional image in, 49
BSS Plus solution, for intraocular irriga-
      tion, 1301–1302
Bull's eye maculopathy, 1028, 1030–1031,
      1033t, 1034
  benign, 1025–1035, *1026–1029*
  differential diagnosis of, 1028, 1030–
      1031, 1033t, 1034
  in adult-onset foveomacular pigment
      epithelial dystrophy, 1033t, 1034
  in atrophic maculopathy with heredi-
      tary ataxia, 1033t, 1034
  in central areolar choroidal dystrophy,
      1031, 1033t, 1034
  in central areolar pigment epithelial
      dystrophy, 1031, 1033t
  in chloroquine retinopathy, 1028,
      1033t
  in clofazimine retinopathy, 1030, 1033t
  in cone dystrophy, 1030, 1033t
  in dominant drusen, 1031, 1033t
  in dominant slowly progressive macu-
      lar dystrophy, 1033t, 1034
  in fenestrated sheen macular dystro-
      phy, 1033t, 1034
  in Hallervorden-Spatz syndrome,
      1033t, 1034
  in hydroxychloroquine retinopathy,
      1030, 1033t
  in Leber's congenital amaurosis, 1033t,
      1034
  in pattern dystrophy, 1031, 1033t
  in retinitis pigmentosa, 1031, 1033t
  in rod monochromatism, 942, *944*, 944
  in Spielmeyer-Vogt (Batten-Mayou)
      disease, 1030, 1033t
  in Stargardt's disease, 1030–1031,
      1033t

Bull's eye maculopathy (*Continued*)
  in trichorrhexis nodosa bull's eye,
      1033t, 1034
  in unilateral acute idiopathic maculo-
      pathy, 1033t, 1034
  trichorrhexis nodosa with, 1033t, 1034
Bungee jumping, ocular disorders from,
      841, *841*
Butterfly dystrophy, 1011

CACD. See *Central areolar choroidal dys-
      trophy (CACD)*.
Calcific emboli, in central retinal artery,
      274, *274*
Calcification, intraocular, conditions fea-
      turing, 1145
Calcium, abnormalities of, and hyperten-
      sion, 348
Candidiasis, 772–777
  clinical manifestations of, 772–775
  differential diagnosis of, from crypto-
      coccosis, 783
    from tuberculosis, 803
  endophthalmitis from, 772–777, 1472,
      1472, 1473–1474
    differential diagnosis of, 775
    in children, 774
    in drug abusers, 774–775
    in pregnancy, 509
  in HIV infection, 740
  ocular, 772–777
    choroiditis from, 774, *774*
    diagnosis of, 775
    histopathological features of, 775–
        776, *776*
    in immunocompromised patients,
        775, *775*
    in leukemia, 1199
    retinitis from, 774, *774*
    symptoms of, 772, 774
    treatment of, 776–777
      response to, 777
    vitrectomy for, 777
    white lesions in, 616t
  transmission of, 772
  treatment of, 776–777
Canthaxanthine deposits, differential di-
      agnosis of, 1044
  ocular disorders from, 864–865, *865*
Capillaries, retinal, 8
Capillary angiomas, hyperfluorescence
      of, 36
Capsulotomy, laser, retinal detachment
      and, 1244
Carbon dioxide therapy, for retinal artery
      occlusion, 277–278
Carbonic anhydrase inhibitors, for cys-
      toid macular edema, 247t, 249,
      251t, 251–252
Cardiac valvular diseases, cotton-wool
      spots in, 282t
Cardiovascular disease. See also
      Hypertension.
  diabetic retinopathy and, 319t
  fundus changes in, 345–369
  ocular ischemic syndrome in, 377
Carmustine, toxicity of, 491
Carotid artery, atherosclerosis of, central
      retinal artery occlusion and, 277
    ocular ischemic syndrome from, 372
  dissection of, ocular ischemic syn-
      drome from, 372
  insufficiency of, central retinal vein oc-
      clusion and, 288

Carotid artery (*Continued*)
  obstruction of, differential diagnosis of, from parafoveal telangiectasis, 405
Carotid endarterectomy, for ocular ischemic syndrome, 377–380
Carotid-cavernous sinus fistulas, central retinal vein occlusion and, 288, 292
Catalase, protective effect of, 844
Cataracts, congenital, differential diagnosis of, from retinoblastoma, 1152t, 1157
  epimacular membranes and, 236
    management of, 234, *234, 235*
  from pneumatic retinopexy, 1284
  from radiation therapy, 129, 129t
  from silicone liquid, 1331
  from vitrectomy, 1316
  in acute retinal necrosis, 763
  in bone marrow transplantation, 488
  in diabetic retinopathy, 1425
  in myotonic dystrophy, 932
  in sarcoidosis, 646
  in Stickler syndrome, 924
  in uveitis, intermediate, 601
  in Vogt-Koyanagi-Harada syndrome, 575, 580–581, *581*
  in X-linked retinoschisis, 1014
  macular hole surgery and, 1437, 1443, *1445*
  phacoemulsification of, 1380
  surgery for, cystoid macular edema after, 238–252. See also *Cystoid macular edema.*
    hyperfluorescence after, 37
    in intermediate uveitis, 611
    macular edema after, differential diagnosis of, intermediate uveitis, 606
    photic injury from, 845
    sympathetic ophthalmia and, 569
    uveal effusion in, 663
  sympathetic ophthalmia and, 572
  traumatic, 1379–1382
    case example of, 1391, 1392
Cat-scratch disease, differential diagnosis of, from Leber's idiopathic optic neuroretinitis, 885, 887
Cavernous hemangiomas, differential diagnosis of, from age-related macular degeneration, 97
  from Coats' disease, 395
Cavernous sinus arteriovenous fistulae, uveal pressure in, 659
Cefazolin, for endophthalmitis, 1470
  for traumatic ocular injuries, prophylactic, 1378
Ceftazidime, for endophthalmitis, 1390, 1402, 1468, 1468t, 1471
Cell-mediated immunity, acquired defects in. See *Human immunodeficiency virus (HIV) infection.*
  in cytomegalovirus, 717
  progressive outer retinal necrosis and, 766
  to toxoplasmosis, 682–683
Central areolar choroidal dystrophy (CACD), 949, 951–955, *952–955*
  bull's eye maculopathy in, 1031, 1033t, 1034
  clinical features of, 956t
  differential diagnosis of, 955t
    from serpiginous choroiditis, 561
  electrophysiology of, 951
  fluorescein angiography of, 951, *951–955*

Central areolar pigment epithelial dystrophy, bull's eye maculopathy in, 1031, 1033t
Central retinal artery occlusion, 271–278
  ancillary studies of, 275, *275, 276*
  background of, 271
  cherry-red spot in, 271, *273*
  clinical features of, 271–275, *273, 274*
  combined with central vein, 278–280, *279*, 280t
    aminoglycoside toxicity versus, 280, 280t
    fluorescein angiography of, 279, *279*
  differential diagnosis of, from radiation retinopathy, 483
  electroretinography in, 275, *276*
  emboli in, 274, *274*
  etiology of, 276–277
  fluorescein angiography of, 275, *275*
  from congenital retinal arteriovenous communications, 1172
  from pneumatic retinopexy, 1282
  from syphilis, 795
  histopathological features of, 272
  hypertension and, 276
  hypofluorescence in, *34, 35*
  in sickle cell retinopathy, 442, *444*
  rubeosis iridis and, 271, 274–275
  systemic associations with, 276t–277t, 276–277
  treatment of, 277–278
  visual acuity in, 273
  visual field studies in, 275
Central retinal vein occlusion, 286–296
  cilioretinal artery occlusion and, 280, *281*
  clinical appearance of, 286
  clinical types of, 288–289
  combined with central artery, 278–280, *279*, 280t
  definition of, 286
  differential diagnosis of, from ocular ischemic syndrome, 377, 380t
    from radiation retinopathy, 483
    from shaken baby syndrome, 838
  electroretinopathy of, 294–295
  epidemiology of, 286, 288
  etiology of, 288
  fluorescein angiography of, 293–294
  from oral contraceptives, 863, *863*
  from syphilis, 795
  from tuberculosis, 802
  histopathological features of, 287, 289–292
  in leukemia, 1197t, 1198
  in pregnancy, 508
  in protein C deficiency, *461–463, 462, 463*
  in the young, 288
  initial assessment of, 293, 305
  iris and angle neovascularization in, 286, 292, 299–306, 302t, 303t, *304*
  ischemic, 288, *289–291*
  management of, 295, 305–306
    medical, 295–296
    study of, 299–306
  natural course of, 295
  natural history of, study of, 299–306
  nonischemic, 288–289, *292–294*
  pathophysiology of, 289–292
  predisposing factors for, 288
  prognosis for, 295, 305
  relative afferent pupillary defect in, 288, 292, 293
  slit lamp examination in, 293

Central retinal vein occlusion (*Continued*)
  symptoms of, 292–295
  visual acuity in, 299–306
Central senile areolar choroidal atrophy. See *Central areolar choroidal dystrophy (CACD).*
Cerebroretinal vasculopathy, 405
Ceroid lipofuscinosis, neuronal, 902
C_2F_6 gas, for retinopexy, 1279
Chalcosis, from intraocular foreign bodies, 1402
Chemoreduction, for retinoblastoma, *1148*, 1149
Chemotherapy. See also specific agents.
  bone marrow transplantation retinopathy and, 491
  for choroidal metastasis, 1108, *1108*
  for retinoblastoma, 1148
  immunosuppression from, intraocular lymphomas and, 1204
  ocular disorders from, 868
  radiation retinopathy and, 479
Chemothermotherapy, for retinoblastoma, *1148*, 1148–1149
Cherry-red spot, in central retinal artery obstruction, 271, *273*
  in ocular ischemic syndrome, 372, 375
  in progressive outer retinal necrosis, 767, *769*
Child abuse, shaken baby syndrome and, 838–839
Childhood-onset retinitis pigmentosa, 901–903
Chlorambucil, ocular disorders from, 868
Chloroaluminum sulfonated phthalocyanine (CASPc), 74
Chloroquine, maculopathy from, bull's eye, 1028, 1033t
  in SLE, 525–527, *526*
  ocular disorders from, 856, 858–860, *860–861*
    differential diagnosis of, from retinitis pigmentosa, 910, *912*
    electrophysiology of, *861*, 861
Chlorpheniramine, retinal folds from, 265
Chlorpromazine, ocular disorders from, 858, *859*
  differential diagnosis of, from retinitis pigmentosa, 909
Cholesterol emboli, in central retinal artery, 274, *274*
  in ocular ischemic syndrome, 375
Chondroitinase, for proliferative vitreoretinopathy, 1366
Choriocapillaris, 8, 83
  atrophy of, in choroidal dystrophies, 949
  degeneration of, in Wagner's syndrome, 926, *936*
  lack of blood-ocular barrier in, 347
  multifocal, differential diagnosis of, from AMPPPE, 550
  occlusion of, DIC and, 475
Chorioretinal atrophy, hyperfluorescence in, 38, *38*
  in serpiginous choroiditis, 555, 556
  in Stickler syndrome, 924
  progressive bifocal, hereditary, 975–976
Chorioretinal degeneration, cobblestone, 17–18, *18*
Chorioretinal disorder(s), hereditary, 889–1049. See also individual disorders.
  Alagille syndrome as, 931

Chorioretinal disorder(s) (*Continued*)
  Alport's syndrome as, 930
  benign concentric maculopathy as, 1025–1035
  Best's disease as, 989–1004
  Bietti's crystalline dystrophy as, 974, 975, 1037–1048
  choroidal dystrophy(ies) as, 949–976
    Bietti's crystalline dystrophy as, 974–975, 1037, 1048
    central areolar, 951–955
    choroideremia as, 956, 958, 960
    classification of, 949–951, 951t
    generalized, 956
    gyrate atrophy as, 960, 964, 973–974
    pericapillary, 955–956
    progressive bifocal chorioretinal atrophy as, 975–976
  cone dystrophies as, 942–947
    cone monochromatism in, 942–943
    progressive, 943–946
    rod monochromatism in, 942
  congenital stationary night blindness as, 934–940
  fundus flavimaculatus as, 978–987
  lysosomal storage disorders as, 927–930
  myotonic dystrophy as, 930–931
  pattern dystrophy of RPE as, 1006–1011
  retinitis pigmentosa as, 891–920
    atypical, 896–904
    differential diagnosis of, 908t, 908–917
    molecular genetics of, 917t, 917–920, 918t
    systemic diseases associated with, 904–908
    typical, 891–896
  Stargardt's disease as, 978–987
  vitreoretinal degenerations, 924–927
  X-linked retinoschisis as, 1013–1017
Chorioretinal folds, 256–263
  bilateral, 260t
  causes of, 259–263, 260t, 264t
  clinical evaluation of, 256, *257–258*
  fluorescein angiography of, 256–257, *257*
  in choroidal neovascularization, 150, 261–262
  in hyperopia, 260–261
  in hypotony, 262–263
  in optic disc swelling, 261
  in orbital masses and inflammation, 259–260, *261*
  in posterior scleritis, 262
  in Vogt-Koyanagi-Harada syndrome, 574, *575*
  mechanisms of, 258–259
  ultrasonography of, 257–258
  unilateral, 260t
Chorioretinal granuloma, differential diagnosis of, from uveal melanoma, 1075t, 1081
Chorioretinal heat conduction, 63
Chorioretinal light absorption, 62
Chorioretinal neovascularization, from laser photocoagulation, for diabetic retinopathy, 1420–1421
Chorioretinal rupture, traumatic, 833–834, *835, 1389,* 1389–1390
Chorioretinal scars, from coccidioidomycosis, 779, *780*
  from toxoplasmosis, *678,* 679

Chorioretinitis, differential diagnosis of, from retinitis pigmentosa, 909, *910, 911*
  from cryptococcosis, 782, *782*
  from toxoplasmosis, 675, 677
  in coccidioidomycosis, 778–779
  in Leber's idiopathic optic neuroretinitis, 886
  in sarcoidosis, 646t, 646–647, *647*
  in syphilis, 795, *796, 797*
  multifocal, differential diagnosis of, 589–590
  sclopetaria, 833–834, *835, 1389,* 1389–1390
    management of, 1389
  striata, 553
Chorioretinopathy. See also *Choroiditis.*
  central serous, 206–213
    acute retinal pigment epitheliitis and, 597, 598
    choroidal neovascularization in, 150
    clinical course of, 209–210
    clinical examination for, 206–208, *207,* 207t, *208*
    clinical history of, 206
    complications of, 209
    demography of, 206
    differential diagnosis of, 208–209, 209t
      from age-related macular degeneration, 97
      from choroidal metastasis, 1105
      from macular holes, 222
      from posterior scleritis, 637
      from Vogt-Koyanagi-Harada syndrome, 579
    electrophysiologic studies of, 212
    fluorescein angiography of, *210,* 210–211
      for location of leakages, 210–211
      for number of leakages, 211
      for types of leakages, 210, *210*
    histopathology of, 213
    in older adults, 209
    in pregnancy, 498–500, *499*
    in systemic lupus erythematosus, 520, *521–523*
    in women, 210
    indocyanine green angiography of, 45, *45, 211,* 211–212
    natural history of, 209–210
    optical coherence tomography of, 72, 212
    pathogenesis of, 212–213, 213t
    recurrent, 209
    senile (degenerative) retinoschisis and, 1240–1241
    treatment of, 213
    type I, 206
    type II, 206
    from *Pneumocystis carinii,* 738, *738,* 739
    hypertensive, 348, 360–369
    punctate inner. See *Punctate inner choroidopathy.*
Choriovitreal neovascularization, from laser photocoagulation, for diabetic retinopathy, 1420–1421
Choristomas, osseous, 1097
Choroid, 83
  lack of blood-ocular barrier in, 347
Choroid white lesions, diseases manifesting, 616t–617t
Choroidal abnormalities, in myopia, degenerative, 192, *193*

Choroidal detachment, after scleral buckling for retinal detachment, 1268, *1268*
  differential diagnosis of, from uveal melanoma, 1075t, 1081
  hemorrhagic, differential diagnosis of, 667
  retinal detachment and, pneumatic retinopexy for, 1286
  traumatic, case example of, 1392
Choroidal dystrophy(ies), hereditary, 949–976
  Bietti's crystalline dystrophy as, 974–975
  central areolar, 951–955
  choroideremia as, 956, 958, 960
  classification of, 949–951, 951t
  fluorescein angiography of, 949
  generalized, 956, *961–963*
    differential diagnosis of, 956
    histopathological features of, 956
  gyrate atrophy as, 960, 964, 973–974
  pericapillary, 955–956
  progressive bifocal chorioretinal atrophy as, 975–976
Choroidal flush, in fluorescein angiography, 31
Choroidal granulomas, differential diagnosis of, from choroidal metastasis, 1103
  from coccidioidomycosis, 780
Choroidal hemangioma, 1083–1090
  B-scan ultrasonography of, 53
  circumscribed, 1083–1088
    clinical features of, 1083, *1084*
    computed tomography of, 1084
    diagnosis of, 1083, *1085, 1086*
    differential diagnosis of, from choroidal osteoma, 1095
      from uveal melanoma, 1075t, 1076, *1076*
    fluorescein angiography of, 1083, *1085*
    histopathological features of, 1084, *1087*
    indocyanine green angiography of, 1083, *1086*
    laser photocoagulation for, 1087, *1088*
    magnetic resonance imaging of, 1084, *1087*
    radiation therapy for, 1088, *1088*
    radioactive phosphorus uptake test for, 1084
    treatment of, 1084, 1087–1088, *1088*
    ultrasonography of, 1084, *1086*
  differential diagnosis of, from choroidal metastasis, 1103, 1105
    from intraocular benign reactive lymphoid hyperplasia, 1214
  diffuse, 1088–1090
    clinical features of, 1088–1089, *1089*
    diagnosis of, 1090
    differential diagnosis of, 1088
    histopathological features of, 1090
    laser photocoagulation for, 1090
    radiation therapy for, 1090
    treatment of, 1090
    ultrasonography of, 1090
  hyperfluorescence of, *35, 35,* 36, 37
  in pregnancy, 505
  radiation therapy for, 127
Choroidal hemorrhage, in scleral buckling, 1263
  in subfoveal surgery, 157
  perfluorocarbon liquids for, 1323

Choroidal hypofluorescence, causes of, 31t, *32*, 32–33
  in acute multifocal posterior placoid pigment epitheliopathy, 549
Choroidal infarction, DIC and, 475
Choroidal infiltration, in leukemia, 1197t, 1199
Choroidal melanocytic nevus, neovascularization in, 150
Choroidal melanoma, 1067–1072. See also *Ciliary body melanoma; Uveal melanoma.*
  B-scan ultrasonography of, *52*, 52–53
  choroidal nevus evolving into, 1056
  clinical features of, 1067, *1068*
  diagnosis of, 1067–1070, *1070*, *1071*
  differential diagnosis of, 1074–1082
    from choroidal metastasis, 1103, 1105, 1106
    from choroidal nevus, 1055
    from choroidal osteoma, 1095
    from combined hamartoma of retina and RPE, 1128
    from congenital hypertrophy of RPE, 1058–1059
    from retinal capillary hemangioma, 1160
    from vasoproliferative tumors, 1175, 1176
  fluorescein angiography of, 1067–1069, *1070*
  hyperfluorescence of, *35*, 37
  juxtapapillary, differential diagnosis of, from optic nerve melanocytoma, 1189
  management of, 1070–1072
  mushroom-shaped, 1067, *1068*, 1069, *1071*, 1106
  pathology of, 1067, *1069*, *1070*
  three-dimensional ultrasonography for, 57–58
Choroidal metastasis, 1103–1108
  chemotherapy for, 1108, *1108*
  computed tomography of, 1106
  diagnosis of, 1106–1107
  differential diagnosis of, 1103, 1105–1106
    from choroidal osteoma, 1095
  fine needle aspiration biopsy of, 1106–1107
  incidence of, 1103–1104
  indocyanine green angiography of, 1106
  management of, 1107–1108
  medical history and, 1104
  physical findings in, *1104*, 1104–1105, *1105*
  prognosis for, 1107
  radiation therapy for, *1107*, 1107–1108
  symptoms of, 1104
Choroidal neovascular membrane, in choroidal osteoma, 1095
  laser photocoagulation for, 1101
Choroidal neovascularization (CNV), 79, 137–158, 1449–1457. See also *Macular degeneration, age-related, neovascular.*
  angiogenesis inhibition in, 123–124
  angioid streaks and, 142, *142, 143*, 166, *171, 172, 173, 175*
    treatment results for, 1452, *1453*
  chorioretinal folds in, 150, 261–262
  choroidal osteoma and, 145, 147, *150, 151*
  choroidal rupture and, 145, *149*, 835
  differential diagnosis of, from postsurgical cystoid macular edema, 243

Choroidal neovascularization (*Continued*)
  geographic atrophy and, 89
  hemorrhage from, in age-related macular degeneration, 103
  hereditary dystrophies and, 147–148
  histopathology of, 137
  histoplasmosis and, 138–140, *139*, 178, 180, 183
    surgical treatment of, 1449, 1450, *1450, 1453*
  hyperfluorescence in, *36, 37*
  idiopathic, 140
    surgical treatment results in, 1451, *1451, 1453*
  idiopathic juxtafoveal telangiectasis and, 149, 153–154
  idiopathic polypoid choroidal vasculopathy and, 148, *152*
  in age-related macular degeneration, 94–119
    angiography obscuring, 98, 101, *101, 102*
    classic, 98, *98*
    fading, *102*, 104
    feeder vessels and, *102*, 104, 105
    laser photocoagulation for, 108t, 108–116, 111t
      extrafoveal, 108t, 110, 111t
      juxtafoveal, 108t, 110–112, 111t
      recurrent, 108t, 111t, 116, 117
      subfoveal, 108t, 111t, 112–115
    occult, 98, *99, 100*
    pathogenesis of, 94, 96
    radiation therapy for, 126–130
    risk of fellow eye developing, 116
    surgical treatment results for, *1450*, 1450–1451, *1451, 1453*
  in central serous chorioretinopathy, 209
  in pregnancy, 500
  in sickle cell retinopathy, 442, *443*, 443
  in Vogt-Koyanagi-Harada syndrome, 578, 580, *581*
  indocyanine green angiography of, 39–42, *41–43*, 44–45, 150–151
  infections and, 147
  investigational therapies for, 157–158
  laser treatment of, *137–138*, 150, *151*–157, 155, 156
  macular holes and, 223
  mechanisms of, 123
  multifocal choroiditis and, 142–144, *144, 145*
    surgical treatment for, *1451*, 1451–1452, *1453*
  myopia and, 140–142, *141*, 196–203
    clinical signs of, 196–197, *198, 199*
    fluorescein angiography of, 197–198
    ICG angiography of, 198, *198*
    natural history of, 198
    treatment of, 198–199, *201–203*, 203
    results of, 1452, *1452, 1453*
  optical coherence tomography of, 72–73
  radiation therapy for, 126–130
    adverse effects of, 129t, 129–130
      acute, 129, 129t
      late, 129t, 130
    brachytherapy, 128–129
    characteristics of, 127, *127, 128*
    external beam photon, 128–129
    methods of, 128
    theory of, 126–127
  recurrent, management of, 1453
    prevention of, 1457
  serpiginous choroiditis and, 144, *146*–148

Choroidal neovascularization (*Continued*)
  subfoveal surgery for, 157, 1449–1457
    complications of, 1452–1453
    for recurrence, 1453
    future directions for, 1454, 1456
    patient selection for, *1454*
    results of, 1449–1452, 1450t, *1450–1452*
      interpretation of, *1453*, 1453–1454, *1454*
  subretinal surgery for, *133*, 133–134, *134*
  toxoplasmosis and, 680
  type I, 137
  type II, 137
  underlying disorders in, 1450t
Choroidal nevus, 1053–1057
  amelanocytic, 1053, *1054*
  clinical features of, 1053, *1054*, 1055, *1055*
  diagnosis of, 1055–1056
  differential diagnosis of, 1055
    from choroidal osteoma, 1095
    from combined hamartoma of retina and RPE, 1128
    from congenital hypertrophy of RPE, 1058
    from optic nerve melanocytoma, 1189
    from uveal melanoma, 1074, 1075t, 1076, *1076*
  fluorescein angiography of, 1053, 1055–1056, *1056*
  histopathological features of, 1055, *1055*
  incidence of, 1053
  laser photocoagulation for, 1057
  management of, 1056–1057
  metastasis of, 1056
  prognosis for, 1057
  ultrasonography of, 1056
Choroidal osteoma, 145, 147, *150, 151*, 1092–1101
  clinical features of, 1092, 1094–1095, *1094–1097*
  computed tomography of, 1100, *1101*
  definition of, 1092
  diagnosis of, 1099–1101
  differential diagnosis of, 1095–1097, *1098*
    from intraocular benign reactive lymphoid hyperplasia, 1214
    from serpiginous choroiditis, 561
    from uveal melanoma, 1075t, 1077, *1077*
  fluorescein angiography of, 1095, *1097*, 1099
  histopathological features of, 1093, 1097
  incidence of, 1092
  indocyanine green angiography of, 1099
  laboratory diagnosis of, 1101
  magnetic resonance imaging of, 1100
  management of, 1101
  pathogenesis of, 1097, 1099
  prognosis for, 1101
  radioactive phosphorus uptake of, 1100–1101
  roentgenography of, 1100
  ultrasonography of, 1100, *1101*
Choroidal rupture, 145, *149*, 834–836, *835*
  differential diagnosis of, from age-related macular degeneration, 96
  direct, 835

Choroidal rupture (*Continued*)
  indirect, 835, *835*
  macular holes and, 833
Choroidal tubercles, 802, 803
Choroidal tumors. See also *Choroidal metastasis* and specific tumors.
  chorioretinal folds in, 263
  differential diagnosis of, from age-related macular degeneration, 97
    from posterior scleritis, 637, 637t
  uveal effusion in, 664
Choroidal vascular defects, hypofluorescence in, 31t, 35
Choroidal vasculature, anatomic and physiologic properties of, 345–348
Choroidal vasculopathy, idiopathic polypoid, 148, *152*
Choroideremia, 956, 958, 960
  clinical features of, 956, 958, *964t*, 965–969
  end stage, 958, *969*
  female carriers of, 958, 960, *970–972*
  histopathological features of, 950, 960
  hypofluorescence in, 35
  molecular genetics of, 960
  simulating gyrate atrophy, 958, *968*
  simulating retinitis pigmentosa, 958, *966–967*
  visual function studies in, 958
Choroiditis. See also *Chorioretinopathy.*
  differential diagnosis of, from toxocariasis, 704, 705t
  from blastomycosis, 784–785, *785*
  from candidiasis, 774, *774*
  from coccidioidomycosis, 778, 779, *779*
  from cryptococcosis, 782
  from diffuse unilateral subacute neuroretinitis, 808
  from tuberculosis, 738, *739*
  multifocal, 142–144
    choroidal neovascularization and, surgical treatment for, *1451*, 1451–1452, *1453*
    differential diagnosis of, from AMPPPE, 550
      from chorioretinopathy, central serous, 208
      from intraocular lymphomas, 1207
      from serpiginous choroiditis, 561
    neovascularization in, 142–144, *144*, *145*
    with panuveitis, 614–621, 628, 629. See also *Multifocal choroiditis with panuveitis.*
  neovascularization in infectious, 147
  serpiginous, differential diagnosis of, from AMPPPE, 550
    neovascularization in, 144, *146–148*
Choroiditis areata, 553
Choroidopathy, geographic. See *Serpiginous choroiditis.*
  helicoid, 956, *958*
  hypertensive. See *Hypertensive choroidopathy.*
  lupus, 35
  punctate inner. See *Punctate inner choroidopathy.*
Chronic lymphocytic leukemia, 1194
Chronic myelogenous leukemia, 1194
CHRPE. See *Retinal pigment epithelium, congenital hypertrophy of.*
Cidofovir, adverse effects of, 726
  for cytomegalovirus, 724, 726, 1482
Ciliary body fibrosis, in acute retinal necrosis, 763

Ciliary body granuloma, from blastomycosis, 784
  from tuberculosis, 802
Ciliary body melanoma. See also *Choroidal melanoma; Uveal melanoma.*
  clinical features of, 1067, *1068*
  diagnosis of, 1067–1070, *1070*, *1071*
  differential diagnosis of, 1074–1082
    from nonpigmented ciliary epithelium tumor, 1130
  management of, 1070–1072
  pathology of, 1067, *1069*, *1070*
Ciliary epithelium tumors, nonpigmented, acquired, 1130–1133
  clinical features of, 1130, *1131*
  diagnosis of, 1131–1132, *1132*
  fluorescein angiography of, 1132, *1132*
  histopathological features of, 1130–1131, *1131*, *1132*
  management of, 1132
  prognosis for, 1133
  ultrasonography of, 1132, *1132*
  differential diagnosis of, from uveal melanoma, 1075t, 1079
Ciliary pigment epithelium (CPE), adenoma of, differential diagnosis of, from nonpigmented ciliary epithelium tumor, 1130
  from uveal melanoma, 1079
  congenital hypertrophy of, differential diagnosis of, from uveal melanoma, 1078, *1079*
  reactive hyperplasia of, differential diagnosis of, from uveal melanoma, 1078–1079
  tumors of, differential diagnosis of, from medulloepithelioma, 1135
Ciliochoroidal detachments, from laser photocoagulation, for diabetic retinopathy, *1420*, 1420–1421
  uveal effusion in, 659, 663, *663*
Ciliochoroidal effusion, 658–667. See also *Uveal effusion.*
Cilioretinal artery, central retinal artery occlusion and, 273, *273*
  occlusion of, 278, *280*, 280–281, *281*
    central retinal vein occlusion and, *280*, 281
    fluorescein angiography of, 280, *281*
Cinchonism, 860
Ciprofloxacin, for endophthalmitis, 1470
Circinate choroidal atrophy, 956, *959–960*
Circumpapillary dysgenesis, of pigment epithelium, 553
Cisplatin, ocular disorders from, 868
  toxicity of, 491
Clindamycin, adverse effects of, 690
  for toxoplasmosis, 688, 689t, 690
    in HIV infected, 735
  for traumatic ocular injuries, prophylactic, 1378
Clinical examination of posterior segment, 21–28
Clofazimine, adverse ocular effects of, 741–742, *742*, 842
  retinopathy from, bull's eye maculopathy in, 1030, 1033t
    differential diagnosis of, from retinitis pigmentosa, 911
  salt-and-pepper, 964t
Clostridiopeptidase, for proliferative vitreoretinopathy, 1366
CME. See *Cystoid macular edema (CME).*

Coats' disease, 390–396
  adult-onset, 392, *392*, 393t
  aggressive pediatric form of, 392–393, *393*
  classification of, 390
  clinical presentation of, 390
  congenital, 392
    differential diagnosis of, 392t
  demographics of, 390
  diagnosis of, 394–395
  differential diagnosis of, 392t, 393t, 394t, 394–395
    from familial exudative vitreoretinopathy, 424, 427t, 428
    from retinal capillary hemangioma, 1160
    from retinoblastoma, 394, 1151–1153, 1152t, *1153*
    from toxocariasis, 704, 705t, 706
  etiology of, 390
  fluorescein angiography of, *393–394*, 394, 1152
  histopathological features of, 391, 395, *395*
  history of, 390
  hyperfluorescence of, *35*, 36
  intraocular calcification in, 1145
  management of, 395–396
  ultrasonography of, 1152–1153
  vasoproliferative ocular fundus tumors and, 1077
  vasoproliferative tumors and, 1175, 1176, 1178t
Cobblestone degeneration, 17–18, *18*
Coccidioides immitis, 777–778
  life cycle of, 777–778, *778*
Coccidioidomycosis, 777–781
  clinical manifestations of, 778
  diagnosis of, 780
  differential diagnosis of, 780
    from cryptococcosis, 783
  endophthalmitis from, 778–779, 1473
  histopathological features of, 780
  ocular, 778–780
    in children, 780
  posterior segment disease from, 778–780, *779*, *780*
  systemic, 778
  treatment of, 780–781
Collagen vascular diseases, cotton-wool spots in, 282t
  differential diagnosis of, from parafoveal telangiectasis, 405
Coloboma, differential diagnosis of, from retinoblastoma, 1152t, 1156, *1156*
  vasoproliferative tumors and, 1175, 1178t
Commotio retinae, 836–837, *837*
  choroidal rupture and, 835
  histopathological features of, 832
  macular holes and, 833, *834*
Complement fixing antibody test, for toxoplasmosis, 683t, 684
Computed tomography (CT), of choroidal hemangioma, circumscribed, 1084
  of choroidal metastasis, 1106
  of choroidal osteoma, 1100, *1101*
  of cysticercosis, 711, *711*
  of intraocular foreign bodies, 1372, 1395–1396, *1396*
  of optic disc drusen, 882, *882*
  of posterior scleritis, 637–638, *640*
  of posterior uveal melanoma, 1069–1070

Computed tomography (*Continued*)
  of retinal capillary hemangioma, 1164
  of retinoblastoma, *1140,* 1144, 1144–
    1145
  of toxocariasis, 704
  of traumatic ocular disorders, 1372
Concentric maculopathy, benign, 1025–
    1035
Cone(s), 7–8
Cone dystrophies, bull's eye maculopa-
    thy in, 1030, 1033t
  hereditary, 942–947
    cone monochromatism in, 942–943
    progressive, 943–946, *945, 947*
      differential diagnosis of, 987
    rod monochromatism in, 942, *943,*
      943t, 944
  progressive, differential diagnosis of,
    from central areolar choroidal dys-
    trophy, 956t
Cone monochromatism, 942–943
Cone receptors, congenital loss of, 942,
    943, 943t, 944
Congenital disorder(s). See also *Hereditary*
    chorioretinal disorders.
  achromatopsia as, 942, *943, 943t, 944*
  hypertrophy of RPE as, 1058–1063,
    1116–1118
  retinal arteriovenous communications
    (racemose hemangiomas) as,
    1172–1174
  rubella as. See *Rubella.*
  stationary night blindness as, 934–940
  syphilis as, 793, *794.* See also *Syphilis,*
    congenital.
  toxoplasmosis as, 675–676, 676t. See
    also *Toxoplasmosis, congenital.*
Congenital stationary night blindness
    (CSNB), classification of, 934, 935t,
    936
  complete, 936, 937t
  fundus albipunctatus as, 938–940, *939*
  incomplete, 936, 937t
  with abnormal fundus, 937–938, *938,*
    938t, 939
  with normal fundus, 934–937
    classification of, 936, 937t
    histopathological features of, 936
    modes of inheritance of, 934–935
    molecular genetics of, 936–937
    visual function studies in, 935, *935,*
      936, 936t
Conjunctiva, examination of, in trauma,
    1371
Conjunctival bleb, endophthalmitis and,
    1466, *1472,* 1472–1473
Conjunctival hyperemia, in sympathetic
    ophthalmia, 569
Conjunctival sarcoidosis, 646
Conjunctivitis, from coccidioidomycosis,
    778
  from radiation therapy, 129, 129t
Contact lens, for slit lamp ophthalmos-
    copy, 27, 27–28
Cornea, examination of, in trauma, 1371
Cornea angiogenesis inhibitor (CAI),
    122–123
Corneal abnormalities, from vitrectomy,
    for diabetic retinopathy, 1427
Corneal complications, from vitrectomy,
    early, 1314
  late, 1315–1316
Corneal epithelial edema, proliferative
    vitreoretinopathy and, 1355
Corneal graft rejection, from interferon
    alfa, 864

Corneal laceration, traumatic, case exam-
    ple of, 1391, 1392
Corneal lacerations, traumatic, 1373
Corneal opacity, proliferative vitreoreti-
    nopathy and, 1355
Corneal ulceration, in graft-versus-host
    disease, 488
Cortical blindness, in pre-eclampsia, 506
Cortical vitreous, anatomy of, vitrectomy
    and, 1298, *1299*
Corticosteroids, for acute retinal necrosis,
    764
  for angiostrongyliasis, 818
  for Behçet's disease, 517
  for birdshot retinochoroidopathy, 567
  for candidiasis, 777
  for choroiditis, multifocal, with pan-
    uveitis, 619, 621, 623t
    multiple, 143–144
    serpiginous, 144, 562, 563
  for cystoid macular edema, 247t, 247–
    248, 251t, 251–252
  for diffuse subretinal fibrosis syn-
    drome, 626–627
  for endophthalmitis, 1468t, 1471
  for frosted branch angiitis, 431, 436
  for hyphema, 1379
  for intermediate uveitis, 607–609
    oral and intravenous, 608–609
    periocular injections of, 607, 609
    transdermal, 607
  for ophthalmomyiasis, 814
  for posterior scleritis, 639–640
  for punctate inner choroidopathy, 623t,
    623–624
  for sarcoidosis, 655
  for sympathetic ophthalmia, 572
  for toxoplasmosis, 689t, 690
    in immunocompromised host, 691
  for Vogt-Koyanagi-Harada syndrome,
    579
  rheumatic retinal diseases and, 515
Corynebacterium, endophthalmitis from,
    1472
Cotton-wool spots, *281,* 281–283, *282,*
    282t
  central retinal vein occlusion and, 288
  in bone marrow transplantation reti-
    nopathy, 489–494
    resolution of, 494–495, *495*
  in diabetic retinopathy, 322, 331
  in HIV infection, 282, *714, 716,* 716
  in hypertensive retinopathy, 351, 353,
    356–358, *357*
    fluorescein angiography of, 356, *357*
  in leukemia, 1197t, 1197–1198
  in ocular ischemic syndrome, 375
  in radiation retinopathy, 477, 479, 480,
    482, *482*
  in shaken baby syndrome, 838
  in systemic lupus erythematosus, 523–
    525, *524–525*
CPE. See *Ciliary pigment epithelium (CPE).*
Crohn's disease, frosted branch angiitis
    in, 434
Cryopexy, for giant retinal tears, 1340,
    1344, 1347
  for retinal tears, 833
  pneumatic retinopexy and, for retinal
    detachment, 1272, 1278, 1280–1281
Cryotherapy, for cyclodialysis, 1382
  for familial exudative vitreoretinopa-
    thy, 428
  for hemoglobinopathies, 452, *455*
  for intermediate uveitis, 609–610

Cryotherapy (*Continued*)
  for localization of retinal breaks, 1253–
    1254, *1255,* 1261
  for retinal detachment, 1249, 1267
    pneumatic retinopexy and, 1272
  for retinal horseshoe tears, 1265–1266
  for retinoblastoma, 1146
  for retinopathy of prematurity, 411–412
  for vasoproliferative ocular fundus tu-
    mors, 1180
  prophylactic, for fellow eye of giant
    retinal tear, 1346
  uveal effusion after, 661t, 663–664
Cryptococcosis, 739–740, 781–784
  clinical manifestations of, 781–782
  cultures of, 783
  diagnosis of, 783
  differential diagnosis of, from candidi-
    asis, 775
    from coccidioidomycosis, 780
    from tuberculosis, 803
  endophthalmitis from, 782, 1473
  histopathological features of, 783
  in HIV infection, 739–740, *740,* 781
  neurophthalmic, 782
  ocular, 782–783
  of CNS, 781–782, 783
  posterior segment disease from, *782,*
    782–783
  pulmonary, 781, 783
  systemic, 781–782
  transmission of, 781
  treatment of, 783–784
  white ocular lesions in, 616t
Cryptococcus neoformans, 739–740, 781.
    See also *Cryptococcosis.*
Crystalline dystrophy, 951t, 974–975
  of retina and choroid, 949, 951t, 974–
    975, 1037–1048. See also *Bietti's*
    crystalline dystrophy.
Crystalline lens, displaced, perfluorocar-
    bon liquids for removal of, 1323–
    1324
  examination of, in trauma, 1371
  removal of, for giant retinal tears, 1342
  traumatic subluxated and dislocated,
    1376, 1379–1382, *1380, 1381*
Crystalline retinopathy, classification of,
    975t
  differential diagnosis of, 975t
  drug-induced, 857t, 864–867
CSC. See *Chorioretinopathy, central serous*
    (CSC).
CSNB. See *Congenital stationary night*
    blindness (CSNB).
Cultures, vitrectomy samples for, 1487
Cuterebra, 813
CVO. See *Central retinal vein occlusion.*
Cyclodialysis, traumatic, 1382
Cyclopegics, for hyphema, 1379
Cyclopexy, for cyclodialysis, 1382
Cyclophosphamide, for intermediate
    uveitis, 610
  for posterior scleritis, 640
Cyclosporine, bone marrow transplanta-
    tion retinopathy from, 490
    management of, 494
  for birdshot retinochoroidopathy, 567
  for diffuse subretinal fibrosis syn-
    drome, 626
  for intermediate uveitis, 610
  for posterior scleritis, 640
  for serpiginous choroiditis, 562, 563t
  for Vogt-Koyanagi-Harada syndrome,
    580

Cyclosporine (*Continued*)
 immunosuppression from, intraocular
  lymphomas and, 1204
 rheumatic retinal diseases and, 515
Cyst(s), differential diagnosis of, from
  uveal melanoma, 1075t, 1081
 foveal, in cystoid macular edema, 241
 in medulloepithelioma, 1136
 of *Cysticercus cellulosae*, 710
 of pars plana, *1224*, 1224–1225
 traumatic macular, 833
Cystic retinal tufts (CRT), 9, *10*, 1234–
  1237, *1235–1238*, 1244
 clinical features of, 1234–1236, *1235–
  1238*
 histopathological features of, 1234,
  1235
 history of, 1234
 prognosis and management of, 1235
Cysticercosis, 709–713
 differential diagnosis of, from coccidioidomycosis, 780
 histopathological features of, 710, 712,
  713
 history of, 709
 intraocular and adnexal, *711*, 711–712,
  712
 nonocular, 711, *711*
 parasitology of, 709, *711*
 prophylaxis and treatment of, 713
 white ocular lesions in, 616t
Cysticercus cellulosae, 709
 cysts of, 710
Cystinosis, differential diagnosis of, 1044
 ocular disease in, *929*, 929–930
Cystinuria, retinitis pigmentosa and, 905t
Cystoid degeneration, of retina, 14–15,
  15
 peripheral, 1222, *1223*
  reticular, 15, *15*
  typical, 15, *15*
Cystoid macular edema (CME), biomicroscopy of, 240
 chronic, 240
 conditions associated with, 242t
 differential diagnosis of, 242t, 242–244
  from macular holes, 222, 244
 drug-induced, 857t, 862–863
 from epinephrine, 862–863
 from nicotinic acid, 863
 in birdshot retinochoroidopathy, 566
 in central serous chorioretinopathy, 209
 in retinitis pigmentosa, 893, *894*
 in serpiginous choroiditis, 556
 in subretinal fibrosis and uveitis syndrome, 634
 in syphilis, 795
 in uveitis, intermediate, 599, 600, 602,
  605
 in Vogt-Koyanagi-Harada syndrome,
  580
 multifocal choroiditis with panuveitis
  and, 615
 parafoveal telangiectasis and, 398, 403
 postsurgical, 238–252
  angiographic, 238
  carbonic anhydrase inhibitors for,
   249
  classification of, 238, 240
  clinical examination of, *240*, 240–241
  clinical presentation of, 240–241
  clinically significant, 238, 240
  corticosteroids for, 247t, 247–248
  differential diagnosis of, 242t, 242–
   244

Cystoid macular edema (*Continued*)
  from branch retinal vein occlusion,
   242–243
  from choroidal neovascularization,
   243
  from diabetic macular edema,
   243
  from endophthalmitis, 243
  from hypotonous retinopathy,
   243–244
  from macular hole, 244
  from photic maculopathy, 243
  from retinal detachment, 243
  electrophysiology of, 242
  fluorescein angiography of, *241*, 241
  grid laser photocoagulation for, 249
  histopathological features of, 239,
   242, *242*
  history of, 238
  hyperoxic therapy for, 249–250
  in scleral buckling for retinal detachment, 1269
  inflammation and, 245–246
   mediators of, 245–246, 246t
  intraocular lens removal for, 250–
   251
  light damage and, 246
  Nd:YAG vitreolysis for, 250
  NSAIDs for, 248
  pathogenesis of, 244–246
  prevalence of, 244
  prophylaxis of, 248
  symptoms of, 240
  treatment of, 247t, 247–252
   strategies for, 251t, 251–252
  vitrectomy for, 250
  vitreous incarceration and, 244–245
  vitreous traction and, 244
  vitreous-uveal traction and, 245
 visual acuity in, 238, 240
 vitritis and, in pregnancy, 509
Cytology, vitrectomy samples for, 1489
Cytomegalovirus (CMV), congenital inclusion disease from, 716
 diagnostic vitrectomy for, 1491–1492,
  1493
 in bone marrow transplantation, 488
 retinitis from, diagnosis of, 1491–1492,
  1493
  differential diagnosis of, from acute
   retinal necrosis, 752, 762
   from candidiasis, 774, 775
   from cryptococcosis, 783
   from intraocular lymphomas,
    1207, *1208*
   from progressive outer retinal ne-
    crosis, 768–769
   from retinoblastoma, 1152t, 1156
   from sarcoidosis, 655
   from toxoplasmosis, 681–682
  frosted branch angiitis and, 432t,
   432–433, *434*, 435, 436, 718
  in HIV infection, 432t, 432–433, *434*,
   435, 715, 716–731, 734
  diagnosis of, 717–720, *717–722*
  epidemiology of, 716–717, 1478
  future research on, 731
  pathology of, 719
  prophylaxis for, 726–727
  retinal detachments from, 728–
   730, *731*, *732*, 1478–1483
  treatment of, 720–724, 1478–1483
   local agents for, 724–726, 1482–
    1483
   response to, 727–728, *728–731*

Cytomegalovirus (*Continued*)
   systemic, 720, 722–724, 1482–
    1483
   toxicity of agents for, 722–724
   visual prognosis for, 730
   with other ocular pathogens, 719–
    720, *723*
  in leukemia, 1199
  proliferative vitreoretinopathy and,
   1479
  retinal detachments from, 728–730,
   731, *732*, 1478–1483
   bilateral, 1478
   risk factors for, 1478–1479
   silicone liquid for, 1480–1482
   surgery for, *1479*, 1479–1482, *1480*
 white ocular lesions in, 616t

Dalen-Fuchs nodules, in sympathetic
  ophthalmia, 569, 570, *571*, 572
Darier-Rousy lesions, in sarcoidosis, 645
"Dark-without-pressure" patches, in
  sickle cell retinopathy, 444
ddI, adverse ocular effects of, 742–743,
  862
Deafness, in Stickler syndrome, 924
  syndromes with retinal degeneration
   and, 905t
Deferoxamine retinopathy, differential diagnosis of, from retinitis pigmentosa, 911
Dentate processes, 8–9
Dexamethasone, for endophthalmitis,
  1468t, 1471
  for intermediate uveitis, 607
Dextromethorphan, retinal folds from,
  265
Diabetes mellitus, central retinal vein occlusion and, 286, 288
 endophthalmitis and, 1467
 ocular ischemic syndrome in, 377
 radiation retinopathy in, 478–479
 retinal oxalosis from, 866
 retinopathy in. See *Diabetic retinopathy.*
 type I (IDDM), 318
 type II (NIDDM), 318
Diabetic lenses, in vitrectomy, 1302
Diabetic macular edema, 316, 326t, 329–
  331, *330–336*
 avascular zones in, 330, *330*
 differential diagnosis of, from postsurgical cystoid macular edema, 243
 diffuse leaks in, 330, *330*
 focal leaks in, 330
 laser photocoagulation for, 319, 331,
  334–336
Diabetic maculopathy, choroidal neovascularization in, 150
 differential diagnosis of, from parafoveal telangiectasis, 400, 404
Diabetic retinopathy, 316–341, 1407–1427
 angiogenesis in, 122
 cataracts in, 1425
 clinical guidelines on, 327t, 340t–341t,
  340–341
 clinical trial(s) on, 320t–323t, 320–321
  DCCT, 316, 320–321, 323t, 333, 337,
   1407
  DRS, 316, 320, 320t, 333, 1407, 1413–
   1415, 1414t, 1418, 1421
  DRVS, 316, 320, 322t, 1407, 1423
  ETDRS, 316, 318, 320, 321t, 333,
   1407, 1413, 1414t, 1415, 1416t,
   1418, 1421
  WESDR, 1407

Diabetic retinopathy (*Continued*)
  clinically significant visual loss in, 316
  cotton-wool spots in, 282, 331
  diagnosis of, 321–323
  differential diagnosis of, from ocular
      ischemic syndrome, 377, 380t
    from parafoveal telangiectasis, 405
    from radiation retinopathy, 483
  electrophysiology of, 1412
  electroretinography in, 294, 1412
  epidemiology of, 318–320
  eye examination schedule for, 332–333,
      341t
  fibrovascular membranes in, vitrec-
      tomy for, *1307*, 1307–1308
  fluorescein angiography in manage-
      ment of, 331–333
  follow-up evaluations for, 323t, 326t,
      333
  "four-two-one rule" for, 1409
  future research on, 337–340, 341t
  histopathological features of, 317
  hyphema in, 1425
  in pregnancy, 340–341, 501–504
    fetal well-being and, 504
    macular edema of, 502
    nonproliferative, 502
    optic disc edema in, 504
    pre-eclampsia and, 504
    preproliferative, 502
    progression of, 501–504
      versus nonpregnant women, 503–
          504
    proliferative, 502–503
  intraocular gases for, 1326, 1327t
  intraretinal hemorrhages in, 323, *324*
  intraretinal microvascular abnormali-
      ties in, 323, 1409, *1410*
  iris neovascularization in, 1412–1413,
      1413, 1427
  laser photocoagulation for, 316, 319,
      333–337, 1413–1415, 1418t, 1418–
      1419
    complications of, 340t, 1419t, 1419–
        1421, *1420, 1422*
    performance of, 1421–1423, *1422–
        1424*
    protocols for, 335–337, 340t
    timing of, 333–335, 340t
  lensectomy for, 1425
  levels of, 323t, 325–328
  macular edema in, 316, 326t, 329–331,
      330–336, 1414
  macular holes and, 223
  medical complications of, 319t
  moderate visual loss in, 316
  neovascular glaucoma in, 1316
  neovascularization elsewhere in, 324,
      1410, *1412*
  nonproliferative, 323t, 325–328, 326t,
      327t, *328*
    management of, 327t
    mild, 326, 326t, 327t
    moderate, *323*, 326, 326t, *328*
    severe, 326, 326t, 328
    very severe, 326t, 328, *328*
  optic disc neovascularization in, 324,
      324, 1409, 1410, *1411*, 1415, 1421
  pathophysiology of, 321–322
  pre-eclampsia and, 504
  pregnancy and, 340–341
  proliferative, 319, 323t, 324, *324*, 325,
      326t, 327t, *328*, 328–329, *329*,
      1407–1427, *1408*
    clinical features of, 1408–1413, 1409t,
        1409–1413

Diabetic retinopathy (*Continued*)
  cryosurgery for, 1423
  DRS on, 1413–1415, 1414t
  early, 326t, 328–329
  epidemiology of, 1407–1408, *1409*
  ETDRS on, 1413, 1414t, 1415, 1416t
  high-risk, 326t, 329, *329*
  laser photocoagulation for, 1414–
      1415, 1418t, 1418–1419
    complications of, 1414, 1415, 1419t,
        1419–1421, *1420, 1422*
    performance of, 1421–1423, *1422–
        1424*
  management of, 327t
  perfluorocarbon liquids for, 1321–
      1322, *1322*
  regression of, 1415–1418, 1416t, *1417*
  vitrectomy for, 1423–1425, 1424t,
      1425t
    complications of, 1427, 1427t
    long-term effects of, 1427
    technique of, 1425–1426
  protein kinase C activation in, 338
  radiation therapy exacerbating, 130
  retinal lesions in, 322–325, *323*, 323t,
      324
  retinal microaneurysms in, 322–323,
      323, 1409
  retinal neovascularization in, 324–325,
      325, 1409, *1409*, 1426
  retinal traction detachments in, 325,
      336, 1411, *1412*, 1423–1425, 1426
  rubeosis in, 1412–1413
  silicone liquid for, 1329
  sorbinil for, 337, 341t
  sorbitol accumulation in, 337–338
  terminology in, 316, 318t
  vascular endothelial growth factor and,
      339–340, 1418–1419, 1426
  venous caliber abnormalities in, 323–
      324, *324*
  vitrectomy for, 325, 336, 1423–1427,
      1424t, 1425t
    complications of, 1427, 1427t
  vitreoschisis in, 1426
  vitreous detachment in, 1411
  vitreous hemorrhage in, 1426, 1427
Diacylglycerol (DAG), diabetic retinopa-
      thy and, 338
Diagnostic ophthalmic instruments, pho-
      tic retinopathy from, 847
Diagnostic vitrectomy, 1487–1501. See
      also *Vitrectomy, diagnostic.*
DIC. See *Disseminated intravascular coagu-
      lopathy (DIC).*
Diclofenac sodium, for cystoid macular
      edema, 247t, 248
2′,3′-Dideoxyinosine (ddI), adverse ocular
      effects of, 742–743, 862
Diet, for age-related macular degenera-
      tion prevention, 90, 94, 96
Diffuse subretinal fibrosis syndrome
      (DSF), 624–627
  clinical course and treatment of, 626t,
      626–627, *628*
  clinical features of, 625
  clinical signs of, 625–626
  patient characteristics of, 618t, 625
  visual acuity in, 624t
Diffuse unilateral subacute neuroretinitis
      (DUSN), 806–811
  clinical features of, 808, *809–810*
  diagnosis of, 808–811, *809*
  differential diagnosis of, 808, 809, 811
    from MEWDS, 590

Diffuse unilateral subacute neuroretinitis
      (*Continued*)
    from ophthalmomyiasis, 814
    from sarcoidosis, 655
  electroretinography in, 810
  epidemiology of, 806
  etiology of, 806–807, *807*
  fluorescein angiography of, *809*, 809
  natural course and treatment of, 811
  pathogenesis of, 808
  serologic tests in, 810–811
Digital indocyanine-green videoangiogra-
      phy. See *Indocyanine-green
      angiography.*
Digitalis, ocular disorders from, 867–868
Dilating drops, use of, in pregnancy, 510
Direct agglutination test, for toxoplasmo-
      sis, 683t, 684
Disciform degeneration, hemorrhagic,
      differential diagnosis of, from cho-
      roidal metastasis, 1105
Disciform macular degeneration, 79
Disciform scars, in Coats' disease, 393
  tears of, in age-related macular degen-
      eration, 102–103, *107*
Disseminated intravascular coagulopathy
      (DIC), 473–476
  differential diagnosis of, from
      AMPPPE, 550
  etiology of, 473–474
  in pregnancy, 473, 508–509
  ocular manifestations of, *474*, 474–476,
      475
  pathophysiology of, 474
DNA probes, for endophthalmitis speci-
      mens, 1467
Dominant slowly progressive macular
      dystrophy, bull's eye maculopathy
      in, 1033t, 1034
Drug abusers, candidiasis in, 774–775
  talc retinopathy in, 866–867
Drug-induced ocular disorders, crystal-
      line retinopathy from, 857t, 864–
      867
  cystoid macular edema from, 857t,
      862–863
  differential diagnosis of, from retinitis
      pigmentosa, 909–911
  from aminoglycosides, 864
  from antibiotics, 864
  from canthaxanthine, 864–865, *865*
  from chemotherapeutic agents, 868
  from chloroquine, 856, 858–860, *860–
      861*
  from chlorpromazine, 858, *859*
  from digitalis, 867–868
  from epinephrine, 862–863
  from ergot alkaloids, 864
  from gentamicin, 864
  from hydrochloroquine, 860
  from indomethacin, 862
  from interferons, 864
  from methoxyflurane, 865–866
  from nicotinic acid, 863
  from oral contraceptives, *863*, 863–864
  from phenothiazines, 855, 857–858
  from quinine sulfate, 860–862, *862*
  from talc, 866–867, *867*
  from tamoxifen, 866, *866*
  from thioridazine, 855, *857*, 857–858,
      858
  from tuberculosis treatment, 804
  from vancomycin, 864
  in HIV infection, 741–743, 862
    from clofazimine, 741–742, *742*, 862

Drug-induced ocular disorders (*Continued*)
    from ddI, 742–743, 862
    from ethambutol, 743
    from rifabutin, 742
  myopia from, retinal folds in, 265
  retinal and RPE disruption from, 855–862, 857t
  retinopathies from, 855–868
    classification of, 857t
  salt-and-pepper retinopathy from, 964t
  uveal effusion from, 664
  vascular damage from, 857t, 863–864
Drusen, 79. See also *Maculopathy, age-related.*
  central, differential diagnosis of, from macular holes, 222
  diffuse, 12, *13*
  dominant, bull's eye maculopathy in, 1031, 1033t
  from choroidal nevus, 1053, *1054*
  grading of, 84t
  large, soft, 83, 85–86, *86*
    and geographic atrophy, 88
    fluorescein angiography of, 83
    histopathologic types of, 83
    laser photocoagulation for, 91
  location of, 84t
  morphology of, 84t
  number of, 84t
  of optic disc, 880–883
    clinical features of, 880, *881*
    complications of, 882–883
    diagnosis of, 881–882, *882*
    epidemiology of, 880
    histopathological features of, 882
    ocular associations with, 883
    pathogenesis of, 882
  predominant types of, 84t
  small, hard, 83, *86*
    fluorescein angiography of, 83
DSF. See *Diffuse subretinal fibrosis syndrome (DSF).*
DUSN. See *Diffuse unilateral subacute neuroretinitis (DUSN).*
Dye laser photocoagulators, 64
Dysproteinemias, central retinal vein occlusion and, 288

Eales' disease, 415–420
  angiography of, 419
  biomicroscopic findings in, 418
  clinical findings in, 415–416, 416t, *417–418*
  course of, 417–418
  definitional problems in, 420
  differential diagnosis of, 419
    from chorioretinopathy, central serous, 208
    from intermediate uveitis, 606
    from radiation retinopathy, 483
    from tuberculosis, 804
  etiology of, 419
  pathology of, 419
  presentation of, 417
  prognosis for, 418
  sheathing in, 415–416
  so-called, 416
  stages of, 418–419
  treatment of, 419–420
  vasculitis in, 415–416
  vitritis in, 415–416
Eccentric disciform degeneration, differential diagnosis of, from uveal melanoma, 1080, *1080*

Eckhardt keratophoresis, for trauma, 1375, *1375*
Eclampsia, retinal changes in, 505–506, 506t
Ectopia lensis, B-scan ultrasonography of, 49
Ehlers-Danlos disease, angioid streaks in, 142, 169t
  manifestations of, 169t
Electromagnetic spectrum, 61
Elschnig's spots, 475, 506
Emboli, in central retinal artery, 274, *274*
Embryotoxon, in Alagille syndrome, 932
EMMs. See *Epimacular membranes (EMMs).*
Enclosed ora bay, 9, *9*, 1220–1221, *1221*
Endodiathermy, for CMV-related retinal detachments, 1481
  in vitrectomy, 1311
Endophotocoagulation, for giant retinal tears, 1344–1345
Endophthalmitis, 1466–1475
  acute postoperative, 1466–1471
  conjunctival filtering bleb-associated, 1466, *1472*, 1472–1473
  corticosteroids for, 1468t, 1471
  delayed-onset postoperative, 1466, 1471–1472, *1472*
  diagnostic features of, 1466–1467, *1467*
  differential diagnosis of, from postsurgical cystoid macular edema, 243
    from toxocariasis, 704, 705t
  DNA probes for, 1467
  endogenous, 1466, 1473–1474, *1474*
    differential diagnosis of, from retinoblastoma, 1152t, 1156, *1156*
  epimacular membranes and, 235
  from *Aspergillus*, 1473–1474
  from *Bacillus*, 1390, 1401, 1473
  from blastomycosis, 785, 1473
  from candidiasis, 740, 772–777, *1472*, 1472, 1473–1474
    differential diagnosis of, 775
    in children, 774
    in drug abusers, 774–775
    in pregnancy, 509
  from coccidioidomycosis, 778–779, 1473
  from cryptococcosis, 782, 1473
  from *Fusarium*, 1473
  from gram-negative organisms, 1466–1467
  from histoplasmosis, 1473
  from intraocular foreign bodies, 1473
  from *Mucor*, 1473
  from pneumatic retinopexy, 1284
  from *Propionibacterium acnes*, 1471–1472, *1472*
  from sporotrichosis, 740–741
  from staphylococci, 1390, 1401, 1466, 1472, 1474
  from streptococci, 1466, 1472–1473
  from toxocariasis, 697–707, *699*
  from tuberculosis, 802
  from vitrectomy, 1315
  in bone marrow transplantation, 488
  in diabetics, 1467
  incidence of, 1466
  intraocular antibiotics for, 1467–1468, 1468t
  periocular antibiotics for, 1468t, 1470–1471
  posttraumatic, 1390–1391, 1466, 1473
  prevention of, 1474–1475, *1475*
  systemic antibiotics for, 1468t, 1470

Endophthalmitis (*Continued*)
  tissue plasminogen activator for, 1471
  topical antibiotics for, 1468t, 1471
  vitrectomy for, 1468t, 1468–1470, 1472
  diagnostic, 1467
Enhanced S-cone syndrome, 903–904, *904*
Enteritis, regional, acute multifocal posterior placoid pigment epitheliopathy and, 547
Enucleation, of retinoblastoma, 1145, *1146*
  of uveal melanoma, 1072
Enzyme-linked immunosorbent assay (ELISA), for toxocariasis, 704
  for toxoplasmosis, 683t, 685
  vitrectomy samples for, 1487
Eosinophilia, from toxocariasis, 701, 704
Epidermal nevus syndrome, ichthyosis hystrix variant of, Coats' disease and, 393
Epimacular membranes (EMMs), 230–236
  after scleral buckling, for retinal detachment, 1269, *1269*
  cataracts and, 236
    management of, 234, *234*, 235
  complications of, 235–236
  differential diagnosis of, hamartoma of retina and RPE, 1128
  endophthalmitis and, 235
  etiology of visual loss in, 230
  histopathological features of, 231
  history of, 230
  in cystoid macular edema, 240–241
  in hamartoma of retina and RPE, 1128
  macular holes and, 1433, 1435, *1435*, *1435*, 1446–1447
  management of, 230–235
    for coexistent cataract in, 234, *234*, 235
    for retinal breaks in, 233–234
    in proliferative vitreoretinopathy surgery, 1357
    patient selection for, 230, 232
    results of, 234–235
    vitreomacular traction in, 232, *232*
  optical coherence tomography of, 72
  pathogenesis of, 230
  recurrence of, 235
  recurrence of proliferative vitreoretinopathy in, 235
  removal of, 232–233, *233*
  retinal breaks and, 235
    management of, 233–234
  retinal folds in, 265
  retinal whitening and, 235–236
  rhegmatogenous retinal detachment and, 235
  trauma and, 1375, 1376
  vitrectomy for, *1306*, 1306–1307
Epinephrine, ocular disorders from, 862–863
Epiretinal membranes. See *Epimacular membranes (EMMs).*
Episcleral balloons, for subretinal fluid, 1273–1274
Episcleral plaque brachytherapy, for retinoblastoma, 1146, *1147*
Episcleritis, acute multifocal posterior placoid pigment epitheliopathy and, 545
  from coccidioidomycosis, 778
Epitheliopathy, acute multifocal posterior placoid pigment. See *Acute multifocal posterior pigment epitheliopathy.*

Epithelium villi, of RPE, 4

Equator, 3

Ergot alkaloids, ocular disorders from, 864

Erythema nodosum, acute multifocal posterior placoid pigment epitheliopathy and, 547

Erythropsia, postoperative, 846

Escherichia coli, endophthalmitis from, 1474

Ethambutol, adverse effects of, in HIV infection, 743
  for tuberculosis, 804

Exenteration, for medulloepithelioma, 1137

Exocryotherapy, for retinopathy of prematurity, 412

External beam photon radiotherapy, 128. See also Radiation therapy.

External limiting membrane, of retina, 6

Famciclovir, for acute retinal necrosis, 763

Familial adenomatous polyposis (FAP), 1060, 1062, 1063

Familial exudative vitreoretinopathy. See Vitreoretinopathy, familial exudative (FEVR).

Fat embolism syndrome, ocular disorders from, 840

Favre-Goldmann syndrome, differential diagnosis of, from central areolar choroidal dystrophy, 956t

Fecal-oral transmission, of toxocariasis, 699–700

Fenestrated sheen macular dystrophy, bull's eye maculopathy in, 1033t, 1034

FEVR. See Vitreoretinopathy, familial exudative (FEVR).

FFM. See Fundus flavimaculatus.

Fibrin, pupillary block glaucoma from, 1315

Fibrin(ogen) degradation products (FDPs), 474

Fibrin-platelet thrombi, in central retinal artery, 274, 274

Fibroblast growth factor, basic (bFGF), hemoglobinopathies and, 447

Fibrocytes, migration of, proliferative vitreoretinopathy and, 1350–1351

Fibrous metaplasia, in parafoveal telangiectasis, 401, 402

Fibrovascular membranes, vitrectomy for, 1307, 1307–1308

Fine needle aspiration biopsy, of choroidal metastasis, 1106–1107
  of intraocular lymphoma, 1207–1208
  of posterior uveal melanoma, 1067, 1069
  of uveal neurilemmoma, 1113

FK506, for Vogt-Koyanagi-Harada syndrome, 580

Flavimaculatus flecks, X-shaped macular dystrophy with, 1007, 1010

Flecked retina syndromes, 866, 939, 1045
  differential diagnosis of, from fundus albipunctatus, 939

Flexner-Wintersteiner rosette, in retinoblastoma, 1142, 1143

Fluconazole, for candidiasis, 777
  for cryptococcosis, 740, 784
  for endophthalmitis, 1474

Flucytosine, for candidiasis, 777
  for endophthalmitis, 1473–1474

Fluid-air exchange. See Air-fluid exchange.
  in proliferative vitreoretinopathy, 1359, 1364
  in scleral buckling for retinal detachment, 1261
  in vitrectomy, 1308, 1310, 1326

Fluid-gas exchange, for giant retinal tears, traumatic, 1384

Fluorescein angiography, 29–38, 73–74. See also under specific disorders.
  choroidal filling in, 31
  choroidal flush in, 31
  early arteriovenous phase of, 31
  history of, 29
  hyperfluorescence in, 31, 32t, 34–38, 35–38
  hypofluorescence in, 31, 31t, 32–34, 32–35
  in pregnancy, 509–510
  interpretation of abnormal, 31–38
  late arteriovenous phase of, 31
  normal, 31
  patchy filling in, 31
  properties of dye for, 29–30
  recirculation phase of, 31
  technique of, 30–31

Fluorosilicone, 1331

Flurbiprofen sodium, for cystoid macular edema, 247t

Focal hyperpigmentation, of retinal pigment epithelium, 79, 86, 87

Focal intraretinal periarteriolar transudate (FIPT), 351–353, 354–356
  color of, 358
  differential diagnosis of, 358
  fluorescein angiography of, 354–356, 358
  in hypertensive retinopathy, 351–353, 354–356
  life cycle of, 358
  location of, 358
  pathogenesis of, 358, 358, 359
  resolution of, 358
  shape and size of, 358

Focal (hot) spots, indocyanine-green angiography of, 40, 41–43, 42

Foerster-Fuchs spot, 198

Food-borne disease(s), cysticercosis as, 709, 713
  toxoplasmosis as, 674, 674t

Foralkyl Ac-6, 1321. See also Perfluorocarbon liquids.

Foreign bodies, intraocular, 1395–1404
  case example of, 1392
  chalcosis from, 1402
  computed tomography of, 1372, 1395–1396, 1396
  contact B-scan ultrasonography of, 53–54
  diagnosis of, 1395–1397
  diagnostic vitrectomy of, 1497–1501, 1498, 1500–1501
  endophthalmitis from, 1401, 1401–1402, 1473
  history taking on, 1395
  lens implantation and, 1401
  localization of, 1395–1397, 1396
  magnetic extraction of, 1397, 1399
  magnetic resonance imaging of, 1396
  management of, 1397–1401, 1399t
  mechanisms of, 1397
  metallic, 1397, 1398
  metallosis from, 1402
  perfluorocarbon liquids for removal of, 1323–1324
  prevention of, 1404

Foreign bodies (Continued)
  prognosis for, 1403–1404
  results of treatment of, 1402–1403
  retinal detachments and, 1400–1401
  siderosis from, 1402
  surgery for, 1397–1401
  types of, 1397
  ultrasonography of, 1395, 1396, 1396–1397
    contact B-scan, 53–54
  vitrectomy for, 1341–1342, 1397–1398, 1400, 1400, 1401, 1403
  intraretinal, 1400–1401, 1403

Forsius-Eriksson ocular albinism, 935t, 936

Foscarnet, adverse effects of, 723–724
  for cytomegalovirus, in HIV infected, 720, 722–724
  local therapy with, 724
  for progressive outer retinal necrosis, 757–758
  for varicella-zoster virus, 770

Fovea, anatomy of, 3, 4, 7

Foveal cysts, in cystoid macular edema, 241

Foveal neurosensory detachment, differential diagnosis of, from macular holes, 222

Foveola, anatomy of, 3, 4, 7

Foveomacular pigment epithelial dystrophy, bull's eye maculopathy in, 1034

Frosted branch angiitis, 431–436
  classification of, 431, 432t
  differential diagnosis of, from intraocular lymphomas, 1207
    from cytomegalovirus, 432t, 432–433, 434, 435, 436, 718
    from leukemia, 432t, 433–434
    from retinal phlebitis, 434
  pathophysiology of, 435–436
  primary (idiopathic), 431–432
  secondary, 432t, 432–435

FTA-ABS test, 736, 797–798, 887, 909

Fuchs' heterochromia, toxoplasmosis and, 679

Fuchs' heterochromic iridocyclitis, diagnosis of, 1489
  differential diagnosis of, 606

Fuchs' spots, 140, 198
  histopathological features of, 190

Fundus, ophthalmoscopy of, 21–22

Fundus albipunctatus, 899, 901, 938–940, 939
  differential diagnosis of, 1043, 1045
    from retinitis punctata albescens, 899, 902, 939

Fundus examination, in trauma, 1371

Fundus flavimaculatus, 148, 978–987. See also Stargardt's disease.
  classification of, 982–984
  clinical features of, 978–984, 980, 993
  color vision in, 984
  dark adaptation studies in, 984
  demography of, 978, 980
  differential diagnosis of, 986–987
    from Best's disease, 1002
    from intraocular lymphomas, 1207
    from pattern dystrophy of RPE, 1006
    from retinitis pigmentosa, 914
    from serpiginous choroiditis, 561
  electro-oculography in, 984
  electroretinography in, 984, 984t
  fluorescein angiography of, 980, 981, 983, 984–985, 985

Fundus flavimaculatus (*Continued*)
genetics of, 986
histopathological features of, 979, 985–986
hypofluorescence in, 33
indocyanine green angiography of, 985
pattern dystrophy of RPE and, 1007
prognosis for, 986
retinal function tests in, 984
signs of, 980–984, *981–983*
symptoms of, 980
visual fields in, 984
Fundus photography, technique of, 30–31
Fungal infection(s), 772–787. See also individual fungi.
aspergillosis from, 786–787
blastomycosis from, 784–786
candidiasis from, 772–777
coccidioidomycosis from, 777–781
cryptococcosis from, 739–740, 781–784
diagnostic vitrectomy of, 1492–1495
ocular, in leukemia, 1199
retinitis from, differential diagnosis of, from intraocular lymphomas, 1207
in bone marrow transplantation, 488
sporotrichosis from, 786–787
Fusarium, endophthalmitis from, 1473
FV Q506 mutation, 462

Ganciclovir, adverse effects of, 722–723
for cytomegalovirus, and retinal detachments, 1482–1483
implant therapy with, 724–726, *726*, 1483
in HIV infected, 720, 722–724, 1482–1483
local therapy with, 724
prophylactic use of, 726
for varicella-zoster virus, 734, 769
Ganglion cell, 3, 8
aging of, 11
attrition of, 11
Ganglion cell layer of retina, 7
Gardner's syndrome, 1060, *1062*, 1063
Gas injection, in pneumatic retinopexy, 1272–1286. See also *Pneumatic retinopexy*.
intravitreal, in scleral buckling for retinal detachment, 1260–1261
problems with, 1265
Gases, intraocular, 1325–1329. See also individual gases.
clinical applications for, *1326, 1326t*, 1326–1327, 1327t
complications of, 1328–1329
for giant retinal tears, 1326, 1327t, 1347–1348
for ocular trauma, 1378–1379
for proliferative vitreoretinopathy, 1326, 1327t, 1365
functional role of, 1325–1326
subretinal. See also *intraocular*.
deposits of, 1328
from pneumatic retinopexy, 1281–1282, *1282*
GBR solution, for intraocular irrigation, 1301
Genetic disorders. See also *Hereditary chorioretinal disorders*.
hypertension and, 348
retinal dystrophies associated with systemic, 924–931

Gentamicin, for traumatic ocular injuries, prophylactic, 1378
ocular disorders from, 864
Geographic atrophy, 79, 83
choroidal neovascularization and, 89
grading of, 84t
macular degeneration from, hyperfluorescence of, 36
of retinal pigment epithelium, *87*, 87–89
fluorescein angiography of, 88
soft drusen and, 86, 88
visual acuity in, 88–89
Geographic choroidal dystrophy, classification of, 951t
Geographic choroiditis (choroidopathy). See *Serpiginous choroiditis*.
Geographic helicoid pericapillary choroidopathy. See *Serpiginous choroiditis*.
Giant cell arteritis, ocular ischemic syndrome from, 372
retinal artery occlusion from, 277
Giant retinal tears. See *Retinal tears, giant*.
Glaucoma, angle closure, postoperative, 1314–1315
erythroclastic, 1314, 1315
from intraocular gases, 1328
from laser photocoagulation, for diabetic retinopathy, 1419
from silicone liquid, 1330, 1331
from toxoplasmosis, 680
from vitrectomy, 1314–1315, 1316
ganglion cell aging in, 11
in diabetic retinopathy, 1425
in Vogt-Koyanagi-Harada syndrome, 575, 580
intraocular medulloepithelioma and, 1134, 1135
macular hole surgery and, 1441
neovascular, angiogenesis in, 122
from congenital retinal arteriovenous communications, 1172
from vitrectomy, 1316
in central retinal vein occlusion, 286, 288, 292, 301–302
radiation retinopathy and, 479
pneumatic retinopexy and, 1276
pupillary block, 1315
silicone liquid use and, 1347
surgery for, sympathetic ophthalmia and, 569
sympathetic ophthalmia and, 572
uveal effusion in, 662, 664, 667, *667*
Glial cell(s), 8
migration of, proliferative vitreoretinopathy and, 1350–1351
Globe, rupture of, secrete, 1371
surgery for, 1373
Globular masses. See *Cystic retinal tufts*.
Glutamate, retinal physiology and, 18
Glutathione, for intraocular irrigation, 1301–1302
Gnathostoma spinigerum, 814
Gnathostomiasis, intraocular, 814–817, *818–820*
Goldmann three-mirror lens, 27, *27*
Goldmann-Favre syndrome, 904, 926–927, *927*
differential diagnosis of, from X-linked retinoschisis, 1015
Graft-versus-host disease, in bone marrow transplantation, 488–491
Granular floaters. See *Cystic retinal tufts*.
Granular patch. See *Cystic retinal tufts*.

Granuloma(s), chorioretinal, differential diagnosis of, from uveal melanoma, 1075t, 1081
choroidal, differential diagnosis of, from choroidal metastasis, 1103
from coccidioidomycosis, 780
ciliary body, from blastomycosis, 784
from tuberculosis, 802
from sarcoidosis, 643, 644, 651–652
from toxocariasis, 701
iris, from blastomycosis, 784
nematode, differential diagnosis of, from retinal capillary hemangioma, 1160
retinal, differential diagnosis of, from astrocytic hamartoma, 1182
from retinoblastoma, 1153
from toxocariasis, 702
uveal, from sarcoidosis, 646
from toxocariasis, 703
Granulomatous iridocyclitis, from coccidioidomycosis, 778–779
from tuberculosis, 802
Graves' ophthalmopathy, chorioretinal folds and, 260
Grönblad-Strandberg syndrome. See *Pseudoxanthoma elasticum*.
GRTs. See *Retinal tears, giant*.
Gummata, syphilitic, 794
Gyrate atrophy, biochemical studies in, 964
choroideremia simulating, 958, *968*
clinical features of, 960, 964, *973–974*
differential diagnosis of, from Bietti's crystalline dystrophy, 1045
fluorescein angiography of, 964, *973–974*
hereditary, 960, 964, 973–974
histopathological features of, 950, 964, 973
molecular genetics of, 973–974
treatment of, 964
visual function studies in, 964

Hagberg-Santavuori disease, retinitis pigmentosa and, 905t, 906
Hallervorden-Spatz syndrome, bull's eye maculopathy in, 1033t, 1034
Haltia-Santavuori disease, retinitis pigmentosa and, 905t, 906
Hamartoma, combined, of retina and RPE, 1123–1129. See also *Retinal pigment epithelium, combined hamartoma of*.
differential diagnosis of, from choroidal nevus, 1055
Harada's disease. See also *Vogt-Koyanagi-Harada syndrome*.
choroidal neovascularization in, 150
corticosteroids for, 579
differential diagnosis of, from age-related macular degeneration, 97
from central serous chorioretinopathy, 208
in birdshot retinochoroidopathy, 567
retinal detachments in, *913*
uveal pressure in, 659, 661
uveitis in, 664
Hearing loss. See also *Deafness*.
acute multifocal posterior placoid pigment epitheliopathy and, 547
Heat conduction, laser photocoagulation and, 63
Heerfordt-Waldenström syndrome, 645

Helicoid chorioretinal abiotrophy, 553
Helicoid choroidopathy, 956, *958*
Helicoid degeneration, 553
Helicoid peripapillary chorioretinal atrophy, 553
Helicoid peripapillary chorioretinal degeneration. See *Serpiginous choroiditis.*
HELLP syndrome in, 506
Hemangioma, choroidal, 1083–1090
    retinal capillary, 1159–1166
    retinal cavernous, 1168–1171
Hemoglobin, light absorption by, 62
Hemoglobin AS, 438, 440t
Hemoglobin C trait, 438, 440t
Hemoglobinopathies, 438–456
    clinical features of, *440*, 440–441
    comma sign in, 440, *440*
    cryotherapy for, 452, *455*
    differential diagnosis of, 448–449, 451t
        from parafoveal telangiectasis, 405
    epidemiology of, 438, 440t
    future research on, *455*, 455–456
    histopathological features of, 439
    laser photocoagulation for, 449–451
        feeder vessel, 449–450, 452, 452t, 453t
        scatter, 450, 452t, 453, *454*
    management of, 449–453
    pars plana vitrectomy for, 452–453
    pathophysiology of, *440*, 440–441
    retinal manifestation(s) of, 441–448
        angioid streaks as, 445, *445*
        black sunburst as, 441–442, *442, 443*
        choroidal occlusions as, 443
        hairpin loops as, 442, *444*
        in optic nerve head, 444–445, *445*
        iridescent spots as, 441, *442*
        macular, 443, *444*
        occlusions as, 442, *444*
        proliferative, 445–448, *446*
            Goldberg stage I, 446, *446*
            Goldberg stage II, 446–447, *447*
            Goldberg stage III, 447, *448–450*
            Goldberg stage IV, 447, 450t
            Goldberg stage V, 447–448, *451*
        salmon patch hemorrhage as, 441, *441*
        vascular tortuosity as, 442, *443*
        vitreoretinal interface in, 444
    scleral buckling for, 453–454, 454t
    systemic manifestations of, 438–440
Hemolysis, intravascular, DIC from, 473
Hemorrhage, choroidal. See *Choroidal hemorrhage.*
    intraretinal. See *Intraretinal hemorrhage.*
    macular, in central retinal vein occlusion, 286
    retinal. See *Retinal hemorrhage.*
    splinter, optic disc drusen and, 880
    subarachnoid, in Terson's syndrome, 839
    subconjunctival, acute multifocal posterior placoid pigment epitheliopathy and, 545
    submacular, perfluorocarbon liquids for, 1323
    traumatic, 1386–1387, *1387*
    subretinal. See *Subretinal hemorrhage.*
    suprachoroidal, traumatic, 1387–1389, *1388*
    vitreous. See *Vitreous hemorrhage.*
Hemorrhagic retinal arterial macroneurysms, 383, 385, *386, 387*
Hemorrhagic vascular lesions, differential diagnosis of, from uveal melanoma, 1075t, 1079–1080

Hemostasis, in vitrectomy, 1311
Henle, outer plexiform layer of, 3, 6, *6*
    aging of, 10
Heparin cofactor II deficiency, 465
Hepatic disorders, retinitis pigmentosa and, 905t
Hereditary chorioretinal disorder(s), 889–1049. See also individual disorders.
    Alagille syndrome as, 931
    Alport's syndrome as, 930
    benign concentric maculopathy as, 1025–1035
    Best's disease as, 989–1004
    Bietti's crystalline dystrophy as, 974–975, 1037–1048
    choroidal dystrophy(ies) as, 949–976
        Bietti's crystalline dystrophy as, 974–975, 1037–1048
        central areolar, 951–955
        choroideremia as, 956, *958*, 960
        classification of, 949–951, 951t
        generalized, 956
        gyrate atrophy as, 960, 964, 973–974
        pericapillary, 955–956
        progressive bifocal chorioretinal atrophy as, 975–976
    cone dystrophies as, 942–947
        cone monochromatism in, 942–943
        progressive, 943–946, *945, 947*
        rod monochromatism in, 942, *943*, 943t
    congenital stationary night blindness as, 934–940
    fundus flavimaculatus as, 978–987
    lysosomal storage disorders as, 927–930
    myotonic dystrophy as, 930–931
    pattern dystrophy of RPE as, 1006–1011
    retinitis pigmentosa as, 891–920
        atypical, 896–904
        differential diagnosis of, 908t, 908–917
        molecular genetics of, 917t, 917–920, 918t
        systemic diseases associated with, 904–908
        typical, 891–896
    Sorsby's fundus dystrophy as, 1018–1024
    Stargardt's disease as, 978–987
    vitreoretinal degenerations, 924–927
    X-linked retinoschisis as, 1013–1017
Hereditary dystrophies, choroidal neovascularization and, 147–148
Hereditary retinal dystrophies, differential diagnosis of, from retinitis pigmentosa, 914, *915*
Heredopathia atactica polyneuritiformis (Refsum's disease), 906, 908
Herpes simplex virus (HSV), acute retinal necrosis from, 732–733, 752, 1483–1484
    CMV co-infection with, in HIV infected, 720
    diagnostic vitrectomy for, 1491
    differential diagnosis of, from candidiasis, 774, 775
        from intermediate uveitis, 606
    progressive outer retinal necrosis from, 766, 769, 1483–1484
    white ocular lesions in, 616t
Herpes zoster ophthalmicus, 733
Heterochromia iridis, in retinoblastoma, 1140

Hexameter, 819
"Histo spots," 138, 180, *181*
Histology, of retina, 3–8
    of retinal pigment epithelium, 3–5, *4*
Histoplasma capsulatum, 178
Histoplasmin skin test, 178
Histoplasmosis, endophthalmitis from, 1473
    presumed ocular, 178–187
        choroidal neovascularization and, 138–140, *139*, 178, 180, 183
        choroidal neovascularization in, surgical treatment of, 1449, 1450, *1450, 1453*
        clinical features of, 180, *181, 182*
        differential diagnosis of, from age-related macular degeneration, 96
            from central serous chorioretinopathy, 208
            from choroidal metastasis, 1105
            from choroiditis, 143
            from diffuse unilateral subacute neuroretinitis, 739
            from DUSN, 811
            from ophthalmomyiasis, 814
            from sarcoidosis, 655
            from serpiginous choroiditis, 561
            from tuberculosis, 739
        etiology of, 178
        fluorescein angiography of, 138–139, 180, *181, 182*
        geographic distribution of, 180
        histopathological features of, 179
        history of, 178
        HLA associations with, 183
        in HIV infection, 741
        incidence of, 180–182
        laser photocoagulation for, 139, *139*, 140, 183, *184, 184t*, 184–186, *185*, 186t
        multifocal choroiditis with panuveitis and, 615
        natural history of, 180–182
        pathogenesis of, 183
        prevalence of, 180
        prognosis for, 182–183
        risk to second eye from, 180–181
        submacular surgery for, 186–187
        treatment of, 139–140, 183–187
        white ocular lesions in, 616t
    pseudo-presumed ocular, acute macular neuroretinopathy and, 596
    vasoproliferative tumors and, 1175, 1178t
HIV infection. See *Human immunodeficiency virus (HIV) infection.*
HLA typing, acute retinal necrosis and, 749
    in birdshot retinochoroidopathy, 565
    in histoplasmosis, 183
    in intermediate uveitis, 607
    in sarcoidosis, 645
    in serpiginous choroiditis, 558
    in Vogt-Koyanagi-Harada syndrome, 573
Hodgkin's lymphoma, intraocular involvement in, 1212, 1214
Hollenhorst plaque, in central retinal artery, 274, *274*
Homocystinuria, 465
Horizontal cells, 8
Human immunodeficiency virus (HIV) infection, 714–743
    acute retinal necrosis in, 731–732, 734, 1483–1484

Human immunodeficiency virus (HIV) infection (*Continued*)
bacterial retinitis in, 741
candidiasis in, 740, 772
CMV retinitis in, 432t, 432–433, *434*, 715, 716–731, 734, 1478–1483
diagnosis of, 717–720, *717–722*
epidemiology of, 716–717, 1478
future research on, 731
pathology of, 719
prophylaxis for, 726–727
retinal detachments from, 728–730, *731, 732,* 1478–1483
silicone liquid for, 1480–1482
surgery for, *1479,* 1479–1482, *1480*
treatment of, 720–724
local agents for, 724–726, 1482–1483
response to, 727–728, *728–731*
systemic agents for, 720, 722–724, 1482–1483
toxicity of agents for, 722–724
visual prognosis for, 730
with other ocular pathogens, 719–720, 723
cotton-wool spots in, 282, 714, *716, 716*
cryptococcosis in, 739–740, *740,* 781
drug-induced ocular disorders in, 741–743, 862
from clofazimine, 741–742, *742, 862*
from ddI, 742–743, 862
from ethambutol, 743
from rifabutin, 742
histoplasmosis in, 741
intraocular lymphoma in, 741, 1204, 1211–1212
iridocyclitis in, 741
Pneumocystis carinii in, 737–738, *738, 739,* 1212
progressive outer retinal necrosis in, 732, *733,* 733–734, *734,* 766–770, 1483–1484
retinal and choroidal manifestations of, 714–716
microvascular, 714–716, *716*
retinal detachments in, from CMV retinitis, 728–730, *731, 732,* 1478–1484
silicone liquid for, 1329, 1480–1482
surgical management of, 1478–1484
retinal hemorrhages in, 714, *716*
retinopathy of, 490
differential diagnosis of, 494
sporotrichosis in, 740–741
syphilis in, 735–737, *736, 737,* 796–797
treatment of, 799, 799t
toxoplasmosis in, 671, 680–682, *681,* 734–735, *735,* 1484
tuberculosis in, 738–739, *739,* 801
differential diagnosis of, 803
tumors in, 741
uveal effusion in, 664
uveitis in, 741
Human T-cell leukemia virus (HTLV), diagnostic vitrectomy for, 1492
Hunter's syndrome, retinitis pigmentosa and, 905t
uveal effusion in, 665
Hurler's syndrome, 927–928
retinitis pigmentosa and, 905t
Hutchinson's teeth, 793, *794,* 909
Hyaloid space, gas in, from retinopexy, 1281, *1282*

Hydroxychloroquine, bull's eye maculopathy from, 1030, 1033t
ocular disorders from, 860
differential diagnosis of, from retinitis pigmentosa, 910, *912*
Hyperbaric oxygen therapy, for cystoid macular edema, 249–250
Hypercholesterolemia, in Coats' disease, 390
Hyperemia of optic disc, central retinal vein occlusion and, 288
Hyperfluorescence, in fluorescein angiography, 31, 32t, *34–38,* 35–38
Hyperglycemia, diabetic retinopathy and, 321
Hyperhomocysteinemia, 465
Hyperlipidemia, diabetic retinopathy and, 319t
in hypertensive retinopathy, 359, *361–363*
Hypermetropia, in X-linked retinoschisis, 1014
Hyperopia, chorioretinal folds in, 260–261
Hyperornithenemia, gyrate atrophy and, 964, 974
Hyperoxaluria, retinal oxalosis from, 866
Hyperoxic therapy, for cystoid macular edema, 249–250
Hyperpigmentation, focal, *86, 87*
grading of, 84t
in nongeographic atrophy of RPE, 87, *87*
Hypersensitivity reactions, acute multifocal posterior placoid pigment epitheliopathy and, 548
delayed-type, acute multifocal posterior placoid pigment epitheliopathy and, 548–549
retinal vasculitis and, 435
Hypertension, age-related macular degeneration and, 90
central retinal artery occlusion and, 276
central retinal vein occlusion and, 286, 288
change in lumen size of precapillary arterioles and, 347
change in vascular endothelial function in, 347
choroidopathy in, 348, 360–366. See also *Hypertensive choroidopathy.*
cotton-wool spots and, 282t
diabetic retinopathy and, 319t
fundus changes in, 345–369
in central retinal artery occlusion, 276
in pregnancy, 505–506
cortical blindness in, 506
HELLP syndrome in, 506
retinopathy of, 505–506, 506t
serous retinal detachment in, 506, *507, 508*
intraocular, from acute retinal necrosis, 750, 762
from intraocular gases, 1328
from intravitreal gas injection, 1265
from laser photocoagulation, for diabetic retinopathy, 1419
from vitrectomy, 1314–1315
for diabetic retinopathy, 1427
postoperative, management of, 1314
malignant. See *Malignant hypertension.*
ocular ischemic syndrome in, 377
optic neuropathy in, 348, 366–368. See also *Hypertensive optic neuropathy.*
physiology of, 346, *346*

Hypertension (*Continued*)
retinopathy in, 348, 349–360. See also *Hypertensive retinopathy.*
Hypertensive choroidopathy, 347, 360–369
lesions of, 362–365
pathogenesis of, 362
RPE lesions in, 364
acute focal, *350, 355, 356, 360, 364, 364*
degenerative, 364–365
early, *353, 356, 357,* 364–365
late, *352, 353, 357, 360,* 365
serous retinal detachment in, *350,* 354–356, 360–362, 365, *366*
vascular bed abnormalities from, 362–364, *364*
in acute ischemic phase, 363
in chronic occlusive phase, 363, *365*
in chronic reparative phase, 364
Hypertensive encephalopathy, hypertensive optic neuropathy and, 367, *368*
Hypertensive optic neuropathy, 348, 366–368
angiotensin II and, 368
axoplasmic flow stasis in, 368
dangers of precipitous reduction of blood pressure in, 368
edema in, 367–368
due to raised intracranial pressure, 367
ischemic nature of, 367–368
similar to hypertensive encephalopathy, 367, *368*
lesions of, *350–353, 356, 357, 360, 363,* 366–367
mechanisms of ischemia in, 367, 368
pathogenesis of, 367–368
peripapillary choroid in, 367, 368
Hypertensive retinopathy, 348, 349–360
arteriolar changes in, 349–351, *350–353*
during chronic phase, 350–351, *352, 353*
during early, acute phase, 349–350, *350–351*
capillary changes in, 357, *358*
cotton-wool spots in, 351, 353, 356–358, *357*
color of, 358
differential diagnosis of, 358
fluorescein angiography of, 356, *357*
life cycle of, 358
location of, 358
pathogenesis of, 358
resolution of, 358
differential diagnosis of, from parafoveal telangiectasis, 405
from radiation retinopathy, 483
early and late signs of, 360
edema in, macular, *350,* 354–357, 359, *360–361*
retinal, 359
extravascular lesions in, 359–360
focal intraretinal periarteriolar transudate in, 351–353, *354–356*
color of, 358
differential diagnosis of, 358
fluorescein angiography of, 358
life cycle of, 358
location of, 358
pathogenesis of, 358, *358,* 359
resolution of, 358
shape and size of, 358

Hypertensive retinopathy (*Continued*)
   hemorrhages in, *356, 357,* 359
   in main arterioles, 349–351, *350–353*
   in pre-eclampsia, 505–506, 506t
   in systemic lupus erythematosus, *521–523,* 523
   in terminal arterioles, 351
      dilatation from, 351
      occlusion from, 351
   lipid deposits (macular star) in, 359, *361–363*
   nerve fiber loss in, *356,* 359–361
   vascular lesions in, 349–359
   venous changes in, 358
Hyphema, from vitrectomy, for diabetic retinopathy, 1427
   in diabetic retinopathy, 1425
   traumatic, 1379, *1379*
Hypofluorescence, in fluorescein angiography, 31, 31t, *32–34,* 32–35
Hypoglycemia, serpiginous choroiditis and, 557
Hypopigmentation, grading of, 84t
   in nongeographic atrophy of RPE, 87, *87*
Hypopyon, endophthalmitis and, 1315
Hypopyon uveitis, from rifabutin, 742
   from toxocariasis, 699
Hypotonous maculopathy, chorioretinal folds in, 262–263
Hypotonous retinopathy, differential diagnosis of, from postsurgical cystoid macular edema, 243–244
Hypotony, from vitrectomy, 1316–1317
   ocular, uveal effusion in, 658, 661t, 661–662, *662*
   retinal detachment and, pneumatic retinopexy for, 1286
Hypotrichosis, from interferon alfa, 864

ICG-V. See *Indocyanine-green angiography.*
Idiopathic retinal vasculitis, aneurysms, and neuroretinitis (IRVAN), 526–533, *526–533*
   differential diagnosis of, from Coats' disease, 395
   treatment of, 530, *532–533,* 533
Immune complexes, circulating, and rheumatic diseases, 514
Immunocompromised hosts, candidiasis in, 775, *775*
   cryptococcosis in, 781
   from HIV infection. See *Human immunodeficiency virus (HIV) infection.*
   intraocular lymphomas in, 1204
   toxoplasmosis in, 680–682, *681*
      immune defenses and, 682–683
      management of, 691
Immunosuppressive therapy. See also specific agents.
   for bone marrow transplantation, 488, 489–490
   for diffuse subretinal fibrosis syndrome, 626
   for intermediate uveitis, 610
   for leukemia, 1199
   for posterior scleritis, 640
   for serpiginous choroiditis, 562, 563t
Incontinentia pigmenti, differential diagnosis of, from familial exudative vitreoretinopathy, 427t, 428
Indirect fluorescent antibody test, for toxoplasmosis, 683t, 684
Indirect hemagglutination test, for toxoplasmosis, 683t, 684

Indocyanine green angiography, 39–45, 73–74. See also under specific disorders.
   applications of, 40–45
   for laser photocoagulation, 42, 44
   history of, 39–40
   in age-related macular degeneration, 40, *41–44,* 44–45
   of choroidal neovascularization, 150–151
   of combination lesions, 42, *44,* 44–45
   of focal (hot) spots, 40, *41–43,* 42
   of plaques, 42, *44*
   pharmacology of, 40
   properties of dye for, 39
   technique of, 40
Indocyanine green dye, 39
   pharmacology of, 40
   properties of, 39
   toxicity of, 40
Indomethacin, for posterior scleritis, 639
   for sarcoidosis, 655–656
   ocular disorders from, 862
Infectious disorders, 669–828. See also specific infections.
   choroidal neovascularization from, 147
   diffuse unilateral subacute neuroretinitis from, 806–811
   endophthalmitis from, differential diagnosis of, from toxocariasis, 704, 705t
      from candidiasis, 740, 772–777
      from coccidioidomycosis, 778–779
      from cryptococcosis, 782
      from sporotrichosis, 740–741
      from toxocariasis, 697–707, *699, 702,* 703
      from tuberculosis, 802
   leukemia and, 1199
   myiasis from, 813–827
   of cysticercosis, 709–713
   of fungi, 772–787
      aspergillosis from, 786–787
      blastomycosis from, 784–786
      candidiasis from, 772–777
      coccidioidomycosis from, 777–781
      cryptococcosis from, 781–784
      sporotrichosis from, 786–787
   of HIV infection, 714–743
   of nematodes, 806–811
   of syphilis, 793–799
   of toxocariasis, 697–707
   of toxoplasmosis, 671–692
   of tuberculosis, 801–804
   of viral syndromes, 749–758. See also *Human immunodeficiency virus (HIV) infection.*
      acute retinal necrosis syndrome from, 749–755, 760–764
      progressive outer retinal necrosis syndrome from, 755–758, 766–770
Inflammatory bowel disease, posterior scleritis and, 638
Inflammatory disorder(s), 535–668. See also specific disorders.
   acute macular neuroretinopathy as, 593–596
   acute multifocal posterior placoid pigment epitheliopathy as, 535–551
   acute retinal pigment epitheliitis as, 597–599
   birdshot retinochoroidopathy as, 565–568
   differential diagnosis of, from uveal melanoma, 1075t, 1080–1081

Inflammatory disorder(s) (*Continued*)
   diffuse subretinal fibrosis syndrome as, 624–627
   intermediate uveitis (pars planitis) as, 599–611
   multifocal choroiditis with panuveitis as, 614–621
   multiple evanescent white dot syndrome as, 584–591
   posterior scleritis as, 635–641
   sarcoidosis as, 643–656
   serpiginous choroiditis as, 553–563
   subretinal fibrosis and uveitis syndrome as, 631–634
   sympathetic ophthalmia as, 569–572
   uveal effusion as, 658–667, 661t
   Vogt-Koyanagi-Harada syndrome as, 573–581
Infrared radiation, 61
Inner nuclear layer of retina, 6–7
Inner plexiform layer of retina, 7
Insulin-like growth factor, in central retinal vein occlusion, 292
Intercellular adhesion molecule-1 (ICAM-1), in subretinal fibrosis and uveitis syndrome, 632
Interferon(s), ocular disorders from, 864
Interferon alfa, for antiangiogenesis, 123–124
   for choroidal neovascularization, in AMD, 118–119, 123–124
   ocular disorders from, 864
Interferon gamma, toxoplasmosis and, 682
Interleukin 6, toxoplasmosis and, 682
Interleukin 8, choroidal neovascularization and, 123
Interleukin 12, toxoplasmosis and, 682, 683
Internal limiting membrane (ILM), of retina, 5, 7
   aging and, 14–15
Intranuclear area, 3
Intraocular benign reactive lymphoid hyperplasia, 1214–1215
Intraocular foreign bodies. See *Foreign bodies, intraocular.*
Intraocular gases. See *Gases, intraocular.*
Intraocular hypertension, from acute retinal necrosis, 750, 762
   from intraocular gases, 1328
   from intravitreal gas injection, 1265
   from laser photocoagulation, for diabetic retinopathy, 1419
   from vitrectomy, 1314–1315
      for diabetic retinopathy, 1427
   postoperative, management of, 1314
Intraocular inflammation. See also *Inflammatory disorder(s).*
   chorioretinal folds in, 259–260, *261*
   in cystoid macular edema, 241, 245–246
   mediators of, 245–246, 246t
Intraocular irrigation solution, for vitrectomy, 1301–1302
Intraocular lens (IOL), anterior chamber, in proliferative vitreoretinopathy treatment, 1356
   complications of, from vitrectomy, 1314
   contact B-scan ultrasonography of, 49, *49*
   dislocated, perfluorocarbon liquids for removal of, 1324
   dislocation of, traumatic, 1380
   implantation of, for trauma, 1381–1382
   foreign bodies and, 1401

Intraocular lens (*Continued*)
  opacities of, from intraocular gases,
      1328
    from laser photocoagulation, for dia-
        betic retinopathy, 1419
    from vitrectomy, for diabetic retinop-
        athy, 1427
    in vitrectomy, 1312
  posterior chamber, implantation of,
      1401
    in proliferative vitreoretinopathy
        treatment, 1356
  removal of, for cystoid macular edema,
      250–251
  subluxation of, traumatic, 1380
Intraocular lymphoid tumors, 1204–1215
  benign, *1214, 1214t,* 1214–1215
  malignant, 1204–1214. See also *Lym-
      phoma, intraocular.*
Intraocular medulloepithelioma, 1134–
    1137. See also *Medulloepithelioma,
    intraocular.*
Intraocular pressure, elevated. See *Intra-
    ocular hypertension.*
  in ciliochoroidal effusion, 659
Intraocular traction, management of, in
    proliferative vitreoretinopathy sur-
    gery, 1356–1362, *1357–1362*
Intraretinal hemorrhage. See also *Retinal
    hemorrhage.*
  from radiation retinopathy, 477, 479,
      480, 482, *482*
  in bone marrow transplantation, 488
  in branch retinal vein occlusion, 308
  in diabetic retinopathy, 323, *324*
  in systemic lupus erythematosus, 523–
      525, *524–525*
Intraretinal microvascular abnormalities
    (IRMA), in diabetic retinopathy,
    323, 1409, *1410*
  radiation retinopathy and, 481
IOFBs. See *Foreign bodies, intraocular.*
IRBs. See *Foreign bodies, intraretinal.*
Iridectomy, for proliferative vitreoreti-
    nopathy, 1365, *1365*
Iridescent spots, in sickle cell retinopa-
    thy, 441, *442*
Iridociliary cysts, differential diagnosis
    of, from uveal melanoma, 1075t,
    1081
Iridocyclectomy, for medulloepithelioma,
    1137
  partial lamellar, for adenoma and ade-
      nocarcinoma of RPE, 1122
Iridocyclitis, in HIV infection, 741
Iridodialysis, traumatic, 1382
Iris, artificial, for traumatic injuries, 1376
  atrophy of, from toxoplasmosis, 680
    in acute retinal necrosis, 763
  examination of, in trauma, 1371
  granulomas of, from blastomycosis, 784
  intraocular medulloepithelioma and,
      1134
  masses of, from toxocariasis, 699, 703
  neovascularization of, 275, 278
    from vitrectomy, 1316
    in branch retinal vein occlusion, 312
    in central retinal vein occlusion, 286,
        292, 299–306, 302t, 303t, *304*
    in Coats' disease, 1152, *1153*
    in diabetic retinopathy, 1412–1413,
        1413, 1427
    in retinoblastoma, 1140
  nodules of, from tuberculosis, 802
    in Vogt-Koyanagi-Harada syndrome,
        575, *577*

Iris retractors, in proliferative vitreoreti-
    nopathy treatment, 1355
Iritis, from tuberculosis, 802
IRVAN. See *Idiopathic retinal vasculitis, an-
    eurysms, and neuroretinitis.*
Irvine-Gass syndrome, differential diag-
    nosis of, from parafoveal telangi-
    ectasis, 400
  intermediate uveitis, 606
Ischemic ocular inflammation. See *Ocular
    ischemic syndrome.*
Ischemic oculopathy. See *Ocular ischemic
    syndrome.*
Ischemic syndrome, ocular, 372–381. See
    also *Ocular ischemic syndrome.*
Isoniazid, for serpiginous choroiditis, 562
  for tuberculosis, 804
Itraconazole, for cryptococcosis, 740

Jansky-Bielschowsky disease, retinitis
    pigmentosa and, 905t, 906
Joint contractures, diabetic retinopathy
    and, 319t
Juxtafoveolar retinal telangiectasis, idio-
    pathic, 149, *153–154*
  choroidal neovascularization and,
      149, *153–154*
  differential diagnosis of, from Bietti's
      crystalline dystrophy, 1045
Juxtapapillary choroidal infiltrates, from
    coccidioidomycosis, 779, *779*

Kasabach-Merritt syndrome, 473
Kearns-Sayre syndrome, retinitis pigmen-
    tosa and, 908, 917
Keratic precipitates, in acute retinal ne-
    crosis, *750,* 750, 753, 762
Keratitis, from candidiasis, 774
  from toxocariasis, 699
  from vitrectomy, 1312
  interstitial, in congenital syphilis, 793,
      794
Keratoconjunctivitis, from coccidioido-
    mycosis, 778
Keratopathy, from intraocular gas, 1328
  from silicone liquid, 1330
  from vitrectomy, 1312, 1315
Keratophoresis, for proliferative vitreo-
    retinopathy treatment, 1355
  temporary, for trauma, 1375, *1375*
Keratoplasty, cystoid macular edema af-
    ter. See *Cystoid macular edema.*
  for proliferative vitreoretinopathy
      treatment, 1355
Ketoconazole, for blastomycosis, 786
  for candidiasis, 776
  for coccidioidomycosis, 781
  for cryptococcosis, 740
  for endophthalmitis, 1474
Ketorolac tromethamine, for cystoid mac-
    ular edema, 247t, 248
Klippel-Trénaunay-Weber syndrome, cho-
    roidal hemangioma and, 1088
Krills' disease. See *Retinal pigment epithe-
    liitis, acute.*
Krypton laser photocoagulation. See *La-
    ser photocoagulation.*
Krypton laser photocoagulators, 64
Kufs' disease, retinitis pigmentosa and,
    906
Kveim-Slitzbach test, in sarcoidosis, 652

Lacquer cracks, in degenerative myopia,
    193, 195, *195–197*
  treatment of, 204
Lacrimal gland involvement, in sarcoido-
    sis, 651
Lamellar macular hole, 223, 224
Landers-Foulks keratophoresis, for
    trauma, 1375
Larva migrans, intraocular, differential
    diagnosis of, 827
Laser, coherence in, 61
  effects of, 61–63
  irradiance in, 61
  light absorption and, 62
  light of, 61–62
  light scattering and, 62
  monochromacity of, 61
  short pulse, 75
  thermal effects of, 63
  tissue optics and, 62
  wavelengths of, 61
Laser bypass, for branch retinal vein oc-
    clusion, 315
Laser chorioretinal venous anastomosis,
    for central retinal vein occlusion,
    295
Laser photocoagulation, 61–67
  after scleral buckling, for retinal de-
      tachment, 1261, *1262*
  burn intensity adjustment in, 66
  clinical applications of, 63–67
  delivery systems for, 65
    defocus, 65
    parfocal, 65
  for acute retinal necrosis, 754–755
  for age-related macular degeneration,
      neovascular, 108t, 108–116, 137–
      138
    nonneovascular, 91–92
  for angioid streaks, 142, *171,* 174–175,
      175
  for bone marrow transplantation reti-
      nopathy, 495
  for branch retinal vein occlusion, 312–
      314, *314*
    for macular edema, 312–314
    for retinal neovascularization, 314,
        314
  for chorioretinopathy, central serous,
      213
  for choroidal hemangioma, 1087, *1088,*
      1090
  for choroidal neovascularization, 137–
      138, *150,* 151–157, *155, 156*
    complications of, 157, *158*
    extrafoveal, 108t, 110, 111t, 137
    follow-up schedule for, 155, 157
    in degenerative myopia, 198–199,
        201–203
    in histoplasmosis, 139, *139,* 140
    in myopia, 141–142
    juxtafoveal, 108t, 110–112, 111t
    recurrent, *108t, 110, 111t,* 116, 117
    risks and benefits of, 110–112
    subfoveal, 108t, 111t, 112–115, 137
    wavelength selection for, 109, 152,
        155
  for choroidal nevus, 1057
  for choroidal osteoma, 1101
  for CMV-related retinal detachments,
      1479–1480
  for Coats' disease, 396
  for cyclodialysis, 1382
  for cystoid macular edema, 249
  for diabetic retinopathy, 333–337,
      1413–1415, 1418t, 1418–1419

Laser photocoagulation (*Continued*)
  complications and adverse effects of, 340t
  complications of, 1419t, 1419–1421, *1420, 1422*
  performance of, 1421–1423, *1422– 1424*
  protocols for, 335–337, 340t
  timing of, 333–335, 340t
  for diffuse unilateral subacute neuro-retinitis, 811
  for familial exudative vitreoretinopathy, 428
  for giant retinal tears, 1340, 1344, 1347
  for hemoglobinopathies, 449–451
    feeder vessel, 449–450, *452*, 452t, 453t
    scatter, 450, 452t, 453, *454*
  for histoplasmosis, presumed ocular, 139, *139*, 140, *184*, 184t, 184–186, *185*, 186t
  for intermediate uveitis, 609–610
  for macular edema, in branch retinal vein occlusion, 312–314
  for macular holes, 1434
  for multifocal choroiditis with panuveitis, 621
  for ocular ischemic syndrome, 380–381
  for optic nerve head congenital pits, *878*, 878–879
  for proliferative vitreoretinopathy, 1358–1359, *1359*, 1364
  for punctate inner choroidopathy, 624, *625*
  for radiation retinopathy, 485
  for retinal arterial macroneurysms, 387–388, *388, 389*
  for retinal cavernous hemangioma, 1169
  for retinal detachment, 1267
    after scleral buckling, 1261, *1262*
    pneumatic retinopexy and, 1272
  for retinal horseshoe tears, 1265–1266
  for retinal tears, 833
  for retinoblastoma, 1146, *1147*, 1148
  for retinopathy of prematurity, 412
  for serpiginous choroiditis, 562, 563t
  for sickle cell retinopathy, 449–451
  for toxocariasis, 707
  for toxoplasmosis, 690–691
  for vasoproliferative ocular fundus tumors, 1180
  indocyanine-green angiography for, 42, 44
  ophthalmoscopy and, 65, 66–67
    direct, 66
    indirect, 66
  pneumatic retinopexy and, for retinal detachment, 1272, 1278, 1280–1281
  principles of, 61–63
  prophylactic, for fellow eye of giant retinal tear, 1346
  safety filters for, 67
  safety of, 67
  silicone liquid and, 1329
  sources of, 61–63
  treatment parameters for, 65–66
  uveal effusion after, 661t, 663–664, *664*
  vitrectomy and, 1311
Laser scotometry, for optic disc drusen, 881
Laser-associated photic retinopathy, 846–847
Lattice degeneration, 16–17, *17*, 1227t, *1227–1230*, 1227–1234
  atrophic retinal holes in, *1231–1232*, 1231–1233

Lattice degeneration (*Continued*)
  clinical features of, 1227–1230, *1227– 1230*
  histopathological features of, *1227*, 1227–1230
  history of, 1227
  localization of, for scleral buckling, 1253, *1255*
  pneumatic retinopexy contraindicated in, 1277
  prognosis and management of, in aphakic or pseudophakic fellow eyes, 1233–1234
    in phakic fellow eyes, 1233, 1234t
    in phakic nonfellow eyes, 1232–1233
  retinal detachment and, 1227t, 1244
  scleral buckling for, 1266
  snail track feature in, *1228–1230*, 1230–1231
  white lines in, *1228–1230*, 1230–1231
Laurence-Moon syndrome, retinitis pigmentosa and, 905
Leber's congenital amaurosis, 901, *903*, 1007
  bull's eye maculopathy in, 1033t, 1034
Leber's idiopathic optic neuroretinitis, 885–888
  clinical features of, 885–886, *886*
  demography of, 885
  differential diagnosis of, 887
  etiology of, 887–888
  fluorescein angiography of, 886–887
  history of, 885
  macular star of, 886, *886*
  treatment of, 888
Leiomyoma, differential diagnosis of, from nonpigmented ciliary epithelium tumor, 1130, 1131
    from uveal melanoma, 1075t, 1078, *1078*
  uveal, 1110–1112. See also *Uveal leiomyoma.*
Lensectomy, for cataracts, in epimacular membranes, 234
    in intermediate uveitis, 611
  for diabetic retinopathy, 325, 336, 1425
  for giant retinal tears, 1342, 1347, 1348
  for hamartoma of retina and RPE, 1128
  for hemoglobinopathies, 452–453
  for intermediate uveitis, 610–611
  for intraocular foreign bodies, 1398
  for macular holes, 227
  for retinopathy of prematurity, 1462–1463
  for suprachoroidal hemorrhages, 1388
  for toxoplasmosis, 690–691
  for trauma, 1375
  in proliferative vitreoretinopathy treatment, 1355
  sympathetic ophthalmia after, 569
  vitrectomy with, 1304–1305, *1305*. See also *Vitrectomy.*
    for cataracts, in epimacular membranes, 234
    in intermediate uveitis, 611
    for diabetic retinopathy, 325, 336
    for hamartoma of retina and RPE, 1128
    for hemoglobinopathies, 452–453
    for intermediate uveitis, 610–611
    for macular holes, 227
    for toxoplasmosis, 690–691
    sympathetic ophthalmia after, 569
"Leopard-spot" fundus, in uveal effusion, 660, *660*

Leprosy, differential diagnosis of, from sarcoidosis, 655
Leucovorin, for toxoplasmosis, in HIV infected, 735
Leukemia, acute lymphocytic, 1194–1195
  diagnosis of, 1496
  acute myelogenous, 1195
  choroid findings in, 1197t, 1199
  chronic lymphocytic, 1194
  chronic myelogenous, 1194
  diagnosis of, 1496
  classification of, 1194, 1195
  clinical manifestations of, 1197–1199
  complications of treatment of, *1200, 1201*, 1201–1202
  frosted branch angiitis from, 432t, 433–434
  ophthalmic manifestations of, 1194–1202
    prognosis for, 1199, *1200*, 1201
  opportunistic infections and, 1199
  optic nerve findings in, 1199
  prevalence and incidence of, 1196t, 1196–1197, 1197t
  retinal findings in, 1197t, 1197–1198, *1198*
  vitreous findings in, 1197t, 1198–1199
Leukemic retinopathy, 1201
Leukokoria, from endogenous endophthalmitis, 1156, *1156*
  from myelinated nerve fibers, 1156, *1157*
  from retinoblastoma, 1139, *1140*
  from retinopathy of prematurity, 1157
  from toxocariasis, 702, *703*
Light, absorption of, 62
  scattering of, in lasers, 62
    Mie, 62
    Rayleigh, 62
Light exposure, age-related macular degeneration and, 848
Linkage analysis, 918
  in retinitis pigmentosa, 918
Lipid deposits, in Coats' disease, 395
  retinal (macular stars), in hypertensive retinopathy, 359, *361–363*
Lipofuscin, 5
  in Best's disease, 1000–1002, 1004
  in fundus flavimaculatus, 985
Lipofuscinosis, neuronal ceroid, 902
Lofgren's syndrome, 645
Low-coherence interferometry, 69
Luetic tarsitis, 795
Lung carcinoma, choroidal metastasis and, 1104, 1105, *1105*, 1107
Lupus anticoagulant (LA), ocular manifestations of, 465
Lupus choroidopathy, hypofluorescence in, 35
Lupus pernio, in sarcoidosis, 645
Lyme disease, vs. intermediate uveitis, 606
  vs. Leber's idiopathic optic neuroretinitis, 887
Lymphocytes, in frosted branch angiitis, 435
Lymphoid hyperplasia, intraocular benign reactive, 1214–1215
  diagnosis of, 1215
  differential diagnosis of, 1214, 1214t
Lymphoma, intraocular, 1204–1214
  CNS non-Hodgkin's lymphoma and, 1204, 1207–1210, *1207–1210*, 1209t
  diagnostic vitrectomy for, 1496–1497

Lymphoma (*Continued*)
   differential diagnosis of, from
      birdshot retinochoroidopathy,
      567
     from central serous chorioretinop-
      athy, 208
     from sarcoidosis, 655
   fine needle aspiration biopsy of,
     1207–1208
   histopathological features of, 1205–
     1206
   immunophenotyping of, 1208, *1210*
   in HIV infection, 741, 1204, 1211–
     1212
   rare forms of systemic lymphoma
     and, 1212, 1214, *1214*
   systemic non-Hodgkin's lymphoma
     and, 1210–1212, *1211–1213*
   large cell, differential diagnosis of, in-
     termediate uveitis, 606
   white ocular lesions in, 616t
Lysosomal storage disorder(s), chorioretinal disorders in, 927–930
   cystinosis as, *929*, 929–930
   mucopolysaccharidoses as, 927–928
   oxalosis as, 930, *930*
   sphingolipid storage diseases as, *928*,
     928–929, *929*

Macrophages, migration of, proliferative
   vitreoretinopathy and, 1350–1351
Macroreticular dystrophy, 1011
Macula, anatomy of, 3, 7
   light absorption by, 62
   thinning of, 10–11
   vascular changes in, in sickle cell reti-
     nopathy, 443, *444*
Macular degeneration, age-related, angiogenesis in, 122
   biology of, 122–123
   antiangiogenic therapy for, 122–124
   choroidal neovascularization in, 94–
     119
     angiography obscuring, 98, 101,
       101, *102*
     classic, 98, *98*
     fading, *102*, 104
     feeder vessels and, *102*, 104, 105
     laser photocoagulation for, 108t,
       108–116, 111t
       extrafoveal, 108t, 110, 111t
       juxtafoveal, 108t, 110–112
       recurrent, 108t, 111t
       subfoveal, 108t, 111t, 112–115
     occult, 98, *99*, *100*
     pathogenesis of, 94, 96
     radiation therapy for, 126–130
     risk of fellow eye developing, 116
     surgical treatment results for, *1450*,
       1450–1451, *1451*, *1453*
   classification of, 79
   differential diagnosis of, from Best's
     disease, 1002
     from central areolar choroidal dys-
      trophy, 956t
     from chorioretinopathy, central se-
      rous, 208
     from macular holes, 222
     from parafoveal telangiectasis, 401
     from serpiginous choroiditis, 562
     from uveal melanoma, 1075t, 1079,
      1080, *1080*
   dry (atrophic). See *nonneovascular.*
   grid for classification of, *85*

Macular degeneration (*Continued*)
   indocyanine-green angiography of,
     40, *41*
   light exposure and, 848
   neovascular, 79, 94–119
     classic CNV in, *98*, 98
     clinical features of, 96–97
     differential diagnosis of, 96–97
     disciform scar in, 102–103, *107*
     epidemiologic studies of, 94, 96
     experimental and clinicopathologic
      studies on, 94
     extrafoveal CNV, treatment of,
      108t, 110, 111t
     fading CNV in, 102, *104*
     features and location of, 85t
     feeder vessels in, 102, *104*, *105*
     fluorescein angiography of, 97–
      103, *97–107*
      obscuring CNV, 98, 101, *101–*
       102
     future research for, 117–119
     hemorrhage in, 103
     histopathological features of, 95
     indocyanine green angiography of,
      103, *106–107*
     juxtafoveal CNV, treatment of,
      108t, 110–112, 111t
     laser photocoagulation for, 108t,
      108–116
      risks and benefits, 110–112
      wavelength selection, 109
     loculated fluid in, 102, *106*
     management of, 108t, 108–116
      evaluating extent of laser treat-
       ment, 115
      follow-up evaluations in, 115–
       116
      for recurrent CNV, 116
      pharmacologic interventions for,
       118–119
      photodynamic therapy for, 118
      postoperative, 115–116
      radiation therapy for, 118
      risk of fellow eye developing
       CNV, 116
      submacular surgery for, 117–
       118
     occult CNV in, *98*, 99, 100
     pathogenesis of, 94, 96
     recurrent CNV, management of, 116
      predicting, 116, *117*
     RPE tear in, 102, *106*
     signs of, 96
     subfoveal CNV, treatment of, 108t,
      111t, 112–115, *113*, *114*
     symptoms of, 96
   nonneovascular, 79–92
     antioxidants and, 89–91
     education on, 91–92
     focal hyperpigmentation of RPE
      in, *86*, 87
     geographic atrophy of RPE in, *87*,
      87–89
     histopathological features of, 80–
      81
     light exposure and, 89
     nongeographic atrophy of RPE in,
      87, 87
     photocoagulation for, 91
     treatment of, 89–92
   optical coherence tomography of,
     72–73
   radiation therapy for, 126–130
   standardized grading criteria for, 83,
     84t–85t

Macular degeneration (*Continued*)
   submacular hemorrhage and, per-
     fluorocarbon liquids for, 1323
   subretinal surgery for, 131–136
   wet (exudative). See *neovascular.*
   disciform, differential diagnosis of,
     from choroidal osteoma, 1095,
     1096
   hyperfluorescence in, 37, *37*
Macular depression sign, in sickle cell
   retinopathy, 443, *444*
Macular detachment, in retinal arterial
   macroneurysms, 383, 385
Macular disorder(s), 77–268. See also
   specific disorders.
   age-related degeneration as. See *Macu-*
     lar degeneration, age-related.
   chorioretinal folds as, 256–263
   epimacular membranes as, 230–236
   histoplasmosis, presumed ocular, as,
     178–187
   holes as, 217–227
   myopia as, 189–204
   postsurgical cystoid edema as, 238–
     252
   retinal folds as, 263–265
   subretinal surgery for, 131–136
Macular edema, cystoid. See *Cystoid mac-*
   ular edema.
   diabetic, 316, 326t, 329–331, *330–336*,
     1414
     in pregnancy, 502
     laser photocoagulation for, 319
   from cytomegalovirus, 719, *722*
   from laser photocoagulation, for dia-
     betic retinopathy, 1419–1420,
     1420
   from toxoplasmosis, 678
   hyperfluorescence in, 37
   in bone marrow transplantation, 491,
     494
   in branch retinal vein occlusion, 308
     ischemic, *311*, 311–312
     laser management of, 312–314
     perfused, 310–311, *311*
   in epimacular membranes, 232
   in hypertensive retinopathy, 350, *354–*
     357, 359, *360–361*
   in ocular ischemic syndrome, 375, *379*
   in radiation retinopathy, 477, 479, 480,
     483
   in sympathetic ophthalmia, 569
   ischemic, from branch retinal vein oc-
     clusion, *311*, 311–312
   optical coherence tomography of, 72
   perfused, from branch retinal vein oc-
     clusion, 310–311, *311*
   persistent, in central retinal vein occlu-
     sion, 286, 292
   postsurgical cystoid, 238–252. See also
     Cystoid macular edema.
   traumatic, 833
Macular exudates, in bone marrow transplantation, 491
   in radiation retinopathy, 477, 479, 480,
     482
Macular hemorrhage, in central retinal
   vein occlusion, 286
Macular holes, 217–227, 1432–1447t
   biomicroscopy of, 219–220, 221t
   B-scan ultrasonography of, 50, *50*
   cataracts and, 1437, 1443, *1445*
   clinical characteristics of, 1432
   conditions associated with, 223
   cystoid degeneration theory of, 217

Macular holes (*Continued*)
  differential diagnosis of, 220, 222–223, *223*
    from postsurgical cystoid macular edema, 244
  endophthalmitis and, 1441
  epiretinal membranes and, 1433, 1435, *1435, 1446–1447*
  fellow eyes and, 225–226
  fluorescein angiography of, 1437, *1437, 1438, 1442*
  focal electroretinography of, 225–226
  from congenital retinal arteriovenous communications, 1172
  full-thickness, 223, *224*
    differential diagnosis of, 222, *223*
    management of, *226,* 226–227, 1434–1436, *1434–1436*
    natural history of, 225
  Gass classification of, 219–220, *220,* 221t, 222, 1432
  glaucoma and, 1441
  histopathological features of, 217, 218, 223–224, *224*
  history of, 217
  idiopathic, 11, 218, 1433
  in Best's disease, 997
  in central retinal vein occlusion, 292
  intraocular gases for, 1326, 1327t, 1434
  lamellar, 223, 224, *224*
  laser coagulation for, 1434
  management of, 226–227, 1434–1443
    case selection for, 1441
    complications of, 1441, 1443, *1443–1445*
    extended indications for, 1437, *1440–1441,* 1440–1442
    failure of, 1437, *1439*
    results of, 1436–1437, *1436–1439*
  membrane stripping for, 1441
  natural history of, 224–226, 1433, *1433*
  occult, 219, *222*
  opercula and, 223–224
  optical coherence tomography of, *71,* 71–72, 223
  pathogenesis of, 217, 1432
  perfluorocarbon liquids for, 1323
  photic retinopathy from surgery for, 846
  pneumatic retinopexy and, 1440
  premacular, 219, 223–224
    management of, 227
    natural history of, 224–225
  pseudo, 222
  pseudo-operculum and, 219, 223
  retinal detachments and, 1440, 1441
  retinal tears and, 1441
  silicone-tipped suction cannula for, 1434, *1434*
  stage 1, 219, *220,* 221t, 224–225, 1432
  stage 2, *220,* 221t, 225, 1432
  stage 3, *220,* 221t, 222, 225, 1432, *1433, 1435, 1439*
  stage 4, *220,* 221t, 222, 225, 1432
  traumatic, 217, 833, *834, 1440,* 1440–1441
  vascular theory of, 217
  visual acuity in, 224–225
  vitrectomy for, 1434
  vitreous theory of, 219
Macular neuroretinopathy, acute, 593–596
  differential diagnosis of, 590
  fundus appearance in, 593, *594, 595*
  laboratory testing in, 593–594

Macular neuroretinopathy (*Continued*)
  natural history of, 593, *595*
  ocular disorders associated with, 595–596
  systemic disorders associated with, 594–595
  treatment of, 596
  in pregnancy, 509
Macular nonperfusion, in central retinal vein occlusion, 286
Macular puckers. See *Epimacular membranes (EMMs).*
Macular serpiginous choroiditis. See *Serpiginous choroiditis.*
Macular star, in Leber's idiopathic optic neuroretinitis, 886, *886*
Macular thickening, from branch retinal vein occlusion, 308
Macular trauma, photic, 845
Maculopathy, age-related, 79, 83. See also *Macular degeneration, age-related.*
  definitions of, 82t
  focal hyperpigmentation of RPE in, *86, 87*
  geographic atrophy of RPE in, *87,* 87–89
  grid for classification of, *85*
  nongeographic atrophy of RPE in, *87, 87*
  patterns of, 83–89
  small, hard drusen, 83, *86*
  studies of, 82t
  benign concentric, 1025–1035. See also *Benign concentric maculopathy.*
  cellophane. See *Epimacular membranes.*
  Leber's. See *Leber's idiopathic optic neuroretinitis.*
Madarosis, in syphilis, 795
  in Vogt-Koyanagi-Harada syndrome, 575, *577*
Magnetic extraction, of intraocular foreign bodies, 1397, *1399*
Mainster lens, 28
Malignant hypertension, bone marrow transplantation retinopathy and, 490
  choroidopathy in, 348, 360–366. See also *Hypertensive choroidopathy.*
  fundus changes in, 345–369
    terminology of, 348–349
  optic neuropathy in, 348, 366–368
  pathophysiology of, 348–349
  physiology of, 346, *346*
  retinopathy in, 348, 349–360. See also *Hypertensive retinopathy.*
  uveal effusion in, 661t, 663
Malignant hyperthermia, hypofluorescence in, 35
Marcus Gunn pupil, 1188
Marfan's syndrome, lens in, B-scan ultrasonography of, 49, *49*
Marginal spots, indocyanine-green angiography of, *40, 42,* 44
Maroteaux-Lamy syndrome, uveal effusion in, 665
Masquerade syndrome, differential diagnosis of, intermediate uveitis, 606
MCP. See *Multifocal choroiditis with panuveitis (MCP).*
Medulloepithelioma, 1143
  intraocular, 1134–1137
    clinical features of, 1134–1135, *1135, 1136*
    cysts in, 1136
    diagnosis of, *1135, 1136,* 1136–1137

Medulloepithelioma (*Continued*)
  differential diagnosis of, from non-pigmented ciliary epithelium tumor, 1130, 1131
    from retinoblastoma, 1135, 1136, 1152t, 1154, *1154*
  fluorescein angiography of, 1134, *1135*
  histopathological features of, 1135–1136, *1136, 1137*
  malignant, 1136
  management of, 1137
  prognosis for, 1137
  ultrasonography of, 1134, *1136,* 1137
Melanin, light absorption by, 62
  protective effect of, 844
Melanin pigment granules, 4, *4*
Melanocytoma, of optic nerve, 1188–1192
  clinical features of, 1188–1189, *1189, 1190*
  diagnosis of, 1190, *1190,* 1192
  differential diagnosis of, from combined hamartoma of retina and RPE, 1128
    from malignant melanoma, 1188, 1192
    from uveal melanoma, 1075t, *1077,* 1077–1078
  management of, *1191–1192,* 1192
Melanoma, amelanotic, differential diagnosis of, from uveal leiomyoma, 1110
  choroidal, 1067–1072. See also *Choroidal melanoma.*
  cutaneous, 917
    choroidal metastasis and, 1104, *1105,* 1107
  differential diagnosis of, from age-related macular degeneration, 97
  of ciliary body, 1067–1072. See also *Ciliary body melanoma.*
  optic nerve melanocytoma and, 1188, *1191–1192,* 1192
  posterior uveal, 1067–1072. See also *Uveal melanoma, posterior.*
Membrane delamination, in vitrectomy, 1308, *1309*
Membrane peeling, in vitrectomy, 1305–1307, *1306, 1307*
  silicone liquid and, 1329
Membrane sectioning, in vitrectomy, *1307,* 1307–1308
Membrane stripping, for macular holes, 1441
  for proliferative vitreoretinopathy, 1353
Meningitis, cryptococcal, 740, 783
  in sarcoidosis, 645
Meridional complexes, 9, *9,* 1219–1220, *1220*
Meridional folds, 9, *9,* 1219–1220, *1220*
Mesocercaria infections, 821, 825, *826,* 827
Metabolic disorders, retinitis pigmentosa and, 905t
Metalloproteins, in Sorsby's fundus dystrophy, 1021, 1024
Metallosis, from intraocular foreign bodies, 1402
Metamorphosia, in age-related macular degeneration, 96
Metastases, choroidal, 1103–1108. See also *Choroidal metastasis.*
  contact B-scan ultrasonography of, 53, *53*

Metastases (*Continued*)
differential diagnosis of, from age-related macular degeneration, 97
from chorioretinopathy, central serous, 208
from nonpigmented ciliary epithelium tumor, 1130
from serpiginous choroiditis, 561
from Vogt-Koyanagi-Harada syndrome, 578
uveal. See *Uveal metastasis.*
white ocular lesions in, 616t
Methotrexate, for intermediate uveitis, 610
for intraocular lymphomas, 1209
ocular toxicity of, 1201
Methoxyflurane, ocular disorders from, 865–866
Methylphenidate HCl abuse, 867
Methylprednisolone, for cystoid macular edema, 247t, 249
MEWDS. See *Multiple evanescent white dot syndrome (MEWDS).*
MHA-TP test, 798
Miconazole, for candidiasis, 776–777
for coccidioidomycosis, 781
Microcephaly, pigmented ocular fundus lesions and, 1063
Microfilarial ocular infections, 820–821
Microvitreoretinal (MVR) blade, 132
Mie scattering, 62
Miosis, management of, in proliferative vitreoretinopathy treatment, 1355
Mitochondria, of RPE, 5
Mitochondrial myopathy (Kearns-Sayre syndrome), 908
Mizuo's phenomenon, 944
Monochromatism, cone, 942–943
rod, 94, *942, 943,* 943t
Morning glory disc anomaly, differential diagnosis of, hamartoma of retina and RPE, 1128
Mucopolysaccharide (MPS) storage disorders, 927–928
retinitis pigmentosa and, 905t
uveal effusion in, 665
Müller cells, 5, 6–7, 8, *8*
Multifocal choroiditis with panuveitis (MCP), 614–621, 628, 629
anterior segment signs of, 615
clinical course and treatment of, 617, 619–621, 621–623, 626t
clinical features of, 614–617, 618t
corticosteroids for, 619, 621, 623t
differential diagnosis of, from DUSN, 811
from MEWDS, 589
electroretinography of, 617
fundus findings in, 615, *615*
laser photocoagulation for, 621
patient characteristics of, 614–615, 618t
perimetry signs of, 615, 617, *619–620*
prognosis for, 621
visual acuity in, 624t
Multifocal posterior placoid pigment epitheliopathy. See *Acute multifocal posterior placoid pigment epitheliopathy.*
Multiple evanescent white dot syndrome (MEWDS), 584–591
acute macular neuroretinopathy and, 595
choroiditis and, 143
course of, *587,* 588–589
demography of, 584

Multiple evanescent white dot syndrome (*Continued*)
differential diagnosis of, 589–590
from AMPPPE, 550
from DUSN, 811
electrophysiology of, 588
fluorescein angiography of, 585, *585, 586*
indocyanine green angiography of, 585, *587*
recurrence of, *587,* 588
symptoms and clinical findings in, 584, *585–589*
visual fields in, 584, 589, 590
white ocular lesions in, 617t
Multiple sclerosis, differential diagnosis of, from Eales' disease, 419
intermediate uveitis and, 604, 605
Mycobacterium tuberculosis, 738–739, 801. See also *Tuberculosis.*
Mycosis fungoides, intraocular involvement in, 1212, *1214*
Myelinated nerve fibers, differential diagnosis of, from retinoblastoma, 1152t, 1156–1157, *1157*
Myiasis, 813–827
Alaria mesocercaria as, 821, 825, *826, 827*
intraocular angiostrongyliasis as, 817–819, *820–821*
intraocular ascaridiosis as, 819–820, *822–824*
intraocular gnathostomiasis as, 814–817, *818–820*
ocular onchocerciasis as, 820–821, *824–826*
ophthalmomyiasis as, 813–814, *814–817*
Myopia, 189–204
chorioretinal folds and, 260–261
choroidal neovascularization and, treatment of, results of, 1452, *1452, 1453*
degenerative, 189
atrophic areas in, 192–193, *194*
biomicroscopy of, 191, 193, *195, 196, 196*
choroidal abnormalities in, 192, *193*
choroidal neovascularization in, 196–203
clinical signs of, 196–197, *198, 199*
fluorescein angiography of, 197–198
ICG angiography of, 198, *198*
laser photocoagulation for, 198–199, *201–203*
natural history of, 198
surgery for, 203
treatment of, 198–199, *201–203,* 203
complications of, 195–203
fluorescein angiography of, 192, 193, 197–198
histopathological features of, 190
ICG angiography of, 192, 193, 198, *198*
lacquer cracks in, 193, 195, *195–197,* 204
optic disc abnormalities in, *191,* 191–192
pathophysiology of, 189
posterior retinal detachment and, 195, *197*
posterior staphyloma in, 189, 191, *191*

Myopia (*Continued*)
prevalence of, 189
prevention of, 203–204
retinal abnormalities in, 192, *193*
treatment of, 203–204
vitreous abnormalities in, 192
giant retinal tears and, 1342
in pregnancy, 505
in retinopathy of prematurity, 412
in Stickler syndrome, 924
in Wagner's syndrome, 925
macular holes and, 223
pathologic, choroidal neovascularization and, 140–142, *141*
laser photocoagulation for, 141–142
differential diagnosis of, from age-related macular degeneration, 96
from serpiginous choroiditis, 562
physiologic, 189
retinal detachment and, 1244, 1248
scleral buckling for, 1266–1267
three-dimensional ultrasonography of, 58
Myopic fundus, 189–195
Myotonic dystrophy, hereditary, 930–931

Nanophthalmos, uveal effusion in, 665, *665*
uveal pressure in, 659
Nasal dialysis, 833
Nasaruplase, for central retinal vein occlusion, 295
Nd:YAG laser. See *Neodymium:yttrium-aluminum-garnet (Nd:YAG) laser.*
Necrotizing enteritis, in syphilis, 736, *737*
Necrotizing retinitis, differential diagnosis of, from intraocular lymphomas, 1207, *1209*
focal, from toxoplasmosis, 678, *678*
Needle aspiration biopsy, fine. See *Fine needle aspiration biopsy.*
Nematode endophthalmitis, differential diagnosis of, from medulloepithelioma, 1135
from retinoblastoma, 1153–1154, *1154*
intraocular calcification in, 1145
Nematode granulomas, differential diagnosis of, from retinal capillary hemangioma, 1160
Nematode infection(s), 806–811
diffuse unilateral subacute neuroretinitis from, 806–811
gnathostomiasis as, 814–817
toxocariasis as, 697–707
Neodymium:yttrium-aluminum-garnet (Nd:YAG) laser, 62, 64
cystoid macular edema after, 238, 244. See also *Cystoid macular edema.*
endophthalmitis after, 1472
for cystoid macular edema, 250
for diabetic retinopathy, 1427
frequency-doubled, 64–65
high-repetition-rate Q-switched, 65
retinal detachment and, 1244
sympathetic ophthalmia after, 569
Neonatal photic retinopathy, 848
Neoplasm. See *Tumor(s);* specific neoplasm, e.g., *Lymphoma.*
Neoplastic uveal effusion, 664, *665*
Neosynephrine, for ophthalmoscopy, 21
Nephritis, acute multifocal posterior placoid pigment epitheliopathy and, 547

Neurilemmoma, differential diagnosis of, from nonpigmented ciliary epithelium tumor, 1130, 1131
uveal, 1112–1114. See also *Uveal neurilemmoma.*
Neurologic disorders, retinitis pigmentosa and, 905t
Neuronal cells, 7–8
Neuronal ceroid lipofuscinosis (NCL), 902
retinitis pigmentosa and, 905–906
Neuroretinopathy, acute macular, 593–596. See also *Macular neuroretinopathy, acute.*
Neurosensory detachment, in serpiginous choroiditis, 556
Neurosensory retina, 83
Neurosyphilis, 794. See also *Syphilis.*
in HIV infected, 736
white ocular lesions in, 616t
Nevi, choroidal, 1053–1057. See also *Choroidal nevus.*
differential diagnosis of, from age-related macular degeneration, 97
halo, 1053
Nevus sebaceous syndrome, linear, differential diagnosis of, from choroidal osteoma, 1096–1097
Niclosamide, for cysticercosis, 713
Nicotinic acid, ocular disorders from, 863
Niemann-Pick disease, 928–929, *929*
histopathological features of, 925
Night blindness, congenital stationary, 934–940. See also *Congenital stationary night blindness.*
Nisl's granules, 8
Nitrosureas, ocular disorders from, 868
Nocardiosis, differential diagnosis of, from coccidioidomycosis, 780
Nongeographic atrophy, of retinal pigment epithelium, 87
Non-Hodgkin's lymphoma, CNS, intraocular lymphoma and, 1204, 1207–1210, *1207–1210*, 1209t
differential diagnosis of, from serpiginous choroiditis, 561
in HIV infection, 741
systemic, intraocular lymphoma and, 1210–1212, *1211–1213*
Nonpigmented ciliary epithelium tumors, acquired, 1130–1133
Nonsteroidal anti-inflammatory drugs (NSAIDs), for cystoid macular edema, 245, 248
for posterior scleritis, 640
Norrie's disease, differential diagnosis of, from familial exudative vitreoretinopathy, 427t, 428
from X-linked retinoschisis, 1015
North Carolina macular dystrophy, differential diagnosis of, from central areolar choroidal dystrophy, 956t
Nyctalopia, in Refsum's disease, 906

Occlusive vascular disease, in pregnancy, 506–509
Ocular angina, 373
Ocular blood flow, physiologic properties of, 346
Ocular calcification, contact B-scan ultrasonography of, 53
Ocular disorder(s), traumatic. See *Traumatic ocular disorder(s).*

Ocular fundus tumors, vasoproliferative, 1175–1181
Ocular histoplasmosis syndrome (OHS). See *Histoplasmosis, presumed ocular.*
Ocular ischemic syndrome, 372–381
ancillary studies of, 375–377, 377t, *378–380*
background of, 372
carotid artery studies of, 376
carotid endarterectomy for, 377–380
differential diagnosis of, 377, 380t
from acquired retinal arteriovenous communications, 1174
electroretinography of, 375–376, *380*
etiology of, 372
fluorescein angiography of, 375, 377t, *378–380*
in anterior segment, 373, *373*
in posterior segment, 373–375, 374t, *374–376*
laser photocoagulation for, 380–381
ophthalmodynamometry of, 377
pain of, 373
signs of, 372t, 373–375
symptoms of, 372–373
systemic associations with, 377, *380*
treatment of, 377–381
visual acuity in, 373
visual evoked potentials for, 376–377
visual loss in, 372–373, *374–376*
Ocular massage, for retinal artery occlusion, 277
Oculomotor paralysis, from interferon alfa, 864
Oguchi's disease, 937–938, *938*, 938t, 939, 944
histopathological features of, 939
molecular genetics of, 939
Onchocerciasis, ocular, 820–821, *824–826*
white ocular lesions in, 616t
Operating microscope, photic retinopathy from, 845
Ophthalmomyiasis, 813–814, *814–817*
clinical manifestations of, 813, *814–817*
external, 813
internal, 813
Ophthalmoscopy, direct, 21–22, *22–23*
laser photocoagulation and, 66
photic retinopathy from, 847
indirect, 22–28, *24–26*
laser photocoagulation and, 66
laser photocoagulation and, 66–67
methods of, 21–22
slit lamp, 22, 26
biomicroscopic, 26
contact lens, *27*, 27–28
non-contact lens, *26*, 26–28
Optic atrophy, from thioridazine, 855
in cryptococcosis, 781
in diffuse unilateral subacute neuroretinitis, 808
in mucopolysaccharide storage disorders, 928
in sarcoidosis, 650–651, *652, 653*
in toxoplasmosis, 680
in uveitis, intermediate, 603–604
in Vogt-Koyanagi-Harada syndrome, 581
sympathetic ophthalmia and, 572
Optic disc, coloboma of, macular holes and, 223
drusen of, 880–883
clinical features of, 880, *881*
complications of, 882–883
computed tomography of, 882, *882*

Optic disc (*Continued*)
diagnosis of, 881–882, *882*
differential diagnosis of, from astrocytic hamartoma, 1182
epidemiology of, 880
fluorescein angiography of, 882
histopathological features of, 882
in pseudoxanthoma elasticum, *172*, 172–173
ocular associations with, 883
pathogenesis of, 882
ultrasonography of, 882
edema of, acute multifocal posterior placoid pigment epitheliopathy and, 545
central retinal vein occlusion and, 288
hypertensive optic neuropathy and, 367–368
in bone marrow transplantation, 492
management of, 494
in diabetic retinopathy, in pregnancy, 504
in Leber's idiopathic optic neuroretinitis, 886
in sympathetic ophthalmia, 569, *571*
hemangioma of, differential diagnosis of, 1162
in myopia, degenerative, *191*, 191–192
neovascularization of, 275
in acute retinal necrosis, 750
in CMV infection, 718, *720*
in diabetic retinopathy, 324, *324*, 1409, 1410, *1411*, 1415, 1421
in ocular ischemic syndrome, 374, *376*
in uveitis, intermediate, 603–604
in Vogt-Koyanagi-Harada syndrome, 581
swelling of, chorioretinal folds in, 261
vascular defects of, hypofluorescence in, 31t
Optic nerve, aging of, 11
chorioretinal folds and, 258–259
clinical examination of, 21–28
disorders of, 873–888. See also specific disorders.
drusen of, choroidal neovascularization in, 150
evulsion of, fluorescein angiography of, 838, *838*
traumatic, 838, *838*
granulomas of, from toxocariasis, 702, 703
in cystoid macular edema, 241
intraocular medulloepithelioma and, 1134
leukemia and, 1199
melanocytoma of, 1188–1192
Optic nerve head (ONH), congenital pits of, 875–879
clinical features of, 875, *876–878*
differential diagnosis of, from chorioretinopathy, central serous, 208
eccentric, 875, *876–877*
fluorescein angiography of, 875, *876–877*
laser photocoagulation for, *878*, 878–879
optical coherence tomography of, 73
pericapillary, 875, *876–878*
retinal detachment and, 875–876, *876–878*
retinoschisis and, 876
treatment of, *878*, 878–879

Optic nerve head (*Continued*)
　　visual acuity in, 876–877
　　vitrectomy for, 879
　　drusen of, in retinitis pigmentosa, 893, *894*
　　in sickle cell retinopathy, 444–445
　　lack of blood-ocular barrier, 347
　　mechanisms of ischemia of, in hypertensive optic neuropathy, *367*, 368
　　neovascularization of, from toxoplasmosis, 680
　　vasculature of, anatomic and physiologic properties of, 345–348
Optic nerve melanocytoma, 1188–1192
　　clinical features of, 1188–1189, *1189, 1190*
　　diagnosis of, 1190, *1190*, 1192
　　differential diagnosis of, from combined hamartoma of retina and RPE, 1128
　　　from uveal melanoma, 1075t, *1077, 1077–1078*
　　management of, *1191–1192*, 1192
　　pathology of, 1189, *1190*
Optic neuritis, from oral contraceptives, 864
　　in sarcoidosis, 650–651, *652, 653*
　　in syphilis, 736, 795
　　in toxocariasis, 699
　　in toxoplasmosis, 678, *680*
　　in Vogt-Koyanagi-Harada syndrome, 574
　　sympathetic ophthalmia and, 572
Optic neuropathy, anterior ischemic, differential diagnosis of, from Leber's idiopathic optic neuroretinitis, 887
　　drusen and, 882
　　from hypertension, 348, 366–368
　　from interferon alfa, 864
　　from laser photocoagulation, for diabetic retinopathy, 1421
　　from radiation, 481–483, *484*
　　　prevention of, 485
　　in acute retinal necrosis, 750, 762
Optic neuroretinitis, differential diagnosis of, 887
　　Leber's idiopathic, 885–888. See also *Leber's idiopathic optic neurretinitis.*
Optic pits, retinal detachment from, pneumatic retinopexy for, 1286
Optical coherence tomography (OCT), 69–71, *70*
　　of age-related macular degeneration, 72–73
　　of central serous chorioretinopathy, 72
　　of epiretinal membrane, 72
　　of macular edema, 72
　　of macular holes, 71, *71–72*
Ora bay, enclosed, *9, 9*, 1220–1221, *1221*
　　partially enclosed, 9
Ora pearls, *9, 9*, 1224, *1224*
Ora serrata, 3, 8
　　anatomy of, vitrectomy and, 1298, *1299*
Oral contraceptives, central retinal vein occlusion and, 288
　　ocular disorders from, *863*, 863–864
Orbital exenteration, for uveal melanoma, 1072
Orbital hemorrhage, from vitrectomy, 1314–1315
Orbital masses, chorioretinal folds in, 259–260, *261*
Ornithine aminotransferase, in gyrate atrophy, 964, 973, 974

Ossification, intraocular, 1092. See also *Choroidal osteoma.*
Osteitis deformans, angioid streaks in, 163, 169t, 173
Osteoma, choroidal, 145, 147, 1092–1101. See also *Choroidal osteoma.*
　　differential diagnosis of, from age-related macular degeneration, 97
Outer plexiform layer, of retina, 6, *7–8*
Owl's eye cells, 719
Oxalate maculopathy, 930
Oxalate retinopathy, 866
Oxalosis, differential diagnosis of, from Bietti's crystalline dystrophy, 1044
　　ocular disease in, 930, *930*
　　retinitis pigmentosa and, 905t
Oxygen therapy, for retinal artery occlusion, 277–278
　　for retinopathy of prematurity, 409
Oxyphenbutazone, for sarcoidosis, 655–656

Paget's disease, angioid streaks in, 163, 169t, 173
　　manifestations of, 169t, 173
　　ocular, 173
Panoramic viewing, for giant retinal tears, 1340, 1347
　　traumatic, 1384
　　for laser photocoagulation, for diabetic retinopathy, 1421–1422
　　for proliferative vitreoretinopathy surgery, 1356
　　for traumatic injuries, 1376
Panretinal scatter laser photocoagulation (PRP). See also *Laser photocoagulation.*
　　for intermediate uveitis, 610
Panuveitis, multifocal choroiditis with. See *Multifocal choroiditis with panuveitis.*
Papilledema, chorioretinal folds and, 261
　　choroidal neovascularization in, 150
　　drusen and, 882
　　from cryptococcosis, 781
　　from interferon alfa, 864
　　in shaken baby syndrome, 838
Papillitis, from candidiasis, 774
　　from cytomegalovirus, 719, *722, 723*
　　from syphilis, 795, *796*
　　　in HIV infected, 736, *737*
　　from toxocariasis, 699, *703*
　　from toxoplasmosis, 678, *680*, 706
　　from tuberculosis, 803
　　serpiginous choroiditis and, 560
Paracentesis, anterior chamber, for retinal artery occlusion, 278
Parafoveal area, 3, 6, *6*
Parafoveal telangiectasis, 398–405. See also *Telangiectasis, parafoveal.*
Paraneoplastic syndromes, differential diagnosis of, from retinitis pigmentosa, 915, 917
Parasitic infections, diagnostic vitrectomy of, 1492–1495
Pars ciliaris, anatomy of, vitrectomy and, 1298, *1299*
Pars plana, anatomy of, vitrectomy and, 1298, *1299*
　　clinical examination of, 21–28
　　cysts of, *1224*, 1224–1225
Pars plana vitrectomy. See *Vitrectomy.*
Pars planitis. See *Uveitis, intermediate.*
Pars plicata, 8

Pattern dystrophy of RPE, 1006–1011
　　bull's eye maculopathy in, 1031, 1033t
　　clinical course of, 1006
　　clinical features of, 1006, *1007–1009*
　　clinical variants of, 1006–1007, *1010, 1011*
　　differential diagnosis of, 1031, 1033t
　　electrophysiology of, 1006
　　fluorescein angiography of, 1006, *1008, 1009*
　　molecular genetics of, 1007, 1011
Pavingstone degeneration of the retina, 1222–1224, *1223*
Pearl of ora serrata, *9, 9*, 1224, *1224*
Peau d'orange pigment, in pseudoxanthoma elasticum, *166, 171*, 171
Penicillin, for syphilis, 737, 798–799, 799t
Pentamidine, for *Pneumocystis carinii*, 738
Pentoxifylline, for central retinal vein occlusion, 295
Perfluorocarbon liquids, 1320–1325
　　characteristics of, 1320–1321, 1321t
　　complications of, 1324
　　extended-term intravitreal placement of, 1324–1325
　　for diabetic retinopathy, 1321–1322, *1322*
　　for giant retinal tears, 1322–1323, *1323, 1323*, 1338, 1339t, 1339–1340
　　　surgical techniques with, 1342–1345, *1343–1345*, 1348
　　　traumatic, 1384
　　for macular surgery, 1323
　　for perforating injuries, 1386
　　for proliferative vitreoretinopathy, 1321–1322, *1322*, 1357–1359, *1358–1361*
　　for removal of displaced crystalline lens, intraocular lens, or foreign bodies, 1323–1324
　　for suprachoroidal hemorrhages, 1388–1389
　　for trauma, 1323, 1376, 1378, 1384–1385
　　in combination therapy, 1331–1332
　　in vitrectomy, 1308
　　indications for, 1321t, 1321–1324
　　tolerance of, 1324
Perfluorocarbon-air exchange, in vitrectomy, 1308, 1310
Perfluorodecalin ($C_{10}F_{18}$), 1320–1325
　　properties of, 1321t
Perfluoroethane (C_2F_6), 1325–1329. See also *Gases, intraocular.*
　　characteristics of, 1326t
　　for giant retinal tears, 1346–1347
　　indications for, 1327t
Perfluoroethylcyclohexane (C_8F_{16}), 1320–1325. See also *Perfluorocarbon liquids.*
Perfluoromethane (CF_4), 1325–1329. See also *Gases, intraocular.*
　　characteristics of, 1326t
　　indications for, 1327t
Perfluoro-N-octane (C_8F_{18}), 1320–1325. See also *Perfluorocarbon liquids.*
　　for giant retinal tears, 1339–1340
　　for proliferative vitreoretinopathy, 1357–1359, *1358–1361*
　　for trauma, 1376
　　properties of, 1321t, 1339t, 1339–1340
Perfluorophenanthrene ($C_{14}F_{24}$), 1321–1325. See also *Perfluorocarbon liquids.*
　　properties of, 1321t

Perfluoropropane (C₃F₈), 1325–1329. See also *Gases, intraocular.*
characteristics of, 1326t
for giant retinal tears, 1346–1347
for proliferative vitreoretinopathy, 1364, 1365
for retinopexy, 1279
for traumatic injuries, 1378–1379, 1384–1385
for vitrectomy, 1310
indications for, 1327t
Perfluorotributylamine (C₁₂F₂₇N), 1321
Perfluorotri-N-propylamine, 1321
Pericapillary choroidal dystrophy, hereditary, 951t, 955–956, *957–960*
differential diagnosis of, 960t
Pericapillary edema, in sympathetic ophthalmia, 569
Pericapillary (pericentral) pigmentary degeneration, differential diagnosis of, from retinitis pigmentosa, 914, *916*
Pericentral retinal degeneration, in pregnancy, 505
Perimacular folds, in shaken baby syndrome, 838
Peripapillary choroid, in hypertensive optic neuropathy, *367, 368*
Peripapillary hemorrhages, optic disc drusen and, 880
Peripapillary subretinal neovascularization, differential diagnosis of, from serpiginous choroiditis, 562
Peripheral cystoid degeneration (PCD), 1222, *1223*
Peripheral neuropathy, diabetic retinopathy and, 319t
Peripheral retinal degeneration, acquired, differential diagnosis of, from retinitis pigmentosa, 911, 914, *914*
Peripheral retinal lesions, clinically insignificant, 1219–1226, 1220t
clinically significant, 1219, 1220t, 1227–1245
related to rhegmatogenous retinal detachments, 1219–1245, 1220t. See also specific lesions.
Peripherin/RDS mutations, retinitis pigmentosa and, 919
Peroxidase, protective effect of, 844
Persistent hyperplastic primary vitreous, differential diagnosis of, from familial exudative vitreoretinopathy, 427, 427t
from retinoblastoma, 1151, 1152t, *1153*
from toxocariasis, 704, 705t, 706
intraocular medulloepithelioma and, 1134, 1135
Peutz-Jeghers syndrome, 1061
Phagosomes, of RPE, 5
Phenothiazines, ocular disorders from, 855, 857–858
differential diagnosis of, from retinitis pigmentosa, 909, *911*
Phenylpropanolamine, retinal folds from, 265
Photic maculopathy, differential diagnosis of, from postsurgical cystoid macular edema, 243
Photic retinopathy, 844–848
age-related macular degeneration and, 848
defense mechanisms against, 844–845

Photic retinopathy (*Continued*)
from diagnostic ophthalmic instruments, 847
iatrogenic, *845,* 845–846
prevention of, 846
laser-associated, 846–847
mechanisms of, 844
neonatal, 848
solar, *847,* 847–848, *848*
Photochemical ocular injury, 847. See also *Photic retinopathy.*
Photocoagulation ocular injury, 844. See also *Photic retinopathy.*
Photodynamic therapy (PDT), 74–75
for choroidal neovascularization, 157
in AMD, 118
Photons, 61
absorption of, 62
Photoreceptor cells, 7–8
aging of, 11
Photoreceptor layer, of retina, 6, *6*
Photosensitivity, from sodium fluorescein dye, 29–30
Photosensitizer hematoporphyrin derivative (HPD), 74
Photothermolysis, selective, 75
Phototoxicity, cystoid macular edema and, 246
PHPV. See *Persistent hyperplastic primary vitreous.*
Phthisis bulbi, B-scan ultrasonography of, 54
Phthisis pubis, intraocular ossification and, 1092
PIC. See *Punctate inner choroidopathy (PIC).*
Pigment changes, from sodium fluorescein dye, 29
Pigment epithelial detachment (PED), drusenoid, 101, *103*
fibrovascular, 99, 101
hemorrhagic, 101, *103*
in age-related macular degeneration, 98, *99–102*
in chorioretinopathy, central serous, 207, 212
indocyanine-green angiography of, 42
serous, 101, *102*
Pigmentary retinopathies, unilateral, differential diagnosis of, from retinitis pigmentosa, 917, 917t
Pigmented ocular fundus lesions (POFLs), *1060–1062,* 1060–1063. See also *Retinal pigment epithelium, congenital hypertrophy of.*
familial adenomatous polyposis and, *1060, 1062,* 1063
microcephaly and, 1063
Pigmented paravenous chorioretinal atrophy, differential diagnosis of, from retinitis pigmentosa, 914, *915*
Pilocarpine, macular holes and, 223
Pineoblastoma, 1141, 1144
Plaques, indocyanine-green angiography of, *40, 42,* 44
Plasma protein risk factors, for retinal vascular occlusive disease, 459–471
Plasmin, for proliferative vitreoretinopathy, 1366
Platelet-activating factor, cystoid macular edema and, 246
Plus disease, 410, *410, 411*
Pneumatic retinopexy, 1272–1286
for CMV-related retinal detachments, 1480

Pneumatic retinopexy (*Continued*)
for harsh retinal tears, 1265
for retinal detachment, 833, 1249t, 1272–1286, *1273*
Betadine use in, 1278
case selection for, 1276–1277, 1277t
cataracts from, 1284
central retinal artery occlusion from, 1282
complications of, operative, 1281–1282
postoperative, 1282–1284
cryotherapy and, 1278, 1280–1281
endophthalmitis from, 1284
failure of reattachment in, 1282
for scleral buckling failures, 1285
gas bubble duration and size in, 1279
gas in anterior hyaloid space from, 1281, *1282*
gas injection in, 1278–1279, *1279*
gas selection for, 1279
laser photocoagulation and, 1278, 1280–1281
new retinal breaks from, 1283–1284
paracentesis and, 1278
postoperative care in, 1281
preoperative preparation for, 1277
proliferative vitreoretinopathy from, 1284
pseudophakic, 1266, 1276
repeat procedures for, 1284
special indications in, 1286
steamroller maneuver in, 1280, *1280*
subconjunctival gas from, 1282
subretinal fluid management in, 1272–1274, *1274*
delays in, 1283
subretinal gas from, 1281–1282, *1282*
technique of, 1277–1279
vitreous hemorrhage from, 1282
vitreous incarceration and, 1277, 1282
with multiple breaks, 1277, 1284–1285, *1285,* 1286
for retinal tears, giant, 1346–1347
history of, 1274–1275
literature on, 1275–1276
macular holes and, 223
surgeon and patient requirements for, 1276
Pneumocystis carinii, CMV co-infection with, in HIV infected, 720
differential diagnosis of, from tuberculosis, 803
fluorescein angiography of, 738
in HIV infection, 737–738, *738, 739,* 1212
management of, 738
white ocular lesions in, 616t
POFLs. See *Pigmented ocular fundus lesions (POFLs).*
POHS. See *Histoplasmosis, presumed ocular.*
Poliosis, in Vogt-Koyanagi-Harada syndrome, 575, *577*
Polycythemia, central retinal vein occlusion and, 288
Polydimethylsiloxane. See *Silicone liquid.*
Polymerase chain reaction (PCR), for toxoplasmosis, 683t, 685
for varicella-zoster virus, 769
vitrectomy samples for, 1488, *1488*
Polypoidal vasculopathy, idiopathic choroidal, choroidal neovascularization and, 148, *152*
indocyanine-green angiography for, 45

Porrocaecum, 819
Posterior placoid pigment epitheliopathy, acute multifocal. See *Acute multifocal posterior pigment epitheliopathy.*
Posterior scleritis, 635–641. See also *Scleritis, posterior.*
Posterior segment, clinical examination of, 21–28
  in bone marrow transplantation, 488, 489t
  trauma in, 831–841
    chorioretinitis sclopetaria from, 833–834, *835*
    choroidal rupture from, 145, *149*, 834–836, *835*
    commotio retinae from, 836–837, *837*
    histopathological features of, 832
    direct, 831–838
    epidemiology of, 831
    fat embolism syndrome and, 840
    in bungee jumping, 841, *841*
    indirect, 838–841
    macular holes from, 833, *834*
    optic nerve evulsion from, 838, *838*
    photic retinopathy as, 844–848
    Purtscher's retinopathy from, 839–840, *840*
    retinal detachments from, 831, 833
    retinal dialyses from, 831, 833
    retinal pigment epithelium contusion and tears from, *837*, 837–838
    retinal tears from, 831, 833, *833*
    shaken baby syndrome and, 838–839, *839*
    Terson's syndrome and, 839, *839*
    Valsalva retinopathy from, 840, *840*
    whiplash retinopathy from, 840–841
Posterior uveal bleeding syndrome. See *Choroidal vasculopathy, idiopathic polypoid.*
Posterior vitreoretinal interface, contact B-scan ultrasonography of, 50, *50*
Potassium, abnormalities of, and hypertension, 348
PPRPE. See *Retinal pigment epithelium, preserved para-arteriolar.*
PR, pneumatic. See *Pneumatic retinopexy.*
Precapillary arterioles, change in lumen size of, 347
Prednisolone, for cystoid macular edema, 247, 247t
Prednisone. See also *Corticosteroids.*
  for acute retinal necrosis, 750, 764
  for serpiginous choroiditis, 562
Pre-eclampsia, cortical blindness in, 506
  diabetic retinopathy and, 504
  HELLP syndrome in, 506
  retinal changes in, 505–506, 506t
  retinopathy of, 505–506, 506t
  serous retinal detachment in, 506, *507*, *508*
Pregnancy, amniotic fluid embolism in, 509
  candidal endophthalmitis in, 509
  central serous chorioretinopathy in, 498–500, *499*
  choroidal hemangiomas in, 505
  choroidal neovascularization in, 500
  cystoid macular edema associated with vitritis in, 509
  diabetic retinopathy in, 340–341, 501–504
    fetal well-being and, 504

Pregnancy (*Continued*)
  macular edema of, 502
  nonproliferative, 502
  optic disc edema in, 504
  pre-eclampsia and, 504
  preproliferative, 502
  progression of, 501–504
    versus nonpregnant women, 503–504
  proliferative, 502–503
  DIC in, 473
  dilating drops in, use of, 510
  disseminated intravascular coagulopathy in, 508–509
  fluorescein angiography in, 509–510
  hypertension in, 505–506
    cortical blindness in, 506
    HELLP syndrome in, 506
    retinopathy of, 505–506, 506t
    serous retinal detachment in, 506, *507*, *508*
  macular neuroretinopathy in, 509
  myopia in, 505
  occlusive vascular disease in, 506–509
  ocular toxoplasmosis in, 504–505
  pericentral retinal degeneration in, 505
  pseudoxanthoma elasticum in, 505
  retinal artery occlusion in, 507–508, *508*
  retinal changes associated with disorders of, 505–509
  retinal changes in context of pre-existing retinal disease, 500–505
  retinal changes in normal, 498–500
  retinal detachment surgery in, 505
  retinal diseases in, 498–510
  retinal hemorrhages in, 509
  retinal vein occlusion in, 508
  retinitis pigmentosa in, 505
  sarcoidosis in, 505
  thrombotic thrombocytopenia purpura in, 509
  topical anesthetics in, use of, 510
  toxemia of, differential diagnosis of, from AMPPPE, 550
    hypofluorescence in, 35
    retinal detachments in, *913*
  toxoplasmosis in, 504–505
    management of, 691
    screening for, 692
    serologic tests for, 685–687, 686t
  unilateral acute idiopathic maculopathy in, 500
  uveal melanoma in, 500
  uveitis in, 505
  Valsalva maculopathy in, 509
  Vogt-Koyanagi-Harada syndrome in, 505
Premacular fibroplasia (fibrosis). See *Epimacular membranes (EMMs).*
Prematurity, retinopathy of, 407–412. See also *Retinopathy of prematurity.*
Preretinal membranes. See *Epimacular membranes (EMMs).*
Preretinal neovascularization, in Coats' disease, 392
Presumed ocular histoplasmosis syndrome (POHS). See *Histoplasmosis, presumed ocular.*
Procarbazine, ocular disorders from, 868
Progressive bifocal chorioretinal atrophy, hereditary, 975–976
Progressive cone dystrophy, 943–946, *945*, *947*
  differential diagnosis of, 987

Progressive outer retinal necrosis (PORN), 755–758, 766–770. See also *Acute retinal necrosis (ARN).*
  anterior segment in, 755
  clinical features of, 755, 766–768, *767–769*
  "cracked mud" scarring from, 733, *733*, 755
  diagnosis of, 756
  differential diagnosis of, 734, 767t, *768*, 768–769
    from acute retinal necrosis, 766, 767t, 769
    from toxoplasmosis, 681–682
  epidemiology of, 755
  etiology of, 756, 769, *770*
  histopathological features of, 756–757
  in HIV infection, 732, *733*, 733–734, *734*
  laboratory diagnosis of, 733–734
  posterior segment in, 755–756, *756*, *757*
  prognosis and treatment of, 757–758
  retinal detachments and, 1483–1484
  treatment of, 734, 769–770
  VZV and, 733–734
Proliferative vitreoretinopathy (PVR), 1350–1367
  after scleral buckling, for retinal detachment, 1250, 1251, 1270
  anterior, 1351–1352, *1352*
    surgical management of, 1360–1362, *1361*, *1362*
  classification of, 1352–1353, 1353t, 1354t
  CMV-related retinal detachments and, 1479
  fluid-air exchange in, *1359*, 1364
  from pneumatic retinopexy, 1275, 1284
  giant retinal tears and, 1339, 1341, 1342, *1343*, 1346
    management of, 1342
  in epimacular membranes, 230, 232
    recurrence of, 235
    vitrectomy for, 1306, 1357
  intraocular gases for, 1326, 1327t, 1365
  intraocular tamponade for, 1364
  laser photocoagulation for, 1364
  pathophysiology of, 1350–1352
  perfluorocarbon liquids for, 1321–1322, 1357–1359, *1358–1361*
  pharmacologic prevention of, 1366–1367
  posterior, surgical management of, 1356–1360, *1357–1361*
  relaxing retinotomy/retinectomy for, 1363–1364, *1364*
  retinal folds in, 263, 265
  silicone liquid for, 1329, 1330, 1331, *1365*, 1365–1366
  subretinal membrane dissection for, *1362*, 1362–1363, *1363*
  subretinal strands in, surgery for, 135–136
  surgical management of, 1353–1356
    for closure of retinal breaks, 1354
    for long-term retinal stabilization, 1354
    for reduction of recurrence, 1354
    for relief of traction, 1354
    improving visualization for, *1355*, 1355–1356
    principles of, 1354
    selection of procedure for, 1355
    timing of, 1355

Proliferative vitreoretinopathy (*Continued*)
trauma and, 1375, 1376, 1378, 1387
case example of, 1391
vitrectomy for, 1341–1342, 1356
enzyme-assisted, 1366
Proparacaine hydrochloride, for ophthalmoscopy, 21
Propionibacterium acnes, cultures of, 1487, 1489
endophthalmitis from, 1471–1472, *1472*
Prostaglandin(s), abnormalities of, and hypertension, 348
cystoid macular edema and, 245–246, 246t
E₁, for central retinal vein occlusion, 295
Prostate carcinoma, choroidal metastasis and, 1104
Protein C, activated, resistance to, 459, 460, 464
deficiency of, 459–464
acquired, 459–460
central retinal vein occlusion in, *461–462*, 462
congenital, 459
ocular manifestations of, *460–464, 462–464*
diagnosis of, 463–464
therapy for, 464
Protein kinase C activation, in diabetic retinopathy, 338
Protein S deficiency, ocular manifestations of, 465, *468–469*
Proteinuria, diabetic retinopathy and, 319t
Proteoglycans, uveal effusion and, 665–666
Pseudoaphakia, retinal detachment and, 1233–1234, 1244
Pseudohypopyon, endophthalmitis and, 1474
Pseudomembranous conjunctivitis, in graft-versus-host disease, 488
Pseudo-operculum, 219, 223
Pseudophakia, retinal detachment and, balloon buckles for, 1292–1293, *1295*
pneumatic retinopexy for, 1266, 1276
Pseudoretinitis pigmentosa, 908–920
bilateral, 908t, 909–917
differential diagnosis of, 821
from syphilis, *794*, 795
unilateral, 917, 917t
Pseudotumor cerebri, from oral contraceptives, 864
Pseudoxanthoma elasticum, angioid streaks in, 142, *143*, 168, 169t, 170–173
crystalline bodies in, *167*, 172
fluorescein angiography of, 171, *171, 172*
focal atrophic RPE lesions in, 171–172
in cardiovascular system, 170
in pregnancy, 505
in skin, 168, 170, *170*
indocyanine green angiography of, 171
manifestations of, 168, 169t, 170, *170*
ocular manifestations of, 170–173
optic disc drusen in, *172*, 172–173
peau d'orange pigment in, *166, 171,* 171
Punctate inner choroidopathy (PIC), 621–624, 628–629
clinical course and treatment of, 623–624, 626t
clinical features of, 621
corticosteroids for, 623t, 623–624

Punctate inner choroidopathy (*Continued*)
differential diagnosis of, from AMPPPE, 550
from MEWDS, 589
from sarcoidosis, 655
electroretinography of, 623
laser photocoagulation for, 624, *625*
patient characteristics of, 618t, 621
perimetry signs of, 622–623
posterior segment signs of, 622, *624*
subfoveal surgery for, 624
visual acuity in, 624t
Punctate keratitis, in graft-versus-host disease, 488
Pupillary defect, relative afferent, in central retinal artery obstruction, 271
in central retinal vein occlusion, 288, 292, 293
Pupillary dilation, for ophthalmoscopy, 21
Pupillary reflex, as defense mechanism, 844
Purtscher's retinopathy, 839–840, *840*
bungee jumping and, 841
differential diagnosis of, from bone marrow transplantation retinopathy, 494
from shaken baby syndrome, 838
PVR. See *Proliferative vitreoretinopathy (PVR)*.
PXE. See *Pseudoxanthoma elasticum*.
Pyrimethamine, adverse effects of, 688
for toxoplasmosis, 688, 689t, 690
in HIV infected, 735
in neonates, 691
in pregnancy, 691

Quinine sulfate, ocular disorders from, 860–862, *862*

Racemose hemangioma. See *Retinal arteriovenous communications, congenital*.
Radiation, characteristics of, 127
isodose curves of, 127, *128*
sources of, 127
Radiation retinopathy, 477–486
background, 480–481, 481t
treatment of, 483, 485t
bone marrow transplantation retinopathy and, 490
clinical course of, 483
clinical features of, *479*, 479–481, *480*, 481t, *482*
delivery system and, 478
differential diagnosis of, 483, 485t
from parafoveal telangiectasis, 405
dosages and, 478
epidemiology of, 477–479
etiology of, 477–479
fluorescein angiography of, *479, 480, 481, 482*
from leukemia treatment, 1201
histopathological features of, 483
history of, 477
laser photocoagulation for, 485
pathology of, 481–483
preproliferative, 480, 481, 481t
treatment of, 485, 485t
prevention of, 485–486
prognosis for, 483, *484*
proliferative, 480, 481t
treatment of, 485, 485t

Radiation retinopathy (*Continued*)
risk factors for, 478, 478t
treatment of, 483–485, 485t
Radiation therapy, bone marrow transplantation retinopathy and, 488, 490
for choroidal hemangioma, 1088, *1088,* 1090
for choroidal metastasis, 1107, *1107–* 1108
for choroidal neovascularization, 126–130, 157
adverse effects of, 129t, 129–130
acute, 129, 129t
late, 129t, 130
brachytherapy, 128–129
characteristics of, 127, *127, 128*
external beam photon, 128–129
in AMD, 118
methods of, 128
theory of, 126–127
for retinoblastoma, 1145–1146, *1146*
for uveal melanoma, 1071, *1071*
for vasoproliferative ocular fundus tumors, 1180
Rayleigh scattering, 62
Recirculation phase, of fluorescein angiography, 31
Refsum's disease, retinitis pigmentosa and, 906, 908
Remote spots, indocyanine-green angiography of, *40, 42,* 44
Renal cell carcinoma, choroidal metastasis and, 1104
Renal disorders, retinitis pigmentosa and, 905t
Renin-angiotensin-aldosterone system, abnormalities of, hypertension and, 348
Restriction fragment length polymorphisms (RFLPs), 918
Reticulum cell sarcoma. See *Lymphoma, intraocular*.
Retina, anatomy of, 3, *4*
clinical examination of, 21–28
cystic degeneration of, 14–15, *15*
developmental variations in, 8–10
sensory, 3
Retinal abnormalities, in degenerative myopia, 192, *193*
Retinal angiomatosis, intraocular calcification in, 1145
Retinal arterial macroaneurysms, 383–389
classification of, 387
demography of, 383, 385t
exudative, 383, *387*
fluorescein angiography of, 385, *386*
from congenital retinal arteriovenous communications, 1172
hemorrhagic, 383, 385, *386, 387*
histopathological features of, 383, 384, *388*
laser photocoagulation for, 387–388, *388, 389*
macular detachment in, 383, 385
vitreous hemorrhage in, 383, *386–387*
Retinal arterial microaneurysms, central retinal vein occlusion and, 295
in bone marrow transplantation, 491, *493*
in diabetic retinopathy, 322–323, *323*
in leukemia, 1197t, 1197–1198
in ocular ischemic syndrome, 374, *375*
in radiation retinopathy, 477, 479

Retinal arterial occlusion, 271–283
  branch, 277, 278. See also *Branch retinal artery occlusion.*
  central, 271–278. See also *Central retinal artery occlusion.*
  cotton-wool spots in, *281,* 281–283, *282,* 282t
  in pregnancy, 507–508, *508*
  in systemic lupus erythematosus, 523–525, *524–525*
  of cilioretinal artery, *280,* 280–281, *281*
Retinal arteries, physiology of, 347
  pulsations of, in ocular ischemic syndrome, 375
Retinal arterioles, physiology of, 347
Retinal arteriovenous communications, acquired, 1174
  congenital, 1172–1174
    central retinal vein occlusion and, 292
    classification of, 1174
    clinical presentation of, 1172, 1174, *1174*
    differential diagnosis of, from retinal capillary hemangioma, 1160
    histopathological features of, 1173
    hyperfluorescence of, *35, 36*
    systemic abnormalities associated with, 1172, 1174
    treatment of, 1174
  macular holes and, 223
Retinal astrocytoma, 1182–1187. See also *Astrocytic hamartoma.*
  acquired, 1183–1186
    clinical features of, *1185,* 1185–1186
    diagnosis of, 1186, *1186*
    differential diagnosis of, from vasoproliferative tumors, 1176
    fluorescein angiography of, 1186
    management of, 1186
    pathology of, 1186, *1186*
    ultrasonography of, 1186, *1186*
Retinal breaks. See also *Retinal detachment(s), rhegmatogenous; Retinal tears.*
  asymptomatic, 1243–1244
    clinical features of, 1244
    histopathological features of, 1244
    history of, 1243–1244
    prognosis and management of, 1244
  balloon buckles for localizing, 1292, *1294*
  cystic retinal tufts and, 1234–1235, *1235–1236*
  differential diagnosis of, from enclosed ora bay, 1220–1221
    from white-with-pressure sign, 1225, 1226
  horseshoe, balloon buckles for, 1296t
  in epimacular membranes, 230, 235
    management of, 233–234
  in hemoglobinopathies, 448
  in Stickler syndrome, 924, 926
  large horseshoe, localization of, 1253, *1255*
  localization of, for scleral buckling of detachment, 1253–1254, *1254, 1255*
  new, from pneumatic retinopexy, 1283–1284
  retinal detachment and, 1244
  senile (degenerative) retinoschisis and, 1240–1241, *1241*
  traumatic, 1374, 1376

Retinal capillary hemangioma, 1159–1166
  clinical features of, 1159–1160, *1160–1162,* 1180t
  color Doppler imaging of, 1163
  computed tomography of, 1164
  cryotherapy for, 1165
  diagnosis of, 1163–1164
  differential diagnosis of, 1160, 1162
    from astrocytic hamartoma, 1182
    from retinoblastoma, 1152t, 1155
    from vasoproliferative tumors, 1175, 1176, 1180t
  fluorescein angiography of, *1161–1163,* 1163
  histopathological features of, 1162–1163
  indocyanine green angiography of, 1163
  laser photocoagulation for, 1164, *1165*
  magnetic resonance imaging of, 1164
  management of, 1164–1165, *1165*
    systemic, 1164t, 1165
  pathogenesis of, 1162–1163
  prognosis for, 1165
  radiation therapy for, 1165
  systemic evaluation of, 1164, 1164t
  ultrasonography of, 1163
Retinal cavernous hemangioma, 1168–1171
  clinical features of, 1168, *1169*
  diagnosis of, 1168–1169, *1170*
  differential diagnosis of, from retinal capillary hemangioma, 1160
    from uveal melanoma, 1075t, 1078, *1078*
  fluorescein angiography of, 1168, *1170*
  histopathological features of, 1168, *1170*
  management of, 1169
  ultrasonography of, 1168
Retinal detachment(s), balloon buckles for, 1288–1296
  complications of, 1293
  history of, 1288
  indications for, 1291–1293, *1291–1295*
  pathophysiology of, 1288, *1289*
  results of, 1293, 1296t
  technique of, 1288–1289, *1290*
  breaks and, 831. See also *rhegmatogenous.*
  choroidal metastasis and, 1104
  choroidal nevus and, 1053, *1055*
  contact B-scan ultrasonography of, *51,* 51–52
    traction, 51–52, *52*
  dialyses and, 831
  DIC and, 475
  differential diagnosis of, from postsurgical cystoid macular edema, 243
  from vitrectomy, 1312–1313, *1313,* 1316
  funnel, B-scan ultrasonography of, 51, *51*
  in acute retinal necrosis, 749, 753, 762–763
    prophylaxis for, 754–755, 764
  in Best's disease, 997
  in CMV infection, 718–719, *721,* 728–730, *731–732,* 1478–1483
    epidemiology of, 1478
    risk factors for, 1478–1479
    surgery for, *1479,* 1479–1482, *1480*
  in Coats' disease, 393, 396, 1152, *1153*
  in degenerative myopia, 195, *197*

Retinal detachment(s) (*Continued*)
  in diffuse unilateral subacute neuroretinitis, 808
  in familial exudative vitreoretinopathy, 423t, 424, 425, 427t
  in HIV infected, from CMV, 728–730, *731–732*
    silicone liquid for, 1329
  in nematode endophthalmitis, 1154
  in posterior scleritis, 635, *636*
  in progressive outer retinal necrosis, 734, 758, 779
  in retinopathy of prematurity, 412, 1459–1460, 1462–1463
    at stage 5, 1462–1463
    evolution of, 1459–1460, *1460*
    late surgical intervention for, 1463
  in Stickler syndrome, 924
  in syphilis, 795
  in toxocariasis, 701–702
  in toxoplasmosis, 679, *679,* 681
  in tuberculosis, 803
  in uveitis, intermediate, 603, 605
  in Vogt-Koyanagi-Harada syndrome, 574, *578, 579, 579*
  in X-linked retinoschisis, 1013, *1016*
  intraocular foreign bodies and, 1400–1401
  intraocular gases for, 1326, 1327t
  macular holes and, 1440, 1441
  myopia and, 1244
    scleral buckling for, 1266–1267
  optic nerve head congenital pits and, 875–876, *876–878*
  pathoanatomy and pathophysiology of, 1249–1250, *1250*
  pneumatic retinopexy for, 1272–1286, *1273*
    case selection for, 1276–1277, 1277t
    cataracts from, 1284
    central retinal artery occlusion from, 1282
    complications of, operative, 1281–1282
      postoperative, 1282–1284
    cryotherapy and, 1272, 1280–1281
    endophthalmitis from, 1284
    failure of reattachment in, 1282
    for scleral buckling failures, 1285
    gas bubble duration and size in, 1279
    gas in anterior hyaloid space from, 1281, *1282*
    gas injection in, 1278–1279, *1279*
    gas selection for, 1279
    laser photocoagulation and, 1272, 1280–1281
    new retinal breaks from, 1283–1284
    postoperative care in, 1281
    preoperative preparation for, 1277
    proliferative vitreoretinopathy from, 1284
    repeat procedures for, 1284
    special indications for, 1286
    steamroller maneuver in, 1280, *1280*
    subconjunctival gas from, 1282
    subretinal fluid management in, 1272–1274, *1274*
      delays in, 1283
    subretinal gas from, 1281–1282, *1282*
    technique of, 1277–1279
    vitreous hemorrhage from, 1282
    vitreous incarceration from, 1282
    with multiple breaks, 1284–1285, *1285,* 1286

Retinal detachment(s) (*Continued*)
  proliferative vitreoretinopathy and, 1351–1352, *1352*
  pseudophakic, balloon buckles for, 1292–1293, *1295*
    scleral buckling for, 1266
  recurrent/persistent, after scleral buckling, 1269–1270
  resolution of, differential diagnosis of, from retinitis pigmentosa, 911, *913*
  rhegmatogenous. See also specific disorders featuring.
    asymptomatic, 1243–1244
    asymptomatic breaks and, 1243–1244
    atrophic retinal holes and, *1231–1232*, 1231–1233
    choroidal neovascularization in, 150
    cystic retinal tuft and, 1234–1237, *1235–1238*
    differential diagnosis of, from choroidal metastasis, 1105
      from retinoblastoma, 1152t, 1157
      from uveal melanoma, 1075t, 1082
    epimacular membranes and, 235
    in birdshot retinochoroidopathy, 566
    in familial exudative vitreoretinopathy, 425, 429
    in retinopathy of prematurity, 1460–1461
    lattice degeneration and, 1227t, *1227–1230*, 1227–1234
    multiple risk factors for, 1244–1245
      three, 1245
      two, 1244
    pathoanatomy and pathophysiology of, 1249–1250, *1250*
    peripheral lesions related to, 1219–1245, 1220t. See also specific lesions.
      clinically insignificant, 1219–1226, 1220t
      clinically significant, 1219, 1220t, 1227–1245
    pneumatic retinopexy for, 1272–1286. See also *pneumatic retinopexy for*.
    prognosis and management of, in aphakic or pseudophakic fellow eyes, 1233–1234
      in phakic, fellow eyes, 1233, 1234t
      in phakic, nonfellow eyes, 1232–1233
    scleral buckling for, 1248–1271. See also *scleral buckling for*.
    senile (degenerative) retinoschisis and, 1238–1243, *1239–1242*
    vasoproliferative tumors and, 1175, 1178t
    white lines and, *1228–1230*, 1230–1231
  scleral buckling for, 833, 1248–1271, 1249t
    accessory techniques in, 1260–1261
    air-fluid exchange and, 1261
    altered refractive error after, 1268
    anatomic results of, 1267
    choroidal detachment after, 1268, *1268*
    common causes of detachment, 1265t
    configurations for, 1251–1253, 1252t, *1253*, 1254
    configurations of, 1251–1253, 1252t, *1253–1254*

Retinal detachment(s) (*Continued*)
    favored routine, 1254–1257, *1255, 1256*
    cystoid macular edema after, 1269
    drainage technique in, *1258, 1258–1260, 1259*
      problems with, 1263–1264, *1264*
    encircling, 1256–1257
    final adjustment in, 1260
    for inferior temporal dialysis, 1266
    for large superior horseshoe tear, *1265, 1265–1266, 1266*
    for multiple horseshoe tears and lattice degeneration, 1266
    for myopic detachments, 1266–1267
    intraoperative management of dilemmas, 1261–1265
    intravitreal gas injection and, 1260–1261
      problems with, 1265
    localization and treatment of breaks in, 1253–1254, *1254, 1255*
      dilemmas in, 1261, 1263
    macular pucker after, 1269, *1269*
    management of subretinal fluid in, 1257–1260
    nondrainage techniques in, 1257–1258
    postoperative complications of, 1267–1270
    postoperative laser photocoagulation and, 1261, *1262*
    principles of, 1250–1265
    proliferative vitreoretinopathy after, 1270
    pseudophakic, 1266
    recurrent/persistent detachment, 1269–1270
    scleral buckle/retinal break relationship in, *1264*, 1264
    segmental, 1256
    strabismus after, 1268
    suture placement, problems with, 1263, *1263*
    visual results of, 1267
  serous, acute multifocal posterior placoid pigment epitheliopathy and, 545
    in chorioretinopathy, 207
    in hypertensive choroidopathy, *350, 354–356, 360–362, 365, 366*
    in pre-eclampsia, 506, *507, 508*
  silicone liquid for, 1329
  suprachoroidal hemorrhage and, 1388
  surgery for, pregnancy and, 505
  sympathetic ophthalmia and, 572
  traction, from branch retinal vein occlusion, 312
    in diabetic retinopathy, 325, 1411, *1412*, 1423–1425, 1426
    in hemoglobinopathies, 447–448
    radiation retinopathy and, 479
    treatment of, 485
  traumatic, 831, 833, 1374, 1376, 1382–1385, *1385*
    case example of, 1391
    hemorrhagic, 1386–1387, *1387*
  uveal effusion and, 659–660, *660*, 662, 666
  vasoproliferative ocular fundus tumors and, 1077
Retinal dialysis, giant retinal tears and, 1338, *1339*
  scleral buckling for inferior, 1266
  traumatic, 831, 833

Retinal dialysis (*Continued*)
  vasoproliferative tumors and, 1175, 1178t
  traumatic, 831, 832, 1382–1383
Retinal disruption, drug-induced, 855–862, 857t
Retinal drawing, 25
Retinal dystrophies, systemic genetic disorders associated with, 924–931
Retinal edema, in hypertensive retinopathy, 359
Retinal flaps, giant retinal tears and, management of, 1341–1342
Retinal folds, 263–265
  after surgery, 265
  causes of, 264t, 264–265
  circumferential, proliferative vitreoretinopathy and, 1351, *1352*
  clinical evaluation of, *258*, 263–264, *264*
  fluorescein angiography of, 264
  in drug-induced myopia, 265
  in epiretinal membranes, 265
  in familial exudative vitreoretinopathy, 427t
  in infants and children, 265
  in posterior scleritis, 635, *636*
  in proliferative vitreoretinopathy, 265
  mechanisms of, 264
Retinal granulomas, differential diagnosis of, from astrocytic hamartoma, 1182
  from retinoblastoma, 1153
  from toxocariasis, 702
Retinal hairpin loops, in sickle cell retinopathy, 442, *444*
Retinal hamartoma, astrocytic, differential diagnosis of, from retinal capillary hemangioma, 1160
  from retinoblastoma, 1152t, 1155, *1155*
  from vasoproliferative tumors, 1176
  combined, 1123–1129. See also *Retinal pigment epithelium, combined hamartoma of*.
    clinical features of, 1125–1127, *1126*
    definition of, 1123
    diagnosis of, 1127
    differential diagnosis of, 1128
      from optic nerve melanocytoma, 1189
      from retinoblastoma, 1155, *1155*
    epidemiology of, 1125
    etiology of, 1127
    histopathological features of, 1124, 1125
    history of, 1123, 1125
    systemic associations with, 1127–1128
    treatment of, 1128–1129
Retinal hemangioma, acquired, differential diagnosis of, 1162
  from retinal capillary hemangioma, 1160, 1162
  capillary. See *Retinal capillary hemangioma*.
  presumed acquired. See *Vasoproliferative ocular fundus tumors*.
Retinal hemorrhage. See also *Intraretinal hemorrhage; Subretinal hemorrhage*.
  acute multifocal posterior placoid pigment epitheliopathy and, 545
  DIC and, 475
  from congenital retinal arteriovenous communications, 1172

Retinal hemorrhage (*Continued*)
  from diffuse unilateral subacute neuro-
      retinitis, 808
  from toxoplasmosis, 678, 680
  in bone marrow transplantation, 491,
      492, 494
    management of, 494
  in Eales' disease, 418
  in HIV infection, 714, *716*
  in hypertensive retinopathy, *356, 357,*
      359
  in leukemia, 1197t, 1197–1198, *1200,*
      1201, *1201*
  in ocular ischemic syndrome, 374, *374*
  in pregnancy, 509
  in Purtscher's retinopathy, 839
  in sarcoidosis, 648, *648*
  in shaken baby syndrome, 838
  macular holes and, 833
  perfluorocarbon liquids for, 1323
  subretinal fluid drainage and, 1263
Retinal holes, atrophic, retinal detach-
      ments and, *1231–1232,* 1231–
      1233
  from subretinal fluid drainage, 1263
Retinal hypofluorescence, causes of, 31t,
      32, *32*
Retinal incarceration, from vitrectomy,
      1313–1314
  subretinal fluid drainage and, 1263
  traumatic, 1374, 1384–1385, *1385*
    case example of, 1391
Retinal ischemic spots, internal. See
      Cotton-wool spots.
Retinal microaneurysms, in diabetic reti-
      nopathy, 1409
Retinal necrosis, acute. See *Acute retinal
      necrosis.*
  progressive outer. See *Progressive outer
      retinal necrosis.*
Retinal neovascularization, choroidal os-
      teoma and, 1095
  choroidal rupture and, 835–836
  from operating microscope, 846
  in acute retinal necrosis, 750
  in branch retinal vein occlusion, 312,
      312, 313
    laser management of, 314, *314*
  in candidiasis, 774
  in diabetic retinopathy, 324–325, *325,*
      1409, *1409,* 1426
  in familial exudative vitreoretinopathy,
      423, *423,* 423t, *424,* 427t
  in leukemia, 1197t, 1198
  in ocular ischemic syndrome, 374,
      376
  in radiation retinopathy, 477, 479, 480,
      482
  in sarcoidosis, 648
  in serpiginous choroiditis, 556
  in systemic lupus erythematosus, 523,
      525, *525*
  in toxoplasmosis, 680
  in tuberculosis, 802
  in uveitis, intermediate, 602, 605
  in Vogt-Koyanagi-Harada syndrome,
      574
  parafoveal telangiectasis and, 405
Retinal nerves, fiber loss of, in hyperten-
      sive retinopathy, *356,* 359–361
Retinal occlusive disease, arterial. See
      Retinal arterial occlusion.
  in systemic lupus erythematosus, 523–
      525, *524–525*
  venous. See *Retinal venous occlusion.*
Retinal oxalosis, 866

Retinal periphlebitis, in sarcoidosis, 647,
      647, 648
  in tuberculosis, 804
  serpiginous choroiditis and, 560
Retinal phlebitis, frosted branch angiitis
      from, 434
Retinal phototoxicity, 844–848. See also
      Photic retinopathy.
Retinal pigment epitheliitis, acute, 597–
      598
  differential diagnosis of, 598
    from MEWDS, 589
  electrophysiologic tests in, 598
  fluorescein angiography of, 597–598
  macular lesions in, 597
Retinal pigment epithelium (RPE), ade-
      nocarcinoma of, 1120–1122. See
      also *adenoma of.*
  adenoma of, 1120–1122
    clinical features of, 1120, *1121*
    diagnosis of, 1120–1121, *1121, 1122*
    differential diagnosis of, 1075t, 1079,
        1079
      from combined hamartoma of ret-
          ina and RPE, 1128
      from vasoproliferative tumors,
          1175, 1180t
    histopathological features of, 1120,
        1121
    management of, 1121–1122
    ultrasonography of, 1121, *1121,
        1122*
  aging of, 11
  atrophy of, 12
    geographic, *87,* 87–89
    in central serous chorioretinopathy,
        207, 207, 208, 208
    nongeographic, 87
  black sunburst in, in sickle cell reti-
      nopathy, 441–442, *442, 443*
  blood-retinal barrier in, 347
  bull's eye maculopathy in, 1031, 1033t
  cells of, 4, *4*
  clinical features of, 1180t
  combined hamartoma of, 1118–1120,
      1122, 1123–1129
    associated ocular findings in, 1126–
        1127
    clinical features of, 1119, *1119,* 1125–
        1127
    clinical presentation of, 1125
    diagnosis of, 1119, *1120,* 1127
    differential diagnosis of, 1128
      from melanoma, 1075t, 1079, *1079*
      from optic nerve melanocytoma,
          1189
      from retinoblastoma, 1155, *1155*
    epidemiology of, 1125
    etiology of, 1127
    fundoscopic features of, 1125–1126,
        1126
    histopathological features of, 1119,
        1119, 1124, 1125
    history of, 1123, 1125
    management of, 1119–1120, 1128–
        1129
    prognosis for, 1128
    systemic associations with, 1127–
        1128
    visual acuity in, 1125
  congenital hypertrophy of, 1058–1063,
      1116–1118, 1122
    clinical features of, 1058, *1059,* 1116–
        1117, *1117*
    diagnosis of, 1117

Retinal pigment epithelium (*Continued*)
    differential diagnosis of, 1058–1059,
        1059, 1128
      from choroidal nevus, 1055
      from uveal melanoma, 1078, *1079*
    electrophysiology of, 1059
    familial adenomatous polyposis and,
        1060, *1062*
    fluorescein angiography of, 1058,
        1117
    histopathological features of, 1059–
        1060, 1117
    molecular genetics of, 1063
    multifocal, 1116–1117, *1117*
    pigmented ocular fundus lesions
        and, *1060–1062,* 1060–1063
    solitary, 1116, *1117*
    systemic diseases associated with,
        1060
    vasoproliferative tumors and, 1175,
        1178t
    visual fields in, 1059
  contusion of, *837,* 837–838
    fluorescein angiography of, 837, *837*
  degeneration of, in central serous cho-
      rioretinopathy, 209
    in choroidal dystrophies, 949
    peripheral, 14
  detachment of. See also *Retinal
      detachment(s).*
    hemorrhagic, differential diagnosis
        of, from uveal melanoma, 1075t,
        1080
    in central serous chorioretinopathy,
        207, *208*
  DIC and, 474
  disruption of, drug-induced, 855–862,
      857t
  focal atrophic lesions of, in pseudoxan-
      thoma elasticum, 171–172
  focal hyperpigmentation of, *86,* 87
  functions of, 5
  hamartoma of, 1123–1129
  histology of, 3–5, *4*
  hyperplasia of, aging and, 13–14, *14,
      17,* 17
    choroidal rupture and, 835
    differential diagnosis of, from optic
        nerve melanocytoma, 1189
    diffuse, 14
    localized, 13–14, *14*
    reactive. See *reactive hyperplasia of.*
  hypertensive choroidopathy and, *350,
      355, 356, 360,* 364, *364*
    degenerative, 364–365
    early, *353, 356, 357,* 364–365
    late, 352, *353, 357, 360,* 365
  hypertrophy of, aging and, 12–14, *13,
      17,* 17
    congenital, 1058–1063. See also *con-
        genital hypertrophy of.*
    differential diagnosis of, from optic
        nerve melanocytoma, 1189
  hypopigmentation of, aging and, 12
  in cystoid macular edema, 241
  in diffuse unilateral subacute neuro-
      retinitis, 808
  in epimacular membranes, 230
  in myopia, degenerative, 189
  in parafoveal telangiectasis, 401
  in pregnancy, 498–499
  in serpiginous choroiditis, 555, 556
  in syphilis, salt-and-pepper, 793, *794*
  in Vogt-Koyanagi-Harada syndrome,
      573–574

Retinal pigment epithelium (*Continued*)
    migration of cells of, proliferative vit-
        reoretinopathy and, 1350–1351
    optical coherence tomography of, 70
    pattern dystrophy of, 1006–1011
        clinical course of, 1006
        clinical features of, 1006, *1007–1009*
        clinical variants of, 1006–1007, *1010,
            1011*
        electrophysiology of, 1006
        fluorescein angiography of, 1006,
            1008, 1009
        molecular genetics of, 1007, 1011
    photic injury and, 844
    preserved para-arteriolar, 903, *904*
    reactive hyperplasia of, 1118, 1122
        clinical features of, 1118, *1118*
        diagnosis of, 1118
        differential diagnosis of, from uveal
            melanoma, 1075t, 1078–1079
        histopathological features of, 1118
    regeneration of, in choroidal neovascu-
        larization treatment, 1454
    subfoveal, subretinal surgery and, 131
    tears of. See also *Retinal tears.*
        in acute retinal necrosis, 763
        in age-related macular degeneration,
            102, *106*
        traumatic, *837*, 837–838
    transplantation of, in choroidal neovas-
        cularization treatment, 1454, 1456
    tumors of, 1116–1122
Retinal tags. See *Retinal tufts.*
Retinal tears, 9, *10.* See also *Retinal
    breaks.*
    contact B-scan ultrasonography of, 50,
        51
    flap ("horseshoe"), scleral buckling for,
        1250
    from vitrectomy, 1312–1313
    giant, background of, 1338–1339
        bilateral, 1338–1339
        definition of, 1338
        fellow eye involvement in, 1338–
            1339
        idiopathic, nontraumatic, 1338
        intraocular gases for, 1326, 1327t,
            1347–1348
        management of fellow eye in, 1346
        panoramic viewing of, 1340
        pathogenesis of, 1339
        perfluorocarbon liquids for, 1322–
            1323, *1323*, 1338, 1339t, 1339–1340
            surgical techniques with, 1342–
                1345, *1343–1345*, 1348
        pneumatic retinopexy for, 1346–1347
        preoperative assessment of, 1340–
            1341
        scleral buckling for, 1338, 1340–
            1341, *1341, 1348*, 1348
        silicone oil for, 1347–1348
        surgery for, 1338–1348
        traumatic, 1383–1384, *1384*
        vitrectomy for, 1338, 1341–1346, 1348
            lens-sparing, 1347
    large superior horseshoe, scleral buck-
        ling for, *1265*, 1265–1266, *1266*
    macular holes and, 1441
    multiple horseshoe, scleral buckling
        for, 1266
    operculated, scleral buckling for, 1250
    retinal detachment and, 1248
    traumatic, 1382–1383
        giant, 1383–1384, *1384*
    zonular traction tufts and, 9–10, *11,*
        1221–1222, *1222*

Retinal telangiectasis, in bone marrow
        transplantation, 491
    in Coats' disease, 390–396
    in radiation retinopathy, 477, 479, 480,
        482
Retinal temperature, laser photocoagula-
    tion and, 63, 65–66
Retinal tufts, 9, *10*
    cystic, 9, *10*, 1234–1237, *1235–1238,*
        1242. See also *Cystic retinal tufts.*
    noncystic, 9, *10*, 1221, *1221*
    zonular traction, 9–10, *11,* 1221–1222,
        1222
Retinal vascular diseases, 269–534. See
    also specific diseases.
    arterial macroneurysms as, 383–389
    arterial occlusion as, 269–283
    bone marrow transplant retinopathy
        as, 488–496
    branch vein occlusion as, 308–315
    central vein occlusion as, 286–296
        natural history and clinical manage-
            ment of, 299–306
    Coats' disease as, 390–396
    diabetic retinopathy as, 316–341
    disseminated intravascular coagulopa-
        thy as, 473–476
    Eales' disease as, 415–420
    familial exudative vitreoretinopathy as,
        421–429
    frosted branch angiitis as, 431–436
    hemoglobinopathies as, 438–456
    hypertensive fundus changes as, 345–
        369
    in pregnancy, 498–510
    ocular ischemic syndrome as, 372–381
    parafoveal telangiectasis as, 398–405
    plasma protein risk factors for occlu-
        sive, 459–471
    radiation retinopathy as, 477–486
    retinopathy of prematurity as, 407–412
    rheumatic, 514–533
Retinal vasculature, 8. See also specific
    vessels.
    anatomic and physiologic properties
        of, 345–348
    blood column of, 348
    tortuosity of, in sickle cell retinopathy,
        442, *443*
Retinal vasculitis, classification of, 431,
    432t
    differential diagnosis of, from intraocu-
        lar lymphomas, 1207
    from cytomegalovirus, 432t, 432–433,
        434
    from leukemia, 432t, 433–434
    from phlebitis, 434
    idiopathic (primary), 431–432
        in rheumatic diseases, 515, *516*
        peripheral, 416
    in acute retinal necrosis, 750, 762
    in Eales' disease, 415–416
    pathophysiology of, 435–436
    secondary, 432t, 432–435
Retinal vasculitis, aneurysms, and neuro-
    retinitis. See *Idiopathic retinal vas-
    culitis, aneurysms, and neuroretinitis.*
Retinal veins, changes in, in hypertensive
    retinopathy, 358
Retinal venous occlusion, branch. See
    Branch retinal vein occlusion.
    central. See *Central retinal vein
        occlusion.*
    differential diagnosis of, from acquired
        retinal arteriovenous communica-
        tions, 1174

Retinal venous occlusion (*Continued*)
    from toxoplasmosis, 680
    in pregnancy, 508
Retinal whitening, diseases manifesting,
    616t–617t
    epimacular membranes and, 235–236
    in Purtscher's retinopathy, 839, *840*
    in sickle cell retinopathy, 444
Retinectomy, for proliferative vitreoreti-
    nopathy, 1363–1364, *1364*
    silicone liquid and, 1329
Retinitis, from blastomycosis, 784–785
    from candidiasis, 774, *774*
    from cytomegalovirus. See *Cytomegalo-
        virus, retinitis of.*
    from syphilis, 795
    necrotizing, in acute retinal necrosis,
        750, *751*, 760, *762*
    recurrent central. See *Chorioretinopathy,
        central serous.*
Retinitis pigmentosa, 891–920
    atypical, 896–904
    autosomal dominant, 896, 897, 898,
        917t, 919
        peripherin/RDS mutations and, 919
        rhodopsin mutations and, 919
        type I, 893
        type II, 893
    autosomal recessive, *896*, 917t, 919–
        920
    Bardet-Biedl syndrome and, 905
    Bassen-Kornzweig syndrome and, 906,
        907
    bull's eye maculopathy in, 1031, 1033t
    candidate gene approach to, 918t, 918–
        919
    childhood-onset, 901–903
    choroideremia simulating, 958, 966–
        967
    "cone-rod," 894, 917t
    differential diagnosis of, 821, 908t,
        908–920
        from acquired peripheral retinal de-
            generation, 911, 914, *914*
        from 4-aminoquinoline retinopathy,
            910–911, *912*
        from bilateral pseudoretinitis pig-
            mentosa, 908t, 909–917
        from chorioretinal inflammations,
            909, *910, 911*
        from clofazimine retinopathy, 911
        from deferoxamine retinopathy, 911
        from drug-induced disorders, 909–
            911
        from DUSN, 811
        from hereditary retinal dystrophies,
            914, *915*
        from paraneoplastic syndromes, 915,
            917
        from pericapillary (pericentral) pig-
            mentary degeneration, 914, *916*
        from phenothiazine retinopathy, 909,
            911
        from pigmented paravenous chorio-
            retinal atrophy, 914, *915*
        from retinal detachment resolution,
            911, *913*
        from Stargardt's disease, 987
        from unilateral pigmentary retinopa-
            thies, 917, 917t
        from X-linked retinoschisis, 1015–
            1016
    digenic inheritance of, 917t, 920
    electro-oculogram of, 894, *899*
    electroretinogram of, 893–894, *898*

Retinitis pigmentosa (*Continued*)
  enhanced S-cone syndrome and, 903–
    904, *904*
  implicit times in, 896, *898*
  in pregnancy, 505
  Kearns-Sayre syndrome and, 908
  Laurence-Moon syndrome and, 905
  Leber's congenital amaurosis and, 901,
    903
  linkage analysis in, 918
  metabolic disorders associated with,
    905t
  molecular genetics of, 917–920
  neurologic disorders associated with,
    905t
  neuronal ceroid lipofuscinosis and,
    905–906
  preserved para-arteriolar RPE and,
    903, *904*
  Refsum's disease and, 906, 908
  renal or hepatic disorders associated
    with, 905t
  "rod-cone," 894
  salt-and-pepper retinopathy in, 964t
  sector, 914–915, *916*
  segmental, differential diagnosis of,
    from central serous chorioreti-
    nopathy, 208
  sine pigmento, 896, 898, *900*
  systemic diseases associated with, 904–
    908
  typical, 891–896
    clinical features of, 891, 893, *893–895*
    electrophysiology of, 893–896, *898,*
      899
    fluorescein angiography of, 893, *895*
    histopathological features of, 892
    psychophysics of, 893, *896, 897*
    Usher's syndrome and, *895,* 904–905,
      905t, 917t
    vasoproliferative tumors and, 1175,
      1178, 1178t
    ocular fundus, 1077
  X-linked recessive, 896, *899,* 917t
Retinitis punctata albescens, 898–901,
    901, 902
  differential diagnosis of, 1043, 1045
    from fundus albipunctatus, 899, *902*
Retinoblastoma, 1139–1149
  chemoreduction for, *1148,* 1149
  chemotherapy for, 1148
  chemothermotherapy for, *1148,* 1148–
    1149
  clinical features of, 1139–1142, *1140,*
    1141
  computed tomography of, 1140, *1144,*
    1144–1145
  cryotherapy for, 1146
  diagnosis of, 1143–1145
  differential diagnosis of, 1145, 1151–
    1158, 1152t
    classification of, 1152t
    from astrocytic hamartoma, 1182
    from Coats' disease, 394, 1151–1153,
      1152t, *1153*
    from coloboma, 1152t, 1156, *1156*
    from combined hamartoma of retina
      and RPE, 1152t, 1155, *1155*
    from congenital cataracts, 1152t,
      1157
    from congenital cytomegalovirus ret-
      initis, 1152t, 1156
    from congenital toxoplasmic retinitis,
      1152t, 1155
    from developmental disorders, 1152t,
      1156–1157

Retinoblastoma (*Continued*)
    from dominant exudative vitreo-
      retinopathy, 1152t, 1157
    from endogenous endophthalmitis,
      1152t, 1156, *1156*
    from hereditary conditions, 1152t
    from inflammatory conditions, 1152t,
      1155–1156
    from intermediate uveitis, 1152t,
      1156
    from medulloepithelioma, 1135,
      1136, 1152t, 1154, *1154*
    from myelinated nerve fibers, 1152t,
      1156–1157, *1157*
    from neoplastic disorders, 1152t,
      1154–1155
    from ocular toxocariasis, 1152t,
      1153–1154, *1154*
    from persistent hyperplastic primary
      vitreous, 1151, 1152t, *1153*
    from retinal astrocytic hamartoma,
      1152t, 1155, *1155*
    from retinal capillary hemangioma,
      1152t, 1155, 1160
    from retinopathy of prematurity,
      1152t, 1157
    from rhegmatogenous retinal detach-
      ment, 1152t, 1157
    from toxocariasis, 704, 705t
    from vitreous hemorrhage, 1152t,
      1157
  diffuse infiltrating, 1140
  endophytic, 1139, *1141,* 1142–1143
  enucleation of, 1145, *1146*
  episcleral plaque brachytherapy for,
    1146, *1147*
  exophytic, 1139, *1141,* 1143
  fluorescein angiography of, *1143,* 1144
  genetic counseling on, 1149
  laser photocoagulation for, 1146, *1147,*
    1148
  magnetic resonance imaging of, 1145,
    1145
  management of, 1145–1149
  pathology of, *1142,* 1142–1143
  radiation therapy for, 1145–1146, *1146*
  spontaneously regressed, *1142, 1142*
  trilateral, 1141
  ultrasonography of, *1144, 1144*
Retinochoroidal anastomosis, from toxo-
    plasmosis, 680
Retinochoroidal coloboma, vasoprolifera-
    tive tumors and, 1175, 1178t
Retinochoroiditis. See *Chorioretinitis.*
Retinocytoma, 1141–1142
Retinopathy, acute macular neural, 593–
    596
  chorio. See *Chorioretinopathy.*
  diabetic. See *Diabetic retinopathy.*
  drug-induced. See *Drug-induced ocular*
    disorders.
  hypertensive, 348, 349–360. See also
    Hypertensive retinopathy.
  photic, 844–848
  radiation. See *Radiation retinopathy.*
  sickle cell, 438–456
  solar, *847,* 847–848, *848*
  surface wrinkling. See *Epimacular*
    membranes.
  vitreo. See *Vitreoretinopathy.*
  whiplash, 840–841
    macular holes and, 833
Retinopathy of prematurity (ROP), 407–
    412, 1459–1464
  angiogenesis in, 122

Retinopathy of prematurity (*Continued*)
  classification of, 409, *409,* 409t, *410*
  differential diagnosis of, from familial
    exudative vitreoretinopathy, 427t,
    427–428
    from retinoblastoma, 1152t, 1157
    from toxocariasis, 704, 705t, 706
    from X-linked retinoschisis, 1015
  examination of neonate for, 1459
  factors associated with, 407–409
  histopathological features of, 408
  intensive care unit light exposure and,
    848
  lensectomy for, 1462–1463
  lens-sparing vitreous surgery for,
    1461–1462, 1464
  retinal detachment in, at stage 5, 1462–
    1463
    evolution of, 1459–1460, *1460*
    late surgical intervention for, 1463
  retinal folds in, 263
  scleral buckling for, 1460–1461
  screening for, 410–411
  stages of, 409t
    4 and 5, 1459–1464
  structural changes after regression of,
    412
  surgery for, 1460–1463
    results of, 1463–1464
  threshold, 411–412
  vasoproliferative tumors and, 1175
  visual fields in, 412
Retinopexy, in epimacular membranes,
    230
  pneumatic, 1272–1286. See also *Pneu-*
    matic retinopexy.
Retinoschisis, 15–17, *16*
  contact B-scan ultrasonography of, 51,
    51
  differential diagnosis of, from central
    serous chorioretinopathy, 208
  juvenile, differential diagnosis of, from
    central areolar choroidal dystro-
    phy, 956t
    from familial exudative vitreo-
      retinopathy, 427t, 428
    vasoproliferative tumors and, 1175
  optic nerve head congenital pits and,
    876
  optical coherence tomography of, 73
  peripheral, 1013, *1014, 1015*
  senile (degenerative), 15–16, *16,* 1238–
    1243, *1239–1242*
    clinical features of, *1239–1241,*
      1239–1242
    differential diagnosis of, from pe-
      ripheral cystoid degeneration,
      1222
      from uveal melanoma, 1075t, 1081
      from white-with-pressure sign,
        1226
    histopathological features of, 1239,
      1239
    history of, 1238–1239
    prognosis and management of,
      1241–1242, 1242–1243
    reticular (bullous), 16, *16,* 1239, *1239*
    retinal detachment and, 1239–1240,
      1242, *1242,* 1243
    "schisis-detachment" in, *1241, 1242,*
      1242–1243
    typical (flat), 15, 1239
  X-linked, 1013–1017
    clinical features of, 1013–1014
    differential diagnosis of, 1015–1017

Retinoschisis (*Continued*)
  electroretinographic features of, 1014, *1016*
  management of, 1014–1015
  ocular features of, 1013–1014, *1014–1016*
Retinotomy, for proliferative vitreoretinopathy, 1363–1364, *1364*
  in subretinal surgery, 132. See also *Subretinal surgery.*
  relaxing, for trauma, 1384
  silicone liquid and, 1329
  small, 131–132
Retrobulbar ischemic optic neuropathy, radiation retinopathy and, 481
Retrolental fibroplasia. See *Retinopathy of prematurity (ROP).*
Rhegmatogenous retinal detachments. See *Retinal detachment(s), rhegmatogenous.*
Rheumatic retinal diseases, 514–533
  clinical features of, 514–515
  idiopathic retinal vasculitis, aneurysms, and neuroretinitis syndrome, 526–533, *526–533*
  idiopathic vasculitis as, 515, *516*
  in Behçet's disease, 515–517, *517–519*
  in sarcoidosis, 515, *517*
  in systemic lupus erythematosus, 517–527, *521–526*
  management of, 515
  steroids for, systemic, 515
  treatment of, 515
Rheumatoid arthritis, juvenile, differential diagnosis of, from intermediate uveitis, 606
  posterior scleritis and, 638
Rhodamine-6G, 64
Rhodopsin mutations, retinitis pigmentosa and, 919
Rifabutin, adverse effects of, in HIV infection, 742
Rifampin, for endophthalmitis, 1470
Riggs-type CSNB, 935, 936t
Ringer's lactate, for intraocular irrigation, 1301–1302
Rod(s), 7–8
Rod monochromatism, *844, 942, 943,* 943t
Rodenstock panfundoscopic contact lens, *27, 28*
ROP. See *Retinopathy of prematurity (ROP).*
Rosette-like formation. See *Cystic retinal tufts (CRT).*
Roth's spots, in sarcoidosis, 648, *648*
Roundworm ocular infections, 819–820
RPE. See *Retinal pigment epithelium (RPE).*
Rubella, congenital, differential diagnosis of, retinitis pigmentosa, 909
  retinopathy of, 909, *911*
  salt-and-pepper retinopathy in, 964t
Rubeosis, in diabetic retinopathy, 1412–1413
Rubeosis iridis, from vitrectomy, 1316
  in central retinal artery obstruction, 271, 274–275
  in ocular ischemic syndrome, 373

Sabin-Feldman dye test, for toxoplasmosis, 683t, 684
Salmon patch hemorrhage, in sickle cell retinopathy, 441, *441*
Salt-and-pepper retinopathy, conditions featuring, 956, 964t
  in choroideremia, 956, 958

Sanfilippo's syndrome, retinitis pigmentosa and, 905t
Sarcoidosis, 643–656
  acute, 645
  acute multifocal posterior placoid pigment epitheliopathy and, 547
  anterior segment disease in, 646, 646t
  BAL test in, 654–655
  biopsies in, 652, *654,* 654t
  branch retinal vein occlusion in, 648, *649*
  cardiac, 645
  choroidal lesions in, 646t, 646–647, *647*
  choroidal neovascularization in, 150
  chronic, 645
  clinical features of, 645–652
  CNS involvement in, 645
  diagnosis of, *647, 649–654,* 652–655, 654t
  differential diagnosis of, 655
    from coccidioidomycosis, 780
    from cryptococcosis, 783
    from DUSN, 811
    from Eales' disease, 419
    from intermediate uveitis, 606
    from intraocular lymphomas, 1207
    from serpiginous choroiditis, 561
    from tuberculosis, 803
    from Vogt-Koyanagi-Harada syndrome, 579
  epidemiology of, 643
  etiology of, 644
  fluorescein angiography of, *647, 649–654,* 655
  gallium citrate scans in, 654
  history of, 643
  hypercalcemia in, 644
  in pregnancy, 505
  Kveim-Slitzbach test in, 652
  lacrimal gland involvement in, 651
  multifocal choroiditis with panuveitis and, 615
  ocular manifestations of, 646t, 646–652, *646–653*
  optic neuritis and atrophy in, 650–651, *652, 653*
  orbital disease in, 646, 646t
  orbital granulomas in, 643, 644, 651–652
  pathogenesis of, 644–645
  pathology of, *644,* 644t, 644–645
  posterior scleritis and, 638
  posterior segment disease in, 646, 646t
  prognosis for, 656, *656*
  proliferative retinopathy in, 648–649, *650*
  retinal diseases in, 515, *517*
  retinal hemorrhages in, 648, *648*
  retinal neovascularization in, 648
  retinal periphlebitis in, *647, 647,* 648
  Roth's spots in, 648, *648*
  serpiginous choroiditis in, 648, *648*
  serum angiotensin-converting enzyme in, 652, 654, 654t
  skin lesions in, 645, *645*
  "string of pearls" in, 648, *648*
  systemic manifestations of, 645
  treatment of, 655–656
  white ocular lesions in, 617t
Scheie' syndrome, 927, 928
  retinitis pigmentosa and, 905t
Schistosomiasis, acute multifocal posterior placoid pigment epitheliopathy and, 548
Schubert-Bornschein CSNB, 935, 936, *936,* 936t

Schwannoma. See *Neurilemmoma.*
Sclera, penetration of, by suture needle, 1263, *1263*
Scleral buckling, 1248–1271
  anatomic and physiologic effects of, 1249–1250
  circumferential, 1254–1257, *1255, 1256,* 1258, 1261
    for horseshoe tears, 1266
    for myopic retinal detachments, 1266–1267
    segmental, 1256
  clinical principles of, 1250–1265
  cystoid macular edema after, 1269
  encircling, 1256–1257
  "fish-mouth phenomenon" and, 1260, 1264, *1264*
  for acute retinal necrosis, 755, 763, 764
  for CMV-related retinal detachments, 1480
  for diabetic retinopathy, 325
  for familial exudative vitreoretinopathy, 428–429
  for giant retinal tears, 1338, 1340–1341, *1341,* 1348, *1348*
  traumatic, 1384
  for retinal detachment, 833, 1248, 1249t
    accessory techniques in, 1260–1261
    air-fluid exchange and, 1261
    altered refractive error after, 1268
    anatomic results of, 1267
    balloon buckles and, 1292
    choroidal detachment after, 1268, *1268*
    common causes of detachment, 1265t
    configurations of, 1251–1253, 1252t, *1253–1254*
      favored routine, 1254–1257, *1255, 1256*
    cystoid macular edema after, 1269
    drainage technique in, *1258,* 1258–1260, *1259*
      problems with, 1263–1264, *1264*
    encircling, 1256–1257
    final adjustment in, 1260
    for inferior temporal dialysis, 1266
    for large superior horseshoe tear, *1265,* 1265–1266, *1266*
    for multiple horseshoe tears and lattice degeneration, 1266
    for myopic detachments, 1266–1267
    intraoperative management of dilemmas, 1261–1265
    intravitreal gas injection and, 1260–1261
      problems with, 1265
    localization and treatment of breaks in, 1253–1254, *1254, 1255*
    dilemmas in, 1261, 1263
    macular pucker after, 1269, *1269*
    management of subretinal fluid in, 1257–1260
    nondrainage techniques in, 1257–1258
    postoperative complications of, 1267–1270
    postoperative laser photocoagulation and, 1261, *1262*
    principles of, 1250–1265
    proliferative vitreoretinopathy after, 1270
    pseudophakic, 1266
    recurrent/persistent detachment after, 1269–1270

Scleral buckling (*Continued*)
  scleral buckle/retinal break relation-
      ship in, *1264,* 1264
  segmental, 1256
  strabismus after, 1268
  suture placement, problems with,
      1263, *1263*
  visual results of, 1267
  for retinopathy of prematurity, 1460–
      1461
  for sickle cell retinopathy, 449
  for traumatic ocular disorders, 1375,
      1377–1378, 1384
  for X-linked retinoschisis, 1015
  history of, 1248–1249
  macular holes and, 223
  pneumatic retinopexy compared with,
      1275
  pneumatic retinopexy for failures of,
      1285
  prophylactic, for fellow eye of giant
      retinal tear, 1346
  radial, 1254
      segmental, 1256
  reattachment forces created by, 1250,
      1251
  retinal folds in, 263, 265
  silicone liquid and, 1329
  uveal effusion in, 664
Scleral depression, in ophthalmoscopy,
      24, *26*
Scleral sutures, placement of, 1263, *1263*
Scleritis, anterior, 635
  from candidiasis, 774
  from coccidioidomycosis, 778
  from toxoplasmosis, 680, *680*
  from tuberculosis, 802
  posterior, 635–641
      chorioretinal folds in, 262
      clinical features of, 635, 637, 637t
      complications of, 640–641, 641t
      computed tomography of, 637–638,
          640
      differential diagnosis of, 637, 637t
          from age-related macular degener-
              ation, 97
          from choroidal osteoma, 1095,
              1096
          from serpiginous choroiditis, 561
          from uveal melanoma, 1075t,
              1080–1081, *1081*
          from Vogt-Koyanagi-Harada syn-
              drome, 578
      fluorescein angiography of, 637, *638,*
          639
      in syphilis, 638, 736
      indocyanine green angiography of,
          637
      magnetic resonance imaging of, 638
      symptoms of, 635
      systemic evaluation of, 638–639,
          640t
      treatment of, 639–640, 640t
      ultrasonography of, 637, *639*
      unilateral versus bilateral, 635
  uveal effusion in, 664
Sclerochoroidal calcification, idiopathic,
      differential diagnosis of, from cho-
      roidal osteoma, 1095, 1096, *1098*
Scleromyxedema, chorioretinal folds in,
      263
Sclerotomy, for suprachoroidal hemor-
      rhages, 1388
  for vitrectomy, 1302
      closure of, 1311

Sclerotomy (*Continued*)
  superonasal, 132
  superotemporal, 132
Sclerouvectomy, partial lamellar, for
      uveal leiomyoma, 1112
  for uveal melanoma, 1071, *1072*
S-cone syndrome, enhanced, 903–904,
      904
Scotomata, from diffuse unilateral sub-
      acute neuroretinitis, 808
  in acute macular neuroretinopathy,
      593, *594*
  in age-related macular degeneration,
      96
  in myopia, 192
SD. See *Stargardt's disease.*
Sea fan neovascularization, in sickle cell
      retinopathy, 445–446, 447, 449, *449*
  hyperfluorescence of, *35,* 36
  management of, 449
Selenium, protective effect of, 844
Semiconductor diode (GaAlAs) laser
      photocoagulation, 64
Senior-Loken syndrome, Coats' disease
      and, 393
Sensory retina, 3, 5–7
  anatomy of, *5,* 5–7, *6*
  nine layers of, *5,* 5–7, *6*
Serologic tests, for candidiasis, 775
  for diffuse unilateral subacute neuro-
      retinitis, 810–811
  for syphilis, 736, 797–798
  for toxoplasmosis, 683t, 683–687
Serpiginous choroiditis, 553–563
  age and, 553
  antibiotics for, 562, 563t
  antivirals for, 562, 563t
  causes of visual impairment in, 556,
      556t
  clinical characteristics of, 553–555
  clinical presentation of, 555–558
  differential diagnosis of, 558, 560–562,
      561t
      from AMPPPE, 558, 560–561
      from birdshot retinochoroidopathy,
          567
      from choroidal neovascularization,
          562
      from degenerative or dystrophic dis-
          orders, 561
      from DUSN, 811
      from infectious disorders, 561
      from infiltrative diseases of choroid,
          561–562
  electrophysiologic studies in, 557–558
  environmental exposures and, 557
  etiology of, 559–560
  fluorescein angiography of, 557, *558*
  histopathological features of, 554
  HLA typing in, 558
  hyperfluorescence in, 38, *38*
  immunologic studies in, 558
  immunosuppressive therapy for, 562,
      563t
  in sarcoidosis, 648, *648*
  indocyanine green angiography of,
      557
  laser photocoagulation for, 562, 563t
  natural history of, 559
  ophthalmoscopic and clinical features
      of, *555,* 555–556, *556*
  pathogenesis of, 559–560
  systemic findings in, 556t, 556–557
  treatment of, 562, 563t
  visual fields in, 557
  white ocular lesions in, 617t

Serum angiotensin-converting enzyme
      (SACE), in sarcoidosis, 652, 654, 654t
Shaken baby syndrome, ocular disorders
      in, 838–839, *839*
  retinal folds in, 265
Sheathing, from diffuse unilateral sub-
      acute neuroretinitis, 808
  in Eales' disease, 415–416
  in familial exudative vitreoretinopathy,
      422, *422*
  in frosted branch angiitis, 435, 436
  in HIV microvascular disease, 714
  in radiation retinopathy, 480
  in rheumatic retinal diseases, 515, *516,*
      517
  in toxoplasmosis, 678, *679*
  in Wagner's syndrome, 926
Sickle cell disease, 438, 440, 440t
  angioid streaks in, 142, *142, 163, 169t,*
      173
  manifestations of, 169t
Sickle cell hemoglobin C, 438, 440, 440t
Sickle cell retinopathy, 438–456. See also
      Hemoglobinopathies.
  differential diagnosis of, from acquired
      retinal arteriovenous communica-
      tions, 1174
      from parafoveal telangiectasis, 405
      from retinal capillary hemangioma,
          1160
Sickle cell thalassemia, 438, 440, 440t
Sickle cell trait, 438, 440t
Sickle disc sign, 444–445, *445*
Siderosis, from intraocular foreign bod-
      ies, 1402
Siedel test, in trauma, 1371
Silicone liquid, 1329–1332
  cataracts from, in HIV infected, 1482,
      1482
  complications of, 1330–1331
  emulsification of, 1330, 1331
  fluorinated derivatives of, 1331
  for CMV-related retinal detachments,
      1480–1482
      complications of, 1482, *1482*
  for giant retinal tears, 1345, 1347–1348
  for ocular trauma, 1378–1379
  for proliferative vitreoretinopathy,
      1329, 1330, 1331, *1365,* 1365–1366
  in combination therapy, 1331–1332
  indications for, 1329t, 1329–1330
  ocular tolerance of, 1330–1331
  properties of, 1330
  pupillary block glaucoma from, 1315
Sjögren-Larsson syndrome, differential
      diagnosis of, from Bietti's crystal-
      line dystrophy, 1044–1045
Sjögren's reticular dystrophy, 1011
Slit lamp ophthalmoscopy, 22, 26
  biomicroscopic, 26
      contact lens, 27, 27–28
      non-contact lens, *26,* 26–28
  photic retinopathy from, 847
Sloan achromatopsia test, 943
Small retinotomy technique, 131–132
Smoking, age-related macular degenera-
      tion and, 90
SO. See *Sympathetic ophthalmia (SO).*
Sodium, abnormalities of, and hyperten-
      sion, 348
Sodium fluorescein dyes, adverse effects
      of, 30, 30t
  leakage of, hyperfluorescence from, 37
  pooling of, hyperfluorescence from, 37,
      37
  properties of, 29–30

Solar retinopathy, *847, 847–848, 848*

Sorbinil, for diabetic retinopathy, 337, 341t

Sorbitol, in diabetic retinopathy, 337–338

Sorsby's fundus dystrophy, clinical features of, 1018, 1019t, *1020–1023,* 1021t
  differential diagnosis of, from serpiginous choroiditis, 561
  family pedigree for, *1019–1021*
  fluorescein angiography of, 1018–1019
  molecular genetics of, 1021, 1024
  neovascularization in, 148, 1021, 1021t
  prognosis and treatment of, 1019, 1021
  visual function in, 1019

Spherocytosis, hereditary, angioid streaks in, 169t
  manifestations of, 169t

Sphingolipid storage disorders, ocular disease in, *928,* 928–929, *929*

Spielmeyer-Vogt (Batten-Mayou) disease, bull's eye maculopathy in, 1030, 1033t
  retinitis pigmentosa and, 905–906

Spiramycin, for toxoplasmosis, 689t, 690
  in pregnancy, 691

Splinter hemorrhages, optic disc drusen and, 880

Sporotrichosis, 786–787
  in HIV infection, 740–741

Sporotrichum schenckii, 786

Squint response, as defense mechanism, 844

Staphylococcus aureus, endophthalmitis from, 1390, 1401, 1466, 1472, 1474

Staphylococcus epidermidis, endophthalmitis from, 1390, 1401, 1466, 1472

Staphylomas, B-scan ultrasonography of, 54, *54*
  equatorial, retinal detachment and, pneumatic retinopexy for, 1286
  posterior, in degenerative myopia, 189, 191, *191*
    treatment of, 204
  three-dimensional ultrasonography of, 58, *58–59*

Stargardt's disease, 978–987. See also *Fundus flavimaculatus.*
  bull's eye maculopathy in, 1030–1031, 1033t
  classification of, 982–984
  clinical features of, 978–984, *980, 993*
  color vision in, 984
  dark adaptation studies in, 984
  demography of, 978, 980
  differential diagnosis of, 986–987
    from Best's disease, 1002
    from central areolar choroidal dystrophy, 956t
    from retinitis pigmentosa, 914, 987
  electro-oculography in, 984
  electroretinography in, 984, 984t
  fluorescein angiography of, *980, 981, 983,* 984–985, *985*
  genetics of, 986
  histopathological features of, 985–986
  indocyanine green angiography of, 985
  prognosis for, 986
  retinal function tests in, 984
  signs of, 980–984, *981–983*
  symptoms of, 980
  visual fields in, 984

Steamroller maneuver, for giant retinal tears, 1341, *1341*
  in pneumatic retinopexy, for retinal detachment, 1280, *1280*

Stellate maculopathy, in X-linked retinoschisis, 1013

Stellate retinopathy, Leber's. See *Leber's idiopathic optic neuroretinitis.*

Stickler's disease, 924, 926, *926*
  differential diagnosis of, from X-linked retinoschisis, 1016–1017
  vasoproliferative tumors and, 1175

Stickler-Wagner syndrome, giant retinal tears in, 1339

Strabismus, after scleral buckling for retinal detachment, 1268
  from retinopathy of prematurity, 412
  from toxocariasis, 702, *703*

Streptococcus, endophthalmitis from, 1390, 1466, 1472

Streptokinase, for hyphema, 1379

Streptomycin, for serpiginous choroiditis, 562, 563t
  for tuberculosis, 804

"String of pearls," in sarcoidosis, 648, *648*

Stroke, ocular ischemic syndrome in, 377

Sturge-Weber syndrome, choroidal hemangioma and, 1088
  uveal pressure in, 659, 663

Subarachnoid hemorrhage, in Terson's syndrome, 839

Subconjunctival hemorrhage, acute multifocal posterior placoid pigment epitheliopathy and, 545
  in protein C deficiency, 462

Subfoveal surgery, for choroidal neovascularization, 157
  complications of, 157
  for punctate inner choroidopathy, 624

Submacular hemorrhage, perfluorocarbon liquids for, 1323
  traumatic, 1386–1387, *1387*

Submacular surgery, 186–187
  for choroidal neovascularization, in AMD, 117–118

Subretinal abscess, from tuberculosis, 802, 803

Subretinal fibrosis, surgery for, 132

Subretinal fibrosis and uveitis syndrome, 631–634
  clinical manifestations of, 631, *632*
  differential diagnosis of, *633,* 633t, 633–634
  electrophysiologic studies of, 633
  fluorescein angiography of, 633
  histopathological features of, 631–632, *632*
  immunopathologic features of, 631–632
  treatment of, 634

Subretinal fluid, drainage of, in giant retinal tears, 1347
  in age-related macular degeneration, 96, 97
  resorption of, in pneumatic retinopexy, 1272–1274, *1274*
    delays in, 1283
    in scleral buckling, for retinal detachment, 1251, 1252t, 1257–1260, 1266

Subretinal fluid (SFR), resorption of, pneumatic retinopexy for, 1272–1274

Subretinal gas. See also *Gases, intraocular.*
  deposits of, 1328
  from pneumatic retinopexy, 1281–1282, *1282*

Subretinal hemorrhage. See also *Retinal hemorrhage.*
  differential diagnosis of, from choroidal nevus, 1055
  in myopia, degenerative, 193
  indocyanine green angiography of, 40, *41,* 42, *43*
  large, mechanical clot extraction in, 135
    surgery for, 135
  surgery for, 134–135
  t-PA assisted clot extraction in, 134–135
  traumatic, 1386–1387

Subretinal infusion, from vitrectomy, 1312

Subretinal layers, clinical examination of, 21–28

Subretinal membrane, dissection of, in proliferative vitreoretinopathy surgery, *1362,* 1362–1363, *1363*

Subretinal neovascularization, in parafoveal telangiectasis, 401–402

Subretinal precipitates, in central serous chorioretinopathy, 207

Subretinal space, 5

Subretinal strands, in proliferative vitreoretinopathy, surgery for, 135–136

Subretinal surgery, 131–136
  approach in, 132–136
    general, 132–133, *133*
  for choroidal neovascularization, *133,* 133–134, *134,* 158
  for hemorrhage, 134–135
    large, 135
    mechanical clot extraction in, 135
    t-PA assisted clot extraction in, 134–135
  for subretinal strands in proliferative vitreoretinopathy, 135–136
  history of, 131
  indications for, 131
  small retinopathy technique in, 131–132

Sulfadiazine, for toxoplasmosis, in HIV infected, 735

Sulfonamides, for toxoplasmosis, 688, 689t, 690
  uveal effusion from, 664

Sulfur hexafluride (SF₆) gas, 1325–1329
  characteristics of, 1326t
  for retinopexy, 1279
  for vitrectomy, 1310

"Sunset glow" fundus, in Vogt-Koyanagi-Harada syndrome, 574, *576,* 580

Superoxide dismutase, protective effect of, 844

Suprachoroidal fluid, drainage of, 1268, *1268*
  in vitrectomy, 1312

Suprachoroidal hematomas, chorioretinal folds in, 263

Suprachoroidal hemorrhage, traumatic, 1387–1389, *1388*

Surgical retina. See also individual procedures.
  balloon buckles for, 1288–1296
  for choroidal neovascularization, 1449–1457
  for detachments in AIDS, 1478–1484
  for diabetic retinopathy, proliferative, 1407–1427
  for endophthalmitis, 1466–1475
  for giant retinal tears, 1338–1348

Surgical retina (*Continued*)
  for intraocular foreign bodies, 1395–
    1404
  for macular holes, 1432–1447
  for proliferative vitreoretinopathy,
    1350–1367
  for retinopathy of prematurity, 1459–
    1464
  for trauma, 1370–1392
  peripheral lesions related to rhegmato-
    genous detachments and, 1217–
    1502, 1219–1245
  pneumatic retinopexy for, 1272–1286
  scleral buckling for, 1248–1271
  vitrectomy for, 1298–1317
    diagnostic, 1487–1501
  vitreous substitutes for, 1502
Sympathetic ophthalmia (SO), 569–572
  differential diagnosis of, from intraocu-
    lar lymphomas, 1207
    from Vogt-Koyanagi-Harada syn-
      drome, 579
    from vitrectomy, 1317
  histopathological features of, 569, 570,
    571, 572
  sequelae of, 572
  treatment of, 572
  uveal pressure in, 659, 661
  uveitis in, 664
Synechiae, in intermediate uveitis, 601
Syphilis, 793–799
  congenital, 793, 794
    differential diagnosis of, retinitis pig-
      mentosa, 909
    salt-and-pepper retinopathy in, 964t
    treatment of, 799t
  CSF analysis in, 797–798
  diagnosis of, 736, 797–798, 909, 909
  differential diagnosis of, 798
    from coccidioidomycosis, 780
    from Leber's idiopathic optic neuro-
      retinitis, 887
    from retinitis pigmentosa, 909
    from tuberculosis, 739, 803
  epidemiology of, 736
  in HIV infection, 735–737, 736, 737,
    796–797
    treatment of, 799, 799t
  natural history of acquired, 793–794
  ocular manifestations of acquired, 794–
    796, 795t, 796–798
  papillitis from, in HIV infected, 736,
    737
  posterior scleritis and, 638, 736
  retinitis from, in HIV infected, 736, 736
  serologic tests for, 736, 797–798
  treatment of, 798–799, 799t
  uveitis in, 664, 736
  vitreoretinal manifestations of ac-
    quired, 795, 795t
Systemic lupus erythematosus (SLE), 514,
    517–527, 521–526
  antiphospholipid antibodies in, 520
  cardiac manifestations of, 520
  central serous chorioretinopathy in,
    520, 521–523
    treatment of, 520
  chloroquine maculopathy in, 525–527,
    526
    treatment of, 527
  clinical features of, 519–520
  CNS manifestations of, 519–520
  differential diagnosis of, from
    AMPPPE, 550
    from Eales' disease, 419

Systemic lupus erythematosus
    (*Continued*)
    from intermediate uveitis, 606
    from parafoveal telangiectasis, 405
    from sarcoidosis, 655
  epidemiology of, 518
  etiology of, 518
  hypertensive retinopathy in, 521–523,
    523
    treatment of, 523
  immune complexes and, 518–519
  laboratory findings in, 520
  lymphocyte dysfunction in, 519
  ocular manifestations of, 465, 466–467,
    520–527
  pathogenesis of, 518–519
  pathology of, 519
  posterior scleritis and, 638
  renal manifestations of, 520
  reticuloendothelial dysfunction in, 519
  skin manifestations of, 519
  vascular occlusive disease in, 523–525,
    524–525
    treatment of, 525, 525

T cell(s), in cytomegalovirus, 717
  progressive outer retinal necrosis and,
    766
  toxoplasmosis and, 682
Taenia solium, 709. See also *Cysticercosis.*
  life cycle of, 709
Talc, ocular disorders from, 866–867,
    867
    differential diagnosis of, from Bietti's
      crystalline dystrophy, 1044
Tamoxifen retinopathy, 866, 866, 868
    differential diagnosis of, from Bietti's
      crystalline dystrophy, 1044
Tamponade. See also *Gases, intraocular;
    Silicone liquid.*
  for proliferative vitreoretinopathy,
    1364–1366
  for subretinal breaks, in scleral buck-
    ling, 1260–1261
Tapetoretinal dystrophy, differential diag-
    nosis of, from onchocerciasis, 820
    from parafoveal telangiectasis, 400
Tay-Sachs disease, 928, 928
Telangiectasis, idiopathic juxtafoveolar,
    149, 153–154
    differential diagnosis of, from Bietti's
      crystalline dystrophy, 1045
  in Coats' disease, 390–396, 398
  parafoveal, 398–405
    differential diagnosis of, from radia-
      tion retinopathy, 483
    group 1 (visible, with exudation),
      398–400
      differential diagnosis of, 400
    group 2 (occult, with minimal exu-
      dation), 400–404, 400–404
      histopathological features of, 403,
        403–404, 404
    group 3 (visible, with capillary oc-
      clusion and minimal exudation),
      404–405
      histopathological features of, 399
    idiopathic. See *group 2 (occult, with
      minimal exudation).*
Temporal arteritis, differential diagnosis
    of, from Eales' disease, 419
  retinal vasculitis and, 435
Temporal retinopathy, straight, 132

Terson's syndrome, differential diagnosis
    of, from shaken baby syndrome,
    838
  in leukemia, 1199, 1200
  retinal folds in, 265
  traumatic ocular disorders in, 839, 839
Thalassemia, angioid streaks in, 142, 169t
  manifestations of, 169t
Thermal ocular injury, 844. See also *Pho-
    tic retinopathy.*
Thermoacoustic damage, laser photoco-
    agulation and, 63
Thermotherapy, transpupillary, for uveal
    melanoma, 1072
Thiabendazole, for diffuse unilateral sub-
    acute neuroretinitis, 811
Thioridazine, ocular disorders from, 855,
    857, 857–858, 858
  salt-and-pepper retinopathy from, 964t
Three-dimensional ultrasonography (3D
    US), 55–59
  area measurement technique in, 57, 57
  clinical experience with, 57–58, 58–59
  in vitro testing with, 57
  limitations and artifacts in, 58–59, 59
  linear measurement technique in, 56–
    57, 57
  system for, 55, 56
  volume measurement technique in, 57
Thrombotic thrombocytopenia purpura,
    in pregnancy, 509
  ocular disorders from, 509
Thyroiditis, acute multifocal posterior
    placoid pigment epitheliopathy
    and, 547
Tie receptors, 124
Tilorone, ocular disorders from, 868
Tin etiopurpurin (SnET2), 74
Tissue plasminogen activator (t-PA), for
    endophthalmitis, 1471
  for fibrin, in proliferative vitreoreti-
    nopathy, 1367
  for hyphema, 1379
  for subretinal hemorrhage, 134–135
Topical anesthetics, use of, in pregnancy,
    510
Total body irradiation (TBI), bone mar-
    row transplantation retinopathy
    and, 488, 490
Toxemia of pregnancy. See *Pregnancy,
    toxemia of.*
Toxocara canis, 697, 699. See also
    Toxocariasis.
  life cycle of, 699–700, 700
Toxocariasis, 697–707
  differential diagnosis of, from coccidi-
    oidomycosis, 780
  ocular, 697–707
    associations of, 697, 699
    clinical features of, 701–703, 702, 703
    diagnosis of, 703–704, 1495–1496,
      1496
    differential diagnosis of, 704–706,
      705t
      from intermediate uveitis, 606
      from retinoblastoma, 704, 705t,
        1152t, 1153–1154, 1154
    diffuse unilateral subacute neuro-
      retinitis from, 807
    histopathological features of, 698
    history of, 697, 699
    pathophysiology of, 700, 700–701
    treatment of, 706–707
    vasoproliferative ocular fundus tu-
      mors and, 1077

Toxocariasis (*Continued*)
  white ocular lesions in, 616t
  pathophysiology of, 699, *700*, 701
  transmission of, 699–700, *700*
  vasoproliferative tumors and, 1175,
    1178t
Toxoplasma gondii, 671–675, *673*. See also
    Toxoplasmosis.
  epidemiology of, 674, 674t
  life cycle of, 671, 673–674
  oocysts of, 673, *673*
  pathogenicity of, 675
  tachyzoites of, 671
  tissue cysts of, 671, *673*
  transmission of, 674t, 674–675
Toxoplasmosis, 671–692. See also *Toxo-
    plasma gondii.*
  acquired, 676–678
    clinical manifestations of, 677t, 677–
      678
  CMV co-infection with, in HIV in-
    fected, 720
  congenital, 675–676, 676t
    clinical manifestations of, 676, 676t
    diagnosis of, 687
    differential diagnosis of, from reti-
      noblastoma, 1152t, 1155
    in HIV infected, 681
    management of, 691
    transmission of, 674, 674t, 675–676
  diagnosis of, 683t, 683–687, 1494
    aqueous humor analysis for, 683t,
      685
    complement fixing antibody test for,
      683t, 684
    direct agglutination test for, 683t,
      684
    ELISA for, 683t, 685, 1494
    in fetus, 687
    indirect fluorescent antibody test for,
      683t, 684
    indirect hemagglutination test for,
      683t, 684
    polymerase chain reaction for, 683t,
      685
    Sabin-Feldman dye test for, 683t,
      684
    serologic tests for, 683t, 683–687
      in pregnancy, 685–687, 686t
    vitrectomy and, 1494–1495
    Western blot for, 683t, 685
  differential diagnosis of, from candidi-
    asis, 774, 775
    from cryptococcosis, 783
    from DUSN, 811
    from intraocular lymphomas, 1207
    from MEWDS, 590
    from retinoblastoma, 1155
    from serpiginous choroiditis, 561
    from toxocariasis, 705t, 706
    from tuberculosis, 739
  epidemiology of, 674, 674t
  histopathological features of, 672
  immune response and self defenses to,
    682, 682–683
  in bone marrow transplantation, 488
  in HIV infection, 671, 680–682, *681*,
    734–735, *735*
  in pregnancy, 504–505
    management of, 691
    screening for, 692
    serologic tests for, 685–687, 686t
  management of, in HIV infected, 735
    in pregnancy, 691
    ocular, 687–688, 689t, 735

Toxoplasmosis (*Continued*)
  ocular, 678–682, *679–681*
    complications of, 679–680, *680*, 680t
    diagnosis of, 683–687
    differential diagnosis of, 681–682
    in HIV infected, 734–735, *735*, 1484
    in immunocompromised host, 680–
      682, *681*, 734–735
    in leukemia, 1199
    management of, 687–688, 689t, 735
      atovaquone for, 689t, 690
      clindamycin for, 688, 689t, 690
      corticosteroids for, 689t, 690
      in HIV infected, 735
      in immunocompromised patients,
        691, 735
      in neonates, 691
      in pregnancy, 691
      laser photocoagulation for, 690–
        691
      pars plana vitrectomy for, 690–
        691
      pyrimethamine for, 688, 689t, 690
      spiramycin for, 689t, 690
      sulfonamides for, 688, 689t, 690
    pathology of, 683
    retinochoroiditis from, 675, 677
    uveitis from, 664, 678
    white ocular lesions in, 616t
  pathogenesis of, 675
  prevention of, 691–692
  screening for, 692
  transmission of, 674t, 674–675
  vasoproliferative tumors and, 1175
TPCD (typical peripheral cystoid degen-
    eration), 15, *15*
Transforming growth factor *beta*, cystoid
    macular edema and, 246
  for macular holes, 227
  proliferative vitreoretinopathy and,
    1351
  toxoplasmosis and, 682
Transmission window defects, hyperflu-
    orescence of, 36
Transmitted fluorescence, *35*, 35
Transplantation, bone marrow. See *Bone
    marrow transplantation.*
  toxoplasmosis from, 674, 674t
Traumatic ocular disorder(s), 829–851
  cataracts as, 1379–1382
  chorioretinitis sclopetaria from, 833–
    834, *835*, *1389*, 1389–1390
  chorioretinopathy from, vasoprolifera-
    tive tumors and, 1175
  choroidal osteoma and, 1098
  choroidal rupture from, 145, *149*, 834–
    836, *835*
  commotio retinae from, 836–837, *837*
    histopathological features of, 832
  complications of, pathophysiology of,
    1373–1374
    surgical tools for, *1375*, 1375–1376,
      1376
  computed tomography of, 1372
  contact B-scan ultrasonography of, 53–
    54, *54*, *54*, 1372
  cyclodialysis from, 1382
  dialyses from, 831, 833
  direct, 831–838
  endophthalmitis from, 1390–1391
  epidemiology of, 831, 1370–1371
  foreign objects and. See *Foreign bodies,
    intraocular.*
  gas vs. silicone liquid tamponade for,
    1378–1379

Traumatic ocular disorder(s) (*Continued*)
  history taking in, 1371
  hyphema from, 1379, *1379*
  in bungee jumping, 841, *841*
  in fat embolism syndrome, 840
  in shaken baby syndrome, 838–839,
    839
  in Terson's syndrome, 839, *839*
  indirect, 838–841
  iridodialysis from, 1382
  macular holes from, 833, *834*, *834*,
    1440, 1440–1441
  magnetic resonance imaging of, 1372
  manifestations of, 831, 833t
  ophthalmic examination in, 1371
  optic nerve evulsion from, 838, *838*
  perfluorocarbon liquids for, 1323, 1378
  perforating (double-penetrating), *1385*,
    1385–1386
  photic retinopathy as, 844–848
  posterior segment manifestations of,
    831–841. See also *Posterior seg-
    ment, trauma in.*
  preoperative diagnostic ancillary tech-
    niques for, 1371–1372
  prophylactic antibiotics for, 1378
  Purtscher's retinopathy from, 839–840,
    840
  retinal detachments from, 831, 833,
    1248, 1382–1385, *1385*
    hemorrhagic, 1386–1387, *1387*
  retinal incarcerations from, 1384–1385,
    1385
  retinal pigment epithelium contusion
    and tears from, *837*, 837–838
  retinal tears from, 831, 833, *833*, 1382–
    1383
    giant, 1383–1384, *1384*
  ruptured globe from, 1373
  scleral buckling for, 1377–1378
  subluxated and dislocated crystalline
    lenses in, 1379–1382, *1380*, *1381*
  subretinal hemorrhages from, 1386–
    1387
  suprachoroidal hemorrhage from,
    1387–1389, *1388*
  ultrasonography of, 1371–1372
  uveal effusion after, 661t, 663
  Valsalva retinopathy from, 840, *840*
  visual evoked potentials of, 1372, 1377
  vitreoretinal surgery for, 1370–1392
    case examples of, 1391–1392
    controversies in, 1377–1379
    early vs. late, 1377
    principles of, 1374–1375
    prognosis for, 1376–1377
  whiplash retinopathy from, 840–841
Treponema pallidum, 736, 793. See also
    Syphilis.
Triamcinolone acetonide, for cystoid
    macular edema, 247t
  for intermediate uveitis, 607
Trichorrhexis nodosa, with bull's eye,
    1033t, 1034
Trifluoperazine, 909
Trimethoprim-sulfamethoxazole, for en-
    dophthalmitis, 1475
  for *Pneumocystis carinii*, 738
  for toxoplasmosis, 688
Tropicamide, for ophthalmoscopy, 21
Troxerutin, for central retinal vein occlu-
    sion, 295
Tuberculin skin test, 804
  acute multifocal posterior placoid pig-
    ment epitheliopathy and, 548–549

Tuberculomas, 738
Tuberculosis, 801–804
    diagnosis of, 804
    differential diagnosis of, 739, 803–804
        from coccidioidomycosis, 780
        from cryptococcosis, 783
        from intraocular lymphomas, 1207
        from sarcoidosis, 655
        from serpiginous choroiditis, 561
    fluorescein angiography of, 803
    in HIV infection, 738–739, 739, 801
        differential diagnosis of, 803
    ocular manifestations of, 801–804,
        802–803
    pathogenesis of, 801
    serpiginous choroiditis and, 556
    treatment of, 804
        drug toxicities from, 804
    ultrasonography in, 803
    white ocular lesions in, 616t
Tuberous sclerosis, Coats' disease and, 393
Tumor(s), 1051–1216. See also individual
        tumors, e.g., Choroidal hemangioma.
    chorioretinal folds and, 259
    choroidal metastatic as, 1103–1108
    contact B-scan ultrasonography of, 52,
        52–53
    diagnostic vitrectomy for, 1496–1497,
        1497
    DIC in, 473
    differential diagnosis of, from central
        serous chorioretinopathy, 208
    in HIV infection, 741
    intraocular lymphoid, 1204–1215
    of nonpigmented ciliary epithelium,
        acquired, 1130–1133
    of ocular fundus, vasoproliferative,
        1175–1181
    of retinal pigment epithelium, 1116–
        1122
        congenital hypertrophy of, 1058–
            1063
        hamartoma of, 1123–1129
    optical coherence tomography of, 73
    three-dimensional ultrasonography of,
        57–58
    white ocular lesions in, 616t
Tumor necrosis factor alpha, toxoplasmo-
        sis and, 682, 683
Turcot's syndrome, 1061
Turner's syndrome, Coats' disease and,
        393
Typical peripheral cystoid degeneration
        (TPCD), 15, 15

Ultrasonography, A-scan, 48, 49
    contact B-scan. See B-scan ultrasonogra-
        phy, contact.
    for toxocariasis, 704
    history of, 47
    principles and technical aspects of, 47–
        48
    three-dimensional, 55–59
        area measurement technique in, 57,
            57
        clinical experience with, 57–58, 58–
            59
        in vitro testing with, 57
        limitations and artifacts in, 58–59, 59
        linear measurement technique in,
            56–57, 57
        system for, 55, 56
        volume measurement technique in,
            57

Ultrasound biomicroscopy, 69
Ultraviolet light, 61
    age-related macular degeneration from,
        89
    cystoid macular edema and, 246
Umbo, 3, 7, 7
Unilateral acute idiopathic maculopathy,
        bull's eye maculopathy in, 1033t,
        1034
    in pregnancy, 500
Unilateral pigmentary retinopathies, dif-
        ferential diagnosis of, from retini-
        tis pigmentosa, 917, 917t
Urokinase, for hyphema, 1379
Usher's syndrome, retinitis pigmentosa
        and, 895, 904–905, 905t, 917t
    subtypes of, 904
Uveal effusion, 658–667
    after photocoagulation or cryotherapy,
        661t, 663–664, 664
    after trauma or surgery, 661t, 663
    classification of, 661t, 661–667
    clinical evaluation of, 658–660, 659,
        660
    differential diagnosis of, 659, 667, 667
        from intraocular benign reactive
            lymphoid hyperplasia, 1214
        from uveal melanoma, 1075t, 1081–
            1082
        from Vogt-Koyanagi-Harada syn-
            drome, 578, 579
    from syphilis, 795
    hydrodynamic, 661–663
    idiopathic, 665–667, 666
    in drug reactions, 664
    in elevated uveal venous pressure, 658,
        661t, 662, 662–663, 663
    in HIV infection, 664
    in malignant hypertension, 661t, 663
    in mucopolysaccharidosis, 665
    in nanophthalmos, 665, 665
    in ocular hypotony, 658, 661t, 661–662,
        662
    in scleral and orbital inflammation,
        658, 664
    in uveitis, 664
    inflammatory, 658, 661t, 663–664
    laboratory diagnosis of, 660–661
    macrophages and, 1489
    neoplastic, 664, 665
    pathophysiology of, 658, 659
    secondary to abnormal sclera, 665–
        667
    ultrasonography of, 660–661, 661
Uveal infusion, in vitrectomy, 1312,
        1312
Uveal leiomyoma, 1110–1112
    clinical features of, 1110, 1111
    diagnosis of, 1110–1111
    differential diagnosis of, 1110
    electron microscopy of, 1112
    fluorescein angiography of, 1111
    management of, 1112
    pathology of, 1111, 1111–1112, 1112
    ultrasonography of, 1111
Uveal melanoma, differential diagnosis
        of, from intraocular benign reac-
        tive lymphoid hyperplasia, 1214
    from myogenic and neurogenic, 1110
    from tuberculosis, 803
    in pregnancy, 500
    posterior, 1067–1072
        clinical features of, 1067, 1068
        computed tomography of, 1069–
            1070

Uveal melanoma (Continued)
    diagnosis of, 1067–1070, 1070, 1071
    differential diagnosis of, 1074–1082,
        1075t
        from adenoma and adenocarci-
            noma of CPE and RPE, 1075t,
            1079, 1079
        from age-related extramacular de-
            generation, 1075t, 1080, 1080
        from age-related macular degener-
            ation, 1075t, 1079, 1080, 1080
        from chorioretinal granuloma,
            1075t, 1081
        from choroidal detachment, 1075t,
            1081
        from choroidal nevus, 1074, 1075t,
            1076, 1076
        from choroidal osteoma, 1075t,
            1077, 1077
        from circumscribed choroidal
            hemangioma, 1075t, 1076, 1076
        from combined hamartoma of
            RPE, 1075t, 1079, 1079
        from congenital hypertrophy of
            RPE, 1075t, 1078, 1079
        from cystic lesions, 1075t, 1081
        from degenerative retinoschisis,
            1075t, 1081
        from hemorrhagic detachment of
            RPE or sensory retina, 1075t,
            1080
        from hemorrhagic vascular le-
            sions, 1075t, 1079–1080
        from inflammatory lesions, 1075t,
            1080–1081
        from iridociliary cysts, 1075t,
            1081
        from leiomyoma, 1075t, 1078,
            1078
        from melanocytoma, of optic
            nerve, 1075t, 1077, 1077–1078
        from neurilemmoma, 1075t, 1078
        from nonpigmented ciliary epithe-
            lium tumors, 1075t, 1079
        from posterior scleritis, 1075t,
            1080–1081, 1081
        from posterior uveal metastasis,
            1075t, 1076, 1076–1077
        from reactive hyperplasia of RPE
            and CPE, 1075t, 1078–1079
        from retinal cavernous heman-
            gioma, 1075t, 1078, 1078
        from retinal detachments, rhegma-
            togenous, 1075t, 1082
        from uveal effusion syndrome,
            1075t, 1081–1082
        from vasoproliferative tumor,
            1075t, 1077, 1077
    enucleation of, 1072
    epidemiology of, 1067
    fine needle aspiration biopsy of,
        1067, 1069
    fluorescein angiography of, 1067–
        1069, 1070
    laser photocoagulation for, 1071
    local resection for, 1071, 1072
    management of, 1070–1072
    observation for, 1071
    orbital exenteration for, 1072
    pathology of, 1067, 1069, 1070
    prognosis for, 1072
    radiotherapy for, 1071, 1071
    transpupillary thermotherapy for,
        1072
    ultrasonography of, 1069, 1070,
        1071

Uveal metastasis, differential diagnosis of, from intraocular benign reactive lymphoid hyperplasia, 1214
  from intraocular lymphomas, 1207
  posterior, differential diagnosis of, from uveal melanoma, 1075t, *1076,* 1076–1077
Uveal neurilemmoma, 1110, 1112–1114
  clinical features of, *1112,* 1113, *1113*
  diagnosis of, *1113,* 1113, *1114*
  differential diagnosis of, from uveal melanoma, 1075t, 1078
  fine needle aspiration biopsy of, 1113
  fluorescein angiography of, 1113, *1113*
  management of, 1114
  pathology of, *1114,* 1114
  ultrasonography of, 1113, *1114*
Uveal syndromes, from tuberculosis, 802
Uveal tumors. See also specific tumors.
  myogenic and neurogenic, 1110–1114
Uveal venous pressure, elevated, 658, 661t, *662,* 662–663, *663*
Uveitis, anterior, acute multifocal posterior placoid pigment epitheliopathy and, 545
  in candidiasis, 774
  serpiginous choroiditis and, 560
  effusion in, 664
  experimental autoimmune, 601
  granulomatous, from sarcoidosis, 646
  from toxocariasis, 703
  in HIV infection, 741
  in pregnancy, 505
  in syphilis, 664, 736, 794–795
  in toxoplasmosis, 664, 678
  in tuberculosis, 738, 802
  intermediate, 599–611
    anterior signs of, 601
    antimetabolite and immunosuppressive therapy for, 610
    cataract extraction and, 611
    clinical course and prognosis for, 604–605
    clinical presentation of, 601–604
    corticosteroids for, 607–609
    cryotherapy for, 609–610
    differential diagnosis of, 605–606
      from birdshot retinochoroidopathy, 567
      from connective tissue diseases, 606
      from Eales' disease, 419, 606
      from infectious diseases, 606
      from medulloepithelioma, 1135
      from parafoveal telangiectasis, 400
      from retinoblastoma, 1152t, 1156
      from sarcoidosis, 655
      from surgical/traumatic diseases, 606
      from toxocariasis, 705t, 706
      from tumors, 606
    epidemiology of, 599
    evaluation of, 606–607, 607t
    from toxocariasis, 697, 699, 702
    histopathological features of, 600
    immunology of, 601
    laser photocoagulation for, 610
    multiple sclerosis and, 604, 605
    pathogenesis of, 599
    pathology of, 601
    posterior signs of, 602–604, *602–605*
    symptoms of, 601
    treatment of, 607–609, *608, 609*
    uveal pressure in, 659
    uveitis in, 664

Uveitis (*Continued*)
    vasoproliferative tumors and, 1175, 1178t
      ocular fundus, 1077
    vitrectomy/lensectomy for, 610–611
  peripheral. See *intermediate.*
  pneumatic retinopexy contraindicated in, 1277
  posterior. See *Choroiditis.*
  subretinal fibrosis and, 631–634. See also *Subretinal fibrosis and uveitis syndrome.*
  sympathetic, differential diagnosis of, from birdshot retinochoroidopathy, 567
  sympathetic ophthalmia and, 569

Vaccination reactions, acute multifocal posterior placoid pigment epitheliopathy and, 549
Valcyclovir, for acute retinal necrosis, 763
Valsalva maculopathy, in pregnancy, 509
Valsalva retinopathy, 840, *840*
Vancomycin, for endophthalmitis, 1390, 1402, 1468, 1468t, 1471, 1472, 1473
  ocular disorders from, 864
Varicella-zoster virus (VZV), acute retinal necrosis from, 732–733, 752, 1483
  CMV co-infection with, in HIV infected, 720
  diagnostic vitrectomy for, 1491
  differential diagnosis of, from candidiasis, 774, 775
    from intermediate uveitis, 606
  in bone marrow transplantation, 488
  progressive outer retinal necrosis from, 733–734, 766–767, 769, *770*
    treatment of, 734
  treatment of, 734
  white ocular lesions in, 616t
Vascular damage, drug-induced, 857t, 863–864
Vascular disease, retinal. See *Retinal vascular diseases.*
Vascular endothelial growth factor (VEGF), central retinal vein occlusion and, 292
  choroidal neovascularization and, 123
  diabetic retinopathy and, 339–340
  hemoglobinopathies and, 447
  in diabetic retinopathy, 1418–1419, 1426
Vascular filling defects, hypofluorescence in, 33, *33,* 35
Vasculitis, retinal. See *Retinal vasculitis.*
Vasoproliferative ocular fundus tumors, 1175–1181
  clinical features of incidence of, 1175–1178, *1178,* 1178t, *1179,* 1179t, 1180t
  control of, 1175, 1176t
  definition of, 1175
  diagnosis of, 1179–1180
  differential diagnosis of, 1176
    from uveal melanoma, 1075t, 1077, *1077*
  fluorescein angiography of, 1179
  incidence of, 1175
  management of, 1180–1181
  ocular conditions associated with, 1176, 1178t
  pathology and pathogenesis of, 1178–1179
  ultrasonography of, 1180

Vasoproliferative retinal tumor. See *Retinal hemangioma, acquired.*
VDRL test, 736, 798, 887, 909
Venous caliber abnormalities, in diabetic retinopathy, 323–324, *324*
Venous stasis retinopathy. See *Ocular ischemic syndrome.*
Venules, postcapillary, 8
Verhoeff's membrane, 5
Vidarabine, for varicella-zoster virus, 734
Videoangiography, digital indocyanine-green. See *Indocyanine-green angiography.*
Viral syndromes, 749–758. See also specific viruses.
  acute multifocal posterior placoid pigment epitheliopathy and, 547–548
  acute retinal necrosis syndrome from, 749–755, 760–764
  diagnostic vitrectomy for, 1491–1492
  progressive outer retinal necrosis syndrome from, 755–758, 766–770
  retinitis, in bone marrow transplantation, 488
Visceral larva migrans, 700. See also *Toxocariasis.*
Visual evoked potentials, for ocular ischemic syndrome, 376–377
  for optic disc drusen, 881–882
Vitamin(s), for age-related macular degeneration prevention, 90, 94, 96
Vitamin A, deficiency of, serpiginous choroiditis and, 557
  for age-related macular degeneration prevention, 90
Vitamin C, for age-related macular degeneration prevention, 94, 96
Vitamin E, for age-related macular degeneration prevention, 90
  protective effect of, 844
Vitelliform dystrophy, adult-onset foveomacular, 1006, 1007, *1010*
Vitelliform lesions, of Best's disease, 991, *992, 994–996, 998–1000, 1002,* 1002
Vitelliform macular degeneration, adult, macular holes and, 223
  differential diagnosis of, from Stargardt's disease, 987
Vitiliginous chorioretinitis. See *Birdshot retinochoroidopathy.*
Vitiligo, in Vogt-Koyanagi-Harada syndrome, 575, *577*
Vitrectomy, 1298–1317
  air-gas exchange in, 1310–1311
  anatomy for, 1298–1299, *1299*
  anesthesia for, 1300–1301
  background for, 1299–1300, *1300*
  basic procedure of, *1303,* 1303–1304, *1304*
  blood removal in, 1311
  cataracts from, 1316
  complications of, 1312–1317
    intraoperative, 1312–1314
    postoperative, 1314–1317
      early, 1314–1315
      late, 1315–1317
  core, 132
  corneal complications from, early, 1314
    late, 1315–1316
  diagnostic, 1487–1501
    for antibody testing, 1487–1488
    for bacterial, fungal, and parasitic infections, 1492–1495, *1494, 1496*
    for cultures, 1487

Index

Vitrectomy (*Continued*)
  for cytology, 1489
  for intraocular foreign bodies, 1497–
      1501, *1498, 1500–1501*
  for intraocular malignancies, 1496–
      1497, *1497*
  for polymerase chain reaction, 1488,
      1488
  for viral infections, 1491–1492, *1493*
  indications for, 1491–1501
  needle aspiration for, 1489
  one-port mechanical, 1489–1490,
      1490
  processing samples from, 1491, 1491t
  techniques for, 1489–1490, *1490*
  three-port mechanical, 1490, *1490*
  elevated intraocular pressure from,
      1314–1315
  endophthalmitis from, 1315
  fluid-air exchange in, 1308, 1310, *1310*
  for acute retinal necrosis, 755, 763, 764
  for candidiasis, 777
  for CMV-related retinal detachments,
      1480–1481
  for cystoid macular edema, 250, 252
  for diabetic retinopathy, 1423–1425,
      1424t, 1425t
    complications of, 1427, 1427t
    long-term effects of, 1427
    technique of, 1425–1426
  for dislocated lenses, 1380–1381, *1381*
  for Eales' disease, 419
  for endophthalmitis, 1468t, 1468–1470,
      1472
    diagnostic, 1467
  for endophthalmitis specimens, 1467
  for epimacular membranes, *232*, 232–
      233
  for familial exudative vitreoretinopa-
      thy, 428–429
  for giant retinal tears, 1340–1346, 1348
    lens-sparing, 1347
    panoramic viewing in, 1340
    traumatic, 1384
    with perfluorocarbon liquids, 1342–
      1345
  for intraocular foreign bodies, 1341–
      1342, 1397–1398, *1400*, 1400, *1401*,
      1403
  for macular holes, *226*, 226–227, 833
  for optic nerve head congenital pits,
      879
  for perforating injuries, *1385*, 1385–
      1386
  for proliferative vitreoretinopathy,
      1341–1342, 1356
    enzyme-assisted, 1366
  for pseudophakic retinal detachment,
      1266
  for retinal detachment, 833, 1249t
    CMV-related, 1480–1481
    pseudophakic, 1266
    rhegmatogenous, 1270t
  for retinopathy of prematurity, lens-
      sparing, 1461–1462, 1464
  for sickle cell retinopathy, 449, 452–453
  for suprachoroidal hemorrhage, 1388–
      1389
  for trauma, 1375, 1377
  for X-linked retinoschisis, 1015
  glaucoma from, 1314–1315, 1316
  hemostasis in, 1311
  hypotony from, 1316–1317
  indications for, 1298, 1299t
  intraocular irrigation solution for,
      1301–1302

Vitrectomy (*Continued*)
  laser photocoagulation and, 1311
  lens complications from, 1314
  lensectomy with, 1304–1305, *1305*
    for cataracts, in epimacular mem-
      branes, 234
    in intermediate uveitis, 611
    for diabetic retinopathy, 325, 336
    for hamartoma of retina and RPE,
      1128
    for hemoglobinopathies, 452–453
    for intermediate uveitis, 610–611
    for macular holes, 227
    for toxoplasmosis, 690–691
    sympathetic ophthalmia after, 569
  membrane delamination and, 1308,
      1309
  membrane peeling and, 1305–1307,
      1306, 1307
  membrane sectioning and, *1307*, 1307–
      1308
  orbital hemorrhage from, 1314–1315
  panoramic viewing in, for giant retinal
      tears, 1340
  patient preparation and draping for,
      1301
  perfluorocarbon liquids and, 1308
  perfluorocarbon-air exchange in, 1308,
      1310
  preoperative instrument check for,
      1300, 1300t
  retinal detachment from, 1312–1313,
      1313, 1316
  retinal incarceration from, 1313–1314
  retinal tears from, 1312–1313
  scleral buckling and, 1302
  sclerotomy for, 1302
    closure of, 1311
  subretinal infusion from, 1312
  sympathetic ophthalmia from, 1317
  techniques for, 1300–1311
  uveal effusion from, 1312, *1312*
  vitreous hemorrhage from, 1316
  vitreous incarceration from, 1313–1314
Vitreitis, acute multifocal posterior plac-
      oid pigment epitheliopathy and,
      545
  in acute retinal necrosis, 750, 762
Vitreomacular traction, B-scan ultraso-
      nography of, 50, *50*
  cataract surgery and, 244
  differential diagnosis of, from macular
      holes, 222
  in cystoid macular edema, 244
  in epimacular membranes, *232*, 232
  optical coherence tomography of, 73
Vitreoretinal adhesions, pneumatic reti-
      nopexy contraindicated in, 1277
  vitrectomy for, 1299
Vitreoretinal degenerations, hereditary,
      924–927
    Goldmann-Favre syndrome as, 926–
      927, *927*
    Stickler's syndrome as, 924, 926, *926*
  retinal detachment in, 1248
Vitreoretinal picks, 1300t
Vitreoretinal surgery. See also specific
      procedures.
  for toxocariasis, 706–707
Vitreoretinopathy, dominant exudative,
      differential diagnosis of, from reti-
      noblastoma, 1152t, 1157
  familial exudative, 421–429
    clinical features of, 421–426, 423t
    differential diagnosis of, 427t, 427–
      428

Vitreoretinopathy (*Continued*)
    from Eales' disease, 419
    from retinal capillary heman-
      gioma, 1160
    from toxocariasis, 704, 705t, 706
    from X-linked retinoschisis, 1016
  fluorescein angiography of, 422, *422*
  genetics of, 426–427
  histopathological features of, 426
  history of, 421
  laser photocoagulation for, 428
  management of, 428–429
  pathogenesis of, 426
  presentation of, *425*, 425–426
  prognosis for, 425–426
  retinal folds in, 263
  stage 1, 421–422, *422*, 423t
  stage 2, 422–424, *423*, 423t, *424*
  stage 3, *424*, 424–425, *425*
  vasoproliferative tumors and, 1175,
      1178t
  proliferative. See *Proliferative
      vitreoretinopathy.*
Vitreoschisis, in diabetic retinopathy,
      1426
Vitreous, clinical examination of, 21–28
Vitreous abnormalities, in degenerative
      myopia, 192
Vitreous base, anatomy of, vitrectomy
      and, 1298, *1299*
Vitreous base contraction, proliferative
      vitreoretinopathy and, 1351
Vitreous biopsies, 1489–1501. See also
      Vitrectomy, diagnostic.
  diluted, 1491, 1491t
  undiluted, 1491, 1491t
Vitreous body, anatomy of, vitrectomy
      and, 1298, *1299*
Vitreous cortex, anatomy of, vitrectomy
      and, 1298, *1299*
Vitreous cutting instruments, 1299–1300,
      1300, 1300t
Vitreous degeneration, in Goldmann-
      Favre syndrome, 926, *927*
  in Stickler syndrome, 924
  in Wagner's syndrome, 926
Vitreous detachment, from toxoplasmo-
      sis, 678
  in diabetic retinopathy, 1411
  posterior, in central retinal vein occlu-
      sion, 292
    in myopia, 192
    retinal horseshoe tears following,
      1265–1266
  retinal detachment following, 1248
Vitreous forceps, 1300t
Vitreous hemorrhage, B-scan ultrasonog-
      raphy of, 49–50
  differential diagnosis of, from retino-
      blastoma, 1152t, 1157
  from vitrectomy, 1316
  in bone marrow transplantation, 488
  in Coats' disease, 392
  in congenital retinal arteriovenous
      communications, 1172
  in diabetic retinopathy, 1426, 1427
  in Eales' disease, 418
  in hemoglobinopathies, 447
  in leukemia, 1197t, 1198–1199
  in radiation retinopathy, 477, 479
    treatment of, 485
  in retinal cavernous hemangioma, 1169
  in Terson's syndrome, 839
  in X-linked retinoschisis, 1013–1014
  optic disc drusen and, 880

Index

Vitreous hemorrhage (*Continued*)
  perfluorocarbon liquids for, 1323
  pneumatic retinopexy and, 1277, 1282
  traumatic, 1374
    case example of, 1391
Vitreous hyaloid, B-scan ultrasonography
    of, 50
Vitreous incarceration, from pneumatic
    retinopexy, 1282
  from vitrectomy, 1313–1314
  in cystoid macular edema, 244–245
  in trauma, 1371
  traumatic, 1374
  vitrectomy for, 1341–1342
Vitreous opacities, contact B-scan ultraso-
    nography of, 49–50, *50*
Vitreous scissors, 1300t
Vitreous substitute(s), 1320–1332. See
    also individual materials.
  intraocular gases as, 1325–1329
  perfluorocarbon liquids as, 1320–
    1325
  silicone liquid as, 1329–1332
Vitreous traction, in cystoid macular
    edema, 244
  in toxocariasis, 701–702, *702*
Vitreous-uveal traction, in cystoid macu-
    lar edema, 245
Vitritis, in Eales' disease, 415–416
  in syphilis, 736, *737*, 795
  in tuberculosis, 803
  serpiginous choroiditis and, 560
Vogt-Koyanagi-Harada syndrome, 573–
    581. See also *Harada's disease.*
  clinical signs of, 574–575, *574–577*
  complications of, 580–581, *581*
  definition of, 573
  diagnostic tests for, 575, *578*, 578–579,
    1489

Vogt-Koyanagi-Harada syndrome
    (*Continued*)
  differential diagnosis of, 579
    from AMPPPE, 550
    from intraocular lymphomas, 1207
    from posterior scleritis, 637
  epidemiology of, 573
  etiology of, 573
  fluorescein angiography of, 575, 578,
    578
  histopathological features of, 573–574
  in pregnancy, 505
  indocyanine green videoangiography
    of, 578
  presenting symptoms of, 574
  prognosis for, 580
  stages of, 574
  treatment of, 579–580
  ultrasonography of, 578–579, *579*
Vogt-Spielmeyer disease, retinitis pig-
    mentosa and, 906
von Hippel-Lindau disease, 1159–1166.
    See also *Retinal capillary
    hemangioma.*
  differential diagnosis of, from vasopro-
    liferative tumors, 1176
  systemic evaluation of, 1164, 1164t
  systemic management of, 1165
  tumors associated with, 1160t

Wagner syndrome, 926, *926*
Waterhouse-Friderichsen syndrome, 473
Wedl cells, radiation therapy and, 129
Wegener's granulomatosis, posterior scle-
    ritis and, 638
Western blot, for toxoplasmosis, 683t, 685
Whiplash retinopathy, 840–841
  macular holes and, 833

Whipple's disease, chorioretinal folds in,
    263
  diagnostic vitrectomy of, 1492
  differential diagnosis of, from sarcoid-
    osis, 655
White dot syndrome, differential diagno-
    sis of, 633t, 633–634
  multiple evanescent, 584–591. See also
    *Multiple evanescent white dot
    syndrome.*
White lesions in retina and choroid, dis-
    eases manifesting, 616t–617t
White lines, retinal detachments and,
    1228–1230, 1230–1231
White-with-pressure sign, 1222, *1225,*
    1225–1226, *1226*
  in senile (degenerative) retinoschisis,
    1239
Window defects, hyperfluorescence of, 36
Witmer quotient, 1487, 1488, 1491, 1494
Wyburn-Mason syndrome, 1172, *1173*
  hyperfluorescence in, *35,* 36

Xanthophyll, light absorption by, 62
  protective effect of, 844

Yellow-orange lipofuscin, 5

Zinc, for age-related macular degenera-
    tion prevention, 90
  protective effect of, 844
Zonula adherens, 5
Zonula occludens, 5
Zonular traction tufts, 9–10, *11,* 1221–
    1222, *1222*

ISBN 0-7216-7607-3

90071

9 780721 676074